Treatment of Dry Skin Syndrome

Marie Lodén • Howard I. Maibach
Editors

Treatment of Dry Skin Syndrome

The Art and Science of Moisturizers

Springer

Editors
Marie Lodén, M.Sc. Pharm.
Eviderm Institute
Solna, Sweden

Howard I. Maibach, M.D.
Department of Dermatology
University of California
San Francisco School of Medicine
San Francisco, California
USA

ISBN 978-3-642-27605-7 ISBN 978-3-642-27606-4 (eBook)
DOI 10.1007/978-3-642-27606-4
Springer Heidelberg Dordrecht London New York

Library of Congress Control Number: 2012937364

Printed on acid-free paper

Springer is part of Springer Science+Business Media (www.springer.com)

Preface

Our desire to apply oily materials to the skin is almost instinctive and may be as old as mankind itself. This is related to our physical and psychological functioning which is facilitated by gentle touch, particularly in terms of reducing stress, relieving pain, and in the improvement of skin characteristics. Moisturizing creams contain a great variety of ingredients that give rise to different sensory and functional effects when applied to the skin. For example, treatment of children with atopic dermatitis may feel soothing and comforting, punitive and intrusive, or functional and neutral. Treatment of normal and diseased skin also shows different effects on the epidermal biochemistry and functional characteristics, with consequences for the outbreak of inflammation, eczema and potentially asthma.

The development of moisturizers is a scientific and artistic discipline, including both formulation technology and consumer insights. This new book aims to bridge the gap between the moisturizers and the skin. The composition and development of moisturizing creams are discussed in the book, including the value of lipids, humectants, natural raw materials, and preservatives. Overviews and updates on dry skin disorders and their treatments are also covered, along with regulatory aspects and claim substantiation. In addition, the exciting sensory systems of epidermal keratinocytes are explained, and new insights into stratum corneum biomechanics, molecular organization, desquamation, and barrier function are discussed. The authors represent a cross section of the international well-known scientists from academia to industrial research.

With the use of the knowledge in this book, we anticipate that cosmetic scientists, researchers and dermatologists will go beyond the traditional thinking of skin care. The readers will have new insights that suggest the properties required for a new generation of moisturizing treatments, improving quality of life.

Solna, Sweden — Marie Lodén,
San Francisco, CA, USA — Howard I. Maibach

Preface

Introduction

Corneobiology and Corneotherapy: A Final Chapter

A. M. Kligman

Reprinted from: *International Journal of Cosmetic Science*, 2011, 33, 197–209 with permission.

The text obtained for this review from Professor Albert Kligman was drawn posthumously from a variety of notes that he had been planning to use to write a review on corneobiology and corneotherapy. It was a review that he had dearly hoped to complete – his final 'magnum opus' with reflections on the subject.

The review is reprinted with permission from Kligman, A.M. Corneobiology and Corneotherapy – a final chapter. *International Journal of Cosmetic Science*, 2011, 33, 197–209.

Introduction

Corneobiology refers to that broad range of experimental studies that are focused on the anatomy, physiology and biology of the stratum corneum, centred particularly on the human horny layer that has features uniquely different from other mammals. Corneobiology has a very broad reach, encompassing studies that deal with immunology, endocrinology, neurobiology and psychology, comprising a network of complex interactions that have connections to the central nervous system. It has attracted the attention of a confederation of scientists from very different disciplines, including molecular biologists, anatomists, physiologists, pharmacologists, geneticists, psychologists and still others. However, it was not until the latter half of the twentieth century that the stratum corneum began to be viewed as much more than a dead, inert passive membrane, a Saran-type wrapping around the integument with the sole function of limiting the movement of substances into and out of the viable tissues, featuring the special functions of preventing diffusional water loss against a hostile, dessicating environment and limiting the penetration of exogenous toxic chemicals with antigens [1].

I have given an historical account of the evolution, one might say revolution, regarding the new appreciation of the horny layer as having multiple, dynamic functions in a previous treatise entitled 'How the dead stratum corneum became alive' [2]. Before then, the established dogma was that the principal biologic mission of the epidermis was to create the impermeable stratum corneum barrier, essentially sealing the body from the outside world, leading some authorities to label the stratum corneum as the ultimate shield against mechanical, chemical and physical external threats. For instance, in 1958, S. Rothman in his seminal text on the *Physiology and Biochemistry of Skin* depicted the stratum corneum as a loose, amorphous mass of keratin filaments, the product of the holocrine degeneration of epidermal keratinocytes, epitomized in dermatologic texts as the 'basket weave' horny layer [3]. This view of the horny layer as a loose collection of filaments separated by wide empty spaces, as seen in H&E-stained histologic specimens, posed a paradox for physiologists who universally held that the stratum corneum constituted a barrier to the penetration of exogenous substances preventing diffusional water loss to a hostile dry environment. The 'basket weave' image turned out to be an artefact of formalin fixation of H&E-stained sections.

In 1964, myself and Enno Christophers showed that the horny layer floated off as thin, tough, transparent membrane when full-thickness specimens of skin were immersed for 1 min in water at 60°C [4]. In unfixed sections swollen by 1 N NaOH, we subsequently demonstrated that the membrane was a coherent tissue composed in most body regions of 14–16 cornified cells, later called corneocytes. These findings showed unequivocally that the stratum was a cellular tissue, not an amorphous filamentous graveyard of degenerated keratinocytes. My 1964 landmark paper, entitled 'The biology of the stratum corneum', marked the inauguration of a new cutaneous discipline, 'Corneobiology', which centred on the structure and function of the horny layer [1]. This paper, however, propagated a serious misconception. The teaching of the time was that the stratum corneum was a dead, inert, passive membrane, a Saran Wrap-like impermeable shroud, encasing the body, protecting it from chemical and physical exogenous threats. In fact, this was but one of many errors regarding the structure and function of the horny layer, which has taken many years to correct, a process of deconstruction that continues to this very day.

No area of cutaneous biology has attracted more investigative attention than the stratum corneum. A multitude of studies in the last few decades have shown that the horny layer is a very complex, dynamic tissue whose formation involves many highly orchestrated metabolic enzymatic functions. The horny layer has become very much alive. It was holy doctrine in major textbooks of dermatology that the sole function of the horny layer was to provide an impermeable 'barrier' to the inward and outward diffusion of substances, especially toxic exogenous chemicals. The synonym for the stratum corneum was the 'barrier', a term which still remains popular. It is now known with certainty that the horny layer has diverse and numerous functions, indispensable for maintaining cutaneous homeostasis.

Corneobiology Enthusiasts

It is appropriate to mention briefly the academicians whose early investigations created the background for the concepts underpinning corneobiology. It was left to many scientists but most notably Professor Elias – the maestro – to articulate the concept that the epidermis had many diverse functions and that most of these localized to the stratum corneum, which in turn had many diverse functions, elevating the stratum corneum as a key player in the many biologic processes of the integument [5]. Elias, in fact, laid down the fundamental principals underlying the science of corneobiology, listing in detail ten major horny layer functions, linking each one to specific constituents, a brilliant, original, systematic exposition. For example, the linkages of each function were first to its basic principal compartment, such as the extracellular matrix or the corneocyte; then the linkage to its structural basis, such as the bilaminar membranes of the extracellular domain, corneodesmosomes, cornified envelopes and keratin filaments and cytosols; next, the chemical basis, specifically ceramides, cholesterol, antimicrobial peptides, barrier lipids, filaggrin derivatives, glycerol and proteases; and finally linkage to regulatory scientists, glucocorticosteroids, etc.

Although it may seem tedious to list individually each of Elias' ten functions, it is exceedingly informative and edifying to grasp the scope and diversity of these functions. These are as follows:

1. Permeability
2. Antimicrobial
3. Antioxidant
4. Cohesion (integrity) – desquamation (shedding)
5. Mechanical/rheological
6. Chemical, exclusion of antigens
7. Psychosensory
8. Hydration
9. Protection against electromagnetic radiation
10. Initiation of inflammation (cytokine activation)

Although the above inventory of multiple functions is impressive, it does not tell the whole story; this is a work in progress. Searching the rapidly expanding literature furnishes further examples of the diversity of functions displayed by the horny layer. To Elias' list, one may add the following:

1. A biosensor of meteorological conditions, especially humidity.
2. Regulator of innate and adaptive immunity.
3. A storage site of chemical mediators, topical drugs, cosmeceuticals, cosmetics.
4. Protection against carcinogenesis and photoageing.
5. An organ of social communication – dry, scaly, rough stratum corneum is unappealing to touch and light, engendering repulsion, inducing anxiety, anger and depression in those afflicted by ichthyotic skin.
6. Generation of natural moisturizing factors, a mixture of low molecular weight substances that are hygroscopic (urea, amino acids, glycerol).

The upshot of these disparate observations is that the conventional view of the stratum corneum as a passive, inert, metabolically lifeless membrane is obviously archaic. The stratum corneum has obviously become very much alive. The recent publication in 2006 by Elias and Feingold, titled *The Skin Barrier*, is obligatory reading, covering every aspect of corneobiology. It is an unparalleled source of references [6].

The scientific basis of corneobiology is experimental quantification and not simply empirical observation, further strengthened by the development of non-invasive methods that allow repeated, sequential observations of the same site without damaging the tissue, as is the case of biopsies. For example, the integument is constantly being deformed by stretching by mechanical forces, about which knowledge is scanty, lacking measurable data. To fill this gap, recent studies show that using a suction device to apply strengths of 400–600 mbar to the forearms results in significant increases in transepidermal water loss (TEWL), signifying increased permeability, and marked decrease in capacitance, signifying less ability to take up and hold water, making the horny layer less resilient [7]. This is echoed by the work of Rawlings et al. [8] further demonstrating in vitro disruption of lipid bilayers with extension of the stratum corneum, resulting in increased water vapour transport rates. These results are rather surprising, considering the rheological stresses that the integument experiences in daily living, not to mention sports, and not everyone concurs with these findings.

Contributors to building the edifice, we now call corneobiology, are a motley, diverse crew of investigators, mainly situated in industry and academia from around the world. These individuals are all individually acknowledged in the delightful, historical, narrative essay by the indefatigable master of masters, Dr. Anthony Rawlings of Great Britain, entitled '50 years' of stratum corneum research and moisturization, laying out decade by decade the most innovative discoveries, starting in the 1950s [9]. Rawlings and his collaborators are best known for their exhaustive, comprehensive works on moisturization, culminating in the Rawlings magnum opus in 2004 on 'Stratum corneum moisturization at the molecular level', which is a must-read for all parvenus to the field of corneobiology, covering in exquisite detail every aspect of moisturization, including the development of an impressive assay of modern multidimensional products for effectively treating the common dry, scaling, ichthyotic conditions, a far cry from our forefathers who advocated such primitive remedies as goose grease, vegetable oils and animal fats [10].

Another distinguished name must be added to those who have made outstanding contributions to corneobiology, namely, Professor Ronald Marks of Cardiff, Wales. Dr. Marks has sponsored six international symposia, focused entirely on the stratum corneum. In 1971, he invented the cyanoacrylate skin surface biopsy technique that enables the microscopic visualization of bacteria, fungi, bacteria and demodectic mites in the superficial, desquamating portion of the stratum corneum [11]. He was also among the first to show that the impermeable dressings with no active pharmacologic agents could clear psoriatic plaques and that supposedly inert ointments, such as petrolatum, could have anti-inflammatory effects [12].

Tagami in Japan realized in 1998 that the stratum corneum was a rich reservoir of cytokines, including IL-8, IL-6, IL-10, TNF-a and others, enabling 'an explosive inflammatory tissue' whenever fragments of the horny layer are extruded into the dermis, heralding the idea that the horny layer could start chronic inflammatory disorders [13]. Tagami immersed a sheet of normal stratum corneum in buffered saline for 2 days and found a large quantity of IL-12 in the supernatant. Marks had earlier demonstrated that a suspension of corneocytes obtained by scrubbing callus tissue initiated a severe, long-lasting, inflammatory granuloma when injected into the dermis [14]. Spontaneous examples of this response occur when epidermal cysts rupture, dumping their contents into the dermis, and also when acne comedones rupture to form papulo-pustules. Frenetic scratching can mimic this phenomenon by dislodging keratinous fragments into viable tissue. Nickoloff and Naidu had also foreseen the potential of the stratum corneum to initiate inflammatory and immune-mediated reactions [15]. They found, by immunostaining biopsied tissue, marked increases in TNF-a, IL-a, IL-16, intercellular adhesion molecules and growth factors as early as 6 h after tape stripping. They were among the first to appreciate that the epidermis vigorously participates in a multitude of homeostatic responses, well beyond producing the horny layer barrier. Nickoloff then went on to show that there was a rapid release of cytokines after topical application of irritants, as well as after application of allergens in sensitized subjects, indicating a common triggering, a pathway after injury to the stratum corneum [16].

It is appropriate to point out that the remarkable advances in our understanding of the horny layer have been made possible by the utilization of highly sophisticated, modern technology, including TEM, SEM, cryofixation, spectroscopy, staining of immunologic markers, optical coherent tomography and histochemical and other non-invasive methodologies. Some recent illuminating studies are worth mentioning.

We have been taught, since the early in vitro diffusional studies of Scheuplein and Blank, that all layers of the stratum corneum contribute to its barrier properties [17]. Now we learn, in a recent paper by Richter et al. of Beiersdorf, Hamburg, Germany, using cryofixation and scanning electron microscopy, that skin specimens immersed in 5–20% salt solutions show three distinct hydration zones within the horny layer [18]. The outermost zone where desquamation occurs shows massive swelling, whereas the innermost zone shows that the granular layer swells to more than double its normal thickness, associated with massive water inclusions between adjacent cell layers. By contrast, the middle zone remains compact, without water pools. The authors conclude that the middle zone constitutes the vaunted permeability barrier, a near heresy to conventional thinking.

An earlier paper by the same group using high-pressure cryofixation compels us to reconsider how our conventional concepts need serious revision [19]. The most surprising finding is that organelles and tonofilaments within the cytoplasm of keratinocytes are not uniformly distributed as usually depicted but instead are organized instead into 'microdomains', clusters of organelles separated by relatively empty spaces, a startling new concept of keratinocyte morphology. New knowledge is occurring so rapidly that we are no longer shocked when our conventional dogmas are overturned. The famous impermeability of the horny layer turns out to be an oversimplification, even to the point where physicists can proclaim boldly that the vaunted barrier may have porous domains.

It is now understood that permeability can be enhanced by a variety of chemical and physical techniques, including simple occlusion. The normal stratum corneum contains widely separated lacunar dilatations in the extracellular domains that can be enlarged to form continuous pore pathways, allowing for the ready penetration of both polar and non-polar molecules attesting to the new awareness of the dynamic nature of the horny layer [20].

Emollients and Moisturizers: The Beginnings of Corneotherapy

It was not long ago when dermatologists were scorned and mocked for their primitive, empirical topical therapies. The therapeutic credo was: 'If it's dry, wet it. If it's wet, dry it'. The ointments followed the rule of the three S's. Their efficacy was thought to be proportionate to the degree to which they *stained, stunk or stung*. However, corneobiology, which has revealed the inner workings of the horny layer barrier, has revolutionized topical therapies, allowing striking improvements, which can be epitomized in a few sentences. They are more effective; safer, using lower concentrations of active agents, with fewer adverse side effects such as stinging, burning and irritancy; free of allergens, fragrances and preservatives; more easily and conveniently applied; more agreeable to use, being colourless and odourless, rubbing in easily and leaving no residue; more stable with a longer shelf life and compatible with other daily treatments such as sunscreens, moisturizers and cleansers. A wave of new topical drugs and cosmeceuticals has entered the market place, whose benefits are more likely to be substantiated by 'evidence-based' medicine.

The use of bland, non-medicated emollients for treating a variety of dermatologic disorders is as old as dermatology itself. Dermatologists in European centres extensively used emollients in the nineteenth and twentieth centuries to treat a variety of chronic, inflammatory disorders. The term 'emollient' (from the Greek, meaning to soften) refers to oily substances, such as ointments and creams, which are used to moderate rough, scaling, xerotic, erythematous, often pruritic conditions to make the skin flexible, soft and agreeable to the touch and sight. More recently, the term 'moisturizers', a creation of Madison Avenue merchandizers, has come into use to denote substances, usually in the form of emulsions, that 'moisten' and hydrate dry skin conditions. The two terms are now used interchangeably to encompass a huge variety of commercial formulations possessing attributes that go well beyond merely moistening and softening. It should be made clear that emollients are not drugs in the FDA sense and technically contain no pharmacologically active substances; nonetheless, they may have drug-like effects and are best classified in the category of cosmeceuticals.

The corneotherapy story begins with some prescient observations by Tree and Marks in a 1975 paper having the provocative title of 'An explanation for the 'placebo' effect of bland ointment bases' [12]. These authors were trying to explain how bland emollients, without pharmacologically active ingredients, could be effective in moderating common inflammatory disorders such as psoriasis and atopic dermatitis. They showed that several bland agents could inhibit and prevent the increased epidermal mitotic rate, which occurred when the skin of hairless mice was tape-stripped. They found that the venerable ointment, petrolatum, exerted the greatest anti-mitotic effect among other creams and pastes. They had no explanation for this.

Penney later proffered the explanation that petrolatum might be acting as an anti-inflammatory agent [21]. He could show, at least in vitro, that petrolatum inhibits the prostaglandin-mediated formation of the pro-inflammatory arachidonic acid. In 1976, Comaish and Greener showed that petrolatum had an inhibitory effect using a quite different model [22]. Their study was based on the renowned Köbner phenomenon in which insults to the uninvolved skin of patients with active psoriasis provoke new psoriatic lesions at the traumatized sites. They provoked the Köbner reaction by making 1-cm-long deep scratches. By pretreating uninvolved skin for 3 weeks before scratching, they found that new lesions were generally inhibited.

In still another model, myself and Lorraine investigated the ability of emollients to inhibit ultraviolet-induced carcinogenesis in hairless mice [23]. The mice were irradiated thrice weekly for 20 weeks with broad-spectrum UVB. The selected emollient was applied just before each irradiation. We found that petrolatum gave almost complete protection against the formation of tumours. Another hydrophobic emollient, lanolin, was only 50% effective. By contrast, tumour formation was greatly enhanced by mineral oil in this animal model, which contains lower molecular weight hydrocarbons than petrolatum, with a potential for irradiation. USP cold cream had no protective effect. Interestingly, a modest protective effect, about 20%, was determined even when petrolatum was applied after each irradiation. It was shown that petrolatum had a negligible sunscreen effect, with an SPF of <2.

In my own studies of bland emollients for the correction of varied xerotic states with defective horny layer barriers, I have found that ancient war horse petrolatum to be highly effective. My assessment of moisturization efficacy was based on the dry skin regression method that determines the time after cessation of a 3-week treatment for skin to return to the original state [24].

The chief complaint against petrolatum, which strongly limits its acceptance, is its greasiness and disagreeable feel. After experimenting with a variety of oil-rich emollients, which are clearly superior to lotions, we have concluded that Aquaphor is second only to petrolatum for repairing defective barriers in chronic dermatoses. Patients have to be taught that once rubbed in, its perceived oiliness mostly disappears.

I proffer the following experimental example of the high efficaciousness of Aquaphor in repairing the markedly defective barrier by oral administration of 13-*cis*-retinoic acid (Accutane). I treated three men with severe acne conglobata of the face and back with 80 mg of *cis*-retinoic acid daily for 4 months with excellent therapeutic results but which resulted in marked scaling, even bruising and purpura after moderate erythema in two, associated with itching and dryness to touch and sight. One dorsal forearm, from the wrist to antecubital space, was treated with Aquaphor b.i.d. for 5 weekdays for 1 month, whereas the opposite forearm served as an untreated control. Dryness, scaling, itching and fragility disappeared completely in 2 weeks. The following measurements were made 3 days after the end of 4 weeks of treatment, expressed in averages. Transepidermal water loss (estimated by Servomed) was 22.3 mg m^2/h on the untreated side and 5.2 mg m^2/h on the treated side, a value within the normal range of the forearm. The number of corneocyte layers determined by the alkali swelling technique on a razor slice biopsy was 6.1 on the untreated side and 10.3 on the treated side, within the normal range. Twelve Scotch tape strips induced purpura on the control side but not on the treated side. Videomicroscopy (by Hi-Scope, ×20) showed near-normal glyphic markings of primary and secondary lines on the treated side with near obliteration of glyphics on the untreated side. Despite the facial sample, the near-normal restoration of the defective barrier by b.i.d. applications of Aquaphor can scarcely be queried.

Subsequently, petrolatum in many reports has been found to be beneficial in a variety of clinical settings, for example, after chemical and laser peels, after dermabrasion, in promoting wound healing and for relieving chronic, inflammatory disorders. A noteworthy effect of petrolatum is enhanced repair of the disrupted horny layer barrier in human skin. For example, Herd and Agner examined the ability of six different moisturizers to repair the horny layer barrier damaged by a 24-h patch test of 0.5% sodium lauryl sulphate, a classic anionic detergent that makes the barrier extremely permeable, increasing TEWL to 20 times normal [25]. All six moisturizers accelerated barrier repair, measured quantitatively by a variety of bioengineering techniques, with petrolatum the best performer. The key finding in that study was that the rate of repair was directly proportioned to the respective oil content of the moisturizers. They recommended this model as a reliable way to estimate efficacy. Although still elusive, we are coming closer to understanding the mechanism by which moisturizers work.

The momentous increase in knowledge of the intricacies of stratum corneum anatomy and physiology has paid off handsomely in the way in which topical drugs are formulated to enhance penetration, thereby increasing efficacy at lower concentrations, also diminishing adverse reactions. Topical drugs can be targeted to preferentially enter follicular pathways in disorders such as acne.

Corneotherapy Is the Basis for a New Wave of Improved Topical Treatments

Corneotherapy refers to therapeutic interventions, usually topical, which are aimed at repairing stratum corneum barriers that are impaired in a wide variety of unrelated dermatologic disorders. Corneotherapy applies most often to the treatment of common chronic inflammatory disorders such as atopic dermatitis and psoriasis but also to a wide spectrum of skin diseases of very different origins, viz. occupational diseases, irritant and allergic contact dermatitis, congenital ichthyotic diseases, keloids and hypertrophic scars, severely premature neonates, the photoaged face because of excessive solar radiation and others, which are classically manifested by dry, xerotic, scaling, often pruritic cutaneous surfaces. A variety of objective non-invasive measurements are available to characterize and quantify these diverse conditions that invariably exhibit increased TEWL and decreased capacity to maintain hydration resulting in viable dry scaly skin among other impairments of the horny layer barrier.

Actually, corneotherapy has been practised unwittingly by dermatologists from the earliest times, encompassing different approaches and basically targeting defective horny layers ranging from traditional ancient approaches such as emollients, occlusive dressings, hydrotherapy (spas), ultraviolet light, natural and artificial, arriving at modern resurfacing strategies for correcting photoaged faces (lasers, chemical peels, dermabrasions, etc.).

Corneotherapy refers to preventive interventions that are primarily directed to the correction and restoration of the stratum corneum barrier that has been rendered defective and impaired by disease, genetics and a variety of mechanical, physical, chemical and psychological exogenous insults and stresses.

Invariable and characteristic features of defective horny layer are marked increases in diffusional TEWL to a hostile dessicating environment; a decreased capacity to take up and retain sufficient water to maintain a supple, soft, resilient, smooth horny layer and a host of structural imperfections, which degrade the ability of the horny layer to carry out its multiple and diverse protective functions.

Great advances in our knowledge of the structure and function of the stratum corneum, the science of corneobiology, have formed the background for a wave of improved, novel products that have recently entered the marketplace for the treatment of common dermatologic conditions. These products cover a wide range, including drugs, moisturizers, cleansers, sunscreens, barrier repair, enhanced wound healing, etc. Big Pharma, until recently, has essentially abandoned dermatology in favour of billion-dollar blockbuster drugs, opening up a marketing need for smaller companies that are dedicated exclusively to dermatology. The result has been a stunning variety of innovative products that have not only improved the efficacy and safety of traditional remedies but have made them more convenient, pleasant and easier to use. These innovations encompass new delivery systems to enhance penetration; new modes of application, including sprays, foams, gels and encapsulation in microspheres; stable, fixed combinations that were formerly incompatible; metered applications that reduce waste; packaging kits that provide complete treatment programs and formulations of active agents, which also reduce disagreeable adverse sensory responses such as itching, burning and stinging, enhancing compliance and even enhancing sleep patterns.

Many of these are available without prescriptions and, being produced by dermatologic companies, have passed the usual toxicity tests for allergic and irritant contact dermatitis, phototoxicity, comedogenicity, etc. The following section provides a selected few informative examples out of a number too great to review in detail.

Coal Tar

Coal tar has been a venerable treatment for plaque-type psoriasis for centuries but suffers from poor compliance because of its bad odour, messiness and dark staining of skin. These disagreeable factors have all been eliminated by its new presentation in a 2% quick-breaking foam that dries rapidly and spreads easily and is at least as effective as calcipotriol, an effective vitamin D derivative.

Region-Specific Products

Corneobiologists have demonstrated that the stratum corneum barrier varies greatly in various body regions, being very thick on the palms and soles, very thin on the eyelids and vulva, and has poor barrier properties of the face to immature corneocytes, mostly because of photoageing. Accordingly, products are now available that are specifically designed for each region; for example, keratolytics, such as salicylic acid, are included for the feet, moisturizers and sunscreens for the face.

Fixed Combinations for ACNE Therapy

Separate applications of a retinoid and benzoyl peroxide are highly effective for the treatment of acne vulgaris. These are incompatible when applied together because the retinoid becomes degraded by the oxidizing activity of benzoyl peroxide. A pharmacologic breakthrough has been released by a fixed combination of 0.1% adapalene and 2.5% benzoyl peroxide in a microsponge formulation. It should be noted that benzoyl peroxide is half the concentration of most stand-alone benzoyl peroxides. This is a synergistic combination of two drugs with different modes of action and has the highly valuable added advantage of lessening adverse sensory reactions (stinging, burning). Once-daily applications are sufficient, which greatly enhance compliance.

Azelaic Acid Gel

A 20% azelaic acid cream has been available for the treatment of rosacea for the last 20 years, often accompanied by irritancy and sensory discomforts. Modern formulations of topical drugs have come to appreciate that in addition to the usual toxicity tests to ascertain safety, also adverse sensory reactions, such as itching, burning and stinging are addressed. Patients will not use products, no matter how effective, if they cause disagreeable sensations. A new formulation (Finacea) containing 15% azelaic acid in the form of a gel is more agreeable to use, spreading easily, leaving no residue, less irritating, with minimal itching and stinging. Like most other dermatologic disorders, monotherapy is not optimal. Greater improvement is achieved by the addition of a mild cleanser and an emollient–moisturizer. The manufacturer is following a new trend, making available Finacea Plus, a packaging kit that includes a moisturizer and cleanser, adequately tested and relieving the consumer of having to buy these separately and having to make choices among scores of competing manufacturers.

5-Fluorouracil (5-FU) for the Treatment of Actinic Keratosis

For many decades, 5% 5-FU cream has been shown to be highly effective for the treatment of actinic keratosis in a 3-week b.i.d. course. A limitation that has greatly restricted its use has been the severe, painful, erosive, crusted, irritating reactions, which all patients experience. An ingenious solution to the intolerable irritancy problem has been the development of a 0.5% 5-FU cream (Carac), which is usually well tolerated, notably because of a tenfold reduction in concentration and because it is a slow-release microsponge formulation that allows a steady release of the drug, greatly reduced toxicity, rather than a sudden burst of; moreover, once-daily application to each head and neck lesion is often sufficient to bring about complete clearing of more than 50% of AKs in 1 week. Treatment of the remaining lesions is continued until clearing in the next week or two, a flexible arrangement. This is an excellent example of employing innovative pharmaceutical knowledge to solve a dreadful problem.

The Scientific Validation of the Efficacy of Glycerine as an Effective Component of Skin Care Formulations

Glycerol is well known to the cosmetic industry as a humectant that can take up three times its weight from a water-saturated atmosphere. It has been used extensively since its discovery in 1799 to improve dry skin conditions, based on empirical observations. Now in an ingenious study, Hora and Verkman have proved conclusively that glycerol is a major determinant of stratum corneum water retention and has other beneficial effects on stratum corneum biophysical properties [26]. This study used aquaporin-deficient mice, but the results doubtless hold for human skin. In brief, the horny layer of these mice had multiple defects manifested by markedly evaluated TEWL, decreased hydration (dryness) and poor elasticity after being deformed by suction and extremely impaired barrier repair after tape stripping. After oral intraperitoneal and topical applications of glycerol, these deficiencies were completely corrected using quantitative, sophisticated and biophysical methods. Another important finding was that glycerol enhanced the biosynthesis of the physiologic lipids that are responsible for barrier function.

Interestingly, corneobiologists, but few others, are unaware that glycerine mediates still other functions beyond its spectacular humectancy, namely, in regulating orderly shedding of corneocytes at the surface, thus keeping the horny layer at a steady state of thickness during desquamation. It accomplishes this by enhancing proteolytic activity and promoting the dissolution of corneodesmosomes near the surface, which are responsible for the cohesion of corneocytes below the surface as shown by Rawlings et al. [27].

Equally, glycerol also has effects on cornified envelopes, a previously unrecognized structural component of the horny layer that provides a new target for cutaneous therapeutics. The famous brick and mortar mould of the structural architecture of the horny layer failed to appreciate the presence of rigid, insoluble structures that surrounded the horny cells (corneocytes) and were composed of a mixture of proteins assembled during differentiation. Hirao et al. in Japan have now demonstrated that cornified envelopes are critical elements in the construction of the barrier and in mediating its functions [28]. These workers collected corneocytes by tape stripping the outermost layers of the stratum corneum and then stained these to determine the degree of maturation of cornified envelopes using Nile red to assay their acquiring hydrophobicity during maturation and anti-involucrin antibodies to evaluate loss of antigenicity during maturation. This ingenious method enabled them to differentiate immature corneocytes, which are fragile and in varying sizes and shapes, from mature ones which are rigid, flat and sturdy.

The findings of this elaborate and ingenious study are groundbreaking and very illuminating. The story begins with the discovery of the common disorders that are characterized by dysfunctional, impaired barriers, such as psoriasis and atopic dermatitis, and immature cornified envelopes were abundant in the outermost stratum corneum in contrast to the normal body areas such as the trunk and extremities where the envelopes were fully mature, whether the subjects were Caucasians, Japanese or Afro-Americans. On the other hand, immature cornified envelopes were frequently found on the face, especially in winter, explained by the fact that the facial horny layer is a poor barrier, thinner and more permeable, qualifying as dysfunctional, an unpractical area exposed to environmental stresses, such as arsenic damage. It is now firmly established that immature fragile corneocytes inevitably signify an impaired barrier [29].

Next, ex vivo incubation of corneocytes from the face in a humidified environment for a few days resulted in a rapid maturation of the corneocyte envelopes. Interestingly, exposure to facial corneocytes to commercial moisturizers accomplished the same degree of maturation, attributable simply to increased water content. To complete this picture, in vivo treatment of the face with a moisturizer had the beneficial effect of eliminating immature corneocyte envelopes, associated with improved barrier functions, such as decreased TEWL [30]. These findings are consistent with those of Rawlings and collaborators who showed that fragile corneocyte envelopes, which are increased in dry skin conditions, are converted into mature, rigid corneocytes by the application of moisturizers to the face [31].

The practical clinical message of this innovative investigation is that corneocyte envelopes should become a target for evaluating the efficacy of moisturizers in promoting the function of the horny layer barrier.

Effect of Emollients on Very Premature Infants

In no other skin disorder is the beneficial effect of an oil-rich, non-medicated emollient so striking on the general parameters of well-being as in very premature infants. Premature infants with an estimated gestational age of less than 33 weeks are born with an extremely impaired horny layer barrier. Transepidermal water loss may be 15 times greater than in the full-term infant, with drastic immediate consequences relating to dehydration, electrolyte imbalance and thermal instability. Topically applied drugs may penetrate the highly permeable stratum corneum so easily as to produce toxic systemic reactions [32]. Monitoring devices such as transcutaneous intravascular lines, urine catheters, chest tubes, etc., lead to nosocomial infection, as high as 30% [33]. Increases in the density of bacterial and fungal microflora may lead to bacteraemia and sepsis.

In a model systematic study, Nupper et al. [34] applied Aquaphor (Beiersdorf) ointment twice daily for 2 weeks to 30 very premature infants while monitoring a matched untreated control group of 30 premature infants. Aquaphor is a hydrophobic ointment that contains no preservatives and is water miscible, whose ingredients consist entirely of petrolatum, lanolin mineral oil and lanolin alcohols. They found that TEWL decreased 67% 30 min after application, greatly enhancing repair of the severely defective barrier throughout the 2-week study in relation to untreated skin. Bacterial cultures of the skin revealed significantly decreased colonization by the resident microflora, chiefly *S. epidermidis*. Positive blood and cerebrospinal cultures were 33% in the treated group and 20.7% in the untreated group. Clinical evaluation of the general condition of the skin showed increased scaling in the control group and no xerosis in the treated group. Mild dermatitis (not defined) was less apparent in the treated group.

My own group has previously conducted a pilot study on eight children with comparable lesions of severe, itchy atopic dermatitis on opposite antecubital spaces, comparing once-daily applications of the vehicle, which was not oil rich, on one side, to Eucerin Cream on the opposite side. At the end of 3 weeks, there were no differences between the two sides in any clinical criteria of improvement. However, there was a marked difference in the time to first relapse when treatment was discontinued. In three of the eight subjects, the relapse time was the same, approximately 2–3 weeks. For the other five, the vehicle-treated side showed a relapse time that was 2 weeks greater on the Eucerin side in three subjects and 3–4 weeks greater in the remaining two. The message here is that relapse times are relevant in comparing efficacy.

Treatments for Atopic Dermatitis

Awareness of the primary role of the stratum corneum in the pathogenesis of chronic inflammatory diseases, of which atopic dermatitis is the best example, has opened up new therapeutic options. Depletion of physiologic lipid, especially ceramides, is a fundamental biochemical marker that accounts for increased TEWL, decreased hydration and the signs of xerotic dry skin [35]. Old-fashioned, traditional moisturizers, such as lanolin and petrolatum, are helpful but remain trapped in the horny layer and do not reach the viable epidermis. The newest formulations by contrast contain physiologic ceramide-dominant lipids that penetrate the viable epidermis, are taken up by keratinocytes and then secreted into the intercellular lipid domains of the stratum corneum, repairing the defective, leaky barrier [36]. 'Barrier repair' creams are now very popular moisturizers, on full display on the shelves of pharmacies [12]. One of these physiologic lipid creams, EpiCeram, containing the correct molar 1:1:1 ratio of ceramides, cholesterol and fatty acids, employed as monotherapy for atopic dermatitis, has been shown to be as effective as a mid-potency corticosteroid fluticortisone (Cuterate) [37]. Another very welcome advantage of these ceramide-dominant creams is their preparation in the form of foams that leave no residue and are pleasant to use, completely avoiding the messiness of ointments.

The historical origins of corneotherapy for this application derive from the numerous, innovative works of Elias and co-workers in San Diego, California. They first laid out this approach in a 2001 paper with this interesting title, 'Does the tail wag the dog?', in which they introduced the concept of 'outside-in therapy', a novel and radical notion in the current age of immunology which holds that in common chronic inflammatory disorders, such as psoriasis, the abnormal T cells in the circulation become trapped in the dermis, which causes derangements in the overlying epidermis and stratum corneum [38]. Which Elias et al. have dubbed the 'inside-out' concept of pathogenesis, the stratum corneum alterations are secondary downstream events [39, 40]. Accordingly, the rational therapeutic approach is the use of anti-inflammatory agents, notably corticosteroids and immunosuppressives, such as calcineurin inhibitors, to suppress the dermal inflammatory reaction that in turn leads to the normalization of the impaired horny layer barrier. By contrast, outside-in therapy assumes that the abnormal horny layer is the primary pathologic event, the correction that mitigates the underlying dermal inflammatory reaction. This turns the conventional anti-inflammatory approach upside down; clinical clearing occurs as a downstream event secondary to restoration of the affected horny layer barrier. Incidentally, this highlights an unusual feature of corneotherapy, which in its form does not require the use of pharmacologically active drugs, a case in point being bland emollients and occlusive dressings. In this sense, corneotherapy is more benign as it avoids atrophogenic events such as atrophy and striae. It should be noted that the inside-out and outside-in approaches are not actually exclusive but are often complimentary in the real world.

Perturbations of the permeability barrier regardless of type, solvents, tape stripping, detergents, burns and mechanical, physical and chemical injuries all result in the stimulation of metabolic responses in the underlying epidermis aimed at normalizing the stratum corneum. The most notable response is the initiation of the cytokine and chemokine cascade, referring to the release of preformed pools of IL-Ia and TNF-b adhesion molecules, including Langerhans cell activation, inducing further downstream effects leading to trapping of circulating inflammatory cells in the dermis, angiogenesis and fibroplasia.

The cytokine cascade can provoke and sustain several important chronic inflammatory dermatoses accompanied by the accumulation of abnormal T cells in psoriasis and atopic dermatitis.

These changes are followed by barrier repair mechanisms, which these workers divide into three types:

1. Dressings containing no active pharmacologic ingredients
2. Non-physiologic lipids such as petrolatum and hydrophobic emulsions (Aquaphor)
3. Physiologic lipids comprising cholesterol, ceramides and free fatty acids in proper proportions

Non-physiologic lipids, for example, hydrophobic emulsions, such as Eucerin or Aquaphor, are indicated in extremely low-birth weight, premature infants, as they entirely lack a lamellar body secretory system and have no way to process physiologic lipids. On the other hand, physiologic lipids are indicated in atopic dermatitis and photoaged skin where depletion of ceramides has been demonstrated. In these cases and other disorders, a deficiency of lipids, application of ceramide-dominant physiologic lipids is the preferred strategy for barrier repair as the mechanism for exocytic processing of lamellar bodies into intercorneocytic bilamellar membranes is already in place.

Defective barriers can arise in a wide range of dermatologic disorders; for example, in bullous diseases, chronologic ageing and phototoxic reactions. Barrier defects associated with immunologic or pathophysiologic changes are common and familiar examples, including psoriasis, irritant and allergic contact dermatitis, hypertrophic scars and keloids, occupational dermatitis and congenital ichthyosis, and, of course, atopic dermatitis has yielded new insights regarding pathogenesis and has suggested novel approaches to treatment.

Originally it was thought that abnormalities of the adaptive immune functions were key features in pathogenesis involving Th1/Th2 cell dysregulation, increased IgE production, dendritic cell (Langerhans) signalling and production of mast cell mediators, resulting in the intense pruritus and chronic inflammatory changes that characterize this disorder. These clinical manifestations have been widely assumed to reflect downstream consequences of the immunologic abnormalities, the basis for the historical 'inside–outside' concept, promoting the use of anti-inflammatory agents to effect clinical clearing [38–40]. This traditional view has been challenged, indeed completely reoriented as a primary disorder of the structure and function of the stratum corneum. Accordingly, the well-known permeability barrier abnormality in AD is not merely an epiphenomenon, a downstream consequence of inflammation, but is in fact the very revision, the driver of disease activity, the newly constructed outside–inside view of pathogenesis. This revision is strengthened by the observation that the barrier abnormality persists years after clinical clearing, both in involved and uninvolved skin, and that specific replacement of the depleted physiologic lipids that are a hallmark feature not only corrects the barrier deficiency but comprises effective anti-inflammatory activities, replacing the use of atrophogenic corticosteroids. Furthermore, the characteristic increase in surface pH, increased serum protease activity, exposure to low environmental relative humidity, increased use of detergents for washing and barrier impairment by psychologic stress all point to weakening of the barrier as a primary factor in pathogenesis. The ascending view is that atopic dermatitis represents a genetically determined broad barrier failure.

These convergent pathologic features create a strong rationale for the deployment of specific strategy to restore barrier function, ranging from a simple reduction in pH (acidification), application of well-described effective moisturizers that have been shown to steroid-sparing application of serine protease inhibitors, culminating in the recent commercial development of ceramide-rich, triple lipid, barrier repair creams, notably EpiCeram (Ceragenix Pharmaceuticals, Denver, Colorado), which has been shown to be therapeutically equivalent to a high-potency corticosteroid, fluticasone [41]. For a more complete discussion of the genetic factors underlying atopic dermatitis, the essay by Michael Cork entitled 'Epidermal barrier dysfunction in atopic dermatitis', is a splendid, highly informative review of current knowledge [42].

Finally, the paper by Voegeli, Rawlings and collaborators on increased stratum corneum protease actively provides a detailed account of recent developments and novel therapeutic options [43]. These investigators demonstrated increased protease activity in atopic dermatitis, including tryptase-like enzyme, plasmin, urokinase and leucocyte elastase, associated with impaired barrier function, irritation and reduced capacitance (hydration). These findings suggest that serine protease inhibitors present a new option for the effective treatment of atopic dermatitis.

The Steroid-Sparing Effects of Emollients

Physicians, including dermatologists, have fallen into the habit, long sanctioned by tradition, of prescribing topical drugs to be applied twice and even three times daily. This is almost a reflex decision, not validated by evidence-based medicine. In no instance is this practice less rational and potentially more harmful than in the case of topical corticosteroids, which are first-line treatments for chronic inflammatory disorders. Recent studies have made it abundantly clear that once-daily applications of corticosteroids alternating with an emollient, usually the vehicle, are therapeutically equivalent to twice-daily applications of the corticosteroid.

Once-daily applications are salutary for two obvious reasons: the savings in cost are considerable, especially for the most potent steroids that are outrageously expensive; additionally, once-daily applications reduce the threat of adverse reactions such as atrophy, striae, rebound flares and inhibition of the pituitary–adrenal axis, especially when long-term use is required. Convincing examples of the benefits of once-daily applications abound, especially for atopic dermatitis.

In 25 children with atopic dermatitis, Lucky et al. compared the efficacy of twice-daily applications of 2.5% hydrocortisone cream to once-daily applications of the steroid alternating with an oil-rich emollient once daily (Eucerin Cream, Beiersdorf) [44]. There were no differences between the two groups at the end of 3 weeks of treatment. Both were equally effective. A high degree of satisfaction was registered by the parents and the investigators for the alternating regimen. Note that the emollient was Eucerin, not the vehicle base of the hydrocortisone cream. The vehicle is generally inferior to a time-tested oil-rich emollient.

In a similar large, multi-centred study in the United Kingdom, Bleehen et al. [45] treated 275 patients with moderate to severe atopic dermatitis, comparing twice-daily applications of 0.05% fluticasone propionate cream to once-daily application of the steroid alternating with the vehicle base. No differences were noted in therapeutic efficacy.

Kanzler treated 24 patients with plaque-type psoriasis, comparing twice-daily applications of 0.1% triamcinolone acetonide cream, a mid-potency corticosteroid, to once-daily application of the steroid alternating with its vehicle base, as in the earlier studies [46]. At the end of 4 weeks and all intervals in between, no differences in efficacy could be discerned. He also made the important observation that emollients alone can improve psoriatic plaques by as much as 25%. He urged, as we and others concur, to break the habit of twice-daily applications of corticosteroids, especially when using high-potency steroids.

Watsky et al. [47], continuing in the same vein, treated 56 male and 40 female psoriatic patients with twice-daily application of a high-potency steroid, betamethasone dipropionate, in comparison with once-daily application of the steroid alternating with once-daily application of an oil-rich emollient (Eucerin Cream; Beiersdorf, Hamburg, Germany) for 4 weeks.

Again, at all intervals, the two regimens gave identical results in respect of all clinical signs and symptoms of plaque-type psoriasis as well as clinical grading. It is noteworthy that the subjects themselves uniformly expressed satisfaction with the alternating regimen. These investigators also showed that the alternating regimen was superior to once-daily betamethasone dipropionate.

Finally, application of a potent steroid under a hydrocolloid dressing (DuoDERM) was determined to be a steroid-sparing strategy par excellence. Volden treated 48 patients with therapy-resistant atopic dermatitis including hand eczema, nummular eczema, prurigenous lichenoid papules and lichenifications, with once-weekly applications of clobetasol propionate cream, under occlusive DuoDERM hydrocolloid patches [48]. Complete clearing was obtained in 44 of the 48 patients, generally by 2 weeks. Volden estimated that the amount of steroid required to obtain these impressive results was one-twentieth to one-hundredth of the amount used in daily unocclusive applications.

The Stratum Corneum as a Depot for Topically Applied Drugs

In 1955, Malkinson and Ferguson, studying the penetration of radiolabelled hydrocortisone in humans, proposed that the stratum corneum might serve as a depot for topical drugs [49]. They suggested, wrongly as it turned out, that the open spaces within the airy 'basket weave' stratum corneum might allow the accumulation of drugs. It was Vickers in 1963 who unequivocally showed, in a series of simple but elegant studies, that the horny layer was a reservoir for topical drugs [50]. He applied the corticosteroids, fluocinoline acetonide and triamcinolone acetonide, under Saran Wrap, an impermeable plastic film, which in less than a day produced visible vasoconstriction, lasting for 10–12 h after removing the film. He then showed that vasoconstriction (blanching) could be recalled for up to 2 weeks by simply reapplying Saran Wrap. This manoeuvre released the steroid stored from within the interstices of the horny layer.

Since then, many examples of the depot effect have been reported using a variety of lipid-soluble drugs. Roberts, Gross and Anissimov have developed rigorous pharmacokinetic models of the various factors, such as partition coefficients and diffusivity, which predict deposition of the drug [51].

One of the earliest examples of the depot effect, not understood at the time, relates to systemic toxicity, including death of newborn babies by using a hexachlorophene-containing detergent to wash the diaper area. Hexachlorophene had been used for decades with no hint of adverse events, having achieved an excellent safety record. It turned out that while single washings were innocuous, repeated washings led to a build-up of hexachlorophene in the stratum corneum. Wetness of the diaper area increased permeability, as is now well known [52].

Unawareness of the depot effect can be harmful. For example, shower and bath oils are now very popular for their convenience in treating dry skin over the whole body. Consumers of these bath oils have been led to believe that these products are unusually safe and are in addition an effective way to deliver oils to combat xerosis. Loden and co-workers, however, have called attention to an unexpected adverse effect especially when used by people with sensitive skin. They applied 10% solutions of eight popular bath oils in Finn chambers for 24 h, followed by rinsing. Surprisingly, four of the oils produced a clear-cut irritant reaction, verified by increased TEWL and increased blood flow by laser Doppler velocimetry. Three other oils had negligible effects similar to a negative water control. They then rubbed some of each undiluted bath oil for 5 s over each rinsed site, followed by another 5 s rinsing with tap water. The sites were then covered with empty Finn chambers for 24 h with the intent of hydrating the skin by preventing TEWL. One of the oils, containing MIPA-laureth sulphate, showed an irritant reaction under the empty chambers. Thus, so-called protective oil films may increase the risk of an irritant by inducing a subclinical, invisible injury [53].

The depot effect may turn up unexpectedly under rather surprising circumstances. For example, the application of 10% lactic acid to the nasalar cheek for 10 min, followed by rinsing, is often used to identify persons with 'sensitive skin', who typically experience stinging, peaking in about 8 min, as originally described by Frosch and Kligman in 1977 [54]. The site was rinsed with tap water at the end of the test to remove the residue. We studied many factors that influence the stinging reaction but did not anticipate one feature that was brought to our attention by some subjects, namely that taking a shower hours after the application of 10% lactic acid resulted in recall of stinging to the original level.

We examined the recall phenomenon more closely in five women who were moderate lactic acid 'stingers'. Recall was provoked at various intervals by covering the site with a 2 square of non-woven cloth (Webril) saturated with water, sealed under impermeable tape for 10 min, thoroughly wetting the site. After a 1-h interval, wet Webril fully restored stinging to the original degree. After 3 h, the stinging was slightly less. By 6 h, stinging was barely perceptible in three of five subjects and was no longer evident by 24 h. In another study of the same five subjects, the lactic acid site was not rinsed off after the 10-min application. In that case, moderate stinging was recalled in four of the five subjects after a 48-h interval but was no longer perceptible after 72 h. Our interpretation is that lactic acid established a depot in the horny layer of the face, known to be more permeable than other body areas. Wetting the site swelled the horny layer, releasing the stored lactic acid.

Knowledge of the storage effect, presently underappreciated, may impact clinical practices. A good example is the use of topical anaesthetics to reduce pain from minor surgical procedures or exposure to lasers. Friedman et al. [55] compared the efficacy of four topical anaesthetics applied for 1 h under occlusion and tested for the degree of induced anaesthesia by pulses from a Q-switched Nd:Yag laser.

Two of the four yielded more anaesthesia at the end of 60 min. The most interesting finding, however, was that the anaesthesia increased with all four when tested 30 min after the 60-min exposure. The authors correctly surmised that a reservoir had been stored in the 'upper skin layers', doubtless the horny layer, supporting the practical suggestion of Arends–Nielson and Bjerring that patients should apply the anaesthetic under occlusion for 1 h at home before going to the office for painful laser treatment [56].

The Effect of Dressings on Disorders in Which the Human Barrier Layer Is Defective

In 1985, R. Shore, a practising dermatologist, made the serendipitous observation that a Band-Aid left in place over a psoriatic plaque for 3 weeks resulted in clinical clearing of the plaque, surprising enough to warrant publication in the *New England Journal of Medicine* [57]. One year later, he looked at various factors that might enable impermeable dressing to resolve psoriatic plaques. He found that:

1. It was best to leave the tapes in place continuously for at least 1 week.
2. Two- to 3-week continuous applications were necessary for complete clearing.
3. Occlusive tapes were more effective than semipermeable ones.
4. Application of a moderately potent corticosteroid under the tapes enhanced efficacy.
5. The occluded sites stayed clear for at least 2 weeks and sometimes as long as 1 year.

Shore could offer no plausible explanation for the effects of occlusion, a mystery that remains mostly unsolved to this very day. Earlier in 1970, Fry et al. [58] had made some preliminary observations that occlusive dressings might cause clearing of psoriatic plaques, but the findings were inconclusive and did not stimulate further work. It is worth noting, for historical accuracy, that Tree and Marks in 1975 had noted incidentally, while trying to explain the placebo effect of bland ointments, that occlusion alone inhibited the increased mitotic rate induced by tape stripping of hairless mice [12].

Interestingly, India-rubber (gutta-percha) dressing, which is occlusive, had been intensively used in the latter half of the nineteenth century in Hebra's clinic in Vienna to treat various dermatologic disorders, apparently with successful outcomes in many cases. India-rubber was eventually abandoned when it was determined that it often induced allergic contact dermatitis.

Actually, it was Winter's classical observations in 1962 that scabs would not form over wounds that were kept moist under semipermeable dressings, warning that complete occlusion might be harmful by inducing maceration [59]. In any case, it is relevant to the thesis of corneotherapy, which we are proposing, that the horny layer barrier is invariably defective in all chronic inflammatory dermatoses, such as atopic dermatitis and psoriasis, and that repair of the barrier by whatever means, pharmacologically or by dressings, is a prerequisite for healing. Furthermore, a great variety of dressing devices have flooded the marketplace, whose efficacy in correcting barrier-impaired dermatoses can no longer be questioned.

My intent in this section is to review the results of various experimenters, including my own group, to exploit the dressing technologies to promote repair of impaired barrier in various disease states. A good place to begin is the extensive studies by Visscher et al. [60] on the effect of semipermeable dressings in superficial, non-ablative wounds, inflicted on forearm skin by partial tape stripping of the stratum corneum. They found that semipermeable dressings provided the optimal water gradient for repair of the defective horny layer, while complete occlusion actually retarded healing as measured by several bioengineering techniques. I strongly recommend close reading of this paper for the insights it provides, especially for bringing forward and elaborating the new concept of 'comfort science'. In this view, the stratum corneum functions as a 'biological smart material important for imparting the visual and tactile sensory signal processing', which determines fabrics that are most comfortable to wear. I have also identified the stratum corneum as a 'smart tissue' that acts as a biosensor of external environmental changes, reacting adaptively to restore homeostatic equilibrium. I note that this is the first paper to use the term 'corneotherapy', borrowed from me, which in this case is an illustration of the practical application of comfort science. The most complete scientific analysis of 'comfort science' is to be found in the publication by Hoath et al. titled 'Sensory transduction and the mammalian epidermis' [61].

The area that has received the greatest amount of experimental attention regarding dressings and which has provided the most information and insights regarding mechanisms relates to the treatment of psoriatic plaques following the footsteps of Shore's Band-Aid discoveries [57]. The 1995 paper by Christophers et al. [62] is perhaps the most informative and revealing regarding problems encountered. They begin at the outset with the frank statement that the mechanisms are unknown. Their focus was on the diverse immunologic events in psoriatic plaques under occlusion therapy for 1 week. They compared occlusion alone, fluocinomide alone for 3 weeks and the combination of the two, finding by global clinical estimation that occlusion alone was just as effective as fluocinomide alone, whereas, of course, the combination of the two was the most effective compared to the untreated control. They used a battery of immunohistologic techniques in a quest to explain the beneficial effects of a 1-week course of occlusive dressings now that it is understood that psoriasis is an activated T-cell dependent, immunologic-mediated disorder. The epidermal immunologic tests included CD4-T cells, CT8-T cells, Langerhans cells, keratinocyte ICAM-I, IL-8 and others. The dermal tests added endothelial E-selections. The startling finding was that none of these tests were effective by any of the three treatment groups, proffering not even a clue to the mode of action.

These findings were mostly an agreement with Gottlieb et al. [63] who after 2 weeks of occlusion could detect no reduction in immunological markers. Likewise, van Vlijmen-Willems et al. [64] found no reduction along epidermal keratinocytes after 3 weeks of occlusion. The startling disparity between clinical clearing and total lack of immunologic changes is a paradox yet to be resolved. In a way, the absence of immunologic changes is consistent with my earlier findings in my thesis of 'Invisible dermatology' that the characteristic histologic changes of psoriasis, acanthosis and lymphocytic infiltrates were still present many months after clearing of psoriatic plaques by potent corticosteroids [65].

The later report by Hwang et al. [66] in 2001 was fortunately more enlightening than the previous negative reports. These workers focused on the effects of prolonged occlusion in calcium gradients that are known to be disturbed in psoriasis, along with histologic changes revealed by electron microscopy. After 7 days of occlusion, they observed dramatic changes in the parameters under study. They found by light microscopy that 7 days of occlusion resulted in markedly decreased parakeratosis, hyperkeratosis and neutrophilic infiltrates. By electron microscopy, utilizing ruthenium staining of the intercellular spaces, they were able to show striking changes, viz. decreased epidermal thickness and decreased lipid droplets in the stratum corneum, and normalization of intercorneocyte lipid layers, which are scanty and dressed in untreated prose. Increased secretion of lamellar bodies was also noted; in short, almost complete restoration of the abnormal TEM changes. Moreover, the markedly distorted loss of the normal calcium gradient was completely restored to the normal gradient in which Ca deposition is very low in the basal cell layer, reaching a peak level in the outer stratum corneum. Thus, normalization of the epidermal calcium gradient appears to be responsible for the correction of the proliferation and differentiation defects in psoriatic plaques. Although immunologic markers may not be altered by occlusive dressings, it has been shown that for 3 weeks of occlusion therapy with hydrocolloid dressings in psoriasis, expression of differentiating markers such as filaggrin and involucrin was normalized. This has important implications in that these two markers are important for the generation of natural moisturizing factors (NMF) that keep the stratum corneum hydrated even in a dry environment.

Occlusive therapy has become a field unto itself and has resulted in the industrial manufacture of a variety of devices, notable among which are hydrocolloid dressings that are not only occlusive but have the special feature of providing hydration.

Effect of Occlusive Dressing on Keloids and Hypertrophic Scars

In studies of the pathogenesis of keloids and hypertrophic scars, investigators have focused almost exclusively on the prominent changes of the dermal matrix, viz. increased deposition of collagen resulting in elevated indurated lesions, increased production of glycosaminoglycans (GAGs) and increased density of mast cells throughout the upper and lower dermis. Mast cells have received particular attention because they secrete a variety of chemical mediators that could explain the symptoms of itching, pain and inflammation associated with these scars. Little thought has been given to the possible role of the epidermis and stratum corneum when the pathologic changes are considered downstream, events secondary to alterations of the dermal matrix.

An alternative view was proposed by Suetake and co-workers in Japan who undertook an analysis of the functional changes of the stratum corneum overlying hypertrophic scars and keloids reported in 1996 [67]. Clinically, the surface seemed rather dry but they found by non-invasive hygrometric measurements that the surface was actually more hydrated than the surrounding skin. They determined that the horny layer was markedly defective as shown by a great increase in TEWL, indicating a leaky, permeable barrier. Moreover, the turnover time of the horny layer was decreased at least twofold, reflecting increased proliferative activity in the basal layer of the epidermis. Unlike other proliferative disorders, such as atopic dermatitis and psoriasis, they found that the water-holding capacity of the horny layer was increased, not decreased, as is usually the case.

Four years later, this same group, intrigued by the observation of a number of researchers that silicone gel sheets flattened and resolved keloid and hypertrophic scars, undertook a functional analysis of the horny layer overlying these scars [68]. Having found that the horny layer over scars was more hydrated than the surrounding skin, they questioned the prevalent idea that water retention induced by occlusion could be a factor in the efficacy of silicone sheets. They compared silicone sheets to an impermeable plastic, Saran Wrap, renewed daily for 1 week, having established that the TEWL of both devices was equal, 0.5 g m^2/h. They first studied two subjects, one on the normal forearm of a young woman and another on a split-thickness donor graft site. They undertook a functional analysis of the stratum corneum on days 1 and 7, using qualitative non-invasive methodologies described by Tagami. The stratum corneum changes were strikingly different for the two impermeable dressings. After 1 day, water uptake (hygroscopicity) was much greater with Saran Wrap than the silicone sheet, indicating increased hydration. After 7 days, the hydration level fell with the silicone sheet and stayed the same with Saran Wrap. After 1 day, TEWL was measured 30 min after removal of the dressings and was much greater with Saran Wrap than with silicone, increasing further after 7 days, staying the same after 7 days and again reflecting greater uptake of water by Saran Wrap. The capacity to hold water (hydrophilicity), revealed by sorption–desorption kinetics, was as expected greater after Saran Wrap than silicone, increasing further after 7 days of Saran Wrap. Additionally, two subjects with hypertrophic scars were subjected to the same analysis of stratum corneum functions, with results comparable to those described previously for normal skin. Interestingly, these investigators likened the Saran Wrap results to those that were characteristic of the changes induced by an effective moisturizer (Tagami).

The conclusion was that silicone sheets maintained a mild level of hydration, falling with continued exposures, compared to excessive hydration and water-holding capacity with Saran Wrap. Clinicians were aware that excessive exposure to water in such occupations as hair tending, cannery workers and dishwashers experienced adverse effects that Kligman described under the heading of 'hydration dermatitis' [69].

Finally, Elias et al. [70] (P.M. Elias, unpublished data) treated six keloid patients with silicone gel sheets for 24 weeks and demonstrated unequivocal benefits in regard to reductions in itching, pain, redness and elevation, already evident by 4 weeks, with steady improvements over 24 weeks, with complete disappearance of itching and pain.

My group performed pilot studies on two young men with extremely dense and elevated hypertrophic scars associated with severe acne conglobata of the upper back. We compared three treatments on 3-in. squares with symmetrical scars: (1) silicone gel sheets changed daily for 4 weeks, except on weekends; (2) Saran Wrap changed every 3 days for 4 weeks, sealed under occlusive Blenderm tape; and (3) water-saturated non-woven cotton pads (Webril) sealed under Blenderm tape, changed every 3 days. By the end of 4 weeks, we estimated a modest flattening of the scars with fading of erythema with silicone sheets, somewhat less so with Saran Wrap. By contrast, we had to stop the wet Webril applications after 6 and 9 days, respectively, owing to a fierce exacerbation of inflammation, pain, exudation, maceration and oedema, signs that slowly resolved after b.i.d. applications of 0.05% clobetasol propionate cream. This was a dramatic illustration of 'hydration dermatitis'.

Perhaps the most instructive finding of the study by Elias et al. [70] (P.M. Elias, unpublished data) was a decreased density of mast cells throughout the upper and lower dermis, revealed by toluidine blue staining. Mast cells are known to secrete a number of chemical mediators, especially histamine and substance P, which presumably explains the relief of itching, pain and redness by silicone sheets, which are valuable not only for treatment but for the prevention of emerging scars after surgical excisions (Fulton).

Elias et al. [70] (P.M. Elias, unpublished data) have synthesized these findings into a plausible hypothesis of the mechanisms by which silicone sheets exert their beneficial effects, starting with the proved demonstration that the horny layers overlying keloid and hypertrophic scars are defective, structurally deranged and functionally more permeable, known also to be a reservoir or storage depot of pro-inflammatory substances. Accordingly, primary cytokines are released that 'stimulate the formation of additional cytokines, resulting in a downstream cascade of additional cytokines, adhesion molecules and other mediators'. Fibroplasia and angiogenesis are subsequently engendered, which lead to increased production of collagen and GAGs, prominent features of scars. The therapeutic end game is restoration of the impaired barrier that would interrupt this pathogenic sequence.

Conclusions

Corneobiology refers to that broad range of experimental studies that are focused on the anatomy, physiology and biology of the stratum corneum, centred particularly on the human horny layer that has features uniquely different from other mammals. Corneobiology has a very broad reach, encompassing studies that deal with immunology, endocrinology, neurobiology and psychology, comprising a network of complex interactions that have connections to the central nervous system. It has attracted the attention of a confederation of scientists from very different disciplines, including molecular biologists, anatomists, physiologists, pharmacologists, geneticists, psychologists and still others. Corneotherapy refers to preventive interventions that are primarily directed to the correction and restoration of the stratum corneum barrier that has been rendered defective and impaired by disease, genetics and a variety of mechanical, physical, chemical and psychological exogenous insults and stresses. Contributors to building the edifice, we now call corneobiology, are a motley, diverse crew of investigators, mainly situated in industry and academia from around the world.

AV Rawlings has recently named me as 'the father of corneobiology' [71], a high tribute that I hope represents the consensus of the world of corneobiologists.

Acknowledgements

The compilation of this review was initiated by Lorraine Kligman in memory of her husband. Dr. AV Rawlings assisted in compiling the document in cooperation with Ms. Anne Rulinski, Department of Dermatology, University of Pennsylvania, USA.

References

1. Kligman AM (1964) The biology of the stratum corneum. In: Montagna W, Lobitz WB (eds) The epidermis. Academic Press, New York, pp 387–433
2. Kligman AM (2006) A brief history of how the dead stratum corneum became alive. In: Elias PM, Feingold KR (eds) Skin barrier. Taylor & Francis, New York, pp 15–24
3. Rothman S (1954) Physiology and biochemistry of skin. University of Chicago Press, Chicago, pp 64
4. Christophers E, Kligman AM (1964) Visualization of the cell layers of the stratum corneum. J Invest Dermatol 42:407–409
5. Elias PM (2005) Stratum corneum defensive functions: an integrated view. J Invest Dermatol 125(2):183–200
6. Elias PM, Feingold KR (2006) Skin barrier. Taylor & Francis, New York
7. Pedersen L, Jemec GB (2006) Mechanical properties and barrier function of healthy human skin. Acta Derm Venereol 86(4):308–311
8. Rawlings AV, Watkinson A, Harding C, Hope J, Scott IR (1995) Changes in stratum corneum lipid structure and water barrier function during mechanical stress. J Soc Cosmet Chem 46:141–151
9. Rawlings A (2009) Fifty years of stratum corneum and moisturisation research. IFSCC Mag 12:169–170

10. Rawlings AV, Scott IR, Harding C, Bowser P (1994) Stratum corneum moisturisation at the molecular level. J Invest Dermatol 103:731–740
11. Marks R (1972) Histochemical applications of skin surface biopsy. Br J Dermatol 86(1):20–26
12. Tree S, Marks R (1975) An explanation for the ‘placebo’ effect of bland ointment bases. Br J Dermatol 92(2):195–198
13. Takematsu H, Ohmoto Y, Tagami H (1990) Decreased levels of IL-1 alpha and beta in psoriatic lesional skin. Tohoku J Exp Med 161(3):159–169
14. Dalziel K, Dykes PJ, Marks R (1984) Inflammation due to intra-cutaneous implantation of stratum corneum. Br J Exp Pathol 65(1):107–115
15. Nickoloff BJ, Naidu Y (1994) Perturbation of epidermal barrier function correlates with initiation of cytokine cascade in human skin. J Am Acad Dermatol 30(4):535–546
16. Nickoloff BJ (1995) Immunological reactions triggered during irritant contact dermatitis. Am J Contact Dermat 9:107–109
17. Scheuplein RJ, Blank IH (1971) Permeability of the skin. Physiol Rev 51(4):702–747
18. Richter T, Peuckert C, Sattler M et al (2004) Dead but highly dynamic – the stratum corneum is divided into three hydration zones. Skin Pharmacol Physiol 17(5):246–257
19. Pfeiffer S, Vielhaber G, Vietzke JP, Wittern KP, Hintze U, Wepf R (2000) High-pressure freezing provides new information on human epidermis: simultaneous protein antigen and lamellar lipid structure preservation. Study on human epidermis by cryoimmobilization. J Invest Dermatol 114(5):1030–1038
20. Menon GK, Elias PM (1997) Morphologic basis for a pore-pathway in mammalian stratum corneum. Skin Pharmacol 10(5–6):235–246
21. Penneys NS, Eaglstein W, Ziboh V (1980) Petrolatum: interference with the oxidation of arachidonic acid. Br J Dermatol 103(3):257–262
22. Comaish JS, Greener JS (1976) The inhibiting effect of soft paraffin on the Kobner response in psoriasis. Br J Dermatol 94(2):195–200
23. Kligman LH, Kligman AM (1992) Petrolatum and other hydrophobic emollients reduce UVB-induced damage. J Dermatolog Treat 3:3–7
24. Kligman AM (1978) Regression method for testing the efficacy of moisturizers. Cosmet Toilet 93:27–36
25. Held E, Sveinsdottir S, Agner T (1999) Effect of long-term use of moisturizer on skin hydration, barrier function and susceptibility to irritants. Acta Derm Venereol 79(1):49–51
26. Hara M, Verkman AS (2003) Glycerol replacement corrects defective skin hydration, elasticity, and barrier function in aquaporin-3-deficient mice. Proc Natl Acad Sci U S A 100(12):7360–7365
27. Rawlings AV, Watkinson A, Hope J, Harding C, Sabin R (1995) The effect of glycerol and humidity on desmosome degradation in stratum corneum. Arch Dermatol Res 36:1936–1944
28. Hirao T, Denda M, Takahashi M (2001) Identification of immature cornified envelopes in the barrier-impaired epidermis by characterization of their hydrophobicity and antigenicities of the components. Exp Dermatol 10(1):35–44
29. Hirao T, Takahashi M, Kikuchi K, Terui T, Tagami H (2003) A novel non-invasive evaluation method of cornified envelope maturation in the stratum corneum provides a new insight for skin care cosmetics. IFSCC Mag 6(2):103–109
30. Kikuchi K, Tagami H (2008) Noninvasive biophysical assessments of the efficacy of a moisturizing cosmetic cream base for patients with atopic dermatitis during different seasons. Br J Dermatol 158(5):969–978
31. Harding CR, Long S, Richardson J et al (2003) The cornified cell envelope: an important marker of stratum corneum maturation in healthy and dry skin. Int J Cosmet Sci 25(4):157–167
32. Barker N, Hadgraft J, Rutter N (1987) Skin permeability in the newborn. J Invest Dermatol 88(4):409–411
33. Gladstone IM, Clapper L, Thorp JW, Wright DI (1988) Randomized study of six umbilical cord care regimens. Comparing length of attachment, microbial control, and satisfaction. Clin Pediatr (Phila) 27(3):127–129

34. Nopper AJ, Horii KA, Sookdeo-Drost S, Wang TH, Mancini AJ, Lane AT (1996) Topical ointment therapy benefits premature infants. J Pediatr 128(5 Pt 1): 660–669
35. Imokawa G, Abe A, Jin K, Higaki Y, Kawashima M, Hidano A (1991) Decreased level of ceramides in stratum corneum of atopic dermatitis: an etiologic factor in atopic dry skin? J Invest Dermatol 96(4):523–526
36. Elias PM (2006) Epilogue: fixing the barrier – theory and rationale deployment. In: Elias PM, Feingold KR (eds) Skin barrier. Taylor & Francis, New York, pp 591–600
37. Sugarman JL (2008) The epidermal barrier in atopic dermatitis. Semin Cutan Med Surg 27(2):108–114
38. Elias PM, Feingold KR (2001) Does the tail wag the dog? Role of the barrier in the pathogenesis of inflammatory dermatoses and therapeutic implications. Arch Dermatol 137(8):1079–1081
39. Elias PM, Hatano Y, Williams ML (2008) Basis for the barrier abnormality in atopic dermatitis: outside-inside-outside pathogenic mechanisms. J Allergy Clin Immunol 121(6):1337–1343
40. Elias PM, Steinhoff M (2008) 'Outside-to-inside' (and now back to 'outside') pathogenic mechanisms in atopic dermatitis. J Invest Dermatol 128(5):1067–1070
41. Sugarman JL, Parish LC (2009) Efficacy of a lipid-based barrier repair formulation in moderate-to-severe pediatric atopic dermatitis. J Drugs Dermatol 8(12):1106–1111
42. Cork MJ, Danby SG, Vasilopoulos Y et al (2009) Epidermal barrier dysfunction in atopic dermatitis. J Invest Dermatol 129(8):1892–1908
43. Voegeli R, Rawlings AV, Breternitz M, Doppler S, Schreier T, Fluhr JW (2009) Increased stratum corneum serine protease activity in acute eczematous atopic skin. Br J Dermatol 161(1):70–77
44. Lucky AW, Leach AD, Laskarzewski P, Wenck H (1997) Use of an emollient as a steroid-sparing agent in the treatment of mild to moderate atopic dermatitis in children. Pediatr Dermatol 14(4):321–324
45. Bleehen SS, Chu AC, Hamann I, Holden C, Hunter JA, Marks R (1995) Fluticasone propionate 0.05% cream in the treatment of atopic eczema: a multicentre study comparing once-daily treatment and once-daily vehicle cream application versus twice-daily treatment. Br J Dermatol 133(4):592–597
46. Kanzler MH, Chui C, Gorsulowsky DC (2001) Once-daily vs twice-daily triamcinolone acetonide cream for psoriasis. Arch Dermatol 137(11):1529–1532
47. Watsky KL, Freije L, Leneveu MC, Wenck HA, Leffell DJ (1992) Water-in-oil emollients as steroid-sparing adjunctive therapy in the treatment of psoriasis. Cutis 50(5):383–386
48. Volden G (1992) Successful treatment of therapy resistant atopic dermatitis with clobetasol propionate and a hydrocolloid occlusive dressing. Acta Derm Venereol Suppl (Stockh) 176:126–128
49. Malkinson FD, Ferguson EH (1955) Percutaneous absorption of hydrocortisone-4-C14 in two human subjects. J Invest Dermatol 25(5):281–283
50. Vickers CF (1963) Existence of reservoir in the stratum corneum. Experimental proof. Arch Dermatol 88:20–23
51. Roberts MS, Cross SE, Anissimov YG (2004) Factors affecting the formation of a skin reservoir for topically applied solutes. Skin Pharmacol Physiol 17(1):3–16
52. Marzulli FN, Maibach HI (1975) The hexachlorophene story. In: Maibach HI (ed) Animal models in dermatology. Charles Livingston, New York, pp 156–159
53. Loden M, Buraczewska I, Edlund F (2004) Irritation potential of bath and shower oils before and after use: a double-blind randomized study. Br J Dermatol 150(6):1142–1147
54. Frosch PJ, Kligman AM (1977) A method of appraising the stinging capacity of topically applied substances. J Soc Cosmet Chem 28:197–209
55. Friedman PM, Fogelman JP, Nouri K, Levine VJ, Ashinoff R (1999) Comparative study of the efficacy of four topical anesthetics. Dermatol Surg 25(12):950–954
56. Arendt-Nielsen L, Bjerring P (1988) Laser-induced pain for evaluation of local analgesia: a comparison of topical application (EMLA) and local injection (lidocaine). Anesth Analg 67(2):115–123
57. Shore RN (1985) Clearing of psoriatic lesions after the application of tape. N Engl J Med 312(4):246

58. Fry L, Almeyda J, McMinn RM (1970) Effect of plastic occlusive dressings on psoriatic epidermis. Br J Dermatol 82(5):458–462
59. Winter GD (1995) Formation of the scab and the rate of epithelisation of superficial wounds in the skin of the young domestic pig. 1962. J Wound Care 4(8):366–367; discussion 368–371
60. Visscher M, Hoath SB, Conroy E, Wickett RR (2001) Effect of semipermeable membranes on skin barrier repair following tape stripping. Arch Dermatol Res 293(10):491–499
61. Hoath SB, Donnelly MM, Boissy RE (1990) Sensory transduction and the mammalian epidermis. Biosens Bioelectron 5(5):351–366
62. Christophers E, Griffiths CEM, Tranfaglia MG (1995) Prolonged occlusion in the treatment of psoriasis. A clinical and immunochemical study. J Am Acad Dermatol 32:618–622
63. Gottlieb AB, Staiano-Coico L, Cohen SR, Varghese M, Carter DM (1990) Occlusive hydrocolloid dressings decrease keratinocyte population growth fraction and clinical scale and skin thickness in active psoriatic plaques. J Dermatol Sci 1(2):93–96
64. van Vlijmen-Willems IM, Chang A, Boezeman JB, van de Kerkhof PC (1993) The immunohistochemical effect of a hydrocolloid occlusive dressing (DuoDERM E) in psoriasis vulgaris. Dermatology 187(4):257–262
65. Kligman AM (1966) Blind man dermatology. J Soc Cosmet Chem 17:505–509
66. Hwang SM, Ahn SK, Menon GK, Choi EH, Lee SH (2001) Basis of occlusive therapy in psoriasis: correcting defects in permeability barrier and calcium gradient. Int J Dermatol 40(3):223–231
67. Suetake T, Sasai S, Zhen YX, Ohi T, Tagami H (1996) Functional analyses of the stratum corneum in scars. Sequential studies after injury and comparison among keloids, hypertrophic scars, and atrophic scars. Arch Dermatol 132(12):1453–1458
68. Suetak T, Sasai S, Zhen YX, Tagami H (2000) Effects of silicone gel sheet on the stratum corneum hydration. Br J Plast Surg 53(6):503–507
69. Kligman AM (1996) Hydration injury to human skin. In: Van der Valk PGM, Maibach HI (eds) The irritant contact dermatitis syndrome. CRC Press, Boca Raton, pp 187–194
70. Elias PM, Ansel JC, Woods LD, Feingold KR (1996) Signaling networks in barrier homeostasis. The mystery widens. Arch Dermatol 132(12):1505–1506
71. Rawlings AV (2008) What is the cutaneous barrier? Nouv Dermatol 27:93–98

Contents

Part I

The Marketplace and Treatment Aspects

1 Moisturizers as Cosmetics, Medicines, or Medical Device? The Regulatory Demands in the European Union

Amy Sörensen, Peter Landvall, and Marie Lodén

1.1 Introduction

Moisturization of the skin is important for both cosmetic and medical purposes. The majority of moisturizing creams on the market are regulated as cosmetics; however, they may also be classified as pharmaceuticals (equivalent to medicinal products) or as a medical device within the European Member States. When they are regulated as pharmaceuticals or medical devices, they can also be marketed for treatment or prevention of diseases, such as atopic eczema, psoriasis, ichthyosis, and other hyperkeratotic skin diseases. There has been an increase in topically applied semi-solid formulations certified as medical devices used for the treatment of skin diseases in recent years [1].

Moisturizing creams contain a number of different ingredients which can affect their suitability for the different types of dry skin conditions. In addition, these products come into close contact with our body, and they are generally used for long periods of time, which makes their compatibility with our body important.

A. Sörensen
Sorensen Consulting, Cosmetic Regulatory Department, Höllviken, Sweden

P. Landvall
Cellwell, Medical Device Regulatory Department, Åkersberga, Sweden

M. Lodén (✉)
Eviderm Institute, Research and Development, Bergshamra Allé 9, SE-17077 Solna, Sweden
e-mail: marie.loden@eviderm.se

The regulatory requirements and the approval processes for the three product categories are not the same; for example, cosmetics, and class I medical devices are not approved by any (outside) external/third party organization or authority before being placed on the market. On the other hand, medical devices class IIa, IIb, and III need third party (Notified Body) verification of fulfilling medical device regulation while pharmaceuticals go through rigorous evaluation and are granted a "marketing authorization".

The present chapter will give an overview of the similarities and differences between the different regulatory categories. The borders will be described to help the reader understand the gray areas in classification between the categories.

1.2 Regulations and Classifications

Cosmetic products are currently regulated under the Cosmetic Directive 76/768/EEC and its amendments [2]. In late 2009, a Cosmetic Regulation was adopted, 1223/2009/EC, which replaces the above directive and comes into force on 11th July 2013, with some elements earlier [3].

Medicinal Products for Human Use (pharmaceuticals) is regulated under Directive 2001/83/EC and its amendments [4].

Medical devices are regulated under the Medical Device Directive 93/42/EEC and its amendments [5].

Other regulations may also be applicable, such as Regulation (EC) 1272/2008, classification,

M. Lodén, H.I. Maibach (eds.), *Treatment of Dry Skin Syndrome*,
DOI 10.1007/978-3-642-27606-4_1, © Springer-Verlag Berlin Heidelberg 2012

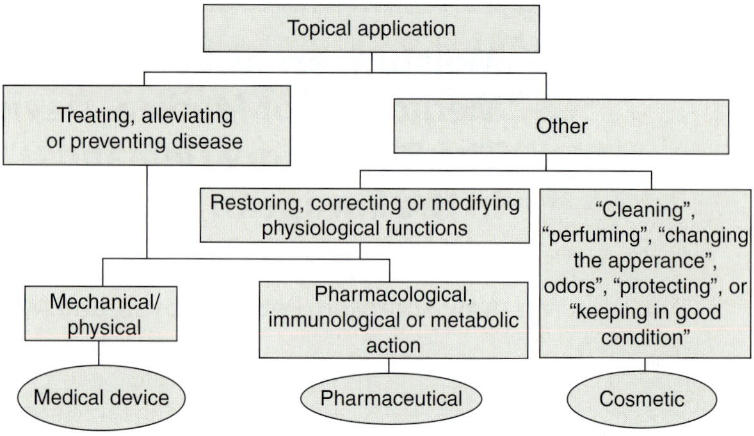

Fig. 1.1 A schematic view on the classification of a medical device, a pharmaceutical and a cosmetic product

labeling and packaging of substances and mixtures, [6] and the General Product Safety Directive 2001/95/EC.

The borderlines between the different product categories may be difficult to demarcate. The intended use, mode of action, composition, physiological properties, and the risks of use are the bases to determine which set of regulations should be applied to a topical formulation, Fig. 1.1 [7, 8].

The definition of a cosmetic product is based on *target* of the application and the *intended function* [3]:

> Any substance or mixture intended to be placed in contact with the various external parts of the human body (epidermis, hair system, nails, lips and external genital organs) or with the teeth and the mucous membranes of the oral cavity with a view exclusively or mainly to cleaning them, perfuming them, changing their appearance and or/correcting body odours and/or protecting them or keeping them in good condition.

The definition is thus based on two cumulative aspects, i.e. the target site of application and the intended main (cosmetic) function.

A "medicinal product" is defined either by virtue of its "presentation" or its "function" [4]. A product constitutes a medicinal product if it falls within either of these two categories:

> Any substance or combination of substances presented as having properties for treating or preventing disease in human beings; or

> Any substance or combination of substances which may be used in or administered to human beings either with a view to restoring, correcting or modifying physiological functions by exerting a pharmacological, immunological or metabolic action, or to making a medical diagnosis.

The terms for the actions are defined according to the following [8]:

"*Pharmacological action*": interaction between the molecules of the substance in question and a cellular constituent, usually referred to as a receptor, which either results in a direct response, or which blocks the response to another agent. Although not a completely reliable criterion, the presence of a dose-response correlation is indicative of a pharmacological effect.

"*Immunological action*": action in or on the body by stimulation and/or mobilisation of cells and/or products involved in a specific immune reaction.

"*Metabolic action*": action which involves an alteration, including stopping, starting or changing the speed of the normal chemical processes participating in, and available for, normal body function. The fact that a product is metabolised by the human body does not necessarily mean that the substance contained in the product has a metabolic action upon the body.

A "Medical Device" is Defined in Article 1(2) of the Medical Device Directive as:

> Any instrument, apparatus, appliance, software, material or other article, whether used alone or in combination, including the software intended by its manufacturer to be used specifically for diagnostic and/or therapeutic purposes and necessary for its proper application, intended by the manufacturer to be used for human beings for the purpose of:
>
> - diagnosis, prevention, monitoring, treatment or alleviation of disease,
> - diagnosis, monitoring, treatment, alleviation of or compensation for an injury or handicap,
> - investigation, replacement or modification of the anatomy or of a physiological process,
> - control of conception,
>
> and which does not achieve its principal intended action in or on the human body by pharmacological, immunological or metabolic means, but which may be assisted in its function by such means.

Medical devices are divided into different classes which are determined by the hazardous use at the *intended use* of the device and *mode of action* [5] (outlined in Annex IX of the Medical Device Directive 93/42/EEC). There are four medical device classes – class I, class IIa, class IIb and class III. The higher the classification, the more hazards are connected to usage for the patient. The classification depends on rules that involve the medical device's duration of body contact, its invasive character, if it has an active substance or not and if it is in connection with the central circulatory system or central nervous system.

Medical devices with a *transient* use are normally intended for continuous use for less than 60 min. Those for *short-term* use are normally intended for continuous use for between 60 min and 30 days, and those for *long-term* use are normally intended for continuous use for more than 30 days. Invasive devices are those which, in whole or in part, penetrate inside the body, either through a body orifice (any natural opening in the body, as well as the external surface of the eyeball) or through a surgical opening of the body. Medical devices can also be denoted as active medical device and active therapeutical device. An active medical device relies on an external source of power (e.g. electrical energy) to exert its function (e.g. laser, photodynamic therapy), whereas the active therapeutical device uses energy, such as electricity, to support, modify, replace, or restore biological functions or structures with a view to treatment or alleviation of an illness, injury, or handicap.

Non-invasive devices, which come into contact with skin, are in class I (low risk), if they are intended to be used as a mechanical barrier, for compression or for absorption of exudates (e.g. simple wound dressings), whereas they belong to class IIb (moderate-high risk), if they are intended to be used principally with wounds which have breached the dermis and can only heal by secondary intent (e.g. chronic ulcerated wounds, dressings for severe burns). Other non-invasive devices are in class IIa (low-moderate risk), including devices principally intended to manage the micro-environment of a wound.

The authorities have clearly stated that a product cannot fall into more than one category. A medical device should not achieve its principal intended action in or on the human body by pharmacological, immunological or metabolic means, but may be assisted in its function by such means. For example, a pharmacological and metabolic action is demonstrated by zinc oxide containing products; for example, it may play a role in enzymatic processes for support of wound granulation. The pharmacological action may, however, be ancillary when the product concerned is primarily a barrier cream. In such cases, the qualification of zinc oxide containing products is defined as medical device taking into account the claims, the intended purpose and the relevant primary mode of action. Hence, the product is regulated in accordance with rule 13 of Annex IX of Directive 93/42/EEC and not in accordance with Article 2(b) of Directive 2001/83/EC. However, medical devices that contain a substance which separately can be considered as a medicinal substance (as defined in Article 1 of Directive 2001/83/EC) belong to class III devices (high risk). For example, corn plasters containing salicylic acid will be considered as a class III medical device due to the analgesic properties of salicylic acid, whereas those containing trichloroacetic acid for the treatment of corns are considered as class IIa devices as this other acid is considered a chemical substance [9].

In case of doubt, where taking into account all product characteristics, and provided that the product in question meets both the definitions of a pharmaceutical and of a medical device, the provisions of Directive 2001/83/EC applies. However, the national Competent Authorities act under the supervision of the national courts which determines, on a case-by-case basis, which regulatory framework applies to a certain product. For that reason, the regulatory status for a certain product may differ between countries.

1.3 Notifications, Registration, and Market Authorizations

Cosmetic products do not require any pre-market authorization (approval). Instead, cosmetic products need only to be notified. This process is typically simple and varies from country to country. The individual country notification systems will be replaced by a single EU Notification System that should go into effect in 2012. This system will be connected to the various Poison Control Centres in the Member States. While no product approval is necessary, cosmetic manufacturers are expected to have a Product Information File (PIF) prepared for each cosmetic product prior to the products placement on the market.

Pharmaceuticals are the most stringently regulated product category. A marketing authorization needs to be granted by the competent authority *before* the product can be placed on the market. Separate approvals are needed for each country, but this process is usually straightforward once an initial marketing authorization has been granted.

A medical device class I does not require pre-market authorization, but is instead guaranteed by a Declaration of Conformity made by the manufacturer/authorized representative. The risks connected with class I devices are low, which allow the manufacturer to take full responsibility to assess the conformity of these devices to the legislation and certify the product. All class I medical devices have to be registered with the assigned national Competent Authority. In addition, a class I medical device that is placed on the market in a sterile condition or that is used to measure a function must apply to a Notified Body for assessment in regards to aspects of these functions.

A Notified Body must be involved at the production stage for class IIa devices, whereas devices with a high-risk potential, classes IIb and III, require inspection by a Notified Body with regard to both the design and manufacture of the device. The Notified Body will issue a certificate verifying that the product fulfills the relevant requirements in the medical device directive. This is not an actual approval, but its issue means that the product is in compliance and can be placed on the market. Medical devices class IIa, IIb, and III are not required to be registered at the national medical device Competent Authority; however, various countries have added rules requiring registration of some or all of these classes.

The national Competent Authority for medical devices conducts regular market surveillance to review products and their documentation. Any nonconformity can mean a marketing ban on the product and withdrawal of the CE mark.

1.4 Manufacturing and Supply

Manufacturing practice plays an important role in the quality of topical products. One important difference between pharmaceuticals and other topical products is the approval process for *both* the manufacturing facility and the manufacturing process prior to the release of the pharmaceutical to the market, Table 1.1.

Cosmetic products do not require any external approvals for the manufacturing process or the facility. Manufacturers should fulfill the appropriate testing and production to ensure that the product is ready for the consumer in accordance with the regulation [3] and the manufacturing standard for cosmetics (ISO 22716:2007).

In contrast, manufacturing units for pharmaceuticals are regularly inspected by the Competent

Table 1.1 Overview of differences and similarities in regulatory requirements for topical products

Parameter	Cosmetics	Pharmaceuticals	Medical devices (Class I non-sterile and non-measuring and Class IIa)
Targeted body regions	Skin, hair, teeth, outer genitalia and mucosa in the mouth	Skin, hair, teeth, inner and outer genitalia/vulva, nasal cavity, mucosa in the mouth, ear canal, and eyes	Skin, hair, teeth, inner and outer genitalia/ vulva, nasal cavity, mucosa in the mouth, ear canal, and eyes
Common formulation types	Emulsions, ointments, liquids, gels	Emulsions, ointments, liquids, gels	Emulsions, ointments, liquids, gels
Marketing, presentation	No reference to diseases is allowed	Treatment and/or prevention of diseases	Treatment and/or prevention of diseases
Pre-market authorization of product	No	Yes	No
Authorization of Good Manufacturing Practice (GMP) by Competent Authority	No	Yes	No
Mode of action of actives	Mainly physical, no significant modification of physiological functions via pharmacological, immunological and/or metabolic action	Changes of physiological functions via pharmacological, immunological and/or metabolic action	Mainly via physical effects, may include changes of physiological functions
Ingredient labeling	All ingredients must appear on the labeling using International Nomenclature of Cosmetic Ingredients (INCI)	All ingredients must appear on the labeling. Excipients should be referred to by their recommended international non-proprietary name (INN), the European Pharmacopoeia name or failing this, their usual common name	Not mandatory to label ingredients considered to be innocuous
Efficacy studies	May be inspected by Competent Authority	Competent Authority approves protocol and receives information on study results	Competent Authority is informed about study protocol and may ban the study based on consideration of public health and safety
Safety studies	Animal experiments on finished product are not allowed, and ban on raw materials testing are being implemented	Studies on animals and humans are performed if considered relevant	Studies on animals and humans are performed if considered relevant
Consumer information on risks for adverse effects	May be labeled, but is available on demand by the affected consumer	Product Information Leaflet (PIL)	In Instructions For Use (IFU)

Authority and receive a Good Manufacturing Practice certificate upon approval of the routines. The manufacturing process is evaluated and reviewed during the approval process.

Medical device manufacturers are regularly assessed by the Notified Body to verify that the manufacturer fulfills the requirements for the production of all classes (except class I non-sterile). The frequency of the assessment depends on the classification of the product.

All three product types have requirements for traceability both at the production stages (where ingredients and components do come from) and in the marketing stage (to whom the products are sold). The new Cosmetic Regulation states that the responsible person needs to identify downstream distributors and that a distributor has to identify its upstream suppliers and the responsible persons. Both are obliged to do so for the 3 years that follow the batch of the cosmetic product being made available to the distributor.

1.5 Labeling and Markings

The Cosmetic Regulation has basic requirements for cosmetic labeling: function of the product, net contents, manufacturer/distributor name and address, and an ingredient listing. Directions are not necessarily required. Warning statements may be required depending on the presence of certain ingredients or to prevent harm to the consumer.

Cosmetic products are required to have a "best used before the end of…" date. If the product has a shelf life greater than 30 months, instead of a "best used before the end of" date, it can carry an open jar symbol together with a number denoting a period of time after opening for which the product can be used – the Period After Opening (PAO) Symbol. The Cosmetic Regulation also allows cosmetic products to carry the same type of symbol as used on medical devices to denote an expiry as opposed to stating, "best used before the end of…", Fig. 1.2.

Product labels may contain a "Hand and Book" symbol to indicate that further information, often in other languages, is contained within the package. Certain products also contain an e-mark, which is a mark appended to the nominal mass or volume printed on pre-packaged goods for sale. Cosmetic products are required to have batch numbers and to state the country of origin (if imported into the EU).

The labels for pharmaceuticals are reviewed and approved by the Competent Authorities prior to product approval. These labels have a prescribed format and content, and the size of the letters should be at least Times New Roman 9 point. Pharmaceuticals also have a Product Information Leaflet (PIL) which is approved by the authorities.

The following is a general list of items that shall appear on the label of a pharmaceutical product.

- Name of the pharmaceutical, followed by strength and pharmaceutical form
- Statement of active substances expressed qualitatively and quantitatively per dosage unit or according to the form of administration for a given volume or weight, using their common names
- Pharmaceutical form and the net contents either by weight, by volume or by number of doses of the product
- List of excipients
- Method of administration and if necessary, the route of administration
- Special warning to store out of reach and sight of children
- Warnings
- Expiry date
- Special storage precautions
- Specific precautions relating to the disposal of unused pharmaceuticals or waste derived from the product

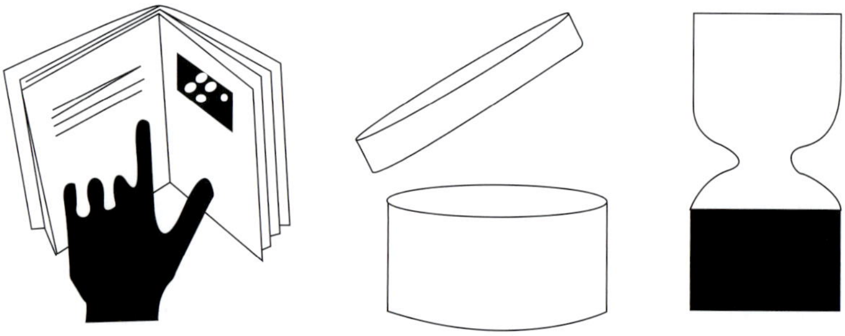

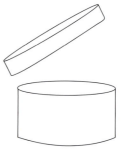

Fig. 1.2 Hand and Book Symbol. Period After Opening (PAO) Symbol. Date of minimum durability

- Name and address of the marketing authorization holder
- The number of the authorization (MT number)
- Batch number
- Instructions for use in the case of non-prescription pharmaceuticals

A medical device presentation (label, Instruction for Use (IFU), packaging) has many of the same basic requirements as the label for a pharmaceutical (trade name, manufacturer and address, batch code/serial number, warnings/precautions, instructions for use and storage, etc.). The major difference between a medical device label and the label of other products is the use of the CE mark and other symbols according to the ISO standard EN 980. Furthermore, ingredients considered to be innocuous do not need to be labeled.

The CE mark guarantees the compliance of the product with the medical device regulations and is placed on the device or its package in a way that it will be separated from other symbols. The CE marking is an assurance by the manufacturer that the device will perform as stated, the product is safe and that the clinical benefit of the device outweighs any side effects when it is used as intended. With few exceptions, medical devices cannot be sold without the CE mark, and the CE mark cannot be affixed unless the product is in compliance with medical device regulation.

Medical devices are also permitted to use other types of international symbols which can be used without any explanation within Europe. There is a special harmonized European Standard (EN 980:2008) which lays out the authorized symbols. Use of these symbols simplifies the labeling, helps to prevent the need for multiple translations, and prevents separate development of different symbols to convey the same information. The use of any other symbols *not* specified in EN 980:2008 has to be explained in the "Instruction for Use."

While the product label for the three categories has distinct differences, there are similar requirements which are handled differently by the regulations. These differences can cause confusion for the consumer. For example, the nomenclature for ingredient labeling is not harmonized for the three regulatory categories of products although there is overlap. Cosmetic products use INCI nomenclature (International Nomenclature Cosmetic Ingredients) while pharmaceuticals typically use International Nonproprietary Names (INN) or the European Pharmacopoeia (Ph Eur) nomenclature, if available. This can make it complicated for the consumers to avoid products with substances for which they have a known contact allergy, such as preservatives [10]. Certain ingredients can also trigger specific warning statements, which may differ between the product categories, Table 1.2.

Table 1.2 Examples of differences in the nomenclature of ingredients in cosmetics, pharmaceuticals, and medical device, and potential mandatory warnings

INCI name	INN/Ph Eur	Wording of warnings on the label
Arachis hypogaea oil	Peanut oil/arachidis oleum	"(Medicinal product) contains arachis oil (peanut oil). If you are allergic to peanut or soya, do not use this medicinal product"[18]
Benzalkonium chloride	-Benzalkonii chloridum	When used in cosmetics "Avoid contact with eyes" [3] (This substance is frequently used as a preservative in products for the treatment of the eyes) When used in pharmaceuticals "Irritant, may cause skin reactions" [18] When used in medical devices, warning is not mandatory
Benzoic acid	Benzoic acid/acidum benzoicum	When used in pharmaceuticals: "Mildly irritant to the skin, eyes and mucous membranes" [18]. (Frequently used as preservative in cosmetics)
Cetyl alcohol	Cetyl alcohol/alcohol cetylicus	When used in pharmaceuticals: "May cause local skin reactions (e.g. contact dermatitis)" [18]. (Frequently used as thickener in cosmetics)

1.6 Responsible and Qualified Persons, and Notified Bodies

Regulations in all three product categories have requirements for specific personnel to take responsibility for some or all aspects of the product.

The new Cosmetic Regulation requires that a legal or natural person be designated as the "Responsible Person" for any cosmetic product placed on the market. The Responsible Person should ensure compliance with the relevant obligations set out in the regulations. This person needs to make sure that the PIF, including the Cosmetic Product Safety Report, is up to date, complete, and accurate. The name of this person will be included in the new notification system that goes into effect in 2012. This person needs to be aware of how the product is sold or distributed in the EU and to be a part of the companies' adverse event reporting system. The Responsible Person is expected to notify the authorities in the event of a serious undesirable event in respect to a cosmetic product and to cooperate with the authorities either when a product presents a risk to human health or when other inquiries are made. For imported products, the Responsible Person needs to be established within the EU. A burden is placed upon this person to ensure compliance, and if they believe the product is not in compliance, they are required to take the appropriate corrective measures to bring the product into compliance, withdraw or recall it, as appropriate.

Pharmaceuticals are required to have Qualified Persons (QP), who fulfill their responsibilities personally and are resident within the European Economic Area. One type of Qualified Person is responsible for ensuring that each batch of the pharmaceutical is manufactured and checked in compliance with applicable laws and in accordance with the marketing authorization. This Qualified Person also ensures that the pharmaceutical imported into the EU has undergone (and passed) the appropriate analytical testing in the importing Member State. Another Qualified Person monitors the safety of the company's product and focuses on the pharmacovigilance system to ensure that information about all suspected adverse reactions is collected and collated in order to be accessible in at least one point within the community. A Responsible Person should also be appointed in each distribution point to ensure that a quality system for Good Distribution Practice of pharmaceuticals is implemented and maintained.

A manufacturer without a registered place of business in a Member State needs to have a European Authorized Representative in accordance with the Medical Device Directive 93/42/EEC and IVD Directive 98/79/EC, if he places products on the market under his own name.

A Notified Body, in the context of medical devices, is a certified organization which a national Competent Authority of a Member State designates to carry out one or more of the conformity assessment procedures described in the Annexes of the Directives [11]. A Notified Body must be qualified to perform all of the functions set out in any annex for which it is designated. Except for a class 1, non-sterile and non-measuring device, a medical device manufacturer is required to use the services of a Notified Body to demonstrate that the device complies with the applicable requirements in the regulation. When a Notified Body is involved in the conformity assessments for a medical device, the manufacturer can only place the CE mark on the product when they receive a certificate from the Notified Body. The identification number assigned to that Notified Body by the Commission will appear below the CE mark.

1.7 Efficacy Testing and Claim Substantiation

New substances and new mode of actions require scientific studies and clinical testing to demonstrate performance and safety. Irrespective of product category, randomized, controlled and blinded studies are the preferred strategy to identify valuable performance and discriminate between products. Human investigations must be performed under the responsibility of a medical practitioner or other qualified person in accordance with the recommendations guiding physicians in biomedical research that was adopted in 1964 by the 18th World Medical Assembly, in Helsinki, Finland, "Helsinki declaration," with later revisions. In addition to international guidelines, human studies should always be performed in compliance with the national regulations of the country where the testing is being conducted. In addition, an ethical committee needs to approve the protocol of the study. Ethics can be considered as a personal attitude towards what is right or wrong, but it must be subordinated to and coordinated with a public norm.

The cosmetic regulation requires substantiation for all claims to be held in the PIF. The extent of testing, if any, depends on the type of product and the claims being made. Data obtained from previous studies may well be applied to new formulations to substantiate their effects. Results from in vitro tests of the "active" cosmetic ingredients in combination with open-label consumer trials of the final product have also gained increased popularity in the marketing of cosmetics. However, in vitro parameters have to be carefully validated for the clinical endpoint in order to make sense for the consumers and not be misleading. Any laboratory conducting clinical tests needs to follow good laboratory practices, but clinical testing of cosmetics does not need approval from any Competent Authority.

The new Cosmetic Regulation requires standards to be set for substantiation of claims. For example, in order to reduce the variability in labeling of sunscreen products, the testing and labeling of sunscreens were recently agreed on by international industry organizations [12] and adopted by the European Commission [13]. Upon request, the substantiation for the claims on a cosmetic product can be reviewed by the Competent Authority. The consumer has no insight into the efficacy data.

The claims allowed for a pharmaceutical are carefully reviewed by the competent authority. The active/product must have demonstrable efficacy and safety (or at least safety with prescribed cautions). If an active has an already well-established use, evidence to support claims may be available in the literature or already accepted by the authorities. In such cases, additional testing *may* not be required, but instead, only data proving the bioavailability of the active substance is needed. New substances, new claims, or new combinations will typically require clinical testing. The clinical testing protocol for a pharmaceutical has to be approved by the Competent Authority prior to commencement of the study. Furthermore, the test results have to be submitted to the authority after completion of the study.

Medical devices, irrespective of their classification, have to present clinical data to comply with the Medical Device Directive [5]. This does not necessarily mean an obligation to accomplish a clinical trial, as citation of published research on identical or similar products which have been clinically tested may be acceptable. The adequacy of the clinical data must be based on scientific evidence from the available literature.

The clinical investigation of a medical device must be performed on the basis of an appropriate plan of investigation (Clinical Investigation Plan, CIP according to standard International Organization for Standardization, ISO, 14155), reflecting the latest scientific and technical knowledge. These investigations must include an adequate number of observations to guarantee the scientific validity of the conclusions and confirm the safety and performance of intended use. The clinical investigations must be performed in circumstances similar to the normal conditions of use of the device. The manufacturer may commence the relevant clinical investigation at the end of a period of 60 days after the notification, unless the Competent Authorities have notified the manufacturer within that period of a decision to the contrary based on considerations of public health or public policy.

There are no restrictions regarding the start of the marketing of cosmetics, whereas marketing of pharmaceuticals is not allowed before authorization. Medical devices may be displayed at trade fairs, exhibitions, demonstrations, etc., provided that a visible sign clearly indicates that such devices cannot be marketed or put into service until they have been made to comply with the valid medical device regulation.

1.8 Safety Assessment and Risk Management

The safety of any finished products is of critical importance; however, the degree of evaluation and substantiation varies between the different categories. Safety is assessed by taking into consideration the toxicological profile of the ingredients, their chemical structure, and the level of exposure.

The toxicological evaluation of ingredients for cosmetics is made challenging by a phase out of animal testing in the 7th Amendment to the Cosmetic Directive [2]. A testing ban on finished cosmetic products has applied since September 2004, and a testing ban on ingredients or combination of ingredients has applied since March 2009. A marketing ban has also been in place since March 2009 which prohibits marketing in the European Union finished cosmetic products or finished products with ingredients which were tested on animals after the cut-off dates. There were exceptions for some of the more complex tests; in this case, the ban will apply step by step as soon as alternative methods are validated and adopted, but with a maximum cut-off date of 10 years after entry into force of the Directive, i.e. March 2013, irrespective of the availability of alternative non-animal tests. A great deal of research into alternative test methods is currently ongoing, and while good progress has been made, there is still work to be done. The Commission is required to determine whether or not validated methods will be available by the 2013 deadline.

In order to increase the safety and to facilitate safety assessment of cosmetics, the Cosmetic Directive has lists of prohibited and restricted substances among the 15,000 chemical substances that are found in the European Inventory of Cosmetic Ingredients. More than 1,000 substances are identified as forbidden and almost 300 substances may be used only in accordance with the restrictions laid down in the regulation in cosmetic products. In addition, approximately 150 colorants, almost 30 ultraviolet filters and almost 60 preservatives are approved to be used in cosmetics [14].

The Cosmetic Regulation helps to clarify the obligations of manufacturers in the product safety assessment process. Safety Assessments for cosmetic products are done by a qualified safety assessor. The Cosmetic Product Safety Report, which includes the Safety Assessment, is included in the PIF and shall be kept for a period of 10 years following the date on which the last batch of the cosmetic product was placed on the market.

The safety assessment of a pharmaceutical has to be approved by the Competent Authority before the product is approved for the market. Actives, excipients, potential impurities, and decomposition products go through an extensive review process. If adequate information already is available on a specific ingredient, no further toxicological tests are needed.

A medical device class I needs to have a risk assessment made according to the Medical Device Directive, Essential Requirements, although there is no requirement for third party review of the assessment. Risk management for medical devices with higher risk classification (class IIa, IIb, and III) is reviewed and verified by the Notified Body prior to certification of conformity.

Manufacturers of pharmaceuticals and medical devices are obliged to try to look into the future to predict possible hazards resulting from all potential uses of their product. "Known or foreseeable hazards" based upon safety characteristics could be listed as well as "reasonably foreseeable misuse" related to the safety of the product. The risk analysis should include an estimation of the risks for each hazard, where the probability, severity, and consequence are analyzed separately. The acceptability of the risks and the possibility to reduce the risk also have to be decided. This process is generally referred to as a Risk Management Plan (RMP) [15] and such an organized approach is essential for good risk management. The organized plan provides the roadmap for risk management, and encourages objectivity and helps prevent essential elements being forgotten.

1.9 Definition of Undesirable Events and Effects

Undesirable effects caused by topical products may lead to acute and chronic suffering, for example, lifelong intolerance to specific substances implying negative consequences for the individual as well as for the health care and social insurance systems. The majority of negative skin reactions from topical products are however transient smarting and stinging reactions in the skin. Other examples of undesirable effects are: irritant and allergic effects, cosmetic acne, phototoxic effects, photosensitivity, anaphylactic shock, and itching.

A cosmetic product must be suitable for its purpose and may not lead to adverse reactions under normal use that are disproportional in relation to the intended effect of the product. An undesirable effect for a cosmetic product is defined as [3]:

> An adverse reaction for human health attributed to the normal or reasonably foreseeable use of a cosmetic product.

In the Cosmetic Regulation, a serious undesirable effect is defined as:

> An undesirable effect which results in temporary or permanent functional incapacity, disability, hospitalisation, congenital anomalies or an immediate vital risk or death

For pharmaceuticals, adverse events are defined as [16]:

> Any untoward medical occurrence that may present during treatment with a medicine but which does not necessarily have a causal relationship with this treatment.

An Adverse Drug Reaction (ADR) is defined as [4, 16]:

> A response which is noxious and unintended, and which occurs at doses normally used in humans for the prophylaxis, diagnosis, or therapy of disease, or for the modification of physiological function.

If the symptoms are covered by the reference safety information, the adverse event may be regarded as expected. A *serious* adverse event is any event that [16]:

- Is fatal
- Is life threatening
- Is permanently/significantly disabling
- Requires or prolong hospitalization
- Causes congenital anomaly/birth defect
- Requires intervention to prevent permanent impairment or damage

In the Medical Devices Directive, the term "incident" is used, which is defined as [5]:

> Any malfunction or deterioration in the characteristics and/or performance of a device, as well as any inadequacy in the labelling or the instructions for use which, directly or indirectly, might lead to or might have led to the death of a patient or user or of other persons or to a serious deterioration in their state of health.

All incidents are events, but not all events are incidents; events may be complaints or something else, for example, unanticipated adverse reactions or unanticipated side effects. Side effects are not covered by the "incident" definition in the directive unless the change in the risk-benefit ratio is considered as a deterioration in the performance of the device.

1.10 Post-marketing Surveillance and Vigilance

Safety for the consumer is of primary importance in all three product categories. No matter the effort put in to evaluate safety before a product is launched, data are inevitably incomplete.

The regulation of a product as a cosmetic, pharmaceutical, or medical device will determine which procedure should be followed for the reporting of an adverse incident. The Cosmetic Regulation requires manufacturers of cosmetic products to maintain data on undesirable effects on human health, resulting from the use of the cosmetic product. The vigilance system for cosmetics does not need any external approvals, but the authorities have the right to audit them.

The new Cosmetic Regulation requires that, in the event of a serious undesirable effect, the Responsible Person should, without delay, notify the Competent Authority in the Member State in which the event occurred. Information on undesirable effects must also be made available to the public upon request. Undesirable effects accessible to the public do not include, for example, those resulting from abuse or misuse of the product and those related to associated items, such as the packaging.

The manufacturer of a pharmaceutical is required to have a pharmacovigilance system in place to track and respond to adverse events. This process is audited and approved by the authorities. Furthermore, the analysis of safety is regulated, and so-called Periodic Safety Update Reports (PSUR) are written and submitted to the medical authorities at specified intervals (2004/27/EC). This report contains a description of the adverse events reported for the product, along with an analysis of the relationship to the product. Furthermore, other types of new information on the drug should also be addressed. Scientific literature and other media should be watched for new findings. Scientific reports, daily press, and web-based search sites (PubMed, Toxnet, etc.) constitutes the base for this information search. The PSUR is submitted every 6 months the first 2 years after placing the product on the market, then once a year, the following 2 years and thereafter at three yearly intervals. Furthermore, the PSUR should be enclosed with each renewal application.

Medical device manufacturers are also obligated to set up and maintain a vigilance system to ensure that any problems or risks associated with use of the device are indentified early, reported and acted upon to thus reduce the likelihood of reoccurrence of an incidence [17]. Such a system maintains records of adverse incident reports received from any source. It also describes how the reports are investigated by competent personnel and the corrective and preventative action processes. An "incident" which meets the reporting criteria will require reporting to the Competent Authority. This is done through an electronic system and depending on the severity of the incident; the report should be made within 2–30 calendar days (in general). Also depending on the severity of the event, a Field Safety Corrective Action (FSCA) may need to be taken; this is typically done to reduce a risk of death or serious deterioration in the state of health associated with the use of the device. FSCAs are communicated to users or customers via a Field Safety Notice (FSN).

The manufacturer of a medical device should also have routines to periodically evaluate, group, and trend product events, adverse effects, and adverse incidents. Trend reports should be written at least annually and presented at a management quality review to discuss, and if appropriate, take necessary action(s). The Notified Body, if involved with the device, would review these reports.

Vigilance for medical devices in the EU is effectively tied together by European Database for Medical Devices (EUDAMED) which in part includes data on vigilance. This in conjunction with a NCAR (National Competent Authority Report) allows communication between Member States to protect human health in the event of a serious incident.

Conclusion

Products for topical use include semi-solid formulation types, such as creams (emulsions), ointments, liquids, and gels. Products may look the same, have similar indications and be placed next to each other on the shelf at pharmacies or drug stores, but their regulatory classifications are different. Moisturizers regulated as pharmaceuticals or medical devices can be marketed for prevention or treatment of dry skin in connection with diseases, such as atopic dermatitis, ichthyosis, and psoriasis. Cosmetics are allowed to be marketed for the treatment of temporary dryness caused by environmental impact, such as low temperature. The users of the products and those approving and recommending the products to patients and consumers should preferably be aware of the regulatory status of the products and the differences in their quality assurance.

Informed product choices should also be facilitated by a transparent system that enables both the consumers and professionals to take part in the scientific evidence regarding the claimed effect of the skin as well as of the safety assessment and potential adverse effects.

Take Home Messages

- The majority of moisturizing creams on the market are regulated as cosmetics although they may also be classified as pharmaceuticals (equivalent to medicinal products) or as medical devices within the European Member States.
- Moisturizers regulated as pharmaceuticals or medical devices are allowed to be marketed for treatment of dry skin in connection with diseases, such as atopic dermatitis, ichthyosis, and psoriasis.
- The efficacy and safety of a cosmetic product is not approved or reviewed by an outside body. The extent of testing, if any, depends on the type of product and the claims being made. An animal testing ban on finished cosmetic products has been applied since 2004, whereas a testing ban on ingredients or combination of ingredients is applied step by step as soon as alternative methods are validated and adopted, but with a maximum cut-off date in March 2013.
- The efficacy and safety of pharmaceuticals must be approved by the Competent Authority before the product is released to the market. Actives, excipients, potential impurities, and decomposition products go through a review process.
- The effectiveness and safety of medical devices with higher risks must be verified by a Notified Body before CE labeling of the product.
- The users of moisturizers and those approving and recommending the products to patients and consumers should be aware of the regulatory status of the product and the differences in quality assurance among different categories. A transparent system that enables both the consumers and professionals to take part in the scientific evidence regarding the claimed effect of the skin, as well as of the safety assessment and potential adverse effect, should facilitate informed product choices.

References

1. Korting HC, Schollmann C (2012) Medical devices in dermatology: topical semi-solid formulations for the treatment of skin diseases. J Dtsch Dermatol Ges 10:103–109
2. Council Directive 76/768/EEC on the approximation of the laws of the Member States relating to cosmetic products (1976) OJ L 262/169. Non-official consolidated version at http://eur-lex.europa.eu/LexUriServ/LexUriServ.do?uri=CONSLEG:1976L0768:20100301:en:PDF. Accessed May 2011
3. Buzek J, Ask B (2009) Regulation (EC) No 1223/2009 of the European Parliament and of the Council of 30 November 2009 on cosmetic products. Official Journal of the European Union, L342/59–L342/209
4. Directive 2001/83/EC of the European Parliament and of the Council on the Community code relating to medicinal products for human use (2001) OJ L 311/67 as amended. Non-official consolidated version at: http://ec.europa.eu/health/documents/eudralex/vol-1/index_en.htm. Accessed May 2011
5. Council Directive 93/42/EEC concerning medical devices (1993) OJ L 169/1 as amended. Non-official consolidated version at: http://eur-lex.europa.eu/LexUriServ/LexUriServ.do?uri=CONSLEG:1993L0042:20071011:en:PDF. Accessed May 2011
6. CLP, Regulation (EC) 1272/2008 of the European Parliament and of the Council on classification, labeling and packaging of substances and mixtures (2008) OJ L 353/1 as amended. http://eur-lex.europa.eu/LexUriServ/LexUriServ.do?uri=OJ:L:2008:353:0001:1355:en:PDF. Accessed May 2011
7. Guidance document on the demarcation between the cosmetic products directive 76/768 and the medicinal products directive 2001/83 as agreed between the commission services and the competent authorities of member states. http://ec.europa.eu/consumers/sectors/cosmetics/files/doc/guidance_doc_cosm-medicinal_en.pdf. Accessed Feb 2012
8. MEDICAL DEVICES (2010) Guidance document. Borderline products, drug-delivery products and medical devices incorporating, as an integral part, an

ancillary medicinal substance or an ancillary human blood derivative. Guidelines relating to the application of: the council directive 90/385/EEC on active implantable medical devices the council directive 93/42/EEC on medical devices. MEDDEV 2. 1/3 rev 3. http://ec.europa.eu/consumers/sectors/medical-devices/files/meddev/2_1_3_rev_3-12_2009_en.pdf. Accessed Feb 2012
9. MHRA (2011) Bulletin no. 17. Medical devices and medicinal products. http://www.mhra.gov.uk/home/groups/es-era/documents/publication/con007498.pdf. Accessed Sept 2011
10. de Groot AC (1990) Labelling cosmetics with their ingredients. BMJ 300(6740):1636–1638
11. MEDDEV 2.10–2 Rev. 1. Designation and monitoring of notified bodies within the framework of EC directives on medical devices. http://ec.europa.eu/health/medical-devices/files/meddev/2_10_2date04_2001_en.pdf. Accessed Sept 2011
12. Gardiner J et al. (2006) International sun protection factor (SPF) test method. Colipa Guideline www.cosmeticseurope.eu/downloads/86.html. Accessed Feb 2012
13. Verheugen G (2006) Commission recommendation of 22 September 2006 on the efficacy of sunscreen products and the claims made relating thereto. Off J Eur Union 265:265/39–265/43
14. SCCS (2010) The SCCS's notes of guidance for the testing of cosmetic ingredients and their safety evaluation, 7th revision. http://ec.europa.eu/health/scientific_committees/consumer_safety/docs/sccs_s_004.pdf. Accessed Feb 2012
15. Medical devices – application of risk management to medical devices. ISO 14971:2007. http://www.iso.org/iso/iso catalogue/catalogue_tc/catalogue_detail.htm?csnumber=38193. Accessed Sept 2011
16. WHO (2002) Safety of medicines – a guide to detecting and reporting adverse drug reactions - why health professionals need to take action. http://apps.who.int/medicinedocs/en/d/Jh2992e/. Accessed Feb 2012
17. MEDDEV 2.12–1 rev 6 (2009) Guidelines on a medical devices vigilance system. http://ec.europa.eu/health/medical-devices/files/meddev/2_12_1-rev_6–12–2009_en.pdf. Accessed Sept 2011
18. Guidelines. Medicinal products for human use. Safety, environment and information. Excipients in the label and package leaflet of medicinal products for human use, in Notice to applicants, E.C.E. directorate-general, Editor. 2003

Design of Claims Support for Moisturizers

2

Judith K. Woodford

2.1 Introduction

One may question the need for an entire chapter devoted to claims support testing. After all, there are many studies and methodologies reviewed in other sections of this book. However, the end goal of claims support testing is inherently different than that of the prior studies. There are many reasons to conduct scientific studies in the moisturization field ranging from the purest basic research to technology and methods development to optimization of treatments and products. In each of these areas, the scientist is either functioning in an exploration mode or is testing hypotheses. The key difference in claims support testing is that the result is already known. The purpose of the claims support test is not to discover if something is true, but rather to demonstrate to a relevant authority that the specific claim being made for the product is true and is adequately supported.

This end goal of claims support testing impacts the details of a suitable study design. The impact may be subtle, and at a high level glance may not even be apparent. But if not recognized and accounted for can lead to rejection of a study and loss of a desirable, compelling claim. The focus of this chapter is not detailed methodology, but rather, the process to design a readily defensible protocol to support the claims that marketing departments believe are key to the commercial success of a moisturizer or other personal care product.

2.2 Claims and Advertising

Before designing a study, it is important to recognize both what is a claim and what is advertising. Advertising is any communication that is intended to convince the consumer to purchase a product or service. Advertising is not limited to the obvious such as television, magazine, or radio. It encompasses all spaces of communication including package, store displays, and digital media as detailed in Table 2.1.

Claims are communicated within the advertising. Claims are not just the benefit the product delivers, such as moisturization. They are much more–they are the specific words, the specific communication of the benefit. Claims concerning the moisturization benefit could include *immediately improves visible dryness, moisturizes all day*, or *hydrates better than…* Claims testing is required to support not just the general benefit but also the specific claim concerning the benefit. Each of the three examples above requires unique data for support.

Advertising laws across the globe typically include a stipulation that advertising not be misleading to the consumer [5–8]. In addition, there may be Advertising Codes governing the implementation of the laws [9–11]. To determine if an advertisement is misleading, one must first establish what claims have been made within the

J.K. Woodford, Ph.D.
Research and Development, Kao Corporation, 2535 Spring Grove Avenue, 45214 Cincinnati, OH, USA
e-mail: judy.woodford@kao.com

M. Lodén, H.I. Maibach (eds.), *Treatment of Dry Skin Syndrome*,
DOI 10.1007/978-3-642-27606-4_2, © Springer-Verlag Berlin Heidelberg 2012

Table 2.1 Advertising venues

Traditional	Digital media	Product/package based
Television	Company website[a]	Packaging
Radio	Facebook	In-store displays
Magazine	Twitter	Brochures
Billboards	YouTube	Coupons
Advertorials	Email blasts	Direct mailers/ sampling

[a]UK (United Kingdom) – under ASA (Advertising Standards Authority) remit as of March 2011 [1, 2]; USA (United States of America) – FDA (Food and Drug Administration) views as part of package label if the website is declared on the label [3, 4]

Table 2.2 Television preclearance and self-regulatory agencies

Country	TV preclearance	Self-regulatory agency
US	Individual networks	NAD
UK	Clearcast	ASA
Canada	ASC; MIJO	ASC
Australia	CAD	ACB; ACCC; FTCPA

NAD National Advertising Division of the Better Business Bureau, *ASA* Advertising Standards Authority, *ASC* Advertising Standards Canada, *MIJO* MIJO Corporation, formerly Broadcast Clearance Advisory, *CAD* Commercials Advice Pty Limited, *ACB* Advertising Claims Board of Advertising Standards Bureau, *ACCC* Australian Competition and Consumer Commission, *FTCPA* Fair Trading and Consumer Protection Agencies

advertisement. One way to group claims is by explicit and implicit classification. Explicit are direct, straightforward claims: *moisturizes for 8 hours*. Implicit, or implied, claims are subjective and open to interpretation. For example, *now made with aloe, moisturizes even longer*, can be interpreted as either two distinct explicit claims or the two explicit claims plus a third implied claim. The explicit claims are *now made with aloe* and *now moisturizes even longer*. The implied claim is *the addition of the aloe makes the moisturization last longer*. If this implied claim is factual and supported, there is no problem. But, if the longer duration is instead due to an increase in glycerin level, then the claim is not supported and is misleading to the consumer.

2.3 Authorities Examining Claims Support Testing

Various external agencies may examine claims support data. The purpose typically falls into one of four categories: advertising preclearance, in-market advertising challenge, routine regulatory review, and regulatory investigation of a specific issue.

2.3.1 Advertising Preclearance

Preclearance is predominantly utilized for television advertising, Table 2.2. However, there are several magazines in the United States of America (USA) that also routinely request claims support prior to running print ads. The USA television approval process is unique in that the individual television networks review the data and approve the ad, requiring approval by multiple agencies. In contrast, in the United Kingdom (UK), Canada, and Australia, a single approval is sufficient to air on all networks. In the UK and Australia, there is a single option available, Clearcast and CAD (Commercials Advice Pty Limited), respectively. In Canada, the agencies are private companies, and at least two are currently in operation; Advetising Standards Canada and MIJO Corporation (formerly Broadcast Clearance Advisory).

Another difference between the four regions is the level of scrutiny given to the claims support. Canada is the least rigorous. In this case, the authorities require a letter of attestation as assurance that the company has done due diligence in supporting the claims. In special cases, such as linking a claim to a single ingredient, the agencies will request submission of the supporting data. In the USA and Australia, the agencies desire to assure themselves that the claims have been adequately supported and will require submission of the study methods and results. Clearcast, in the UK, is the strictest. Inclusion of all study support and information is requested with the initial submission of the script. Clearcast rigorously reviews the methodology in relation to the specific claim and takes a conservative stance that the support portfolio should be robust enough to withstand any challenge and preferably would not give rise to a challenge in the first place.

2.3.2 In-Market Advertising Challenge

As detailed in Table 2.2, there are self-regulatory agencies in place in the USA, the UK, Canada, and Australia to handle complaints of false or misleading advertising. If a complaint is investigated, it is expected that the advertiser provide the agency with the relevant data to support the claims in question. The NAD (National Advertising Division of the Better Business Bureau), in the USA, is staffed entirely by lawyers. NAD decisions are published at www.NADreview.org. It is clear from the detail within the descriptions that the team reviews the submitted data and methodology in detail, and though not scientists themselves, apply a strict logic to their decisions. The NAD will make educated determinations concerning implied claims and will ensure the study design matches the actual claim. The FTC (Federal Trade Commission) is the federal agency in the USA with oversight of false and misleading advertising. The two agencies have a working relationship and the NAD refers cases to the FTC if the advertiser declines to participate. Similar to the NAD, the ASA (Advertising Standards Authority) in the UK will review the data and determine the applicability to the claim. However, there are two key differences from the USA: (1) clearcast will also be in front of the ASA, defending their decision to approve the ad, and (2) ASA has been noted for applying a more extensive interpretation of implied claims. The Advertising Codes in the UK stipulate that implied claims are those that the average consumer would take away [9, 10]. In a report published by the ASA after a review of their processes in 2010, the agency indicated that they would be more clear in regard to misleading claims in that the claim in dispute must be likely to mislead as opposed to having a slight chance of misleading [12]. ASA adjudications are reported at www.asa.org.uk.

Advertising Standards Canada (ASC) relies on a volunteer board of representatives from the public alongside senior members of the advertising industry. Council decisions are reported at www.adstandards.com. Australia's complaint system differs from the others in that there are multiple agencies involved. Competitive complaints are reviewed by the Advertising Claims Board of the Advertising Standards Bureau. The Board is comprised of lawyers and their case reports are listed at www.adstandards.com.au. Additionally, misleading claims may be investigated by either the Australian Competition and Consumer Commission (ACCC) or individual territory Fair Trading and Consumer Protection Agencies.

2.3.3 Regulatory Review

Review by a governmental regulatory agency can be divided into two groups. The first includes routine reviews. In the EU (European Union) and the ASEAN (Association of Southeast Asian Nations) regions, there are regulations in place for postmarket surveillance of personal care products [13, 14]. In both regions, there is a requirement that POEs (Proof of Effect documents) be made available at the request of the designated competent authority. As these agencies are conducting routine monitoring, their primary purpose is to receive assurance that the company has used due diligence in supporting the relevant claims. As such, high level descriptions of the data are typically sufficient.

In contrast, nonroutine investigations are typically initiated because the authorities are concerned about the product in question. Common reasons for concern include safety and drug/cosmetic issues. In these cases, the agency will be looking for the full details of the claims support. In the case of the FDA (Food and Drug Administration) in the USA, the agency can request complete files related to the product, extending beyond the testing intended to support the claims. Similarly, if involved within a court case, the discovery process will result in disclosure of all material, not just the studies the company wishes to divulge. Understanding these agencies and instances where data may be shared externally helps to shape the design in conjunction with the two elements detailed in the next section.

2.4 Analysis Prior to Study Design

Prior to completing the study design, two additional elements need to be evaluated. First, the wording of the specific claim should be examined for both explicit and implicit claims. The company making the claims is responsible to support all the claims, not just those that the marketing department intended to convey. As will be detailed in the section below, the way the claim is worded will impact the study design.

Secondly, the product itself should be characterized. As stated in the Introduction, the results of a claims support study should already be known prior to the execution of the protocol. The support study is not intended to discover what the product can do, it is intended to provide a demonstration that a specific claim is true under conditions tailored to the wording of the claim. Therefore, a solid knowledge of the product is important. For example, consider:

- Details such as how the product is applied and how the application is communicated to the consumer through the package instructions.
- Where the product is applied, the intended usage.
- By what mechanism the benefit is delivered.
- Is the product providing hydration, exfoliating the surface, or masking imperfections with colored or light diffusing pigments?
- What is the temporal relationship between the application of the product and measurable delivery of the benefit?

Represented in Fig. 2.1 are three products with three different temporal patterns. The black arrows along the top indicate product application timepoints. The product represented by the solid black line delivers the benefit immediately after a single application. The dashed-line product also delivers the benefit after a single application, but the benefit development is delayed by a few hours. The last sample product, dotted line, requires repeated application prior to measurable benefit delivery. Responses to the questions above will factor into the study design.

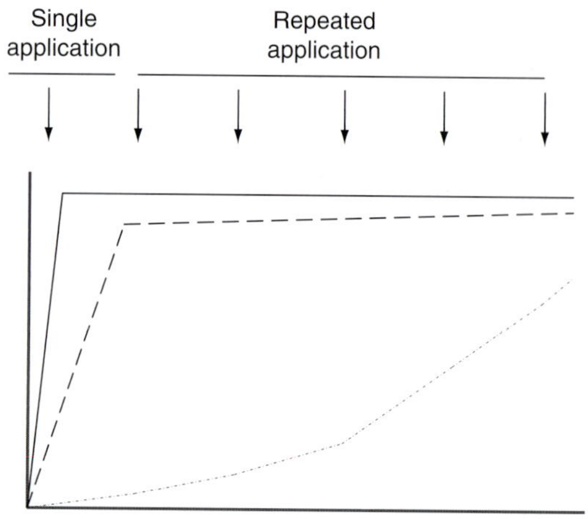

Fig. 2.1 Representation of timecourse for delivery of benefit in relation to product application. The *black line* illustrates a product which delivers the benefit "immediately" after a single application. The *dashed line* illustrates a product which delivers the benefit after a single application; however, the delivery is delayed by period of hours. The *dotted line* illustrates a product which does not deliver the benefit until after repeated application

2.5 Study Design for Claims Support Testing

With the product and claims information in hand, the study design can be tailored to the wording of the claim. The elements of the design are the same as for other types of product testing and are listed in Table 2.3.

2.5.1 Measurement Details

There are often multiple tools available to measure a benefit. However, the appropriate tool for claims support may be dependent upon the specific wording of the claim. Shown in the example in Table 2.4 are four methods to examine dry skin and two hypothetical claims for a product. While all four provide valid measures, the first claim, *visibly reduces dryness*, requires a method that addresses the visible aspect of the condition. Likewise, the second claim, *increases hydration*,

Table 2.3 Elements of a claims support study

Measurement	Product application	Control site
Tools	Test site	Untreated
Frequency	Method	Placebo
Timing	Frequency	Competitor
	Timing	Established positive

Table 2.4 Picking an appropriate measurement tool. Match the tool to the wording of the claim

Tool	"Visibly reduces dryness"	"Increases hydration"
Observer dryness scoring	√	
Digital imaging	√	
Conductance		√
Raman spectroscopy		√

Table 2.5 Selecting a suitable time for postapplication measures[a]. Match the timing to the wording of the claim

Claim	Time lapse between application and measure
Instantly moisturizes	None[b]
Moisturizes all day	8 h
24 hour moisturization	24 h
Improved moisture in just 1 week	1 week[c]

[a]For purposes of this illustration, a single postapplication measure is assumed.

[b]As close to application as feasible, taking into account potential artifacts from limitations of the measurement device.

[c]Assumes repeated application over the 1 week period.

is most appropriately supported with data generated by a technique that either directly or indirectly measures the water content of the skin.

The timing of the measurement(s) may also be dependent on the wording of the claim. In the example detailed in Table 2.5, it is assumed that there is a single postapplication measurement available. The most appropriate timepoint for this measurement is listed for each hypothetical claim. The two explicit claims, *24 hour moisturization* and *improved moisture in just 1 week*, are easy to assign – the timepoint is stated within the claim. The other two claims are not as straightforward. *Instantly moisturizes* appears to be explicit; however, the actual timepoint may be impacted by the limitations of the device taking the measurement. Observer dryness scoring may be conducted immediately, but an instrumental measure such as conductance will require a short delay to avoid artifacts from product residue on the skin. The last example, *moisturizes all day*, would typically require statistical significance at least 8 h after application, although longer timepoints may be chosen.

The frequency of application prior to measurement is also impacted. Claims such as *instantly moisturize* or *24 hour moisturization*, without additional context, imply the benefit is delivered with a single product application. On the other hand, the claim of *moisturizes in just 1 week* would typically require daily or repeated applications. The context of the claim should make it clear to the consumer the expected frequency of application to achieve the benefit.

2.5.2 Product Application Details

As mentioned in Sect. 2.4, the details of product application will be determined by the characteristics of the product and the wording of the claim. The four elements of product application include the site, the frequency, the timing in relation to the measurements to be taken, and the application process.

Ideally, the test site will be at the intended site of application by the consumer. However, there may be occasion where an alternate site would be acceptable. For example, facial moisturizers could be applied on the volar forearms in support of a qualitative moisturization claim. This strategy allows for multiple samples to be tested in a single panel.

The frequency and timing of application should follow the package instructions as closely as possible while bearing in mind the actual claim. Consider the example of an undereye product which claims *lightly moisturizes from the first use* on the back panel of the package and *wake up to diminished dark circles* prominently on the front panel. The instructions read *apply liberally before bed for visible results in just 1 week*. The frequency of application will be different for the two claims. For the moisturization claim, a single application is sufficient, while for the dark circle claim, repeated application over 1 week will be required following package instructions. For the repeated application study, there is also the question of how many applications per day. In this example, a single daily application would be most appropriate as the common consumer practice is to go to bed a single time each day.

The timing of the application may also be different between the two studies. In the case of the dark circle claim, the product should be applied in the evening as close to bed as possible. The wording *wake up to diminished dark circles* adds a time element to the claim. The consumer has been promised that the product will work overnight with results visible upon rising in the morning. In contrast, the moisturization claim does not include any time elements, and it may be acceptable to conduct the single application study during daytime hours which are more convenient to the subjects and the testing facility.

The method of application must also be considered. While it is ideal to follow package instructions as closely as possible, it may also be advantageous to control the exact amount of product applied and other factors such as time. For example, hand and body lotions may have simple instructions such as *apply daily* or *apply liberally to dry areas*. In a consumer usage study utilizing self-application, this level of instruction may be sufficient. But in a clinical setting, it is advisable to have a clinician apply a standard dosage and to rub the product in for a set amount of time. Especially if the product is to be compared to anything other than an untreated control.

2.5.3 Suitable Study Controls

The most common types of controls in claims studies are untreated, placebo, or positive controls, Table 2.6. The positive control is necessary in instances when it must be established that the individual subjects within the panel are responsive to the benefit to be measured. Assume a new product has been developed to provide skin conditioning benefits similar to alpha-hydroxy lotions but without irritation. The inclusion criteria for the panel require dry skin and poor texture associated with aging. Observer erythema scoring and self-assessed discomfort ratings are the measurement tools chosen. In the absence of a positive control, there is a glaring vulnerability if the study is exposed externally. An astute reviewer will immediately question whether the individual subjects would be capable of developing erythema or experiencing discomfort. In contrast, if an alpha-hydroxy lotion was included as a positive control and the subjects reacted at that site, there would be no question of the suitability of the panel.

Table 2.6 Suitable study controls

Control type	Typical applications
Positive control	Demonstrate subjects within panel are capable of developing the attribute to be measured
Placebo control	Benefit within the claim is attributed to a single or to a limited group of ingredients
Placebo control	To blind subjects to the "untreated" site if self-assessments are measured
Untreated control	To measure effect of external and periodic factors in extended duration studies

A placebo control is necessary in situations where a benefit is ascribed specifically to one or a limited group of ingredients within a product. In the case of the claim *rich shea butter softens and conditions skin*, the appropriate study design will include a placebo lotion containing all but the shea butter. To support the claim, the lotion with shea butter would need to provide statistically improved softness and skin conditioning compared to the placebo. In contrast, the claim *Rich lotion softens and conditions skin. Made with shea butter* does not state that the shea butter is providing the benefit, but rather that the full lotion is. Therefore, the study design in that case would not require the placebo control.

Another situation in which a placebo control is relevant is a study design where subjects are providing a self-assessment and need to be blinded as to which site is "untreated." Assume the subjects are to rate their lower legs for the appearance of dryness or roughness. The test products can be masked during application with the actual moisturizer applied by a clinician to one leg and a gelled water applied to the other leg. The subject will not know which leg had the actual test product applied and should not be biased to rate that leg better than the other.

An untreated control is suitable for most claims studies and is necessary in studies of long duration. For example, the dryness level on the lower legs is not anticipated to change much within 1–2 h if a short-term single application study is to be conducted under controlled conditions. If instead the study is to be conducted over several weeks, there is a high probability that the dryness level will change due to external factors such as washing and climatic changes. Even over a period of a day or 24 h, there may be either diurnal rhythms or environmental factors impacting the measures. Therefore, an untreated control is necessary to demonstrate the changes measured are due to the product applied and not due to the environment. Represented in Fig. 2.2 are illustrative charts for two hypothetical studies of 4 weeks duration. As seen by the solid lines, the product-treated site was substantially improved by the end of both studies. However, only the data in study (a) supports the desired claim *improved skin condition within 4 weeks*. The data in study (b) does not support the claim because it is seen that the values at the untreated control site, dashed line, changed to the same extent as at the product-treated site – the observed change was due to an external factor.

The untreated control site is commonly "untouched" for the duration of the study. However, there are several points to take into consideration. If the study is of long duration, it is important that any other products applied to the untreated site are the same as at the treated site. For example, the same cleanser should be used throughout and the same cleansing device (hands, sponge, washcloth). Additionally, if the test product is intended to be applied using a specialized applicator, such as with a massaging ball, the specific claim must be evaluated to determine if the untreated site should also be treated with a massaging ball. For example, consider the case of an undereye product that is applied from a container with a ball applicator.

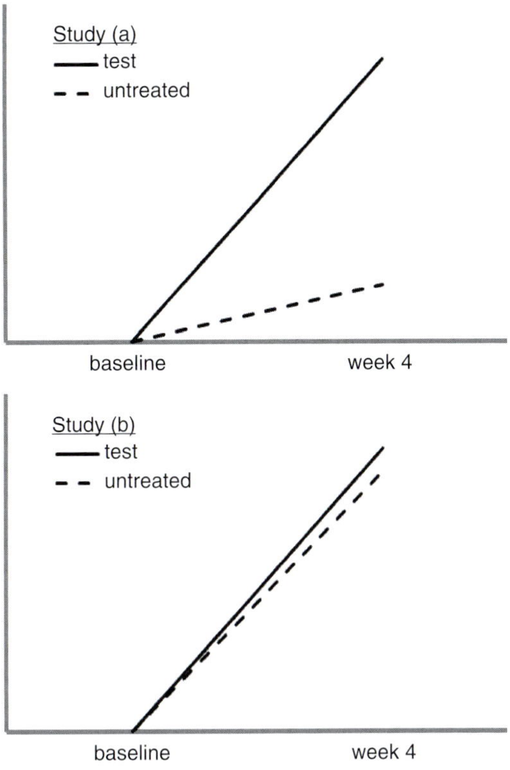

Fig. 2.2 Results from two hypothetical 4-week skin condition studies. The results at the product-treated site are represented by *solid lines*. The results at the untreated control site are represented by *dashed lines*. The results of study (**a**) support the desired claim *improved skin condition within 4 weeks*. The claim is not supported for the product in study (**b**) as the results at the untreated site are comparable to those at the product-treated site

If the stated claim is *lightweight formula diminishes dark circles*, testing would require the ball be applied at the untreated site to isolate the measured difference to the "formula." In contrast, the alternate claim *daily application of ultra eye tonic diminishes dark circles* could be supported by comparison to an untouched, untreated site as the claim specifies the "application" diminishes the dark circles and the "application" includes both the massaging and the lotion.

Conclusion

In today's regulatory and advertising environment, claims support study design is diverging from that of basic research and formulation development. Prior to planning the claims support study, it is key to understand what exactly is being communicated to the consumer – both explicitly and implied. The support portfolio must cover all claims being made, not just those intended to be conveyed. The details of product application, measurement, timing, and study control should be based on the claims in the advertisement, application instructions to the consumer, and practical considerations of the measurement method. The depth of the support portfolio will also be influenced by the intended purpose. External authorities that may be examining the study data range in their expectations and in how deeply the study details will be scrutinized.

Take Home Messages

- All claims, both explicit and implied, require support.
- Authorities that may be examining support data include governmental regulatory agencies, advertising preclearance agencies and advertising self-regulatory agencies.
- Claims support methods should be tailored to the specific wording of the claim.
- Suitable measurement tools should be chosen based on the specific benefit communicated.
- The timing of the measurements should be based on any temporal elements within the claim and upon the action of the product.
- Application of the product should be as close to package instructions as possible with the frequency and timing in relation to the measurement being determined by the specifics of the claim.
- Potential study controls should include an untreated site, a placebo-treated site, and/or a positive-control-treated site. The suitability of the control is determined by both the claim and the study design.

Abbreviations

ACB	Advertising Claims Board of Advertising Standards Bureau (Australia)
ACCC	Australian Competition and Consumer Commission (Australia)
ASA	Advertising Standards Authority (UK)
ASC	Advertising Standards Canada (Canada)
ASEAN	Association of Southeast Asian Nations
CAD	Commercials Advice Pty Limited (Australia)
EU	European Union
FDA	Food and Drug Administration (USA)
FTC	Federal Trade Commission (USA)
FTCPA	Fair Trading and Consumer Protection Agencies (Australia)
MIJO	MIJO Corporation, formerly Broadcast Clearance Advisory (Canada)
NAD	National Advertising Division of the Better Business Bureau (USA)
USA	United States of America
UK	United Kingdom

References

1. United Kingdom Committee of Advertising Practice (2010) ASA digital remit extension: we have the answers. http://www.copyadvice.org.uk/News/2010/Digital-remit-extension.aspx. Accessed 2 Sept 2010
2. United Kingdom Advertising Standards Authority (2010) Landmark agreement extends ASA's digital remit. http://asa.org.uk/Media-Centre/2010/ASA-digital-remit-extension.aspx. Accessed 2 Sept 2010
3. United States Food & Drug Administration (2009) Warning Letter Nestle USA. http://www.fda.gov/ICECI/EnforcementActions/WarningLetters/ucm194122.htm. Accessed 23 Mar 2010
4. United States Food & Drug Administration (2010) Warning Letter Unilever, Inc. http://www.fda.gov/ICECI/EnforcementActions/WarningLetters/ucm224509.htm. Accessed 8 Sept 2010
5. United States Federal Trade Commission (2001) Advertising practices frequently asked questions answers for small business. http://business.ftc.gov/documents/bus35-advertising-faqs-guide-small-business. Accessed 28 Sept 2009
6. European Union Parliament (2008) Statutory instruments 2008 No. 1277 Consumer Protection. The consumer protection from unfair trading regulations 2008

7. Health Canada (2006) Guidelines for cosmetic advertising and labelling claims. http://www.hc-sc.gc.ca/cps-spc/pubs/indust/cosmet/index-eng.php. Accessed 31 July 2008
8. Australian Government ComLaw (1974) Trade Practices Act 1974 No. 51, 1974. http://www.comlaw.gov.au/Details/C2004A00109. Accessed 5 Nov 2008
9. United Kingdom Committee of Advertising Practice (2010) The UK code of non-broadcast advertising, sales promotion and direct marketing (CAP Code). http://www.cap.org.uk/The-Codes/CAP-Code.aspx. Accessed 30 Nov 2010
10. United Kingdom Committee of Advertising Practice (2010) The UK code of broadcast advertising (BCAP Code). http://www.cap.org.uk/The-Codes/BCAP-Code.aspx. Accessed 6 May 2011
11. Advertising Standards Canada (2007) Canadian code of advertising standards. http://www.adstandards.com/en/Standards/theCode.aspx. Accessed 13 July 2010
12. Advertising Standards Authority (2010) More effective, efficient, cost-effective and in tune with our stakeholders. The ASA's Preliminary Response to the Process Review. http://www.asa.org.uk/Media-Centre/2010/ASA-update-on-process-review.aspx. Accessed 24 June 2010
13. European Parliament (2009) Regulation (EC) No 1223/2009 of the European Parliament and of the Council of 30 November 2009. J Euro Union 52:59–209
14. Association of Southeast Asian Nations (2003) Agreement on the ASEAN harmonized cosmetic regulatory scheme. http://www.aseansec.org/20705.htm. Accessed 12 Jan 2010

Educational Interventions for the Management of Children with Dry Skin

3

Steven J. Ersser and Noreen Heer Nicol

3.1 Introduction

Dry skin or xerosis is a common and important problem of children. Dry skin often reveals a disruption to the protective skin barrier, increasing its vulnerability, and is often accompanied by uncomfortable symptoms. The skin is often underrated in regard to its vital roles as a barrier, foundation and calorie reserve, as well as those of temperature regulation, sensation, insulation, psychosocial impact and self-image [26]. Xerosis contributes to the development of epithelial microfissures, which favours the entry of microbial organisms, irritants and allergens. This problem can become aggravated during the dry winter months and in certain living environments.

Dry skin management includes basic proper daily skin care including appropriate bathing and use of cleansers and emollients [7, 22]. If educational approaches are to be effective in managing dry skin in children, especially if of a chronic nature, then attention needs to be given to the parent's and child's knowledge and behaviour. Lack of knowledge and skills lead to poor treatment adherence and ineffective therapy, and this may in turn compound the problem as treatments are erroneously abandoned as ineffective [25]. Further examination of treatment adherence is discussed elsewhere in this text.

This chapter highlights several key themes including the importance of education in the management of dry skin in children, the nature of educational interventions to support effective treatment application, some key evidence related to the educational process and the key resources available. Related issues such as pharmaceutical factors, emollient selection criteria and application effectiveness are discussed elsewhere in this book.

3.1.1 Behavioural Pattern and Management of Dry Skin

The management of chronically dry skin requires addressing a number of factors to sustain effective health behaviour [9]. The factors to be considered include the knowledge, skills and attitudes of both the parent and child, dependent on age, and specifically their health behaviour and adaptive self-management. These require professional

S.J. Ersser, Ph.D. (Lond), RN, CertTHEd (✉)
Faculty of Health and Social Care, University of Hull, Cottingham, Hull, HU6 7RX, UK
e-mail: s.ersser@hull.ac.uk

N.H. Nicol, Ph.Dc., RN, FNP, NEA-BC
Professional Development, Children's Hospital Colorado, Denver, CO, USA

National Jewish Health, Denver, CO, USA

Clinical Sciences, University of Colorado, Denver, CO, USA
e-mail: noreen.nicol@childrenscolorado.org

M. Lodén, H.I. Maibach (eds.), *Treatment of Dry Skin Syndrome*,
DOI 10.1007/978-3-642-27606-4_3, © Springer-Verlag Berlin Heidelberg 2012

Table 3.1 Self-management knowledge and skills related to the management of chronic dry skin

Self-management competence in dry skin management	Knowledge required	Skill required
Manage symptoms and medication use	Demonstrate understanding of symptoms and their triggers	Adapt treatment to change in condition
	Describe beliefs and understanding of treatment	Apply topical treatments effectively
	Use appropriate judgement when treatment is not working	Use prescribed therapies effectively
		Adapt treatment to changes in their condition (e.g. during acute episodes of a chronic skin condition)
		Judge the limits of self-management and when to seek help
Communicate effectively with health professionals	Describe self/family beliefs, understanding, and preferences about their condition and treatment	Adapt treatment to their lifestyle, whilst maintaining effectiveness
		Exercise treatment choices adapted to preferences/lifestyle
	Recognize when to intervene in self-manage and its limitations (when to self-refer)	Communicate preferences and needs to members of the health care team

Adapted from Ersser [9]

assessment and support, especially if the skin problem is moderate to severe.

The severity and chronicity of dry skin will influence the nature and degree to which educational intervention will be required. A key element to achieve effective self-management is the need to be clear about the expectations of the person and their caregivers. Educational intervention needs to be planned and systematically delivered, addressing that which supports the required treatment for the child and parent. It will need to reveal where there are unmet or poorly met educational and support needs, and the assessed limits to self-management or the process of self-care fails.

Table 3.1 outlines some of the knowledge and skills needed to self-manage dry skin effectively. It illustrates some of the complexity of helping patients to use their treatment optimally and the educational and support challenges for health professionals. It also provides an illustration of common areas of educational need that supports self-management for those with chronic skin conditions [9]. These areas of health care need present nurses and other health professionals with significant therapeutic opportunities to support the person and their family to engage actively in the self-management of dry skin.

Patient surveys can provide an indication of patterns of need that practitioners can plan to address; several highlight the difficulties people may find in using topical treatments, for example, [5, 18]. Some of these needs are reflected in Table 3.1. They convey a necessity to understand their condition, those factors that adversely affect and improve it and their treatment. Dissatisfaction with the effectiveness of treatments is a theme running through research findings such as those cited on the management of chronic dermatoses, which are often accompanied by dry skin. This has been validated through recent qualitative evidence, reflecting self-management needs in other areas where management of dry skin is required, as with psoriasis, albeit in adults [10].

Table 3.1 also reflects the fact that effective use of treatment requires an exploration of what the patient understands by their treatment regimen within the consultation. Research evidence suggests that problems of adherence stem more from a disbelief in their efficacy to use prescribed medication effectively than from disease activity [34]. Practitioners also need to explore expectations of treatments to manage dry skin. Qualitative research evidence suggests that dermatology patients may not share precisely the same views with dermatology professionals about what criteria are important in judging treatment effectiveness; as in the case of those living with psoriasis [15]. Also, if a person expects their treatment to work quickly but in practice, the medication is effective only after sustained treatment over a period of time, such as with the application of emollient therapy, there is a high risk that such treatment may be abandoned prematurely. There is a need to give consideration therefore to the range of factors affecting both the patients or carers treatment choice (preference) and use in practice and to recognise the related educational opportunities.

3.2 Daily Skin Care and Hydration

Daily skin care emphasizing prevention and hydration remains a cornerstone to a successful dry skin care. At the US author's centre, 'soak and seal' was developed as a fundamental concept for proper skin care emphasizing use of hydration, moisturizers, cleansers and topicals to help maintain an intact skin barrier [6, 21, 24]. Confusion about how to hydrate and moisturize the skin still exists. Typically, evaporation and microfissuring occur when wet skin is not immediately covered by a protective layer of moisturizer, occlusive or medication. In contrast, the soak-and-seal method leads to rehydration, by sealing in of moisture and assisting the repair of the damaged epidermal barrier.

Bathing or soaking the affected area is recommended once per day for approximately 10–15 min in warm water. A wet washcloth or towel can be used to cover the face, head, neck or body not covered by water to increase hydration. Adding age-appropriate toys will help young children cooperate with the bath. Young children must be supervised during baths. Water temperature should feel comfortable to the patient, as the oft recommended 'tepid' is usually too cool for most patients. Showers may be appropriate in patients with mild xerosis.

Bathing, showering and cleansing may also remove allergens from the skin surface and reduce general colonization by *Staphylococcus aureus*. A Cochrane review of interventions to reduce *S. aureus* in the management of atopic eczema, a common cause of dry skin in children, [4] concluded that they failed to find evidence that commonly used antistaphylococcal interventions are clinically helpful in people with eczema that is not clinically infected. Therefore, their continued use should be questioned in such situations, until better and longer-term studies show clear evidence of clinical benefit.

Guidance on reducing skin irritation is summarised in Appendix 1.

3.2.1 Cleansers

The use of appropriate cleansers plays an important role in managing dry skin conditions. It is important that patients are not using cleansers that have ingredients which are drying or irritating. Cleansers with minimal defatting activity and a neutral pH are preferred. Formulations that are dye-free and fragrance-free are less irritating and more appropriate for dry, sensitive skin. Patients should be instructed not to scrub with a washcloth/flannel.

3.3 Emollients and Moisturizer Usage

Studies have shown that patients fail to receive adequate explanation of the causes and triggers of dry skin or are not taught how to apply topicals, even though instruction and practical demonstrations may be associated with dramatic improvement in the treatment outcomes [22].

Patients frequently do not understand the various vehicles of skin care products such as ointments, creams, lotions and oils and how they can affect treatment outcomes. In general, ointments are more effective sealants and can be the most hydrating when used after bathing; they are also formulated with the fewest additives. Since they are the most occlusive, in a hot, humid environment, they may trap perspiration, which may result in increased pruritus. Lotions and creams may be irritating due to added preservatives or fragrances. In addition, lotions contain more water than creams and may have a drying effect due to evaporation. While oils may go on easily, they are often less-effective moisturizers. Patients should be encouraged to carry moisturizers in small tubes with them at all times and to keep a separate supply in the day care, school or work environment.

Topical therapy to replace abnormal epidermal lipids, improve skin hydration, and decrease skin barrier dysfunction may be useful therapeutically [23]. Recommending the use of moisturizers together with hydration may help re-establish and preserve the skin barrier. Patients, caregivers as well as health care providers all over the world acknowledge they are frequently confused about which moisturizer or emollient to use and how to best use it [13].

Following hydration of the skin, patients should gently pat away excess water with a soft towel and apply the appropriate topical moisturizer or medication to prevent evaporation, which completes the "soak and seal" process. Application of appropriate moisturizers or medications should occur within 3 min ("3 minute rule"). This rule has been promoted to patients by organizations such as the National Eczema Association (www.nationaleczema.org) in the USA.

Moisturizers should be obtained in the largest size available (typically 500 g/one pound jars or pump packs) since they typically need to be applied several times each day on a chronic basis. Plastic spoons or wooden tongue depressors (sticks) can be used to remove the product, especially ointments or creams from large jars to avoid contamination. Commonly recommended emollients and moisturizers which are available in a 500 g/one pound jar or tub include *Aquaphor® Ointment, Vanicream®, CeraVe® Cream, Cetaphil® Cream and Eucerin® Crème*. The availability of these products of course varies across countries; all are available in the USA. In the UK, commonly used moisturizers (or emollients) include *aqueous cream, emulsifying ointment, diprobase ointment* or *cream, doublebase gel, E45 cream, Epaderm, Balenum plus* and *Eucerin*. Health professionals are advised to consult the latest edition of their national formulary, such as the *British National Formulary* or *Nurse Prescribers' Formulary* in the UK, to obtain up to date information on suitable on availability and formulation.

Patients and caregivers need to understand that petroleum jelly is a good occlusive preparation to seal in water; it should be used *after* hydrating the skin. Of note, even young patients can be taught to apply these products, which allow them to participate in their skin care and develop skills in self-management.

3.4 Key Educational Challenges for Emollient and Moisturizer Use

Emollients are important for promoting skin health, especially in vulnerable groups such as the very young and very old, and for treating dry skin diseases such as eczema and psoriasis. A survey of the literature indicates that there is little primary evidence as to how emollients should be effectively used [13]. The advice and common practice that have arisen are reflected in the clinical literature (e.g. see summary in [13]); key issues and guidance sources are highlighted in this chapter. Emollient issues that the healthcare practitioners need to answer for patients are dependent on individual patient need, for example, how dry the skin is and the size of the person. The teaching encompasses all the important dimensions of what, when, where how, and why. Table 3.2 below outlines some of the key point areas related to emollient and moisturizer usage.

Direct demonstration of effective skin care includes the use topical application of agents [6, 23, 24]. Demonstration should be followed up with observation of the patient doing a self-application. This will allow confidence and performance accomplishment to be achieved by the individual. Watching the patient's or caregiver's current technique often reveals fundamental errors which may give providers valuable insights into why a patient may not be showing the expected therapeutic response. A typical example is that of the patient who was observed to apply a very small quantity of medication from a small-sized

Table 3.2 Key points to consider when teaching about emollient or moisturizer use

What product to choose (difference between types)
When to apply emollients (best after bath or shower)
Where to apply emollients or other topical s (order of application)
How to and how much emollient (ensuring continuous and adequate supply)
How to change application with a change in symptoms
When and why to liaise with a health professional

tube over a large area. On examination of their dispensed medication, the tube which should have lasted for only 2 weeks still remained partially full at the 3-month period [25]. This type of educational interaction provides a teaching opportunity to discuss these practical points.

3.4.1 Promoting Adherence Through Concordance

The effective use of treatments requires adherence which conforms to best evidence on their optimal application. This includes ensuring that the emollient appropriate to the dryness of the skin is used; emollients of adequate quantity are plied using an appropriate technique. Therefore, there is a need to demonstrate to patients the correct method of application. For emollients, this includes application in a downward direction, in the direction of hair growth to prevent folliculitis [13]. For many people living with chronic dermatoses, often associated with dry skin, they have to manage a number of medications which they have been recommended for use. If they fail to utilize their treatment effectively; this may be due to a lack of knowledge, skill, confidence or motivation. Patients are often unclear or unaware of the different properties of emollients and the importance of their (and their child's) preference to choose specific emollients that will be utilised.

To improve adherence, the consultation must involve actively engaging with the person or parent and child based on a negotiation about medication between health care professional and patient that respects patients' beliefs and wishes [29].

Table 3.3 Dry skin education and communication for caregivers within consultations

Spend time listening to the patient and/or the parent beliefs and expectations
Deal sensitively with patient's emotions and concerns
Individualize treatment
Explain the nature of the condition and clarify the goal is control
Demonstrate the technique and how much to apply various topical agents (e.g. emollients, sealers, medications)
Reinforce the need to use emollients frequently and liberally
Explain how skin infection (bacterial or viral) can cause deterioration in condition and teach the signs and symptoms of skin infection
Provide written recommendations with step care moving up and down regarding all therapies including bathing and/or showering
Include written instructions for prescription as well as over-the-counter products
Distribute carefully selected patient education brochures – individualise information where necessary
Check patient's understanding and commitment to recommendations
Recommend psychosocial support or counselling as appropriate

Adapted from Nicol and Ersser [25], p. 378

To achieve concordance, the patient and health care professional must actively negotiate an agreement on the nature of the problem (illness) and the treatment plan that draws on the experiences, beliefs and wishes of the patient to decide when, how and why to use medicines [19]. It is essential and crucial to take account of the views of the child and parents when making decisions about what is suitable for use to ensure a match to their preferences and lifestyle. Through this approach treatment adherence, and therefore treatment effectiveness, is more probable. The following strategies can assist the process of negotiation within a consultation (Table 3.3).

Atopic eczema is a common source of dry skin in children [6]. Treatment adherence problems are a common cause of apparent treatment failure. These include factors such as the patient or parental carer having a poor understanding of disease [17]. In this context, there may be an educational discussion to enhance the parent's capacity to avoid or manage trigger factors, managing the child's sleep disturbance (dry skin may be more pruritic) or finding better ways of communicating with professionals regarding treatment. Consideration needs to be given to the parent's and, in some cases, the child's ability to manage successfully topical applications such as emollients, antibiotic and steroid creams.

3.5 The Nature of Educational Interventions

When considering educational interventions to manage dry skin in children, it is helpful to address the various dimensions – what is an optimal and minimal therapeutic approach in terms of (1) '*how*' – the format of how best to deliver the information and promote understanding, (2) considering the '*what*' – the content of the messages; (3) '*when*' – the timing of the education, which includes consideration of frequency and duration; (4) '*who*' delivers the education; (5) '*why*' – providing some rationale for the educational episode, which underpins each of the rationales given for the foregoing, 1–4; and finally (6) '*where*' education is best delivered. Consideration is needed of some of the key 'content' or review of what dimensions have been discussed above, to ensure that key messages help develop the necessary skill and confidence in the parent and or the child. As such, this section will focus on the format of delivery and its timing, with reference to multi-professional involvement.

3.5.1 How: Educational Formats

Educational material for managing problem skin is now available in multiple formats, ranging from the conventional paper pamphlet to now technologically based material, which ranges from patient advice websites to hard copy in the form of DVDs or CDs to the use of smartphones.

Educational resources come in a variety of format, but are essentially either paper-based or are technological in nature; the latter is a developing area. An illustrative outline of the range of resources available are summarised in Table 3.4.

Parents have to potentially deal with a large range of information of dry skin and related problems such as eczema from wide range of sources, the media, industry, popular magazines, the internet and social networking sources, patient support group leaflets as well as formal information that may be available from health services. Information may also come from family and friends, all of which may influence their decision-making. Ersser [9] has highlighted that the task of identifying reliable information sources of quality information is a challenge for patients who can become bombarded with information sources. The quality of information from health-related websites has been found to be a problem from a systematic review of studies reviewing such sites, with the finding that in 70% of cases, the quality of information was a problem [16]. The complexity of the process by which parents need to establish if the source of information is reliable and beneficial or not in helping them to manage their child's eczema has been highlighted by Surridge's [33] investigation.

Some programmes have been established to assist consumers in the difficult process of navigating the complexity of information directed at eczema and sensitive skin patients and to evaluate the myriad of personal care and household products on the market. One such example is the *Eczema & Sensitive-Skin Education (EASE) Program* (see: www.easeeczema.org). This is a patient empowerment program that is intended to improve patient outcomes and the quality of life for millions of persons who suffer from eczema and severe sensitive skin conditions. It provides educational tools and resources relating to the care and treatment of eczema and sensitive skin.

A key consideration when using pre-prepared educational material is the need to ensure that the generic material presented address the individualized need for the parent/child. Key messages and variations need to be highlighted. Standard materials can be supplemented with a brief written or annotated sheet of key points relevant to the particular child.

Careful attention is needed to the ways in which patients are guided to information sources and how best to utilise resources due to the high

Table 3.4 Educational resources related to managing chronically dry skin: examples

Websites
Dermatology professionals:
British Association of Dermatologists information sheets www.bad.org.uk/public/leaflets/
International widely regarded dermatology sites (advanced): www.dermnet.org.nz/
Generic sites: National Health Service (UK) NHS Direct www.nhsdirect.nhs.uk/
Condition specific sites:
National Eczema Society (UK)*: www.eczema.org/ email info@eczema.org
National Eczema Association (USA) www.nationaleczema.org/ email info@nationaleczema.org
www.eczema.org/abouteczema.html
Psoriasis Association (UK)*: www.psoriasis-association.org.uk/
National Psoriasis Foundation (USA): www.psoriasis.org/home/
Ichthyosis: www.ichthyosis.org.uk/
Printed materials
Dermatology professionals: *American Academy of Dermatology*: www.aad.org/forms/pamphlets/default.aspx: produce a catalogue of patient education resources including a leaflet on *Dry skin and Keratosis Pilaris* (www.aad.org/)
Patient groups: materials can be ordered from many organisations (see above)*
Pharmaceutical companies make some materials and so may have commercial influences; as such, these require careful review before use. However, useful unbiased resources can still be found, for example, some companies' do produce useful tear-off pads depicting and explaining the maintenance of the skin barrier using emollients. Material also comes in other formats, such as posters, for example, depicting emollients – to highlight the range and different types available
Guidebooks, for example, *Eczema and your child: a parent's guide* by Mitchell et al. [20], although over 10 years old, this book remains a popular resource in the UK
Audiovisual materials
These are limited. Again, pharmaceutical companies make some materials and so these may have commercial influences, unless independently verified and endorsed
Podcasts – these are underdeveloped at present; however, they are likely to expand, for example, now available from the Psoriasis Association: www.psoriasis-association.org.uk/ (November 2008)

volumes of education material of variable quality. There is a need to assess the parent's and child's educational needs, and ideally their preferred methods of learning and the means of access (paper versus technological) and the level and complexity of information required. It would seem to be commonplace to indiscriminately hand out of generic information leaflets is invariably ineffective and may well be misleading since it may lack necessary modification for the individual. Furthermore, evaluation of the educational material is needed during follow-up – assessing the effectiveness of the source material given as part of a package of care. This may be done in follow-up clinics or possibly telephone consultations to review learning, remaining areas of help needed and changing educational needs.

It is essential to ensure that educational opportunities are planned and individually tailored; however, resource efficiencies can be gained by considering the common learning needs that can be efficiently delivered in a group context. This can provide the added benefit of group support and vicarious learning from others and how they adapt to their condition and treatment. Group support and learning may apply to, say, parents of children with eczema, who will learn from each other. To ensure time is used efficiently, learning needs should be identified. Educational aids may be used such as the appropriate use of a video, discussion time, and time for practical demonstrations and for questions.

A major web-based educational development and evaluation initiative is being undertaken by Santer et al. [30] in the UK within a study entitled, 'Supporting parents and carers of children with eczema: development of a web-based intervention and pilot RCT', which is funded by the National Institute for Health Research (UK). Building on qualitative research, an intervention is being developed; it supports parents of children with eczema, and so dry skin, which is mediated by the web and will then be subsequently evaluated.

3.5.1.1 Smartphones and Mobile Computers

Various mobile or mHealth devices, such as Mobile (cell) phones, smartphones, smart watches, wireless tablets, laptops, e-mail, text and USB drives, are increasingly being used by patients and providers to store and exchange health information [35]. Tessier argues that their value is in their ability to access, record and transmit data anyplace, anytime and by anyone. Health professionals are using them to improve their productivity and service users (or their carers) to manage their conditions effectively, such as those with diabetes or in this context those with eczema, experiencing chronically dry skin. Increasingly, applications are being developed on smartphones to promote effective self-management, and this is likely to include dermatological care.

In the case of dry skin management, Pena-Robichaux et al.'s study [28] has demonstrated how text messages (TMs) may be used as a reminder aid and educational tool in for both adults and adolescents with atopic dermatitis; as such, these may have potential use for the parents of children with chronic dry skin. Daily TMs provided medication reminders and AD education. The study found that user feedback on the TM system was positive with the vast majority of participants reporting that the reminder TMs and educational TMs were helpful. They concluded that the study participants were receptive to using TMs as a reminder aid and educational tool and that this lays the ground work for further studies needed to elucidate the full potential of this simple and cost-effective intervention.

3.5.2 When: Temporal Factors, Timing, Duration, Key Messages, Staging Information

Key issues in the education of parents of children or the child themselves with dry skin are those related to timing of the education. This includes when best to deliver education and under what conditions. This will depend on the child's developmental stage and readiness to engage in learning. The issues include those of what opportunities there are for education and the balance of the timing of professional-led education and service-user-led education at home. Consideration is also needed of the timing of education for the parent alongside or with the child and the duration and frequency of the education process, which will vary with different health systems. The Cochrane review of educational interventions for childhood eczema revealed that temporal issues were a key variant in the delivery of education, which in turn may influence its effectiveness [12]. These are primarily issues of what duration of education is possible. These issues will be shaped by the severity of the dry skin, whether a transient encounter being managed in the community by say a community pharmacist or a practice nurse or a more complex case in which the child has a severe chronic dermatoses, such as atopic eczema, where more intensive education will be needed and opportunities present themselves for interaction with other health professionals, such as specialist nurses.

3.5.3 Who

Patients, parents and even healthcare providers may have difficulty evaluating what constitutes solid, reliable dermatological information to guide routine practices, such as skin moisturization [14]. Parents have to potentially deal with a large range of information of dry skin and related problems such as eczema from wide range of sources. Who delivers this information and the process of validation is a key consideration. In the clinic context, nurses are often well placed to deliver structured education within nurse-led clinics, allowing time for clarification and follow-up. Whichever professional takes this on, they will require planned and structured opportunities to ensure education is effective and evaluated. This is highlighted further under the rationale Sect. 3.5.4.

Sources of information often arise from outside of the health care setting, namely, via the media, industry, popular magazines, the internet and social networking sources, patient support group leaflets as well as formal information that may be available from health services. Information may also come from family and friends, all of which may influence their decision-making. The task of identifying reliable information sources of quality information is a challenge for patients who can become bombarded with information sources has been highlighted [9]. The quality of information from health-related websites has been found to be a problem from a systematic review of studies reviewing such sites, with the finding that in 70% of cases, the quality of information was a problem [16].

3.5.4 Why

The effectiveness of educational intervention for the management of dry skin in children can be assisted by some theoretical considerations. Again, this has most relevance when dealing with chronically dry skin that requires sustained management over time and integration with the parent-child's lifestyle. One key set of ideas are those regarding the parent's belief in their ability to help their child self-manage and how they may learn from one another in social groups to enhance the effectiveness of learning.

For the parent managing a child with chronically dry skin, there is a need to build confidence in their and perhaps their child's self-management ability. Self-efficacy is an important concept which is similar to but technically distinct from that of confidence. It provides a key motivational force, which health professionals need to support. Bandura [1, 2] defined self-efficacy as 'an individual's belief in their capacity to successfully execute a health-related behaviour'. It is based on Bandura's Social Learning Theory [1], which indicates that people learn by observing the behaviour of others within a social context. Practically, this would be relevant when planning perhaps group education for parents who are trying to manage their child's chronically dry skin and the way in which they may learn from each other, how best to apply emollients or say manage the pruritus that can result from dry skin. In this context, the self-efficacy concept predicts that the parent or child is more likely to engage in certain behaviours when they believe they are capable of carrying them out successfully, that is, when they have high self-efficacy developed through the acquisition of the mastery or acquisition of self-management skills.

During the educational process, it is important to note that learning may or may not result in behavioural change. For example, a parent may be taught to apply their topical treatments; however, they may not have the confidence to apply them or, say, the skill to effectively apply a wrapping bandage. It is fundamental for the carer to have sufficient degree of self-belief by the person in their capacity to act as well as knowledge, skill and indeed motivation. Education needs to be directed to enhancing the parent's or child's capacity to make choices in managing their dry skin to help them to adapt effectively. Self-efficacy is recognised as a key basis for effective self-care ability for those with chronic conditions.

Bandura [3] summarises strategies to enhance or provide sources of self-efficacy.

Their practical application will now be illustrated within the context of a dermatology consultation.

1. *Personal accomplishment and verbal persuasion*: can lead to stronger efficacy beliefs than other strategies of influence. This involves reinforcing (acknowledging and encouraging) instances when patients effectively engage in successful health behaviour, such as managing to apply topical medications in the correct order. It is important to assess the patient's self-management ability and to give them performance feedback, including verbal persuasion to encourage them to build on what they are already doing well.
2. *Vicarious experience or social modelling:* highlights the importance of opportunities for parents or children to learn from others. The importance of demonstrating has been highlighted earlier in this chapter. This may include health professionals demonstrating effective practices, such as a wet wrapping technique by a parent or creating group-learning opportunities where there is sharing of

good practice by a patient or parental carer with others in a similar social learning situation.

3. *Regulation of emotional behaviour*: Bandura [3] highlights how emotional and physical arousal, such as anxiety and stress, may interfere with the performance of a desired behaviour. Chronically dry skin may be stressful for parent and child, especially if accompanied by regular scratching and damage to the skin. The patient can be directed to strategies to help them manage stress and anxiety more effectively through pursuing relaxation opportunities, such as returning to social hobbies which have been curtailed due to a lack of self-esteem or engaging them in the use of relaxation methods.

Work is at an advanced stage of developing and testing measure of parental, self-efficacy in managing their child's eczema, through the development of the *Parental Self-Efficacy with Eczema Self-Care Index* (PASECI tool), which will be published in due course [11].

3.5.5 Where

Consideration needs to be given to the optimal environments for the education of the parent and child; however, there may be very limited opportunities to provide effective support. Furthermore, many parents will have limited consultation times with health professionals and so will need to be guided to sources of remote education and support, such as through the internet or being guided to read approved educational resources such as leaflets or a DVD at home. This may include telephone consultation, the use of e-mail and other internet-mediated contact, such as Skype and smartphone. In some facilities, the available physical space for consultation may be an issue, to ensure that the educational process is not disrupted.

3.6 Outline of Evidence on the Effectiveness of Educational Intervention

There are a small but growing number of studies developing and testing interventions to support the management of specific dermatology conditions – some of which are subject to systematic reviews. A Cochrane systematic review of psychological and educational interventions to manage childhood atopic eczema [12] identified only four educational studies that met the inclusion criteria on methodological rigour, which included those of [8, 27, 32, 31]. For each of these studies, the intervention was an adjunct to conventional therapy, not a substitute for it. It was not possible to synthesise the data due to the variation in the type of data available, especially its heterogeneity. However, it was possible to provide an extensive critical appraisal of the included studies.

The studies by Niebel et al. [27] and Staab et al. [31, 32] identified that education can lead to an improvement in clinical severity and in parental quality of life [31], but only marginal improvement was seen in the latter within [8] study. For each study, a systematic approach to education was implemented using one of two models of service delivery, either (1) an eczema school – multidisciplinary approach, which are more typical in Germany or (2) nurse-led clinics that are more typical in the UK. The focus of all four studies was directed towards parental education. It was concluded that the Eczema School model was much more likely to be resource intensive compared to the nurse-led clinic model [12], although no comparative studies have been undertaken as yet of their relative effectiveness. Education was delivered in both hospital outpatient settings (Niebel and both Staab studies) and in primary care (Chinn) and with and without the use of technology. The use of technology was revealed in Niebel's study where video-assisted education was used and found to be more effective in improving severity than direct education and the control (discussion) ($p<0.001$). The most rigorous study found to date was that of Staab et al. [31], which evaluated long-term outcomes. Significant improvements were found in both disease severity (3 months to 7 years, $p=0.0002$; 8–12 years, $p=0.003$; 13–18 years, $p=0.0001$) and parental quality of life (3 months to 7 years, $p=0.0001$; 8–12 years $p=0.002$) for children with atopic eczema. The [12] review is being updated in 2012.

As a limited number of studies to date address the effectiveness of educational approaches to improve dry skin conditions in children, such as atopic dermatitis, the authors recommend that an international priority be given to assessing the impact of patient and parental education by nurses and other care providers for children with skin diseases with a dry skin component in children. Research studies designed to address the common weaknesses of existing randomized studies should be utilized. International collaboration will help to establish greater clarity on developing more effective evidence-based models for delivering dry skin education and support by healthcare teams for children living with chronically dry skin across differing health systems [25].

Appendix 1

Guidance on reducing skin irritation through effective skin care
Wash all new clothes before wearing them. This removes irritating chemicals, such as formaldehyde
Add a second rinse cycle to ensure removal of detergent. Residual laundry detergent, particularly accompanying perfume or dye, may be irritating when it remains in the clothing. Changing to a liquid and fragrance-free, dye-free detergent may be helpful. Some liquid detergents are branded as being suitable for 'sensitive skin' but such claims needed to be tested in practice for the individual
Wear garments that allow air to pass freely to your skin. Open weave, loose-fitting, cotton-blend clothing may be most comfortable
Work and sleep in comfortable surroundings with a fairly constant temperature and humidity level. Adequate ventilation is important
Fingernails should be kept very short and smooth to help prevent damage due to scratching
Carry a small tube of moisturizer/sunscreen at all times. Such a separate supply of moisturizer enables regular access for application throughout the day when at school or work. For young children, other carers, such as those at play group, need to be instructed in effective application
Shower or bathe after swimming in chlorinated pool or using hot tub using a gentle cleanser to remove irritating chemicals and then apply moisturizer

Adapted from National Jewish Atopic Dermatitis Program Step-Care 'AD Action' Plan. ([24], p. 8)

Take Home Messages

- Behaviour of the parent and their child who have dry skin has a significant impact on the effectiveness of moisturizer use, especially when the condition is chronic.
- Consumers with dry skin are often unsure how to effectively manage their condition.
- Planned and systematic education is an essential preparation for the effective self-management to ensure parents and or their children with dry skin have the knowledge, skill and confidence that underpins effective treatment adherence.
- Generic information invariably needs to be adapted for the individual child and family.
- Management of dry skin, especially when chronic, requires moisturization to become a part of routine skin care and hygiene.
- Effective adherence to the use of moisturizers depends on the adoption of a concordance approach to consultations in which patient beliefs and preferences are taken into account in the decision-making process.
- Educational interventions vary according to how they are delivered (format), when, why and where this takes palace. Each element requires consideration within the planning of the educational process.
- Parent's self-efficacy, akin to confidence in the management process, is an important factor affecting their effective use of moisturisers.
- Evidence on the educational process related to moisturiser use is limited – but indicates the different models by which health professionals can deliver education and variation on the components described above (how, when, etc.). Attention needs to be given to the importance in the variation of these components (e.g. technological versus paper-based) and a comparison of different service delivery models within the health system, when managing chronic dry skin.

References

1. Bandura A (1977) Social learning theory. Prentice Hall, Englewood Cliffs
2. Bandura A (1989) Human agency in social cognitive theory. Am Psychol 44(9):1174–1184
3. Bandura A (1997) Self-efficacy: the exercise of control. Freeman, New York
4. Bath-Hextall FJ, Birnie AJ, Ravenscroft JC, Williams HC (2010) Interventions to reduce *Staphylococcus aureus* in the management of atopic eczema: an updated Cochrane review. Br J Dermatol 163(1):12–26
5. Beresford A (2002) Psoriasis Association Members Questionnaire Survey. Psoriasis Association, Northampton
6. Boguniewicz M, Nicol NH (2008) General management of patients with atopic dermatitis. In: Reitamo S, Luger TA, Steinhoff M (eds) Textbook of atopic dermatitis. Informa UK Ltd, Andover, pp 147–164
7. Boguniewicz M, Nicol NH, Kelsay K, Leung DYM (2008) A multidisciplinary approach to evaluation and treatment of atopic dermatitis. Semin Cutan Med Surg 27(2):115–127
8. Chinn DJ, Poyner T et al (2002) Randomized controlled trial of a single dermatology nurse consultation in primary care on the quality of life of children with atopic eczema. Br J Dermatol 146(3):432–439
9. Ersser SJ (2010) Helping patients make the most of their treatment. In: Penzer R, Ersser SJ (eds) Principles of skin care: a guide for nurses and other health care professionals. Wiley-Blackwell, Oxford
10. Ersser SJ, Cowdell F, Latter SM, Healy E (2010) Self-management experiences in adults with mild-moderate psoriasis: an exploratory study and implications for improved support. Br J Dermatol 163(5):1044–1049
11. Ersser SJ, Farasat H, Jackson K, Dennis H, Hind M (2011) Parental Self-Efficacy with Eczema Self-care Index (PASECI tool), Unpublished document. University of Hull, Hull, UK
12. Ersser SJ, Latter S et al (2007) Psychological and educational interventions for atopic eczema in children. Cochrane Database Syst Rev (3), Art. No.: CD004054. doi: 10.1002/14651858. CD004054.pub2
13. Ersser SJ, Maguire S, Nicol N, Penzer R, Peters J (2009) Best practice in emollient therapy; a statement for health care professionals, 2nd edition. Dermatol Nurs (Suppl) 8(3):1–22
14. Ersser SJ, Nicol NH (2010) The challenges of evidence-based practice for the dermatology nurse: when should you believe what is being presented? Dermatol Nurs 22(1):1–3
15. Ersser SJ, Surridge H et al (2002) What criteria do patients use when judging the effectiveness of psoriasis management? J Eval Clin Pract 8(4):367–376
16. Eysenbach G, Till J (2001) Ethical issues in qualitative research on internet communities. Br Med J 323(7321):1103–1105
17. Fischer G (1996) Compliance problems in paediatric atopic eczema. Australas J Dermatol 37(Suppl 1): S10–S13
18. Krueger G, Koo J et al (2001) The impact of psoriasis on quality of life – Results of a 1998 National Psoriasis Foundation Patient-Membership Survey. Arch Dermatol 137(3):280–284
19. Medicines Partnership (2003) Medicines partnership project evaluation toolkit. Medicines Partnership, London
20. Mitchell T, Paige D, Spowart K (1998) Eczema and your child: a parent's guide. Class Publishing, London
21. Nicol NH (1987) Atopic Dermatitis: The (wet) wrap-up. Am J Nurs 87:1560–1563
22. Nicol NH (2005) Use of moisturizers in dermatologic disease: The role of healthcare providers in optimizing treatment outcomes. Cutis 76(suppl 6):26–31
23. Nicol NH (2011) Efficacy and safety considerations in topical treatments for atopic dermatitis. Pediatric Nursing 37(6):295–302
24. Nicol NH, Boguniewicz M (2008) Successful strategies in atopic dermatitis management. Dermatol Nurs (Suppl):3–18
25. Nicol NH, Ersser SJ (2010) The role of the nurse educator in managing atopic dermatitis. In: Boguniewicz M (ed) Immunology and Allergy Clinics of North America: atopic dermatitis. Saunders/ Elsevier, Philadelphia, 30(3):369–383
26. Nicol NH, Huether SE (2010) Alterations of the integument in children. In: McCance KL, Huether SE, Brasher VL, Rote NS (eds) Pathophysiology – the biologic basics for disease in adults and children, 6th edn. Mosby-Year Book, Inc, St. Louis, pp 1573–1607
27. Niebel G, Kallweit C et al (2000) Direct versus video-based parental education in the treatment of atopic eczema in children. A controlled pilot study [Direkte versus videovermittelte Elternschulung bei atopischem Ekzem im Kindesalter als Erganzung facharztlicher Behandlung. Eine Kontrollierte Pilotstudie]. Hautarzt 51:401–411
28. Pena-Robichaux V, Kvedar JC, Watson AJ (2010) Text messages as a reminder aid and educational tool in adults and adolescents with atopic dermatitis: a pilot study. Dermatol Res Pract Article ID: 894258:6 doi: 10.1155/2010/894258
29. Royal Pharmaceutical Society of Great Britain (1997) From compliance to concordance: achieving shared goals in medicine taking. Report of the working group at the Royal Pharmaceutical Society which enquired into the causes of medicine taking problems, RPSGB, London
30. Santer M, Little P, Yardley L, Lewis-Jones S, Ersser SJ et al (2011-ongoing) National Institute for Health Research (UK) funded study (unpublished) proposal. Supporting parents and carers of children with eczema: development of a web-based intervention and pilot RCT. University of Southampton, UK

31. Staab D, Diepgen TL et al (2006) Age related structured educational programmes for the management of atopic dermatitis in children and adolescents: multicentre randomised controlled trial. Br Med J 332: 933–938
32. Staab D, von Rueden U et al (2002) Evaluation of a parental training program for the management of atopic dermatitis. Pediatr Allergy Immunol 13: 84–90
33. Surridge HR (2005) Exploring parental needs and knowledge when caring for a child with eczema. *Exchange*. The National Eczema Society, London
34. Taal E, Rasker E et al (1993) Health status, adherence with health recommendations, self -efficacy and social support in patients with rheumatoid arthritis. Patient Educ Couns 20:63–76
35. Tessier C (2010) Management and security of health information on mobile devices. AHIMA Press, Chicago

4 Dry Skin in Childhood and the Misery of Eczema and Its Treatments

Susan Lewis-Jones

4.1 Dry Skin in Childhood Eczema

Dry skin is a general term used to describe the clinical appearance of superficial scaling, peeling and fissuring of the skin that may be associated with a build-up of scales and hyperpigmentation. It is seen almost universally in eczema, psoriasis and ichthyosis, although the abnormal epidermal structural and immunopathological changes differ. The term xerosis is often used to describe mildly dry skin in eczema, and although there may not be overt clinical signs of inflammation, it has been shown that there are functional as well as biochemical abnormalities which reflect a subclinical inflammation [1]. Dry skin in eczema represents a breakdown of normal epidermal barrier function caused by complex gene-environmental interactions. The end result is cellular dehydration and loss of the lipid bilayer with a resultant increase in trans-epidermal water loss and reduction in the functional integrity of the cornified cell envelope forming the outer skin barrier [2, 3]. Defective barrier function permits penetration of irritants, allergens and microbiological agents into the epidermis causing an inflammatory immune response with the potential for allergic sensitisation [4]. However, O'Regan and colleagues have suggested that 'the sequence of biologic, physicochemical, and aberrant regulatory events that constitute the transition from an inherited barrier defect to clinical manifestations of inflammatory eczematous lesions and susceptibility to related atopic disorders' is still largely unknown' [4].

4.2 Skin Barrier Structure and Function

The epidermal barrier performs a large number of functions including physical and immunological protection, absorption of substances, regulation of heat and water loss and sensory messaging. Importantly, it is the most visual body organ, and obvious disruption of the skin barrier may affect psychosocial functioning which is a particular problem for eczema sufferers.

At a very simplistic level, the integrity of the skin barrier is maintained by the corneocyte cell envelope, a network of mature corneocytes linked together by corneodesmosomes and lying within a complex lipid bilayer. An essential balance is maintained between the formation of new epidermal cells at the basement layer and desquamation of surface corneocytes aided by proteases which break down the corneodesmosomal connections. The initial cuboidal shape of basal epidermal cells is maintained by a cytoskeleton of keratin filaments but during migration of the cells through the epider-

S. Lewis-Jones, FRCP, FRCPCH
Department of Dermatology,
Ninewells Hospital and Medical School,
Dundee, Tayside, Scotland DD1 9SY, UK
e-mail: sue.lewis-jones@nhs.net

M. Lodén, H.I. Maibach (eds.), *Treatment of Dry Skin Syndrome*,
DOI 10.1007/978-3-642-27606-4_4, © Springer-Verlag Berlin Heidelberg 2012

mis towards the *Stratum corneum* alignment, and aggregation of the keratin filaments occurs by action of the structural protein filaggrin (FLG), resulting in flattening of the cells [5]. The nucleus is lost at this stage, and other complex changes occur in the cell envelope to form mature corneocytes or squames. FLG is subsequently further metabolised to produce natural moisturising substance which is part of the lipid bilayer essential to normal skin barrier function [5]. Many other epidermal proteins are known to be vital for normal skin barrier function and integrity. For a more detailed description of the function and structure of epidermis, see Chaps. 8–14.

4.2.1 Genetic Factors Implicated in Atopic Dry Skin

The *FLG* gene is located on chromosome 1q21 at the site of a large gene cluster known as the epidermal differentiation locus. Genetic studies suggest that inheritance of loss-of-function (null) mutations of the *FLG* gene is a major cause of impaired skin barrier function, is responsible for the clinical manifestations of ichthyosis vulgaris [5] and carries a high risk of the development of atopic eczema [6]. There is mounting evidence that possession of *FLG* null mutations is associated with early-onset eczema [3] persistent in to adulthood [7] and an increased risk of allergic sensitisation [4]. A report of another single nucleotide polymorphism independent of the *FLG* risk alleles but with a strong association with atopic eczema suggests that it may be 'multiplicative in its effect' [8]. Genetic and environmental factors that govern enhanced protease activity and decreased synthesis of the lipid lamellae are also recognised to play a part in eczema causation [2], but their role and that of others governing inflammation, cytokine release and IgE function are not fully elucidated [9]. A recent review provides a fuller account of the current state of knowledge and future goals of eczema genetics [9].

For a more detailed account of the role of filaggrin in dry skin, see Chapter 9.

4.2.2 Environmental Factors Causing Dry Skin in Eczema

It seems self-evident that physical factors such as mechanical friction, exposure to chemicals, thermal damage or ultraviolet light should impair epidermal barrier integrity, but there is currently scant confirmatory evidence to support the majority of environmental factors which have been suggested as a trigger for eczema [10, 11]. The risk of developing eczema seems to be increased in urban compared with rural areas [12], suggesting a role for environmental pollution. Schmitt et al. [13] have performed a systematic review on the effectiveness and safety of interventions on breastfeeding, controlling house-dust mite levels, corticosteroids, dietary exclusion of eggs or cow's milk, elementary diets, emollients, essential fatty oils, few-foods diet, multivitamins, pimecrolimus, probiotics, pyridoxine, reducing maternal dietary allergens, tacrolimus, vitamin E and zinc supplements [13]. The role of soaps and detergents remains unproven [10], although alkaline soaps dissolve the lipid bilayer and increased pH results in up-regulation of serine protease activity and an increase in epidermal cell desquamation and dryness [2], so the use of soap substitutes seems sensible despite a lack of confirmatory evidence [14]. Hard water has been thought to be a cause of dry skin and eczema, but a recent UK study [Softened Water Eczema Trial [SWET]] on the use of water softeners in hard water areas did not show any overall statistical significance to justify their use in treating eczema [15].

4.2.3 The Role of Emollients in Dry Skin

Emollients are used to hydrate the skin to improve the appearance of dryness, to reduce itching [16] and have a cooling effect through evaporation in the case of water-based emollients. They are used in all types of dry skin conditions as wash or bath products and as leave on emollients. Guidelines for the care of eczema such as those by the National Institute for Clinical Excellence [NICE] [17, 18], the European ETFAD/EADV eczema task force [19], SIGN [Scottish Intercollegiate Guidelines network] [20] and the American Academy of Dermatology Association [21] *all recommend the regular daily use of emollients in the treatment of eczema even during periods of disease quiescence to prevent flares.*

The choice of emollient is largely patient-centred, but generally speaking, water-based creams or lotions are helpful for acutely hot, inflamed eczema because of the cooling effect from evaporation, whereas greasy ointments are used for very dry skin. Fissuring is common in severely dry skin, especially in the creases of the digits, wrists, ankles and heels, and clinical experience suggests that the use of greasy emollients under occlusion is beneficial in these sites. Emollients are thought to have antioxidant, anti-protease, anti-inflammatory activity and aid in restoring the natural balance of lipids in atopic eczema, thus restoring barrier function [22]. They vary greatly in their types of base (see Chap. 24) and other constituents (excipients/additives), and this affects their action, water-retaining potential and patient acceptability. See also Chaps. 21, 22, 23, 24, 25, 26, 27, 28, 29, 30, 31, 32, 33, 34, 35, 36, 37, 38 and 39 on 'Ingredients and treatment effects'. Emollient treatment has been demonstrated to significantly reduce the use of high-potency topical corticosteroids by 40–50% in infants with atopic eczema compared to controls, [16, 23]. In one small study on eczema, the response to treatment with topical corticosteroids seemed to be enhanced by an emollient containing urea [24]. Another study on the use of emollients to treat eczema in 48 children concluded that the liberal usage of emollients and bathing cleanser alone does not seem to alter disease severity or trans-epidermal water loss within 2 weeks, implying that additional treatments are necessary to manage atopic eczema [25]. There is little published evidence to show the superior effect of one emollient over another in the treatment of eczema, and it is vital to take into account patients personal preference in order to encourage treatment adherence [17, 18]. The GREAT [Global Resource of EczemA Trials] database lists all recent randomised controlled trials [RCTs] for eczema and contains a short list of those involving emollient therapy in eczema [26].

A current UK pilot study into the use of emollients on healthy skin of infants to prevent the development of atopic eczema in high-risk groups is almost complete, and the results are shortly to be published (Williams HC, personal communication to the author).

4.2.4 Harmful Effects of Emollients in Eczema (See also Chap. 26)

Occasionally, the effects of emollients are not beneficial, especially to children with eczema. Excipients such as preservatives in creams and lotions often cause stinging which affects patient acceptability. Other excipients often included for their humectant effect are glycerol, propylene glycol, sorbitol and others. Significant absorption of additives such as urea or lactic acid can lead to dangerous toxicity if used over large body surface areas in younger children, particularly neonates and preterm infants who have a much thinner immature epidermis. This is exaggerated in atopic eczema because of impaired epidermal barrier function. In preterm infants, use of emollients should be confined to simple paraffin-based products without preservatives. Ointments generally lack preservatives and are therefore less likely to cause irritancy and stinging, but they may cause folliculitis, particularly if used under occlusion [27].They are unsuitable for pump dispensation and are usually supplied in open containers such as tubs. These can easily become secondarily contaminated with microbes from repeated finger application, and theses may be one possible reason for recurrent episodes of bacterial infection in eczema (Cork M, personal communication to author). To prevent contamination, children and their parents/carers should be counselled to use a clean implement to remove sufficient ointment for their needs from the container and warned not to return any residual unused preparation to the container. Ointments have been reported to solidify and block plumbing in cold weather (patients personal communications to author).

Emollient creams or lotions are water-based and contain preservatives making them more likely to cause irritant contact eczema or more rarely allergic sensitisation, either of which may not be recognised in chronic eczema. It is therefore vital to patch test all young children with chronic eczema or inexplicable flares and including emollients in the series [28]. There are a few reports of cutaneous allergy occurring in children from the use of emollients containing food proteins such as oatmeal [29]. There has been concern about the use of such emollients in infants at high risk of food allergy, but at this time, there is insufficient evidence to recommend avoiding such products routinely in young infants with eczema. Those emollients containing arachis oil should be avoided in cases of peanut allergy or if there is a family history of it, and it would seem wise to avoid topical use of any nut oil in nut allergy sufferers. It should be remembered that many families use 'over the counter' (OTC) emollients for treating eczema that often contain perfumes or other excipients which may cause contact eczema. Many of the fashionable so-called natural products contain plant extracts which may sensitise, especially in those with atopic eczema. There is a cultural preference in many communities for using olive oil to treat eczema; however, it has been shown to cause both irritant and allergic contact eczema, especially if used under occlusive bandages [30].

Some excipients used in emollients may actually damage epidermal barrier function. Commonly used 'aqueous cream' was designed as a wash product but is frequently used as a 'leave on' emollient. It usually contains sodium lauryl sulphate (SLS), a known skin irritant. Recent work has shown that application of aqueous cream reduces *Stratum corneum* thickness and increases the rate of trans-epidermal water loss (TEWL) during tape stripping [31] and is associated with reduced maturity and size of corneocytes and increased desquamatory and inflammatory protease activity [32].

A recent review of comparison and suitability of emollients used in young children suggested that emollients should be chosen to minimise the risk of contact sensitisation. The authors noted that emulsifiers can promote skin dryness by emulsification of the endogenous epidermal lipids [33].

4.3 The Misery of Living with Eczema

4.3.1 The Psychosocial Effects of Eczema on Children and Their Families

Children with eczema and their families have a miserable time whenever the eczema flares [34–37], and this may be a constant feature in the more severe and chronic cases. Data taken directly from children and their parents [34, 35] and many subsequent quality of life studies suggest that eczema affects all aspects of their lives and may cause psychological disturbance in the child or its family unit [38].

Sleep Disturbance: The inflammatory nature of eczema causes intense pruritus and often intractable scratching which affects sleep in between 66% and 80% of children compared to less than 45% of 'normal' children [35, 39–41]. It also affects family members of younger children with eczema, especially siblings, and parents may lose an average of 2.5 h of sleep per night during flares [39]. Sleep disturbance can manifest as an increase in sleep latency (getting to sleep) and increased frequency and length of night-time wakening and restlessness during sleep. Sleep disturbance occurs in 39% of normal infants, but eczema causes a pattern of much more severe night-time wakening and reduced sleep efficiency [42]. Pruritus causing sleep loss and tiredness is amongst the most important problems relating to eczema according to children and their parents [34, 35, 43]. The use of sedating antihistamines for pruritus or to aid sleep may further increase day-time tiredness and impair concentration [37]. Sleeping with parents (co-sleeping) is normal in many societies, but even in those where it is uncommon, parents often take the affected child into their bed with consequent negative effects on their own sleeping patterns [44].

Physical Effects [34, 36, 37]: These include itching, burning, tiredness, loss of concentration, etc. Excoriations often sting with treatment application or when exposed to chlorinated water, so children often refuse treatment or to go swimming. Painful fissuring is seen in hand and foot dermatitis, and children report problems with writing, unscrewing bottle tops, riding their bikes, handling sports equipment and wearing sports shoes or activities involving running or jumping. Parents report problems with discomfort and pain in infants during bathing or dressing [35].

Performance and Schooling: The resultant tiredness from sleep deprivation causes irritability and mood swings which may affect concentration, school performance and sporting activities [34]. In infants, tiredness leads to an increase in tantrum behaviour [36]. Time lost from schooling is a problem for those with the more severe or chronic spectrum of disease, and school avoidance sometimes occurs, especially if there has been teasing or bullying [37]. A US Study on parents of over 400 children up to age 15 years reported difficulties with schooling, daily, social and leisure activities in 60% [45]. Ultimately, having chronic eczema may affect career choices, for example, having to avoid wet work because of the risk of hand eczema in the catering, hairdressing or medical professions or in manual occupations such as the mechanical or building trades.

Embarrassment and Psychosocial Reactions to Eczema [34, 37, 38, 45]: The visual nature of eczema causes loss of confidence even if comments or questions are kindly meant. Teasing and bullying are common and may lead to peer group ostracisation resulting in anxiety, mood swings, sadness, anger and depression. Occasionally, other psychological problems arise, including behavioural problems and school avoidance. Embarrassment about their appearance when undressing in front of others, especially for communal changing such as for sporting activities, is a frequently mentioned problem so that children seek to avoid such situations. They also have to contend with the necessity of wearing different clothes from their peers, either as cover to hide the eczema or because certain materials such as synthetics which may cause increased sweating and irritation. Eczema of the face or hands is a particular embarrassment because it is difficult to conceal, and using make-up for camouflage often irritates or stings. Embarrassment about the shiny/greasy appearance of skin or clothes due to emollient use may contribute to treatment refusal.

Other Social Aspects [34, 35]: Bedding and clothes are frequently soiled or bloodied from scratching or the use of greasy emollients and require frequent washing and replacement. This is often quoted as a reason for avoiding hotel holidays or overnight stays at friend's houses. Those with real or suspected food allergy may also have problems away from home, especially at parties or eating out with the family. Other things of major concern to children are the restriction on owning or having contact with furry pets or other animals, and this may also prevent visits to relatives or friends houses. In one small utility study in younger children when asked about their favourite things, children specified their pet as one of the top three items demonstrating the importance children place on pet ownership [46]. In family studies, parents reported that not being able to own a pet affected other family members [35].

Mealtime and Dietary Problems: Parents frequently blame foods as a cause of eczema, often with no confirmation of true allergy, and as a result a significant majority report increased time spent shopping, preparing food and difficulty at mealtimes as major problems [35]. They also frequently spend money on 'Allergy tests' on the High Street or increasingly on the internet, although there is no evidence of the benefit of these [17]. Children on food-restricted diets have especial problems at parties, when staying with friends or at school. True food allergy occurs mainly in infants, usually those with moderate to severe eczema cases where foods may be a triggering factor for eczema in about a third of cases [17]. Mild eczema occurs in 80% of cases, and food allergy in these cases is much less likely to be a triggering factor. Milk, egg and peanut allergy account for about 75% of food allergy cases triggering eczema, and although milk and egg allergy usually remit in early childhood, peanut allergy tends to persist throughout life in the majority [17]. Food allergy should be suspected in those infants with gastrointestinal disturbance such as reflux, vomiting, colic and diarrhoea and should alert physicians to possible food allergy [17]. Unfortunately, some children suffer from severe restriction of their diet, often unnecessarily. It is therefore vital that suspected cases are properly investigated so that appropriate advice can be given where indicated and unnecessary dietary restriction avoided in those not requiring it. In particular, a few infants on long-term unsupervised milk-free or other restricted diets may develop 'faltering growth' [17], and there are occasional reports of severe nutritional deficiency and the development of rickets [47]. A Cochrane review of nine randomised controlled trials concluded that there is no benefit from the use of a milk- or egg-free diet, elemental or few-foods diet in *unselected patients* with atopic eczema [48]. Those children with proven food allergy should be referred for paediatric dietetic advice, and all prepubertal children with moderate to severe eczema should be monitored for growth on a regular basis [17].

4.3.2 Psychological Impairment in Children with Eczema and Their Parents

A study of 30 preschool children with severe atopic eczema compared with 20 matched controls found that minor behaviour problems and parenting distress were important features of severe atopic eczema in early childhood [40]. The levels of stress were much higher (85%) in those with more severely affected children. The authors found significantly higher levels of behavioural problems in 23%, dependency/clinginess in 50% and fearfulness in 40%, but no difference between the two groups in the security of attachments. Mothers felt particularly stressed in relation to their parenting and less efficient in their disciplining of the affected child, although they did not display negative attitudes towards their child. Only 1/3 of mothers in the eczema group felt socially supported compared to 2/3 of controls [40]. A German study on the psychological adjustment in parents of young children found high rates of psychological distress that were directly related to the severity of the eczema [49]. However, although Titman also found chronic eczema to cause higher levels of psychological distress in both parents and children compared to those in a general paediatric population, this did not relate to the eczema severity [50]. In this study, the child's rating of the impact of eczema on their QoL was significantly related to their psychological symptoms. In an Australian study, maternal stress in caring for children with eczema was found to be equivalent to that associated with the care of children with severe developmental and physical problems [51].

In contrast Absolon et al. found levels of mental distress to be no greater in mothers of children with eczema than in parents of the control group. However, they did find twice the rate of psychological disturbance in children with moderate to severe eczema compared to the control group, but not in those with mild eczema [52]. There was no difference in the degree of social support experienced by the eczema families in this study. A small study from India ($n=22$) found that an increased number of mothers of affected children, 59%, were submissive when compared to 10% in the control group ($p<0.01$) [53].

In adults, Schmitt et al. found that eczema was independently associated with affective and stress-related behaviour, and in particular, the risk of developing schizophrenic disorders had an odds ratio (OR) of 2.12 (95%, CI 1.22–3.71) [54]. These risks increased with the number of physician attendances, suggesting a higher risk for those with severe disease [54]. Since eczema in children with severe eczema often persists into adult life, it is vitally important to search for and treat any psychological disturbances early in life to try to prevent problems in adulthood.

4.3.3 The Effect of Eczema on Family Life and Members

Eczema is a chronic disease affecting the functioning of the whole family so that the impact on the child cannot be viewed in isolation. In ethnographic interviews of 33 families [35] with young children with atopic eczema, 11 main domains of life were reported to be affected in descending order of frequency, see Table 4.1. Over 90% of families reported on the practical difficulties of caring for a child with eczema, and this was one of their major concerns [35]. Other problems

Table 4.1 The effects of eczema on family functioning

Practical care problems, for example, time pressures to apply treatments and for nurse/family doctor/hospital visits, increased washing of clothes/bedding, house-dust avoidance measures, preparing special foods for food allergic children, shopping for cotton clothing/bedding, etc.
Psychological and physical pressures, for example, stress, anxiety about child's future and worry about treatment side effects, depression, frustration, anger, coping with child problems, exhaustion from sleep loss and extra housework
Alteration in family life style, for example, unable to keep pets, restriction of family diet if child has food allergy, restriction of visits to houses with furry pets
Sleep disturbance from sleep latency and frequent night-time wakening causes parents to lose an average of 2 h per night during eczema flares causing physical and mental exhaustion and poor performance and may affect sleep patterns of siblings
Schooling problems include child care problems when children are off school because of the eczema and time lost from work for parents. Children may develop school phobia especially if teased or bullied. Siblings and affected child school performance may be affected by sleep loss
Coping with child's behavioural problems, for example, increased crying and tantrums in infants, refusal to cooperate with treatment application, difficulties at mealtimes and bath times, negative or difficult behaviour
Social life of family members, for example, too tired to go out, difficulty in finding babysitters, fear of leaving child with eczema with others
Interpersonal relations, for example, increased stress, reported as a major cause of marriage break down in 2/33 families
Practical support, for example, lack of help or support from other family members or outside agencies including the medical profession
Holiday difficulties, for example, avoiding sunny holidays because of heat worsening the eczema or anxiety about staying in hotels or with friends because of special diets or ruining bedclothes
Financial problems in this UK study were not of great concern except for two single parent families where it was a major problem. However, many 'hidden costs' caused by having a child with eczema were reported

Adapted from the DFI [35]
These data were used to develop the Dermatitis Family Impact score (DFI©)

encountered included the physical effects of tiredness and exhaustion from lack of sleep, psychological pressures such as anxiety, guilt, frustration, resentment and helplessness and even depression occurred in 71%. Two thirds of families said that they did not have a normal lifestyle because of restrictions on owning pets, foods, household products and interference with holidays, and a third reported that they rarely went out socially because of tiredness, difficulty in obtaining a babysitter and fear of leaving a child with eczema. Twenty-nine percent felt that having a child with eczema affected their interpersonal relationships.

Parents describe being disheartened and frustrated about the management of eczema and complain of lack of knowledge and information with resultant confusion over the use of treatments [35]. Only 24% of patients and caregivers feel confident they can manage AD flares adequately. Seventy-five percent of caregivers and patients feel that being able to effectively control AD would be the single most important improvement to their or their child's quality of life [35]. Insufficient support from medical and social support, conflicting advice from friends, relatives and healthcare workers all increase the anxiety and guilt [35, 41, 45, 55]. Time taken to treat eczema may amount to as much as 2–3 h per day and is a significant drain on parents time [56] and energy. Parental loss of sleep can cause a deterioration of work-related performance, and they may miss time off work to cover child care during eczema flares [57]. Negative comments from others about a child's appearance and fears of possible contagion from eczema are very distressing to parents, and blame is often felt to be apportioned by their spouse or relatives [55].

Financial Costs: Having a child with eczema places a large burden on the family and healthcare resources [56–60]. Costs to managing eczema are overt and hidden and are higher if it is severe and require frequent hospital visits [56]. Su et al. [56]

showed that this cost was higher than that for asthma, but equivalent to caring for a child with diabetes. Other factors influencing costs include the type of healthcare system and local, religious or ethnic preferences or beliefs about health care. Where health care is free, there is less impact on the family budget, and therefore, cost is a lower priority in terms of need in many cases, but even in the UK, a utility study demonstrated that to single parent families, the cost related to eczema may be an important negative factor [35]. In countries without free medical aid, low income families can have major problems in paying for consultation or hospital fees, tests and drugs and some will be unable to afford them at all [57]. Hidden costs to eczema care include travel costs for health care, which rise with eczema severity, reducing the allergen load by increased house cleaning or purchase of hypoallergenic bedding. Clothes and bedding soiled or damaged from blood or emollients require increased washing or replacement. Emollients also speed up the perishing of washing machine seals causing extra repair bills. Buying cotton clothes and bedding or special foods for food allergy sufferers all add to the cost, and many parents report spending on over the counter preparations, alternative therapies or 'High Street allergy testing'. One study found that family costs accounted for 36% of total costs for eczema [60]. A UK community-based study took into account these multiple factors including visits to health professionals, time lost off work or paying for childcare during eczema flares. It found that the cost to both family and community of managing eczema was equivalent to the cost of treating chronic venous leg ulcers at that time [61]. A recent European study on the costs of treating eczema concluded that the mean annual healthcare costs and family costs varied considerably in six identified studies, but in their study, substituting a specialised nurse practitioner for follow-up rather than using dermatologists was both cost-saving and cost-effective [62]. The avoidable secondary economic cost of AD has been estimated at 2 billion Euros per year across the European Union [63]. Carroll et al. [59] estimated the personal and medical costs of eczema in the USA as 1 billion dollars per annum in 2005.

4.4 Quality of Life Measurement in Children with Eczema

A definition of QoL in children suggests that it can be defined as how a child views their life and their reasonable expectations of how they would like it to be [64]. This is dependent upon many factors including age, gender, education, cognitive ability, culture and ethnicity, and psychosocial adaptation to life experiences [38]. HRQoL scales are widely used as outcome measures for assessing disease severity, treatment effects and monitoring disease control, both in the clinical setting and in clinical studies. They usually contain a mixture of objective measures which focus on physical ability and subjective measures which reflect on the meaning to the individual [65]. Used correctly HRQoL measures can give additional information to that from clinical measures of disease activity alone and provide great insight into a person's perspective of their disease and the practical and emotional life problems that they face. They are now considered to be a key consideration in the management of eczema [65], and use of HRQoL measures in children and their families suggests that eczema has a negative effect on all aspects of their lives [38]. Although some studies have shown a reasonably good correlation between objective measures of disease severity in eczema and impact on QoL [66], they are not always well correlated. This is because two individuals with the same objective disease severity may have very different subjective perceptions [38]. The impact of a disease is also dependent upon a child's (and their parents') adaptation to the disease or 'coping ability' so that a child with chronic severe life-long eczema who copes well may appear to suffer less measurable impact of their HRQoL than a child with mild eczema who has an occasional sudden exacerbation to which they are poorly adapted [38]. Measurement of coping ability is not the same as HRQoL assessment, and more research of the two is essential to our understanding of patient's perceptions and adaptation to their disease. One study using a structural educational programme in the management of eczema found a greater improvement in children's coping behaviour and the parents ability to handle the children compared to the control group [67].

4.5 Types of Quality of Life Measures

It is essential that all HRQoL questionnaires should be correctly validated for content, construct and criterion and tested for reliability, repeatability and internal consistency for use in the study population [38]. In young children or those with cognitive impairment, proxy measures are often employed, using responses from another person such as the parent/carer or the attending medical professional. In addition to the factors affecting response listed in the preceding section, the ratings in proxy measures will be influenced by the proxy provider's own psychosocial circumstances and beliefs [38]. When comparing a child's rating versus that of their parent/carer, they demonstrate much more agreement on physical ability rather than on emotional response, for example, they will usually agree on the effect that disease has on a child's ability to do a sport but may differ widely on a child's subjective assessment about their emotional responses to their disease [65]. Generic and specialty-specific measures are useful for disease comparison but give less detailed information than a disease-specific measure, so often, more than one type is employed in a particular study. HRQOL measurement in eczema shows that it may affect most aspects of a child's life and have a more major impact than many other chronic childhood diseases [43]. In a comparative study, the impact of eczema was greater than that of enuresis, epilepsy, diabetes, asthma and equivalent to renal disease and cystic fibrosis [43]. Another study found the disease burden of atopic diseases was greater than all other childhood diseases [68].

There are several validated eczema-specific QOL scales for use in childhood eczema including the Infants Dermatitis Quality of Life score (IDQoL)* [36], the Dermatitis Family Impact score (DFI)* [35], The Children's Atopic Dermatitis Impact Score (CADIS) [55], the Parent's Index of Quality of Life in atopic Dermatitis (PIQoL-AD) [69].

The Children's Dermatology Life Quality Index (CDLQI)* [34] is a dermatology-specific scale (completed by the child) which can be used to compare eczema with any other dermatological disease. It is also available in cartoon format [70] (Table 4.2).It is a simple 10-question validated scale that has been the most widely used in dermatology and is currently translated into 24 languages. A high score indicates a greater negative impact on QoL. It was designed from data taken from children themselves about the problems they encountered from having a skin disease. These problems are described more fully under 'the psychosocial effects of eczema'. It has been used in clinical settings as a monitor for disease impact and the effect of treatment and as an outcome measure in many clinical and research trials on eczema (38SL-J).

Eczema causes many and various effects on a child's quality of life. Use of the CDLQI shows

Table 4.2 Validated HRQoL scales used in studies of childhood eczema

Eczema specific
Infants Dermatitis Quality of Life (IDQoL©)[a] [36]: A 10-item scale for infants up to the age of 4 years, includes 1 question on eczema severity as perceived by the parent/carer and scored separately. Translated into 20 languages
Dermatitis Family Impact (DFI©)[a] [35]: A 10-item scale measuring the impact of eczema on families. Translated into 14 languages
The Children's Atopic Dermatitis Impact Score (CADIS) [55]: A 45-item scale validated for use in the United States for parents and children up to age 6 years [4 child subscales; 4 family subscales]
Parent's Index of Quality of Life in Atopic Dermatitis (PIQoL-AD) [69]: Constructed and validated from data of several European countries for use in commercial studies on pimecrolimus in the treatment of eczema
Specialty specific
Children's Dermatology Life Quality Index (CDLQI©)[a] [34]: A 10-item scale for children aged 4–16 years which can be used for all childhood skin diseases. It is now translated into 40 languages. The cartoon version is available in 5 languages

[a]The IDQoL, DFI and CDLQI can be downloaded at www.dermatology.org.uk/

that the highest scoring questions pertain to itch, sleep loss, difficulties with or loss of schooling and difficulties with treatment. A good correlation between eczema severity and HRQoL impairment has been seen in several studies using the CDLQI, and one study showed that every 1 unit change in SCORAD was associated with a 0.12 change in the CDLQI score [66]. Amongst common childhood skin diseases, eczema has been shown to cause the most impact on quality of life, although other itchy dermatoses such as scabies and urticaria also score highly [34]. In clinical trials on the use of eczema treatments, the CDLQI has shown to be sensitive to clinical change proving its use as an outcome measure [38].

4.5.1 Infantile Eczema and Quality of Life Impairment

*The Infants Dermatitis QoL[IDQoL©]** [36] is a 10-question scale similar to the CDLQI but with an additional but separately scored question on the parental perception of eczema severity. It has demonstrated particular problems in infants with eczema with itching and sleeping, bathing and mood changes such as tantrums. Use of the IDQoL for monitoring showed that consultation with a physician led to significantly increased quality of life for the infant with eczema and their parents [71]. It has also been used successfully in many clinical trials [38]. In a study by Beattie et al., the highest IDQoL scores were for itching, scratching, bath-time problems and time taken to fall asleep, and those in the DFI were for tiredness/exhaustion, sleep loss and emotional distress [71]. These domains correlated well with the severity of eczema. Children were seen by a dermatologist, and majority also had face to face nurse consultation or via telephone. Those with the most severe eczema (median score 14) improved the most by 64%, and the domains showing the greatest improvement were 'time to get to sleep', and 'meal-time difficulties'. For the parents, the most improved domains were 'tiredness and exhaustion' and 'emotional distress'. Statistical significance of improvement between visits was $p=0.0001$.

4.5.2 Health-Related Quality of Life Family Measures

*The Dermatitis Family Impact Scale (DFI©)** [35] is a 10-item scale focussing on the effect of eczema on the family (Table 4.1). It was constructed from data obtained by ethnographic and brainstorming techniques and showed good correlation between clinical eczema severity and impact on family QoL [35]. It is often used in conjunction with the IDQoL scale [36] as an outcome measure in clinical practice and research. It is now translated into 14 languages. Using the DFI, Ben Gashir and colleagues found family life to be affected in 45% of children with eczema [72], which related to objective eczema severity, and this has been confirmed in other studies [73]. The PIQol-AD was validated for use in multicentre European studies on pimecrolimus in the treatment of eczema [69]. Use of the PIQol-AD found positive but low levels of association between the QoL scores and disease severity and showed that family QoL improved the greatest in the pimecrolimus-treated group [69]. In the USA, Chamlin and colleagues developed a scale for young children with eczema and their parents using directed focus sessions which provided 181 specific QoL effects that related to either the child or the family. These were used to develop a conceptual framework containing domains of physical and emotional health and functioning [55]. In their further validation studies, they also showed a correlation between eczema severity and HRQoL impairment [74].

4.5.3 Utility Studies

Whilst utility measures are much favoured by health economists because they give information on patient preferences, they are difficult to perform even in older children, and there are no reported studies on their use in children with eczema. There is one small study in normal young children who were asked to list their three favourite things which

* author declaration of interest: co-copyright holder of these measures

they reported as their pet, playing with friends and their favourite toy [46]. Parents are particularly keen for their child to be able to cope with their eczema, and in a utility study amongst families, they scored it as the first most important factor after coping with the practical difficulties and having satisfactory family relationships [35]. These findings are borne out by the ISOLATE study (International Study of Living with Atopic Eczema) where eczema sufferers also rated being able to cope with their eczema as their most important goal [63]. Utility studies in adults with chronic severe eczema found that they were willing to pay up to £80 per month for a 'cure' [75].

More detailed accounts of QoL measurement in children with eczema are found elsewhere [37, 38] and a list of reference of their use at www.dermatology.org.uk/.

4.6 Difficulties Associated with Using Topical Treatments in Eczema

4.6.1 Problems with Adherence to Therapy

The problem of lack of use of treatments is complex and encompasses incorrect use. There is little doubt amongst dermatologists that failure to adhere to therapy is the main cause of poor control of eczema and is likely to lead to a state of disease chronicity. However, very little is known about adherence to therapy in childhood eczema since most studies have been conducted with adults. One study in children using a method of 'stealth monitoring' suggested that adherence to eczema therapies in childhood eczema is very poor [76].

Bradley looked at adherence to oral therapy in adults and devised the concept of the 'rule of thirds', i.e. one third of patients take their treatment correctly, one third take it intermittently but to some effect and one third do not take it at all, suggesting that only 50% of patients take oral treatments effectively [77]. A review on the use of dermatological therapies in adults concluded that poor adherence was seen in at least 35–40% of patients and is also associated with self-reported psychiatric morbidity [78]. In an objective assessment of compliance with psoriasis therapy amongst adults, non-compliance was associated with being male, single, unemployed, drinking alcohol, smoking, paying for treatment, side effects of therapy, twice-daily treatment and oral therapy [79]. The same group studied compliance with acne treatments and found that non-compliance was associated with a younger age, higher impairment with QoL and smoking and alcohol abuse, whereas good compliance was seen in married females, those in employment and where there were no treatment costs [80]. Carroll et al. showed that compliance in psoriasis therapy gradually reduced over an 8-week period from 84.6% to 51%, although there was slightly better adherence in older females [81]. They used three methods of adherence monitoring and found that electronic monitoring caps were more accurate for assessing actual treatment usage than medication logs or medication usage by weight. Another small study used electronic monitors to compare adherence in psoriatics to that observed in clinical trials of hand eczema and atopic eczema. Adherence was shown to be better around the time of office visits or during clinical trials with close follow-up [82].

4.6.2 Lack of Knowledge About Treatments and How to Use Them

The most fundamental problem is lack of knowledge by parents, children, healthcare professionals and the general public about eczema and its treatment and the necessity for provision of adequate support and follow-up [41, 83]. Lack of knowledge often leads to conflicting and misleading advice that heightens parental and child anxiety and causes confusion. Parents and adults with eczema report that they want easy access to more understandable information [41, 63]. It is vital that information should be available in a language understood by the family. Eczema treatments are often prescribed by healthcare professionals who have little knowledge about the practicalities of their use, and parents rarely receive any instructions on their use. In a study by the National Eczema Society, only 53% of responders were given advice on daily cleansing and moisturising routine, and only 25% of those who were prescribed emollients had been given demonstrations of their use [41].

Problems with use of treatments (see also problems associated with emollient usage, 4.2.4)

- *Adverse Reactions:* Children often refuse to use cream or lotion preparations which sting or cause irritation because of the preservative content, and in a minority, there may be actual allergic contact dermatitis. Absorption of products through the skin is commoner in children, especially neonates and premature infants. Urea and lactic acid in some emollients may cause toxicity or, in the case of topical corticosteroids, excessive absorption causing cushingoid features or thinning of the skin and telangiectasia. Evidence from a study on anti-retroviral therapy showed that those who suffered adverse events were 12.8 times less likely to maintain a 95–100% adherence [84].
- *Anxiety About Potential Side Effects*: Especially of topical corticosteroids is also a major problem for non-adherence [85]. In the ISOLATE study, 66% of patients used steroids as a last resort, and 39% used them less frequently than recommended because of a the fear of side effects [63]. Beattie found that parental knowledge of the potency of topical corticosteroids was very poor [83]. Steroid phobia is not confined to patients, and ignorance and over-exaggeration of side effects are common in all types of healthcare professionals. There may also be dislike of conventional therapy and preference for 'natural' products or alternative therapies.
- *Lack of Time:* The necessity of using topical therapy on a regular basis in skin diseases such as eczema causes problems for children that are not seen in other common chronic childhood diseases such as diabetes, asthma or epilepsy [43]. Topical therapy is time-consuming to apply and is cited as a major problem, particularly if the parent is single or both parents are working [35, 43]. There is often little time in the morning before work or school, and older children are often late home because of outside activities.
- *Lack of Availability of Treatments:* Parents often run out of treatment for many reasons that include laziness, lack of time, inability to pay for treatment, forgetting to order the medication or to take it if staying away from home. Children living in more than one home require enough therapy at each abode. Medication may be lost or damaged or out of date. *Healthcare professional often fail to prescribe sufficient quantities* [86]. *This is a particular problem with emollients which are sometimes viewed as non-essential therapy.* A community study looked at dispensed prescriptions for topical corticosteroid preparations and emollients in over 25,000 children in Tayside aged ≥6 years over a 17-month period. It found that 22.8% of children were supplied with a prescription for a topical corticosteroid, but half of these (50.6%) were not prescribed any emollients [87]. Parents are also much less likely to pay for treatments such as emollients when the disease is quiescent leading to poor disease control.
- *Child Refusal:* Children and their parents frequently complain that treatments are messy, often sting and take too long to apply [34, 35]. Refusal may be due to stinging, fear of side effects, dislike of the texture or it may represent a behavioural problem. Children are also embarrassed by the appearance of the greasy effect of emollients on skin and clothes and do not like to draw attention to their disease or apply treatments in front of others. Children may also refuse therapy for gain in order to avoid school or sports or to get attention, and some learn that they can punish or control parents by scratching to maintain disease activity [88].
- *Failure to Maintain Therapy During Remission:* Eczema is a chronic problem which is often not perceived as such by patients but also many healthcare professionals so that therapies are stopped as soon as the eczema clears. This reflects what has been observed in asthma where good adherence is associated with understanding the disease and accepting its chronic nature, whereas poor

adherence is found in those who perceive that 'no symptoms means no disease' and view asthma as an episodic rather than a chronic disease [89]. It has been suggested that education of patients and parents/carers to accept eczema as a chronic disease and that dryness represents the early occult stages should lead to better control of disease flares and possibly to prevention if used early in life in high-risk patients. *This underscores the necessity of using emollient therapy on a regular daily basis as the mainstay treatment for childhood eczema, even when the eczema is clear* [17, 18].

- *Loss of Faith in Treatment and/or Physician:* Good doctor-patient relationships are essential in the treatment of eczema [90], but unfortunately parents and children often lose faith in treatments and also faith in the healthcare professional [41]. This may be partly due to the fact that many family doctors and other health care professions know very little about eczema and its treatment and fail to follow-up after an initial consultation.

4.6.3 Failure to Control Eczema Despite Adequate Treatment Compliance

Sometimes, appropriate treatments seem ineffective because there is failure to increase the corticosteroid potency when the eczema worsens. It must be clearly explained that treatment should be stepped up when eczema flares [17, 18]. Alternatively, it may be due to the provision of too weak a potency of a topical corticosteroid in cases of severe eczema. There may be additional complications such as secondary infection, scabies infestation or the development of contact irritancy or allergy. In infants with severe eczema who fail to respond to adequate therapy, food allergy should be considered as a possible triggering factor [17, 18]. In severe cases, it is important to review the diagnosis particularly if there is evidence of severe recurrent infection or faltering growth that might reflect an underlying immunodeficiency. Sometimes, it is due to behavioural problems [88], and such cases require assessment by a clinical psychologist. There are, however, a small minority of children with extremely severe atopic eczema who may require systemic therapies.

4.7 Factors Thought to Improve Treatment Adherence

If treatment is perceived to be effective and safe and patients understand how to use it correctly, then they are more likely to use it. Patient satisfaction with care seems to be an important factor [91]. According to Kjellgren, providers and patients felt that factors affecting adherence to dermatological therapy were: patients' expectations and experiences of therapeutic effect, patients taking an active part in treatment decisions and the mode of administration and type of medication [92]. A Japanese study showed that the most important factor in compliance with therapy was a good doctor-patient relationship and the willingness to use therapies [90]. A review on adherence to therapy concluded that major determinants of good adherence are a good doctor-patient interaction and good patient satisfaction [78].

Feldman et al. concluded that 'frequent follow-up visits in clinical trials increase patients' adherence to medications'. They proposed the use of a follow-up visit shortly after initiating treatment as an effective way to boost patients' use of their medication with the object of achieving better treatment outcomes [82].

Studies on demonstration of treatments by a specialist nurse have shown the benefit of this [93–96]. Carroll et al. [59] suggested that the cost of treating eczema could be reduced by 'targeting parents and caregivers with education and psychosocial support' that might decrease family and personal burden'. The most comprehensive study reported on education used a structured education programme for parents and children with eczema and showed that the intervention group did better than the control group, an effect maintained at 12 months [97]. They concluded that 'Education must therefore underpin all management for eczema for treatment to be successful' [97]. An international collaboration of paediatric dermatologists 'OPENED' has collated educational tools from different centres used for eczema patients in an attempt to share knowledge Stalder et al. [98]. See also a Cochrane review on RCTs of psychological and education interventions in eczema [99].

A Key recommendation from the NICE guidelines states 'provide information in verbal and written forms with practical demonstrations that cover

- How much treatment to use
- How often to apply treatments
- When and how to step treatment up or down
- How to treat atopic eczema'

There is also a recommendation on treating flares which suggests that 'treatment should be started as soon as signs and symptoms appear. Continue for 48 h after symptoms subside'. Older children should be encouraged to do their own treatment, but parents/carers should oversee this initially to ensure it is being done and especially if treatment starts to fail.

If the management of eczema is to progress favourably, then more investigation is required in the field of patients' needs and education, especially on the complex reasons for failure of adherence to treatment.

Take Home Messages

- Eczema is caused by a complex interplay of genetic and environmental factors leading to a breakdown in epidermal barrier function.
- Ichthyosis vulgaris, the main cause for dry skin in eczema, is due to loss-of-function mutations in the protein filaggrin that is essential for normal epidermal cell maturation.
- Possession of *FLG* null mutations is highly associated with early-onset severe eczema often persisting into adult life.
- Eczema may have a profoundly negative effect on the quality of life and psychosocial functioning of children and their families, preventing a normal lifestyle.
- Quality of life studies in children show that eczema has an effect equal to or greater than the impact caused by diabetes, asthma or epilepsy.
- Psychological distress due to eczema has been found to be higher than 'normal' in children and their mothers and is significantly related to disease severity in most cases.
- Emollients of a patient's own choice should be used regularly in eczema and during periods of disease remission to prevent flares.
- Education is essential for patients, parents and healthcare workers involved in the management of eczema to improve adherence to therapy and improve outcomes.
- Patients and parents of children with eczema need simple, clear information on eczema and its treatments in a verbal and written format with practical demonstrations on applying treatments.
- Patient satisfaction and a good patient-physician rapport are essential for good adherence to therapies.
- Patients should be followed up soon after initial consultation to improve adherence to therapy.

References

1. Tagami H, Kobayashi H, O'goshi K, Kikuchi K (2006) Atopic xerosis: employment of noninvasive biophysical instrumentation for the functional analyses of the mildly abnormal stratum corneum and for the efficacy assessment of skin care products. J Cosmet Dermatol 5(2):140–149
2. Cork MJ, Danby SG, Vasilopoulos Y, Hadgraft J, Lane ME, Moustafa M, Guy RH, Macgowan AL, Tazi-Ahnini R, Ward SJ (2009) Epidermal barrier dysfunction in atopic dermatitis. J Invest Dermatol 129(8):1892–1908, Epub 2009 Jun 4
3. Flohr C, England K, Radulovic S, McLean WH, Campbel LE, Barker J, Perkin M, Lack G (2010) Filaggrin loss-of-function mutations are associated with early-onset eczema, eczema severity and

transepidermal water loss at 3 months of age. Br J Dermatol 163(6):1333–1336
4. O'Regan GM, Sandilands A, McLean WH, Irvine AD (2008) Filaggrin in atopic dermatitis. J Allergy Clin Immunol 122(4):689–693, Epub 2008 Sep 5
5. Smith FJ, Irvine AD, Terron-Kwiatkowski A, Sandilands A, Campbell LE, Zhao Y, Liao H, Evans AT, Goudie DR, Lewis-Jones S, Arseculeratne G, Munro CS, Sergeant A, O'Regan G, Bale SJ, Compton JG, DiGiovanna JJ, Presland RB, Fleckman P, McLean WH (2006) Loss-of-function mutations in the gene encoding filaggrin cause ichthyosis vulgaris. Nat Genet 38(3):337–342
6. Palmer CN, Irvine AD, Terron-Kwiatkowski A, Zhao Y, Liao H, Lee SP, Goudie DR, Sandilands A, Campbell LE, Smith FJ, O'regan GM, Watson RM, Cecil JE, Bale SJ, Compton JG, Digiovanna JJ, Fleckman P, Lewis-Jones S, Arseculeratne G, Sergeant A, Munro CS, El Houate B, McElreavey K, Halkjaer LB, Bisgaard H, Mukhopadhyay S, McLean WH (2006) Common loss-of-function variants of the epidermal barrier protein filaggrin are a major predisposing factor for atopic dermatitis. Nat Genet 38(4): 441–446, Epub 2006 Mar 19
7. Barker JN, Palmer CN, Zhao Y, Liao H, Hull PR, Lee SP, Allen MH, Meggitt SJ, Reynolds NJ, Trembath RC, McLean WH (2007) Null mutations in the filaggrin gene (FLG) determine major susceptibility to early-onset atopic dermatitis that persists into adulthood. J Invest Dermatol 127(3):564–567, Epub 2006 Sep 21
8. O'Regan Gráinne M, Campbell Linda E, Cordell Heather J, Irvine Alan D, Irwin McLean WH, Brown Sara J (2010) Chromosome 11q13.5 variant associated with childhood eczema: an effect supplementary to filaggrin mutations. J Allergy Clin Immunol 125(1–4): 170–174
9. Brown SJ, McLean WHI (2009) Eczema genetics: current state of knowledge and future goals. J Invest Dermatol 129:543–552
10. Langan SM, Williams HC (2006) What causes worsening of eczema? A systematic review. Br J Dermatol 155(3):504–514
11. Langan SM, Silcocks P, Williams HC (2009) What causes flares of eczema in children? Br J Dermatol 161(3):640–646, Epub 2009 Jun 5
12. Shams K, Grindlay DJ, Williams HC (2011) What's new in atopic eczema? An analysis of systematic reviews published in 2009–2010. Clin Exp Dermatol 36(6): 573–577. doi:10.1111/j.1365–2230.2011.04078.x;quiz 577–8. Epub 2011 Jul 1
13. Schmitt J, Apfelbacher CJ, Flohr C (2011) Eczema. Clin Evid (Online) pii:1716
14. Blume-Peytavi U, Cork MJ, Faergemann J, Szczapa J, Vanaclocha F, Gelmetti C (2009) Bathing and cleansing in newborns from day 1 to first year of life: recommendations from a European round table meeting. J Eur Acad Dermatol Venereol 23(7):751–759
15. Thomas KS, Koller K, Dean T, O'Leary CJ, Sach TH, Frost A, Pallett I, Crook AM, Meredith S, Nunn AJ, Burrows N, Pollock I, Graham-Brown R, O'Toole E, Potter D, Williams HC (2011) A multicentre randomised controlled trial and economic evaluation of ion-exchange water softeners for the treatment of eczema in children: the Softened Water Eczema Trial (SWET). Health Technol Assess 15(8):v–vi, 1–156
16. Lucky AW, Leach AD, Laskarzewski P, Wenck H (1997) Use of an emollient as a steroid sparing agent in the treatment of mild to moderate atopic dermatitis in children. Pediatr Dermatol 14:321–324
17. NHS (2007) NICE guidelines on management of atopic eczema in children from birth up to the age of 12 years, CG057, http://guidance.org.uk/CG57, Dec 2007
18. Lewis-Jones S, Mugglestone MA, Guideline Development Group (2007) Management of atopic eczema in children aged up to 12 years: summary of NICE guidance. BMJ 335(7632):1263–1264
19. Darsow U, Wollenberg A, Simon D, Taïeb A, Werfel T, Oranje A, Gelmetti C, Svensson A, Deleuran M, Calza AM, Giusti F, Lübbe J, Seidenari S, Ring J, European Task Force on Atopic Dermatitis/EADV Eczema Task Force (2010) ETFAD/EADV eczema task force 2009 position paper on diagnosis and treatment of atopic dermatitis. J Eur Acad Dermatol Venereol 24(3):317–328, Epub 2009 Aug 31
20. SIGN: Management of atopic eczema in primary care SIGN guideline 125. http://sign.ac.uk/guidelines/fulltext/125/index.html 2011 accessed 31.1.12
21. Hanifin JM, Cooper KD, Ho VC, Kang S, Krafchik BR, Margolis DJ et al (2004) Guidelines of care for atopic dermatitis, developed in accordance with the American Academy of Dermatology (AAD)/American Academy of Dermatology Association "Administrative Regulations for Evidence-Based Clinical Practice Guidelines". J Am Acad Dermatol 50:391–404
22. Frankel A, Sohn A, Patel RV, Lebwohl M (2011) Bilateral comparison study of pimecrolimus cream 1% and a ceramide-hyaluronic acid emollient foam in the treatment of patients with atopic dermatitis. J Drugs Dermatol 10(6):666–672
23. Grimalt R, Mengeaud V, Cambazard F, Study Investigators' Group (2007) The steroid-sparing effect of an emollient therapy in infants with atopic dermatitis: a randomized controlled study. Dermatology 214(1): 61–67
24. Kantor I, Milbauer J, Psoner M, Weinstock IM, Simon A, Thormahlen S (1993) Efficacy and safety of emollients as adjunctive agents in topical corticosteroid therapy for atopic dermatitis. Today Ther Trends 11: 157–166
25. Hon KL, Wang SS, Lau Z, Lee HC, Lee KK, Leung TF, Luk NM (2011) Pseudoceramide for childhood eczema: does it work? Hong Kong Med J 17(2):132–136
26. Global Resource of EczemA Trials (GREAT database) 2000–2011. www.greatdatabase.org.uk/
27. Beattie PE, Lewis-Jones MS (2004) A pilot study on the use of wet wraps in infants with moderate atopic eczema. Clin Exp Dermatol 29:348–353

28. Fonacier LS, Aquino MR (2010) The role of contact allergy in atopic dermatitis. Immunol Allergy Clin North Am 30(3):337–350
29. Boussault P, Léauté-Labrèze C, Saubusse E, Maurice-Tison S, Perromat M, Roul S et al (2007) Oat sensitization in children with atopic dermatitis: prevalence, risks and associated factors. Allergy 62:1251–1256, Allergy (2008) 63:781–782
30. Kränke B, Komericki P, Aberer W (1997) Olive oil-contact sensitizer or irritant? Contact Dermatitis 36(1): 5–10
31. Tsang M, Guy RH (2010) Effect of Aqueous Cream BP on human stratum corneum in vivo. Br J Dermatol 163(5):954–958
32. Mohammed D, Matts PJ, Hadgraft J, Lane ME (2011) Influence of Aqueous Cream BP on corneocyte size, maturity, skin protease activity, protein content and transepidermal water loss. Br J Dermatol 164(6):1304–1310
33. Wolf G, Höger PH (2009) Hypoallergenic and non-toxic emollient therapies for children. J Dtsch Dermatol Ges 7(1):50–60
34. Lewis-Jones MS, Finlay AY (1995) The children's dermatology life quality index (CDLQI): initial validation and practical use. Br J Dermatol 132:942–949
35. Lawson V, Lewis-Jones MS, Finlay AY, Reid P, Owens RG (1998) The family impact of childhood atopic dermatitis: the dermatitis family impact questionnaire. Br J Dermatol 138:107–113
36. Lewis-Jones MS, Finlay AY, Dykes P (2001) The infants' dermatitis quality of life index (IDQOL). Br J Dermatol 144:104–110
37. Lewis-Jones S (2006) Quality of life and childhood atopic dermatitis: the misery of living with childhood eczema. Int J Clin Pract 60(8):984–992
38. Lewis-Jones MS, Charman CR (2011) Atopic Dermatitis: scoring severity and quality of life assessment. In: Irvine A, Hoeger P, Yan A (eds) Harper's textbook of pediatric dermatology (third Edition) Vol 1 chapter 29 pp 29.9-29.16 Publisher Wiley-Blackwell
39. Reid P, Lewis-Jones MS (1995) Sleep disturbance in preschoolers with atopic eczema. Clin Exp Dermatol 20:38–41
40. Daud LR, Garralda ME, David TJ (1993) Psychosocial adjustment in preschool children with atopic eczema. Arch Dis Child 69(6):670–676
41. Long CC, Funnell CM, Collard R, Finlay AY (1993) What do members of the National Eczema Society really want? Clin Exp Dermatol 18(6):516–522
42. Stores G, Burrows AB, Crawfors C (1998) Physiological sleep disturbance in children with atopic eczema: a case controlled study. Pediatr Dermatol 15:264–268
43. Beattie PE, Lewis-Jones MS (2006) A Comparative study of impairment of Quality of Life (QoL) in children with skin disease and children with other chronic childhood diseases. Br J Dermatol 155:145–151
44. Chamlin SL, Mattson CL, Frieden IJ, Williams ML, Mancini AJ, Cella D, Chren MM (2005) The price of pruritus: sleep disturbance and cosleeping in atopic dermatitis. Arch Pediatr Adolesc Med 159(8): 745–750
45. Paller AS, McAlister RO, Doyle JJ, Jackson A (2002) Perceptions of physicians and pediatric patients about atopic dermatitis, its impact, and its treatment. Clin Pediatr (Phila) 41(5):323–332
46. Aledan M, Gonzales M, Finlay AY (2000) Utility measures for children with skin disease. J Eur Acad Dermato Venereol 14(S1):281 (Abstract)
47. Carvalho NF, Kenney RD, Carrington PH, Hall DE (2001) Severe nutritional deficiencies in toddlers resulting from health food milk alternatives. Pediatrics 107(4):E46
48. Bath-Hextall FJ, Delamere FM, Williams HC. Dietary exclusions for established atopic eczema. Cochrane Database of Systematic Reviews 2008, Issue 1. Art. No.: CD005203. DOI: 10.1002/14651858.CD005203.pub2. Published Online:8 OCT 2008
49. Warschburger P, Buchholz HT, Petermann F (2004) Psychological adjustment in parents of young children with atopic dermatitis: which factors predict parental quality of life? Br J Dermatol 150(2):304–311
50. Titman PS, Barker C, Smith CH (2001) The psychological impact of chronic eczema on children and their families. Br J Dermatol 145(S59):128–129 (Abstract)
51. Faught J, Bierl C, Barton B, Kemp A (2007) Stress in mothers of young children with eczema. Arch Dis Child 92(8):683–686, Epub 2007 Apr 5
52. Absolon C, Cottrell D, Eldridge S, Glover M (1997) Psychological disturbance in atopic eczema: the extent of the problem in school aged children. Br J Dermatol 137:241–245
53. Sarkar R, Raj L, Kaur H, Basu S, Kanwar AJ, Jain RK (2004) Psychological disturbances in Indian children with atopic eczema. J Dermatol 31(6):448–454
54. Schmitt J, Romanos M, Pfennig A, Leopold K, Meurer M (2009) Psychiatric comorbidity in adult eczema. Br J Dermatol 161(4):878–883, Epub 2009 Jul 14
55. Chamlin SL, Cella D, Frieden IJ, Williams ML, Mancini AJ, Lai JS, Chren MM (2005) Development of the Childhood Atopic Dermatitis Impact Scale: initial validation of a quality-of-life measure for young children with atopic dermatitis and their families. J Invest Dermatol 125(6):1106–1111
56. Su J, Kemp A, Varigos G, Nolan T (1997) Atopic eczema: its impact on the family and financial cost. Arch Dis Child 76(2):159–162
57. Lapidus CS, Kerr PE (2001) Social impact of atopic dermatitis. Med Health R I 84(9):294–295
58. Balkrishnan R, Housman T, Carroll C, Feldman S, Fleischer A (2003) Disease severity and associated family impact in childhood atopic dermatitis. Arch Dis Child 88(5):423–427
59. Carroll CL, Balkrishnan R, Feldman SR, Fleischer AB Jr, Manuel JC (2005) The burden of atopic dermatitis: impact on the patient, family, and society. Pediatr Dermatol 22(3):192–199

60. Emerson R, Williams HC, Allen BR (2001) What is the cost of atopic dermatitis in preschool children? Br J Dermatol 144:514–522
61. Herd RM, Tidman MJ, Prescott RJ, Hunter JA (1996) The cost of atopic eczema. Br J Dermatol 135(1):20–23
62. Schuttelaar ML, Vermeulen KM, Coenraads PJ (2011) Costs and cost-effectiveness analysis of treatment in children with eczema by nurse practitioner vs. dermatologist: results of a randomized, controlled trial and a review of international costs. Br J Dermatol 165(3): 600–611
63. Zuberbier T, Orlow SJ, Paller AS, Taïeb A, Allen R, Hernanz-Hermosa JM, Ocampo-Candiani J, Cox M, Langeraar J, Simon JC (2006) Patient perspectives on the management of atopic dermatitis. J Allergy Clin Immunol 118(1):226–232
64. Collier J, MacKinlay D, Phillips D (2000) Norm values for the Generic Children's Quality of Life Measure (GCQ) from a large school-based sample. Qual Life Res 9(6):617–623
65. Eiser C, Morse R (2001) Can parents rate their child's health-related quality of life? Results of a systematic review. Qual Life Res 10(4):347–357
66. Ben-Gashir MA, Seed PT, Hay RJ (2004) Quality of life and disease severity are correlated in children with atopic dermatitis. Br J Dermatol 150(2):284–290
67. Kupfer J, Gieler U, Diepgen TL, Fartasch M, Lob-Corzilius T, Ring J, Scheewe S, Scheidt R, Schnopp C, Szczepanski R, Staab D, Werfel T, Wittenmeier M, Wahn U, Schmid-Ott G (2010) Structured education program improves the coping with atopic dermatitis in children and their parents-a multicenter, randomized controlled trial. J Psychosom Res 68(4): 353–358
68. Emerson RM, Williams HC, Allen BR (1997) How much disability does childhood atopic eczema cause compared to other childhood problems. Br J Dermatol 137:19 (Abstract)
69. McKenna SP, Whalley D, Dewar AL, Erdman RA, Kohlmann T, Niero M, Baró E, Cook SA, Crickx B, Frech F, van Assche D (2005) International development of the Parents' Index of Quality of Life in Atopic Dermatitis (PIQoL-AD). Qual Life Res 14(1):231–241
70. Holme SA, Man I, Sharpe JL, Dykes PJ, Lewis-Jones MS, Finlay AY (2003) The Children's Dermatology Life Quality Index: validation of the cartoon version. Br J Dermatol 148(2):285–290
71. Beattie PE, Lewis-Jones MS (2006) An audit of the impact of a consultation with a paediatric dermatology team on quality of life in infants with atopic eczema and their families: further validation of the Infants' Dermatitis Quality of Life Index and Dermatitis Family Impact score. Br J Dermatol 155(6): 1249–1255
72. Ben-Gashir MA, Seed PT, Hay RJ (2002) Are quality of family life and disease severity related in childhood atopic dermatitis? J Eur Acad Dermatol Venereol 16(5): 455–462
73. Aziah MS, Rosnah T, Mardziah A, Norzila MZ (2002) Childhood atopic dermatitis: a measurement of quality of life and family impact. Med J Malaysia 57(3):329–339
74. Chamlin SL, Lai JS, Cella D, Frieden IJ, Williams ML, Mancini AJ, Chren MM (2007) Childhood Atopic Dermatitis Impact Scale: reliability, discriminative and concurrent validity, and responsiveness. Arch Dermatol 143(6):768–772
75. Lundberg L, Johannesson M, Silverdahl M, Hermansson C, Lindberg M (1999) Quality of life, health-state utilities and willingness to pay in patients with psoriasis and atopic eczema. Br J Dermatol 141(6):1067–1075
76. Krejci-Manwaring J, Tusa MG, Carroll C, Camacho F, Kaur M, Carr D, Fleischer AB Jr, Balkrishnan R, Feldman SR (2007) Stealth monitoring of adherence to topical medication: adherence is very poor in children with atopic dermatitis. J Am Acad Dermatol 56(2):211–216, Epub 2006 Nov 13
77. Bradley C (1999) Compliance with drug therapy. Prescribers J 39(1):44–50
78. Serup J, Lindblad AK, Maroti M, Kjellgren KI, Niklasson E, Ring L, Ahlner J (2006) To follow or not to follow dermatological treatment – a review of the literature. Acta Derm Venereol 86(3):193–197
79. Zaghloul S, Goodfield M (2004) Objective assessment of compliance with psoriasis treatment. Arch Dermatol 140:408–414
80. Zaghloul S, Cunliffe W, Goodfield M (2005) Objective assessment of compliance with treatments in acne. Br J Dermatol 152(5):1015–1021
81. Carroll CL, Feldman SR, Camacho FT, Manuel JC, Balkrishnan R (2004) Adherence to topical therapy decreases during the course of an 8-week psoriasis clinical trial: commonly used methods of measuring adherence to topical therapy overestimate actual use. J Am Acad Dermatol 51(2):212–216
82. Feldman SR, Camacho FT, Krejci-Manwaring J, Carroll CL, Balkrishnan R (2007) Adherence to topical therapy increases around the time of office visits. J Am Acad Dermatol 57(1):81–83, Epub 2007 May 10
83. Beattie PE, Lewis-Jones MS (2003) Parental Knowledge of topical therapies used in the treatment of atopic dermatitis. Clin Exp Dermatol 28:549–553
84. Ickovics JR (2002) Consequences and determinants of adherence to antiretroviral medication. Antivir Ther 7(3):185–193
85. Charman C, Williams H (2003) The use of corticosteroids and corticosteroid phobia in atopic dermatitis. Clin Dermatol 21(3):193–200
86. Long C, Finlay AY (1993) Perceived under prescription of topical therapy. Br J Gen Pract 43:305
87. Santer M, Lewis-Jones S, Fahey T (2006) Appropriateness of prescribing for childhood eczema: evidence form a community-based study. Clin Exp Dermatol 31:671–673
88. Vaughan V (1966) Emotional undertones in eczema in children. J Asthma Res 3:193

89. Halm EA et al (2006) No symptoms, no asthma: the acute episodic disease belief is associated with poor self-management among inner-city adults with persistent asthma. Chest 129:573–580
90. Ohya Y, Williams H, Steptoe A, Saito H, Iikura Y, Anderson R, Akasawa A (2001) Psychosocial factors and adherence to treatment advice in childhood atopic dermatitis. J Invest Dermatol 117(4):852–857
91. Renzi C et al (2001) Factors associated with patient satisfaction with care among dermatological outpatients. Br J Dermatol 145(4):617–623
92. Kjellgren KI, Ring L, Lindblad AK, Maroti M, Serup J (2004) To follow dermatological treatment regimens-patients' and providers' views. Acta Derm Venereol 84(6):445–450
93. Broberg A, Kalimo K, Lindblad B, Swanbeck G (1990) Parental education in the treatment of childhood atopic eczema. Acta Derm Venereol 70(6):495–499
94. Cork MJ, Britton J, Butler L, Young S, Murphy R, Keohane SG (2003) Comparison of parent knowledge, therapy utilization and severity of atopic eczema before and after explanation and demonstration of topical therapies by a specialist dermatology nurse. Br J Dermatol 149(3):582–589
95. Gradwell C, Thomas KS, English JS, Williams HC (2002) A randomized controlled trial of nurse follow-up clinics: do they help patients and do they free up consultants' time? Br J Dermatol 147(3): 513–517
96. Moore EJ, Williams A, Manias E, Varigos G, Donath S (2009) Eczema workshops reduce severity of childhood atopic eczema. Australas J Dermatol 50(2): 100–106
97. Staab D et al (2006) Age related, structured educational programmes for the management of atopic dermatitis in children and adolescents: multicentre, randomised controlled trial. BMJ 332(7547):933–938
98. Stalder JF, Bernier C, Ball A, De Raeve L, Gieler U, Deleuran M, Marcoux D, Eichenfield L, Lio P, Lewis-Jones S, Gelmetti C, Takaoka R, Chiaverini C, Misery L, Barbarot S, for the Oriented Patient-Education Network in Dermatology (OPENED) (2011) Therapeutic patient education on atopic dermatitis: worldwide experiences. Br J Dermatol http://opened-dermatology.com/ (accessed 31.1.12)
99. Ersser SJ, Latter S, Sibley A, Satherley PA, Welbourne S. Psychological and educational interventions for atopic eczema in children. Cochrane Database of Systematic Reviews 2007, Issue 3. Art. No.:CD004054. DOI: 10.1002/14651858.CD004054.pub2. Published Online: 21 JAN 2009

Use of Moisturizers in Patients with Atopic Dermatitis

5

Kam Lun Ellis Hon and Alexander K.C. Leung

5.1 Atopic Dermatitis: An Overview

Atopic (Greek *atopos*, meaning "strange" or "unusual") dermatitis (AD) is a chronically relapsing dermatosis characterized by pruritus, erythema, vesiculation, papulation, exudation, excoriation, crusting, scaling, and sometimes lichenification [1–5]. Atopic eczema (Greek *ekzema*, meaning "erupt" or "boil over") is synonymous with atopic dermatitis. The prevalence of atopic dermatitis has increased two- to threefolds over the past three decades in industrialized countries, and there is evidence to suggest that this prevalence is continuing to increase [1, 3, 6–8]. The increase in prevalence may be due to increased access to medical care, improved recognition, better epidemiological reporting, or increased environmental allergens due to industrialization and pollution. AD affects 10–20% of children and 1–3% of adults in the United States [3, 9–12]. AD occurs more frequently in temperate rather than tropical areas [13] and is more prevalent in children that belong to advantaged socioeconomic classes, smaller family sizes, and families with overzealous hygiene [14]. Approximately 30–50% of children with one affected parent and 50–80% with two affected parents develop the disorder [15]. In terms of disease burden, it is the most common chronic skin disease in new referrals and requires the most frequent follow-ups [16]. Secondary bacterial infection, most commonly with *Staphylococcus aureus*, is the main complication of atopic dermatitis [3, 17]. Purulent oozing, honey-color crusting, folliculitis, and pyoderma indicate secondary infection with *S. aureus*. The anterior nares are an important reservoir of *S. aureus* [17].

AD is uncomfortable and distressing to patients because of the associated pruritus and unsightly lesions [13]. Children with AD may suffer from lack of sleep, irritability, daytime tiredness, emotional stress, lowered self-esteem, and psychological disturbance [18, 19]. The disruption of school, family, and social interactions can severely impair the quality of life and extends beyond the child [18, 20–22]. Parents may experience guilt, frustration, resentment, exhaustion, and helplessness due to their child's condition [8]. There are also considerable economic costs associated with caring for children with AD [8].

AD most often presents in infancy or early childhood [2, 3]. Approximately 60% of children

K.L.E. Hon, M.B.B.S., M.D., FAAP, FCCM (✉)
Department of Pediatrics, The Chinese University of Hong Kong, Prince of Wales Hospital, Shatin, Hong Kong
e-mail: ehon@hotmail.com

A.K.C. Leung, M.B.B.S., FRCPC, FRCP(UK & Irel), FRCPCH, FAAP
Department of Pediatrics, The University of Calgary, Alberta Children's Hospital, Calgary, Alberta, Canada
e-mail: aleung@ucalgary.ca

M. Lodén, H.I. Maibach (eds.), *Treatment of Dry Skin Syndrome*,
DOI 10.1007/978-3-642-27606-4_5, © Springer-Verlag Berlin Heidelberg 2012

with AD manifest the disease by the first year of life and an additional 30% before the age of 5 years [1, 2, 23]. In infants, the eruption often affects the face and scalp, although the extensor surfaces of the extremities and the trunk may also be affected [2, 24]. In older children and adolescents, the neck and antecubital and popliteal fossae usually display the eruption [2, 24].

Lesions are classified as acute, subacute, or chronic and are usually symmetrical [25]. Acute lesions are intensely pruritic, erythematous papules, papulovesicles, or weeping lesions [25]. Subacute lesions are erythematous scaling papules or plaques [1]. Chronic lesions are characterized by prominent scaling, excoriations, and lichenification in affected body areas [1]. Exacerbations and remissions are common and to be expected [1].

The diagnosis of AD is predominantly clinical, based on a constellation of clinical features. Firm criteria to define atopic dermatitis were first established by Hanifin and Rajka [3, 26].

AD involves defective cell-mediated immunity related, in part, to an imbalance in two subsets of CD4 T cells that creates a predominance of T-memory cells in the T-helper 2 pathways and preferential apoptosis of interferon-gamma-producing T-helper 1 memory and effector T cells [2, 27, 28]. T-helper 2 cells express a set of cytokines (interleukin-4, -5, -6, -10, and -13) [27, 29]. These cytokines stimulate the proliferation and differentiation of B lymphocytes, upregulate the expression of adhesion molecules on endothelial cells, and contribute to the hypereosinophilia, high serum IgE levels, sustained cutaneous inflammation, histamine release, and pruritus characteristic of AD [13].

5.2 The Pathogenesis of Dry Skin

Xerosis or dry skin results from reduced amount of ceramides in the skin with enhanced transepidermal water loss. It is seen in 67–98% of patients with AD [30]. Xerosis predisposes to the development of microfissures and cracks in the epithelium which favor the entry of allergens and microorganisms [11].

The pathogenesis of AD involves complex interactions between susceptible genes, immunological factors, skin barrier defects, infections, neuroendocrine factors, and environmental factors [3]. There is a strong genetic predisposition, as evidenced by the familial nature of the disease and the high concordance in monozygotic twins [3, 31]. It has been shown that loss-of-function mutations in the filaggrin (*FLG*) gene predispose to AD [32–34]. Five *FLG* null mutations, namely, R501X, 2282del4, R2447X, S2554X, and S2889X, are some of the more popular mutations identified in Caucasian and Japanese populations [35].

Impairment of the barrier function of the skin is an important etiologic factor in the pathogenesis of AD [3]. FLG, an epidermal barrier protein, plays an important role in the barrier function of the skin [36]. FLG protein is present in the granular layers of the epidermis, and the keratohyalin granules in the granular layers are predominantly composed of profilaggrin [37]. FLG proteins aggregate the keratin cytoskeleton system to form a dense protein–lipid matrix that is cross-linked by transglutaminases to form a cornified cell envelope [36, 37]. The latter prevents epidermal water loss and impedes the entry of allergens, infectious agents, and chemicals [36]. It is believed that defective epidermal function is related to the downregulation of the *FLG* gene and reduced ceramide levels [38].

A reduced content of ceramides has been noted in both normal and affected skin of patients with AD [39]. The reduction in ceramides may result from increased sphingomyelin deacylase activity and reduced production of ceramides by keratinocytes [27]. Ceramides serve as important water-holding molecules in the extracellular space in the horny layer [7]. A deficiency in ceramides results in enhanced transepidermal water loss, dry skin, and increased permeability to environmental irritants and allergens [27]. In addition, keratinocyte-derived antimicrobial peptides known as cathelicidins and β-defensins are deficient in the skin of patients with AD [40]. These peptides help in the host defense against bacteria, viruses, and fungi.

5.3 Assessment of Severity of Atopic Dermatitis and Psychosocial Impact

Physicians in their busy clinics often claim to be able to take a glance at the patients and be able to determine the disease severity by their experience. This is neither objective nor evidence based. There are many scoring systems and indices for the assessment of disease severity in children with AD. However, many of these scales have not been adequately tested [41]. These scores are often used to objectively evaluate therapeutic efficacy of both topical and systemic treatments. The SCORing Atopic Dermatitis (SCORAD) system is a comprehensive index utilized extensively in Europe as a research tool for the assessment of AD severity. It is the only severity index for which published data could be found on validity, reliability, sensitivity, and acceptability, although problems occur with interobserver variation [41]. SCORAD consists of observations of signs and the assessment of symptoms and takes approximately 10 min to perform by trained physicians who recognize the various components of this score. The SCORAD (score range, 0–103) measures the extent, intensity, pruritus, and sleep loss over the preceding 3 days [42]. It uses a body diagram to record the extent and area of involvement. It also records the intensity of six signs, namely, erythema/darkening, edema/papulation, oozing/crust, excoriation, lichenification/prurigo, and dryness. It is a weighted index, with less weight on the extent (by multiplying a factor of 0.2) but more emphasis on symptomatology of pruritus and sleep loss (by multiplying a factor of 1), and the intensity (by multiplying a factor of 3.5) [42]. The SCORAD is weighted toward pediatric populations and is a rather complex tool not regularly used by the general practitioners. Although not the gold standard, SCORAD has been validated and widely quoted as a reliable research and clinical tool for the assessment of AD severity [42]. Scratching and sleep disturbance are subjective symptoms that are difficult to study. Some scoring systems, therefore, have bypassed the assessment of sleep loss and pruritus and adopt a more objective approach. Kunz and coworkers, for instance, suggested that a modified SCORAD index (without the pruritus and sleep-loss components) is more objective and accurate in defining the disease severity of AD [43].

The Nottingham Eczema Severity Score (NESS) is a three-part score developed for population-based research in the United Kingdom and has the advantage of being very easy to perform [44, 45]. It is a less comprehensive scoring system and only gives a final grading of the severity of AD as being mild, moderate, or severe. There are good agreement and correlation among the NESS scores, severity grades, and the SCORAD scale [45, 46]. The self-administered questionnaire measures disease severity over a 12-month period. The disease severity is determined by evaluating three elements, namely, clinical course, disease intensity, and extent of the examined lesion. Equal weighting is applied to the three parameters; each carries a score of 1–5. A final score is achieved by adding each score to produce a possible range of scores from 3 to 15, with higher scores indicating more severe disease [44]. The NESS is simple and quick to use.

The eczema and severity index (EASI) incorporates body surface area involvement into the measurement. The index assigns proportionate values to four body regions, namely, head (10%), trunk (30%), upper limbs (20%), and lower limbs (40%) in patients 8 years and older, and is slightly modified for younger patients [47, 48]. The six signs of AD, namely, erythema, edema/induration/papulation, excoriation, oozing/weeping/crusting, scaling, and lichenification, are graded on a 4-point scale, ranging from absent (0) to severe [3]. The EASI score ranges from 0 (clear) to 72 (very severe).

Scratching lacks objectivity and is difficult to study. Limb-worn digital accelerometers have been shown to be a useful and practical way of assessing nocturnal scratching in the patient's own home [49, 50]. It has been shown that nocturnal wrist activities measured with DigiTrac® wrist motion monitor (IM Systems, Baltimore, MD, USA) were closely correlated with the objective clinical scores and serum levels of chemokine markers [50]. Sleep efficiency is also reduced in patients with AD and can be objectively demonstrated [51].

In recent years, skin hydration and transepidermal water loss (TEWL) have been objectively measured in various sites including the antecubital fossae, forearm, face, abdomen, and the leg [52–59]. The biophysical properties of skin have been extensively studied in patients with AD. Lodén et al. characterized the biophysical properties of noneczematous skin at three locations in atopics and nonatopics using noninvasive physical methods [60]. Skin friction was measured with a sliding friction instrument, the degree of hydration was measured with a capacitance meter (Corneometer CM 820), and the TEWL was determined using an Evaporimeter model EP1 (Servomed Inc., Stockholm, Sweden). The areas examined (dorsum of the hand, volar forearm, and lower back) showed lower values of friction and capacitance in the atopic patients than did corresponding sites in the normal controls. The TEWL was increased in atopic skin, but TEWL seemed to correlate neither to friction nor to capacitance [60]. Sakurai et al. studied normal-appearing skin in patients with active AD and suggested that an impaired barrier function often seen in normal-appearing skin in AD patients was secondary to subclinical eczematous change in the area [61]. Nevertheless, skin barrier function is not disturbed in patients with completely healed AD [62]. The study of these epidermal biophysical parameters not only helps throw lights on the understanding of the pathophysiology of AD but also allows investigators to gauge the therapeutic efficacy of various topical and systemic treatment modalities.

There is no unified opinion as to which of these sites should be standardized for evaluation. Among the sites evaluated, the antecubital flexural area has often been suggested to show the most consistent correlations with disease severity. However, the flexural surface is angulated, uneven and not ideal for measurement in children. Hon et al. demonstrated that standardized measurements of skin hydration and TEWL can be made at the right antecubital fossa [63]. These measurements are useful for clinical trials especially involving topical treatment. Indeed, Hon et al. proposed a holistic evaluation approach to study the efficacy of any treatment to include severity scores, quality of life assessment, biophysiological measurements (skin hydration, TEWL, scratching activities), surrogate seromarkers, and amounts of concomitant topical and systemic medications [63–65].

A number of indices have been designed to measure the impact of the disease on the quality of life of affected children and the parents. Although some studies have shown a positive correlation between children's and parents' quality of life and disease severity on cross-sectional and over-time observation [22, 66], there is not necessarily a direct relation between the severity of atopic dermatitis and its impact on quality of life [67]. The quality of life measurement provides additional information to the objective clinical scoring systems [66]. The Children's Dermatology Life Quality Index (CDLQ1) for patients 3–16 years of age is a self-administered validated simple tool to measure the impact of a skin condition on the quality of life over the past 7 days [66]. The index covers 16 areas including effects on emotions, social development, sleep disturbance, schooling, hobbies, and treatment issues [68]. The score range is 0–30; a high score indicates diminished life quality [66]. The refined version of Childhood Atopic Dermatitis Scale (CADIS) consists of a five-scale framework, namely, family and social function scale, emotion scale, sleep scale, symptom scale, and activity limitations and behavior scale [69]. It has 45 items and a score ranging from 0 to 180. The CADIS which assesses the impact of AD on both the child and the parent in the same measure has been developed to assess outcome in clinical studies [70].

The Parents' Index of Quality of Life in Atopic Dermatitis (PIQoL-AD) is a quality of life instrument specific to parents of children with atopic dermatitis [71, 72]. It has 28 items, covering a range of parental needs that can be influenced by a child with AD, such as need for rest and relaxation, need for self-respect, need for independence, and need for personal space and time [71].

This scale is particularly useful in those studies in which study participants are too young to provide information about their quality of life [70]. Suffice to say, the scoring systems for assessment of disease severity and psychosocial impact have often been used to assess outcomes in clinical trials [73, 74]. They are rarely used in clinical practice.

5.4 Optimal Skin Care: Moisturizers and Emollients for Atopic Dermatitis

AD is frustrating to both patients and caregivers. The pruritus can be intractable, and the disease has important physical and psychological implications. Because of associated emotional stress and sleep disruption, the impact on the quality of life of patients and families can be significant [3, 19, 64]. Successful treatment requires a holistic approach that consists of avoidance of triggering factors, optimal skin care, pharmacotherapy during acute exacerbations, and education and of patients/caregivers [3]. Although there is no cure, control is possible in most patients with optimal skin care, pharmacotherapy, and adherence to preventive measures [65, 75]. Pharmacotherapy usually consists of topical application of corticosteroids or calcineurin inhibitors [3]. In a subgroup of children with severe AD, the disease is recalcitrant to conservative and topical therapy alone. These children may require systemic treatments such as oral antihistamines, antibiotics, leukotriene receptor antagonists, and systemic immunosuppressants [3]. Emotional stress often exacerbates the skin lesions of AD. If avoidance is not possible, coping mechanisms should be tried [2, 3].

Dry skin is more prone to itch and chapping and hence secondary infection and subsequent perpetuation of AD. Hydration of the skin increases drug penetration as hydration causes swelling of the stratum corneum rendering it more permeable to drug molecules. The key to management of AD and dry skin conditions, especially in-between episodes of flare-ups, is the frequent use of an appropriate moisturizer [1]. Hydration of the skin helps to improve the dryness, reduce the pruritus, and restore the disturbed skin's barrier function and is of paramount importance both in the prevention and management of patients with AD [3, 38]. In the brick-and-mortar hypothesis, the stratum corneum, the outermost layer of the epidermis, normally consists of fully differentiated corneocytes surrounded by a lipid-rich matrix containing cholesterol, free fatty acids, and ceramide; the structure of this matrix closely resembles that of bricks and mortar in a wall. In AD, lipid metabolism is abnormal, causing a deficiency of ceramide that leads to transepidermal water loss [5, 76, 77]. The underlying genetic deficit might be due to null mutation in the filaggrin gene [34].

Hydration of the skin can be achieved by daily baths in lukewarm (not hot) water for approximately 5–10 min, followed by patting the body dry with a towel [1, 3]. Fragrance-free soap and cleansers are preferred [3]. The use of shampoo, bubble bath, and dishwater detergent to cleanse the body should be avoided [3]. Rubbing should also be avoided as such maneuver may precipitate the sensation of pruritus.

Regular topical application of a moisturizer is key in the management of patients with AD. A moisturizer or emollient should be applied within 3 min to prevent evaporation and keep the skin soft and flexible, which helps to prevent the penetration by bacteria, irritants, and allergens [1, 3, 78]. This "soak and seal" method helps to improve the integrity of the skin barrier and prevents the penetration by bacteria, irritants, and allergens. Bathing without the use of moisturizer may compromise skin hydration [79].

The use of moisturizers helps the skin maintain a defensive barrier effect, which is defective in AD [80]. Moisturizers can be in the form of creams, emollients, lotions, or ointments [81–83]. Creams are semisolid emulsions (mixtures of oil and water). Creams are either water-miscible and readily washed off, or oily and not so easily washed off. They are divided into two types: oil-in-water creams which are composed of small droplets of oil dispersed in a continuous phase, and water-in-oil creams which are composed of small droplets of water dispersed in a continuous oily phase. Oil-in-water creams are more comfortable and cosmetically acceptable as they are less greasy and more easily washed off using water. Water-in-oil creams are more difficult to handle, but many drugs which are incorporated into creams are hydrophobic and will be released more readily from a water-in-oil cream than an oil-in-water cream. Water-in-oil creams are also more moisturizing as they provide an oily barrier which reduces water loss from the stratum corneum. Barrier creams often contain water-repellent substances such as dimethicone or other silicones that protect against irritation or repeated hydration. They are useful in the treatment of napkin rash and bedsores. They are the preferred forms of treatment for exudative dermatoses. Creams are often massaged on the affected area twice daily in patients with AD and xerosis. They can be used with other topical agents such as corticosteroids to enhance penetration. Creams contain water and are liable to fungal and bacterial contaminations, and therefore, preservatives are usually added. Commonly used preservatives in creams are chlorocresol and hydroxybenzoates; both of which may cause skin allergy.

Emollients are fats or oils in a two-phase system (one liquid is dispersed in the form of small droplets throughout another liquid). Emollients soften the skin by forming an occlusive oil film on the stratum corneum, preventing drying by evaporation from the deeper layers of skin and rendering it more pliable in dry eczema, ichthyosis, and psoriasis. Emollients minimize dryness and are the mainstay in treating mild AD. There is a wide range of emollients with different greasiness available, and it is important to find the one that the patient is most willing to use. The rule is to use emollients thinly and frequently, and not thickly and occasionally. It is believed that regular and frequent use of emollients can reduce 10–20% of the amount of topical steroid used in the treatment of AD. Some emollients contain lanolin that may sensitize skin.

Lotions are aqueous solutions or suspensions that cool diffusely inflamed unbroken skin by evaporation. They should be applied frequently. Lotions are also used to apply drugs to the skin when only a thin layer of the preparation is intended to apply over a large surface area.

Ointments are semisolid substances that are greasy, normally anhydrous, and insoluble in water. The most commonly used ointment bases consist of soft paraffin or a combination of soft paraffin with liquid paraffin and hard paraffin. Due to their anhydrous nature, ointments do not require any preservatives. They have the advantages of being more moisturizing, more occlusive than creams and form a protective film over the skin. Because of their marked occlusive effect, ointments are not suitable for acute weeping, crusting skin conditions, particularly in the intertriginous areas. Today, there are ointments that possess both hydrophilic and lipophilic proprieties so that they become water-soluble and can be washed off readily. Ointments are very useful particularly for chronic dry skin.

A number of topical preparations are available in the market. The actual ingredients in most of these products are a commercial secret of individual pharmaceutical companies. However, the active ingredients are quoted in the packaging. These products include Ego Skin cream, Keri lotion, Lactacyd, Lacticare, QV cream, QV skin lotion, Sebamed, Urederm, Urecare, Cetaphil, Glaxal base, and many more. The commonly used and inexpensive moisturizers include aqueous cream, emulsifying ointment, and urea cream. Aqueous cream BP contains emulsifying wax (9%), white soft paraffin (15%), liquid paraffin (6%), phenoxyethanol (1%), and purified water to make up to 100%. It is an oil-in-water emulsion with phenoxyethanol as the preservative. Emulsifying ointment BP contains white soft paraffin (50%), emulsifying wax (30%), and liquid paraffin (20%). Urederm (urea cream 10%) contains 10% by weight of urea with carbomer 934, paraffin (light liquid), glycerol, cetostearyl alcohol, mixed parabens, white soft paraffin, cetomacrogol, triethanolamine, and purified water. In general, ointments are most effective but messy; creams are often better tolerated. The type of moisturizer or emollient should be tailored to the individual skin conditions as well as the child's needs and preferences [15, 67].

AD is associated with dry skin, and skin hydration correlates with disease severity. It is thus sensible to encourage patients to use moisturizers regularly [9, 75]. The skin condition may improve significantly with the liberal use of moisturizers such that the use of topical corticosteroids or calcineurin inhibitors could be minimized. Patients should be given practical advice in their daily skin care. In areas rich with sebaceous glands such as the face, formulations should contain less oil than on other body areas [15]. Lotions, which have a high water and low oil content, can worsen xerosis via evaporation and should therefore be avoided. A dye-free, fragrance-free moisturizer should be used [38]. Frequent applications of moisturizers throughout the day help to maintain a high level of hydration in the stratum corneum [3]. Moisturizers containing urea, alpha-hydroxy acids, glycyrrhetinic acids, hyaluronic acids or, ceramides have been shown to improve the integrity of stratum corneum [76, 78, 84–86]. Moisturizers should always be used, even when the skin is clear of active lesions, recognizing that normal-appearing skin in patients with AD may not be immunologically normal [67].

Proper moisturizer therapy can reduce the frequency of flares and reduce the demand of topical corticosteroids or topical calcineurin inhibitors [12, 87–90]. In an open, randomized, prospective, parallel group study, Lodén et al. compared the time to relapse of AD during treatment with a barrier-strengthening moisture (5% urea) with no treatment (no medical or non-medicated preparations) in 53 patients with successfully treated AD affecting the hands [87]. The median time to relapse was 20 days in the moisturizer group compared with 2 days in the no treatment group ($p = 0.04$). In addition, Lodén et al. conducted a parallel, double-blind, randomized, clinical trial on 44 patients with a recent relapse of AD affecting the hands [88]. In this study, twice daily application of a strong corticosteroid cream (betamethasone valerate 0.1%) was compared with once daily application, where a urea-containing moisturizer was substituted for the corticosteroid cream in the morning. The investigator scored the presence of AD, and the patients judged the health-related quality of life (HRQoL) using the Dermatology Life Quality Index (DLQI), which measures how much the patient's skin problem has affected his/her life over the past week. The patients also judged the severity of AD daily on a visual analogue scale. The authors found that both groups improved in terms of AD and DLQI. However, the clinical scoring demonstrated that once daily application of corticosteroid and a urea-containing moisturizer was superior to twice daily application of corticosteroid in diminishing AD, especially in the group of patients with lower AD scores at inclusion. Frankel et al. evaluated the short-term effectiveness and appeal of a ceramide-hyaluronic acid emollient foam as compared to pimecrolimus cream 1% in the treatment of AD within a wide age group of subjects with active AD at baseline [89]. In this study, both pimecrolimus cream and the ceramide-hyaluronic acid emollient foam exhibited efficacy in mild-to-moderate AD. Primary efficacy was measured by Investigator's Global Assessment. After 4 weeks of treatment with the ceramide-hyaluronic acid emollient foam, 82% of target lesions were scored clear or almost clear compared to 71% of target lesions under the pimecrolimus arm. The authors concluded that ceramide-hyaluronic acid emollient foam and pimecrolimus cream 1% work well in the treatment of AD in both children and adults with no associated adverse effects.

5.5 Measurement of Efficacy of Moisturizer Therapy

A number of studies have been done to demonstrate how the efficacy of moisturizer therapy can be objectively measured. Chamlin et al. assessed the efficacy of a newly developed, ceramide-dominant, physiologic lipid-based emollient, when substituted for currently used moisturizers, in 24 children who were also receiving standard therapy for stubborn-to-recalcitrant AD [76]. All subjects continued prior therapy (e.g., topical tacrolimus or corticosteroids), only substituting the barrier repair emollient for their prior moisturizer. Follow-up evaluations, which included SCORAD values and several biophysical measures of stratum corneum function, were performed every 3 weeks for 20–21 weeks. SCORAD values improved significantly in 22 of 24 patients by 3 weeks, with further progressive improvement in all patients between 6 and 20 or 21 weeks. TEWLs, which were elevated over involved and uninvolved areas at entry, decreased in parallel with SCORAD scores and continued to decline even after SCORAD scores plateaued. Both stratum corneum integrity (cohesion) and hydration also improved slowly but significantly during therapy. Finally, the ultrastructure of the stratum corneum, treated with ceramide-dominant emollient, revealed extracellular lamellar membranes, which were largely absent in baseline stratum corneum samples. The authors concluded that a ceramide-dominant, barrier repair emollient represents a safe, useful adjunct to the treatment of childhood AD, and TEWL is at least as sensitive an indicator of fluctuations in AD disease activity as are SCORAD values. The study supports the outside-inside hypothesis as a component of pathogenesis in AD and other inflammatory dermatoses that are accompanied by a barrier abnormality. In this study, no quality of life or global assessment of acceptability of treatment was documented.

Son et al. demonstrated that the regular application of a moisturizer for 2 weeks would improve SCORAD, skin hydration, TEWL, and other cutaneous parameters [59]. The authors rightly addressed the problem that wide variation in outcome methodology could make the interpretation of patient outcomes confusing and the comparison of the results of different studies almost impossible, and that it was important to objectively measure and record the severity of AD for routine clinical practice and research. The authors evaluated whether morphological study of skin surface contours might be helpful to objectively quantify the severity of AD. Thirty patients with AD (12 females, 18 males) participated in this study. Moisturizer was applied twice daily for 2 weeks. Bioengineering methods such as D-Squame, corneometer, evaporimeter, and spectrophotometer were measured at the start of the study and after 1 and 2 weeks. In addition, the authors assessed moisturizer effects after 3 h of moisturizer application. The stereoimage optical topometer based on a new concept of stereoimage was applied for this study. The authors compared stereoimage optical topometer, other bioengineering methods, and the SCORAD index. After 3 h of application with moisturizer, the results measured by stereoimage optical topometer, conventional optical profilometer, D-Squame, and corneometer showed significant differences ($p<0.05$). After 1 and 2 weeks, there were significant changes in the results measured by stereoimage optical topometer, conventional optical profilometer, D-Squame, corneometer, spectrophotometer, and SCORAD index. The authors observed a significant correlation between bioengineering methods and the SCORAD index ($p<0.05$) and concluded that morphological study of skin surface contours is useful in the evaluation of AD severity. They further suggested that a combination of methods to evaluate the physiologic changes and those such as stereoimage optical topometer to measure the morphological changes of skin surface could evaluate more objectively and quantitatively the severity of AD. In this study, however, quality of life, patient global acceptability of treatment, quality and quantity of the moisturizer used were not assessed.

Rosmarinic acid (α-*o*-caffeoyl-3,4-dihydroxyphenyl lactic acid), a naturally occurring hydroxylated compound, is known to have anti-inflammatory and immunomodulatory activities [91]. A double-blind, vehicle-controlled, randomized trial was performed to evaluate the clinical effects of a cream containing 0.3% rosmarinic acid on patients with AD over an 8-week period [91]. Rosmarinic acid (0.3%) cream was topically applied to the elbow flexures of 21 patients (14 females and 7 males, aged 5–28 years) twice a day. Cream without 0.3% rosmarinic acid was applied to the elbow flexures of control subjects twice a day. The mean SCORAD index decreased from 7.37 ± 0.32 before treatment to 3.27 ± 0.21 after treatment with rosmarinic acid-containing cream for 8 weeks ($p<0.05$). However, in the control group, no significant change of SCORAD score was observed. Transepidermal water loss of the antecubital fossa was significantly reduced at 8 weeks compared to before treatment ($p<0.05$). In this study, the outcome measures only included SCORAD and TEWL with a very small number of patients. No assessment of quality of life or global acceptability of treatment was documented.

EpiCeram consists of a specific combination of ceramides, cholesterol, and fatty acids (in the ratio of 3:1:1) that mimics those naturally found in the skin [92, 93]. Recent studies have shown that EpiCeram has similar efficacy compared to a mid-potency topical corticosteroid but has a favorable safety profile [92, 93]. However, these studies did not report objective measurements to demonstrate efficacy of treatment.

Atopiclair, also known as MAS063DP or Zarzenda, a hydrolipidic cream, has been found effective in the treatment of mild-to-moderate AD in both children and adults [94, 95]. The cream contains *Vitis vinifera* (grapevine) extract with antioxidant and antiprotease activity, glycyrrhetinic acid with antipruritic and anti-inflammatory properties, and hyaluronic acid which helps to moisturize the epidermis and restore barrier function [12, 94, 95]. Patrizi et al. conducted a multicenter, randomized, double-blind, vehicle-controlled clinical study to evaluate the efficacy and safety of MAS063DP in 60 pediatric patients affected by AD, aged between 2 and 17 years [95]. Using the Investigator's Global Assessment score for AD, patients with a score of 2 (mild) or 3 (moderate) were enrolled in the study. Patients were randomly assigned to receive MAS063DP (20 patients), MAS060 (20 patients, a similar formulation with lower key ingredients' concentration and no preservatives), or vehicle (20 patients).The study consisted in a treatment period of 43 days, with clinical evaluations at baseline (day 1), days 8, 15, 22, 29, and 43, at which time the treatment was stopped. MAS063DP showed nearly 80% improvement in Investigator's Global Assessment score at day 22, compared with 16.6% and 26.3% with the MAS060 and vehicle, respectively. A statistically significant difference was found by comparing MAS063DP with MAS060 ($p < 0.0001$); a similar result was evidenced comparing MAS063DP and vehicle ($p = 0.001$). By contrast, no significant difference was found between MAS060 and vehicle. A statistically significant difference was sustained until the end of the study. The authors concluded that MAS063DP may be considered as one of the available regimens effective in the treatment of mild-to-moderate AD in children and adolescents. Although it was a randomized trial, the sample size was small, and only Investigator's Global Assessment score was used.

In another randomized, double-blind, vehicle-controlled clinical study, Boguniewicz et al. administered MAS063DP ($n = 72$) or vehicle ($n = 70$) cream to 142 patients aged 6 months to 12 years 3 times per day to affected areas and sites prone to develop AD [94]. The primary endpoint for efficacy was the Investigator's Global Assessment at day 22. Secondary endpoints included Investigator's Global Assessment at other time-points, patient's/caregiver's assessment of pruritus, onset, duration of itch relief, EASI, patient's/caregiver's assessment of global response, and need for rescue medication in the event of an AD flare. The authors found that MAS063DP cream was statistically more effective ($p < 0.0001$) than vehicle cream for the primary endpoint and all secondary endpoints. Treatment discontinuation as a result of an adverse event occurred in 9.9% of patients using MAS063DP cream and 16% of patients using vehicle cream. The authors concluded that MAS063DP cream is effective and safe as monotherapy for the treatment of mild-to-moderate AD in infants and children.

Increased TEWL and downregulated antimicrobial peptides are observed in patients with AD. Park et al. investigated the relationship between antimicrobial and barrier factors by measuring the changes of TEWL and antimicrobial peptides after topical application of tacrolimus and ceramide-dominant emollient in patients with AD [96]. A total of three patients with AD were treated with tacrolimus in one lesion and ceramide-dominant emollient in another lesion for 4 weeks. RT-PCR and Western blotting revealed that the mRNA and protein expression levels of hBD-2 and LL-37 were increased on both study sites. Immunohistochemical analysis showed significant increase of antimicrobial peptides and interleukin-1α, while interleukin-4 was decreased on both study sites. The mean changes of TEWL and antimicrobial peptides showed no statistical difference between both sites. The authors concluded that tacrolimus and ceramide-dominant emollient influence on both TEWL and antimicrobial peptides expression in patients with AD. It should be noted that in this study, the sample size was small, and outcome measurements were focused.

Hon et al. evaluated whether the amount of emollient and skin cleanser used correlates with eczema severity, skin hydration, or TEWL, and whether liberal usage alters disease severity, skin hydration, and TEWL [65]. The authors studied skin hydration and TEWL at three common measurement sites on the forearm (antecubital flexure, 20 mm below the antecubital flexure, mid-forearm) and determined the SCORAD score, NESS, CDLQI, and the amount of emollient and cleanser usage over a 2-week period in consecutive new patients seen at the pediatric skin clinic of a teaching hospital in Hong Kong. In total, 48 subjects and 19 controls were recruited. Patients with AD had significantly higher TEWL and lower skin hydration in the studied sites. Emollient and cleanser usage was significantly higher ($p=0.001$ and $p=0.041$, respectively) in patients with AD than in controls. The amount of emollient usage was correlated with NESS, SCORAD, CDLQI, TEWL, and mid-forearm skin hydration. No such correlation was found with cleanser usage. Regardless of SCORAD, prescribing 130 g/m^2/week of emollient met the requirement of 95.8% of patients, and 73 g/m^2/week of emollient met that of 85.4%. As far as the cleanser is concerned, prescribing 136 g/m^2/week met the requirement of 91.7% of patients. Although both skin dryness and skin hydration were improved, there was no significant improvement in SCORAD or TEWL after 2 weeks. In terms of global acceptability of treatment, three-quarters of patients with AD and controls rated the combination of cream and cleanser as "good" or "very good." The authors concluded that adequate amounts of emollient and bathing cleanser should be prescribed to patients with AD. These amounts can be conveniently estimated based on body surface area instead of the less readily available tools for disease severity, degree of skin hydration, or skin integrity. However, liberal usage of emollients and bathing cleanser alone does not seem to alter disease severity or TEWL within 2 weeks, implying that additional treatments are necessary to manage AD. Hence, liberal amounts of moisturizers should be used which can be conveniently estimated based on body surface area instead of the less readily available tools for disease severity, degree of skin hydration, or skin integrity [65]. The outcome measures in this study included clinical scores, skin hydration, TEWL, and global assessment of treatment measurements. In addition, the amount of emollient usage per unit body surface area per unit time was also assessed.

In another study, Hon et al. recruited 33 patients (mean age 12 years, SD 4 years) with AD to study the clinical and biophysiological effects of twice-daily application of a pseudoceramide-containing cream [97]. Four weeks following the use of the pseudoceramide cream, the skin hydration significantly improved [mean (SD) from 30 (15) to 38 (15), $p=0.039$]. There was no deterioration in TEWL, eczema severity, or quality of life in these patients. The pseudoceramide cream improved the skin hydration but not the severity or quality of life over a 4-week usage. In this study, skin hydration and TEWL, disease severity (SCORAD index), CDLQI, amount of topical corticosteroid usage, and a global assessment of treatment score were used as outcome measurements [97].

In recent years, aqueous cream has been studied by a number of investigators. Aqueous cream BP is widely prescribed to patients with AD to relieve skin dryness. The formulation contains sodium lauryl sulfate, a chemical that is a known skin irritant and a commonly used excipient in personal care and household products. Tsang et al. characterized and assessed skin barrier function of healthy skin after application of aqueous cream BP and studied the physical effects of the formulation on the stratum corneum [98]. In this study, the left and right volar forearms of six human volunteers were each separated into treated and control sides. The treated sides of each forearm were subjected to twice daily applications of aqueous cream BP for 4 weeks at the end of which concomitant tape stripping and TEWL measurements were made. The untreated sides of the forearms were not exposed to any products containing sodium lauryl sulfate during the study period. Changes in stratum corneum thickness, baseline TEWL, and rate of increase in TEWL during tape stripping were observed in skin treated with aqueous cream BP. The mean decrease in stratum corneum thickness was 1.1 μm (12%) ($p=0{\cdot}0015$), and the mean increase in baseline TEWL was 2.5 g/m^2/h (20%) ($p<0.0001$). Reduced stratum corneum thickness and an increase in baseline TEWL, as well as a faster rate of increase in TEWL during tape stripping, were observed in 16 out of 27 treated skin sites. The investigators concluded that the application of aqueous cream BP, containing approximately 1% sodium lauryl sulfate, reduced the stratum corneum thickness of healthy skin and increased its permeability to water loss, and called into question the continued use of this emollient on the already compromised barrier of atopic skin [98].

Aqueous cream BP is known to induce sensitivity in certain patients and also to decrease the thickness of the stratum corneum [99]. Mohammed and colleagues investigated changes in corneocyte size, corneocyte maturity, selected protease activities, protein content, and TEWL in normal skin after a 28-day application of aqueous cream BP [99]. In this study, the left and right mid-volar forearms of six healthy female volunteers were selected as the study sites. Aqueous cream BP was applied twice daily to treated sites for 28 days. At the end of this period, the site was tape-stripped and corneocyte maturity, corneocyte size and protease activity of the desquamatory kallikrein proteases, KLK5, KLK7, inflammatory proteases tryptase, and plasmin were measured. Protein content and TEWL measurements were also recorded. The authors found that corneocyte maturity and size decreased with increasing number of tape strips and were significantly lower in treated sites compared with untreated sites. Protease activity and TEWL values were higher ($p<0.05$) for the treated sites compared with untreated sites. The amount of protein removed from deeper layers of treated sites was significantly lower than from untreated sites. The authors concluded that treatment with aqueous cream BP is associated with increased desquamatory and inflammatory protease activity. Changes in corneocyte maturity and size are also indicative of accelerated skin turnover induced by chronic application of this emollient. The authors question firmly the routine prescription of this preparation as a moisturizer in patients with AD. No clinical scores are used in this study.

Conclusion

Usage of moisturizers is a very important albeit often neglected components of AD management, and the relevant advice is often not evidence based [100]. Investigators should use both clinical as well as biophysiological tools to evaluate efficacy of moisturizers. Aqueous cream is appropriate for use as a soap substitute but is a less effective emollient than white petroleum [101, 102], emulsifying ointment, or white soft paraffin mixed with liquid paraffin [103]. Physicians should assist patients with AD and their parents to establish a good routine as to the use of an appropriate type and amount of moisturizer. Regular assessment of compliance to its use is crucial.

Take Home Messages

- Frequent and proper application of skin moisturizers is a very important albeit often neglected components of AD management, and the relevant advice is often not evidence based.
- Both clinical and biophysiological tools should be used to evaluate efficacy of moisturizers.
- Physicians should assist patients with AD and their parents to establish a good routine as to the use of an appropriate type and amount of moisturizer.
- Regular assessment of compliance to its use is crucial.

References

1. Leung AK, Hon KL (2011) Atopic dermatitis: a review for the primary care physician. Nova Science Publishers, Inc., New York, pp 1–111
2. Leung AKC, Barber KA (2003) Managing childhood atopic dermatitis. Adv Ther 20(3):129–137
3. Leung AK, Hon KL, Robson WL (2007) Atopic dermatitis. Adv Pediatr 54:241–273
4. Leung DY (1995) Atopic dermatitis: the skin as a window into the pathogenesis of chronic allergic diseases. J Allergy Clin Immunol 96(3):302–318
5. Sehra S, Tuana FM, Holbreich M, Mousdicas N, Tepper RS, Chang CH et al (2008) Scratching the surface: towards understanding the pathogenesis of atopic dermatitis. Crit Rev Immunol 28(1):15–43
6. Williams HC (1992) Is the prevalence of atopic dermatitis increasing? Clin Exp Dermatol 17(6): 385–391
7. Leung DY, Boguniewicz M, Howell MD, Nomura I, Hamid QA (2004) New insights into atopic dermatitis. J Clin Invest 113(5):651–657
8. Grillo M, Gassner L, Marshman G, Dunn S, Hudson P (2006) Pediatric atopic eczema: the impact of an educational intervention. Pediatr Dermatol 23(5):428–436
9. Leung R, Wong G, Lau J, Ho A, Chan JK, Choy D et al (1997) Prevalence of asthma and allergy in Hong Kong schoolchildren: an ISAAC study. Eur Respir J 10(2):354–360
10. Wong GW, Hui DS, Chan HH, Fok TF, Leung R, Zhong NS et al (2001) Prevalence of respiratory and atopic disorders in Chinese schoolchildren. Clin Exp Allergy 31(8):1225–1231
11. Leung DY, Nicklas RA, Li JT, Bernstein IL, Blessing-Moore J, Boguniewicz M et al (2004) Disease management of atopic dermatitis: an updated practice parameter. Joint task force on practice parameters. Ann Allergy Asthma Immunol 93(3 Suppl 2):S1–S21
12. Simpson EL (2010) Atopic dermatitis: a review of topical treatment options. Curr Med Res Opin 26(3):633–640
13. Abramovits W (2005) Atopic dermatitis. J Am Acad Dermatol 53(1 Suppl 1):S86–S93
14. Simpson EL, Hanifin JM (2005) Atopic dermatitis. J Am Acad Dermatol 53(1):115–128
15. Roos TC, Geuer S, Roos S, Brost H (2004) Recent advances in treatment strategies for atopic dermatitis. Drugs 64(23):2639–2666
16. Hon KL (2004) Skin diseases in Chinese children at a Pediatric Dermatology Center. Pediatr Dermatol 21(2):109–112
17. Hon KL, Lam MC, Leung TF, Kam WY, Li MC, Ip M et al (2005) Clinical features associated with nasal *Staphylococcus aureus* colonisation in Chinese children with moderate-to-severe atopic dermatitis. Ann Acad Med Singapore 34(10):602–605
18. Chamlin SL, Frieden IJ, Williams ML, Chren MM (2004) Effects of atopic dermatitis on young American children and their families. Pediatrics 114(3):607–611
19. Hon KL, Leung TF, Wong K, Chow C, Chuh A, Ng P et al (2008) Does age or gender influence quality of life in children with atopic dermatitis? Clin Exp Dermatol 33(6):705–709
20. Ben Gashir MA, Seed PT, Hay RJ (2002) Are quality of family life and disease severity related in childhood atopic dermatitis? J Eur Acad Dermatol Venereol 16(5):455–462
21. Ben Gashir MA (2003) Relationship between quality of life and disease severity in atopic dermatitis/eczema syndrome during childhood. Curr Opin Allergy Clin Immunol 3(5):369–373
22. Ben Gashir MA, Seed PT, Hay RJ (2004) Quality of life and disease severity are correlated in children with atopic dermatitis. Br J Dermatol 150(2):284–290
23. Rudikoff D, Lebwohl M (1998) Atopic dermatitis. Lancet 351(9117):1715–1721
24. Kristal L, Klein PA (2000) Atopic dermatitis in infants and children. An update. Pediatr Clin North Am 47(4):877–895
25. Eigenmann PA (2001) Clinical features and diagnostic criteria of atopic dermatitis in relation to age. Pediatr Allergy Immunol 12(Suppl 14):69–74
26. Hanifin JMRG (1980) Diagnostic features of atopic dermatitis. Acta Derm Venereol (Stockh) 2:44–47
27. Leung DY, Jain N, Leo HL (2003) New concepts in the pathogenesis of atopic dermatitis. Curr Opin Immunol 15(6):634–638
28. Leung DY, Bieber T (2003) Atopic dermatitis. Lancet 361(9352):151–160
29. Hon K, Leung TF (2010) Seromarkers in childhood atopic dermatitis. Expert Rev Dermatol 5(3):299–314
30. Hanifin JM (1982) Atopic dermatitis. J Am Acad Dermatol 6(1):1–13
31. Leung TF, Ma KC, Hon KL, Lam CWK et al (2003) Serum concentration of macrophage-derived chemokine may be a useful inflammatory marker for assessing severity of atopic dermatitis in infants and young children. Pediatr Allergy Immunol 14(4):296–301
32. Marenholz I, Nickel R, Ruschendorf F, Schulz F, Esparza-Gordillo J, Kerscher T et al (2006) Filaggrin loss-of-function mutations predispose to phenotypes involved in the atopic march. J Allergy Clin Immunol 118(4):866–871
33. Palmer CN, Irvine AD, Terron-Kwiatkowski A, Zhao Y, Liao H, Lee SP et al (2006) Common loss-of-function variants of the epidermal barrier protein filaggrin are a major predisposing factor for atopic dermatitis. Nat Genet 38(4):441–446
34. Sandilands A, Terron-Kwiatkowski A, Hull PR, O'Regan GM, Clayton TH, Watson RM et al (2007) Comprehensive analysis of the gene encoding filaggrin uncovers prevalent and rare mutations in ichthyosis vulgaris and atopic eczema. Nat Genet 39(5):650–654
35. Ching G, Hon KL (2009) Filaggrin null mutations in childhood atopic dermatitis among the Chinese. Int J Immunogenet 36(4):251–254
36. Enomoto H, Hirata K, Otsuka K, Kawai T, Takahashi T, Hirota T et al (2008) Filaggrin null mutations are

associated with atopic dermatitis and elevated levels of IgE in the Japanese population: a family and case-control study. J Hum Genet 53(7):615–621
37. Candi E, Schmidt R, Melino G (2005) The cornified envelope: a model of cell death in the skin [Review, 142 refs]. Nat Rev Mol Cell Biol 6(4):328–340
38. Krakowski AC, Eichenfield LF, Dohil MA (2008) Management of atopic dermatitis in the pediatric population. Pediatrics 122(4):812–824
39. Hara J, Higuchi K, Okamoto R, Kawashima M, Imokawa G (2000) High-expression of sphingomyelin deacylase is an important determinant of ceramide deficiency leading to barrier disruption in atopic dermatitis. J Invest Dermatol 115(3):406–413
40. Ong PY, Ohtake T, Brandt C, Strickland I, Boguniewicz M, Ganz T et al (2002) Endogenous antimicrobial peptides and skin infections in atopic dermatitis [see comment]. N Engl J Med 347(15):1151–1160
41. Charman C, Williams H (2000) Outcome measures of disease severity in atopic eczema. Arch Dermatol 136(6):763–769
42. (1993) Severity scoring of atopic dermatitis: the SCORAD index. Consensus Report of the European Task Force on Atopic Dermatitis. Dermatology 186(1):23–31
43. Kunz B, Oranje AP, Labreze L, Stalder JF, Ring J, Taieb A (1997) Clinical validation and guidelines for the SCORAD index: consensus report of the European Task Force on Atopic Dermatitis. Dermatology 195(1):10–19
44. Emerson RM, Charman CR, Williams HC (2000) The Nottingham Eczema Severity Score: preliminary refinement of the Rajka and Langeland grading. Br J Dermatol 142(2):288–297
45. Hon KL, Ma KC, Wong E, Leung TF, Wong Y, Fok TF et al (2003) Validation of a self-administered questionnaire in Chinese in the assessment of eczema severity. Pediatr Dermatol 20(6):465–469
46. Sturgill S (2004) Atopic dermatitis update. Curr Opin Pediatr 16(4):396–401
47. Rajka G, Langeland T (1989) Grading of the severity of atopic dermatitis. Acta Derm Venereol 144:13–14
48. Hanifin JM, Thurston M, Omoto M, Cherill R, Tofte SJ, Graeber M (2001) The eczema area and severity index (EASI): assessment of reliability in atopic dermatitis. EASI Evaluator Group. Exp Dermatol 10(1): 11–18
49. Benjamin K et al (2004) The development of an objective method for measuring scratch in children with atopic dermatitis suitable for clinical use. J Am Acad Dermatol 50(1):33–40
50. Hon KL, Lam MC, Leung TF, Kam WY, Lee KC, Li MC et al (2006) Nocturnal wrist movements are correlated with objective clinical scores and plasma chemokine levels in children with atopic dermatitis. Br J Dermatol 154(4):629–635
51. Hon KL, Leung TF, Ma K, Li A, Wong Y, Yin JA et al (2005) Resting energy expenditure, oxygen consumption and carbon dioxide production during sleep in children with atopic dermatitis. J Dermatolog Treat 16(1):22–25
52. Pinnagoda J, Tupker RA, Agner T, Serup J (1990) Guidelines for transepidermal water loss (TEWL) measurement. A report from the Standardization Group of the European Society of Contact Dermatitis. Contact Dermatitis 22(3):164–178
53. Serup J (1992) Characterization of contact dermatitis and atopy using bioengineering techniques. A survey. Acta Derm Venereol 177:14–25
54. Kim DW, Park JY, Na GY, Lee SJ, Lee WJ (2006) Correlation of clinical features and skin barrier function in adolescent and adult patients with atopic dermatitis. Int J Dermatol 45(6):698–701
55. Proksch E, Nissen HP, Bremgartner M, Urquhart C (2005) Bathing in a magnesium-rich Dead Sea salt solution improves skin barrier function, enhances skin hydration, and reduces inflammation in atopic dry skin. Int J Dermatol 44(2):151–157
56. O'goshi K, Serup J (2005) Inter-instrumental variation of skin capacitance measured with the Corneometer. Skin Res Technol 11(2):107–109
57. Seidenari S, Giusti G (1995) Objective assessment of the skin of children affected by atopic dermatitis: a study of pH, capacitance and TEWL in eczematous and clinically uninvolved skin. Acta Derm Venereol 75(6):429–433
58. Choi SJ, Song MG, Sung WT, Lee DY, Lee JH, Lee ES et al (2003) Comparison of transepidermal water loss, capacitance and pH values in the skin between intrinsic and extrinsic atopic dermatitis patients. J Korean Med Sci 18(1):93–96
59. Son SW, Park SY, Ha SH, Park GM, Kim MG, Moon JS et al (2005) Objective evaluation for severity of atopic dermatitis by morphologic study of skin surface contours. Skin Res Technol 11(4):272–280
60. Lodén M, Olsson H, Axell T, Linde YW (1992) Friction, capacitance and transepidermal water loss (TEWL) in dry atopic and normal skin. Br J Dermatol 126(2):137–141
61. Sakurai K, Sugiura H, Matsumoto M, Uehara M (2002) Occurrence of patchy parakeratosis in normal-appearing skin in patients with active atopic dermatitis and in patients with healed atopic dermatitis: a cause of impaired barrier function of the atopic skin. J Dermatol Sci 30(1):37–42
62. Matsumoto M, Sugiura H, Uehara M (2000) Skin barrier function in patients with completely healed atopic dermatitis. J Dermatol Sci 23(3):178–182
63. Hon KL, Wong KY, Leung TF, Chow CM, Ng PC (2008) Comparison of skin hydration evaluation sites and correlations among skin hydration, transepidermal water loss, SCORAD index, Nottingham eczema severity score, and quality of life in patients with atopic dermatitis. Am J Clin Dermatol 9(1):45–50
64. Hon KL, Kam WY, Lam A et al (2006) CDLQI, SCORAD and NESS: are they correlated? Qual Life Res 15:1551–1558

65. Hon KL, Ching GK, Leung TF, Choi CY, Lee KK, Ng PC (2010) Estimating emollient usage in patients with eczema. Clin Exp Dermatol 35(1):22–26
66. Holm E, Wulf HC, Stegmann H, Jemec GBE (2006) Life quality assessment among patients with atopic eczema. Br J Dermatol 154(4):719–725
67. Baumer JH (2008) Atopic eczema in children, NICE. Arch Dis Child Educ Pract 93(3):93–97
68. Lewis-Jones MS, Finlay AY (1995) The Children's Dermatology Life Quality Index (CDLQI): initial validation and practical use. Br J Dermatol 132(6):942–949
69. Chamlin SL, Cella D, Frieden IJ, Williams ML, Mancini AJ, Lai JS et al (2005) Development of the Childhood Atopic Dermatitis Impact Scale: initial validation of a quality-of-life measure for young children with atopic dermatitis and their families. J Invest Dermatol 125(6):1106–1111
70. McKenna SP, Doward LC (2008) Quality of life of children with atopic dermatitis and their families. Curr Opin Allergy Clin Immunol 8(3):228–231
71. McKenna SP, Whalley D, Dewar AL, Erdman RA, Kohlmann T, Niero M et al (2005) International development of the Parents' Index of Quality of Life in Atopic Dermatitis (PIQoL-AD). Qual Life Res 14(1):231–241
72. Meads DM, McKenna SP, Kahler K (2005) The quality of life of parents of children with atopic dermatitis: interpretation of PIQoL-AD scores. Qual Life Res 14(10):2235–2245
73. Drake L, Prendergast M, Maher R, Breneman D, Korman N, Satoi Y et al (2001) The impact of tacrolimus ointment on health-related quality of life of adult and pediatric patients with atopic dermatitis. J Am Acad Dermatol 44(1 Suppl):S65–S72
74. Whalley D, Huels J, McKenna SP, van Assche D (2002) The benefit of pimecrolimus (Elidel, SDZ ASM 981) on parents' quality of life in the treatment of pediatric atopic dermatitis. Pediatrics 110(6):1133–1136
75. Hon KL, Leung T, Wong Y, Li A, Fok T et al (2005) A survey of bathing and showering practices in children with atopic eczema. Clin Exp Dermatol 30(4): 351–354
76. Chamlin SL, Kao J, Frieden IJ, Sheu MY, Fowler AJ, Fluhr JW et al (2002) Ceramide-dominant barrier repair lipids alleviate childhood atopic dermatitis: changes in barrier function provide a sensitive indicator of disease activity. J Am Acad Dermatol 47(2): 198–208
77. Maintz L, Novak N (2007) Getting more and more complex: the pathophysiology of atopic eczema. Eur J Dermatol 17(4):267–283
78. Dohil MA, Eichenfield LF (2005) A treatment approach for atopic dermatitis. Pediatr Ann 34(3): 201–210
79. Lancaster W (2009) Atopic eczema in infants and children. Community Pract 82(7):36–37
80. Tarr A, Iheanacho I (2009) Should we use bath emollients for atopic eczema? BMJ 339:b4273
81. Cork M (1998) Complete emollient therapy. The National Association of Fundholding Practices Official Yearbook, London, pp 159–168
82. Cork MJ, Danby S (2009) Skin barrier breakdown: a renaissance in emollient therapy. Br J Nurs 18(14): 872–877
83. Cork MJ, Danby SG, Vasilopoulos Y, Hadgraft J, Lane ME, Moustafa M et al (2009) Epidermal barrier dysfunction in atopic dermatitis. J Invest Dermatol 129(8):1892–1908
84. Bissonnette R, Maari C, Provost N, Bolduc C, Nigen S, Rougier A et al (2010) A double-blind study of tolerance and efficacy of a new urea-containing moisturizer in patients with atopic dermatitis. J Cosmet Dermatol 9(1):16–21
85. Miller DW, Koch SB, Yentzer BA, Clark AR, O'Neill JR, Fountain J et al (2011) An over-the-counter moisturizer is as clinically effective as, and more cost-effective than, prescription barrier creams in the treatment of children with mild-to-moderate atopic dermatitis: a randomized, controlled trial. J Drugs Dermatol 10(5):531–537
86. Chamlin SL, Frieden IJ, Fowler A, Williams M, Kao J, Sheu M et al (2001) Ceramide-dominant, barrier-repair lipids improve childhood atopic dermatitis. Arch Dermatol 137(8):1110–1112
87. Lodén M, Wirén K, Smerud K, Meland N, Honnas H, Mork G et al (2010) Treatment with a barrier-strengthening moisturizer prevents relapse of hand-eczema. An open, randomized, prospective, parallel group study. Acta Derm Venereol 90(6):602–606
88. Lodén M, Wirén K, Smerud KT, Meland N, Hønnås H, Mørk G et al (2011) The effect of a corticosteroid cream and a barrier-strengthening moisturizer in hand eczema. A double-blind, randomized, prospective, parallel group clinical trial. J Eur Acad Dermatol Venereol. doi:10.1111/j.1468-3083.2011.04128.x
89. Frankel A, Sohn A, Patel RV, Lebwohl M (2011) Bilateral comparison study of pimecrolimus cream 1% and a ceramide-hyaluronic Acid emollient foam in the treatment of patients with atopic dermatitis. J Drugs Dermatol 10(6):666–672
90. Grimalt R, Mengeaud V, Cambazard F, Study Investigators' Group (2007) The steroid-sparing effect of an emollient therapy in infants with atopic dermatitis: a randomized controlled study. Dermatology 214(1):61–67
91. Lee J, Jung E, Koh J, Kim YS, Park D (2008) Effect of rosmarinic acid on atopic dermatitis. J Dermatol 35(12):768–771
92. Draelos ZD (2008) The effect of ceramide-containing skin care products on eczema resolution duration. Cutis 81(1):87–91
93. Madaan A (2008) Epiceram for the treatment of atopic dermatitis. Drugs Today 44(10):751–755
94. Boguniewicz M, Zeichner JA, Eichenfield LF, Hebert AA, Jarratt M, Lucky AW et al (2008) MAS063DP is effective monotherapy for mild to moderate atopic dermatitis in infants and children: a multicenter,

randomized, vehicle-controlled study. J Pediatr 152(6):854–859
95. Patrizi A, Capitanio B, Neri I, Giacomini F, Sinagra JL, Raone B et al (2008) A double-blind, randomized, vehicle-controlled clinical study to evaluate the efficacy and safety of MAS063DP (ATOPICLAIR) in the management of atopic dermatitis in paediatric patients. Pediatr Allergy Immunol 19(7):619–625
96. Park KY, Kim DH, Jeong MS, Li K, Seo SJ (2010) Changes of antimicrobial peptides and transepidermal water loss after topical application of tacrolimus and ceramide-dominant emollient in patients with atopic dermatitis. J Korean Med Sci 25(5):766–771
97. Hon KL, Wang SS, Lau Z, Lee HC, Lee KK, Leung TF et al (2011) Pseudoceramide for childhood eczema: does it work? Hong Kong Med J 17(2):132–136
98. Tsang M, Guy RH (2010) Effect of aqueous cream BP on human stratum corneum in vivo. Br J Dermatol 163(5):954–958
99. Mohammed D, Matts PJ, Hadgraft J, Lane ME (2011) Influence of aqueous cream BP on corneocyte size, maturity, skin protease activity, protein content and transepidermal water loss. Br J Dermatol 164(6):1304–1310
100. Hoare C, Li Wan PA, Williams H (2000) Systematic review of treatments for atopic eczema. Health Technol Assess (Winchester, England) 4(37):1–191
101. Raimer SS (2000) Managing pediatric atopic dermatitis. Clin Pediatr 39(1):1–14
102. Tofte SJ, Hanifin JM (2001) Current management and therapy of atopic dermatitis. J Am Acad Dermatol 44(1 (Part 2)):S13–S16
103. Fischer G (1996) Compliance problems in paediatric atopic eczema. Australas J Dermatol 37(Suppl 1): S10–S13

Part II

Skin Essentials

Sensory Systems of Epidermal Keratinocytes

6

Mitsuhiro Denda

6.1 Introduction

Epidermal keratinocytes have long been recognized to form the water-impermeable stratum corneum, and this barrier function is critical, especially for terrestrial animals. However, recent findings have dramatically changed the picture of epidermal keratinocytes, placing them at the forefront of the sensory system [39].

The traditional view of the skin surface sensory system for environmental factors, such as temperature and chemical stimuli, has been focused on C fibers, which penetrate into the epidermis. In the case of mechanical stimuli, other peripheral nerve endings, such as Merkel cells or Pacinian capsules or Meissner capsules, were thought to act as sensors in the skin [98]. However, over the past two decades, it has become apparent that keratinocytes contain sensory systems for a variety of environmental factors. Thus, epidermal keratinocytes may play a key role in skin surface perception [39]. This idea has been supported by the recent cloning of a series of receptors, which are activated by temperature, mechanical stress, osmotic pressure and chemical stimuli, and the subsequent demonstration that at least some of them are expressed in epidermal keratinocytes (Fig. 6.1).

M. Denda, Ph.D.
Shiseido Research Center,
Yokohama, Japan
e-mail: mitsuhiro.denda@to.shiseido.co.jp

Moreover, we have shown that a variety of environmental factors, including visible light, sound, and external electrical potential, influence epidermal permeability barrier homeostasis [21, 22, 23, 24, 34]. These results led us to hypothesize that epidermal keratinocytes might sense these environmental factors. Indeed, we found that photoreceptor proteins, which are expressed in retina, are also expressed in epidermal keratinocytes [107]. In addition, voltage-gated calcium channels are expressed in keratinocytes [38]. These proteins might be associated with other unknown sensory systems of epidermal keratinocytes.

Information derived from the environment is transferred by afferent nerve fibers to the central nervous system, and processed in the brain, with the aid of a series of neurotransmitters and specific receptors. We have shown that a variety of neurotransmitter receptors, originally found in the central nervous system, are also expressed in epidermal keratinocytes [39]. Interestingly, many of them also influenced epidermal permeability barrier homeostasis. Epidermal keratinocytes also generate various messenger molecules, such as neurotransmitters, neuropeptides, and hormones. Thus, it is reasonable to consider the possibility that epidermal keratinocytes sense environmental factors, process the information, and pass messages to the central nervous system.

In this chapter, I would like to focus on the various sensory systems of epidermal keratinocytes and to discuss the potential role of the epidermis as the border between the living system and the environment.

M. Lodén, H.I. Maibach (eds.), *Treatment of Dry Skin Syndrome*,
DOI 10.1007/978-3-642-27606-4_6, © Springer-Verlag Berlin Heidelberg 2012

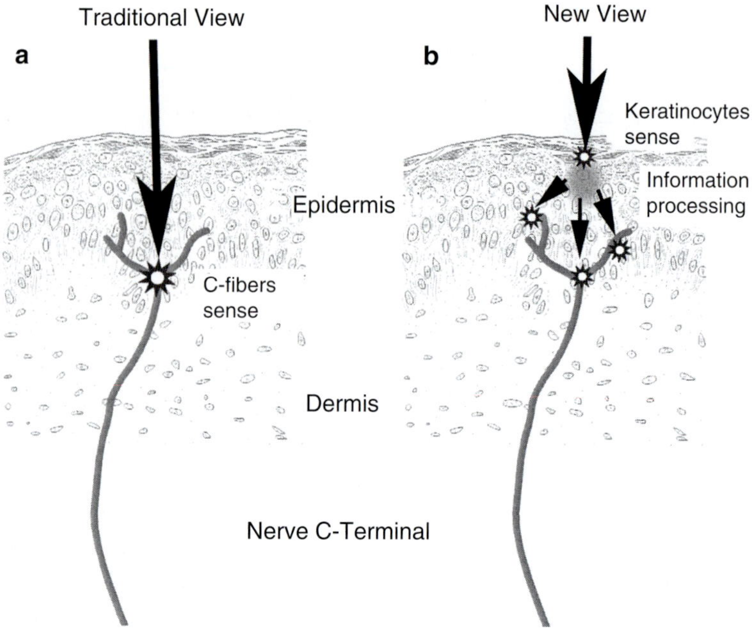

Fig. 6.1 Schematic illustration of the hypothetical skin surface sensory system. (**a**) Traditional view, with C fibers at the forefront of the sensory system. (**b**) Proposed new view, with epidermal keratinocytes at the forefront of the sensory system. A signal is sensed by keratinocytes, processed, and transferred to C-fiber terminals (Arranged from figure by Sakura Kogeisha Co. Ltd)

6.2 Humidity

Seasonal changes affect the condition of normal skin and may trigger various cutaneous disorders [96, 119]. Abundant indirect evidence indicates that decreased humidity precipitates these disorders, whereas, in contrast, increased skin hydration appears to ameliorate these conditions. However, the mechanisms by which alterations in relative humidity might influence cutaneous function and induce cutaneous pathology are poorly understood.

We have evaluated the effects of low environmental humidity on skin pathology [18]. We first demonstrated that low humidity stimulates epidermal DNA synthesis and amplifies the hyperproliferative response to barrier disruption [28]. Stratum corneum morphology was also influenced by a dry environment [27, 94], and abnormal desquamation was observed under low humidity [93]. When animals were kept in a dry condition for more than 1 week, the barrier function was enhanced [27]. On the other hand, a drastic decrease of environmental humidity induced barrier abnormality [95], and a decrease in the water retention capacity of the stratum corneum [67]. Ashida et al. demonstrated an increase of IL-1α in the epidermis [4] and an increase of histamine and mast cells in the dermis [3] in a dry environment. Hosoi et al. demonstrated that the allergic response was enhanced by low environmental humidity [55]. These studies provide evidence that changes in environmental humidity contribute to the seasonal exacerbations/amelioration of cutaneous disorders, such as atopic dermatitis and psoriasis, which are characterized by a defective barrier, epidermal hyperplasia, and inflammation (Table 6.1).

The signaling system through which environmental humidity influences epidermal homeostasis is not yet clear. We previously demonstrated that calcium propagation plays a crucial role in epidermal homeostasis when the epidermis is exposed to a dry environment [45]. We further showed that calcium propagation was induced by air exposure of cultured human keratinocytes [20]. A transient increase of intracellular calcium concentration appeared, followed by a wave-like increase in adjacent unexposed keratinocytes, showing oscillations with a frequency that varied from cell to cell. The increase of calcium concentration did not appear when calcium was removed from the medium or when suramin, a purinergic receptor antagonist, was added. The ATP concentration also increased immediately after keratinocytes were exposed to air. Thus, we speculated that

ATP is secreted from keratinocytes on exposure to air and induces an increase of intracellular calcium concentration. Calcium propagation and ATP secretion in epidermal keratinocytes might be associated with the signaling system of epidermis in response to environmental low humidity [109].

The sensor of the environment humidity was not identified. But, as discussed below, TRPV4 (transient receptor potential subtype V4) is activated by osmotic pressure and so might serve as a sensor of environmental humidity.

6.3 Transient Receptor Potential (TRP) Family

In the last decade, a series of receptors, which are activated at defined temperatures, have been cloned. They were named the transient receptor potential (TRP) family. These polymodal receptors were discovered mainly in the nervous system, where some of them act as sensors of temperature or other physical or chemical factors [43]. However, various thermosensitive TRP receptors were found to be expressed in epidermal keratinocytes [25] (Table 6.2). We first discovered the expression and function of TRPV1 (VR1) in epidermal keratinocytes [33, 61]. TPRV1 is activated by heat (>43°C), acidic conditions (pH<6.6), and capsaicin [13, 104]. Subsequently, expression of TRPV3 and TRPV4 in keratinocytes was also reported [14, 91]. TRPV3 is activated by heat (around 30°C) mechanical stress, camphor, and 2-aminoethoxydiphenyl borate. TRPV4 is activated by heat (around 30°C), osmotic pressure, and 4α-phorbol 12,13-didecanone (4α-PDD) [56, 103, 121].

Previous studies have also identified cold-sensitive proteins, TRPA1 and TRPM8, that are activated by low temperature (<22°C) in peripheral nerve cells [90, 102]. Recently, expression of TRPA1, which is activated by low temperature (<17°C), was also found in epidermal cells [6]. We demonstrated that exposure of cultured human keratinocytes to low temperature induced elevation of intracellular calcium [108]: as the temperature of the medium was reduced, elevation of intracellular calcium was observed at 17–22°C. The extent of elevation was greater in nondifferentiated cells than in differentiated cells. Application of ruthenium red (a nonselective TRP blocker) and HC030031 (a specific antagonist of TRPA1) reduced the elevation. These results suggested that TRPA1 serves as a functional cold-sensitive calcium channel in human epidermal keratinocytes. We also established that TRPM8 was expressed in epidermal keratinocytes, by means of immunohistochemical study and RT-PCR [41].

Table 6.1 Effects of dry environment (low humidity) on skin pathophysiology

Amplification of hyperproliferative response to barrier disruption [28]
Abnormal desquamation of the stratum corneum [93]
Elevation of DNA synthesis in basal layer of the epidermis [92]
Enhancement of barrier function [27]
Appearance of abnormal skin surface morphology [94]
Amplification of allergic reaction [55]
Elevation of IL-1α mRNA and protein [4]
Amplification of proliferative response induced by surfactant [19]
Decrease of water-holding capacity and free amino acid content in stratum corneum [67, 94]
Abrupt decrease in environmental humidity induces abnormalities in barrier homeostasis [95]
Alteration of calcium distribution in epidermis [45]
Increase of mast cell number and histamine content in dermis [3]

Table 6.2 Thermosensitive transient receptor potential proteins expressed in keratinocytes

Name	Activator (s)	References
TRPV1	>43°C, low pH (<6.6), capsaicin, etc.	[33, 61]
TRPV2	>52°C	[111]
TRPV3	> around 30°C, camphor, eugenol, etc.	[90]
TRPV4	> around 30°C, osmotic pressure, mechanical stimuli, etc.	[14]
TRPA1	<17°C, allyl isothiocyanate, cinnamaldehyde, etc.	[6, 108]
TRPM8	<22°C, menthol, etc.	[41]

Previously, we had found that calcium dynamics was associated with epidermal permeability barrier homeostasis [35]. The thermosensitive TRPs described above are cation-permeable channels. Thus, we hypothesized that activation of these TRPs might influence barrier homeostasis. To evaluate the influence of these receptors on the barrier homeostasis, we kept both hairless mouse skin and human skin at various temperatures immediately after tape stripping. At temperatures from 36°C to 40°C, the barrier recovery was accelerated in both cases compared with that at 34°C. At 34°C or 42°C, the barrier recovery was delayed. Topical application of 4αPDD, a specific agonist of TRPV4, accelerated the barrier recovery, while ruthenium red, a blocker of TRPV4, delayed the barrier recovery. Capsaicin, an activator of TRPV1, delayed the barrier recovery, while capsazepine, an antagonist of TRPV1, blocked this delay. 2-Aminoethoxydiphenyl borate and camphor, TRPV3 activators, did not affect the barrier recovery rate. Since TRPV4 is activated at about 35°C and above, while TRPV1 is activated at about 42°C and above, these results suggest that TRPV1 and TRPV4 both play important roles in skin permeability barrier homeostasis. Previous reports suggest the existence of a water flux sensor in the epidermis, and as TRPV4 is known to be activated by osmotic pressure, our results indicate that it might be this sensor [40].

We also examined the effects of topical application of agonists of TRPA1 and brief cold exposure on the barrier recovery rate after barrier disruption [42]. Topical application of a TRPA1 agonist, allyl isothiocyanate or cinnamaldehyde, accelerated the barrier recovery after tape stripping. The effect of both agonists was blocked by HC030031, an antagonist of TRPA1. Brief exposure (1 min) to cold (10–15°C) also accelerated the barrier recovery, and this acceleration was also blocked by HC030031. Electron-microscopic studies indicated that brief cold exposure accelerated lamellar body secretion between stratum corneum and stratum granulosum, while pretreatment with HC030031 inhibited the secretion. These results suggest that TRPA1 is associated with epidermal permeability barrier homeostasis.

We next examined the effect of topical application of TRPM8 modulators on epidermal permeability barrier homeostasis [41]. Topical application of TRPM8 agonists, menthol and WS12, accelerated barrier recovery after tape stripping. The effect of WS12 was blocked by a nonselective TRP antagonist, ruthenium red, and a TRPM8-specific antagonist, BTCT. Topical application of WS12 also reduced epidermal proliferation associated with barrier disruption under low humidity, and this effect was blocked by BTCT. Our results indicate that TRPM8 or a closely related protein in epidermal keratinocytes plays a role in epidermal permeability barrier homeostasis and epidermal proliferation after barrier insult.

It has long been recognized that peripheral nerve fibers play a major role in cutaneous thermosensation. However, as described above, multiple thermosensitive TRP receptors are expressed in epidermal keratinocytes. Thus, keratinocytes may be the main thermosensory cells for detecting skin surface temperature. Moreover, some of the receptors were associated with epidermal permeability homeostasis. Other studies also indicated that TRPs were related to keratinocyte differentiation, proliferation, and inflammation [25]. The TRP family might play an important role not only as a thermosensory system but also in the pathology and physiology of the epidermis.

6.4 Mechanical Stress

The traditional view of tactile perception has been that the key sensors are the peripheral nerve endings and fibers [118]. However, the terminals of the nerve fibers are quite sparse. For example, the pressure points, which detect mechanical stimuli, are localized at distances of millimeters from each other [98]. The skin can detect pattern on a much smaller scale [64, 85, 113, 114] than would be expected on the basis of sampling theory if the nerve terminals were the only sensors [76].

We recently demonstrated that female fingertip can recognize micron-level randomness as unpleasant [81]. We studied the ability of the human fingertip to distinguish three different micron-level patterns (which were not distinguishable with the naked eye) on plastic plates. There were two ordered patterns of 1 × 10 μm and 3 × 30 μm ripples, and one random pattern (randomly mixed 1 × 10 μm and 3 × 30 μm ripples). All 10 female subjects reported the random pattern, but not the regular patterns, as unpleasant, while the majority of the male subjects did not. Nine out of ten female subjects continued to report the random pattern as unpleasant even after their fingertip had been coated with a collodion membrane. The frictional coefficients of the three patterns did not differ greatly. The mechanism of the recognition of ordered and disordered patterns is unknown. Yamada et al. reported a model of artificial finger skin having ridges [123] and presented a simulation of shear strain distribution inside the ridges. The principal component of the shear strain was concentrated in a smaller area than the ridges. There are Merkel terminals at the bottom of the epidermis. With the aid of the ridges, finger skin could detect pattern at a scale smaller than the separation distance of the C-terminals. In our study, however, almost all of the females could detect the disordered pattern even when the ridges were covered with a collodion film. This result implied that the appreciation of fine surface structure in humans cannot be explained only in terms of the mechanoreceptors beneath the fingerprint structure, but must involve some additional mechanism.

In our study, we did not define the velocity of fingertip stroking. All subjects stroked a 10-cm pattern for 0.5–1.0 s per stroke. In the whole 10-cm pattern, 10,000 ripples of 10 μm exist, so stroking the 1 × 10 μm pattern might generate a 10–20-kHz vibration, while the 3 × 30 μm pattern might generate a 3.3–6.7-kHz vibration. Pacinian corpuscles in the dermis can recognize up to kilohertz-order vibration [116], but it is not yet well known whether they can distinguish ordered and random vibrations. A system that is able to recognize randomness might require highly sophisticated information processing.

Among the TRP family members, some were reported to act as sensors of mechanical stress [43]. Thus, we hypothesized that epidermal keratinocytes might contribute to the skin tactile sensory system. To further examine this idea, we investigated the intracellular calcium responses of cultured keratinocytes to external hydraulic pressure [51]. First, we compared the responses of undifferentiated and differentiated keratinocytes with those of fibroblasts, vascular endothelial cells, and lymphatic endothelial cells. Elevation of intracellular calcium was observed after application of pressure to keratinocytes, fibroblasts, and vascular endothelial cells. The calcium propagation extended over a larger area and continued for a longer period of time in differentiated keratinocytes, as compared with the other cells. The response of the keratinocytes was dramatically reduced when the cells were incubated in medium without calcium. Application of a nonselective TRP (transient receptor potential) channel blocker, ruthenium red, also attenuated the calcium response. These results suggest that differentiated keratinocytes are sensitive to external pressure and that TRP might be involved in the mechanism of their response.

We also evaluated the mechanism of calcium propagation induced by mechanical stress [112]. Before differentiation, mechanical stress induced a calcium wave over a limited area, and this was completely blocked by apyrase, which degrades ATP. In the case of differentiated keratinocytes, the calcium wave propagated over a larger area, and application of apyrase did not completely inhibit the wave. Thus, in differentiated cells, induction of calcium waves might involve not only ATP but also another factor. Immunohistochemical study indicated that connexins 26 and 43, both components of gap junctions, were expressed in the cell membrane of differentiated keratinocytes. Application of octanol or carbenxolone, which blocks gap junctions, significantly reduced calcium wave propagation in differentiated keratinocytes. These results suggest that signaling via gap junctions might be involved in the induction of calcium waves in response to mechanical stress at the upper layer of the epidermis.

If epidermal keratinocytes act as a sensory system for external mechanical stress, the signal should be transferred to the peripheral nerve system. Several reports have demonstrated indirect

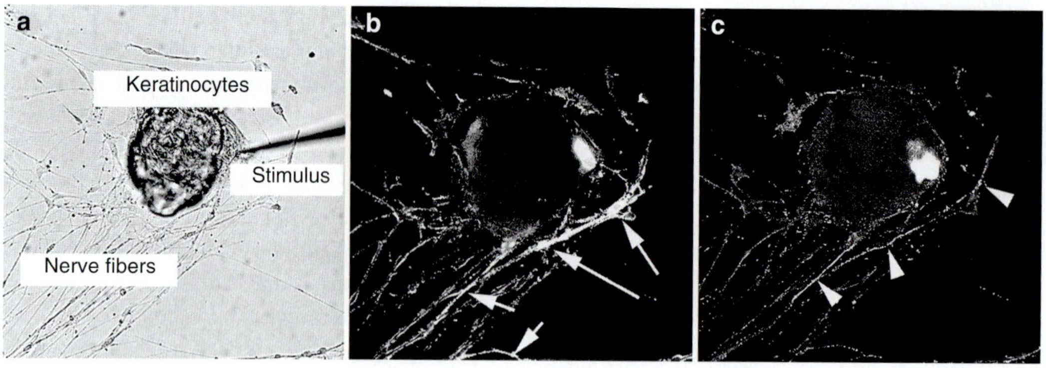

Fig. 6.2 Calcium imaging of keratinocytes and DRG-cell co-culture system. (**a**) Image of keratinocyte aggregates before mechanical stimulation. (**b**) Immediately after mechanical stimulation. Mechanical stimulation induced calcium propagation in keratinocyte aggregates and nerve fibers (*arrows*). (**c**) Image of the same area in the presence of apyrase before mechanical stimulation (*arrowheads*) [110]

or direct communication between keratinocytes and nerve cells. Koizumi and his coworkers demonstrated that mechanical stimulation of cultured keratinocytes induced calcium waves, and the calcium propagation was also transferred to co-cultured nerve cells [72]. In their study, they indicated that ATP, which is secreted from keratinocytes, played a crucial role in the signal transmission, because the calcium propagation was completely blocked by the application of apyrase, an enzyme that degrades ATP. On the other hand, we recently demonstrated that the calcium wave, which was induced in differentiated keratinocytes, resulted in elevation of intracellular calcium in co-cultured nerve cells, and the signal transmission was not completely blocked by apyrase (Fig. 6.2) [110]. Huang and his coworkers demonstrated that prostaglandin E2 played an important role in the signal transmission between keratinocytes and nerve cells [58]. These results suggested that a variety of factors might indirectly or directly mediate signal transmission between keratinocytes and the peripheral nerve system.

The series of study described above suggested that each keratinocyte in the epidermis could contribute to tactile perception. That is, each cell might serve as a sensor for mechanical stress, and so the potential resolution of tactile sensation might reach cellular dimensions, i.e., micrometer order. This speculation could account for the observed tactile resolution of human skin.

In our study [81], female subjects readily recognized a random pattern as unpleasant in the absence of other information, and so it appears that the micron-level random pattern provided a specific signal to the skin, and this signal affected emotional judgment, i.e., pleasant or unpleasant. Thus, invisible tactile patterns could influence human emotion in daily life. This might be consistent with Damasio's idea that the human mind is generated by interaction between brain and body physiology [17]. Epidermal keratinocytes might play an important role as a skin tactile sensory system, which could influence our emotional state at the subconscious level.

6.5 Sound

The frequency range of audible acoustic sound for adult humans is approximately 20–16,000 Hz [54]. However, Oohashi and his coworkers demonstrated that ultrasound at a frequency above 20,000 Hz (20 kHz) influences human brain electrical activity and systemic hormonal levels [69, 87, 88, 122]. Interestingly, these effects did not occur via the ears [88]. On the other hand, a recent study demonstrated that a slight, inaudible air puff on the skin influenced auditory perception [50]. These findings suggested that an unknown system that is responsive to ultrasound exists at the human body surface. Based on the above findings, we speculated that audible or inaudible sound frequencies might influence epidermal barrier homeostasis.

To test this idea, we first evaluated the effects of 5, 10, 20, and 30 kHz sound on intact skin of hairless mice [24]. We disrupted the permeability barrier by tape stripping and immediately exposed the skin to sound for 1 h. The speaker cone lightly touched one side of the flank, and we attached a silent speaker cone to the other flank as a control. Application of sound at a frequency of 10, 20, or 30 kHz accelerated the barrier recovery, while 5 kHz sound had no effect. The effects on barrier recovery were observed 23 h after cessation of the sound application.

To determine whether the effect was induced by sound or skin vibration, we next placed the speaker 1 or 3 cm away from the skin surface. In this case too, significant acceleration of the barrier recovery by sound was observed. The sound pressure levels were as follows: 0 cm, 83 dB; 1 cm, 78 dB; and 3 cm, 70 dB.

We also evaluated the effect of different sound pressures on the barrier recovery rate. The sound source was placed 1 cm away from the skin surface, and the frequency was 20 kHz. The barrier recovery rate increased with increasing sound pressure. An electron-microscopic study indicated that exposure to sound at a frequency of 20 kHz accelerated lamellar body secretion between stratum corneum (SC) and stratum granulosum (SG)

Oohashi and his coworkers demonstrated that inaudible sound was sensed at the body surface, excluding the ears, and influenced brain electrical activity [88], but the mechanism involved is still unknown. Feldmann has suggested that a structure in human eccrine gland has the ability to detect very high frequency (gigahertz) sound [46]. However, we used hairless mice, which do not have eccrine glands, and much lower frequency sound. Another study demonstrated that human epidermis had a piezoelectric sensory system [5]. As described above, individual keratinocytes showed elevation of intracellular calcium elevation in response to external mechanical stress [51, 112]. Thus, they could sense sound, an oscillating mechanical stress. Moreover, several neurotransmitters, such as ATP, dopamine, and nitric oxide, are generated and secreted by keratinocytes [34, 49, 59]. Thus, sound might be sensed by keratinocytes, and the signals might be processed and then transferred to the nervous system directly or via neurotransmitters. Inaudible sound might be sensed by epidermal keratinocytes and influence the endocrine system or emotional state.

6.6 Visible Light

The effects of ultraviolet or infrared radiation on skin are well known, but only a few reports describe the effect of visible light.

We previously demonstrated that visible light influenced the epidermal barrier recovery rate after disruption [21]. The effects of visible light on epidermal permeability barrier recovery were evaluated by using light-emitting diodes as light sources. The flank skin of hairless mice was tape-stripped and immediately exposed to blue (430–510 nm), green (490–560 nm), red (550–670 nm), or white (400–670 nm) light (20 W each) for 1 h, followed by measurement of transepidermal water loss. Control mice were kept in a dark box during the experiments. During the irradiation, the skin surface temperature was kept constant at 37°C in all mice. Irradiation with red light significantly accelerated the barrier recovery, while irradiation with blue light delayed it, compared with the control. White or green light did not affect the barrier recovery rate. We next carried out a study using hairless mouse skin organ culture. The permeability barrier was disrupted by means of acetone treatment, then each section was incubated afloat on the medium (37°C) and irradiated with blue, red, or white light (20 w) for 1 h. Immediately after the end of irradiation, we evaluated the barrier function. Again, red light accelerated the barrier recovery, while blue delayed it. An electron-microscopic study suggested that red light accelerated lamellar body secretion, while blue light blocked it. These results indicate that visible radiation affects skin barrier homeostasis. That is, epidermal keratinocytes appear to have a sensory system for visible radiation.

Rhodopsin is a well-known photosensitive protein found in rod cells of the retina and detects light/dark contrast. Cone opsins are also photosensitive receptors in the cone cells of the retina and detect color. We carried out immunochemical studies using antirhodopsin and antiopsin antibodies on human skin [107]. Both mouse retina and human epidermis showed clear immunoreactivity with each antibody. Interestingly, immunoreactivity against longer-wavelength opsin antibody was observed in the basal layer of the epidermis, while immunoreactivity against rhodopsin and shorter-wavelength opsin was observed in the upper layer. PCR analysis confirmed the expression of rhodopsin- and opsin-like genes in both human retina and skin. These results suggest that a series of proteins, which play a crucial role in visual perception, are expressed in human epidermis.

In retina, transducin and phosphodiesterase 6 play key roles in signal transmission. Thus, we hypothesized that these proteins might exist in epidermal keratinocytes and be associated with barrier homeostasis. Immunohistochemical studies and reverse transcription-PCR assays confirmed the expression of both transducin and phosphodiesterase 6 in epidermal keratinocytes [52]. Topical application of 3-isobutyl-1-methylxanthine, a nonspecific phosphodiesterase inhibitor, blocked the acceleration of the barrier recovery by red light. Topical application of zaprinast, a specific inhibitor of phosphodiesterases 5 and 6, also blocked the acceleration, while T0156, a specific inhibitor of phosphodiesterase 5, had no effect. Red-light exposure reduced the epidermal hyperplasia induced by barrier disruption under low humidity, and the effect was blocked by pretreatment with zaprinast. These results indicate that phosphodiesterase 6 is involved in the recovery-accelerating effect of red light on the disrupted epidermal permeability barrier and that epidermal keratinocytes have a similar energy conversion system to the retina.

In our studies described above, we focused only on the effect of visible light on epidermal barrier homeostasis. However, several other reports have described nonvisual photoreceptors. Reptiles have photoreceptors in the brain, and they form the parietal eye [99]. Several photoreceptors were found in pineal body of chicken and rat [86, 125]. However, in humans, the pineal body is located in a deeper area of the brain. On the other hand, exposure to bright light was shown to influence the circadian rhythm of blind patients [16]. This result suggested the existence of a photosensitive system on the surface of the human body. Thus, visible light might influence endocrinological condition via photoreceptor proteins and the energy transduction system in epidermal keratinocytes.

6.7 Electrical Potential

Nishimura demonstrated that cultured human keratinocytes migrate to the negative pole in direct-current electrical fields [84]. This result suggested that keratinocytes might have a sensory system for the external electrical field. Thus, we hypothesized that external electrical potential would influence epidermal barrier homeostasis. We applied negative and positive electrical potential (0.5 V) to the hairless mice flank skin immediately after barrier disruption for 1 h and evaluated barrier recovery by the measurement of transepidermal water loss. At the area where negative potential was applied, the barrier recovery rate was significantly accelerated, while the recovery was delayed at the area where positive potential was applied [22].

Subsequently, we demonstrated that several interfacial electrical conditions also affect barrier homeostasis. For example, topical application of barium sulfate or aqueous solution of ionic polymers formed an electrical double layer on the skin surface and affected the barrier recovery rate [37, 48]. Moreover, the barrier recovery was accelerated just by placing metals on the skin surface after barrier disruption, presumably because free electrons were supplied from metal to the skin surface [23]. When chemically different materials are in contact, electrochemical phenomena, such as formation of an electrical double layer, would be induced. We previously demonstrated that voltage-gated calcium channels are expressed in the upper layer of the epidermis [38]. Thus, when the skin touches other materials, physiological phenomena might be induced.

The mechanism through which skin surface electrical potential influences epidermal permeability barrier homeostasis was not clarified. However, one of the important steps of the barrier recovery is the phase transition of the lipid bilayer when the lamellar bodies fuse with the cell membrane. The electrical field at the surface of the skin might affect the phase transition.

On the other hand, skin surface electrical potential is considered to reflect the pathophysiological condition of the epidermis [70]. Skin surface electrical potential has long been recognized as a parameter of emotional state [82], and it was believed that sweat glands generated the potential [115]. However, Baker et al. reported that not only sweat glands but also epidermis produced the potential [7]. Moreover, we observed skin surface electrical potential in a hairless skin organ culture, which does not have any sweat glands [32], and we showed that the potential was influenced by modulators of ion pumps and channels [32]. These results indicated that ion dynamics in the epidermis generates the skin surface potential.

Maintenance of an ion gradient, especially of calcium, is strongly associated with epidermal homeostasis [45]. The concentration of calcium is highest in the uppermost region of the epidermis (the epidermal granular layer) in healthy normal skin, and the gradient disappears immediately after barrier disruption in mice and humans [30, 78]. Abnormal calcium gradients in the epidermis have been observed in a variety of skin diseases [47]. Thus, we hypothesized that skin surface electrical potential might be a good indicator of calcium gradation in the epidermis. In healthy skin, calcium ions were localized in the uppermost epidermis, and the calcium gradient disappeared upon tape stripping. Skin surface potential also disappeared after tape stripping. Moreover, environmental humidity affected the potential, whereas temporary hydration of the stratum corneum had no effect. These results suggest that the skin surface electrical potential may be an indicator of the pathophysiology of the living layer of epidermis, and thus may be useful as a new parameter to evaluate skin condition [70]. Further, the calcium gradient in the epidermis disappears in aged skin [36, 47] and in experimentally induced dry skin [48, 68]. We recently demonstrated that aging and surfactant treatment also influence skin surface electrical potential [71]. The skin surface electrical potential was significantly increased after sodium dodecyl sulfate treatment, and the alteration was much more marked than that of transepidermal water loss (TEWL). Further, a significant difference in skin surface electrical potential was observed between young and aged volunteers, whereas there was no significant difference in TEWL between the two groups. These results are all consistent with the idea that skin surface electrical potential may be a good indicator of the pathophysiological state of the living layer of epidermis.

6.8 Oxygen

Keratinocytes express proteins that influence the level of erythropoietin synthesis. Hypoxia-inducible factor (HIF) recognizes the level of oxygen, and when the level of oxygen is decreased, erythropoietin synthesis is increased. Von Hippal–Lindau factor (VHL) perturbs the function of HIF. Keratinocyte-specific HIF knockout mice have a decreased level of erythropoietin in the blood, while VHL knockout mice have an increased level of erythropoietin in the blood [10]. Thus, the level of erythropoietin, i.e., the number of red blood cells in the blood, is influenced not only by respiration but also by the oxygen level at the surface of the skin. Another study confirmed that keratinocytes synthesize erythropoietin [97].

Thus, epidermal keratinocytes might sense the environmental concentration of oxygen and be involved in appropriately modulating the number of red blood cells in the blood.

6.9 Endogenous Factors

Epidermal keratinocytes are also influenced by endogenous factors, such as hormones. Previously, we demonstrated that emotional stress delayed epidermal permeability barrier recovery after disruption [29, 31]. In that study, we also demonstrated that glucocorticoid in the serum plays an important role as a mediator of emotional stress. Another "stress hormone," testosterone, delayed the barrier recovery [66]. We also demonstrated that topical application of sex hormones influenced barrier homeostasis [105]. Application of androgen (testosterone or androsterone) delayed the barrier recovery, and the delay was overcome by application of beta-estradiol. Progesterone also delayed the barrier recovery, but in this case, the delay was enhanced by beta-estradiol. These results indicated that epidermal keratinocytes might have sensory systems that respond to hormones.

As described above, skin surface electrical potential is influenced by emotional condition [82]. Thus, we hypothesized that signals from the brain or peripheral nervous system might affect the skin surface potential. To test this idea, we evaluated the skin surface electric potential of cultured skin of hairless mouse [32] and demonstrated that application of substance P and corticotropin-releasing factor influenced the potential. These results suggested that hormones from the brain and/or peptides from the nervous system might be sensed by epidermal keratinocytes.

The epidermis is the interface between the environment and body systems, and since epidermal keratinocytes can sense not only environmental factors but also endogenous factors, they may broadly responsive to, and reflective of, our whole body physiology and emotional condition.

6.10 Chemical Stimuli

As described above, many TRPs are activated by chemical stimuli. TRPV1 is activated by protons (pH<5.4) and capsaicin [104]. TRPV3 in epidermal keratinocytes is activated by oregano, thyme, and clove-derived flavor components, such as carvacrol, eugenol, and thymol [121]. Interestingly, TRPV3 in epidermal keratinocytes is activated by camphor, whereas TRPV3 in sensory neurons is not [80]. Thus, TRPV3 in epidermal keratinocytes might be a sensor of these herbal extracts. TRPM8 was activated by menthol [90], and TRPA1 was activated by allyl isothiocyanate and cinnamaldehyde [8, 65]. TRPA1 was also activated by acidicity and alkalinity [44].

We previously demonstrated that a variety of neurotransmitter receptors, originally found in the nervous system, are expressed in epidermal keratinocytes [39]. Several amino acids, e.g., glutamate, glycine, serine, and alanine, are agonists of these receptors. That is, keratinocytes can sense amino acids.

6.11 Pain and Itching

Recently, many reports have suggested that TRP family members might be strongly associated with pain and/or itching. In particular, TRPV1 and TRPA1 have attracted attention as potential target of pain relief strategies [89]. As described above, TRPV1 was activated by heat, low pH, and capsaicin [103]. That study was carried out with nerve cells, but epidermal keratinocytes also have these receptors (Fig. 6.3). For example, activation of TRPV1 by the agonist capsaicin induced dose-dependent increases of cyclooxygenase-2, interleukin-8, and prostaglandin 2 expression in HaCaT

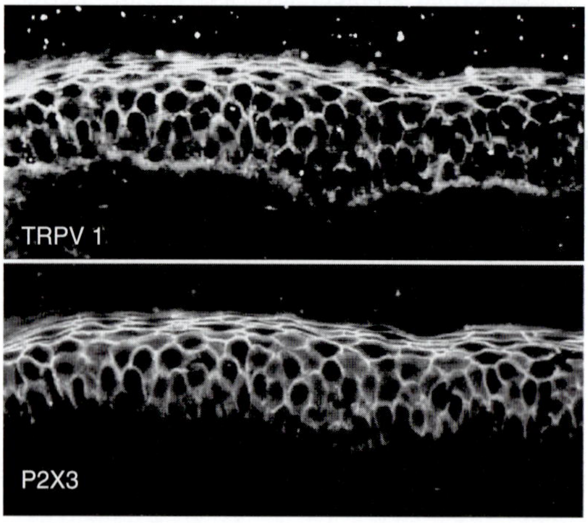

Fig. 6.3 Expressions of "pain" receptors in human epidermis. TRPV1 is strongly expressed in the uppermost and basal layers of the epidermis. P2X3 is strongly expressed in the upper area of the epidermis (Denda 2001c) [34]

keratinocytes, and these increases were blocked by capsazepine, a specific antagonist of TRPV1 [100]. Matrix metalloproteinase-1 (MMP-1) induces collagen degradation and inflammatory responses. Activation of TRPV1 by heat induced MMP-1 mRNA and protein in a temperature-dependent manner in human keratinocytes [75]. This response was blocked by capsazepine. Moreover, knockdown of TRPV1 decreased MMP-1 expression in keratinocytes. Thus, TRPV1 might be associated with skin inflammatory responses. Ultraviolet (UV) radiation appears to induce the expression of TRPV1 in human epidermal keratinocytes [73]; acute UV radiation increased TRPV1 in human skin, and moreover, TRPV1 expression in sun-exposed skin was significantly higher than that in sun-protected skin. They also demonstrated that UV radiation induced matrix metalloproteinase-1 in cultured HaCaT cells [74].

TRPA1 was activated by low temperature and by a variety of pungent chemicals such as isothiocyanate (present in horseradish and mustard), allicin (present in garlic), and bradykinin [8, 65, 77]. Moreover, TRPA1 mediated aldehyde-evoked pain [9, 79]. Although these studies carried out in nerve cells, we recently demonstrated that application of isothiocyanate and cinnamaldehyde in cultured human keratinocytes induced elevation of intracellular calcium [108]. Thus, epidermal keratinocytes might be associated with pain induced by pungent compounds.

Previous study demonstrated that there was a significant difference in brain processing of histamine-induced itch between patients with atopic dermatitis and healthy subjects [63]. The result suggested that brain activity of acute itch in atopic dermatitis might be different from in healthy subject. Recent study demonstrated that TRPA1 and mas-related G-protein-coupled receptor were associated with histamine-independent itch [120]. Studies of these receptors would be necessary for the understanding of histamine-independent itch such as acute itch of atopic dermatitis.

Steinhoff and Biro suggested that TRPV3 might play an important role in itching [101]. A previous study had suggested that TRPV3 was involved in inflammatory responses, pain, and itching sensation [124]. Asakawa et al. showed that mutation at Gly573 in the TRPV3 gene is associated with defective hair growth and dermatitis in mice [2]. It has been speculated that TRPV3^{Gly573Ser} mutation is a cause of pruritus and dermatitis [124].

We reported that topical application of unsaturated fatty acid induced abnormal keratinocyte differentiation and barrier dysfunction [68]. We also found that application of unsaturated fatty acid to cultured human keratinocytes induced elevation of intracellular calcium. Hu et al. showed that elevation of intracellular calcium was induced by unsaturated fatty acids in TRPV3-expressing oocytes [57]. TRPV3 might be associated with abnormal keratinization induced by unsaturated fatty acids, such as comedogenesis.

Another interesting receptor was also found in epidermal keratinocytes. In the nervous system, two distinct families of ATP receptors exist [11]. One is the P2X family, the members of which are ligand-gated ion channels, and the other is the P2Y family of metabotropic, heptahelical G-protein-coupled receptors. P2X3 was first demonstrated as a pain receptor in the peripheral nervous system [15]. In the case of tissue injury, ATP is released and activates P2X3 receptors. Thus, P2X3 was first recognized as a pain receptor in the case of inflammation. We found that P2X3 is expressed in human epidermal keratinocytes (Fig. 6.2). The expression of P2X3 was greater in the upper area of the epidermis. We demonstrated that P2X3 was produced at the terminal differentiation state in a keratinocyte culture system [62]. Thus, at the uppermost layer of the epidermis, P2X3 might play an important role as a mediator of pain or itching induced by ATP secreted from inflammatory tissue.

Recent work suggested that protease-activated receptors in peripheral nerves might be associated with itching [1]. On the other hand, another study demonstrated that protease-activated receptor 2 was expressed in epidermal keratinocytes and was associated with permeability barrier homeostasis [53]. We previously demonstrated that topical application of a serine-type protease inhibitor accelerated barrier recovery and also prevented epidermal hyperplasia induced by repeated barrier disruption [26]. Modulation of proteases in the epidermis might be another target to treat itching or sensitive skin.

As described above, a variety of receptors, considered to be mediators of pain or itching, are expressed in epidermal keratinocytes. Thus, epidermal keratinocytes might be strongly associated with unpleasant skin sensations, and further research on such receptors in keratinocytes might be important for clinical dermatology.

6.12 Peripheral Circulation

We recently demonstrated that epidermal keratinocytes influence the peripheral circulation [60]. The source of nitric oxide (NO) in the cutaneous circulation remains controversial. We have found that barrier disruption induced NO secretion from epidermis [59]. Thus, we hypothesized that epidermal cells might generate NO in response to mechanical stimulation [60]. In hairless mouse skin organ culture, mechanical stimulation resulted in NO release, which declined within 30 min after cessation of stimulation. Similar NO release occurred from a reconstructed skin model containing only keratinocytes and fibroblasts and was suppressed after detachment of the epidermal layer. Moreover, the stimulation-induced NO release was significantly lower in skin organ culture of neuronal NO synthase knockout (nNOS-KO) mice, compared with wild-type (WT) mice. Mechanical stimulation of skin organ cultures of HR-1, nNOS-KO, endothelial NOS-KO (eNOS-KO), and WT mice caused enlargement of cutaneous lymphatic vessels. The enlargement was significantly lower after detachment of the epidermal layer than for normal skin samples and was significantly lower for nNOS-KO than for WT mice. Skin blood flow in nNOS-KO mice after stimulation was significantly lower than in WT mice. eNOS-KO mice also showed lower responses than WT mice, and the difference was similar to that in the case of nNOS-KO mice. These results are consistent with the idea that NO generated by epidermal nNOS plays a significant role in the cutaneous circulatory response to mechanical stimulation.

6.13 Multilayered Organization of Epidermal Keratinocytes

As mentioned above, differentiated keratinocytes were more sensitive to mechanical stimuli [51]. Moreover, cell-cell connection via gap junctions was more marked at the upper layer of the epidermis [112]. On the other hand, sensitivity to ATP, an important second messenger in the epidermis, was higher in undifferentiated keratinocytes in the culture system and at the bottom layer of the epidermis in skin slices [106]. Those results suggested that the superficial layer of the epidermis is a good sensor of external mechanical stimuli, while signals such as ATP released from the upper layer of the epidermis are sensed more efficiently at the bottom layer of the epidermis, where peripheral nerve endings are located.

As regards low temperature, undifferentiated keratinocytes were more sensitive to cold than differentiated cells [108]. On the other hand, there was no significant difference between the responses of undifferentiated and differentiated keratinocytes to high temperature [111]. These results indicate that, although the superficial layer of the epidermis might be less sensitive to low temperature than the deeper layer, the response to high temperature is homogeneous throughout the epidermis. TRPV1 is activated not only by high temperature but also by low pH or chemical stimuli, such as capsaicin [13, 104]. Thus, TRPV1 might function throughout the epidermis as a multimodal sensor. On the other hand, TRPA1 might be involved in homeostasis of internal organs, and this would be consistent with localization in a deeper layer of the epidermis.

Generally, expression levels of proteins in the upper layer of the epidermis are different from those in the bottom layer, i.e., keratinocytes express different proteins, or at least different levels of proteins, depending on their differentiation state. Thus, epidermis is not a homogeneous tissue but is a multilayered organ, like the brain. One of its functions is to form a water-impermeable barrier. However, the variation of sensitivity to external or endogenous factors with depth in the epidermis suggests that the multilayer

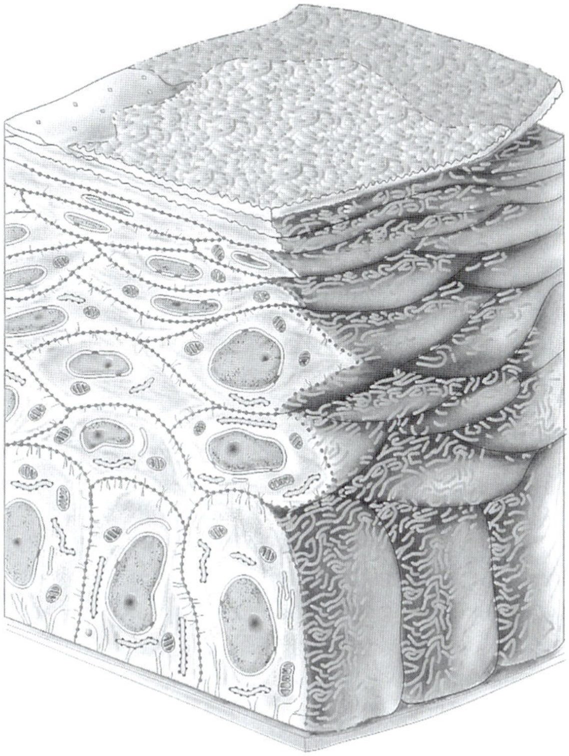

Fig. 6.4 Multilayered organization of epidermal keratinocytes. The uppermost layer of the epidermis might be more sensitive to mechanical stimuli than the deeper layer [51], and there is cell-cell communication via gap junctions at the upper layer of the epidermis [112]. On the other hand, the deeper layer of the epidermis is more sensitive to ATP than the upper layer [106]. The deeper layer of the epidermis might be more sensitive to cold than the upper layer [108] (Arranged from figure by Sakura Kogeisha Co. Ltd)

structure would provide a sophisticated and flexible sensory system (Fig. 6.4).

6.14 Potential Sensory Functions of Epidermal Keratinocytes

As described above, epidermal keratinocytes have a variety of sensory systems for environmental factors. Thus, they might play an important role in regulating whole body homeostasis in a constantly changing environment, especially considering that they cover the whole body. Moreover, epidermal keratinocytes are constantly being renewed. That is, their sensory systems might be well maintained at consistent levels of sensitivity.

Epidermal keratinocytes also have a series of neurotransmitter receptors, which play a crucial role in information processing in the brain and nervous systems [39]. In the brain, information processing is carried out via excitation and inhibition processes. Similar processes have also been observed in epidermal keratinocytes [49]. Although the meaning and role of these processes in keratinocytes remain to be fully clarified, the epidermis seems to have the potential for high-level information processing.

Epidermal keratinocytes also generate a variety of neurotransmitters, neuropeptides, and hormones. It has been long recognized that many of these molecules are produced in the brain. For example, a recent study indicated that the neuropeptide hormone oxytocin influences human emotion [83]. Originally, oxytocin was thought to be generated in the hypophysis cerebri. However, we recently discovered that epidermal keratinocytes also generate oxytocin (Denda, unpublished data). Thus, stimulation of the epidermis, e.g., massage, might induce oxytocin release and influence human emotional state.

Cortisol is well known as a stress hormone and plays an important role in suppression of the immune system. It has been long recognized that cortisol is produced by the adrenal gland. Under stress conditions, corticotropin-releasing hormone is released from hypothalamus and induces secretion of adrenocorticotropic hormone (ACTH). However, it was recently demonstrated that epidermal keratinocytes also produce cortisol [117]. Tissue injury and IL-1beta secretion trigger cortisol generation in the epidermis. Thus, epidermal injury might induce the same physiological response as emotional stress.

The functions of the brain include information sensing, processing, and regulation of the whole body system via neuropeptides and hormones. On the other hand, epidermal keratinocytes have a variety of sensory systems, neurotransmitter receptors, and the ability to generate neurotransmitters, neuropeptides, and hormones. Thus, one could consider that the epidermis is an extension of the brain to the surface of our body.

Life is a nonequilibrium, open system. At the border between the living body and the environment, energy flow and information flow are controlled to maintain homeostatic processes [12] and to maintain high-order architecture and function in the body. For multicellular animals, the skin, and in particular the epidermis, forms the boundary of the body. Therefore, it seems to be a reasonable hypothesis that epidermal keratinocytes contain a variety of sensory systems that can respond to the ever-changing environment, and that the resulting information would be processed in the epidermis via a series of neurotransmitters and receptors, and passed to the brain and central nervous system to contribute to whole body homeostasis and modulation of emotional state. Indeed, there is accumulating evidence that this is the case. It seems likely that further research will continue to extend the range of sensory and functional capabilities of epidermal keratinocytes and the skin.

Take Home Messages

- Epidermal keratinocytes express a series of thermo-activated receptors, called the transient receptor potential (TRP) family.
- The TRP proteins in epidermal keratinocytes may serve as sensors not only of environmental temperature but also of humidity, mechanical stress, and chemical stimuli.
- Photoreceptor proteins (rhodopsin and opsin) and energy-transfer proteins (transducin and phosphodiesterase 6), which are expressed in retina, are also expressed in keratinocytes and appear to influence epidermal barrier homeostasis.
- Epidermal barrier homeostasis is influenced by sound in the 10–30 kHz range.
- External electrical potential and materials that produce an electrical double layer influence barrier homeostasis.
- Epidermal keratinocytes are involved in peripheral circulation and red blood cell generation.
- Epidermal barrier homeostasis is influenced by several sex hormones.
- Itching or skin sensitivity may be caused by interaction between keratinocytes and the peripheral nervous system.

References

1. Akiyama T, Carstens MI, Carstens E (2010) Enhanced scratching evoked by PAR-2 agonist and 5-HT but not histamine in a mouse model of chronic dry skin itch. Pain 151:378–383
2. Asakawa M, Yoshioka T, Matsutani T et al (2006) Association of a mutation in TRPV3 with defective hair growth in rodents. J Invest Dermatol 126:2664–2672
3. Ashida Y, Denda M (2003) Dry environment increases mast cell number and histamine content in dermis in hairless mice. Br J Dermatol 149:240–247
4. Ashida Y, Ogo M, Denda M (2001) Epidermal IL-1 alpha generation is amplified at low humidities: implications for the pathogenesis of inflammatory dermatoses. Br J Dermatol 144:238–243
5. Athenstaedt H, Claussen H, Schaper D (1982) Epidermis of human skin: pyroelectric and piezoelectric sensor layer. Science 216:1018–1020
6. Atoyan R, Shander D, Botchkarvera NV (2009) Non-neural expression of transient receptor potential type A1 (TRPA1) in human skin. J Invest Dermatol 129:2312–2315
7. Baker AT, Jaffe LE, Vanable JW (1982) The glabrous epidermis of cavies confaius a powerful battery. Am J Physiol 242:R358–R366
8. Bandell M, Story GM, Hwang SW, Viswanath V, Eid SR, Petrus MJ, Earley TJ, Patapoutian A (2004) Noxious cold ion channel TRPA1 is activated by pungent compounds and bradykinin. Neuron 41:849–857

9. Bang S, Kim KY, Yoo S, Kim YG, Hwang SW (2007) Transient receptor potential A1 mediates acetaldehyde-evoked pain sensation. Eur J Neurosci 26: 2516–2523
10. Boutin AT, Weidemann A, Fu Z, Mesropian L, Gradin K, Jamora C, Wiesener M, Eckardt KU, Koch CJ, Ellies LG, Haddad G, Haase VH, Simon MC, Poellinger L, Powell FL, Johnson RS (2008) Epidermal sensing of oxygen is essential for systemic hypoxic response. Cell 133:223–234
11. Burnstock G, Williams M (2000) P2 purinergic receptors: modulation of cell function and therapeutic potential. J Pharmacol Exp Ther 295:862–869
12. Camazine S, Deneubourg JL, Franks NR, Sneyd J, Theraulaz G, Bonabeau E (2001) Characteristics of self-organizing systems. In: Anderson PW et al (eds) Self-organization in biological systems. Princeton University Press, Princeton, pp 29–46
13. Caterina MJ, Schumacher MA, Tominaga M, Rosen TA, Levine JD, Julius D (1997) The capsaicin receptor: a heat-activated ion channel in the pain pathway. Nature 389:816–824
14. Chung MK, Lee H, Caterina MJ (2003) Warm temperatures activate TRPV4 in mouse 308 keratinocytes. J Biol Chem 278:32037–32046
15. Cockayne MJ, Hamilton SG, Zhu QM, Dunn PM, Zhone Y, Novakovic S, Malmberg AB, Cain G, Berson A, Kassotakis L, Hedley L, Lachnit WG, Burnstocks G, McMason SB, Ford APDW (2000) Urinary bladder hyporeflexia and reduced pain-related behavior in P2X3-deficient mice. Nature 407:1011–1015
16. Czeisler CA, Shanahan TL, Klerman EB, Martens H, Brotman DJ, Jonathan SE, Klein T, Rizzo JF (1995) Suppression of melatonin secretion in some blind patients by exposure to bright light. N Eng J Med 332:6–11
17. Damasio AR (1994) The body-minded brain. In: Descartes' error. Emotion, reason, and the human brain. Penguin Putnam, New York, pp 223–243
18. Denda M (2000) Influence of dry environment on epidermal function. J Dermatol Sci 24(Suppl 1):S22–S28
19. Denda M (2001) Epidermal proliferative response induced by sodium dodecyl sulphate varies with environmental humidity. Br J Dermatol 145:252–257
20. Denda M, Denda S (2007) Air-exposed keratinocytes exhibited intracellular oscillation. Skin Res Technol 13:195–201
21. Denda M, Fuziwara S (2008) Visible radiation affects epidermal permeability barrier recovery: selective effects of red and blue light. J Invest Dermatol 128:1335–1336
22. Denda M, Kumazawa N (2002) Negative electric potential induces epidermal lamellar body secretion and accelerates skin barrier recovery after barrier disruption. J Invest Dermatol 118:65–72
23. Denda M, Kumazawa N (2010) Effects of metals on skin permeability barrier recovery. Exp Dermatol 19:e124–e127
24. Denda M, Nakatani M (2010) Acceleration of permeability barrier recovery by exposure of skin to 10–30 kilohertz sound. Br J Dermatol 162:503–507
25. Denda M, Tsutsumi M (2011) Roles of transient receptor potential proteins (TRPs) in epidermal keratinocytes. In: Islam MS (ed) Transient receptor potential channels. Advances in experimental medicine and biology, vol 704. Springer, Berlin, pp 847–860
26. Denda M, Kitamura K, Elias PM, Feingold KR (1997) Trans-4-(aminomethyl)cyclohexane carboxylic acid (t-AMCHA), an anti-fibrinolytic agent, accelerates barrier recovery and prevents the epidermal hyperplasia induced by epidermal injury in hairless mice and humans. J Invest Dermatol 109:84–90
27. Denda M, Sato J, Masuda Y, Tsuchiya T, Kuramoto M, Elias PM, Feingold KR (1998) Exposure to a dry environment enhances epidermal permeability barrier function. J Invest Dermatol 111:858–863
28. Denda M, Sato J, Tsuchiya T, Elias PM, Feingold KR (1998) Low humidity stimulates epidermal DNA synthesis and amplifies the hyperproliferative response to barrier disruption: implication for seasonal exacerbations of inflammatory dermatoses. J Invest Dermatol 111:873–878
29. Denda M, Tshuchiya T, Hosoi J, Koyama J (1998) Immobilization-induced and crowded environment-induced stress delay barrier recovery in murine skin. Br J Dermatol 138:780–785
30. Denda M, Hosoi J, Ashida Y (2000) Visual imaging of ion distribution in human epidermis. Biochem Biophys Res Commun 272:134–137
31. Denda M, Tsuchiya T, Elias PM, Feingold KR (2000) Stress alters cutaneous permeability barrier homeostasis. Am J Physiol 278:R367–R372
32. Denda M, Ashida Y, Inoue K, Kumazawa K (2001) Skin surface electric potential induced by ion-flux through epidermal cell layers. Biochem Biophys Res Commun 284:112–117
33. Denda M, Fuziwara S, Inoue K, Denda S, Akamatsu H, Tomitaka A, Matsunaga K (2001) Immunoreactivity of VR1 on epidermal keratinocyte of human skin. Biochem Biophys Res Commun 285:1250–1252
34. Denda M, Inoue K, Fuziwara S et al (2002) P2X purinergic receptor antagonist accelerates skin barrier repair and prevents epidermal hyperplasia induced by skin barrier disruption. J Invest Dermatol 119:1034–1040
35. Denda M, Fuziwara S, Inoue K (2003) Influx of calcium and chloride ions into epidermal keratinocytes regulates exocytosis of epidermal lamellar bodies and skin permeability barrier homeostasis. J Invest Dermatol 121:362–367
36. Denda M, Tomitaka M, Akamatsu H, Matsunaga K (2003) Altered distribution of calcium in facial epidermis of aged adults. J Invest Dermatol 21: 1557–1558
37. Denda M, Nakanishi K, Kumazawa N (2005) Topical application of ionic polymers affects skin permeability barrier homeostasis. Skin Pharmacol Physiol 18:36–41
38. Denda M, Fuziwara S, Hibino T (2006) Expression of voltage-gated calcium channel subunit αC1 in epidermal keratinocytes and effects of agonist and antagonists of the channel on skin barrier homeostasis. Exp Dermatol 15:455–460

39. Denda M, Nakatani M, Ikeyama K, Tsutsumi M, Denda S (2007) Epidermal keratinocytes as the forefront of the sensory system. Exp Dermatol 16:157–161
40. Denda M, Sokabe T, Tominaga T, Tominaga M (2007) Effects of skin surface temperature on epidermal permeability barrier homeostasis. J Invest Dermatol 127:654–659
41. Denda M, Tsutsumi M, Denda S (2010) Topical application of TRPM8 agonists accelerates skin permeability barrier recovery and reduces epidermal proliferation induced by barrier insult: the role of cold-sensitive TRP receptors in epidermal permeability barrier homeostasis. Exp Dermatol 19:791–795
42. Denda M, Tsutsumi M, Goto M, Ikeyama K, Denda S (2010) Topical application of TRPA1 agonists and brief cold exposure accelerate skin permeability barrier recovery. J Invest Dermatol 130:1942–1945
43. Dhaka A, Viswanath V, Patapoutian A (2006) TRP ion channels and temperature sensation. Annu Rev Neurosci 29:135–161
44. Dhaka A, Uzzell V, Dubin AE, Mathur J, Petrus M, Bandell M, Patapoutian A (2009) TRPV1 is activated by both acidic and basic pH. J Neurosci 29:153–158
45. Elias PM, Ahn SK, Denda M, Brown BE, Crumurine D, Kinutai LK, Komuves L, Lee SH, Feingold KR (2002) Modulations in epidermal calcium regulate the expression of differentiation-specific proteins. J Invest Dermatol 119:1128–1136
46. Feldman Y, Puzenko A, Ben Ishai P et al (2008) Human skin as arrays of helical antennas in the millimeter and submillimeter wave range. Phys Rev Lett 100:128102
47. Forslind B, Werner-Linde Y, Lindberg M, Pallon J (1999) Elemental analysis mirrors epidermal differentiation. Acta Derm Venereol 79:12–17
48. Fuziwara S, Ogawa K, Aso D, Yoshizawa D, Takata S, Denda M (2004) Barium sulfate with a negative ζ potential accelerates skin permeable barrier recovery and prevents epidermal hyperplasia induced by barrier disruption. Br J Dermatol 151:557–564
49. Fuziwara S, Suzuki A, Inoue K, Denda M (2005) Dopamine D2-like receptor agonists accelerate barrier repair and inhibit the epidermal hyperplasia induced by barrier disruption. J Invest Dermatol 125:783–789
50. Gick B, Derrick D (2009) Aero-tactile integration in speech perception. Nature 462:502–504
51. Goto M, Ikeyama K, Tsutsumi M, Denda S, Denda M (2010) Calcium ion propagation in cultured keratinocytes and other cells in skin in response to hydraulic pressure stimulation. J Cell Physiol 224:229–233
52. Goto M, Ikeyama K, Tsutsumi M, Denda S, Denda M (2011) Phosphodiesterase inhibitors block the acceleration of skin permeability barrier repair by red light. Exp Dermatol 20:568–571
53. Hachem JP, Houben E, Crumrine D, Man MQ, Schurer N, Roelandt T, Choi EH, Uchida Y, Brown BE, Feingold KR, Elias PM (2006) Serine protease signaling of epidermal permeability barrier homeostasis. J Invest Dermatol 126:2074–2086
54. Heffner RS (2004) Primate hearing from a mammalian perspective. Anat Rec A Discov Mol Cell Evol Biol 281:1111–1122
55. Hosoi J, Hariya T, Denda M, Tsuchiya T (2000) Regulation of the cutaneous allergic reaction by humidity. Contact Dermatitis 42:81–84
56. Hu HZ, Gu Q, Wang C, Colton CK, Tang J, Kinoshita-Kawada M, Lee LY, Wood JD, Zhu MX (2004) 2-aminoethoxydiphenyl borate is a common activator of TRPV1, TRPV2, and TRPV3. J Biol Chem 279: 35741–35748
57. Hu HZ, Xiao R, Wang C et al (2006) Potentiation of TRPV3 channel function by unsaturated fatty acids. J Cell Physiol 208:201–212
58. Huang SM, Lee H, Chung MK et al (2008) Overexpressed transient receptor potential vanilloid 3 ion channels in skin keratinocytes modulate pain sensitivity via prostaglandin E2. J Neurosci 28:13727–13737
59. Ikeyama K, Fuziwara S, Denda M (2007) Topical application of neuronal nitric oxide synthase inhibitor accelerates cutaneous barrier recovery and prevents epidermal hyperplasia induced by barrier disruption. J Invest Dermatol 127:1713–1719
60. Ikeyama K, Denda S, Tsutsumi M, Denda M (2010) Neuronal nitric oxide synthase in epidermis is involved in cutaneous circulatory response to mechanical stimulation. J Invest Dermatol 130:1158–1166
61. Inoue K, Koizumi S, Fuziwara S, Denda S, Inoue K, Denda M (2002) Functional vanilloid receptors in cultured normal human keratinocytes. Biochem Biophys Res Commun 291:124–129
62. Inoue K, Denda M, Tozaki H, Fujishita K, Koizumi S, Inoue K (2005) Characterization of multiple P2X receptors in cultured normal human epidermal keratinocytes. J Invest Dermatol 124:756–763
63. Ishiuji Y, Coghill RC, Patel TS, Oshiro Y, Kraft RA, Yosipovitch G (2009) Distinct patterns of brain activity evoked by histamine-induced itch reveal an association with itch intensity and disease severity in atopic dermatitis. Br J Dermatol 161:1072–1080
64. Johansson RS, Trulsson M, Olsson KA, Westberg K-G (1988) Mechanoreceptor activity from the human face and oral mucosa. Exp Brain Res 72:204–208
65. Jordt SE, Bautista DM, Chuang HH, McKemy DD, Zygmunt PM, Högestätt ED, Meng ID, Julius D (2004) Mustard oils and cannabinoids excite sensory nerve fibres through the TRP channel ANKTM1. Nature 427:260–265
66. Kao JS, Garg A, Mao-Qiang M, Crumrine D, Ghadially R, Feingold KR, Elias PM (2001) Testosterone perturbs epidermal permeability barrier homeostasis. J Invest Dermatol 116:443–451
67. Katagiri C, Sato J, Nomura J, Denda M (2003) Changes in environmental humidity affect the water-holding property of the stratum corneum and its free amino acid content, and the expression of filaggrin in the epidermis of hairless mice. J Dermatol Sci 31:29–35
68. Katsuta Y, Iida T, Inomata S et al (2005) Unsaturated fatty acids induce calcium influx into keratinocytes

and cause abnormal differentiation of epidermis. J Invest Dermatol 124:1008–1013
69. Kawai N, Honda M, Nakamura S et al (2001) Catecholamines and opioid peptides increase in plasma in humans during possession trances. Neuroreport 12:3419–3423
70. Kawai E, Nakanishi J, Kumazawa N, Ozawa K, Denda M (2008) Skin surface electric potential as an indicator of skin condition: a new, non-invasive method to evaluate epidermal condition. Exp Dermatol 17: 688–692
71. Kawai E, Kumazawa N, Ozawa K, Denda M (2011) Skin surface electrical potential as an indicator of skin condition: observation of surfactant-induced dry skin and middle-aged skin. Exp Dermatol 20:757–759
72. Koizumi S, Fijishita K, Inoue K, Shigemoto-Mogami Y, Tsuda M, Inoue K (2004) Ca2+ waves in keratinocytes are transmitted to sensory neurons: the involvement of extracellular ATP and P2Y2 receptor activation. Biochem J 380:329–338
73. Lee YM, Kim YK, Chung JH (2009) Increased expression of TRPV1 channel in intrinsically aged and photoaged human skin in vivo. Exp Dermatol 18:431–436
74. Lee YM, Kim YK, Kim KH et al (2009) A novel role for the TRPV1 channel in UV-induced matrix metalloproteinase (MMP)-1 expression in HaCaT cells. J Cell Physiol 219:766–775
75. Li WH, Lee YM, Kim JY et al (2007) Transient receptor potential vanilloid-1 mediates heat-shock-induced matrix metalloproteinase-1 expression in human epidermal keratinocytes. J Invest Dermatol 127: 2328–2335
76. Loomis JM, Collins CC (1978) Sensitivity to shifts of a point stimulus; an instance of tactile hyperacuity. Percept Psychophys 24:487–492
77. Macpherson LJ, Geierstanger BH, Viswanath V, Bandell M, Eid SR, Hwang S, Patapoutian A (2005) The pungency of garlic: activation of TRPA1 and TRPV1 in response to allicin. Curr Biol 15:929–934
78. Mauro T, Bench G, Sidderas-Haddad E et al (1998) Acute barrier perturbation abolishes the Ca2+ and K+ gradients in murine epidermis: quantitative measurement using PIXE. J Invest Dermatol 111:1198–1201
79. McNamara CR, Mandel-Brehm J, Bautista DM, Siemens J, Deranian KL, Zhao M, Hayward NJ, Chong JA, Julius D, Moran MM, Fanger CM (2007) TRPA1 mediates formalin-induced pain. Proc Natl Acad Sci USA 104:13525–13530
80. Moqrich A, Hwang SW, Earley TJ et al (2005) Impaired thermosensation in mice lacking TRPV3, a heat and camphor sensor in the skin. Science 307:1468–1472
81. Nakatani M, Kawasoe T, Denda M (2011) Sex difference in human fingertip recognition of micron-level randomness as unpleasant. Int J Cosmet Sci 33: 346–350
82. Neuman E, Blanton R (1970) The early history of electrodermal research. Psychophysiology 6: 453–475
83. Neumann ID (2007) Oxytocin: the neuropeptide of love reveals some of its secrets. Cell Metab 5:231–233
84. Nishimura KY, Isseroff RR, Nuccitelli R (1996) Human keratinocytes migrate to the negative pole in direct current electric fields comparable to those measured in mammalian wounds. J Cell Sci 109:199–207
85. Nordin M (1990) Low threshold mechanoreceptive and nociceptive units with unmyelinated (C) fibres in the human supraorbital nerve. J Physiol 426: 229–240
86. Okano T, Yoshizawa T, Fukada Y (1994) Pinopsin is a chicken pineal photoreceptive molecule. Nature 372:94–97
87. Oohashi T, Nishina E, Honda M et al (2000) Inaudible high-frequency sounds affect brain activity: hypersonic effect. J Neurophysiol 83:3548–3558
88. Oohashi T, Kawai N, Nishina E et al (2006) The role of biological system other than auditory air-conduction in the emergence of the hypersonic effect. Brain Res 1073–1074:339–347
89. Patapoutian A, Tate S, Woolf CJ (2009) Transient receptor potential channels: targeting pain at the source. Nat Rev Drug Discov 8:55–68
90. Peier AM, Moqrich A, Hergarden AC et al (2002) A trp channel that senses cold stimuli and menthol. Cell 108:705–715
91. Peier AM, Reeve AJ, Andersson DA, Moqrich A, Earley TJ, Hergarden AC, Story GM, Colley S, Hogenesch JB, McIntyre P, Bevan S, Patapoutian A (2002) A heat-sensitive TRP channel expressed in keratinocytes. Science 296:2046–2049
92. Sato J, Denda M, Ashida Y, Koyama J (1998) Loss of water from the stratum corneum induces epidermal DNA synthesis in hairless mice. Arch Dermatol Res 290:634–637
93. Sato J, Denda M, Nakanishi J (1998) Dry condition affects desquamation of stratum corneum in vivo. J Dermatol Sci 18:163–169
94. Sato J, Yanai M, Hirao T, Denda M (2000) Water content and thickness of stratum corneum contribute to skin surface morphology. Arch Dermatol Res 292:412–417
95. Sato J, Denda M, Chang S, Elias PM, Feingold KR (2002) Abrupt decreases in environmental humidity induce abnormalities in permeability barrier homeostasis. J Invest Dermatol 119:900–904
96. Sauer GC, Hall JC (1996) Seasonal skin diseases. In: Sauer GC, Hall JC (eds) Manual of skin diseases. Lippincott-Raven, Philadelphia, pp 23–28
97. Scheidemann F, Löser M, Niedermeier A, Kromminga A, Therrien JP, Vogel J, Pfützner W (2008) The skin as a biofactory for systemic secretion of erythropoietin: potential of genetically modified keratinocytes and fibroblasts. Exp Dermatol 17:481–488
98. Shephered GM (1994) The somatic senses. In: Shephered GM (ed) Neurobiology. Oxford University Press, Oxford, pp 265–293

99. Solessio E, Engbretson GA (1993) Antagonistic chromatic mechanisms in photoreceptors of the parietal eye of lizards. Nature 364:442–445
100. Southall MD, Li T, Gharibova LS et al (2003) Activation of epidermal vanilloid receptor-1 induces release of proinflammatory mediators in human keratinocytes. J Pharmacol Exp Ther 304:217–222
101. Steinhoff M, Bíró T (2009) A TR(I)P to pruritus research: role of TRPV3 in inflammation and itch. J Invest Dermatol 129:531–535
102. Story GM, Peier AM, Reeve AJ et al (2003) ANKTM1, a TRP-like channel expressed in nociceptive neurons, is activated by cold temperatures. Cell 112:819–829
103. Tominaga M, Caterina MJ (2004) Thermosensation and pain. J Neurobiol 61:3–12
104. Tominaga M, Caterina MJ, Malmberg AB, Rosen TA, Gilbert H, Skinner K, Raumann BE, Basbaum AI, Julius D (1998) The cloned capsaicin receptor integrates multiple pain-producing stimuli. Neuron 21:531–543
105. Tsutsumi M, Denda M (2007) Paradoxical effects of beta-estradiol on epidermal permeability barrier homeostasis. Br J Dermatol 157:776–779
106. Tsutsumi M, Denda S, Inoue K, Ikeyama K, Denda M (2009) Calcium ion gradients and dynamics in cultured skin slices of rat hind-paw in response to stimulation with ATP. J Invest Dermatol 129:584–589
107. Tsutsumi M, Ikeyama K, Denda S, Nakanishi J, Fuziwara S, Aoki H, Denda M (2009) Expressions of rod and cone photoreceptor-like proteins in human epidermis. Exp Dermatol 18:567–570
108. Tsutsumi M, Denda S, Ikeyama K, Goto M, Denda M (2010) Exposure to low temperature induces elevation of intracellular calcium in cultured human keratinocytes. J Invest Dermatol 130:1945–1948
109. Tsutsumi M, Kitahata H, Nakata S, Sanno Y, Nagayama M, Denda M (2010) Mathematical analysis of intercellular calcium propagation induced by ATP. Skin Res Technol 16:146–150
110. Tsutsumi M, Goto M, Denda S, Denda M (2011) Morphological and functional differences in co-culture system of keratinocytes and dorsal root ganglion-derived cells depending on time of seeding. Exp Dermatol 20:464–467
111. Tsutsumi M, Kumamoto J, Denda M (2011) Intracellular calcium response to high temperature is similar in undifferentiated and differentiated cultured human keratinocytes. Exp Dermatol 20:839–840
112. Tsutusmi M, Inoue K, Denda S, Ikeyama K, Goto M, Denda M (2009) Mechanical-stimulation-evoked calcium waves in proliferating and differentiated human keratinocytes. Cell Tissue Res 338:99–106
113. Vallbo A, Olausson H, Wessberg J, Norrsell UA (1993) System of unmyelinated afferents for innocuous mechanoreception in the human skin. Brain Res 628:301–304
114. Vallbo AB, Olausson H, Wessberg J (1999) Unmyelinated afferents constitute a second system coding tactile stimuli of the human hairy skin. J Neurophysiol 81:2753–2763
115. Venables PH, Martin I (1967) The relation of palmar sweat gland activity to level of skin potential and conductance. Psychophysiology 3:302–311
116. Verrillo RT (1979) Change in vibrotactile thresholds as a function of age. Sens Processes 3:49–59
117. Vukelic S, Stojadinovic O, Pastar I, Rabach M, Krzyzanowska A, Lebrun E, Davis SC, Resnik S, Brem H, Tomic-Canic M (2011) Cortisol synthesis in epidermis is induced by IL-1 and tissue injury. J Biol Chem 286:10265–10275
118. Wang L, Hillinges M, Jernberg T, Wiegleb-Edstrom D, Johansson O (1990) Protein gene product 9.5-immunoreactive nerve fibres and cells in human skin. Cell Tissue Res 261:25–33
119. Wilkinson JD, Rycroft RJ (1992) Contact dermatitis. In: Burton JL, Ebling FJG (eds) Champion relative humidity, 5th edn, Textbook of dermatology. Blackwell Scientific Publications, Oxford, pp 614–615
120. Wilson SR, Gerhold KA, Bifolck-Fisher A, Liu Q, Patel KN, Dong X, Bautista DM (2011) TRPA1 is required for histamine-independent. Mas-related G protein-coupled receptor-mediated itch. Nat Neurosci 14:595–602
121. Xu H, Delling M, Jun JC et al (2006) Oregano, thyme and clove-derived flavors and skin sensitizers activate specific TRP channels. Nat Neurosci 9:628–635
122. Yagi R, Nishina E, Honda M et al (2003) Modulatory effect of inaudible high-frequency sounds on human acoustic perception. Neurosci Lett 351:191–195
123. Yamada D, Maeno T, Yamada Y (2002) Artificial finger skin having ridges and distributed tactile sensors used for grasp force control. J Robot Mechatronics 14.140–146
124. Yoshioka T, Imura K, Asakawa M et al (2009) Impact of the Gly573Ser substitution in TRPV3 on the development of allergic and pruritic dermatitis in mice. J Invest Dermatol 129:714–722
125. Zhao X, Haeseleer F, Fariss RN, Huang J, Baehr W, Milam AH, Palczewski K (1997) Molecular cloning and localization of rhodopsin kinase in the mammalian pineal. Vis Neurosci 14:225–232

7 Sensitive Skin: Intrinsic and Extrinsic Contributors

Miranda A. Farage and Michael K. Robinson

7.1 Introduction

Manufacturers of moisturizers and emollients conduct extensive premarket testing to confirm product efficacy and safety, including the potential for these products to irritate the skin. Such goals represent a significant challenge, as today's consumers are a global audience with substantial variability in gender, age, ethnicity, skin type, living environments, and cultural habits. Testing is performed, therefore, with a wide variety of test subjects and conditions to ensure skin compatibility for all consumers. Despite rigorous premarket safety testing, however, some consumers consistently report unpredicted and unpleasant sensory effects related to product use. These purely sensory perceptions, furthermore, influence product sales: 78% of consumers who experience these transient sensory effects report avoiding some products because of the negative sensations evoked [1].

M.A. Farage, Ph.D. (✉)
Clinical Sciences, The Procter & Gamble Company,
Winton Hill Business Center,
6110 Center Hill Rd, P.O. Box 136,
Cincinnati, OH 45224, USA
e-mail: farage.m@pg.com

M.K. Robinson, Ph.D.
Global Biotechnology Division,
Miami Valley Innovation Center,
11810 East Miami River Road,
Cincinnati, Ohio 45252-1038, USA

This phenomenon, originally believed to be an abnormal response to common products afflicting only a small minority of product users, was termed *sensitive skin*, a term defined at that time, as any unpleasant sensory reaction to cosmetics, soaps, lotions, toiletries, or other products upon contact with skin [2]. Although mild and transient physical signs (e.g., erythema, dryness, wheals, or scaling) [3–5] could occasionally accompany the adverse sensory response, more often, the sensations occurred in the absence of any visible signs of irritation [6]. The problem of sensitive skin was therefore viewed with skepticism by many dermatologists and labeled early on as a "princess and the pea" phenomenon, exacerbated by ubiquitous advertising and modern culture and without any real physiological origin [7].

Epidemiological investigations worldwide, however, observe a substantial and steadily increasing prevalence of sensitive skin in the industrialized world (Table 7.1). Currently, the majority of women surveyed believe that they have sensitive skin. The finding of a very similar prevalence in women in two studies on separate continents (69% in the USA [11] compared to 64% in Greece [16]) suggests a genuine physiological disorder. Although the etiology of the disorder is still murky, and meaningful diagnostic tests remain elusive, continuing research is beginning to unravel the physiological basis of this widespread phenomenon. Sensitive skin is now largely recognized as a genuine dermatological condition, one of physiological origin [17] and long duration. A survey of 1,039 subjects found

M. Lodén, H.I. Maibach (eds.), *Treatment of Dry Skin Syndrome*,
DOI 10.1007/978-3-642-27606-4_7,

Table 7.1 Prevalence of sensitive skin perception in women in the industrialized world

Population(s) studied	Population characteristics	Definition of sensitive skin	Percentage of women who claimed sensitive skin	References
Japan, USA, Europe (1992) questionnaire	15,000 men and women	Unusual skin reactivity to specific insult	50% (25% very sensitive skin)	[8]
France (2000) interview	319 women	Cutaneous discomfort in the absence of clinical and histologic evidence of skin lesions	90% (23% very sensitive skin)	[9]
England (2001) questionnaire	3,300 women	Intolerance to cosmetics and toiletries, including both sensory and visible signs	51% (6% very sensitive skin)	[10]
USA (San Francisco) (2002) interview	800 women	Sensitive facial skin	52%	[1]
USA (Cincinnati) (2009) questionnaire	869 women	Sensitive skin	69%	[11]
France (2008) questionnaire	18 women	Sensitive skin	50%	[12]
France (2008) questionnaire	400 women	Sensitive skin	85%	[13]
France (2005) questionnaire	1,006 men and women	Sensitive skin	59%	[14]
France (2006) questionnaire	5,074 women	Sensitive skin	61%	[15]
Greece (2008) questionnaire	25 women	Sensitive skin	64%	[16]

that 53% of those who self-reported sensitive skin claimed duration of more than 5 years [18].

In the quest to understand the physiological mechanisms behind sensitive skin, testing has involved three basic endpoints of chemical exposure: neurosensory response (sensory reactivity tests), visible cutaneous signs of irritation (irritant reactivity tests), and structural and physiological changes in the skin as indicators of irritant effect (dermal function tests) [19] (Table 7.2). Sensory reactivity tests focus on the neurosensory response to a known irritant; most popularly lactic acid (although capsaicin, ethanol, menthol, sorbic acid, and benzoic acid have also been employed) is applied to the skin [21].

Tape stripping, a procedure that removes the stratum corneum, is sometimes performed before irritants are applied [22]. Irritant reactivity tests attempt to measure objective signs of irritation following application of a known irritant, most commonly sodium lauryl sulfate (SLS), a primary irritant which damages skin by direct cytotoxic action, without prior sensitization [23].

Other irritants employed have included dimethyl sulfoxide (DMSO), benzoic acid, trans-cinnamic acid, acetic acid, octanoic acid, decanol, sodium dodecyl sulfate (SDS), and vasodilators and many others of commercial interest [24].

Mechanical irritation methods evaluate irritation from products like paper or tissue products. All forms of irritant reactivity testing often rely on exaggerated exposure testing to achieve chemical or product differentiation. Dermal function tests measure structural or physiological changes in the skin that can be associated with the neurosensory responses in sensitive skin.

Despite a variety of testing strategies, progress in understanding sensitive skin has been hampered by several issues. The condition is, by definition, based on subjective sensory perceptions, which can be defined as stinging, itching, or burning and which may range from very mild and transient to intense. These subjective reports of negative sensations may or may not be accompanied by a diverse assortment of objective signs of irritation. In addition, no consistent correlation of

Table 7.2 Methodological approaches to understanding sensitive skin

Name	Assessment methodology	Provocative agent	Advantages	Disadvantages
Sensory reactivity tests				
Surveys	Questionnaire	Varies by subject report	Useful for large-scale epidemiological studies, no instrumentation required	Time-consuming, self-reported data
Stinger test	Questionnaire	Lactic acid[a]	Quick, easy, no instrumentation required	Often nonreproducible, not predictive of general sensitivity, subjective and difficult to quantify response, not correlatable to objective irritation
Irritant reactivity tests				
Visual erythema	Visual scoring	SLS[a]	Relatively inexpensive, fast, require no instrumentation	Subjective, often not reproducible, not able to correlate with sensory responses
Laser Doppler velocimetry	Skin irritation by blood flow	SLS[a]	Noninvasive, objective	Requires expensive instrumentation, indirect measure, less sensitive than TEWL, minimally quantitative, not relevant to irritation by some agents (NaOH, dithranol)
Color reflectance	Colorimeter	SLS[a]	Noninvasive, objective, accurate, reproducible, allows quantitative comparison within and between individuals	Requires expensive instrumentation, indirect measure, less sensitive than TEWL
TEWL, Irritation by changes in barrier integrity	Evaporimeter	SLS[a]	Biochemical indicator of skin damage, quantitative	Requires expensive instrumentation, requires stringent conditions, easily confounded by temperature, humidity, host factors
Electrical capacitance, irritation by skin hydration	Corneometer	SLS[a]	Quantitative, relatively fast	Units arbitrary, difficult to standardize, confounded by skin surface features and salt content, little correlation with irritant testing
Structural sensitivity testing				
Ultrasound	Skin thickness	SLS[a]	Quantitative, quick highly accurate, noninvasive, suitable for any anatomical site	Requires expensive instrumentation
Light microscopy	Skin thickness	SLS[a]	Quantitative, highly accurate, requires no expensive instrumentation	Labor intensive, invasive, not suitable for any site
Confocal light microscopy	Skin thickness	SLS[a]	Quantitative, accurate, allows direct measurement on skin, allows assessment below surface	Requires specialized expensive instrumentation
UV light	Skin penetrability	SLS[a]	Correlates well with skin sensitivity, permits analysis	Requires specialized expensive instrumentation

Source: Berardesca et al. [20]

NaOH sodium hydroxide, *SLS* sodium lauryl sulfate, *TEWL* transepidermal water loss, *UV* ultraviolet

[a]Most common

objective signs of irritation with a person's subjective perceptions has been defined [4, 25, 26]. Many people who profess sensitive skin do not predictably experience visible signs of the sensations reported, while some who describe themselves as nonsensitive react strongly to tests of objective irritation [27].

For example, an irritant dose in one study that was observed to cause no perception or sign of irritation in 99 subjects caused pronounced irritation in the hundredth; in another study which tested three irritants in 200 subjects, 197 subjects reacted to at least one of three irritants, yet 3 subjects did not respond at all [28].

In addition, the severity of individual response to irritants tested varies tremendously [6], even among chemicals with similar modes of action and/or equivalent overall irritancy profiles. Significant variation in response occurs within the same individual [29] or at different anatomical sites [23, 30].

The existence of significant interpersonal and intrapersonal variation with regard to the perception of sensitive skin implies that both intrinsic and extrinsic factors play a significant role in the development of skin sensitivity. Numerous intrinsic and extrinsic factors affect sensory responses [6] (Table 7.3). A substantial body of research has now evaluated the contributions of both intrinsic factors (e.g., gender, age, ethnicity, anatomical site, concomitant disease) and extrinsic (cultural and environmental factors) to the phenomenon of sensitive skin. This chapter will review what is currently known with regard to contributors to sensitive skin.

7.2 Intrinsic Contributors

7.2.1 Gender

Epidemiological studies across the industrialized world consistently find that women self-report sensitive skin more often than do men with reported prevalence ranging from 30% to 64% in men as compared to 50–69% in women (Table 7.4). Men were less likely to report sensitivity specific to the face (31.9% vs 21.4%, $p=0.004$) or genitals (58.1% vs 41.9%, $p=0.001$) than women [17] and were less likely to report changes in sensitivity over time ($p=0.0263$) [18]. Even in populations where men and women claimed equal prevalence of sensitive skin, men were observed to be much less likely to consider skin sensitivity in buying decisions (67.5% vs 47.2%, $p<0.0001$) or to look specifically for products that claimed to be safe for sensitive skin (3.7% vs 13.1%, $p=0.0006$) [17].

Many gender-based physiological differences in skin have the potential to influence skin sensitivity. Men's and women's skin differs in hormone metabolism, hair growth, sweat rate, sebum production, surface pH, fat accumulation [49], and collagen content [50]; men's skin is thicker [51]. Women, in specimens of skin directly overlying the infraorbital nerve foramen, were observed to have double the nerve fiber density of men [52]. However, no gender differences were observed in the integrity of the skin barrier or time to recovery after tape stripping [53]. Estrogen also acts to increase skin thickness, increase collagen production, inhibit collagen breakdown, decrease sebum production, increase skin hydration, increase vasodilation, increase elasticity, and decrease cellular immune response [54]. Many dermatological conditions are affected by estrogen levels [55].

The menstrual cycle represents an additional gender-related contributor to sensitive skin. The cyclical variations of progesterone and estrogen that define the menstrual cycle represent a major biological influence on the female body. Estrogen receptors are found on virtually every tissue in the female body [54], and it is known that fluctuating levels of sex hormones over the menstrual cycle have the potential to affect both skin and immune function. Response to irritants was observed to peak at the beginning of the menstrual cycle, when estrogen levels are low [56, 57].

Allergic responses to nickel have been demonstrated to be significantly more intense during the luteal phase, when estrogen levels are falling [58]. Mast cell degranulation is increased around the point of ovulation, when estrogen levels are

Table 7.3 Potential contributors to sensitive skin

Intrinsic factors			
Factor	Parameter	Risk factor	References
Genetic	Gender	Female	[10]
	Skin pigmentation	Light-skinned	[31, 32]
	Skin type	Susceptibility to blushing and/or flushing	[10]
Physiologic	Age	Youth	[30]
	Hormonal status	High estrogen levels (neurosensory pathway), low estrogen levels (immunogenic pathway)	[33–35]
	Stratum corneum thickness	Thin stratum corneum	[3, 36]
	Stratum corneum hydration	Dehydration	[37, 38]
	Stratum corneum integrity	Disruption of stratum corneum	[3]
		High baseline TEWL	[23]
	Skin components	Increased epidermal innervation	[39]
		Increased number of sweat glands	[31]
		Increased neutral lipids and decreased sphingolipids	[40]
		Decreased lipids	[41]
	Anatomical site	Vulvar	[35]
		Facial	[39]
	Concomitant disease	Contact allergies	[42, 43]
		Atopic dermatitis	[3, 10, 44]
		Rosacea	[45]
Extrinsic factors			
Environmental	Weather	Cold weather	[46]
		Warm weather	[18, 47]
		Wind	[1]
	Personal products	Cosmetics and hygiene products	[18]
	Fabric and paper	Rough fabric	[46]
Psychosocial		Stress	[46]
		Marketing and advertising	[18, 48]

TEWL transepidermal water loss

Table 7.4 Comparison of prevalence of sensitive skin in men and women in the industrialized world

Population(s) studied	Population characteristics	Definition of sensitive skin	Percentage of subjects who claimed sensitive skin	References
Japan, USA, Europe (1992) questionnaire	15,000 men and women	People whose skin reacts to particular insults more than the majority of people	50% women 30% men	[8]
England (2001) questionnaire	500 men and 3,300 women	Intolerance to cosmetics and toiletries, including both sensory and visible signs	51% women 38% men	[10]
USA (Cincinnati) (2009) questionnaire	1,039 men and women	Sensitive skin	69% women 64% men	[11]
France (2005) questionnaire	1,006 men and women	Sensitive skin	59% women 4% men	[14]
France (2006) questionnaire	8,522 men and women	Sensitive skin	61% women 32% men	[15]

highest [33]. In general, an increased reactivity to antigen is observed in the premenstrual phase, with inhibition of antigen reactivity in the follicular phase and at ovulation [59]. Although specific investigations into the effect of fluctuating levels of estrogen over the menstrual cycle and the perception of pain have been relatively few and collectively nonconclusive, there has been some evidence that pain perception may increase in the periovulatory period [34].

Specific sensory and irritant reactivity tests have been ambiguous. A 2003 facial sting test in men and women demonstrated a trend toward increased sensitivity in women, but no differences were observed at any specific facial site [39, 60]. Although no gender differences were observed in one study with respect to reactivity to 11 different irritants (including SLS) [30], a compilation of results from multiple skin irritation studies demonstrated an increase in reactivity in older subjects (significant in some studies) to four commonly used irritants in patch testing, with male subjects either directionally or significantly more reactive [25].

7.2.2 Ethnicity

Ethnic differences in skin structure and function are an important consideration in the formulation of moisturizers, cosmetics, and skin hygiene products, as distinct differences in skin have been associated with ethnicity and skin coloration (Table 7.5). Most of the large-scale epidemiological surveys of sensitive skin have either focused on Caucasian skin or failed to address the issue of skin type and sensitivity. Two large-scale studies that did investigate racial differences found no different in self-reports of product sensitivity [1, 10].

Structural differences based on skin color which may influence sensitivity have been observed. Epidermal thickness has been observed to be associated with pigmentation ($p=0.0008$) [79]; Blacks and Asians have higher baseline transepidermal water loss (TEWL) values than Caucasians [64], although in another study, no differences in barrier function between Caucasian and Asians were observed [31]. Percutaneous absorption of benzoic acid, caffeine, and acetylsalicylic acid was demonstrated to be higher in Asians as compared with Caucasians but lower in Blacks [31]. Reduced skin penetration in Black skin is likely responsible for a reduced susceptibility to skin irritants and allergens in Blacks vs Caucasians [80].

Sensory and irritant response testing has also revealed ethnic differences. Tristimulus colorimeter assessment of skin reflectance showed that skin pigmentation was inversely associated with susceptibility to irritation, supported by the finding that irritant susceptibility to SLS is decreased after ultraviolet B (UVB) exposure (tanning) [23]. Asians have been reported to complain of unpleasant sensory responses more often than Caucasians, with higher dropout rates in testing due to adverse events [31]. Asian subjects can also be shown to respond significantly more vigorously or rapidly to chemical probes; however, this is often subtle and not always reproducible from study to study [25, 81, 82].

While the overall prevalence of skin sensitivity is similar across skin types and ethnic groups, recent studies have observed differences with regard to what causes discomfort and how sensitivity is expressed. Asians had higher sensitivity to spicy food, and Hispanics had relatively less reactivity to alcohol than Caucasian individuals [1]. Euro-Americans were found to have higher susceptibility to wind relative to other ethnic groups [1]. Caucasian-Americans were more likely to report visual effects related to product use (19% of subjects), while African-Americans (27% of subjects) were more likely to report sensory effects ($p=0.053$) [18]. Although the relative numbers were inadequate to demonstrate statistical significance, Hispanics reported sensory effects much less frequently (5%) than the population as a whole (17%); Asians reported sensory effects much more frequently (32% as compared to 17%) [18]. In addition, African-Americans of both genders were more likely to report sensitivity in the genital area than other groups (66.4% of African-Americans vs 52.4% of white Americans ($p=0.0008$)) [11, 17], although the racial disparity was more pronounced in men.

Table 7.5 Comparison of skin properties in Caucasian and in Black skin

Comparison	Skin property	References
Higher in Black skin	Number of cell layers in stratum corneum	[61]
	Stratum corneum resistance to stripping	[61]
	Lipid content in stratum corneum	[62]
	Electrical resistance of stratum corneum	[37]
	Desquamation of stratum corneum (twofold)	[38]
	Variability of structural parameters of stratum corneum	[61]
	UV protection factor of epidermis (three- to fourfold, 13.4 vs 3.4)	[63]
	Baseline TEWL	[64, 65]
	Reactivity to SLS (measured by TEWL)	[20]
Lower in Black skin	Amount of ceramides in stratum corneum	[66]
	Spectral remittance (above 300 nm, two- to threefold)	[67]
	UVB transmission through epidermis fourfold (7.4 vs 29.4)	[63]
	Stratum corneum UVB transmission (30.0 vs 47.6)	[63]
	Topical application of anesthetic mixture	[68]
	In vivo penetration of C-labeled dipyrithione (34% lower)	[69]
	In vivo penetration of cosmetic vehicle	[69]
	Methylnicotinate-induced vasodilation	[64, 70, 71]
	Reactivity to dichlorethylsulfide (1%) (measured by erythema, 15% vs 58%)	[72]
	Reactivity to 0-chlorobenzylidene malonitrile	[73]
	Reactivity to dinitrochlorobenzene	[74]
	Stinging response	[75]
No observed difference	Stratum corneum thickness trend toward equalization after removal of stratum corneum	[36, 76]
	Corneocyte size	[38]
	In vitro penetration of water	[77, 78]

SLS sodium lauryl sulfate, *TEWL* transepidermal water loss, *UV* ultraviolet, *UVB* ultraviolet B

Interesting patterns of specific sensory responses associated with ethnicity also emerged [18]. Caucasian subjects listed weather-related factors as a principal irritant, with 25% claiming weather sensitivity as compared to only 19% reporting sensitivity to product exposure. Only 19% of African-Americans, on the other hand, reported weather sensitivity. Although the number of Asians tested was much smaller, 32% claimed sensory effects to topical products as their chief complaint [18].

7.2.3 Age

Dramatic changes in the structure and functional capacity of skin occur with age that would presumably predispose the skin toward an increased susceptibility to irritation. The skin becomes thinner, drier, and replaces itself more slowly. The skin of the elderly is also characterized by an increase in permeability but reduction in elasticity, tensile strength, cellularity, and vascularization [83].

Clinical assessments of the erythematous response in older people, however, suggest that susceptibility to skin irritation generally decreases with age, as does the capacity to produce visible physiological signs of cutaneous irritation [30]. A compilation of the results of skin-patch tests conducted among older people over a period of 4 years demonstrated a trend toward lower reactivity to four common irritants in the elderly as compared to younger subjects [25, 60]. However, as is common to sensitive skin complaints, no correlation was observed between the severity of a visual response after exposure to an irritant showed and the subject's perceptions of skin sensitivity [25, 60]. In a large Italian study that performed lactic-acid sting tests on more than 100 elderly subjects, the intensity of the stinging response was inversely proportional to age [84]. In fact, elderly subjects were also shown by different authors to have decreased cutaneous innervation as well as sensory nerve function [85].

Epidemiological studies, however, have found that older subjects who experience skin sensitivity report that their sensitivity has increased over time [18, 46]. A study of sensory perceptions of sensitive skin conducted on 1,039 individuals in Ohio, USA, stratified subjects into four age groups (subjects under 30, subjects in their 30s, subjects in their 40s, and those over 50) and found that those in the over-50 group were more likely to claim sensitive skin than younger adults and more likely to perceive genital skin (to the exclusion of other body sites) to be more sensitive [46]. Men older than 50 years of age, however, were less likely to report general skin sensitivity than younger males, making the gender-associated difference in the prevalence of sensitive skin highest in older people, with 78.6% of women over 50 reporting general skin sensitivity as compared to only 52.9% of men. Sensitivity of genital skin was also reported at significantly lower proportions in younger men (less than 40) than in women [17]. Additionally, it was observed that older subjects who claimed skin sensitivity were more likely to have medically diagnosed skin allergies than younger subjects and more likely to name hot weather and use of antiperspirants as a contributing factor to sensitive skin; younger individuals were more likely to name cold weather and stress as triggers [46].

7.2.4 Anatomic Site

An epidemiological study which surveyed 1,039 people with regard to perceptions of sensitive skin in general and at specific body sites (face, body, and genital area) found that, while overall 68.4% of the subjects questioned claimed general skin sensitivity, 77.3% felt that their facial skin was sensitive, 60.7% claimed sensitivity of the trunk or limbs, and 56.3% claimed genital sensitivity [11]. In a representative study of a French population, 44.2% reported experiencing skin sensitivity of the scalp [86].

The structure and physiology of the skin do differ among body sites. Structurally, the stratum corneum is thickest on the palms and soles and thinnest in the region of the genitalia [87]. Replacement of the stratum corneum is faster on the face than in other anatomical regions [26]. Surprisingly large variations in skin sensitivity have been observed associated with specific anatomical sites, most notably, a patch test using SLS which tested the irritant on identical locations on both arms and found differences in irritant response on the respective limbs in 47% of the subjects tested [23].

Most sensory reactivity testing has focused on the facial skin. Marriott et al. evaluated different areas of the face to determine which regions experienced the greatest stinging response to the application of lactic acid as an irritant. Ten percent lactic acid was applied to the nasolabial fold, forehead, chin, and cheek of 45 volunteers under both occluded and nonoccluded conditions for 8 min. The nasolabial fold was observed to be the most sensitive region of the facial area, followed by the malar eminence, chin, forehead, and upper lip, respectively [39]. Subjects who experienced stinging on the nasolabial fold did not necessarily experience stinging in other areas [39]. Green observed order of magnitude differences in sensory reactivity of the face and forearm to capsaicin and methanol, with face being much more susceptible [88].

SLS-sensitivity testing found that sensitivity increased from the wrist to the cubital fossa area [23]. Interestingly, although a study performed in women with preexisting dermatologist-identified vulvar irritation found no increased genital sensitivity to sanitary pads as compared to normal controls, women with vulvar erythema did report increased facial erythema with the use of cosmetics, reflecting possibly the higher visibility of facial skin [89].

Besne et al. evaluated the effect of age and anatomical site with regard to the density of sensory innervation in the epidermis using biopsy samples from 82 patients ranging in age from 20 to 93. Specimens were taken from either the face (upper eyelid and preauricular areas) or the abdomen and mammary areas. Facial specimens had significantly increased epidermal innervation than did the truncal areas evaluated, with highest density of epidermal nerve fibers occurring on the upper eyelid [85].

Genital skin differs from exposed skin in being dramatically thinner [87] and to varying degrees nonkeratinized and occluded. These differences may make the genital area in women more permeable than exposed keratinized skin [2].

There have been reported differences with regard to race and its influence on the perception of sensitive skin in the genital area. African-Americans report the sensitivity of genital skin at a higher frequency than do Caucasian-Americans, a difference more pronounced in men [17, 90]. However, younger men report genital skin sensitivity much less frequently than older men [17]. It was also observed that women are more likely to report an increase in the sensitivity of the genital skin as they age than are their male counterparts, ($p=0.12$) [46].

7.2.5 Sensitive Skin and Concomitant Disease

Several research groups have found an association between sensitive skin and atopy and allergy. Individuals with contact allergies have higher rates of skin sensitivity, implying the possibility of an underlying immune component; similar cytokines have been found in the development of skin irritation and contact allergy [42]. In a study in the Midwest USA, 1,039 subjects who claimed skin sensitivity were demonstrated to be significantly more likely (five times more likely) to have medically diagnosed skin allergies as well. In addition, those who claimed sensitive skin were 3.5 times more likely to report a family member that also had sensitive skin, implying a genuine physiological cause [91].

Loffler et al. also observed a significant association between the perception of sensitive skin and nickel allergy but, in contrast, found no differences between those who claimed sensitive skin as compared to controls with regard to physiological indicators such as skin hydration, skin blood flow, and TEWL analysis [43].

Atopic dermatitis (AD) was implicated early on as a potential contributor to skin sensitivity [10]. The density of cutaneous nerves has been demonstrated to be higher in atopic skin than in normal skin [45], and an association has been made between AD and positive response to the sting test [3]. Also, baseline TEWL in uninvolved skin in AD patients, which is higher than that of normal subjects, was shown to predict susceptibility to irritants in other sites [44].

An initial study compared women with clinically diagnosed AD to a group of women with other dermatological diseases and found that atopic individuals were significantly more likely to describe their skin as very or moderately sensitive, describing weather-related factors, rough fabric, personal-hygiene products, laundry products, perfumes, and stress as significant triggers. A statistical association was observed between clinically diagnosed atopic dermatitis and self-perceived skin sensitivity. Atopy was also associated with genital sensitivity to hygiene pads. Patients with AD were also significantly more likely to report family history of sensitive skin, ($p=0.004$). Interestingly, 48% of patients with AD reported that their sensitive skin had been present as long as they could remember, a response absent completely from the control group. Of the AD patients, 80% said that the sensitive skin had been present all of their adult life, while only 20% of non-AD subjects reported that long of a duration [16].

Recently, our research group administered a nine-item skin questionnaire on self-perceived skin sensitivity to two groups of dermatological patients: one with clinically diagnosed AD and one with unrelated dermatological complaints (25 subjects in each group). We observed an association between AD and sensitive skin in that self-perceived skin sensitivity, preference for hypoallergenic products, and avoidance of alpha-hydroxy acids were highly predictive of AD. Those three factors correctly classified 88% of the patients with prior AD and 92% of patients without AD [92].

Incontinence, with its chronic exposure to known irritants in urine, could be expected to be associated with skin sensitivity. Extremely common in elderly women, it has a variety of potential dermatologic ramifications, including irritation leading to various forms of dermatitis [93]. It was expected that women with urinary incontinence (UI) may report more sensitivity in the genital area. Twenty Nine (29) women aged at least 50 years old and suffering from mild urinary incontinence filled out questionnaires designed to evaluate their perceptions of sensitive skin. Surprisingly, although significantly more women with UI perceived themselves to have sensitive skin in general, those women were no more likely than controls to report sensitivity of the genital area in particular [90].

A possible link between sensitive skin and rosacea has also been postulated. In one study of rosacea patients, 64% were found to respond positively to a sting test; additionally, pulsed-dye laser treatment of rosacea was demonstrated to result in decreased stinging [45].

7.3 Extrinsic Contributors

The concept of sensitive skin arose primarily out of unexpected reactions to cosmetics, personal cleansers, and other personal care products but grew to include a wide variety of other consumer products including fabrics, household cleaners, paper products, sanitary napkins, and topical medications. It has been demonstrated that long-term use of personal care products, particularly medicaments containing corticosteroids, can produce allergenic sensitivity; [3] chronic use of topical medications has been observed to be the origin of up to 20% of vulvar dermatitis [94].

The vulva is exposed to other products such as sanitary napkins and hygienic wipes that may contribute to skin sensitivity as well. Although the vulvar skin differs from exposed skin in ways that would imply a potential for increased susceptibility to irritation (nonkeratinized, occluded skin), the use of various sanitary napkin designs has demonstrated a negligible occurrence of visual signs of irritation, with only a low frequency of mild and transient sensory effects associated with their use [95]. A study evaluating wet wipes asked 180 women, both pre- and postmenopausal, to use wet wipes in lieu of toilet tissue for 4 weeks. No evidence of vulvar skin irritation was observed [96]. In a study that recruited eight subjects with specifically self-declared sensitive skin who reported adverse skin responses to everyday products and/or clothing, sanitary napkins were patch tested on the forearm for four consecutive 24-h periods. No difference in erythema between the test pads and physiological saline was observed [97].

Environmental factors are consistently reported as a primary trigger for sensitive skin, particular weather-related issues such as cold temperatures, wind, heat, and sun exposure [1, 3]. Subjects in a French study (77%) described themselves as experiencing at least some skin sensitivity related to warm weather, with 87% reporting at least some sensitivity related to winter weather [47]. Our research confirmed environmental triggers as a major contributor to sensitive skin in a group of 1,039 subjects, both male and female, who believed themselves to have sensitive skin. Severe weather was the most common contributor reported in this group, claimed by 24% of respondents as a factor in their skin sensitivity [18].

It has been proposed by research scientists that the increasing incidence of sensitivity represents a cultural phenomenon wherein it has become culturally fashionable to claim sensitive skin. The percentage of people surveyed who perceive themselves to have sensitive skin has risen steadily over the decade of existing epidemiological research, particularly among men [17]. The fact that the majority of women in the industrialized world now claim sensitive skin defies its initial perception as a minority complaint and tends to support at least some cultural component, as does its more dramatic rise among men, a rise observed to be parallel to the increase in marketing of sensitive skin products for men (ostensibly creating a more culturally acceptable climate for male self-identification) [18].

A recent epidemiological study in Europe would seem to confirm a cultural component.

A comparison of self-reported skin sensitivity in eight European countries found dramatic differences between genetically similar national populations (Portugal, Italy, and Spain, e.g., reporting 80–90% of their population as experiencing at least some sensitivity, while Germany, Belgium, and Switzerland reported just a little more than half). The authors attributed these unexpected findings to substantially more fashion and beauty-related advertising in the countries where self-reports of sensitive skin were also high [48].

7.4 The Relationship Between Irritation and Sensitivity

The relationship between irritant stimulation and sensory response has been an area of strong research interest, as a consistent correlation between objective indications of irritation and subjective sensory perceptions has been elusive.

Our laboratory has sought to explore this enigma through more sensitive methodology. One testing approach tested catamenial products in the popliteal fossa (behind the knee or BTK approach) and observed a correlation between the magnitude of the irritation score (an objective measure) and sensory reports of irritation in 13 out of 15 participants [98]. Another study included participants with sensitive and normal skin in the evaluation of facial tissues and found that sensory effects were most reliable indicator of product differences, as opposed to measures of erythema and dryness [22]. Another approach has employed enhanced visual scoring of erythema using cross-polarized light [99]. Use of enhanced visual scoring enabled detection of subclinical irritation that was not apparent using traditional scoring [100]. Use of the BTK method as well as the enhanced visual scoring allowed detection of erythema that distinguished between products in a way that mirrored consumer feedback on the product, a goal formerly unobtainable through traditional testing [99].

7.5 Conclusions

It is clear that certain individuals have exaggerated sensitivity to specific sensory and physical irritants. There is now widespread agreement that sensitive skin is a genuine condition with physiological origin [26] and which can significantly impact quality of life [101]. Nonetheless, meaningful correlation between sensory perceptions and physical signs of irritation are weak and any underlying pathophysiology poorly understood. Sensitive skin appears to represent an abrogation of the skin's tolerance threshold [48] which may stem from several different pathological processes. It is likely that the phenomenon of sensitive skin, when unraveled, will prove to be an umbrella classification comprised of distinct subgroups of clinical sensitivities with different physiological mechanisms. Pons-Guiraud has proposed three subgroups as follows: *very sensitive skin*, reactive to a wide variety of both endogenous and exogenous factors with both acute and chronic symptoms and a strong psychological component; *environmentally sensitive*, comprised of clear, dry, thin skin with a tendency to blush or flush and reactive to primarily environmental factors; and *cosmetically sensitive skin*, transiently reactive to specific and definable cosmetic products [3]. Muizzuddin et al. defined three subgroups somewhat differently. His classifications include *delicate skin*, characterized by easily disrupted barrier function not accompanied by a rapid or intense inflammatory response; *reactive skin*, characterized by a strong inflammatory response without a significant increase in permeability; and *stingers*, characterized by a heightened neurosensory perception to minor cutaneous stimulation [102].

Subclinical irritation may be the key to understanding sensitive skin. The lack of correlation between sensory and visual physiological response may be at least practically temporal: sensory perceptions of irritation occur almost immediately, while physiological sequelae will take time to develop. Visual irritation tests by definition measure lasting effects, while sensory effects are immediate. Methodologies with the capacity to detect subclinical irritation have demonstrated better correlation between objective and subjective parameters of sensitive skin than earlier testing.

7.6 Future Directions

Understanding the pathophysiology of sensitive skin is essential for the development of diagnostic criteria and treatment options. An additional need is a classification system for sensitive skin that meaningfully synthesizes intrinsic and extrinsic factors, thereby laying a foundation for effective treatments.

The most promising research has involved the development of enhanced methodological tools that are capable of detecting very subtle, subclinical skin effects related to skin sensitivity and which focus specifically on subjects found to have sensitive skin. Larger study populations composed specifically of those who believe they have sensitive skin are required to overcome the substantial level of individual variability and therefore produce meaningful results. Another important research goal would be the development of methodological tools that can further exaggerate exposures, enhance ability to clinically score irritation (visually or via instrumentation), and identify new objective endpoints for subjective sensory effects [103, 104]. For maximal usefulness, developed methods will need to be cost efficient, minimally invasive, and consistently reproducible.

Ultimately, the goal of research into sensitive skin will be to synthesize data involving the skin, the nervous system, intrinsic components of sensitive skin, as well as the patient's environment, lifestyle, and culture in order to meaningfully describe the currently mysterious relationship between sensitive skin, sensory responses, and objective evidence of irritation.

Take Home Messages

- A majority of consumers in industrialized countries report "sensitive skin": unpleasant sensations related to the use of certain consumer products, despite extensive premarket testing demonstrating a lack of irritant effect.
- An understanding of this phenomenon has been hampered by the diversity of both sensory perceptions and signs reported and a lack of correlation between subjective sensory perceptions and objective signs.
- A variety of physiological factors have been associated with the consumer experience of sensitive skin.
- A variety of external exposures have been reported as provoking irritant reactions.
- Cultural factors such as advertising appear to influence consumer perceptions of skin sensitivity.
- Improved testing methods are beginning to reveal the physiological mechanisms which underlie the consumer experience of sensitive skin.
- Sensitive skin may ultimately prove to be comprised of subgroups of exaggerated sensitivity stemming from different physiological mechanisms.

Abbreviations

AD	Atopic dermatitis
BTK	Behind the knee
DMSO	Dimethyl sulfoxide
SDS	Sodium dodecyl sulfate
SLS	Sodium lauryl sulfate
TEWL	Transepidermal water loss
UI	Urinary incontinence
UVB	Ultraviolet B

References

1. Jourdain R, de Lacharrière O, Bastien P, Maibach HI (2002) Ethnic variations in self-perceived sensitive skin: epidemiological survey. Contact Dermatitis 46(3):162–169
2. Farage MA, Katsarou A, Maibach HI (2006) Sensory, clinical and physiological factors in sensitive skin: a review. Contact Dermatitis 55(1):1–14

3. Pons-Guiraud A (2004) Sensitive skin: a complex and multifactorial syndrome. J Cosmet Dermatol 3(3): 145–148
4. Marriott M, Holmes J, Peters L, Cooper K, Rowson M, Basketter DA (2005) The complex problem of sensitive skin. Contact Dermatitis 53(2):93–99
5. Farage MA (2005) Are we reaching the limits or our ability to detect skin effects with our current testing and measuring methods for consumer products? Contact Dermatitis 52(6):297–303
6. Farage MA, Maibach HI (2008) Sensitive skin syndrome: sensory response and classification. Cosmet Toil 123(7):26–30
7. Farage MA, Maibach HI (2010) Sensitive skin: closing in on a physiological cause. Contact Dermatitis 62(3):137–149
8. Johnson A, Page D (1992) Making sense of sensitive skin. Congress of the International Federation of Society of Cosmetic Chemists, Yokohama, Poster 700
9. Morizot F, Guinot C, Lopez S, Le Fur I, Tschachler E, Wood C (2000) Sensitive skin: analysis of symptoms, perceived causes and possible mechanisms. Cosmet Toil 115:83–89
10. Willis CM, Shaw S, De Lacharrière O, Baverel M, Reiche L, Jourdain R, Bastien P, Wilkinson JD (2001) Sensitive skin: an epidemiological study. Br J Dermatol 145(2):258–263
11. Farage MA (2009) How do perceptions of sensitive skin differ at different anatomical sites? An epidemiological study. Clin Exp Dermatol 38(8):e521–e530
12. Querleux B, Dauchot K, Jourdain R, Bastien P, Bittoun J, Anton J, Burnod Y, de Lacharrière O (2008) Neural basis of sensitive skin: an fMRI study. Skin Res Technol 14(4):454–461
13. Saint-Martory C, Roguedas-Contios AM, Sibaud V, Degouy A, Schmitt AM, Misery L (2008) Sensitive skin is not limited to the face. Br J Dermatol 158(1):130–133
14. Misery L, Myon E, Martin N, Verrière F, Nocera T, Taieb C (2005) Sensitive skin in France: an epidemiological approach. Ann Dermatol Venereol 132(5): 425–429
15. Guinot C, Malvy D, Mauger E, Ezzedine K, Latreille J, Ambroisine L, Tenenhaus M, Préziosi P, Morizot F, Galan P et al (2006) Self-reported skin sensitivity in a general adult population in France: data of the SU. VI.MAX cohort. J Eur Acad Dermatol Venereol 20(4):380–390
16. Farage MA, Bowtell P, Katsarou A (2008) Self-diagnosed sensitive skin in women with clinically diagnosed atopic dermatitis. Cli Med Dermatol 2:21–28
17. Farage MA (2010) Does sensitive skin differ between men and women? Cutan Ocul Toxicol 29(3):153–163
18. Farage MA (2008) Perceptions of sensitive skin: changes in perceived severity and associations with environmental causes. Contact Dermatitis 59(4):226–232
19. Farage MA, Maibach HI (2008) Sensitive skin syndrome: methodological approaches. Cosmet Toil 123(9): 28–33
20. Berardesca E, Cespa M, Farinelli N, Rabbiosi G, Maibach H (1991) In vivo transcutaneous penetration of nicotinates and sensitive skin. Contact Dermatitis 25(1):35–38
21. Robinson MK, Perkins MA (2001) Evaluation of a quantitative clinical method for assessment of sensory skin irritation. Contact Dermatitis 45(4):205–213
22. Farage MA (2005) Assessing the skin irritation potential of facial tissues. Cutan Ocul Toxicol 24(2):125–135
23. Lee CH, Maibach HI (1995) The sodium lauryl sulfate model: an overview. Contact Dermatitis 33(1): 1–7
24. Basketter DA, York M, McFadden JP, Robinson MK (2004) Determination of skin irritation potential in the human 4-h patch test. Contact Dermatitis 51(1): 1–4
25. Robinson MK (2002) Population differences in acute skin irritation responses. Race, sex, age, sensitive skin and repeat subject comparisons. Contact Dermatitis 46(2):86–93
26. Farage MA, Maibach HI (2008) Sensitive skin syndrome: relationships among factors. Cosmet Toil 123(11):28–31
27. Farage M, Maibach HI (2004) The vulvar epithelium differs from the skin: implications for cutaneous testing to address topical vulvar exposures. Contact Dermatitis 51(4):201–209
28. Basketter DA, Wilhelm KP (1996) Studies on non-immune immediate contact reactions in an unselected population. Contact Dermatitis 35(4):237–240
29. Robinson MK (2001) Intra-individual variations in acute and cumulative skin irritation responses. Contact Dermatitis 45(2):75–83
30. Cua AB, Wilhelm KP, Maibach HI (1990) Cutaneous sodium lauryl sulphate irritation potential: age and regional variability. Br J Dermatol 123(5):607–613
31. Aramaki J, Kawana S, Effendy I, Happle R, Löffler H (2002) Differences of skin irritation between Japanese and European women. Br J Dermatol 146(6): 1052–1056
32. Berardesca E, Maibach HI (1988) Racial differences in sodium lauryl sulphate induced cutaneous irritation: black and white. Contact Dermatitis 18(2): 65–70
33. Kalogeromitros D, Katsarou A, Armenaka M, Rigopoulos D, Zapanti M, Stratigos I (1995) Influence of the menstrual cycle on skin-prick test reactions to histamine, morphine and allergen. Clin Exp Allergy 25(5):461–466
34. Farage MA, Osborn TW, Maclean AB (2008) Cognitive, sensory, and emotional changes associated with the menstrual cycle: a review. Arch Gynecol Obstet 278(4):299–307
35. Britz MB, Maibach HI, Anjo DM (1980) Human percutaneous penetration of hydrocortisone: the vulva. Arch Dermatol Res 267(3):313–316
36. Thomson ML (1955) Relative efficiency of pigment and horny layer thickness in protecting the skin of Europeans and Africans against solar ultraviolet radiation. J Physiol 127(2):236–246
37. Johnson LC, Corah NL (1963) Racial differences in skin resistance. Science 139(3556):766–767

38. Corcuff P, Lotte C, Rougier A, Maibach HI (1991) Racial differences in corneocytes. A comparison between black, white and oriental skin. Acta Derm Venereol 71(2):146–148
39. Marriott M, Whittle E, Basketter DA (2003) Facial variations in sensory responses. Contact Dermatitis 49(5):227–231
40. Lampe MA, Burlingame AL, Whitney J, Williams ML, Brown BE, Roitman E, Elias PM (1983) Human stratum corneum lipids: characterization and regional variations. J Lipid Res 24(2):120–130
41. Seidenari S, Francomano M, Mantovani L (1998) Baseline biophysical parameters in subjects with sensitive skin. Contact Dermatitis 38(6):311–315
42. Loffler H (2006) Contact allergy and sensitive skin. In: Berardesca E, Fluhr J, Maibach H (eds) Sensitive skin syndrome. Taylor and Francis, New York
43. Löffler H, Dickel H, Kuss O, Diepgen TL, Effendy I (2001) Characteristics of self-estimated enhanced skin susceptibility. Acta Derm Venereol 81(5):343–346
44. Effendy I, Loeffler H, Maibach HI (1995) Baseline transepidermal water loss in patients with acute and healed irritant contact dermatitis. Contact Dermatitis 33(6):371–374
45. Lonne-Rahm S, Berg M, Mårin P, Nordlind K (2004) Atopic dermatitis, stinging, and effects of chronic stress: a pathocausal study. J Am Acad Dermatol 51(6):899–905
46. Farage MA (2010) Perceptions of sensitive skin with age. In: Farage MA, Miller KW, Maibach HI (eds) Textbook of aging skin. Springer, Berlin, Heidelberg
47. Misery L, Myon E, Martin N, Consoli S, Nocera T, Taieb C (2006) Sensitive skin: epidemiological approach and impact on quality of life in France. In: Berardesca E, Fluhr JW, Maibach HI (eds) Sensitive skin syndrome. Taylor & Francis, New York
48. Misery L, Boussetta S, Nocera T, Perez-Cullell N, Taieb C (2009) Sensitive skin in Europe. J Eur Acad Dermatol Venereol 23(4):376–381
49. Giacomoni PU, Mammone T, Teri M (2009) Gender-linked differences in human skin. J Dermatol Sci 55(3):144–149
50. Wines N, Willsteed E (2001) Menopause and the skin. Australas J Dermatol 42(3):149–8; quiz 159
51. Leong PL (2008) Aging changes in the male face. Facial Plast Surg Clin North Am 16(3):277–279, v
52. Mowlavi A, Cooney D, Febus L, Khosraviani A, Wilhelmi BJ, Akers G (2005) Increased cutaneous nerve fibers in female specimens. Plast Reconstr Surg 116(5):1407–1410
53. Reed JT, Ghadially R, Elias PM (1995) Skin type, but neither race nor gender, influence epidermal permeability barrier function. Arch Dermatol 131(10):1134–1138
54. Farage MA, Neill S, MacLean AB (2009) Physiological changes associated with the menstrual cycle: a review. Obstet Gynecol Surv 64(1):58–72
55. Farage MA, Berardesca E, Maibach H (2010) The possible relevance of sex hormones on irritant and allergic responses: their importance for skin testing. Contact Dermatitis 62(2):67–74
56. Agner T, Damm P, Skouby SO (1991) Menstrual cycle and skin reactivity. J Am Acad Dermatol 24(4):566–570
57. Agner T (1992) Noninvasive measuring methods for the investigation of irritant patch test reactions. A study of patients with hand eczema, atopic dermatitis and controls. Acta Derm Venereol Suppl (Stockh) 173:1–26
58. Rohold AE, Halkier-Sørensen L, Andersen KE, Thestrup-Pedersen K (1994) Nickel patch test reactivity and the menstrual cycle. Acta Derm Venereol 74(5):383–385
59. Farage MA, Berardesca E, Maibach HI (2009) The effect of sex hormones on irritant and allergic response: possible relevance for skin testing. Br J Dermatol 160(2):450–451
60. Robinson MK (2006) Age and gender as influencing factors in skin sensitivity. In: Berardesca E, Fluhr J, Maibach H (eds) Sensitive skin syndrome. Taylor & Francis, New York
61. Weigand DA, Haygood C, Gaylor JR (1974) Cell layers and density of Negro and Caucasian stratum corneum. J Invest Dermatol 62(6):563–568
62. Reinertson RP, Wheatley VR (1959) Studies on the chemical composition of human epidermal lipids. J Invest Dermatol 32(1):49–59
63. Kaidbey KH, Agin PP, Sayre RM, Kligman AM (1979) Photoprotection by melanin – a comparison of black and Caucasian skin. J Am Acad Dermatol 1(3):249–260
64. Kompaore F, Marty JP, Dupont C (1993) In vivo evaluation of the stratum corneum barrier function in blacks, Caucasians and Asians with two noninvasive methods. Skin Pharmacol 6(3):200–207
65. Wilson D, Berardesca E, Maibach HI (1988) In vitro transepidermal water loss: differences between black and white human skin. Br J Dermatol 119(5):647–652
66. Sugino K, Imokawa G, Maibach H (1993) Ethnic difference of stratum corneum lipid in relation to stratum corneum function. J Invest Dermatol 100:587 [Abstract 594]
67. Anderson RR, Parrish JA (1981) The optics of human skin. J Invest Dermatol 77(1):13–19
68. Hymes J, Spraker M (1986) Racial differences in the effectiveness of a topically applied mixture of local anesthetics. Reg Anesth 11:11–13
69. Wedig JH, Maibach HI (1981) Percutaneous penetration of dipyrithione in man: effect of skin color (race). J Am Acad Dermatol 5(4):433–438
70. Guy RH, Tur E, Bjerke S, Maibach HI (1985) Are there age and racial differences to methyl nicotinate-induced vasodilatation in human skin? J Am Acad Dermatol 12(6):1001–1006
71. Berardesca E, Maibach HI (1990) Racial differences in pharmacodynamic response to nicotinates in vivo in human skin: black and white. Acta Derm Venereol 70(1):63–66
72. Marshall E, Lynch V, Smith H (1919) Variation in susceptibility of the skin to dichlorethylsulfide. J Pharmacol Exp Ther 12:291–301
73. Weigand D, Mershon M (1970) The cutaneous irritant reaction to agent O-chlorobenzylidene malonitrile

(CS); quantitation and racial influence in human subjects. Edgewood Arsenal 4332
74. Weigand DA, Gaylor JR (1974) Irritant reaction in Negro and Caucasian skin. South Med J 67(5):548–551
75. Frosch P, Kligman A (1981) A method for appraising the stinging capacity of topically applied substances. J Soc Cosmet Chem 28:197–209
76. Freeman R, Cockerell E, Armstrong J et al (1962) Sunlight as a factor influencing the thickness of epidermis. J Invest Dermatol 39:295–298
77. Berardesca E, Maibach H (1996) Racial differences in skin pathophysiology. J Am Acad Dermatol 34(4): 667–672
78. Bronaugh RL, Stewart RF, Simon M (1986) Methods for in vitro percutaneous absorption studies. VII: use of excised human skin. J Pharm Sci 75(11):1094–1097
79. Sandby-Møller J, Poulsen T, Wulf HC (2003) Epidermal thickness at different body sites: relationship to age, gender, pigmentation, blood content, skin type and smoking habits. Acta Derm Venereol 83(6):410–413
80. Robinson MK (1999) Population differences in skin structure and physiology and the susceptibility to irritant and allergic contact dermatitis: implications for skin safety testing and risk assessment. Contact Dermatitis 41(2):65–79
81. Rapaport MJ (1984) Patch testing in Japanese subjects. Contact Dermatitis 11(2):93–97
82. Robinson MK (2000) Racial differences in acute and cumulative skin irritation responses between Caucasian and Asian populations. Contact Dermatitis 42(3):134–143
83. Farage MA, Miller KW, Elsner P, Maibach HI (2008) Intrinsic and extrinsic factors in skin ageing: a review. Int J Cosmet Sci 30(2):87–95
84. Sparavigna A, Di Pietro A, Setaro M (2005) 'Healthy skin': significance and results of an Italian study on healthy population with particular regard to 'sensitive' skin. Int J Cosmet Sci 27(6):327–331
85. Besné I, Descombes C, Breton L (2002) Effect of age and anatomical site on density of sensory innervation in human epidermis. Arch Dermatol 138(11):1445–1450
86. Misery L, Sibaud V, Ambronati M, Macy G, Boussetta S, Taieb C (2008) Sensitive scalp: does this condition exist? An epidemiological study. Contact Dermatitis 58(4):234–238
87. Tagami H (2002) Racial differences on skin barrier function. Cutis 70(6 Suppl):6–7; discussion 21–23
88. Green B (1996) Regional and individual differences in cutaneous sensitivity to chemical irritants: capsaicin and menthol. Cutan Ocul Toxicol 15:277–295
89. Farage M, Bowtell P, Katsarou A (2006) The relationship among objectively assessed vulvar erythema, skin sensitivity, genital sensitivity, and self-reported facial skin redness. J Appl Res 6:272–281
90. Farage MA (2009) Perceptions of sensitive skin: women with urinary incontinence. Arch Gynecol Obstet 280:49–57, Epub 2008 Dec 14
91. Farage MA (2008) Self-reported immunological and familial links in individuals who perceive they have sensitive skin. Br J Dermatol 159(1):237–238
92. Farage MA, Bowtell P, Katsarou A (2010) Identifying patients likely to have atopic dermatitis: development of a pilot algorithm. Am J Clin Dermatol 11(3):211–215
93. Farage MA, Miller KW, Berardesca E, Maibach HI (2008) Psychosocial and societal burden of incontinence in the aged population: a review. Arch Gynecol Obstet 277(4):285–290
94. Farage MA, Miller KW, Ledger WJ (2008) Determining the cause of vulvovaginal symptoms. Obstet Gynecol Surv 63(7):445–464
95. Farage MA, Katsarou A, Tsagroni E, Bowtell P, Meyer S, Deliveliotou A, Creatsas G (2005) Cutaneous and sensory effects of two sanitary pads with distinct surface materials: a randomized prospective trial. Cutan Ocul Toxicol 24:227–241
96. Farage MA, Stadler A, Chassard D, Pelisse M (2008) A randomized prospective trial of the cutaneous and sensory effects of feminine hygiene wet wipes. J Reprod Med 53(10):765–773
97. Farage MA, Stadler A (2005) Cumulative irritation patch test of sanitary pads on sensitive skin. J Cosmet Dermatol 4(3):179–183
98. Farage MA, Santana M, Henley E (2005) Correlating sensory effects with irritation. Cutan Ocul Toxicol 24(1):45–52
99. Farage MA (2009) Detecting skin irritation using enhanced visual scoring: a sensitive new clinical method. In: Barel AO, Paye M, Maibach HI (eds) Handbook of cosmetic science and technology, 3rd edn. Informa Healthcare, New York
100. Farage MA (2009) Sensory effects and irritation: a strong relationship. In: Barel A, Paye M, Maibach H (eds) Handbook of cosmetic science and technology. Informa Healthcare USA, Inc, New York
101. Misery L, Myon E, Martin N, Consoli S, Boussetta S, Nocera T, Taieb C (2007) Sensitive skin: psychological effects and seasonal changes. J Eur Acad Dermatol Venereol 21(5):620–628
102. Muizzuddin N, Marenus KD, Maes DH (1998) Factors defining sensitive skin and its treatment. Am J Contact Dermat 9(3):170–175
103. Perkins MA, Osterhues MA, Farage MA, Robinson MK (2001) A noninvasive method to assess skin irritation and compromised skin conditions using simple tape adsorption of molecular markers of inflammation. Skin Res Technol 7(4): 227–237
104. Perkins MA, Osterhues MA, Vogelpohl S, Robinson MK (2000) A clinical skin sampling approach to assess sensory skin irritation. Toxicological Sciences 54:146

Electron Tomography of Skin

8

Lars Norlén

8.1 Introduction

The native structure of skin can be visualized at molecular resolution with *c*ryo-transmission *e*lectron *m*icroscopy (CEMOVIS) and *to*mography (TOVIS) of *vi*treous *s*ections [1–3, 13, 14]. Micrographs of vitrified native skin obtained by CEMOVIS not only show more detail but sometimes also differ dramatically from those obtained by conventional methods (Figs. 8.1 and 8.2). The reason is a better structure preservation and the absence of a plastic embedding medium in the native cryo-preserved skin samples.

When CEMOVIS is combined with tomography (TOVIS), molecular resolution 3D reconstructions may be obtained [12, 15]. However, in electron tomography, both data acquisition and data analysis are far from trivial. This limits the practical applications of TOVIS in skin science and in particular its widespread usage within dermatology and cosmetology. Here we outline the major difficulties and how they are presently dealt with. We will also propose some future applications of TOVIS for skin science.

L. Norlén
Department of Cellular and Molecular Biology (CMB), Medical Nobel Institute, Karolinska Institute, Stockholm, Sweden

Dermatology Clinic, Karolinska University Hospital, Stockholm, Sweden
e-mail: lars.norlen@ki.se

8.2 Cryo-Electron Microscopy of Vitreous Skin Sections

A major drawback with conventional *e*lectron *m*icroscopy (EM) is the need for complete specimen dehydration. Skin dehydration results in partial loss of material, and remaining structures are subject to aggregation. Further, because of the significant background noise derived from the plastic embedding medium, conventional EM uses heavy metal staining in order to increase image contrast. It is thus not the biological material per se that is observed in the micrographs but stain deposited on aggregated biological remnants.

When preparing skin for CEMOVIS, the samples are fixed by ultra rapid (~20 ms) cooling (below −140°C) under high pressure (~2,000 bar) [4]. The high-pressure frozen, vitrified skin sample is then cut into ultrathin (25–50 nm) sections in a cryo-microtome and finally observed in a cryo-electron microscope. In this way, the molecular organization of skin can be studied in its native state, without any treatment such as chemical fixation, dehydration or staining.

8.3 Electron Tomography

In *e*lectron *t*omography (ET), a series of electron microscopy images recorded at different tilt angles is used to three-dimensionally (3D) reconstruct a sample. Single-axis tilting is the most common data acquisition geometry. The vitrified

M. Lodén, H.I. Maibach (eds.), *Treatment of Dry Skin Syndrome*,
DOI 10.1007/978-3-642-27606-4_8, © Springer-Verlag Berlin Heidelberg 2012

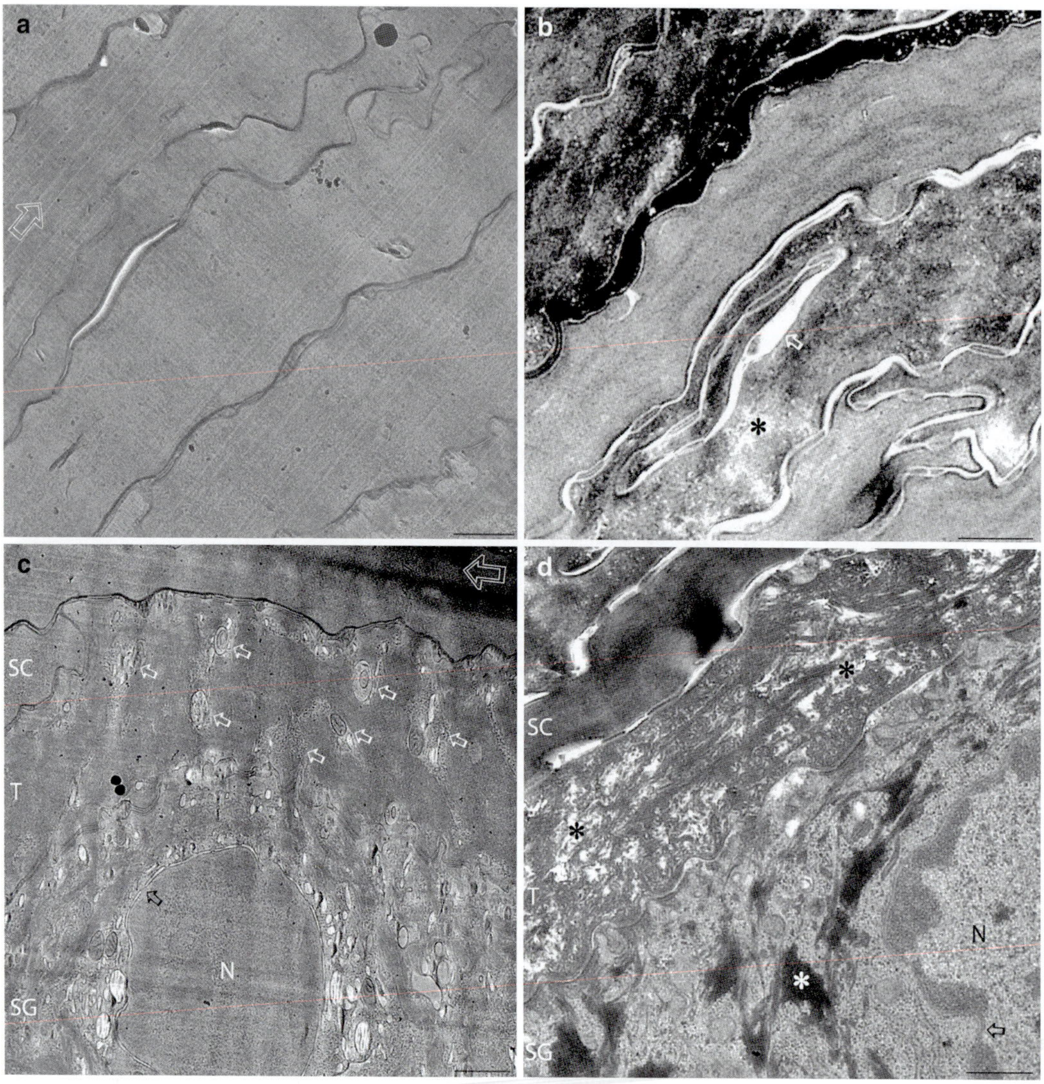

Fig. 8.1 Conventional sample preparation for electron microscopy results in important losses of epidermal biomaterial. Low magnification transmission electron micrographs of human epidermis at the interzone between viable and cornified cell layers (**a**, **b**: lowermost stratum corneum; **c**, **d**: uppermost stratum granulosum). (**a**, **c**) Cryo-electron micrographs of vitreous sections of native epidermis. (**b**, **d**) Conventional electron micrographs of resin-embedded sections. In the vitreous cryo-fixed epidermis (**a**, **c**), cellular as well as intercellular space appears densely packed with organic material, while, in the conventionally fixed epidermis (**b**, **d**), the distribution of biomaterial is characteristically inhomogeneous. Loss of biomaterial appears to have taken place in (**b**, **d**), both in the cytoplasmic (*black asterix*) and intercellular (*white arrow*) space. Large portions of the biomass of the viable cells appear as aggregated, heavily stained clusters, so-called keratohyalin granules (**d**, *white asterix*). Furthermore, the rich variety of cytoplasmic organelles and multigranular structures present in the stratum corneum/stratum granulosum transition (T) cells of native epidermis (**c**) (*white arrows*) are replaced by empty space in resin-embedded samples (**d**) (*black asterix*). Inner and outer nuclear envelopes and nuclear pores are clearly distinguished in the native cryo-fixed non-stained specimen (**c**) (*black arrow*) while they are difficult to distinguish in the conventionally fixed stained specimen (**d**) (*black arrow*). Electron dense single spot in (**a**) and double spot in (**c**) correspond to surface ice contamination. *SG* uppermost stratum granulosum cell, *T* transition cell, *SC* lowermost stratum corneum cell, *N* nucleus, open white double arrow. (**a**, **c**) Section cutting direction. Section thicknesses: ~100 nm (**a**, **c**), ~50 nm (**b**, **d**). Scale bars: 500 nm (**a**–**d**) (Adapted from [13] with permission)

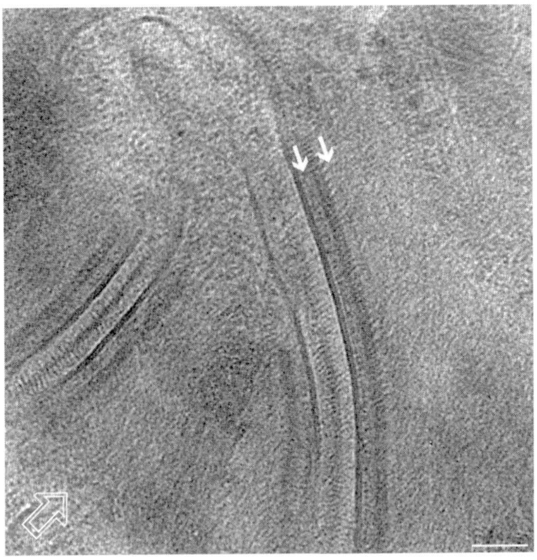

Fig. 8.2 High magnification cryo-electron micrograph of desmosomes at the midportion of the viable part of human epidermis. The plasma membranes appear as ~4 nm thick high-density bilayers. The extracellular core domain is ~33 nm thick and contains transverse electron dense lines with an ~5 nm periodicity corresponding to cadherin adhesion molecules. On the cytoplasmic side, an ~11 nm thick zone of medium electron density separates the electron dense plasma membrane from two parallel electron dense layers, situated ~7 nm apart and interconnected by traversing electron dense lines with an ~6 nm periodicity. Thin *white arrows*: very weak electron dense lines associated with the desmosome cytoplasmic plaque, open *white double-arrow*: section cutting direction. The imaging conditions were identical to those given in Fig. 8.1. Section thickness: ~50 nm. Scale bar: 50 nm (Adapted from [3] with permission)

skin sample is here rotated around a single axis. The rotation angle range is usually ±60°. The ±30° missing region in a single-axis ±60° tilt series results in an about 50% loss of resolution along the beam direction in the 3D reconstruction [18], something that has to be taken into account when interpreting tomographic 3D reconstructions.

Also, there are several problems associated with the calculation of the scattering potential of the specimen from the tilt-series electron micrographs. The main limitation is the low signal-to-noise ratio in tomographic low-dose cryo-electron micrographs. Another problem is that the ±30° missing region in the tilt-series data prevents stable inversion [16]. This leads to instability in the 3D reconstruction procedure. Furthermore, one cannot exactly reconstruct an object's scattering potential as only a subregion of the cryo-section (i.e. the region of interest (ROI)) is exposed to electrons. As the section is tilted, scattered electrons from outside the ROI enter the ROI images. Consequently, one must make assumptions regarding the scattering potential of the section outside the ROI when reconstructing an object inside the ROI [15].

The missing tilt-angle problem, the scattering from outside the ROI and the low signal-to-noise ratio make the 3D reconstruction in skin TOVIS difficult. This is presently dealt with by reconstructing only some information about the specimen that can be stably retrieved or by the introduction of prior information about the specimen into the reconstruction scheme [15].

The first approach is exemplified by filtered and weighted back-projection methods (FBP and WBP) [19, 20, 27] (Fig. 8.3a), in which regularization is simply achieved by low-pass filtering, and in the simultaneous iterative reconstruction technique (SIRT) [10], where it is achieved by stopping the iteration after a limited number of cycles and by not allowing the predicted changes to be fully used between the iterations. The approach taken by the recently introduced Λ-tomography technique [17] is to reconstruct only the information about the sample that can be stably retrieved. This is achieved by only reconstructing the boundaries of the scattering potential, which in turn provide the shape of the boundaries of the molecules in the specimen [15].

The second approach is to stabilize the 3D reconstruction algorithm in ET by introducing additional a priori information. An example is the variational regularization methods [22] (Fig. 8.3b), which are defined as the solution to an optimization problem, and, more recently, l_1-regularization and the associated total variation (TV) regularization [6–8] where the principle is to choose the 3D structure that is as sparse as possible [15].

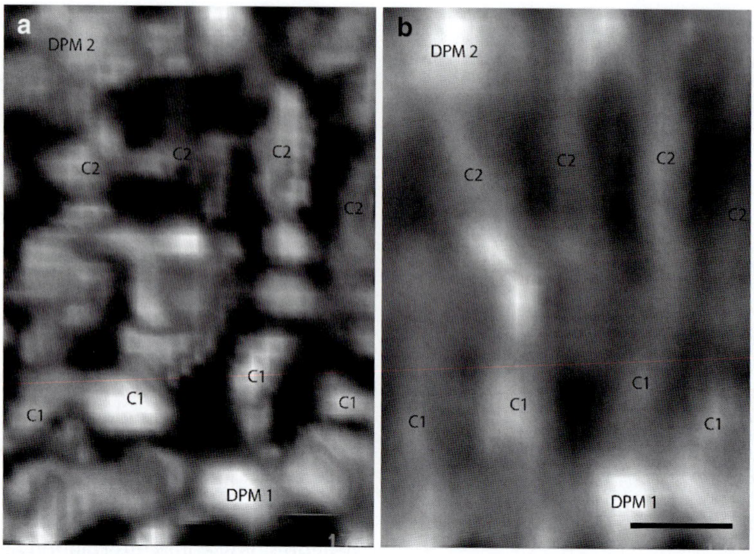

Fig. 8.3 Molecular skin TOVIS in situ 3D reconstruction with weighted back projection (**a**) and refinement with COMET regularization (**b**) of individual cadherin adhesion molecules inside the extracellular domain of a desmosome inside native human epidermis. The 3D reconstructions were obtained from the area marked by a *white box* in Fig. 8.3. The quality of the 3D reconstructions (**a**, **b**) was not sufficient to deduce the native 3D arrangement of the desmosomal cadherins, essentially because of smearing in the z-direction secondary to the missing data (limited tilt angle) problem. We used a single-axis GATAN model 626 cryo-holder (GATAN, Pleasanton, CA) at −180°C. Tilt series were collected at 200 kV in a FEG CM200 FEI microscope, equipped with a cooled slow scan 2,048 × 2,048 TemCam-F214 CCD camera (pixel size 14 μm) and software for automated data collection (TVIPS, Gauting, Germany). The images were recorded at −4 μm defocus (first CTF zeros at 3.1 nm) at the dose of approximately 60 electrons/nm^2 per image (total dose 3,900 electrons/nm^2) and a total magnification of 25,000× (pixel size corresponds to 5.63 Å in the specimen). The tilt series was collected with two-degree increments covering the range from −50° to +60°. The images were displayed in the XPIX program and fiducial marker positions determined in a semi-automated way. A least-squares procedure was used to align the images. The average alignment error was 1.467 pixels (0.825 nm), as estimated from the mean deviation of measured marker positions from positions predicted from the geometry of the tilts. The 3D reconstructions were made using weighted back projection (**a**) and analysed in either the BOB (available at http://www.3tag.com/bobicol.html) or XTV programs. The COMET reconstruction (**b**) was performed using the COMET software version 4.5. The reconstructed volume obtained by weighted back projection (**a**) and low-pass filtered to a resolution of 7 nm was used as the prior. The amplitude contrast ratio was set to 0.15 and the defocus to −4 μm. *DPM1* desmosome plasma membrane of the lower cell, *DPM2* desmosome plasma membrane of the upper cell, *C1* cadherin molecule belonging to the lower cell, *C2* cadherin molecule belonging to the upper cell. Scale bar: 5 nm (Adapted from [15] with permission)

8.4 Immuno-tomography

CEMOVIS and TOVIS allow for structure determination in skin at near-native conditions. They are however costly, time-consuming and technically demanding. Freeze-substitution ET may therefore constitute an attractive complement for questions not requiring molecular resolution. The advantages of freeze-substitution ET are that the signal-to-noise ratio is better as the tissue samples are stained and that higher electron doses are tolerated. Freeze-substitution ET is also much less technically demanding and allows for routine acquisition of dual-tilt series, which reduces the missing tilt-angle problem. However, the most significant advantage of freeze-substitution ET is that it is compatible with immuno-labelling and thus allows for immuno-ET. Electron tomography of antibody-labelled tissues and cells makes it possible to reconstruct antibody–antigen complexes in 3D in situ with a resolution of a few nm [11] (Fig. 8.4). The major practical problem is that contaminating antibodies usually cluster around the gold particle conjugated to the secondary IgG antibody and thereby sometimes obscure the structural

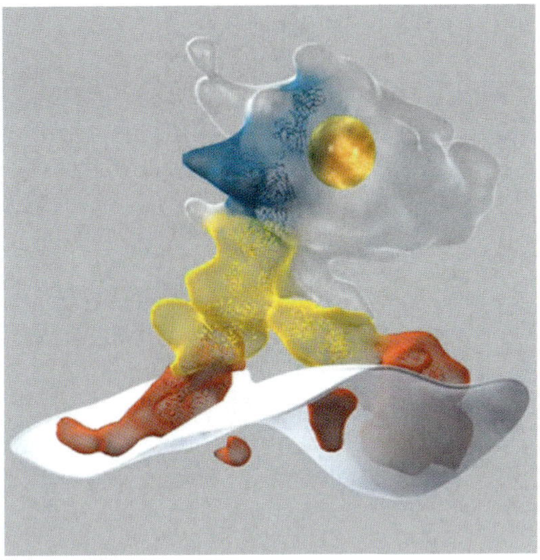

Fig. 8.4 Molecular 3D immuno-EM tomography reconstruction of an epidermal growth factor receptor–antibody complex on the cell surface of a squamous carcinoma (A431) cell prepared by the Tokuyasu technique. *Yellow sphere* represents a 6-nm colloidal gold particle conjugated to a goat anti-human IgG antibody (Adapted from [11] with permission)

details of the primary antibody–antigen interaction. Another limitation is that antibodies only identify antigens that protrude from the section surface and therefore require fairly high antigen concentrations in the freeze-substituted specimen. For antigens that are less abundant, Tokuyasu sample preparation [25] may constitute an alternative to freeze substitution, as antibodies then to some extent may bind antigen also inside the sections. Tokuyasu-prepared samples are however less well preserved and express a lower signal-to-noise ratio than corresponding freeze-substituted samples. A combination of TOVIS and immuno-ET based on both freeze-substituted and Tokuyasu-prepared samples may therefore be optimal for many applications in skin science.

8.5 Analysis of Tomograms

8.5.1 Segmentation

As mentioned above, interpretation of tissue ET reconstructions is not trivial. Extraction of biologically meaningful information is not only complicated by the noisy and incomplete data, but also by the three-dimensional image complexity and the lack of efficient visualization tools for distinguishing overlapping structural components. To facilitate interpretation, certain features can be extracted from the 3D reconstructions and analysed separately via image segmentation. Manual segmentation is still predominantly used. It is, however, of low reproducibility. Computer-based image segmentation algorithms have therefore been developed among which crisp segmentation, i.e., assigning each voxel in the image either to the background or to the object based exclusively on grey-level information, is the most widely used [5, 28]. Crisp segmentation is, however, complicated by the absence of a distinct border between object and background in the low-contrast skin TOVIS setting. An alternative approach is segmentation based on fuzzy set theory, using both grey-level and shape information. Here each voxel is assigned a membership value describing to what degree it belongs to an object [9, 24].

8.5.2 Docking of X-Ray Data into Segmented ET Data

Docking of x-ray crystallography data or atomic models into segmented electron tomography data could aid biological interpretation of skin TOVIS experiments. Presently, rigid docking procedures dominate. A major problem here is that these do not work well in the presence of conformational variation and molecular flexibility. However, flexible docking procedures based on molecular dynamics simulation that bring deviating global molecular features into register while preserving the crystal structure locally have recently been developed [26, 29].

8.5.3 Electron Microscopy Simulation

A new tool to identify and characterize biological structures in cryo-electron images is electron microscopy simulation [23]. It consists of a phantom generator that generates an atomic model of a biological structure adapted for simulation and a transmission electron microscope simulator that calculates the electron–specimen interaction, the electron optics in the microscope and a noise model that includes detector noise. A simulator can be used to find structures in electron images, as well as assist in the docking of x-ray data into segmented ET data. It can further be used to test whether a proposed atomic model of a biological structure is in agreement with the features observed in the electron micrographs.

8.6 Future Applications of ET in Skin Science

The combination of CEMOVIS, TOVIS and immuno-ET with molecular modelling and electron microscopy simulation allows for the identification and structure determination in native skin in situ down to a resolution of about 1–5 nm. The more ordered the target molecules are, the more suitable they will be for analysis. Highly ordered molecular assemblies like membrane structures [cf. 3, 14], cytoskeletal components like keratin filaments [cf. 13] and cell adhesion components such as desmosomal cadherins [cf. 1, 2] are therefore well-disposed target structures. Scientific studies of the molecular mechanisms underlying skin diseases involving skin barrier deficiency, such as atopic dermatitis; scaling diseases, such as dry skin, the ichtyoses and psoriasis; as well as blistering diseases may all benefit from ET in the not too distant future. Further, molecular aspects of skin penetration of drugs as well as local drug skin-target interactions and the effect on skin structure of different topical applications, such as skin moisturizers, are other foreseeable applications.

Take Home Messages

- The three-dimensional structure of native skin can be studied by electron tomography of vitreous skin sections (TOVIS) down to a molecular resolution in situ.
- Electron tomography of antibody-labelled tissues (immuno-ET) allows direct molecular 3D reconstruction in situ of antibody-labelled proteins in skin, in addition to determining their intracellular localization to a resolution of about 2–3 nm.
- Presently, electron tomography, and especially TOVIS, is practically very difficult, very costly and very time-consuming and therefore not suited for scientific routine work. However, in the near future, TOVIS (and hopefully soon immuno-ET) data collection and data treatment will be made on a contract basis in specialized national/international electron microscopy centre facilities. This will make the access to the above-mentioned techniques relatively simple, fast and cheap for any researcher or clinician.
- TOVIS is particularly well suited for the study of the stratum corneum, dry skin and desquamation as both the ceramide-enriched extracellular, the keratin-enriched intracellular and the cadherin-enriched cell adhesion compartments are highly structured.

References

1. Al-Amoudi A, Castaño-Dieza D, Devosa DP, Russell RB, Johnson GT, Frangakis A (2011) The three-dimensional molecular structure of the desmosomal plaque. PNAS 108(16):6480–6485
2. Al-Amoudi A, Dıez DC, Betts MJ, Frangakis AS (2007) The molecular architecture of cadherins in native epidermal desmosomes. Nature 450:832–837
3. Al-Amoudi A, Dubochet J, Norlén L (2005) Nanostructure of the epidermal extracellular space as observed by cryo-electron microscopy of vitreous sections of human skin. J Invest Dermatol 124:764–777
4. Al-Amoudi, A. Norlén, L. Dubochet, J (2004) Cryo-electron microscopy of vitreous sections of native biological cells and tissues. J Struct Biol. 148(1):131–5
5. Baker ML, Yu Z, Chiu W, Bajaj C (2006) Automated segmentation of molecular subunits in electron cryo-microscopy density maps. J Struct Biol 156:432–441

6. Candès EJ (2006) Compressive sampling. Proc. Int. Congress Math, Madrid, Spain, pp 1–20
7. Cipra BA (2006) l_1-magic. SIAM News 39(9)
8. Fanelli D, Öktem O (2008) Electron tomography: a short review with an emphasis on the absorption potential model for the forward problem. Inverse Problems 24 013001 (51 pp)
9. Garduno E, Wong-barnum M, Vilkmann N, Ellisman MH (2008) Segmentation of electron tomographic data sets using fuzzy set theory principles. J Struct Biol 162:368–379
10. Gilbert PFC (1972) Iterative methods for the three-dimensional reconstruction of an object from projections. J Theor Biol 36:105–117
11. Lammerts van Bueren JJ, Bleeker WK, Brännström A, von Euler A, Jansson M, Peipp M, Schneider-Merck T, Valerius T, van de Winkel JBJ, Parren PWHI (2008) The antibody zalutumumab inhibits epidermal growth factor receptor signaling by limiting intra- and intermolecular flexibility. PNAS 105(16):6109–6114
12. Masich S, Östberg T, Norlén L, Shupliakov O, Daneholt B (2006) A procedure to deposit fiducial markers on vitreous cryo-sections for cellular tomography. J Struct Biol 156:461–468
13. Norlén L, Al-Amoudi A (2004) Stratum corneum keratin structure, function, and formation: the cubic rod-packing and membrane templating model. J Invest Dermatol 123(4):715–732
14. Norlén L, Al-Amoudi A, Dubochet J (2003) A cryo-transmission electron microscopy study of skin barrier formation. J Invest Dermatol 120:555–560
15. Norlén L, Öktem O, Skoglund U (2009) Molecular cryo-electron tomography of vitreous tissue sections: current challenges. J Microsc 235:293–307
16. Penczek PA, Frank J (2006) Resolution in electron tomography, Chapter 10. In: Frank J (ed) Electron tomography – methods for three-dimensional visualization of structures in the cell, 2nd edn. Springer, New York, pp 307–330
17. Quinto ET, Öktem O (2008) Local tomography in electron microscopy. SIAM J Appl Math 68(5):1282–1303
18. Radermacher M (1988) Three-dimensional reconstruction of single particles from random and nonrandom tilt series. J Electron Microsc Tech 9:359–394
19. Radermacher M (1992) Weighted back-projection methods. In: Frank J (ed) Electron tomography – three-dimensional imaging with the transmission electron microscope, Chapter 5. Plenum Press, New York
20. Ramachandran GN, Lakshminarayanan AV (1971) Three-dimensional reconstruction from radiographs and electron micrographs: application of convolutions instead of Fourier transforms. Proc Natl Acad Sci USA 68:2236–2240
21. Rullgård H (2008) A new principle for choosing regularization parameter in certain inverse problems. arXiv:0803.3713v2
22. Rullgård, H. Öktem, O. Skoglund, U (2007) A componentwise iterative relative entropyregularization method with updated prior and regularization parameter. Inverse Problems 23:2121–2139
23. Rullgård, H. Öfverstedt, L-G. Masich, S. Daneholt, B. Öktem, O (2011) Simulation of transmission electron microscope images of biological specimens. J. Microscopy 243(3):234–256
24. Svensson S (2007) A decomposition scheme for 3D fuzzy objects based on fuzzy distance information. Pattern Recognit Lett 28:224–232
25. Tokuyasu KT (1973) A technique for ultracryotomy of cell suspensions and tissues. J Cell Biol 57:551–565
26. Trabuco LG, Villa E, Mitra K, Frank J, Schulten K (2008) Flexible fitting of atomic structures into electron microscopy maps using molecular dynamics. Structure 16(5):673–683
27. Vainshtein BK (1970) Finding the structure of objects from projections. Krystallograftya 15:894–902; Vainshtein BK (1970) Crystallography 15:781–787 (Transl. in Soviet Physics)
28. Volkmann N (2002) A novel three-dimensional variant of the watershed transform for segmentation of electron density maps. J Struct Biol 138:123–129
29. Wriggers W (2004) Spanning the length scales of biomolecular simulation. Structure 12(1):1–2

9 Filaggrin Gene Defects and Dry Skin Barrier Function

Martin Willy Meyer and Jacob P. Thyssen

9.1 Filaggrin: The Multifunctional Protein

Filaggrin (**fil**ament-**aggr**egating prote**in**) has an important function in epidermal differentiation and barrier function, but the relative importance of the different functions of filaggrin proteins remains to be elucidated.

The filaggrin gene encodes a large insoluble polyprotein called profilaggrin [3]. Profilaggrin is cleaved to produce multiple filaggrin peptides [7]. Within the cytoskeleton of keratinocytes, filaggrin aggregates keratin 1, keratin 10 as well as other intermediate filaments and forms macrofibrils [3]. The protein-lipid cornified cell envelope forms an important permeability barrier against water and other environmental agents such as microbes, irritants and allergens. Filaggrin is a major component of this barrier function [19].

Filaggrin is producing a mixture of hygroscopic acids that may contribute to epidermal barrier function by retaining water. Among others, histidine is released by filaggrin proteolysis. It helps to maintain the pH gradient of the epidermis by being converted to transurocanic acid. This acid is then undergoing photoisomerization and has local and systemic immunosuppressive effects [3]. A pool of hydrophilic amino acids, including urocanic acid, alanine, and pyrrolidone carboxylic acid, their metabolites, and various ions make up the so-called natural moisturizing factor (NMF) [20]. The N-terminal portion of profilaggrin is a calcium-binding domain. It may be involved in the regulation of calcium-dependent events during epidermal differentiation [3].

In 2006, in Dundee, Scotland, Smith et al. reported that two common loss-of-function mutations within the filaggrin gene, R501X and 2282del4, were associated with ichthyosis vulgaris. Using improved sequencing strategies, they were finally able to report what had been long suspected [24]. The same year, Palmer et al. showed that these loss-of-function genetic variants were very strong predisposing factors for atopic dermatitis. They were detected by using long-range sequencing and multiple alignment techniques, revealing a semidominant pattern of inheritance with incomplete penetrance [18].

Approximately 9% of people of European origin are carrying these variants [18, 27]. More than 40 loss-of-function mutations within the filaggrin gene have now been reported [30]. Each is predicting nonsense or out-of-frame deletion/insertion mutations, with population-specific patterns emerging worldwide [17]. Five null mutations are prevalent within the European population. This strikingly high prevalence of filaggrin null mutations suggests a possible heterozygote advantage [3]. "Natural vaccination" mediated by the mildly perturbed skin barrier in heterozygotes has been hypothesized. Hereby atopy could be a modern plague that is enriched among the survivors of ancient bacterial plagues [11, 23].

M.W. Meyer, M.D. (✉) • J.P. Thyssen, M.D., Ph.D.
Department of Dermato-Allergology, Gentofte Hospital, Niels Andersens Vej 65, 2900 Hellerup, Denmark
e-mail: martinwmeyer@hotmail.com

M. Lodén, H.I. Maibach (eds.), *Treatment of Dry Skin Syndrome*,
DOI 10.1007/978-3-642-27606-4_9, © Springer-Verlag Berlin Heidelberg 2012

9.2 Skin Dryness

It has been suggested that filaggrin may play a role in determining the degree of skin dryness. This is based on filaggrin repeat number polymorphisms. A polypeptide that has a variable number of genetically determined filaggrin-repeat units (10, 11, or 12 repeats) is encoded by the profilaggrin gene. The repeat copy number was correlated with self-perceived episodes of dry skin in one study. It revealed that the filaggrin gene might serve as a genetic marker for dryness of the skin, because of an inverse association between the 12-repeat allele and perceived dryness. Individuals with an absence of the 12-repeat profilaggrin were over four times more likely to report skin dryness than those who carried one or two 12-repeat alleles [8]. The natural moisturizing factor comprises a mixture of amino acids, derived primarily from the degradation of filaggrin. It has been suggested that these acids serve as humectants and maintain hydration as well [20].

9.3 Ichthyosis Vulgaris

Ichthyosis vulgaris, a member of the ichthyosis family of diseases, is the most common inherited disorder of keratinization and is one of the most frequent single-gene disorders. It is an autosomal semidominant disease with incomplete penetrance ($\approx$ 90% in homozygotes). The incidence is approximately 1 in 250. Ichthyosis vulgaris has some phenotypic characteristics: palmar hyperlinearity, keratosis pilaris, and fine scaly skin [13].

Homozygous or compound heterozygous mutations R501X and 2282del4 in filaggrin is the cause of moderate to severe icthyosis vulgaris. The study of Smith et al. showed that heterozygotic individuals displayed mild scaling or no phenotype at all, whereas homozygotic or compound heterozygotic individuals had a severe form of icthyosis vulgaris (dry, scaly skin and an altered skin barrier function) [3, 13, 24].

A diagnosis of icthyosis vulgaris is primarily based on clinical observations including family history, but also by histopathological demonstration and now mutation analysis of the filaggrin gene [13].

9.4 Atopic Dermatitis

Atopic dermatitis is a common, chronic, and relapsing skin disease. It is particularly common during infancy and childhood. Scaly, itchy, and dry skin with excoriations is typically observed clinically. Furthermore, cutaneous infections frequently occur. Atopic dermatitis is often seen together with asthma and/or allergic rhinitis. Atopic dermatitis has a strong genetic predisposition but also a significant environmental component. A major predisposing genetic factor includes null mutations in the filaggrin gene [13, 18]. Palmer et al. showed that atopic dermatitis was manifested in heterozygous carriers of the above mentioned filaggrin null mutations with a relative risk for atopic dermatitis of 3.1, implying a causal relationship [18]. Several European countries as well as China and Japan have demonstrated that filaggrin null mutations in their populations are associated with atopic dermatitis following the initial findings by Palmer et al. [13]. Other studies have shown that null mutations in the filaggrin gene predispose to early-onset atopic dermatitis which persist into adulthood [1] and increase the risk of developing allergic sensitization as well as allergic rhinitis [28]. Despite the most widely and strongest replicated genetic risk for atopic dermatitis is filaggrin null mutations, 50% of patients with moderate to severe atopic dermatitis do not have these null mutations, and 60% of all carriers of filaggrin-null alleles have never had atopic dermatitis. Finally, individuals with null mutations often outgrow their disease [16]. There seem to be other important candidate genes for atopic dermatitis, and furthermore the findings underscore that atopic dermatitis is caused both by a deficient skin barrier and also by an elevated or skewed immune response [13].

A recent comprehensive meta-analysis on filaggrin null mutations showed that filaggrin haploinsuffiency is associated with severe atopic dermatitis and strongly increases the risk of atopic dermatitis [21]. It is evident that environmental factors, modifier genes, and other primary gene defects are relevant for the variable manifestations of atopic dermatitis in different individuals [13]. Another hypothesis is that individuals carrying null mutations in more than one candidate gene have a multiplicative or additive effect. Approximately, 50% of moderate-severe cases may be attributed at least in part to filaggrin null mutations. Of the mild-severe cases, only 15% may be explained by filaggrin on a population scale [3].

The filaggrin story is of great importance of the subcategorization of different forms of atopic dermatitis. The discovery of structural protein gene mutations in atopic dermatitis is groundbreaking and deviate our understanding from the previous immune centric view [13].

9.5 Psoriasis

Psoriasis is a chronic inflammatory skin disease with a strong genetic background.

Genome-wide scans of psoriasis patients have suggested an association with the epidermal differentiation complex (EDC) on chromosome 1q21. The EDC is a cluster of many genes, including filaggrin, which is expressed during epithelial differentiation. Psoriasis susceptibility locus 4 (PSORS4) linked psoriasis to this region located at 1q21 [5, 13].

Despite this potential link, several studies have concluded that there is no association of filaggrin null alleles (particularly R501X and 2282del4) and psoriasis (or psoriatic arthritis). The studies also conclude that the genetic background underlying the epidermal barrier defect in psoriasis is distinct from that found in atopic dermatitis and remains unknown [10, 29, 31]. A study from Taiwan confirms previous findings but finds an association between P478S polymorphism of the filaggrin gene and psoriasis [5].

It appears that the EDC psoriasis gene, PSORS4, is not filaggrin [31]. However, the filaggrin gene may still be a modifier gene contributing to the susceptibility for psoriasis [5].

9.6 Hand Eczema

Chronic hand eczema (CHE) is a common persistent noninfectious eczematous skin inflammation restricted to the hands. The pathogenesis of CHE is multifactorial and involves both endogenous predisposition and environmental triggers. CHE has various risk factors of which atopic dermatitis is known to be one of the most important. Also, wet work and contact allergy are known risk factors. Since a deficient skin barrier function increase the risk of CHE, null mutations in filaggrin might also contribute to CHE. Several studies have investigated whether certain filaggrin variants might be associated with CHE in general. Some also investigated certain CHE subtypes [4, 9, 12, 14, 26].

Probably the most convincing evaluation of the possible association between hand eczema and filaggrin null mutations was provided by a recent general population study including 3,471 adults. It showed that subjects with atopic dermatitis and filaggrin null mutation status had a significantly higher prevalence of hand eczema, as well as earlier onset of disease and higher persistence of disease when compared with subjects who did not report atopic dermatitis and who had wild-type filaggrin status [26]. Carlsen et al. found no association between, respectively, nickel allergy, polysensitization, hand eczema at first appearance or occurrence of dermatitis, and filaggrin null mutations [4]. Molin et al. found that heterozygosity for null mutations in the filaggrin gene may contribute to the manifestation and maintenance of a particular CHE subtype that is characterized by the combination of allergic and irritant contact dermatitis [14]. In a small twin study, Lerbaek et al. found no association between the filaggrin null alleles and hand eczema or contact allergy [12]. Yet another study found that filaggrin null alleles were associated with increased susceptibility to chronic irritant contact dermatitis [6].

It remains unclear whether or not filaggrin gene null mutations increase the overall risk of hand eczema or only increase the risk of hand eczema in subjects with atopic dermatitis. A typical phenotype of hand eczema in subjects with the filaggrin null genotype has been defined based on a small case series [25]. These patients tend to have palmar hyperlinearity, absence of palmar dermatitis, and presence of dermatitis on the dorsal aspects of the hands.

9.7 Allergic Contact Sensitization

Contact allergy is one of the most frequent dermatological problems. It is a delayed type hypersensitivity reaction caused by cutaneous exposure to metals and chemicals. Contact allergy affects 15–20% of the general population and is a persistent condition. Few studies have investigated a possible association between contact allergy and the filaggrin null genotype. Novak et al. showed that filaggrin gene null mutations were associated with nickel sensitization and self-reported nickel dermatitis in a general population study [15]. Thyssen et al. later refined these findings when they showed that a positive association could only be detected in subjects without ear piercing [27]. This finding was explained by the "bypass theory" which suggest that ear piercing is a much stronger risk factor for nickel allergy than filaggrin genotype [15, 22, 27]. In further analyses, Thyssen et al. showed that fragrance allergy was more prevalent in subjects with self-reported atopic dermatitis and the filaggrin null genotype when compared to subject without atopic dermatitis and with the filaggrin wild genotype [26]. Finally, a study based on dermatitis patients with contact allergy found no association between nickel allergy, polysensitization, hand eczema at first appearance or occurrence of dermatitis, and filaggrin null mutations [4].

9.8 Alopecia Areata

Alopecia areata is a common dermatological disease that affects up to 2% of the general population. Alopecia areata has been suggested to be associated with filaggrin null mutations. Examination of a large cohort showed that in patients with atopic dermatitis, filaggrin null mutations were associated significantly with occurrence of alopecia areata. It also showed that filaggrin null mutations might serve as a modifier of the clinical presentation of alopecia areata because mutations were associated with the more severe form of alopecia areata. However, there is no evidence to suggest that filaggrin null mutations cause alopecia areata [2].

9.9 Filaggrin Haploinsuffiency: A Potential Therapeutic Target

The discovery of filaggrin null mutations has been a major breakthrough, but it has not been translated into therapeutic advances for patients with dermatitis or other skin diseases yet. The wild-type allele carried by heterozygotic individuals might be upregulated by small molecules acting on pathways controlling filaggrin gene expression and therefore theoretical have a potential therapeutic target [3].

Most of the null mutations identified so far in the filaggrin gene are premature termination codons causing nonsense mutations. These conditions are potential targets for treatment that enable "read through" of stop codons and permit translation of a full-length protein. This type of treatment is already being tested in other diseases such as Duchenne's muscular dystrophy and cystic fibrosis but will be even more suitable in atopic dermatitis and ichthyosis vulgaris because of the possibility of topical application [13].

Take Home Messages

- Filaggrin has an important function in epidermal differentiation and skin barrier function
- Null mutations within the filaggrin gene cause ichthyosis vulgaris
- Null mutations are very strong predisposing factors for atopic dermatitis
- Null mutations are associated with hand eczema and alopecia areata in atopics but not with psoriasis
- ≈9–10% of people of European origin are carrying these variants
- The discovery of filaggrin genotyping has been a major breakthrough for dermatology, but it has not been translated into therapeutic advances yet

References

1. Barker JN, Palmer CN, Zhao Y, Liao H, Hull PR, Lee SP, Allen MH, Meggitt SJ, Reynolds NJ, Trembath RC, McLean WH (2007) Null mutations in the filaggrin gene (FLG) determine major susceptibility to early-onset atopic dermatitis that persists into adulthood. J Invest Dermatol 127:564–567
2. Betz RC, Pforr J, Flaquer A, Redler S, Hanneken S, Eigelshoven S, Kortum AK, Tuting T, Lambert J, De WJ, Hillmer AM, Schmael C, Wienker TF, Kruse R, Lutz G, Blaumeiser B, Nothen MM (2007) Loss-of-function mutations in the filaggrin gene and alopecia areata: strong risk factor for a severe course of disease in patients comorbid for atopic disease. J Invest Dermatol 127:2539–2543
3. Brown SJ, McLean WH (2009) Eczema genetics: current state of knowledge and future goals. J Invest Dermatol 129:543–552
4. Carlsen BC, Johansen JD, Menne T, Meldgaard M, Szecsi PB, Stender S, Thyssen JP (2010) Filaggrin null mutations and association with contact allergy and allergic contact dermatitis: results from a tertiary dermatology clinic. Contact Dermatitis 63:89–95
5. Chang YC, Wu WM, Chen CH, Hu CF, Hsu LA (2008) Association between P478S polymorphism of the filaggrin gene and risk of psoriasis in a Chinese population in Taiwan. Arch Dermatol Res 300: 133–137
6. de Jongh CM, Khrenova L, Verberk MM, Calkoen F, van Dijk FJ, Voss H, John SM, Kezic S (2008) Loss-of-function polymorphisms in the filaggrin gene are associated with an increased susceptibility to chronic irritant contact dermatitis: a case–control study. Br J Dermatol 159:621–627
7. Gan SQ, McBride OW, Idler WW, Markova N, Steinert PM (1991) Organization, structure, and polymorphisms of the human profilaggrin gene. Biochemistry 30:5814
8. Ginger RS, Blachford S, Rowland J, Rowson M, Harding CR (2005) Filaggrin repeat number polymorphism is associated with a dry skin phenotype. Arch Dermatol Res 297:235–241
9. Giwercman C, Lerbaek A, Bisgaard H, Menne T (2008) Classification of atopic hand eczema and the filaggrin mutations. Contact Dermatitis 59:257–260
10. Huffmeier U, Traupe H, Oji V, Lascorz J, Stander M, Lohmann J, Wendler J, Burkhardt H, Reis A (2007) Loss-of-function variants of the filaggrin gene are not major susceptibility factors for psoriasis vulgaris or psoriatic arthritis in German patients. J Invest Dermatol 127:1367–1370
11. Irvine AD, McLean WH (2006) Breaking the (un) sound barrier: filaggrin is a major gene for atopic dermatitis. J Invest Dermatol 126:1200–1202
12. Lerbaek A, Bisgaard H, Agner T, Ohm KK, Palmer CN, Menne T (2007) Filaggrin null alleles are not associated with hand eczema or contact allergy. Br J Dermatol 157:1199–1204
13. McGrath JA, Uitto J (2008) The filaggrin story: novel insights into skin-barrier function and disease. Trends Mol Med 14:20–27
14. Molin S, Vollmer S, Weiss EH, Ruzicka T, Prinz JC (2009) Filaggrin mutations may confer susceptibility to chronic hand eczema characterized by combined allergic and irritant contact dermatitis. Br J Dermatol 161:801–807
15. Novak N, Baurecht H, Schafer T, Rodriguez E, Wagenpfeil S, Klopp N, Heinrich J, Behrendt H, Ring J, Wichmann E, Illig T, Weidinger S (2008) Loss-of-function mutations in the filaggrin gene and allergic contact sensitization to nickel. J Invest Dermatol 128:1430–1435
16. O'Regan GM, Irvine AD (2010) The role of filaggrin in the atopic diathesis. Clin Exp Allergy 40:965–972
17. O'Regan GM, Sandilands A, McLean WH, Irvine AD (2009) Filaggrin in atopic dermatitis. J Allergy Clin Immunol 124:R2–R6
18. Palmer CN, Irvine AD, Terron-Kwiatkowski A, Zhao Y, Liao H, Lee SP, Goudie DR, Sandilands A, Campbell LE, Smith FJ, O'Regan GM, Watson RM, Cecil JE, Bale SJ, Compton JG, DiGiovanna JJ, Fleckman P, Lewis-Jones S, Arseculeratne G, Sergeant A, Munro CS, El HB, McElreavey K, Halkjaer LB, Bisgaard H, Mukhopadhyay S, McLean WH (2006) Common loss-of-function variants of the epidermal barrier protein filaggrin are a major predisposing factor for atopic dermatitis. Nat Genet 38:441–446
19. Presland RB, Coulombe PA, Eckert RL, Mao-Qiang M, Feingold KR, Elias PM (2004) Barrier function in transgenic mice overexpressing K16, involucrin, and filaggrin in the suprabasal epidermis. J Invest Dermatol 123:603–606
20. Rawlings AV, Harding CR (2004) Moisturization and skin barrier function. Dermatol Ther 17(Suppl 1): 43–48
21. Rodriguez E, Baurecht H, Herberich E, Wagenpfeil S, Brown SJ, Cordell HJ, Irvine AD, Weidinger S (2009) Meta-analysis of filaggrin polymorphisms in eczema and asthma: robust risk factors in atopic disease. J Allergy Clin Immunol 123:1361–1370
22. Ross-Hansen K, Menne T, Johansen JD, Carlsen BC, Linneberg A, Nielsen NH, Stender S, Meldgaard M, Szecsi PB, Thyssen JP (2011) Nickel reactivity and filaggrin null mutations - evaluation of the filaggrin bypass theory in a general population. Contact Dermatitis 64:24–31
23. Sandilands A, Terron-Kwiatkowski A, Hull PR, O'Regan GM, Clayton TH, Watson RM, Carrick T, Evans AT, Liao H, Zhao Y, Campbell LE, Schmuth M, Gruber R, Janecke AR, Elias PM, van Steensel MA, Nagtzaam I, van GM, Steijlen PM, Munro CS, Bradley DG, Palmer CN, Smith FJ, McLean WH, Irvine AD (2007) Comprehensive analysis of the gene encoding

filaggrin uncovers prevalent and rare mutations in ichthyosis vulgaris and atopic eczema. Nat Genet 39:650–654
24. Smith FJ, Irvine AD, Terron-Kwiatkowski A, Sandilands A, Campbell LE, Zhao Y, Liao H, Evans AT, Goudie DR, Lewis-Jones S, Arseculeratne G, Munro CS, Sergeant A, O'Regan G, Bale SJ, Compton JG, DiGiovanna JJ, Presland RB, Fleckman P, McLean WH (2006) Loss-of-function mutations in the gene encoding filaggrin cause ichthyosis vulgaris. Nat Genet 38:337–342
25. Thyssen JP, Carlsen BC, Johansen JD, Meldgaard M, Szecsi PB, Stender S, Menne T (2010) Filaggrin null-mutations may be associated with a distinct subtype of atopic hand eczema. Acta Derm Venereol 90:528
26. Thyssen JP, Carlsen BC, Menne T, Linneberg A, Nielsen NH, Meldgaard M, Szecsi PB, Stender S, Johansen JD (2010) Filaggrin null mutations increase the risk and persistence of hand eczema in subjects with atopic dermatitis: results from a general population study. Br J Dermatol 163:115–120
27. Thyssen JP, Johansen JD, Linneberg A, Menne T, Nielsen NH, Meldgaard M, Szecsi PB, Stender S, Carlsen BC (2010) The association between null mutations in the filaggrin gene and contact sensitization to nickel and other chemicals in the general population. Br J Dermatol 162(6):1278–1285
28. van den Oord RA, Sheikh A (2009) Filaggrin gene defects and risk of developing allergic sensitisation and allergic disorders: systematic review and meta-analysis. BMJ 339:b2433
29. Weichenthal M, Ruether A, Schreiber S, Nair R, Voorhees JJ, Schwarz T, Kabelitz D, Christophers E, Elder JT, Jenisch S (2007) Filaggrin R501X and 2282del4 mutations are not associated with chronic plaque-type psoriasis in a German cohort. J Invest Dermatol 127:1535–1537
30. Zhang H, Guo Y, Wang W, Shi M, Chen X, Yao Z (2011) Mutations in the filaggrin gene in Han Chinese patients with atopic dermatitis. Allergy 66(3): 420–427
31. Zhao Y, Terron-Kwiatkowski A, Liao H, Lee SP, Allen MH, Hull PR, Campbell LE, Trembath RC, Capon F, Griffiths CE, Burden D, McManus R, Hughes R, Kirby B, Rogers SF, Fitzgerald O, Kane D, Barker JN, Palmer CN, Irvine AD, McLean WH (2007) Filaggrin null alleles are not associated with psoriasis. J Invest Dermatol 127:1878–1882

Molecular Organization of the Lipid Matrix in Stratum Corneum and Its Relevance for the Protective Functions of Human Skin

10

Mila Boncheva

10.1 Introduction

Despite the age-old awareness of the skin as a sheath protecting the living organism from its environment, the first studies that pinpointed its topmost layer, the stratum corneum (SC), as the most crucial element in this defense appeared only in the 1940s [1, 2]. Our understanding of the structure and function of the SC has come a long way from the early notions of a passive, physical barrier against desiccation, xenobiotics, and pathogens [3–5]. The current view of the SC is that it is a complex, dynamic tissue capable of adapting its composition, organization, and activity in response to environmental pressures, thus ensuring the homeostasis of the skin. In addition to protecting against loss of water, entry of chemicals, and microorganisms, it protects the underlying living tissues from oxidative and UV damage, provides a constantly renewing barrier of high mechanical integrity, flexibility, and cohesive strength, participates in the psychosensory and neurosensory interface of the organism, and is involved in the initiation of inflammation and in the regulation of innate and adaptive immunity [5, 6].

The diverse protective tasks performed by the SC typically localize in one of its two principal structural compartments – the terminally differentiated cells, corneocytes, or the extracellular, predominantly lipidic, matrix surrounding them [7–10]. A number of defensive properties are enabled solely by the chemical identity of the responsible ingredients; examples include the antimicrobial activity of peptides, ceramides, and fatty acids [11], the retention of water by the components of the natural moisturizing factor (NMF) and glycerol [12], and the triggering of inflammatory and immune-mediated reactions by cytokines [13]. The molecular properties and quantities of the SC constituents alone, however, cannot explain its formidably low permeability to exogenous chemicals, its ability to adjust the rate of evaporation of water in response to the ambient humidity and temperature, its resistance to normal and sheer stress, or its impaired functionality in disease; these characteristics exist largely because of the unique three-dimensional (3D) organization of the extracellular SC domain. Thus, understanding the molecular details of the organization within the SC lipid matrix is essential both for understanding the biophysics and physiology of skin and for the development of efficient therapies for disorders and diseases of skin.

This chapter will summarize the current knowledge of the composition and molecular organization of the lipids found in the SC, review the evidence connecting the structure of the lipid matrix with the efficient performance of the SC, and outline possibilities to improve the functionality of SC by modulating the 3D organization of its lipids.

M. Boncheva
Corporate R&D Division, Firmenich SA,
Route des Jeunes 1, P.O. Box 239, CH-1211 Geneva 8,
Geneva, Switzerland
e-mail: mila.boncheva@firmenich.com

M. Lodén, H.I. Maibach (eds.), *Treatment of Dry Skin Syndrome*,
DOI 10.1007/978-3-642-27606-4_10, © Springer-Verlag Berlin Heidelberg 2012

Table 10.1 The ceramides of human stratum corneum

Fatty acid / Sphingoid base	Non-hydroxy fatty acid [N]	α-hydroxy fatty acid [A]	Esterified ω-hydroxy fatty acid [EO]
Dihydrosphingosine [DS]	CER [NDS]	CER [ADS]	CER [EODS]
Sphingosine [S]	CER [NS] (Cer 2)	CER [AS] (Cer 5)	CER [EOS] (Cer 1)
Phytosphingosine [P]	CER [NP] (Cer 3)	CER [AP] (Cer 6)	CER [EOP] (Cer 9)
6-hydroxy sphingosine [H]	CER [NH] (Cer 8)	CER [AH] (Cer 7)	CER [EOH] (Cer 4)

Cer [NDS]

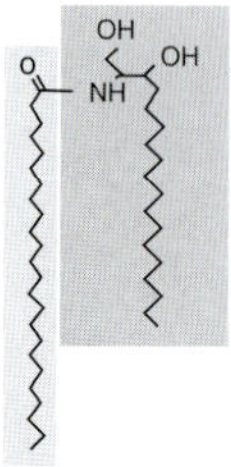

Modified with permission from [18]. The ceramide subclasses are indicated according to the classification of Motta et al. [21] (in capital letters) and according to the earlier classification based on chromatographic mobility (in parentheses). Each ceramide molecule contains one sphingoid and one fatty acid residue, amide-linked as shown next to the table for Cer [NDS]

10.2 Composition of the Lipid Matrix in SC

The lipids of the SC intercellular matrix differ considerably from those typical of the membranes in viable mammalian cells [14, 15]. Three classes of lipid molecules account for over 85–95% of the dry mass of SC matrix: ceramides (about 50% by mass), fatty acids (10–20% by mass), and cholesterol (about 25% by mass). In addition to this approximately equimolar lipidic mixture, the SC contains also several minor lipid ingredients – cholesterol sulfate (0–7%, playing an important role in the processes of desquamation), cholesteryl esters (0–20%), and small amounts of di- and triglycerides, probably of sebaceous origin [16]. The phospholipids typical of the membranes of viable cells are notably absent.

The ceramide composition of the lipid matrix is extremely complex [15, 17–20]. These long-chain lipid molecules consist of fatty acids amide-linked to sphingoid bases. Twelve ceramide subclasses have been identified so far in the extracellular space of SC. Table 10.1 summarizes the known sphingoids and fatty acids that constitute the SC ceramides. The SC ceramides display a distribution of lengths in both the base and the acid chains; this variety results in the existence of over 340 different ceramide species [15, 17, 18]. Most often, the short (sphingoid) hydrocarbon chain comprises 18–20 carbon atoms. The length distribution of the long (fatty acid) chains is broader: it varies between 20 and 32 carbon atoms and peaks at 24 carbons [15]. The majority of the ceramide classes are extractable, i.e., they exist unattached to other molecular species. Most of the ω-hydroxy ceramides, however, are covalently linked to proteins of the corneocyte envelope by esterification of their ω-hydroxyl groups or of one of the hydroxyl groups on the long-chain base moiety [14, 22]; approximately one-third of the Cer [EOS] moiety (and probably also some Cer [EOP] and Cer [EOH]) is present in the interior of the bilayer lamellae [23]. The fatty acid esterified to the ω-hydroxyl groups of Cer [EOS] is most often linoleic acid, occasionally replaced by oleic and stearic acid residues [24]. In principle, the ceramide molecules can adopt three different conformations, depending on their environment (mixed or pure crystals) and the degree of hydration of their head groups [25, 26]: hairpin, with the two hydrocarbon chains pointing in the same direction; splayed, with the two hydrocarbon chains pointing in opposite directions away from the head group; and V-shaped, with the two hydrocarbon chains forming an angle of approximately 60° with the head group positioned at the angle origin. The conformations existing in the native SC lipid matrix are still under debate.

Several structural features of the SC ceramides make them uniquely well-suited for their role as barrier lipids: (1) The asymmetry and the polydispersed lengths of the hydrocarbon chains facilitate the intermolecular mixing between different ceramide subclasses and between ceramides, free fatty acids, and cholesterol [27], and enable the formation of regions of high chain mobility without affecting the head group packing [28]. (2) The presence of unsaturated fatty acid esterified to the long (up to 34 carbon atoms) ω-hydroxy fatty acids in the [EO] ceramides permits the formation of disordered (liquid-crystalline) phases and lamellar structures with large repeat distances. (3) The polar head groups are small and match closely the cross-section of the hydrocarbon chains and thus enable the formation of bilayer lamellar structures. (4) The small size of the functional groups in the head group region precludes its excessive hydration and loss of rigidity in conditions of high humidity. (5) The presence of both donor and acceptor groups in the ceramide head groups enables the formation of extended network of hydrogen bonding between molecules located within the same and within neighboring bilayer leaflets, thus enhancing the impermeability and stability of the lamellae [29–31].

The free fatty acids present in SC (i.e., those existing as individual molecules, and not as a part of the ceramide species) have a fairly broad distribution of chain lengths (between 20 and 30 carbon atoms), peaking at the length of 22–26 carbons – a value unusually high for most biological membranes [32]. They are exclusively nonbranched and saturated. These structural features have important physiological consequences for the performance of the lipid matrix: they ensure lower permeability than lipid membranes comprising unsaturated or branched hydrocarbon chains, and a broader range of phase-transition temperatures than membranes comprising a single chain length [32–34].

The presence of cholesterol in the SC lipid matrix is hardly surprising. This lipid – ubiquitous in biological membranes – is known for its role in regulating the packing density of lipid membranes [35–37] and, thereby, their permeability [33]. Despite considerable research effort over almost a century [38], the exact molecular mechanism by which cholesterol exerts its action is still debatable [39]. Cholesterol also broadens the region of phase-transition temperature, favors intermixing of different lipid species, and, at high concentrations, promotes the formation of lamellar structures [40, 41].

The precursors of the three major SC lipid classes are synthesized locally, in the epidermis, with the notable exception of the essential fatty acids included in the [EO] ceramides; by definition, these unsaturated fatty acids cannot be synthesized in the body and have to be obtained from dietary sources [42]. The extent to which extracutaneous sources (nutritional or from topical application) contribute to the lipid pool in the cells in the stratum granulosum and the extent to which they can modulate or replace the epidermal sources are not clearly determined, although such a possibility clearly exists [43].

10.3 Molecular Organization of the SC Lipids

The lamellar organization of the lipid matrix, later identified as stacked lipid bilayers roughly parallel to the large faces of the corneocytes, has been known since the 1970s [44–47]. Despite the enormous activity in the field, and the exciting progress achieved since then, however, the molecular details of the lipid organization within and across the lamellar planes have not yet been proven unequivocally and are still a hot topic in SC research (reviewed in [48]). The field built upon the extensive knowledge and *savoir-faire* accumulated in more than a century of studies in the biophysics and physical chemistry of cellular and subcellular membranes, based for the most part on model systems derived from phospholipids [49]. The exceptional composition of the lipid matrix and the existence of steep gradients of water, pH, and cations in it, however, preclude assuming direct analogy with other biological membranes and lipid structures; relying on such analogies can be grossly misleading.

A vast array of complementary experimental techniques has been applied to determine the organization of the lipids in SC. These include electron diffraction [9, 50], small- and wide-angle X-ray diffraction [9, 51], neutron diffraction [26, 52, 53], electron microscopy [54–58], Raman [59, 60] and IR spectroscopy [31, 61–64], differential scanning calorimetry [60, 62], ^{2}H NMR spectroscopy [27, 65], electron paramagnetic resonance [66, 67], fluorescence microscopy [68], and atomic force microscopy [69]. The different sensitivity of these techniques to the lipid arrangement in the plane of the lamellae and normal to it, the different level of detail that they can provide, the different propensity they have to artifacts related to sample preparation, the different time and length scales in which they can operate, and the different possibility to apply them in vivo or in vitro clearly indicate that in structural studies, it is preferable to use them in combination rather than to rely exclusively on any single one.

10.3.1 Lateral Molecular Organization

Figure 10.1 shows schematically the possible chain conformations and lateral packing arrangements that are believed to exist in lamellar lipid bilayers (reviewed in [63]). In the most densely packed, orthorhombic phase (OR), the lipid chains adopt *all-trans* conformation and are organized in a rectangular crystalline lattice with no rotational or translational mobility. In the hexagonal (also denoted as gel or L_β) phase (HEX), the *all-trans* lipid chains are tilted in respect to the crystal plane and form a less dense, hexagonal lattice; the lipid molecules have some rotational mobility along their long axis, but their translational mobility is restricted. In the liquid-crystalline (also denoted as L_α) phase (LIQ), the chains exhibit a high degree of *gauche* isomerization, and the lateral organization is entirely lost; the lipid molecules have high rotational and translational mobility in the bilayer plane.

All three lipid phases are present in the SC lipid lamellae, with a marked prevalence of the OR phases. Their coexistence was demonstrated in vitro (in mixtures of extracted SC lipids or their synthetic analogues [70–73]), ex vivo (in isolated SC and in SC flakes removed by tape-stripping [50, 62, 74, 75]), and in vivo (in human volunteers [76]). The abundance of crystalline OR phases in the SC lipids lamellae is in stark contrast with the predominance of LIQ phases in the plasma membranes of living cells [77, 78]; this difference in phase composition reflects the different requirements to the permeability of the two types of lipid structures and the different environmental pressures to which they are exposed.

The amount of extracellular lipids and the relative content of the three phases are not homogeneous throughout the SC thickness. The amount of lipids is highest at the SC surface and progressively decreases toward the inner layers [61]. The topmost SC layers often contain disordered phases, a consequence of the intermixing of sebum and endogenous SC lipids [61, 79, 80]. The middle layers have the highest extent of OR phases [50, 76], and the innermost layers have a lower degree of lateral order than the middle ones, possibly as a result from the incomplete structural reorganization of lipids close to the interface between the stratum corneum and stratum granulosum [16, 81]. In human SC, the lipid content and the depth profiles of the lateral organization do not correlate with age or gender.

The molecular composition of the three lipid phases is still debatable (see also the next section). There are indications that the majority of the free fatty acids and ceramides participate in one and not in several different OR phases; most probably, only a small fraction of the free fatty acids phase-separates into pure OR domains [82]. Phase-separated, crystalline cholesterol frequently exists along with the mixed crystalline phases [83, 84]. The unsaturated linoleate moiety of Cer

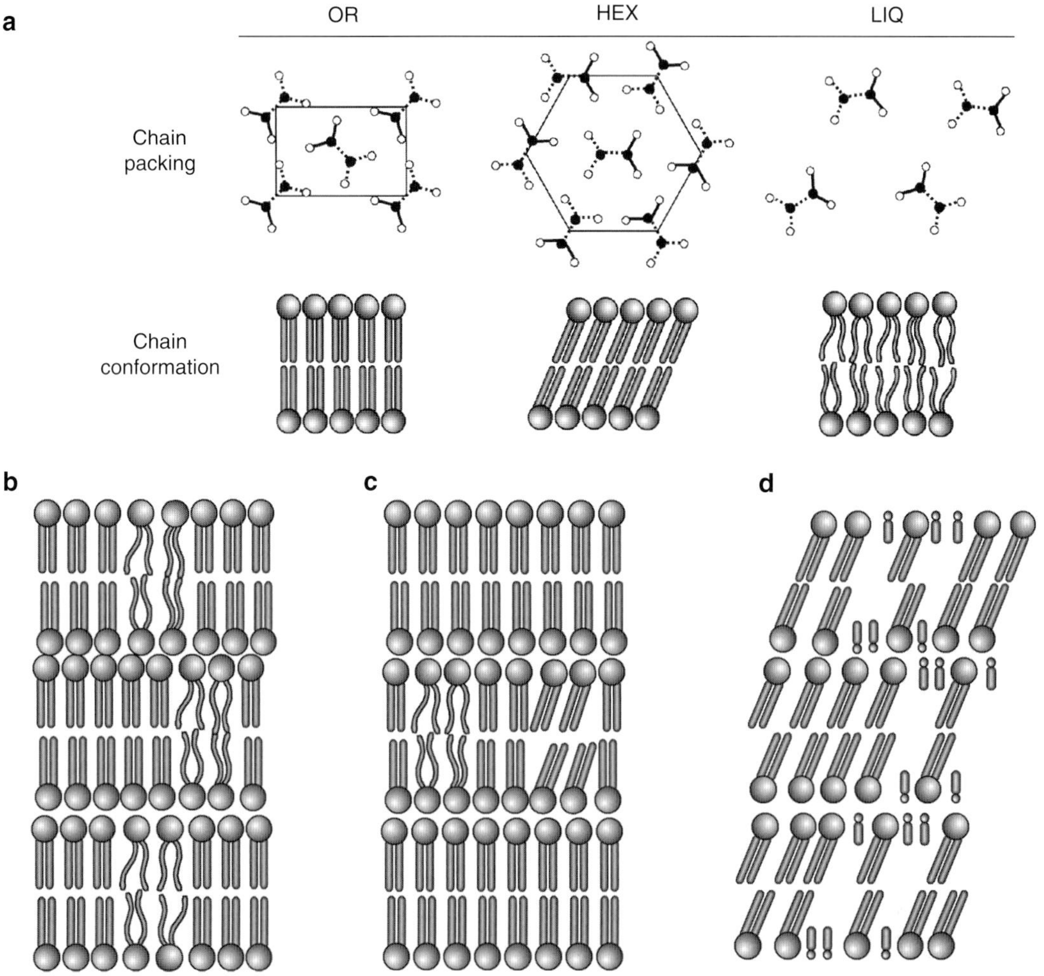

Fig. 10.1 Lateral molecular organization of SC lipids. (**a**) Scheme of the lateral chain packing (*top row*) and chain conformation (*bottom row*) in orthorhombic (*OR*), hexagonal (*HEX*), and liquid-crystalline (*LIQ*) phases of long-chain lipids. (**b**–**d**) Models of the molecular organization of the SC lipid matrix displaying different content and distribution of the lipid phases. The schemes illustrate the domain mosaic model (**b**), the sandwich models (**c**), and the single gel-phase model (**d**). Ceramides and fatty acids are represented with the schematic drawing of long-chain lipids used in (**a**); the presence of cholesterol is explicitly shown only in (**d**) by the smaller of the *two symbols*. The different lipid phases are represented by the conformational order of the long hydrocarbon tails as indicated in (**a**)

[EOS] is most probably located in the highly disordered LIQ phase [82, 85]. Despite its high conformational disorder, however, this fatty acid chain has none of the translational mobility characteristic for a LIQ phase (because of its covalent attachment to the fatty acid chain of the ceramide), and thus, in its presence the phase has the modified characteristics of a "pseudo-fluid" one [82].

Because of the complex composition of the SC lipid matrix and the impossibility to vary systematically its composition in vivo, the role that the different lipid species play in the lateral organization is still not fully understood. Extensive work using simplified model lipid mixtures, however, has helped to establish several important correlations: (1) The presence of Cer [EOS] stabilizes the OR phase regardless of the degree of saturation in the esterified ω-hydroxy fatty acid [86]. (2) A reduction of the content of free fatty acids to less than approximately equimolar with ceramides and cholesterol results in decreased content of OR phases [87]. (3) The length of the alkyl chains of the free fatty acids is important for the type of lipid phases that can form: mixtures of ceramides, cholesterol, and fatty acids with long chains (i.e., having 22 and 24 carbon atoms) form prevalently OR phases (together with some LIQ phases), while similar mixtures containing fatty acids with short chains (i.e., having 16 and 18 carbon atoms) form exclusively HEX phases [48, 88]. (4) The architecture of the ceramide head group is important for the chain packing: the propensity of sphingosine ceramides to form OR domains induces the alkyl chains of the free fatty acids to pack in OR domains; in contrast, the propensity of phytosphingosine ceramides to form domains of more open HEX structure entails the same HEX organization in the alkyl chains of the free fatty acids [30, 82]. (5) The type of fatty acid linked to the ceramide base can also influence the chain packing, as the additional hydroxyl group in the α-hydroxy compared to nonhydroxy fatty acids is also located in the head group region [82].

10.3.2 Lamellar Molecular Organization

In the direction normal to the surface of the corneocytes, the lipid bilayers are stacked on top of each other and form a repeating pattern of structural units (lamellae). Two types of lamellar structures exist in the SC lipid matrix, which differ in their characteristic repeat distance, that is, their thickness: one with a thickness of approximately 13 nm, denoted long periodicity phase (LPP), and another with a thickness of approximately 6 nm, denoted short periodicity phase (SPP). Most often, the LPP is found between the large, flat surfaces of adjacent corneocytes and the SPP – close to their edges [89]. In electron micrographs, the LPP lamellae appear as centrosymmetric stacks of broad-narrow-broad bands [14].

There is still no general consensus concerning the localization and the arrangement of the lipid molecules within the lamellae. Obtaining data with high resolution from native, isolated SC is not straightforward, and their interpretation (especially in the case of diffraction experiments) is sometimes not trivial. Numerous studies have attempted to circumvent these problems by using simplified model mixtures containing only a few lipid species. Despite the undoubted usefulness of this approach, however, it is important to keep in mind that systems of *extremely* simplified composition represent only a rough approximation of the rich molecular variety existing in the native SC and, thus, cannot be expected to give more than a rough approximation of the native molecular organization. For experimental convenience, the selection of the molecules comprising these mixtures has often been limited to species of well-known behavior (such as phospholipids and fatty acids with short chains) or easily available ones (such as those isolated from animal instead of human SC and those commercially available) instead of those most abundant and characteristic for the SC.

The currently existing models proposed for the molecular organization of the SC lipids can be grouped in three major categories according to the presence and the distribution of the main lipid phases: (1) The domain mosaic model of Forslind [90, 91] describes the lipid matrix as a two-phase system in which discontinuous crystalline domains (OR) are embedded in a continuous gel (HEX) or liquid-crystalline (LIQ) phase (Fig. 10.1b), and each lamellar layer contains laterally adjacent impermeable and permeable domains. The molecular transport across the lamellae proceeds by diffusion through disordered phases situated around the borders of the OR domains. Further refinements of this model suggested that both the penetrable and impenetrable SC domains are heterogeneous and comprise lipidic and proteinaceous elements [92, 93]. (2) The sandwich-type models of Bouwstra et al. [94], Swartzendruber et al. [55], Wertz et al. [89], and McIntosh [95] describe the lipid matrix as a multiphase system in which the lamellae contain a central zone of higher mobility (HEX or LIQ, in some models forming a discontinuous phase in an OR matrix) sandwiched between two zones of lower lipid mobility (OR, gel, or ordered liquid phase) (Fig. 10.1c). The molecular transport across the lamellae is slowed by the preferential lateral diffusion of the molecules within the central zone of higher mobility. (3) The single gel-phase model of Norlén [96] describes the lipid matrix as a single and coherent gel phase with no true phase separation in either direction but containing cholesterol-rich domains (organized in closely packed, liquid-crystalline structures) of high permeability and cholesterol-poor domains of low permeability (Fig. 10.1d). Some crystalline domains may form in the upper layers of the SC as a result of the processes of desquamation. Despite its attractive simplicity, however, this model does not accommodate the irrefutable experimental evidence for the existence of highly ordered OR domains within the SC lipid lamellae in vivo and in vitro; thus, its validity is questionable.

Several sandwich-type models exist for the molecular distribution and organization within the LPP. In the model of Bouwstra et al. (first proposed in [94] and refined subsequently), the centrosymmetric unit cell comprises three lipid bilayers of very similar thicknesses – 4.5, 4.0, and 4.5 nm (Fig. 10.2a). The long alkyl chains of ceramides and free fatty acids form tightly packed (OR) outer bilayers, while the unsaturated linoleate chains of Cer [EOS] – slightly interdigitating – form domains with high mobility of the lipid chains (HEX or pseudo-fluid ones) located in the middle bilayer [82]. The ceramides adopt hairpin conformation, with the hydrocarbon chains interdigitating partially (in the outer bilayers) or fully (in the middle bilayer). Cholesterol is most probably asymmetrically enriched in the outer lipid bilayers. There is a gradual change of the chain mobility across the thickness of each LPP lamella.

In the model proposed by Swartzendruber et al. [55] and later refined by Wertz et al. [34, 89], the unit cell comprises three lipid bilayers of uniform (4.3 nm) thickness (Fig. 10.2b). The two outer bilayers are organized in relatively rigid, gel, or liquid-ordered phases. The unsaturated linoleate chains of ceramides [EO] are situated in the middle, relatively fluid (possibly LIQ) bilayer. The ceramides (with the exception of Cer [EO]), free fatty acids, and cholesterol are distributed randomly within the subunits. In all three subunits, the lipid chains do not interdigitate. It is possible that some of the ceramide molecules adopt splayed conformation, with one aliphatic chain inserting in each of a pair of adjacent lamellae. An extended conformation for Cer [AP] is supposed to serve as an armature-like reinforcement preventing the expansion of the lipid bilayers in the course of hydration; Kiselev et al. later suggested that this ceramide undergoes chain-flip transitions between its splayed conformation in partially hydrated SC and hairpin conformation in excessively hydrated SC [97].

The model proposed by McIntosh [95] differs from the previously described ones in that the centrosymmetric unit cell comprises only two lipid bilayers of uniform (4.7 nm) thickness (Fig. 10.2c). Each of these bilayers has a symmetric arrangement of most of the SC ceramides but an asymmetric arrangement of Cer [EOS] (with the linoleate moiety situated in the inner leaflets of the bilayers) and cholesterol (enriched in the outer leaflets of the bilayers). It is possible that some of the ceramides adopt a splayed conformation. The model also suggests a water layer next to the head groups of the outer leaflets of the bilayers.

At present, it is very difficult to affirm unequivocally the superiority of *all* features of one over the other models. Notwithstanding the different interpretations of the experimental data, and the lack of sufficient molecular detail in the resolved structures, the lipid systems that served to develop the models differ considerably in both their composition and their preparation. The models described here have undergone substantial development and revision since their original versions owing to the development of better extraction protocols for native SC lipids, the broader availability of synthetic analogues of the native SC ceramides, and the use of more advanced techniques for structure determination. Undoubtedly, detailed studies of the lamellar molecular organization of the SC lipids continuing in these and other groups will greatly contribute to advance our understanding of the system.

The existence and the structure of the LPP are extremely sensitive to the lipid composition. Ceramides and cholesterol can form an LPP in absence of free fatty acids or in presence of short-chain free fatty acids, but it lacks domains with OR organization [87]. In absence of acylceramides, and, in particular, of Cer [EOS], the

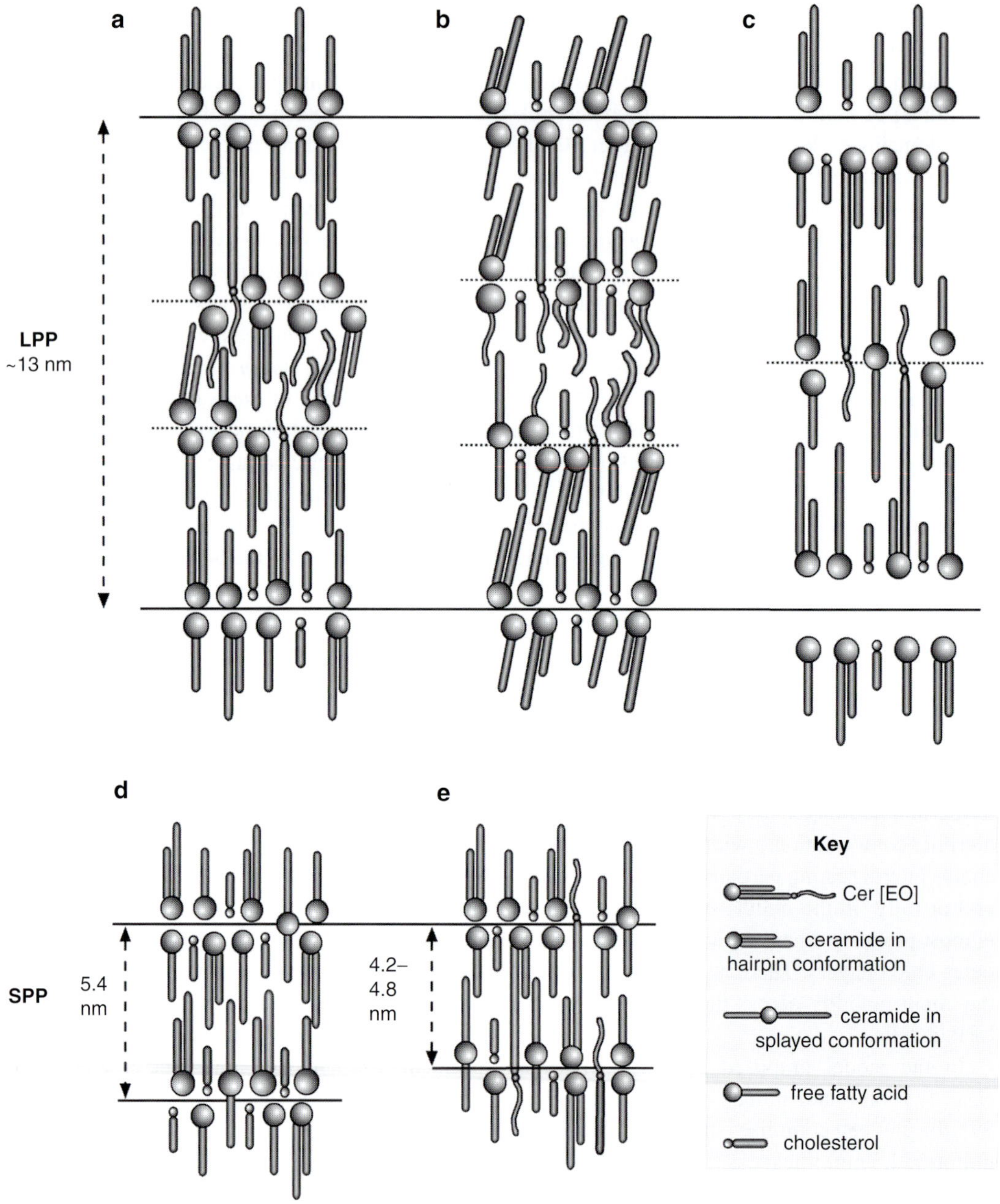

Fig. 10.2 Lamellar molecular organization of the SC lipids. Schematic drawings of the models proposed for the long periodicity phase (*LPP*; **a**–**c**) and the short periodicity phase (*SPP*; **d**, **e**); see the text for a discussion of the main features of the models. The *solid lines* indicate the borders of one lamella, the *dashed arrows* indicate the characteristic periodic repeat distances of the phases, and the *dotted lines* delimit the individual lipid bilayers

fraction of lipids forming the LPP is extremely small [85, 98]. The replacement of the linoleic with saturated residue in the Cer [EOS] molecule prevents the formation of LPP, indicating that the formation of LPP necessitates a fraction of lipids capable of forming a phase of high mobility [86]. Lack of variety in the architecture of the head groups in the ceramide molecules and a narrow distribution of the lengths of the lipid chains reduce the ability to form LPP reproducibly [52, 82].

Several recent studies focused on the structural features of the other lamellar phase present in the SC, the short periodicity phase (SPP). A report by Bouwstra et al. described the formation of SPP in an equimolar mixture of synthetic ceramides (Cer [NS], Cer [NP], and Cer [AS]), cholesterol, and fatty acids (comprising 16–26 carbon atoms, in a ratio typical for human SC) [99]. Cer [EOS] was not included in the lipid mixture because of its prominence in the LPP. In the molecular model of SPP proposed in this work (Fig. 10.2d), the unit cell has a repeat distance of 5.4 nm and comprises one lipid bilayer. The ceramides have a symmetric arrangement in a splayed or hairpin conformation, with interdigitating acyl chains in the middle of the bilayer. The majority of the ceramides, cholesterol, and fatty acids are mixed homogeneously, with only a small fraction of phase-separated cholesterol. The SPP is weakly hydrated and probably contains two water molecules per lipid head group.

Neubert et al. also reported the formation of phases of short periodicity in quaternary lipid mixtures composed of Cer [AP], Cer [EOS], cholesterol, and a fatty acid comprising 16, 22, 24, or 26 carbon atoms [52, 100], or composed of Cer [AP], cholesterol, cholesterol sulfate, and palmitic (C16) or behenic (C22) acid [26, 101]. The unit cells of the observed SPPs contained one bilayer and had repeat distances of 4.2–4.8 nm (Fig. 10.2e). Not surprisingly, even the mixtures containing Cer [EOS] did not form LPP, as they lacked the characteristic for SC polydispersity in the lengths of the fatty acids and in the architectures of the ceramide head groups. The molecular arrangement proposed for the SPP consists of one bilayer in which the Cer [AP] molecules adopt splayed conformation and connect leaflets of adjacent bilayers or adopt hairpin conformation within one bilayer leaflet, and the linoleate moiety of Cer [EOS] protrudes into the adjacent bilayer. The model based on behenic acid allows for interdigitation of the hydrocarbon chains in the middle of the bilayer, and the model based on palmitic acid does not. In both these model systems, a small fraction of the cholesterol phase-separates. Clearly, only further work using model systems with composition approaching the molecular diversity of the endogenous SC lipids will shed more light on the molecular organization and composition of the SPP in healthy SC.

10.4 Self-Assembly of the Lipid Matrix

The 3D organization of the lipid lamellae is a result of hierarchical, templated self-assembly processes that occur at the border between the topmost layer of viable epidermal cells, the stratum granulosum, and the inner layers of SC. The exact sequence of events in the cascade of processes leading to the formation of the lipid lamellae and the concomitant terminal differentiation of the keratinocytes is not yet fully understood [102]; new participants and effectors in this cascade are still being identified [103]. In broad, simplified terms, the lamellar assembly proceeds through the following steps: The precursors of the main SC lipids – glucosyl-ceramides, sphingomyelin, cholesterol, and phospholipids – are synthesized in the keratinocytes of stratum spinosum. There, they are organized in flattened, short bilayer stacks within lamellar bodies (LB) – secretory granules that contain in addition an array of catabolic enzymes, antimicrobial peptides, and other proteins [10, 104–107]. The lamellar bodies are stored in the keratinocytes of stratum spinosum and stratum granulosum. While under basal conditions they are secreted at low rates, an acute barrier disruption generates a number of signals (e.g., changes in the concentration gradients of cations and water [108, 109]) for rapid enhancement of their secretion and the induction of terminal differentiation of corneocytes [103]. In response to these signals, the keratinocytes secrete the content of the LB in the extracellular space surrounding the corneocytes of SC, and it anchors onto the desmosomes [102]. The ω-hydroxy ceramides that are covalently bound to the corneocyte envelope (in particular Cer [OS]) play an important role in templating the proper orientation and alignment of the bilayer stacks. Following their alignment at the corneocyte surface, the short lipid stacks fuse into long lamellae and are processed by the enzymes coextruded from the LB into the ultimate SC lipids of considerably higher hydrophobicity [30, 102, 110]. Driven by the spontaneous organization of the intercellular lipids, the proteinaceous portion of the LB content is displaced toward the hydrophilic loci represented by the extracellular portions of the corneodesmosomes; thus, the newly formed lipid lamellae indirectly aid the colocalization of the SC enzymes and their substrates [111].

The interactions that hold together the final 3D structure of the lipid lamellae are van der Waals forces existing between the long hydrocarbon chains of ceramides and fatty acids in the plane normal to the lamellae, and hydrogen bonds existing between the polar head groups of the ceramides in the lateral plane of the lamellae and between neighboring lamellae [25, 29, 30, 112]. During the formation of the lamellae, hydrophobic interactions (i.e., those combining van der Waals interactions with the enthalpic and entropic consequences of restricting the hydrogen bonding of water in the vicinity of the apolar lipid chains) provide additional contribution to the driving forces involved in the lipid self-assembly. All these reversible, noncovalent interactions are relatively weak and comparable in strength to the ~2.5 kJ/mol of thermal energies (e.g., the van der Waals attraction between two small alkane molecules in water is approximately 10 kJ/mol, and most hydrogen bonds contribute between 10 and 40 kJ/mol [113–115]); nonetheless, they compound in the extensive lipid lamellae to give a robust structure.

It is important to emphasize that the 3D structure of the SC lipids represents a static self-assembled structure and not a dynamic one, as sometimes assumed [96, 116]. By definition, this distinction refers to the energetics of the *structures* resulting from self-assembly processes and not to the *process* itself. Thus, static self-assembled structures are equilibrium ones, existing in global or local energy minima; in contrast, dynamic self-assembled structures are nonequilibrium, energy dissipating ones that are maintained in a steady state by constant supply of energy [117, 118]. Following their formation, the lipid lamellae do not need an influx of energy to maintain their molecular order which corresponds to the minimum thermodynamic potential of the system; in other words, the lipid organization in an appropriately preserved, isolated sheet of SC and in the same SC still attached to a living body (i.e., to a source of energy) would not differ, provided the temperature and humidity conditions are the same. Furthermore, subjected to minor (e.g., thermal) perturbations, the system will tend to return to its initial state and assume its initial molecular organization. The fact that the molecular organization within the lipid matrix corresponds to a (global or local) thermodynamic minimum indicates that it is possible to reproduce it in model systems by mixing and equilibrating the components and that it is possible to study lipid biophysics in isolated SC sheets ex vivo.

Despite the extensive research effort during the last few decades, the thermodynamics of the processes leading to the formation of the intricate 3D structure of the lipid matrix is not fully understood [62]. Because of the low strength of the molecular interactions between the SC lipids, the enthalpies of the interactions holding together the matrix structure are relatively weak (if compared, for example, to those of the covalent bonds binding the ω-hydroxy ceramides to the corneocyte envelope); the interplay between enthalpy and entropy during the self-assembly process is, therefore, significant and should not be ignored. As the self-assembly can be driven by purely enthalpic effects, purely entropic effects, or a combination of both, the relative contributions of both to the reduction of the overall free energy of the system must be considered [113].

10.5 Correlation Between the Molecular Organization of the Lipid Matrix and the SC Performance

In numerous skin conditions (e.g., dry, environmentally stressed, and chronologically aged skin) and diseases (e.g., type 2 Gaucher's disease, Niemann-Pick disease, many ichthyoses, atopic dermatitis, psoriasis, and essential fatty acid deficiency), the lipid composition and quantities differ from those in healthy SC due to perturbations in the synthesis, delivery, or extracellular processing of one or several classes of SC lipids [10, 104, 119]. The way that the abnormal lipid composition translates into impaired SC functionality, however, has been investigated in detail only in few cases, for example in dry skin and in skin from patients with atopic dermatitis, lamellar ichthyosis, and psoriasis (reviewed in [8] and [9]). These studies have clearly demonstrated the importance of the molecular organization of the SC lipids in the etiology of the diseases.

10.5.1 Permeability of the SC

In general terms, the key parameters that determine the permeability of the SC to a given molecule are the partition coefficient of the molecule between its external (e.g., topically applied drug formulation) or internal (e.g., highly hydrated cells of the viable tissue) reservoir and the structural components of the SC (the corneocytes and the lipid matrix), the diffusion coefficient of the molecule within the SC, and the length of the diffusional pathway [120]. All three parameters depend heavily on the molecular organization of the lipid lamellae. Depending on their physicochemical properties (e.g., molecular size and shape, lipophilicity, polarity, and hydrogen bonding ability), molecules cross the SC at different rates and following different pathways [121–123]; as a consequence, different aspects of the molecular organization can be expected to be important for the penetration of small, polar, hydrophilic molecules like water and the penetration of large, apolar, lipophilic molecules like many cosmetic ingredients and topical drugs. While in some cases the skin permeability for *both* hydrophilic and lipophilic molecules is abnormally high (e.g., in skin diseases related to failure in the formation of LB like harlequin ichthyosis [16]), the two are not necessarily identical; thus, the SC permeability to water measured as transepidermal water loss (TEWL) does not always reflect the SC permeability to other molecular species [124].

The well-known correlation between the conformational ordering of the hydrocarbon chains in phospholipid membranes and the membrane permeability has been examined in human SC both ex vivo and in vivo [125–130]. These studies have clearly established that an increase in the content of disordered phases in the SC correlates with increased molecular diffusion. In addition, a recent in vivo study demonstrated the existence of a direct linear correlation between the lateral molecular organization of the SC lipids and the efficacy of SC as a barrier to water transport: the higher the fraction of lipids involved in OR phases, the lower the TEWL [76]. In principle, the direction of transport – outside-in or inside-out – should not influence the SC permeability to a given class of molecules [131]; thus, it would be very interesting to examine if the same correlation holds for topically applied, small hydrophilic molecules.

The relative importance of the lamellar and the lateral molecular organization of the SC lipids for its permeability to molecules of medium and high lipophilicity is not yet well understood. There are strong indications that the LPP which is present in the SC of all species investigated to date plays an important role in SC permeability [9]. In the SC of patients with lamellar ichthyosis, a disease characterized by abnormally high skin permeability, the periodicity of the LPP is decreased, and its general appearance is significantly altered; concomitantly, the content of Cer [EOS], the ceramide crucial for the formation of the LPP, is reduced (reviewed in [9]). A study with synthetic SC membranes demonstrated that in the absence of LPP, the permeability of the membranes to molecules of medium hydrophobicity increased twofold compared to the one observed in the presence of LPP. This observation indicates that at least a part of the SC barrier of the diseased skin is due to a reduced LPP content [132]. It is, however, difficult to separate the effect of the lamellar and lateral lipid organization in these cases: besides having abnormal lamellar structure, atopic SC also has a markedly reduced content of OR, and in SC of skin with lamellar ichthyosis, the HEX content is predominant, possibly together with nonlamellar LIQ phases [133]. A recent work elaborated further on the relative contributions of the lamellar and the lateral lipid organization to the permeability of the SC for small hydrophobic molecules by comparing the activation energies for the penetration of benzoic acid across synthetic SC analogues containing or lacking the LPP [53]. The study showed that the presence of LPP probably leads to an increase of the activation energy of the transport of benzoic acid across the lipid matrix. It will be very interesting to examine the importance of the LPP with molecules having different physicochemical characteristics, while following in detail the effect that these molecules exert on the lateral lipid molecular organization during their transit through the lipid layers. The role of SPP in maintaining the barrier efficiency is not yet fully understood [134].

10.5.2 Integrity and Cohesion of the SC

The maintenance of a competent barrier across the SC requires that it has the capacity to resist minor external insults, a property denoted as integrity. In addition, the homeostasis of the SC barrier necessitates the maintenance of a gradient of intercellular cohesion within the SC, ranging from strong in the inner SC layers (to ensure the mechanical stability of the tissue) to weak in the surface layers (to ensure the normal desquamation of terminally differentiated corneocytes) [135, 136]. Integrity and cohesion are often not discriminated in the literature and are measured experimentally by the damage – expressed as the change of TEWL (integrity) or as the amount of removed protein (cohesion) – caused by tape-stripping.

The current understanding of the role of SC lipids, and especially of their molecular organization, for the integrity and cohesion of SC is incomplete. The difficulty in investigating this correlation stems from the fact that several common factors – that is, the local concentrations of water, Ca^{2+}, and cholesterol sulfate, and the pH – influence both the lamellar organization of the SC lipids and the activity of the hydrolytic enzymes responsible for corneodesmosomal degradation [136–140]; it is not easy to disentangle the relative contributions of the lipidic and the proteinaceous components of the SC to the perturbed cohesion and integrity in topically stressed and diseased skin [119, 135]. Thus, for example, a sustained increase of pH of the skin surface causes the formation of incomplete lamellae and accelerates the degradation of corneodesmosomes [139, 141], while elevated levels of cholesterol sulfate (e.g., those observed in recessive X-linked ichthyosis) provoke abnormal appearance of the lamellae and abnormally high cohesion in the superficial layers of SC [104]. In vitro studies using SC models have shown that a pH of 7.4 and relatively high content of cholesterol sulfate, two conditions typical for the inner SC layers, promote the formation of the LPP phase; their drop in the superficial SC layers may help to destabilize the lipid lamellar organization, thus facilitating desquamation [134, 142].

Several mechanisms might explain how an altered lipid organization can lead to abnormal desquamation and loss of integrity in SC [104]; these include abnormal hydrogen bonding between the SC ceramides [66], abnormal Ca^{2+}-mediated ionic interactions [143], abnormally high content of phase-separated lipids [134], and abnormal ratio of ordered and disordered lipid phases. The experimental evidence connecting the phase content of the lipid matrix and the integrity and cohesion of SC is still incomplete. As discussed earlier, the presence of some lipids adopting LIQ organization is necessary for the formation of the LPP phase and for maintaining its elasticity; in the absence of disordered phases, the lamellae might be unable to follow closely the contours of the corneocytes, thereby weakening the intercellular cohesion [134]. Studies of the mechanical properties of isolated SC, however, have shown that the lipid disordering is not enough to weaken the intercellular cohesion [144]. The extent of lipids participating in OR phases correlates well with the degree of integrity (measured by the change of basal TEWL following tape-stripping) but does not correlate with the degree of cohesion (measured by the protein content of the tapes) in healthy human skin in vivo [145]. Most probably, this observation reflects a different, indirect mechanism by which the lipid molecular organization can impact the integrity and cohesion of SC: by enabling the diffusion of the SC enzymes and of their respective activators and inhibitors to their substrates [105, 136], such as proteolytic enzymes necessary for degradation of the corneodesmosomes [111, 146] and lipid hydrolases necessary to transform precursors secreted form the LB into SC components [104].

10.6 Skin Therapies Based on Topical Modulators of the SC Lipid Organization

The direct correlation between the organization of the lipid matrix and key properties of SC such as permeability and integrity implies that topically applied chemicals, capable of admixing with the endogenous SC lipids and changing their 3D organization, can be used to influence the performance of the SC. Both reduction and enhancement of the SC permeability are therapeutically relevant. Efficient strategies for barrier strengthening are important in a number of circumstances [147, 148]: (1) in the treatment of skin diseases linked to misbalance of the main SC lipids and consequent defective barrier properties; (2) in acquired dermatoses resulting from occupational hazards (e.g., frequent contact with water and detergents), sustained exposure to moisture and elevated pH (e.g., in infants and incontinent adults), and extreme or quickly changing environmental conditions; (3) to remedy immature and underdeveloped skin (e.g., the skin of infants and preterm babies) and chronologically aged skin; and (4) to assist the healing of severely damaged skin (e.g., resulting from burns or other wounds). Strengthening the SC barrier to limit penetration of exogenous chemicals also offers an interesting alternative for the design of topical products intended to prevent the systemic absorption of harmful pollutants, toxins, irritants, sensitizers, and warfare agents. The exceptional impermeability of the healthy SC has also a downside: beneficial topically applied chemicals also have limited access to the inner SC layers and the underlying viable tissues. Thus, in addition to strengthening, the inverse effect – overcoming the SC barrier to penetration – is of enormous interest for the dermal and transdermal delivery of drugs, local anesthetics, vaccines, and cosmeceuticals [149, 150].

10.6.1 Strengthening the SC Barrier

The topical application of lipids – nonphysiologic, occlusive ones, or ones similar to those typically found in healthy SC – has long been the therapy of choice for strengthening the barrier to penetration in diseased and damaged skin and in accelerating its formation in underdeveloped and wounded skin [10, 151–154]. Because of the equimolar ratio between ceramides, fatty acids, and cholesterol necessary to achieve and maintain the 3D organization of the lipid matrix in healthy SC, the types and relative contents of the lipids are of paramount importance for the efficiency of the therapy. In diseases in which this ratio is abnormal (e.g., the characteristic for atopic dermatitis ceramide deficiency and enhanced cholesterol levels, the complete absence of polyunsaturated fatty acid moieties in the ceramide molecules in essential fatty acid deficiency, and the reduced content of free fatty acids in lamellar ichthyosis [155]), the composition of the topically applied lipids is most efficient when it compensates for the imbalance [147]. In other words, "cure-all" creams for barrier repair cannot be expected to – and do not – work equally well on skin with all kinds of barrier damage [148].

The efficient performance of the SC as a barrier to water evaporation strongly depends on its state of hydration. This correlation is at the origin of the initiation and perpetuation of the vicious cycle of dry skin, one of the most common skin disorders: a drop in the SC barrier efficiency and a lessening of its integrity lead to a reduction of the SC hydration, which in turn enhances further the SC permeability for water [140]. Besides having a cosmetically unpleasing appearance and reduced flexibility and resistance, dry SC is chronically inflamed, is prone to attacks from pathogenic microorganisms, and often provides decreased protection against the penetration of chemicals [105]. Importantly, improving the SC barrier efficiency to permeation of water can interrupt the cycle of dry skin at any stage [156]. With the increasing occurrence of this disorder, the search for more efficient strategies for skin moisturization is intense.

Traditionally, moisturizers were thought to act either by their ability to penetrate the SC and retain moisture in its inner layers (a mechanism attributed to small and highly hygroscopic polyhydroxy molecules like glycerol, glycols, glucose, and sorbitol) or by their ability to form an occlusive film at the skin surface (a mechanism attributed to long-chain – typically containing 15–40 carbon atoms – lipophilic molecules like the hydrocarbon mixtures in mineral oil and petrolatum). The finding of a correlation between the molecular organization of the SC lipids and the permeability of SC for water led to the discovery of a novel mechanism for improving the SC hydration – by creating an occlusive effect *within* the SC, termed "internal occlusion" [157]. As discussed earlier, the OR phases have the lowest permeability for water among the lipid phases present in the SC matrix [9], and their content determines the water loss due to TEWL [76]; the mechanism of internal occlusion consists in stabilizing the OR phases within the SC lipid matrix, and thereby increasing its water content by reduction of TEWL. This effect was first described for isostearyl and isopropyl isostearate, lipophilic molecules capable of penetrating the SC in vivo without visibly changing the general appearance of the lamellar lipid phases. These molecules incorporate partially within the LPP phase, promote its formation at the expense of SPP, and partition between the OR phase formed by SC lipids and a pure disordered phase [158, 159]. Their presence increases the thermotropic stability of the OR phases and makes them capable of persisting at temperatures above 30 °C, the phase-transition temperature between the OR and HEX phases observed in the endogenous SC lipids. The molecular mechanism of this stabilization is not well understood; it is possible that internally occluding molecules broaden the extent of the OR phase by partitioning in it and/or by facilitating the incorporation of free fatty acids into the OR domains [160]. Nonetheless, their efficacy in increasing the water content of SC is evident; indeed, chemicals of similar structure have been long used empirically as ingredients in moisturizing formulations [157].

The further development of moisturizers that act solely by this mechanism has, however, to take into account the change of the overall content of OR phases in the SC needed for the required change in TEWL. The correlation between the two parameters observed in normal, healthy skin indicates that to reduce the TEWL by 5 g/m^2h, the content of OR phases has to increase by approximately 50% [76]; depending on the degree of damage to the SC barrier for water, it is possible that the most efficient products for improving the SC moisturization would be those that make use of all three mechanisms – water retention, external occlusion, and internal occlusion – acting simultaneously. It is also important to consider that the content of OR phase is not the only factor contributing to TEWL: together with the water permeability of the SC lipid matrix, the presence of fully matured corneocytes [111, 146] and water-retaining constituents of NMF [156] also contribute to the sustaining of SC hydration. Furthermore, it is generally accepted that the presence of the LPP is important for maintaining an efficient barrier to the transport of exogenous chemicals across the SC. Importantly, the proper formation of the LPP necessitates a fraction of lipids organized in LIQ phases [73]; the relative content of OR and LIQ lipid phases thus has to be properly balanced to maintain the homeostasis of the SC barrier.

This mechanism for strengthening the barrier to evaporation of water through the SC cannot, unfortunately, be generalized as *the* universal solution to making the SC impermeable to *all* types of molecules. As discussed earlier, different aspects of the molecular organization of the SC lipids can be expected to govern the SC permeability to molecules of different physicochemical properties; it is far from certain that the extent of OR phases correlates with the penetration of molecules of moderate to high lipophilicity.

Another possible way to reinforce the SC barrier might be to change the pattern of lateral hydrogen bonding between the ceramides in a way that renders the lamellae more compact without necessarily augmenting the content of OR phases [161]. This mechanism of action was suggested to explain the effect of retarding the penetration of other chemicals observed for one structural analogue of Azone [162] and several oxazolidone derivatives [163]. Despite the broad potential applications of penetration retardants – ranging from localized targeting of therapeutic agents, sunscreen products, and insect repellents in the superficial SC layers to protection from systemic absorption of chemical warfare, toxic spills, and pesticides – not many studies have investigated possible mechanisms to retard the penetration through SC [164–168].

10.6.2 Overcoming the SC Barrier

In addition to strategies for overcoming the SC barrier based on physical disruption, heat, formulation effects, and providing external driving forces for the penetration, the use of chemical enhancers capable of disrupting the highly ordered SC lipids has been widely explored. The majority of the chemical penetration enhancers developed so far act either by insertion in the bilayers or by extracting lipids from them. Extensive research effort has been dedicated to screening potential candidates and to attempting to build structure-activity relationships to understand their action and to facilitate their rational design [169]. The biggest hurdle to the wide practical application of chemical enhancers, however, is not their insufficient enhancement potency but the fact that high enhancement potency typically correlates with high irritation potency [149]; the scope of molecules capable of strongly disorganizing the SC lipids without penetrating into the viable tissues is extremely limited. Recent studies have demonstrated that synergistic combinations of chemical enhancers can exhibit significantly higher potency in enhancement and yet cause lower irritation than their individual ingredients [170, 171]; this approach is now being actively pursued.

10.7 Conclusions and Outlook

The molecular organization of the SC lipid matrix has been an extremely active field of research during the last few decades. The continuing interest in this area comes from two powerful sources: one is our fascination with the unsolved riddles in lipid biophysics and, in general, in molecular self-assembly [172, 173], and the other one – the paramount importance of the SC lipids for maintaining the homeostasis of human skin and the therapeutic relevance of enhancing or reducing its barrier efficiency. The picture that we now have of the extracellular lipids as an intricate, 3D ensemble with modular composition, organization, and functionality has a level of detail closer to reality than the early concept of a homogeneous mortar holding together corneocyte bricks. Despite the progress achieved so far, however, quite a few elements in this picture remain obscure or at best incomplete: (1) Our knowledge of the composition of the SC lipid matrix is still not definite, as illustrated by the uninterrupted stream of newly identified molecules present in SC. (2) With few exceptions, the role that the individual subclasses of the SC lipids play in achieving an optimally functional 3D structure of the lipid matrix is not definitely established; thus, our understanding of the correlation between SC functionality, composition, and structure in healthy and diseased skin remains incomplete. (3) The role played by the minor ingredients of the intracellular space (e.g., cholesterol sulfate and other cholesteryl esters) which are essential for the correct SC function in the organization of lipids is largely unknown. (4) There are still considerable gaps in our understanding of the 3D structure of the lipid matrix. Overall, it appears that both crystalline and disordered lipid phases are present in SC, but the way they are organized within the lipid lamellae is yet to be established beyond reasonable doubt. (5) The extent of compositional and structural variations within the lamellae due to body site, gender, age, race, and depth within the SC is, for the most part, unknown [174–176].

Model systems of simplified lipid composition have proven to be extremely useful in studies designed to elucidate the molecular organization of the native SC lipid matrix and to determine the role of the individual SC lipid subclasses in it. Their preparation is relatively easy, they can readily accommodate both synthetic and endogenous SC lipids, and, provided appropriate composition and preparation protocol, they can reproduce the native molecular organization of SC with fair fidelity. Compared to working with isolated SC, they offer the advantages of precisely controlled chemical identity of the ingredients, uniform thickness, reproducibility, and ease of interpretation of the data. Their undoubted usefulness aside, using these systems in structural studies always carries the inherent danger that the data obtained from such simplified systems may be irrelevant to the native SC, which displays an amazingly broad spectrum of different chemical species. Limiting the number of ceramide species and narrowing the distribution of chain lengths in both ceramides and fatty acids seriously impede the ability to reproduce the native organization of the SC lipid matrix. Thus, conclusions based of systems of extremely simplified composition should always be checked against data obtained from more complex systems or, ideally, from native SC. Despite their attractively ready availability and low cost, lipids isolated from animal skin are not always the best alternative to model the polydispersity in chain lengths and head groups of the human SC lipids and, therefore, to reproduce their organization. Properly composed and formed, however, synthetic SC models and substitutes will continue to be of great use for future structural studies. In view of the high cost, inherent high inter-individual variability, and body-site dependence of the permeability of excised human skin, their use in high-throughput screening of effectors of the skin penetration would be extremely valuable.

While it is, in principle, possible to advantageously modulate the SC performance by manipulating the molecular organization of its lipids with topical products, the details – and, often, the nature – of the correlation between the structure of the lipid matrix and the SC properties are largely unknown. When designing such topical effectors, it is extremely important to keep in mind the complex interconnections that exist between the defensive functions of the SC and to remember that the same parameter might influence several properties in opposing directions [10]. Thus, for example, an exceedingly high content of densely packed lipid phases might improve the skin moisturization by reducing the loss of water through the SC; at the same time, however, the diffusion of corneodesmolytic enzymes to their substrates in such densely packed lipid matrix would be extremely difficult and might result in impaired SC desquamation. An appropriate ratio between the lipid phases present in the SC is apparently vital for the performance of key functions of the SC, ranging from permeability to flexibility to normal desquamation, but the limits within which the phase ratio can vary while still assuring proper SC performance are yet to be defined. Establishing the timescale and reversibility of reformation following structural perturbation is also of utmost importance for the design of effectors of the molecular organization; in addition to being efficient and harmless for the viable tissues, the modifiers of SC permeability have to exert only transient and reversible effect to avoid subsequent entry of undesirable substances and microorganisms in the layers beyond the SC. Work in this direction is in its early stages [75, 177].

Besides influencing the SC health and cosmetic appearance from the outside, using topically applied products, the possibility to manipulate these characteristics from the inside, through nutrition, is clearly indicated [178, 179]. Systematic studies and solid epidemiologic evidence correlating the nutrition and the optimal performance of the SC, however, exist for only a handful of ingredients. Further work in the development of products specifically targeting the SC barrier (i.e., the lipids of the SC extracellular matrix) is warranted to realize the full potential for health promotion and disease prevention of functional foods and neutraceuticals designed for the skin.

In addition to its primary objective – tackling the correlation between lipid composition, structure, and performance of the SC – the research in model and native SC membranes can, potentially, also benefit the understanding of the formation, properties, and functionality of lipid rafts in plasma membranes. Lipid rafts are membrane domains enriched in sphingolipids and cholesterol, proposed to be important for lipid and protein transport across the membranes, in intracellular signaling, and in regulating the activity of membrane-associated proteins [180, 181]. Paralleling the essential problems in the SC lipid organization, the questions of the role of the acyl chain packing and cholesterol in membrane stabilization, the preferential association between different lipid classes, the coexistence of lipid phases, and the formation of domains are central to understanding the formation and stability of structures such as fluctuating raft assemblies [182, 183]. Despite the obvious differences in the composition and the local environment of the lipid lamellae in SC and the lipid rafts in plasma membranes, they illustrate two sides of the general question of how the living organisms use lipids to control composition, structure, and functionality.

The lipid matrix of the stratum corneum is yet another example in the long list of intricate functionality achieved by molecular self-assembly in biological systems [184]. Further extension of our understanding of the correlation between its molecular organization and its meso- and macroscopic properties will doubtlessly be beneficial for establishing the molecular bases of skin health and disease; in addition, it has the potential to contribute to the design of synthetic biomimetic smart materials and systems [172, 185, 186], such as advanced encapsulating materials for slow release of drugs and cosmeceuticals [187, 188], protective cover layers for biomedical applications [189] and wound healing [190], selectively permeable membranes for molecular separations [191], and artificial cells [192].

Take Home Messages

- The extracellular matrix of stratum corneum participates actively in the defensive performance of human skin.
- The unique lamellar organization of the lipids, resulting from their exceptional composition, ensures the low permeability of the skin for xenobiotics, limits the loss of water from the living tissues, and contributes to the formation of a barrier layer of high mechanical integrity, flexibility, and cohesive strength.
- Both crystalline and disordered lipid phases exist in the lamellae, but their 3D organization remains to be definitely established.
- Understanding the correlation between composition, molecular organization, and properties of the lipid matrix helps to elucidate the etymology of skin diseases and disorders and offers the potential to develop new, efficient skin therapies.

Abbreviations

3D	three-dimensional
HEX	hexagonal phase
LB	lamellar body
LIQ	liquid-crystalline phase
LPP	long periodicity phase
NMF	natural moisturizing factor
OR	orthorhombic phase
SC	stratum corneum
SPP	short periodicity phase
TEWL	trans-epidermal water loss

References

1. Winsor T, Burch GE (1944) Differential roles of layers in human epigastric skin on diffusion rate of water. Arch Intern Med 74:428–435
2. Blank IH (1952) Factors which influence the water content of the stratum corneum. J Invest Dermatol 18:433–440
3. Elias PM (2004) The epidermal permeability barrier: from the early days at Harvard to emerging concepts. J Invest Dermatol 122:xxxvi–xxxix
4. Kligman AM (2006) A brief history of how the dead stratum corneum became alive. In: Elias PM, Feingold KR

(eds) Skin barrier. Taylor and Francis, New York, pp 15–24
5. Kligman AM (2011) Corneobiology and corneotherapy – a final chapter. Int J Cosm Sci 33: 197–209
6. Elias PM (2006) Defensive functions of the Stratum corneum: Integrative aspects. In: Elias PM, Feingold KR (eds) Skin barrier. Taylor and Francis, New York, pp 5–14
7. Brody I (1966) Intercellular space in normal human stratum corneum. Nature 209:472–476
8. Harding CR (2004) The stratum corneum: structure and function in health and disease. Dermatol Ther 17:6–15
9. Bouwstra JA, Ponec M (2006) The skin barrier in healthy and diseased state. Biochim Biophys Acta-Biomembranes 1758:2080–2095
10. Elias PM (2005) Stratum corneum defensive functions: an integrated view. J Invest Dermatol 125:183–200
11. Di Nardo A, Gallo RL (2006) Cutaneous barriers in defense against microbial invasion. In: Elias PM, Feingold KR (eds) Skin barrier. Taylor and Francis, New York, pp 363–378
12. Rawlings AV (2006) Sources and role of Stratum corneum hydration. In: Elias PM, Feingold KR (eds) Skin barrier. Taylor and Francis, New York, pp 399–426
13. Nickoloff BJ, Stevens SR (2006) What have we learned in dermatology from the biologic therapies? J Am Acad Dermatol 54:S143–S151
14. Wertz PW, van der Bergh B (1998) The physical, chemical, and functional properties of lipids in the skin and other biological barriers. Chem Phys Lipids 91:85–96
15. Wertz PW, Downing DT (1991) Epidermal lipids. In: Goldsmith LA (ed) Physiology, biochemistry, and molecular biology of the skin. Oxford University Press, Oxford, pp 205–236
16. Feingold KR (2007) The role of epidermal lipids in cutaneous permeability barrier homeostasis. J Lipid Res 48:2531–2546
17. Wertz PW, Swartzendruber DC, Madison KC et al (1987) Composition and morphology of epidermal cyst lipids. J Invest Dermatol 89:419–425
18. Masukawa Y, Narita H, Shimizu E et al (2008) Characterization of overall ceramide species in human stratum corneum. J Lipid Res 49:1466–1476
19. Harding CR, Moore DJ, Rawlings AV (2010) Ceramides and the skin. In: Baran R, Maibach HI (eds) Textbook of cosmetic dermatology. Informa Healthcare, New York, pp 150–164
20. van Smeden J, Hoppel L, van der Heijden R et al (2011) LC/MS analysis of stratum corneum lipids: ceramide profiling and discovery. J Lipid Res 52: 1211–1221
21. Motta S, Monti M, Sesana S et al (1993) Ceramide composition of the psoriatic scale. Biochim Biophys Acta 1182:147–151
22. Wertz PW, Madison KC, Downing DT (1989) Covalently bound lipids of human stratum corneum. J Invest Dermatol 92:109–111
23. Hill J, Paslin D, Wertz PW (2006) A new covalently bound ceramide from human stratum corneum – ω-hydroxyacylphytosphingosine. Int J Cosmet Sci 28:225–230
24. Wertz PW, Miethke MC, Long SA et al (1985) The composition of the ceramides from human stratum corneum and from comedones. J Invest Dermatol 84:410–412
25. Dahlén B, Pascher I (1979) Thermotropic phase behaviour of tetracosanoylphytosphingosine. Chem Phys Lipids 24:119–133
26. Kiselev MA, Ryabova NY, Balagurov AM et al (2005) New insights into the structure and hydration of a stratum corneum lipid model membrane by neutron diffraction. Eur Biophys J 34:1030–1040
27. Brief E, Kwak S, Cheng JTJ et al (2009) Phase behavior of an equimolar mixture of *N*-palmitoyl-d-erythro-sphingosine, cholesterol, and palmitic acid, a mixture with optimized hydrophobic matching. Langmuir 25:7523–7532
28. O'Malley B, Moore DJ, Noro M, et al. (2005) Towards a mechanical model of skin: Insights into Stratum corneum mechanical properties from hierarchical models of lipid organization. Mat Res Soc Symp Proc 844: Y5.7
29. Pascher I (1976) Molecular arrangements in sphingolipids: conformation and hydrogen bonding of ceramide and their implication on membrane stability and permeability. Biochim Biophys Acta 455: 433–451
30. Rerek ME, Moore DJ (2007) Skin lipid structure: Insight into hydrophobic and hydrophilic driving forces for self-assembly using IR spectroscopy. In: Rhein LD, Schlossman M, O'Lenick A, Somasundran P (eds) Surfactants in personal care products and decorative cosmetics. CRC Press, Boca Raton, Surfactant science series, pp 189–209
31. Mendelsohn R, Rerek ME, Moore DJ (2000) Infrared spectroscopy and microscopic imaging of stratum corneum models and skin. Phys Chem Chem Phys 2:4651–4657
32. Norlén L, Nicander I, Lundsjö A et al (1998) A new HPLC-based method for the quantitative analysis of inner stratum corneum lipids with special reference to the free fatty acid fraction. Arch Dermatol Res 290:508–516
33. Fettiplace R, Haydon DA (1980) Water permeability of lipid membranes. Physiol Rev 60:510–550
34. Wertz PW (1996) Integral lipids in hair and Stratum corneum. In: Jolles P, Zahn H, Hocker H (eds) Hair: Biology and structure. Birkhauser Verlag, Basel, pp 227–238
35. Daly TA, Wang M, Regen SL (2011) The origin of cholesterol's condensing effect. Langmuir 27: 2159–2161

36. de Meyer F, Smit B (2009) Effect of cholesterol on the structure of a phospholipid bilayer. Proc Natl Acad Sci USA 106:3654–3658
37. Maxfield FR, Tabas I (2005) Role of cholesterol and lipid organization in disease. Nature 438:612–621
38. Leathes JB (1925) Croonian lectures on the role of fats in vital phenomena. Lancet 205:853–856
39. Róg T, Pasenkiewicz-Gierula M, Vattulainen I et al (2009) Ordering effects of cholesterol and its analogues. Biochim Biophys Acta 1788:97–121
40. Takahashi H, Sinoda K, Hatta I (1996) Effects of cholesterol on the lamellar and the inverted hexagonal phases of dielaidoylphosphatidylethanolamine. Biochim Biophys Acta 1298:209–216
41. McMullen TPW, McElhaney RN (1995) New aspects of the interaction of cholesterol with DPPC bilayers as revealed by high-sensitivity differential scanning calorimetry. Biochim Biophys Acta 1234:90–98
42. Feingold KR (2009) The outer frontier: the importance of lipid metabolism in the skin. J Lipid Res 50:S417–S422
43. Krahn-Bertil E, Hazane-Puch F, Lassel T et al (2009) Skin moisturization by dermonutrition. In: Rawlings AV, Leyden JJ (eds) Skin moisturization. Informa Healthcare USA, Inc., New York, pp 411–425
44. Martinez RI, Peters A (1971) Membrane-coating granules and membrane modifications in keratinizing epithelia. Am J Anat 130:93–120
45. Lavker RM (1976) Membrane coating granules: the fate of the discharged lamellae. J Ultrastruct Res 55:79–86
46. Elias PM, Goerke J, Friend DS (1977) Mammalian epidermal barrier layer lipids: composition and influence on structure. J Invest Dermatol 69:535–546
47. Madison KC, Swartzendruber DC, Wertz PW et al (1987) Presence of intact intercellular lamellae in the upper layers of the stratum corneum. J Invest Dermatol 88:714–718
48. Bouwstra JA (2009) Lipid organization of the skin barrier. In: Rawlings AV, Leyden JJ (eds) Skin moisturization. Informa Healthcare USA, Ins, New York, pp 17–40
49. van Meer G, Voelker DR, Feigenson GW (2008) Membrane lipids: where they are and how they behave. Nature Rev Molec Cell Biol 9:112–124
50. Pilgram GSK, Engelsma-van Pelt AM, Bouwstra JA et al (1999) Electron diffraction provides new information on human stratum corneum lipid organization studied in relation to depth and temperature. J Invest Dermatol 113:403–409
51. Friberg SF, Osborne DW (1985) Small angle X-ray diffraction patterns of stratum corneum and a model structure for its lipids. J Dispers Sci Technol 6:485–495
52. Schroeter A, Kessner D, Kiselev MA et al (2009) Basic nanostructure of stratum corneum lipid matrices based on ceramides [EOS] and [AP]: a neutron diffraction study. Biophys J 97:1104–1114
53. Groen D, Poole D, Gooris GS et al (2011) Is an orthorhombic lateral packing and a proper lamellar organization important for the skin barrier function? Biochim Biophys Acta 1808:1529–1537
54. Swartzendruber DC (1992) Studies of epidermal lipids using electron microscopy. Semin Dermatol 11:157–161
55. Swartzendruber DC, Wertz PW, Kitko DJ et al (1989) Molecular models of the intercellular lipid lamellae in mammalian stratum corneum. J Invest Dermatol 92:251–257
56. Schreiner V, Gooris GS, Pfeiffer S et al (2000) Barrier characteristics of different human skin types investigated with X-ray diffraction, lipid analysis, and electron microscopy imaging. J Invest Dermatol 114:654–660
57. Norlén L (2010) Molecular cryo-electron tomography of skin. Open Derm J 4:46–47
58. Al-Amoudi A, Dubochet J, Norlén L (2005) Nanostructure of the epidermal extracellular space as observed by cryo-electron microscopy of vitreous sections of human skin. J Invest Dermatol 124: 764–777
59. Percot A, Lafleur M (2001) Direct observation of domains in model stratum corneum lipid mixtures by Raman microspectroscopy. Biophys J 81:2144–2153
60. Wegener M, Neubert RHH, Rettig W et al (1997) Structure of stratum corneum lipids characterized by FT-Raman spectroscopy and DSC. III. Mixtures of ceramides and cholesterol. Chem Phys Lipids 88:73–82
61. Bommannan D, Potts RO, Guy RH (1990) Examination of stratum corneum barrier function in vivo by infrared spectroscopy. J Invest Dermatol 95:403–408
62. Babita K, Kumar V, Rana V et al (2006) Thermotropic and spectroscopic behavior of skin: relationship with percutaneous permeation enhancement. Curr Drug Deliv 3:95–113
63. Mendelsohn R, Flach CR, Moore DJ (2006) Determination of molecular conformation and permeation in skin via IR spectroscopy, microscopy, and imaging. Biochim Biophys Acta 1758:923–933
64. Boncheva M, Damien F, Normand V (2008) Molecular organization of the lipid matrix in intact stratum corneum using ATR-FTIR spectroscopy. Biochim Biophys Acta 1778:1344–1355
65. Kitson N, Thewalt J, Lafleur M et al (1994) A model membrane approach to the epidermal permeability barrier. Biochemistry 33:6707–6715
66. Rehfeld SJ, Plachy WZ, Williams ML et al (1988) Calorimetric and electron spin resonance examination of lipid phase transitions in human stratum corneum: molecular basis for normal cohesion and abnormal desquamation in recessive X-linked ichthyosis. J Invest Dermatol 91:499–505
67. Queiros MP, Sousa Neto D, Alonso A (2005) Dynamics and partitioning of spin-labelled stearates into the lipid domain of stratum corneum. J Control Release 106:374–385

68. Norlén L, Placsencia I, Bagatolli LA (2008) Stratum corneum lipid organization as observed by atomic force microscopy, confocal and two-photon excitation fluorescence microscopy. Int J Cosmet Sci 30:391–411
69. Norlén L, Plasencia Gil I, Simonsen A et al (2007) Human stratum corneum lipid organization as observed by atomic force microscopy of Langmuir-Blodgett films. J Struct Biol 158:386–400
70. Lafleur M (1998) Phase behaviour of model stratum corneum lipid mixtures: an infrared spectroscopy investigation. Can J Chem 76:1501–1511
71. Moore DJ, Rerek ME, Mendelsohn R (1997) FTIR spectroscopy studies of the conformational order and phase behavior of ceramides. J Phys Chem B 101: 8933–8940
72. Moore DJ, Rerek ME (2000) Insight into the molecular organization of lipids in the skin barrier from infrared spectroscopy studies of stratum corneum lipid models. Acta Derm Venereol Supp 208:16–22
73. Bouwstra JA, Gooris GS, Ponec M (2002) The lipid organization of the skin barrier: liquid and crystalline domains coexist in lamellar phases. J Biol Phys 28:211–223
74. Bouwstra JA, de Graaff A, Gooris GS et al (2003) Water distribution and related morphology in human stratum corneum at different hydration levels. J Invest Dermatol 120:750–758
75. Pensack RD, Michniak BB, Moore DJ et al (2006) Infrared kinetic/structural studies of barrier reformation in intact stratum corneum following thermal perturbation. Appl Spectrosc 60:1399–1404
76. Damien F, Boncheva M (2010) The extent of orthorhombic lipid phases in the stratum corneum determines the barrier efficiency of human skin in vivo. J Invest Dermatol 130:611–614
77. Gennis RB (1989) Biomembranes: molecular structure and function. Springer-Verlag Inc., NY
78. Mukherjee S, Maxfield FR (2000) Role of membrane organization and membrane domains in endocytic lipid trafficking. Traffic 1:203–211
79. Nicolaides N (1974) Skin lipids: their biochemical uniqueness. Science 186:19–26
80. Yagi E, Sakamoto K, Nakagawa K (2006) Depth dependence of stratum corneum lipid ordering: a slow-tumbling simulation for electron paramagnetic resonance. J Invest Dermatol 127:895–899
81. Madison KC (2003) Barrier function of the skin: "La raison d'être" of the epidermis. J Invest Dermatol 121:231–241
82. Janssens M, Gooris GS, Bouwstra JA (2009) Infrared spectroscopy studies of mixtures prepared with synthetic ceramides varying in head group architecture: coexistence of liquid and crystalline phases. Biochim Biophys Acta 1788:732–742
83. Garson J-C, Doucet J, Lévêque J-L et al (1991) Oriented structures in human stratum corneum revealed by X-ray diffraction. J Invest Dermatol 96:43–49
84. Bouwstra JA, Gooris GS, Salomons-de Vries JA et al (1992) Structure of stratum corneum as a function of temperature and hydration: a wide-angle X-ray diffraction study. Int J Pharm 84:205–216
85. Bouwstra JA, Gooris GS, Dubbelaar FER et al (2002) Phase behavior of stratum corneum lipid mixtures based on human ceramides: the role of natural and synthetic ceramide 1. J Invest Dermatol 118:606–617
86. Sousa Neto D, Gooris GS, Bouwstra JA (2011) Effect of ω-acylceramides on the lipid organization of stratum corneum model membranes evaluated by X-ray diffraction and FTIR studies (Part I). Chem Phys Lipids 164:184–195
87. Bouwstra JA, Gooris GS (2010) The lipid organization in human stratum corneum and model systems. Open Derm J 4:10–13
88. Caussin J, Gooris GS, Janssens M et al (2008) Lipid organization in human and porcine stratum corneum differs widely, while lipid mixtures with porcine ceramides model human stratum corneum lipid organization very closely. Biochim Biophys Acta 1778: 1472–1482
89. Hill JR, Wertz PW (2003) Molecular models of the intercellular lamellae from epidermal stratum corneum. Biochim Biophys Acta 1616:121–126
90. Forslind B (1994) A domain mosaic model of the skin barrier. Acta Derm Venereol 74:1–6
91. Forslind B, Engstrom S, Engblom J et al (1997) A novel approach to the understanding of human skin barrier function. J Dermatol Sci 14:115–125
92. Potts RO, Francoeur ML (1991) The influence of stratum corneum morphology on water permeability. J Invest Dermatol 96:495–499
93. Kitson N, Thewalt JL (2000) Hypothesis: the epidermal permeability barrier is a porous medium. Acta Derm Venereol Supp 208:12–15
94. Bouwstra JA, Dubbelaar FER, Gooris GS et al (2000) The lipid organization in the skin barrier. Arch Dermatol Res Supp 208:23–30
95. McIntosh TJ (2003) Organization of skin stratum corneum extracellular lipid lamellae: diffraction evidence for asymmetric distribution of cholesterol. Biophys J 85:1675–1681
96. Norlén L (2001) Skin barrier structure and function: the single gel phase model. J Invest Dermatol 117:830–836
97. Kiselev MA (2007) Conformation of ceramide 6 molecules and chain-flip transitions in the lipid matrix of the outmost layer of mammalian skin, the stratum corneum. Crystallogr Rep 52:525–528
98. McIntosh TJ, Stewart ME, Downing DT (1996) X-ray diffraction analysis of isolated skin lipids: reconstitution of intercellular lipid domains. Biochemistry 35:3649–3653
99. Groen D, Gooris GS, Barlow DJ et al (2011) Disposition of ceramide in model lipid membranes determined by neutron diffraction. Biophys J 100: 1481–1489
100. Kessner D, Kiselev MA, Dante S et al (2008) Arrangement of ceramide [EOS] in a stratum corneum lipid model matrix: new aspects revealed by neutron diffraction studies. Eur Biophys J 37:989–999
101. Schroeter A, Kiselev MA, Hauss T et al (2009) Evidence of free fatty acid interdigitation in stratum corneum model membranes based on ceramide [AP]

by deuterium labeling. Biochim Biophys Acta 1788: 2194–2203
102. Menon GK (2002) New insights into skin structure: scratching the surface. Adv Drug Deliv Rev 54 (suppl 1):S3–S17
103. Roelandt T, Giddelo C, Heughebaert C et al (2009) The "caveolae brake hypothesis" and the epidermal barrier. J Invest Dermatol 129:927–936
104. Menon GK, Ghadially R, Williams ML et al (1992) Lamellar bodies as delivery systems of hydrolytic enzymes: implications for normal and abnormal desquamation. Br J Dermatol 126:337–345
105. Rawlings AV, Matts PJ (2005) Stratum corneum moisturization at the molecular level: an update in relation to the dry skin cycle. J Invest Dermatol 124:1099–1110
106. Hachem J-P, Houben E, Crumrine D et al (2006) Serine protease signaling of epidermal permeability barrier homeostasis. J Invest Dermatol 126:2074–2086
107. Voegeli R, Rawlings AV, Doppler S et al (2007) Profiling of serine protease activities in human stratum corneum and detection of a stratum corneum tryptase-like enzyme. Int J Cosmet Sci 29:191–200
108. Grubauer G, Elias PM, Feingold KR (1989) Transepidermal water loss: the signal for recovery of barrier structure and function. J Lipid Res 30:323–333
109. Feingold KR, Schmuth M, Elias PM (2007) The regulation of permeability barrier homeostasis. J Invest Dermatol 127:1574–1576
110. Landmann L (1986) Epidermal permeability barrier: transformation of lamellar granule-disks into intercellular sheets by a membrane-fusion process, a freeze-fracture study. J Invest Dermatol 87:202–209
111. Haftek M, Teillon M-H, Schmitt D (1998) Stratum corneum, corneodesmosomes and ex vivo percutaneous penetration. Microsc Res Tech 43:242–249
112. Loefgren H, Pascher I (1977) Molecular arrangement of sphingolipids: the monolayer approach. Chem Phys Lipids 20:273–284
113. Whitesides GM, Mathias JP, Seto CT (1991) Molecular self-assembly and nanochemistry: a chemical strategy for the synthesis of nanostructures. Science 254:1312–1319
114. Atkins PW (1997) Physical Chemistry. Oxford University Press, Oxford, UK
115. Bishop KJM, Wilmer CE, Soh S et al (2009) Nanoscale forces and their uses in self-assembly. Small 5:1600–1630
116. Norlén L (2002) Does the single gel phase exist in stratum corneum? J Invest Dermatol 118:899–901
117. Whitesides GM, Grzybowski B (2002) Self-assembly at all scales. Science 295:2418–2421
118. Grzybowski BA, Wilmer CE, Kim J et al (2006) Self-assembly: from crystals to cells. Soft Matter 5:1110–1128
119. Williams ML, Elias PM (1987) The extracellular matrix of stratum corneum: role of lipids in normal and pathological function. CRC Crit Rev Therap Drug Carrier Syst 3:95–122
120. Mitragotri S, Anissimov YG, Bunge AL et al (2011) Mathematical models of skin permeability: an overview. Int J Pharm 418:115–129
121. Bunge AL, Cleek RL (1995) A new method for estimating dermal absorption from chemical exposure. 2. Effect of molecular weight and octanol-water partitioning. Pharm Res 12:88–95
122. Guy RH (2010) Predicting the rate and extent of fragrance chemical absorption into and through the skin. Chem Res Toxicol 23:864–870
123. Mitragotri S (2003) Modeling skin permeability to hydrophilic and hydrophobic solutes based on four permeation pathways. J Control Release 86:69–92
124. Levin J, Maibach HI (2005) The correlation between transepidermal water loss and percutaneous absorption: an overview. J Control Release 103:291–299
125. Golden GM, McKie JE, Potts RO (1987) Role of stratum corneum lipid fluidity in transdermal drug flux. J Pharm Sci 76:25–28
126. Golden GM, Guzek DB, Kennedy AH et al (1987) Stratum corneum phase transitions and water barrier properties. Biochemistry 26:2382–2388
127. Potts RO, Francoeur ML (1990) Lipid biophysics of water loss through the skin. Proc Natl Acad Sci USA 87:3871–3873
128. Potts RO, Mak VHW, Guy RH et al (1991) Strategies to enhance permeability via stratum corneum lipid pathways. Adv Lipid Res 24:173–210
129. Naik A, Guy RH (1997) Infrared spectroscopic and differential scanning calorimetric investigations of the Stratum corneum barrier function. In: Potts RO, Guy RH (eds) Mechanisms of transdermal drug delivery. Marcel Dekker, NY, pp 87–162
130. Naik A, Kalia YN, Pirot F et al (1999) Characterization of molecular transport across human Stratum corneum in vivo. In: Bronaugh RL, Maibach HI (eds) Percutaneous adsorption. Marcel Dekker, Inc., NY, pp 149–175
131. Imhof RE, Xiao P, De Jesus MEP et al (2009) New developments in skin barrier measurements. In: Rawlings AV, Leyden JJ (eds) Skin moisturization. Informa Healthcare USA, Inc., New York, pp 463–479
132. de Jaeger M, Groenink W, Bielsa i Guivernau R et al (2006) A novel in vitro percutaneous penetration model: evaluation of barrier properties with p-aminobenzoic acid and two of its derivatives. Pharm Res 23:951–960
133. Pilgram GSK, Vissers DCJ, van der Meulen H et al (2001) Aberrant lipid organization in stratum corneum of patients with atopic dermatitis and lamellar ichthyosis. J Invest Dermatol 117:710–717
134. Bouwstra JA, Gooris GS, Dubbelaar FER et al (1999) Cholesterol sulfate and calcium affect stratum corneum lipid organization over a wide temperature range. J Lipid Res 40:2303–2312
135. Milstone LM (2004) Epidermal desquamation. J Dermatol Sci 36:131–140
136. Harding CR, Watkinson AC, Rawlings AV et al (2000) Dry skin, moisturization and corneodesmolysis. Int J Cosm Sci 22:21–52
137. Fluhr JW, Elias PM (2002) Stratum corneum pH: formation and function of the 'acid mantle'. Exogenous Dermatol 1:163–175
138. Fluhr JW, Kao JS, Jain M et al (2001) Generation of free fatty acids from phospholipids regulates stratum

corneum acidification and integrity. J Invest Dermatol 117:44–51
139. Hachem J-P, Crumrine D, Fluhr J et al (2003) pH directly regulates epidermal permeability barrier homeostasis, and stratum corneum integrity/cohesion. J Invest Dermatol 121:345–353
140. Rawlings AV, Harding CR, Watkinson AC et al (2002) Dry and xerotic skin conditions. In: Leyden JJ, Rawlings AV (eds) Skin moisturization. Marcel Dekker, Inc., New York, N.Y, pp 119–143
141. Hachem J-P, Man M-Q, Crumrine D et al (2005) Sustained serine protease activity by prolonged increase in pH leads to degradation of lipid processing enzymes and profound alterations of barrier function and stratum corneum integrity. J Invest Dermatol 125:510–520
142. Arseneault M, Lafleur M (2007) Cholesterol-sulfate and Ca^{2+} modulate the mixing properties of lipids in stratum corneum model mixtures. Biophys J 92: 99–114
143. Epstein EHJ, Williams ML, Elias PM (1981) Steroid sulfatase, X-linked ichthyosis and stratum corneum cell cohesion. Arch Dermatol 117:761–763
144. Wu KS, van Osdol WW, Dauskardt RH (2006) Mechanical properties of human stratum corneum: effects of temperature, hydration, and chemical treatment. Biomaterials 27:785–795
145. Berthaud F, Boncheva M (2011) Correlation between the properties of the lipid matrix and the degrees of integrity and cohesion in healthy human stratum corneum. Exper Dermatol 20:255–262
146. Brandner JM, Haftek M, Niessen CM (2010) Adherens junctions, desmosomes and tight junctions in epidermal barrier function. Open Derm J 4:14–20
147. Elias PM (2008) Skin barrier function. Curr Alergy Asthma Rep 8:299–305
148. Elias PM (2010) Therapeutic implications of a barrier-based pathogenesis of atopic dermatitis. Ann Dermatol 22:245–254
149. Prausnitz MR, Mitragotri S, Langer R (2004) Current status and future potential of transdermal drug delivery. Nature Rev Drug Disc 3:115–124
150. Prausnitz MR, Langer R (2008) Transdermal drug delivery. Nature Biotech 26:1261–1268
151. Loden M, Anderson A-C (1996) Effect of topically applied lipids on surfactant-irritated skin. Br J Dermatol 134:215–220
152. Darmstadt GL, Mao-Qiang M, Chi E et al (2002) Impact of topical oils on the skin barrier: possible implications for neonathal health in developing countries. Acta Paediatr 91:546–554
153. Menon GK, Duggan M (2006) Strategies for improving the skin barrier by cosmetic skin care treatments. In: Wille JJ (ed) Skin delivery systems: Transdermals, dermatologicals, and cosmetic actives. Blackwell Publishing, Ames, pp 25–42
154. Jelenco C 3rd, McKinley JC (1976) Studies in burns: XV. Use of a topical lipid in treating human burns. Am Surg 42:838–848
155. Lavrijsen AP, Bouwstra JA, Gooris GS et al (1995) Reduced skin barrier function parallels abnormal stratum corneum lipid organization in patients with lamellar ichthyosis. J Invest Dermatol 105:619–624
156. Rawlings AV, Harding CR (2004) Moisturization and skin barrier function. Dermatol Ther 17 (suppl 1):43–48
157. Wiechers JW, Dederen JC, Rawlings AV (2009) Moisturization mechanisms: Internal occlusion by orthorhombic lipid phase stabilizers–a novel mechanism of action of skin moisturization. In: Rawlings AV, Leyden JJ (eds) skin moisturization. Informa Healthcare USA, Inc., New York, pp 309–321
158. Caussin J, Gooris GS, Groenink W et al (2007) Interaction of lipophilic moisturizers on stratum corneum domains in vitro and in vivo. Skin Pharmacol Physiol 20:175–186
159. Caussin J, Rozema E, Gooris GS et al (2009) Hydrophilic and lipophilic moisturizers have similar penetration profiles but different effects on SC water distribution in vivo. Exper Dermatol 18:954–961
160. Caussin J, Gooris GS, Bouwstra JA (2008) FTIR studies show lipophilic moisturizers to interact with stratum corneum lipids, rendering them more densely packed. Biochim Biophys Acta 1778:1517–1524
161. Hadgraft J, Finnin BC (2006) Fundamentals of retarding penetration. In: Smith EW, Maibach HI (eds) Percutaneous penetration enhancers. Taylor and Francis, Boca Raton, pp 361–371
162. Hadgraft J, Peck J, Williams DG et al (1996) Mechanisms of reaction of skin penetration enhancers/retardants: azone and analogues. Int J Pharm 141:17–25
163. Peck JV, Minaskanian G, Hadgraft J (2000) Topical compositions useful as skin penetration retardants. US patent 6,086,905
164. Kaushik D, Batheja P, Kilfoyle B et al (2008) Percutaneous penetration modifiers: enhancement versus retardation. Expert Opin Drug Deliv 5:517–529
165. Kim N, El-Khalili M, Henary MM et al (1999) Percutaneous penetration enhancement activity of aromatic S, S-dimethyliminosulfuranes. Int J Pharm 187:219–229
166. Brain KR, Watkinson AC, Walters KA (1999) Reduction of the skin penetration of xenobiotics using chemical penetration retarders. In: Sohns T, Voicu VA (eds) NBC risks: Current capabilities and future perspectives for protection, NATO Science Series: Disarmament Technologies. Kluwer Academic Publishers, Dordrecht, pp 271–277
167. Li N, Su Q, Tan F et al (2010) Effect of 1,4-cyclohexanediol on percutaneous absorption and penetration of azelaic acid. Int J Pharm 387:167–171
168. Braue EH Jr, Doxzon BF, Lumpkin HL et al (2006) Military perspectives in chemical penetration retardation. In: Smith EW, Maibach HI (eds) Percutaneous penetration enhancers. Taylor and Francis, Boca Raton, pp 385–398

169. Smith EW, Maibach HI (eds) (2006) Percutaneous penetration enhancers. Taylor and Francis, Boca Raton
170. Mitragotri S (2000) Synergistic effects of enhancers for transdermal drug delivery. Pharm Res 17: 1354–1359
171. Karande P, Jain A, Ergun K et al (2005) Design principles of chemical penetration enhancers for transdermal drug delivery. Proc Natl Acad Sci USA 102:4688–4693
172. Whitesides GM (1995) Self-assembling materials. Sci Am 273:146–149
173. Lehn J-M (2004) Supramolecular chemistry: from molecular information towards self-organization and complex matter. Rep Prog Phys 67:249–265
174. Lampe MA, Burlingame AL, Whitney J et al (1983) Human stratum corneum lipids: characterization and regional variations. J Lipid Res 24:120–130
175. Gunathilake R, Schurer N, Shoo BA et al (2009) pH-regulated mechanisms account for pigment-type differences in epidermal barrier function. J Invest Dermatol 129:1719–1729
176. Meidan VM, Roper CS (2008) Inter- and intra-individual variability in human skin barrier function: a large scale retrospective study. Toxicol In Vitro 22:1062–1069
177. Moore DJ, Snyder RG, Rerek ME et al (2006) Kinetics of membrane raft formation: fatty acid domains in stratum corneum lipid models. J Phys Chem B 110:2378–2386
178. Boelsma E, Hendriks HFJ, Roza L (2001) Nutritional skin care: health effects of micronutrients and fatty acids. Am J Clin Nutr 73:853–864
179. McDaniel JC, Beluri M, Ahijevych K et al (2008) Omega-3 fatty acids effect on wound healing. Wound Rep Reg 16:337–345
180. Munro S (2003) Lipid rafts: elusive or illusive? Cell 115:377–388
181. Lingwood D, SImons K (2010) Lipid rafts as membrane-organizing principle. Science 327:46–50
182. Dietrich C, Bagatolli LA, Volovyk ZN et al (2001) Lipid rafts reconstituted in model membranes. Biophys J 80:1417–1428
183. London M, London E (2004) Ceramide selectively displaces cholesterol from ordered lipid domains (rafts): Implications for lipid raft structure and function. J Biol Chem 279:9997–10004
184. Boncheva M, Whitesides GM (2005) Making things by self-assembly. MRS Bull 30:736–742
185. Alivisatos AP, Barbara PF, Castelman AW et al (1998) From molecules to materials: current trends and future directions. Adv Mater 10:1297–1336
186. Boncheva M, Whitesides GM (2004) The biomimetic approach to the design of functional self-assembling systems. In: Schwarz JA, Contescu CI, Putyera K (eds) Dekker encyclopedia of nanoscience and nanotechnology, vol 1. CRC Press, Boca Raton, pp 287–294
187. Schaefer-Korting M, Mehnert W, Korting H-C (2007) Lipid nanoparticles for improved topical application of drugs for skin diseases. Adv Drug Deliv Rev 59:427–443
188. Mueller RH, Petersen RD, Hommoss A et al (2007) Nanostructured lipid carriers (NLC) in cosmetic dermal products. Adv Drug Deliv Rev 59:522–530
189. Castner DG, Ratner BD (2002) Biomedical surface science: foundations to frontiers. Surf Sci 500: 28–60
190. Martin P (1997) Wound healing – aiming for perfect skin regeneration. Science 276:75–81
191. Ball P (2002) Natural strategies for the molecular engineer. Nanotechnology 13:R15–R28
192. Noireaux V, Maeda YT, Libchaber A (2011) Development of an artificial cell, from self-organization to computation and self-reproduction. Proc Natl Acad Sci USA 108:3473–3480

11 Desquamation: It Is Almost All About Proteases

Rainer Voegeli and Anthony V. Rawlings

11.1 Introduction

A principal biological mission of the epidermis is to create the stratum corneum (SC) to protect the body from the outside world. The SC is a coherent tissue composed in most body regions of approx. 15 corneocyte layers corresponding to a thickness of 10–20 μm. No area of cutaneous biology has attracted more investigative attention than the SC. A multitude of studies in the last few decades have shown that the SC is a very complex, dynamic tissue whose formation involves many highly regulated metabolic enzymatic functions maintaining cutaneous homeostasis [1]. The epidermis has many diverse functions, and a variety of these are localized to the SC, elevating the SC as a key player in the many protective processes of the integument [2].

In the viable epidermis, several mechanisms are initiated to generate the SC. The final step in these processes is the transformation from keratinocytes to corneocytes. During this maturation, major changes in cell morphology occur. At the transition phase between the stratum granulosum (SG) and the SC, the final stages of programmed cell death await the epidermal keratinocytes. This necessary step results in the production of corneocytes and the integration of the cornified envelope (CE) with the extracellular lipid matrix. This occurs as the lamellar bodies (LBs) are secreted in the extracellular spaces at the SG–SC interface, the nuclei are defragmented, and transglutaminase cross-linked proteins are deposited under the plasma membrane leading to CE formation. This specialized form of cell death in the epidermis is thus intrinsic and programmed [3].

The terminally differentiated corneocytes that are shed from the skin surface are continuously replaced from underneath by keratinocytes. Thus, under normal conditions, there is a delicate balance between basal cell proliferation and shedding of corneocytes (desquamation) maintaining an epidermis of a constant thickness [4]. Roughly estimated, every day one new cell layer appears in the deeper SC, and one old layer is lost off its surface. In other words, every day we lose 2 m^2 of skin without recognizing it. During a lifetime, this accounts for the area of about 6 football fields.

Unlike the keratinocytes in the viable epidermis, the corneocytes of the SC are no longer able to synthesize new proteins, but enzymes, particularly transglutaminases, are involved in anabolic processes. Moreover, several highly specialized and dynamic metabolic activities continue or even start to occur in the SC, due to the presence of numerous enzymes and their substrates that are produced prior to keratinization. The extent

R. Voegeli (✉)
DSM Nutritional Products Ltd.,
Bldg. 203-4/86, P.O. Box 2676, Basel CH-4002, Switzerland
e-mail: rainer.voegeli@dsm.com

A.V. Rawlings
AVR Consulting Ltd.,
26 Shavington Way, Kingsmead, Northwich Cheshire CW9 8FH, UK
e-mail: tonyrawlings@aol.com

M. Lodén, H.I. Maibach (eds.), *Treatment of Dry Skin Syndrome*,
DOI 10.1007/978-3-642-27606-4_11, © Springer-Verlag Berlin Heidelberg 2012

of the changes and their speed are autoregulated and rather constant under physiological conditions, but the environment still has some influence, e.g., through modification of the SC hydration or a disruption of the SC barrier with the subsequent repair-related changes [5].

The SC has a depth-dependent dynamic structure in which multiple enzymatic reactions are balanced to ensure its mechanistic, cohesive, and desquamatory properties are maintained [6]. However, still little is understood of the molecular activation mechanisms of enzymes within the SC. Obviously pH, water, and Ca^{2+} gradients as well as barrier competence influence enzymatic activities. Proteases play important roles in the keratinization process but are also involved in tissue remodeling, lipid barrier homeostasis, and inflammatory conditions. As a consequence, the activity of certain proteases is increased in skin disorders in which the epidermal barrier is impaired. It has also been generally acknowledged that the appearance of dry skin is mainly the result of an alteration in the desquamatory process of the normal SC maturation.

In this chapter, we review the structure, function, and formation of the SC, how it is perturbed in a variety of conditions, as well as the proteases and their inhibitors that play a role in desquamation of healthy and pathological skin.

11.2 Cell–Cell Junctions in the Stratum Corneum

11.2.1 Corneodesmosomes and Their Highly Orchestrated Digestion

11.2.1.1 The "Iron Rods": Molecular Rivets in the Brick and Mortar Construction

Corneodesmosomes are modified desmosomes found in the SC, the uppermost layers of the epidermis. Here they mediate strong intercellular cohesion to provide enough tensile strength to resist shearing forces that is crucial for the physical barrier function of the epidermis. Ultimately, the final stages of corneodesmosomal degradation occur at the time of desquamation [7]. Michaels [8] and later Elias [9] visualized the SC as being similar to a brick wall, with the corneocytes analogous to bricks, and the lipid lamellae acting as mortar. However, lipids are not the major cohesive forces holding corneocytes together [10]. Extending this model, the corneodesmosomes may be thought of as analogous to iron rods that act as molecular rivets between the bricks to give the wall its tensile strength [11]. The term corneodesmosome was first proposed 20 years ago by Serre, Haftek, and coworkers [12], and the same group found that corneodesmosomes contain a unique adhesive glycoprotein in their extracellular space, known as corneodesmosin (CDSN) [13].

11.2.1.2 Structures and Molecules of (Corneo)Desmosomes

Constant formation and removal of desmosomes is required to allow the keratinocytes to move from the epidermal basal layer to the granular layer. The differentiation-dependent composition of desmosomes coincides with the increase of their mechanical stability. In the basal layer, desmosomes are infrequent and small; their size and number rise significantly in the spinous layers and decrease subsequently in the granular compartment [14]. Desmosomes have round or oval, button-like structures with a diameter of 0.2–1 μm [15]. The morphology of desmosomes changes dramatically during the transition from the SG to the SC (Fig. 11.1) [5]. The intercellular portion of the junction loses its electron-dense central band flanked by symmetric light band and becomes homogeneous, whereas the intracellular plaque becomes embedded within the cross-linked CE. Products resulting from proteolysis and from the dispersion of keratohyalin granules fill the interior of corneocytes tightly and make the remnants of keratin cytoskeleton disappear, so even the points of insertion of keratin bundles into desmosomal plaque become invisible. Such a drastic modification of the desmosome structure once made the desmosomal "plugs" between corneocytes to be considered as nonfunctional remnants [5].

There is a clear direct relationship between the number of corneodesmosomes and the strength of cellular cohesion [12]. In the stratum disjunctum,

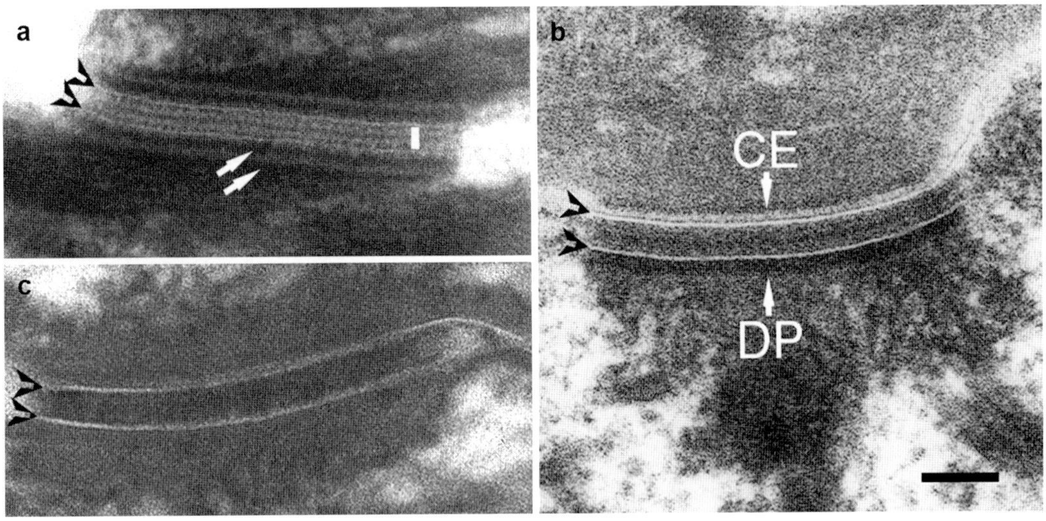

Fig. 11.1 Comparison of the ultrastructure of the spinous layer desmosome (**a**) and a corneodesmosome (**c**). Transition from the granular layer to the SC is shown in (**b**) with a corneodesmosome showing asymmetrical intracellular features. *Arrowhead* points to the cell membranes or lipid cell envelopes in the living and cornified keratinocytes, respectively. *White arrows* in (**a**) point to the internal and external desmosomal plaques, the latter being associated with keratin filaments. The *white rectangle* spans the extracellular portion of the junction – the desmosome core. Bar 100 nm [5]. *DP* desmosomal plaque, *CE* cornified envelope (Reproduced with permission of TAYLOR & FRANCIS GROUP LLC)

fewer corneodesmosomes are present compared to the stratum compactum [16, 17]. In the stratum compactum, one finds one corneodesmosome per μm² on average. This means that there exist approx. 400–600 corneodesmosomes per corneocyte and per site [18].

The (corneo)desmosome proteins originate from three major gene families [19–21]:

- Cadherins (desmogleins, desmocollins)
- Armadillo proteins (plakoglobin, plakophilins)
- Plakins (desmoplakin, envoplakin, periplakin, plectin)

Analogous to the desmosomes mediating keratinocyte cohesion, corneodesmosomes maintain corneocyte adhesion via a Ca^{2+}-dependent interaction in their extracellular space between the two cadherin families: the desmogleins and the desmocollins. To date, four isoforms of desmogleins (DSG1–4) and three isoforms of desmocollins (DSC1–3) have been identified in the human epidermis [20]. The transmembranal cadherins are linked to the keratin intermediate filaments by the armadillo proteins, which are in turn attached to desmoplakin that is essential for linkage to the intermediate filaments (Fig. 11.2) [22].

As keratinocytes are pushed to the surface layers of the skin, they constantly form and retrieve desmosomes at the cell periphery. During this turnover, the cadherins that compose the junctions are also constantly replaced even without physical dissociation of the structure. According to the level of keratinocyte differentiation, DSG2 and DSG3 from the lower epidermal compartment are progressively substituted by DSG1 and DSG4 in the upper viable epidermal layers. In the same way DSC3 is replaced by DSC1 (Fig. 11.3) [14]. Thus, DSC1, DSG1, and DSG4 are strongly associated with terminally differentiating layers, while the remaining isoforms are associated with the lower, proliferating cell layers, suggesting that this differentiation-specific pattern may regulate epidermal development and differentiation [23].

11.2.1.3 Peripheral and Nonperipheral Corneodesmosomes

The process of SC desquamation is complex and is only apparent at the surface of the skin. However, desquamation is not simply a process that spontaneously occurs in the upper layers of the SC, but is a self-regulating process that is

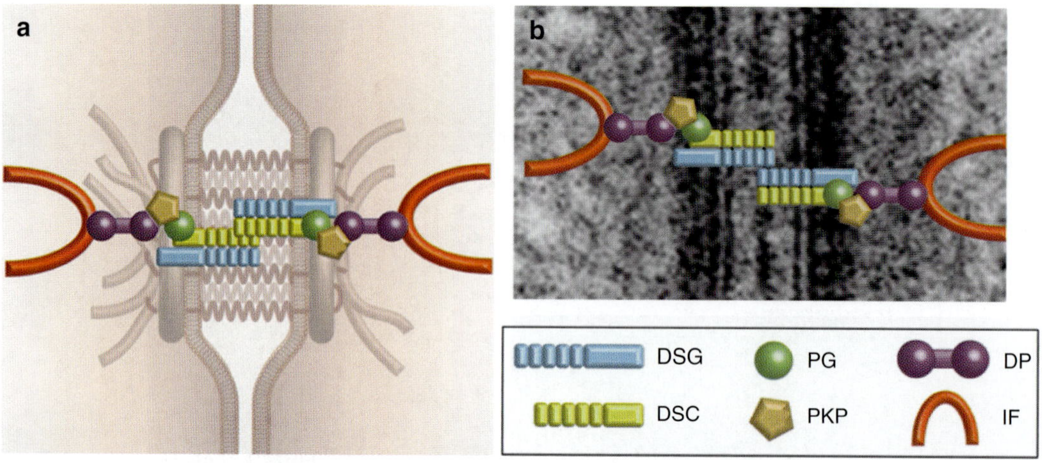

Fig. 11.2 (**a**) Schematic illustration of a desmosome and (**b**) electron micrograph onto which are super-imposed the major desmosomal protein constituents from three families. Transmembrane cadherins, DSG and DSC, bind plakoglobin (*PG*), which in turn anchors desmoplakin (*DP*) and plakophilin (*PKP*). The cytoplasmic plaque, which is further stabilized by lateral interactions among these proteins, anchors the intermediate filaments (*IF*) cytoskeleton to the desmosome [20] (Reprinted with permission from Macmillan Publishers Ltd: J Invest Dermatol 127(11): p. 2499–2515, copyright (2007))

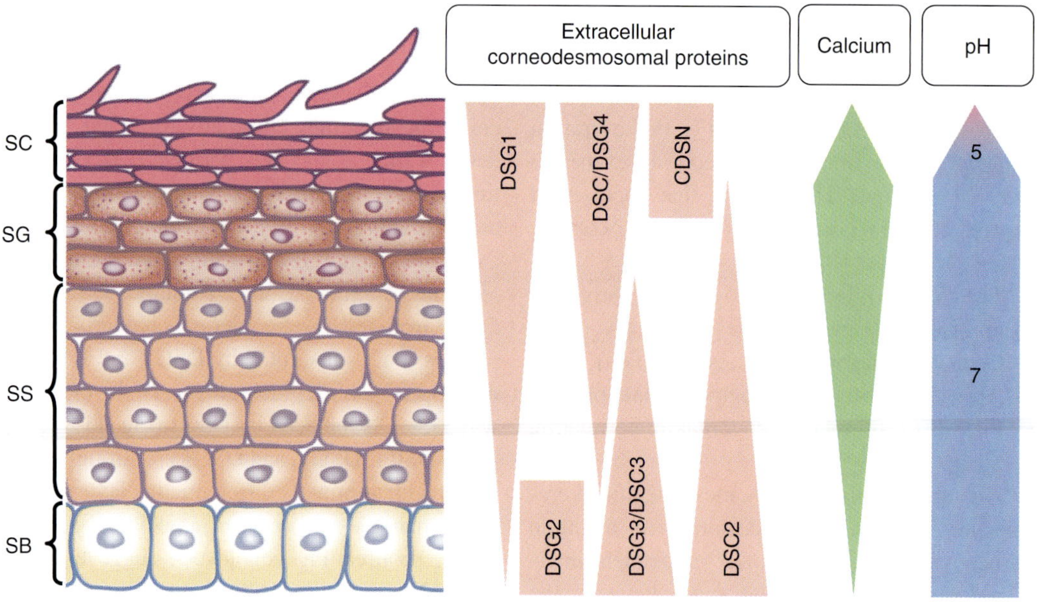

Fig. 11.3 Expression gradients of extracellular corneodesmosomal proteins, calcium, and pH in the epidermis (*SC* stratum corneum, *SG* stratum granulosum, *SS* stratum spinosum, *SB* stratum basale (Modified from [14, 20, 22, 171])

initiated in the lower layers of nonpalmoplantar SC [24] except for the face which appears to be mediated more superficially [25]. Desquamation very likely occurs via a regulated multistep proteolysis. Corneodesmosomes interconnect the corneocytes through the intercorneocyte spaces which themselves are occupied largely by self-organizing lamellar lipids. Once degraded these areas become very hydrophilic due to the presence of amino acids and peptides derived from the original corneodesmosomal proteins. In the uppermost granular layer, the LBs secrete a cocktail of serine, cysteine, and aspartic proteases into the intercellular space between SG and SC [5]

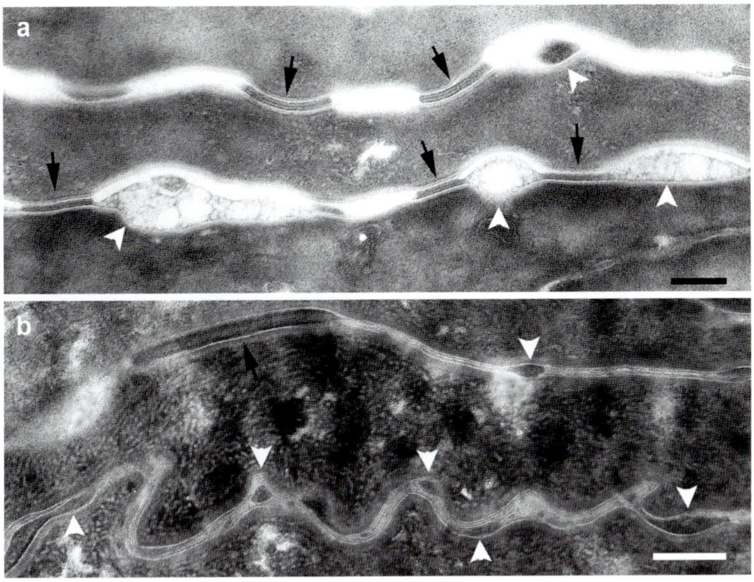

Fig. 11.4 Hydration of the SC promotes the lateral displacements, coalescence, and increase in volume of the extracellular hydrophilic microdomains, leading to the increased frequency of their association with corneodesmosomes (RuO_4 staining). (**a**) In the occluded skin, the well-hydrated SC shows voluminous hydrophilic lacunae (*white arrowheads*) in the proximity of corneodesmosomes (*black arrows*). (**b**) The nonoccluded SC also contains hydrophilic lacunae embedded in the intercellular lipids, but these domains are more discrete. The hydrophilic nature of the intercellular lacunae is compatible with the presence of extracellular enzymes involved in the processes of maturation and desquamation of the SC. Bars = 200 nm [5] (Reproduced with permission of TAYLOR & FRANCIS GROUP LLC)

(Fig. 11.4). This region is a zone of enormous metabolic activity [26–28]. Central, nonperipheral corneodesmosomes in the stratum compactum are initially hydrolyzed resulting in retention of corneodesmosomes only at peripheral edges of corneocytes in the stratum disjunctum [16]. This results in reduced cohesion in the perpendicular plane of the skin, but it still has tremendous resistance to shearing forces in the horizontal plane. The retained peripheral corneodesmosomes in the stratum disjunctum are degraded later, leading to ordered corneocyte shedding at the skin surface. Reasons for the preferential digestion of nonperipheral corneodesmosomes may include:

- A higher impact of shearing forces on junctions between flat rigid surfaces, when applied to the skin or naturally occurring during changes of the corneocyte volume due to variations in the water content
- Easier access for the enzymes, displaced by self-organizing lipid bilayers, when compared to the convoluted lateral intercorneocyte spaces
- An additional protection from degradation of the peripheral junctions by supplementary structures, like remnants of strategically placed tight junctions cross-linked to CEs at the periphery of corneocytes [14]

A change in frequency and size of corneodesmosomes is obvious between the deeper and the more superficial layers of the SC. On nonpalmoplantar SC, corneodesmosomes occupy approximately 30% of the cell surface in the stratum compactum, but represent less than 7% of the cell surface in the stratum disjunctum [29]. The situation is quite different in palmoplantar SC, where more than 50% of the intercellular spaces are occupied by corneodesmosomes up to the upper SC.

11.2.1.4 Importance of Controlled Desquamation for SC Homeostasis

The process of the gradual disappearance of corneodesmosomes in the stratum disjunctum [16, 30] and the parallel disappearance of desmogleins, desmocollins, and CDSN [31, 32] during desquamation is not completely understood. Nevertheless, a growing number of enzymes have been identified and linked to this process [26]. It appears likely that in certain diseases or after external impairment to the skin, the physiologic cascade of desquamation is altered [33–38]. Yet the physiological role and the endogenous targets of the majority of these proteases have not been identified; the conditions required for activation, precise localization, and interdependence still await clarification.

Persistence of peripheral corneodesmosomes can be related to several hyperkeratotic conditions like certain ichthyoses, xerotic diseases, senile dry skin, and winter and soap-induced xerotic skin. The lack of the proteolytic degradation of DSC1, DSG1, and CDSN is a key event in these skin disorders [39–44].

Tight junctions (TJs) have only been described in the superficial granular layer until recently [45, 46]. By ultrastructural examination, Haftek et al. [47] demonstrated that TJs become cross-linked to the cornified envelopes during the process of cornification and thus contribute to the compartmentalization of the intercorneocyte spaces in the SC. The authors hypothesize that such TJ-derived rivets distributed at the corneocyte periphery may significantly delay protease access to peripheral corneodesmosomes when compared to the unprotected junctions located in between the successive layers of SC cells. Therefore, peripheral corneodesmosomes remain relatively intact up to the skin surface. Indeed, Igawa et al. [48] observed persistence of these TJ-like structures up to the eighth deepest cornified layers. Immunoelectron microscopy also detected clusters of the TJ marker proteins occludin and claudin-1 at the corneocyte periphery, whereas kallikrein 7 (KLK7) immunolabeling was found outside of TJ-derived structures in the extracellular space of the lower cornified layers.

According to Wepf et al., corneocytes are held in position not only by corneodesmosomes but also by hook-like structures at the periphery of the cells [10] (Fig. 11.5). Hyperhydrated SC exposes large water inclusions between the single corneocyte layers. These water inclusions disrupt the corneodesmosomes and resist longest at the hook-like structures. These structures are only disrupted if the tension increases and finally also the hook-like structures can be dismantled. Within the hook-like rims, extended corneodesmosomal structures are found, which seem to be the last docking point of a corneocyte during desquamation.

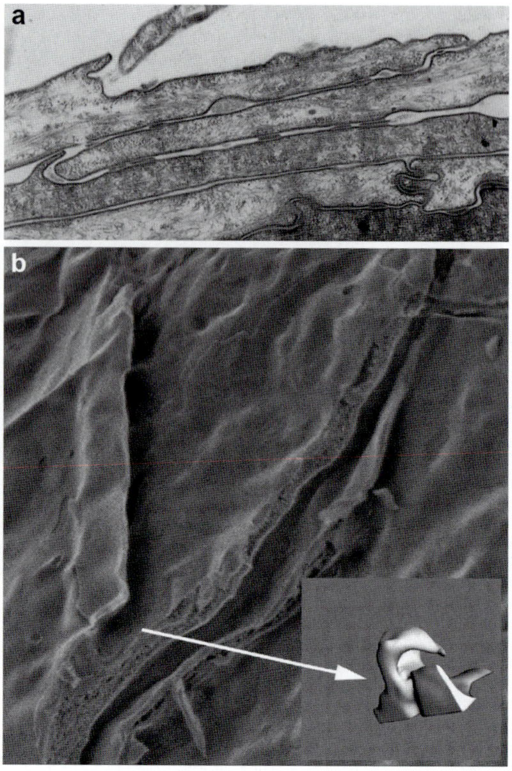

Fig. 11.5 Hook and clip-like structures of the corneocytes in the SC [10]. (**a**) transmission electron micrograph of the outer layer of the SC with corneodesmosomes (*arrows*), (**b**) raster electron microscopic top view on a corneocyte in the medial SC with clip-like hooks (Reproduced with permission of INFORMA HEALTHCARE)

11.3 pH of the Stratum Corneum: Its Important and Misinterpreted Role

The pH is a critical factor regulating skin barrier homeostasis and controls lipid interactions, enzymatic activities, corneodesmosomal degradation, and microbial defense [49]. However, the SC is not an aqueous solution, and the definition of pH should not be directly applied for its acidity measurement. The pH of the epidermis is suggested to follow a sharp gradient across the SC

(Fig. 11.3), which seems to play an important role in controlling the enzymatic activities involved in cellular metabolism and renewal [50].

The outermost layer of the SC exhibits an acidic surface pH. The surface pH measured with a flat electrode on normal human skin ranges between 4 and 5.5, whereas the pH at its base approaches neutrality. From a biological point of view, a change in pH of about 2 units over a tiny distance as 10–20 μm is an important event [51]. However, what is measured at the skin surface is in fact an apparent pH due to extracted material from the SC diffusing into water applied at the surface. pH values recorded at the surface of the semihydrophobic milieu of the SC should be interpreted with great caution because it is obvious that hydrogen ions are not in a pure solution at the surface of the skin [50]. Newer, high-resolution microscopic methods could not confirm the existence of a pH gradient. The measured change in pH in tape-stripping experiments must therefore be viewed as a result of injury to the epidermal permeability barrier, removing part of the acidic compartment and leading to loss of components from the neutral SG, resulting in a mixed or diluted pH measured [52].

Three classes of molecules have been suggested as the most likely source of hydrogen ions in normal SC [2, 50]:

- Certain NMFs including amino acids and filaggrin-related breakdown products, such as urocanic acid and pyrrolidone carboxylic acid
- Alpha-hydroxy acids, such as lactic acid and hydroxybutyric acid, which are present in sweat
- Acidic lipids, such as cholesterol sulfate and free fatty acids derived from sebum, ceramide, and phospholipid hydrolysis

However, Na^+/H^+ exchanger (NHE1) in human and mouse epidermis has been identified as the crucial source of SC acidity at the SG/SC interface [52, 53]. NHE1 is the only Na^+/H^+ antiporter isoform in keratinocytes and epidermis and has been shown to regulate intracellular pH. A novel function for NHE1 demonstrated that it also controls acidification of extracellular microdomains in the SC that are essential for activation of pH-sensitive enzymes and the formation of the epidermal permeability barrier. Fluorescence lifetime imaging studies revealed that SC acidification does not occur through a uniform gradient, but through the progressive accumulation of acidic microdomains. These findings not only visualize the spatial distribution of the SC pH gradient but also demonstrate a role for NHE1 in the generation of acidic extracellular domains of the lower SC, thus providing the acidification of deep SC interstices necessary for both lipid processing and barrier homeostasis and putting this pathway at the center of establishing and maintaining SC pH and epidermal permeability function [52].

It remains suggestive if the pH or its gradient within the SC exerts a major influence on desquamation, either via effect on corneodesmosomes or via activation of serine proteases in the SC [27, 54].

11.4 The Calcium Gradient in the Epidermis

In the epidermis, an increasing extra- and intracellular Ca^{2+} gradient is established toward the SG, after which it declines in the SC (Fig. 11.3). As already mentioned, cadherins maintain corneocyte adhesion via a Ca^{2+}-dependent interaction in their extracellular space. Thus, the elevated extracellular calcium levels in the upper epidermis (Fig. 11.3) certainly contribute to the desmosome stabilization [14]. In addition, the activity of several cysteine and serine proteases requires the presence of Ca^{2+} [55]. High concentration of extracellular Ca^{2+} has been shown induced KLK5 and KLK7 expression on mRNA and protein levels in cultured normal human keratinocytes [56].

When the epidermal permeability barrier is disrupted, the extracellular concentration of Ca^{2+} decreases in the outer epidermis. This process mimics the decrease in the concentration of Ca^{2+} in intact SC and triggers the LBs to extrude their content into the intercellular space to initiate repair [57]. However, barrier disruption also leads to increased serine protease activity, which results in activation of proteinase-activated receptor-2 (PAR2) and influx of Ca^{2+}, thereby counteracting and regulating LB secretion and reestablishing cornification [58, 59].

11.5 Epidermal Proteases Involved in Desquamation

The proteases mentioned in this section are mainly reviewed in respect of their activities in desquamation only although they exert many other biological roles in the body.

An interest in proteases in skin arose with the realization of the important role of proteolysis in many biological phenomena. Early work of Sexsmith and Petersen in 1918 [60] showed that there is considerable proteolytic activity in human skin. Since then huge efforts have been made to characterize the pattern of the proteolytic enzymes and the pathways of proteolysis in normal and pathological skin.

Proteases are currently classified into six groups:

- Serine proteases
- Cysteine proteases
- Aspartate proteases
- Metalloproteases
- Threonine proteases
- Glutamic acid proteases

Of 699 proteases in man, 178 are serine proteases and 138 of them belong to the trypsin protease family. Abundance of these proteases suggests the protein fold presents a selective advantage relative to other proteases [61].

Proteases are often activated through highly orchestrated proteolytic cascades. Due to the irreversible nature of proteolytic activation, these cascades are tightly regulated through a series of feedback loops and inhibitors. Proteolytic regulatory mechanisms are critical in preventing deleterious effects due to uncontrolled protease activation [62]. A cocktail of proteases is secreted at the SG–SC interface to facilitate the breakdown of corneodesmosomes [26–28]. Inactive protease precursors are activated and regulated by a complementary cocktail of protease inhibitors [32]. The enzymes responsible for the cleavage of corneodesmosomal proteins and their regulation are still not well characterized. However, serine, cysteine, and aspartic acid proteases have been identified in the SC and might play a central role in desquamation. Involvement of proteases in desquamation was first postulated in 1987 by Bisset et al. who reported that topical application of trypsin or the protease inhibitor phenylmethylsulfonyl fluoride to pig and human SC greatly accelerated or inhibited the rate of desquamation, respectively [63]. Subsequently, Egelrud and Lundström initiated studies on the SC proteases that greatly contributed to the current understanding of the role of proteases in desquamation [64–70].

11.5.1 Serine Proteases

The serine protease family uses a highly conserved catalytic triad in the substrate-binding pocket (Ser, His, Asp) to hydrolyze peptide bonds. Based on their substrate specificity, serine proteases can be subdivided into three groups [55]:

- The trypsin-like proteases (cleavage preferred at the basic amino acids Arg and Lys)
- The chymotrypsin-like proteases (cleavage preferred at aromatic or bulky nonpolar amino acids, such as Trp, Phe, Tyr, and Leu)
- The elastase-like proteases (cleavage preferred at small to medium hydrophobic amino acids, such as Ala)

11.5.1.1 Kallikreins

Kallikreins are serine proteases expressed by a wide range of tissues and are implicated in a great number of physiological functions, among many others in skin desquamation [62] where they represent the most intense investigated protease family. Between 1994 and 2001, the kallikrein family expanded from 3 to 15 genes, and a complete description of the human kallikrein locus was reported. Kallikreins represent the largest contiguous cluster of protease genes in the human genome. The newly discovered kallikreins all map to the same chromosomal region (19q13.4) as the three classical ones (KLK1, KLK2, and KLK3) [71].

Each of the 15 kallikreins is synthesized as a single-chain preproenzyme, containing each a signal presequence of 16–30 amino acids that is cleaved from the N-terminus prior to secretion [72]. Prodomains are short peptide sequences, i.e., 37 amino acids in proKLK5 and 4–9 amino acids in the other kallikreins, and are cleaved

Table 11.1 Enzymatic classification of the 15 kallikreins

Chymotrypsin-like	Trypsin-like
	KLK1
	KLK2
KLK3	
	KLK4
	KLK5
	KLK6
KLK7	
	KLK8
KLK9	
	KLK10
	KLK11
	KLK12
	KLK13
KLK14	**KLK14**
KLK15	

The proteases that have been found in the SC are blue shaded in bold

upon activation [62]. KLK3, KLK7, KLK9, and KLK15 have chymotrypsin-like activity, and the rest shows trypsin-like activity. KLK14 exerts a high catalytic efficiency and is the only member that cleaves both trypsin-like and chymotrypsin-like peptide substrates (Table 11.1). With chromogenic peptide substrates, essentially all chymotrypsin-like kallikrein activity in the SC can be ascribed to KLK7. On the other hand, at most 50% of the total trypsin-like kallikrein activity in SC extracts was due to KLK5, whereas a major part of the remaining activity was associated with KLK14 [73, 74].

Komatsu et al. performed the most extensive studies on kallikreins in the SC and in sweat. The following eight kallikreins were identified in SC and in sweat extracts by ELISA: KLK5, KLK6, KLK7, KLK8, KLK10, KLK11, KLK13, and KLK14 [75, 76]. They found that the relative proportions of each kallikrein in sweat were similar to those in the SC, suggesting that kallikrein expression in sweat and SC could be regulated via a shared mechanism [76]. Sweat might be a fluid facilitating transport of kallikreins toward the skin surface [76]. As kallikreins have also been identified in sebaceous glands, these could contribute to the kallikrein levels in sweat samples [36]. KLK5, KLK7, KLK8, and KLK14 are the only kallikreins currently known to be present in active forms in SC [27, 34, 37, 38, 54, 68, 70, 73, 74, 76, 77].

The proteolytic activity of kallikreins seems to be cascade mediated and may crosstalk with other proteases. These cascades are highly regulated through a series of feedback loops, inhibitors, (auto)degradation, and internal cleavage. Uncontrolled proteolytic activity of kallikreins is implicated in a large number of pathological conditions [62].

11.5.1.2 Proteases of the Thrombostasis Axis: The Plasminogen System

Like the kallikreins, the trypsin-like serine proteases urokinase (uPA) and plasmin are also involved in many physiological and pathological conditions especially in hemostasis, carcinogenesis, and skin inflammation. Both proteases are secreted as the zymogens plasminogen and pro-uPA. Suzuki et al. first described plasmin and uPA activities in human SC [54]. Although both proteases are present in the SC, they may not necessarily directly be involved in the desquamatory process. To our knowledge, there is no evidence of uPA or plasmin-induced hydrolysis of extracellular components of corneodesmosomes. However, there are indications of activation of certain kallikrein zymogens and vice versa which may lead to aberrant desquamation [78, 79].

pro-uPA contains 411 amino-acid residues arranged in two chains and three domains: the so-called A-chain includes the N-terminal growth-factor-like domain and the central kringle domain, and the B-chain includes the C-terminal catalytic domain. Activation of pro-uPA occurs via the cleavage of the Lys158–Ile159 bond between the A-chain and the catalytic domain containing B-chain, generating a two-chain molecule (HMW-uPA) held together by a single disulfide bond. A further cleavage at Lys135–Lys136 releases the N-terminal growth factor and the kringle domains (amino acids 1–135). The remaining carboxy-terminal region (LMW-uPA, amino acids 136–411) retains full ability to activate plasminogen [80]. A number of serine proteases can activate pro-uPA such as plasmin, cathepsin B, mast cell tryptase, and KLK2 [80, 81]. uPA interacts with the cell surface receptor urokinase-type plasminogen activator receptor (uPAR) [82], which shows affinity for the N-terminal region of uPA only (HMW-uPA). This binding is important for cell-associated plasminogen activation and proteolysis. Like other serine proteases, uPA can be inhibited by plasminogen activator inhibitors (PAIs) [83].

Plasminogen is a single-chain glycoprotein containing 791 amino-acid residues and six structural domains, each with different properties. Its natural activators, one of them is uPA, cleave plasminogen specifically at Arg561–Val562, which gives rise to plasmin, a two-chain molecule linked by two disulfide bonds [81]. uPA-dependent activation is thought to occur primarily in association with the cell surface uPAR. Plasminogen is bound to the cell surface via its lysine-binding sites in a relatively low affinity but high capacity interaction. Cell surface bound plasmin is resistant to inactivation as it is protected from endogenous inhibitors [84].

On the contrary, uPA is expressed predominantly in basal keratinocytes [85, 86] and is the predominant plasminogen activator in epidermal extracts of normal skin [87]. uPA activity was also found to be present in the SC, as well as the basal layer after barrier disruption by tape-stripping and sodium lauryl sulfate [88, 89]. Recently it was shown that uPA activation might occur in the SC itself [88]. uPA and uPAR were reported to be synthesized and secreted in human keratinocytes exposed to UVB [90, 91]. uPA, uPAR, and plasmin-mediated proteolysis are also reported to be increased by proinflammatory cytokines, interleukin-1β, and tumor necrosis factor-α, which are known to be synthesized and secreted in UVB-exposed skin [92].

The plasminogen system in the epidermis is thought to be the major protease activity involved in the delay of barrier recovery [58, 88, 89]. Repeated barrier disruption induces epidermal hyperplasia and is thought to lead to dry skin.

11.5.1.3 Other Serine Proteases

Matriptase is a transmembrane serine protease that is very unusual for a trypsin-like serine protease in that it undergoes efficient autoactivation and therefore has the capacity to initiate proteolytic cascade reactions. It has been shown that matriptase is an efficient activator of epidermal prokallikreins [93]. Therefore, its participation in the cleavage of corneodesmosomes cannot be ruled out. Indeed, matriptase-deficient mice die within 48 h after birth as a consequence of severe loss of the epidermal and oral barrier [94]. Abnormal filaggrin processing, LB disorganization, and impaired desquamation have been described [95, 96].

Furin is a calcium-dependent serine endoprotease. It is enriched in the Golgi apparatus, where it efficiently cleaves downstream precursor proteins at their basic amino-acid target sequence. Furin is a key enzyme for intracellular LEKTI processing [97] (cf. inhibitor chapter below).

11.5.2 Cysteine and Aspartic Acid Proteases and Other Enzymes

Cathepsins are a class of globular lysosomal proteases, most of which contain an active-site cysteine or aspartic acid residue. Although most studies of desquamation have concentrated on serine proteases especially kallikreins, other classes of proteases have also been identified in the SC. Among these are the two cysteine proteases cathepsin L2 (CTSL2) and cathepsin L-like (CTSL-like), and the aspartic acid protease cathepsin D (CTSD).

Synthesized as proenzymes, cathepsins undergo proteolytic maturation, sometimes in an autocatalytic way, and are active in an acidic environment. CTSD and CTSL2 are secreted by LBs into the extracellular spaces around corneodesmosomes in the SC [28, 98]. CTSD has been localized in plantar SC [99]. Although CTSD is associated with the final stage of desquamation [100], its role in corneodesmosomal degradation remains uncertain, and other cathepsins are likely to compensate for CTSD deficiency. Further investigations are necessary to provide a clear understanding of the role of each of these proteases in keratinization and desquamation.

Desquamation is also regulated by an interaction of proteases and glycosidases. Bernard et al. identified an endoglycosidase, heparanase 1, that can play a preproteolytic role toward glycosylated moieties protecting corneodesmosomal proteins [101].

11.6 Endogenous Protease Inhibitors in the Epidermis

The wide-ranging impact of SC protease activities on barrier function and structure, including desquamation, means that regulation of their activity is crucial. The activities of these proteases are regulated by several protease inhibitors localized to the extracellular spaces of the SC. Some of them are involved in the regulation of desquamation-associated proteolysis. Disturbance of the delicate protease/inhibitor balance may have dramatic consequences. To date, a great variety of endogenous inhibitors with physiological significance in the activity regulation of proteases are known. They range from single metal ions to large protein complexes of more than 700 kDa [102].

11.6.1 Metal Ions

The activity of several serine proteases is regulated by endogenous cations. Interestingly, alkali and alkaline earth ions tend to stimulate protease activity at distinct binding sites. Zn^{2+} is a metal ion with manifold functions in living organisms and is present in about 300 human enzymes. It may play a dual role in some activity regulation and inhibit other ones. Strikingly, for KLK5, KLK7, KLK8, and KLK14, inhibition by Zn^{2+} in the low μM range has been reported repeatedly [73, 103–105]. Thus, Zn^{2+} should be considered as an "attenuator" of KLK activity, which binds in a reversible manner to the targets possibly for fine tuning of their proteolytic action [102].

11.6.2 Cholesterol Sulfate

Topically applied cholesterol sulfate inhibits proteases that are involved in desquamation. SC thickness was increased in cholesterol-sulfate-treated mice, and the number of desmosomes was higher than in the vehicle-treated group. Cholesterol sulfate also inhibited the protease-induced cell dissociation of human SC sheets. These results indicate that cholesterol sulfate retards desquamation by acting as a serine protease inhibitor [106] or affects lipid phase behavior that then impacts protease activity.

11.6.3 Relevant Epidermal Proteinaceous Protease Inhibitors

11.6.3.1 LEKTI-1, LEKTI-2, and LEKTI-3

The lymphoepithelial Kazal-type 5 serine protease inhibitor (LEKTI-1) is encoded by the serine protease inhibitor Kazal-type 5 gene (SPINK5). LEKTI-1 is expressed in the granular layer of the epidermis and is composed of 15 serine protease inhibitory domains (D1–D15) [107, 108]. The full-length protein is an inactive inhibitor for kallikreins but inhibits trypsin, plasmin, and elastase [71] and is rapidly cleaved via a furin-mediated intracellular reaction into active single and multidomains that are delivered in LBs into the intercellular space of the SG–SC interface. Here, it is colocalized with kallikreins where the pH is near neutral. Under these conditions, LEKTI-1 domains are potent inhibitors of KLK5, KLK7, and KLK14 [97]. As the pH becomes more acidic (Fig. 11.3), the inhibitory potential of LEKTI-1 is diminished. In the superficial layers of the SC, inhibition by LEKTI-1 is sufficiently reduced to support localized desquamation. Therefore, LEKTI-1 is an important, pH-dependent, regulator of desquamation.

To date, LEKTI-1 is the only known protease inhibitor thought to physiologically target epidermal trypsin-like kallikrein inhibition. Several recombinant LEKTI-1 domains showed inhibitory activity for members of the kallikrein family [97, 109–111]. For instance, recombinant LEKTI-1 domains D5, D6, D8–D11, and D9–D15 exhibited specific and differential inhibition of KLK5, KLK7, and KLK14. Further studies demonstrate the selective efficiency of recombinant LEKTI-1 domains D6–D9 and D9–D12 in inhibiting KLK5 and KLK14. A significant finding is that the LEKTI-1 domain D1–D6 is the most potent inhibitory fragment for all the kallikreins tested. Furthermore, LEKTI-1 D12–D15 was selective in inhibiting only KLK5. The ability of all LEKTI-1 domains (except D1) to strongly inhibit KLK5 confirms that KLK5 is a major protease target of LEKTI-1 in human SC.

Recently LEKTI-2 has been discovered in palmar and plantar SC [112, 113] and LEKTI-3 in SG at various anatomical localizations [114]. The proteins are encoded by SPINK9 and SPINK6 gens, respectively, and are highly homologous to LEKTI-1, but contain only one Kazal-type domain. Recombinant LEKTI-2 inhibited KLK5 only, whereas LEKTI-3 inhibited KLK5, KLK7, and KLK14. Other serine proteases including trypsin, plasmin, and thrombin are not inhibited. Thus, the authors suggest that LEKTI-2 and LEKTI-3 contribute to the regulation of the desquamation process in human skin.

11.6.3.2 SLPI and Elafin

Secretory leukocyte protease inhibitor (SLPI) and elafin are detected in the upper layers of the epidermis and have been shown to prevent the detachment of corneocytes from human plantar epidermis in vitro and to inhibit KLK7 activity in synthetic substrates [115, 116]. Elafin has been shown to covalently bind to corneocytes [117]. Interestingly, SLPI can be cleaved and inactivated by members of the cathepsin family in vitro [118], suggesting the possibility of retrocontrol of KLK7 activity by these proteases. In vitro elafin and SLPI inhibit chymotrypsin-like KLK7, but not trypsin-like KLK5, KLK13, and KLK14 activities [109]. Although elafin is a weak but efficient inhibitor of KLK7, it significantly reduces corneocyte shedding in vitro [32]. SLPI is may be a major physiological inhibitor of KLK7 in the epidermis, but it is also likely to be involved in the innate immune function of the SC [115].

11.6.3.3 α2-Macroglobulin-Like 1

α2-Macroglobulin-like 1 (A2ML1) is a recently discovered member of the α2-macroglobulin protease inhibitor family, which is specifically expressed in the epidermis. A2ML1 is located within the extracellular space between the uppermost granular layer and the SC, and can form specific complexes with KLK7 in vitro [119]. With a preferential inhibition toward the chymotrypsin-like and cysteine proteases, A2ML1 could count cathepsins among its physiological targets and may represent an important regulator of desquamation in vivo.

11.6.3.4 Plasminogen Activator Inhibitor-2

Plasminogen activator inhibitor-2 (PAI-2) is a fast-acting inhibitor of urokinase. PAI-2 is considered an important regulatory element of the plasminogen activation cascade controlling tissue remodeling and fibrinolysis [120]. PAI-2 is the predominant epidermal plasminogen activator inhibitor throughout the normal epidermis [121]. It is localized predominantly in the SG, which implies a possible role in the terminal differentiation of epidermis [122] and that it is a precursor protein for the CE. Therefore, it is speculated that PAI-2 is involved in the pathogenesis of certain cornification disorders, namely, congenital ichthyosis [120].

11.6.3.5 Cystatin M/E

Finally, human epidermis contains specific cysteine protease inhibitors, particularly cystatin M/E, whose expression is restricted to the skin. Importantly, cystatin M/E and CTSL2 are separately transported in LBs and colocated on corneodesmosomes [98].

11.6.3.6 Pathological Inhibitor Deficiency: Netherton Syndrome

Failure of these inhibitory systems can lead to certain pathophysiological conditions. One of the most prominent examples is the Netherton syndrome, which is caused by mutations in the SPINK5 gene [123, 124] leading to dysfunctional domains of LEKTI-1 which fail to appropriately regulate kallikreins in the SC, and consequently to unrestricted kallikrein activity [102]. Interestingly, a strong overexpression of PAI-2 has been found in patients with Netherton syndrome [120]. The Netherton syndrome is an autosomal recessive ichthyotic skin disorder characterized by severe SC barrier dysfunction with SC loss, chronic skin inflammation, atopic features, and hair shaft defects. This enhanced protease activity results in premature corneodesmosome degradation and overdesquamation [125]. All the central manifestations of Netherton syndrome in LEKTI-1-deficient mice depend on the epidermal expression of matriptase [93]. These studies suggest that protease inhibitors other than LEKTI-1 may only have a minor role to play in the control of desquamation.

11.7 Regulation of Desquamation by Proteolytic Cascades Within the Stratum Corneum

The turnover of the epidermis normally proceeds in about four weeks. During that time, cells are part of the SC for about two weeks. The normal physiology of the skin requires both the proper formation and the controlled desquamation of the cornified layers. This tightly regulated equilibrium is regulated in a way to give a cell shedding from the skin surface which balances de novo production of the SC without interfering with the barrier functions of the tissue. The normal appearance of the skin surface requires orderly shedding of outermost corneocytes as single cells in an invisible manner, whereas the integrity of the cornified layers depends on the competency of the barrier lipids and the corneodesmosomes [126]. The continuous process of keratinocyte proliferation, migration, differentiation, cell death, and shedding of corneocytes ensures a permanent regeneration and a constant thickness of the epidermis. Hydrolytic activities of proteases are essential in several parts of this cycle.

Regulation of protease activity in the living organism is a highly complex task that involves all levels of cellular organization. Control and timing of protease activity starts with gene expression, transcription, and translation, and continues with protein targeting and zymogen activation. Once activated, the protease is often kept in check by endogenous inhibitors, while the last steps of protease regulation may be limited proteolysis and final degradation [102].

Prokallikreins are very likely activated in a stepwise manner involving an activation cascade, in which the active form of one kallikrein catalyzes activation of the next zymogen (Fig. 11.6) [127]. The occurrence of such a cascade in the skin is supported by the coexpression of multiple kallikreins in upper epidermal layers and sweat at varying concentrations, and by the ability of some of these kallikreins to autoactivate and activate other prokallikreins [73, 128]. A kallikrein may take on the role of initiator, propagator, and/or executor within the cascade, depending on its concentration, specificity, and activity level. However, minute amounts of the initiator are sufficient to trigger the whole process owing to its catalytic nature [127]. Initially, kallikrein actions in the skin were exclusively attributed to KLK5 and KLK7. In 1988, Lundström and Egelrud first suggested that corneocyte shedding is mediated by an endogenous enzyme-catalyzed reaction [65, 69, 70] and that this process is accompanied by endogenous degradation of DSG1, which was inhibited by application of serine protease inhibitors (Fig. 11.7) [67]. Furthermore, CDSN was found to be progressively modified and proteolyzed by serine proteases during SC turnover [13, 32, 129], whereas CDSN is thought to protect DSC1 and DSG1 against premature proteolysis [41]. Convincing data generated by many investigators led to the conclusion that proteolytic degradation of cadherins and CDSN by serine proteases is a prerequisite for desquamation to occur.

However, wider kallikrein roles in the skin were identified as the concept of a catalytic activation cascade emerged. At the close-to-neutral pH of the deepest layers of the SC, KLK5 undergoes autoactivation or activation by other proteases such as KLK14. Active KLK5 starts to activate proKLK7 at a rate, which, due to the pH tolerance of this reaction, is maintained throughout the SC [73]. Due to the slow rate of KLK7 activation, significant amounts of proKLK7 will remain also in layers close to the skin surface [27]. As a consequence, there will be a concentration gradient of active KLK7 between deep and superficial layers of the SC, and hence also an increase in the rate of degradation of intercellular cohesive proteins as the corneocytes move toward the skin surface [73]. Yoon et al. characterized comprehensively the activation cascade

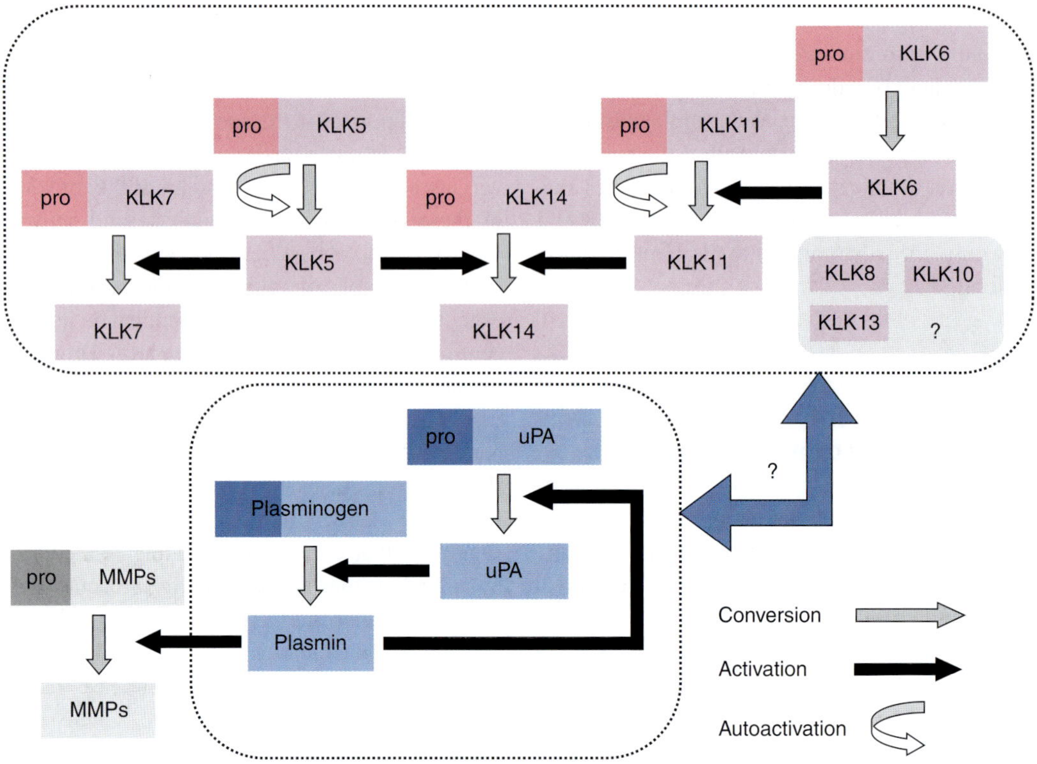

Fig. 11.6 Activation cascades of kallikreins (*pink*) and the plasminogen system (*blue*). Plasmin can activate zymogens of KLK5, KLK6, KLK7, KLK8, KLK11, KLK13, and KLK14 and MMPs (*gray*). On the other side, KLK5 can activate both pro-uPA and plasminogen. However, not much is known about the interaction of desquamatory kallikreins and proteases of the thrombostasis axis

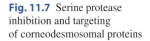

Fig. 11.7 Serine protease inhibition and targeting of corneodesmosomal proteins

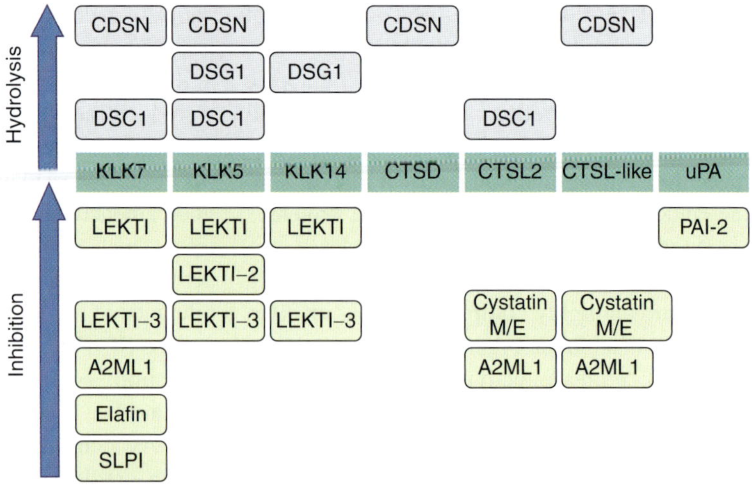

of the kallikrein family [128] upon examining the hydrolysis of 15 prokallikreins by 12 activated kallikreins, excluding KLK9, KLK10, and KLK15. Their novel findings allow expansion of the epidermal kallikrein activation cascade to include two additional kallikrein members known to be expressed in the SC, KLK6 and KLK11, in which proKLK11 is activated by itself and KLK6, and proKLK14 is activated by KLK11 (Fig. 11.6) [127].

Since at least eight kallikreins are present in human SC and sweat, more crosstalk among kallikreins and/or other epidermal proteins may occur, as yet undisclosed. The contribution of KLK8, KLK10, and KLK13 to the skin activation cascade remains to be elucidated. Furthermore, the characterization of initiators, propagators, and executors in the kallikrein proteolytic activation cascade poses a challenge that remains to be solved, although KLK5 is believed to be the cascade initiator [73, 76].

Proteases of the thrombostasis family can efficiently activate specific prokallikreins, demonstrating the potential for important regulatory interactions between these two major serine protease families. Plasmin can activate zymogens of KLK5, KLK6, KLK7, KLK8, KLK11, KLK13, and KLK14 [78]. On the contrary, KLK12 (not present in the SC) can activate uPA [62], and KLK5 can activate both pro-uPA and plasminogen [79].

In vitro CTSL2 appears to be able to cleave DSC1 [28, 98], and CTSL-like has been shown to cleave CDSN [99, 130].

11.7.1 Selection of Protease Activities Beside Desquamation

11.7.1.1 Kallikreins

Certain kallikreins have been shown in vitro to selectively activate protease-activated receptor (PAR) signaling. PARs are a family of four G-protein-coupled cell-surface receptors (PAR1–PAR4) that are activated by serine proteases. PAR signaling has been implicated in a variety of physiological processes, including regulation of muscle contraction, inflammation, cell adhesion, metastasis, and proliferation along with apoptosis. The evidence that kallikreins are functionally associated and interact with specific cell-surface receptors raises the possibility that they may be able to regulate their own expression through these signal transduction pathways [34, 71]. KLK5, KLK6, and KLK14, but neither KLK7 nor KLK8, induced PAR2 signaling [127, 131]. KLK14 also activates PAR4 and disharms/inhibits PAR1, whereas KLK5 and KLK6 do not [127, 132].

11.7.1.2 Plasminogen System

It is proposed that one of the functions of epidermal uPA is to promote keratinocyte proliferation, e.g., by activation of growth factors or by promoting vertical migration of basal keratinocytes into the suprabasal layers, thereby aiding in tissue remodeling that must accompany epidermal hyperproliferation [86, 121].

Plasmin is a relatively unspecific protease. Once activated, it performs a number of functions important in tissue remodeling. Plasmin degrades several components of the extracellular matrix including fibrin, fibronectin, laminin, and proteoglycans [81]. In addition, plasmin can activate its own activator uPA itself as well as a number of latent matrix metalloproteases (proMMPs) leading to collagen degradation (Fig. 11.6) [80].

11.7.1.3 Cathepsin D

CTSD is crucially involved in the activation of transglutaminase 1 and reduced protein levels of the cornified envelope proteins involucrin and loricrin during epidermal differentiation, which results in dry skin and hyperkeratosis [133].

11.8 Detection of Proteases in Healthy and Pathological Skin

SC integrity and cohesion are inversely related to desquamation and are pH-dependent functions. Although a large family of serine proteases is present in SC, KLK5 and KLK7 appear to be the important mediators of the final stages of desquamation [2]. Both proteases show maximal enzymatic activity at pH 8–9 in vitro [54, 134, 135]; however, they could sustain low rates of desquamation in normal SC at an acidic pH, because these enzymes exhibit residual activity against physiologic substances, where aspartate and cysteine proteases, with acidic pH optima, could become operative. KLK5 and KLK7 would exhibit higher activities when SC pH increases, as in inflammatory dermatoses or by using alkaline

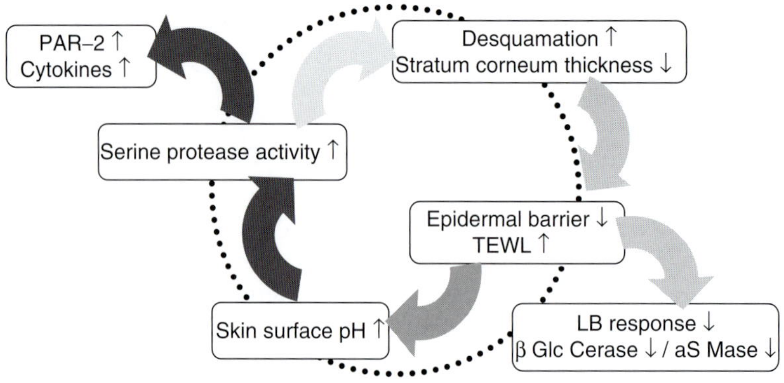

Fig. 11.8 Enhanced serine protease activation and its functional consequences may lead to a vicious circle. An excess of serine protease activity is associated with increased desquamation and SC thinning. Impaired barrier functions are also based on overactivity of serine proteases. Serine proteases suppress the LB secretory responses to acute barrier perturbations. Moreover, two key lipid processing enzymes, β-glucocerebrosidase and acid sphingomyelinase, are degraded by proteolytic attacks. When the SC pH increases and shifts closer to the activity optimum of serine proteases, then the cycle starts again under amplified conditions. Moreover, uncontrolled serine protease activity may lead to an overactivation of PAR-2 and certain cytokines (Modified from [124])

soaps. In the epidermis, proteolytic activity increases 1–2 h [49] following acute barrier disruption [58, 89]. Serine protease activation may as a second signal regulate the LB secretory response. Elevated pH leads to premature degradation of corneodesmosomes, inactivation of the key lipid synthesizing enzymes β-glucocerebrosidase and acidic sphingomyelinase, and subsequent impairment of the epidermal barrier and decrease in SC cohesion [49]. Moreover, uncontrolled serine protease activity may lead to an overactivation of PAR-2 and release of cytokines (Fig. 11.8). It is likely that KLK5 and KLK7 activities dominate at all levels of SC in pathological skin, which is characterized by optimal conditions for serine protease activation, i.e., increased pH, hydration, and Ca^{2+} levels [2]. Furthermore, epidermal overexpression of KLK7 in transgenic mice results in severe pruritus [112, 136].

11.8.1 Healthy Skin

11.8.1.1 Quantification of Kallikreins in the SC: Dependence of Age

Komatsu et al. quantified kallikrein mass and activities in SC extracts of healthy subjects [75, 76]. The concentration ranges are listed in Table 11.2. Total trypsin-like kallikrein mass levels were found to be consistent among different age groups, whereas total chymotrypsin-like kallikrein mass declined with age. On the contrary, overall trypsin-like kallikrein activity did not differ across age groups but was higher in subjects <11 years, and overall chymotrypsin-like activity was not related to age. However, Koyama et al. did find a reduction in SC trypsin-like activity with increasing age [137]. Conversely, in the SC, not only the concentration of each kallikrein but also the overall SC enzymatic activities were highly consistent among body regions, suggesting that the kallikrein expression and the enzymatic activities may be regulated similarly throughout the SC, at least in the body regions studied (forearm,

Table 11.2 Concentration range of kallikreins in SC extracts of forearm and upper arm

Kallikrein	Concentration range(ng/mg dry SC)
KLK5	2–4
KLK6	0.1–0.3
KLK7	7–14
KLK8	6–14
KLK10	0.7–1.0
KLK11	6–14
KLK13	0.02–0.2
KLK14	0.1–0.3

Modified from [75]

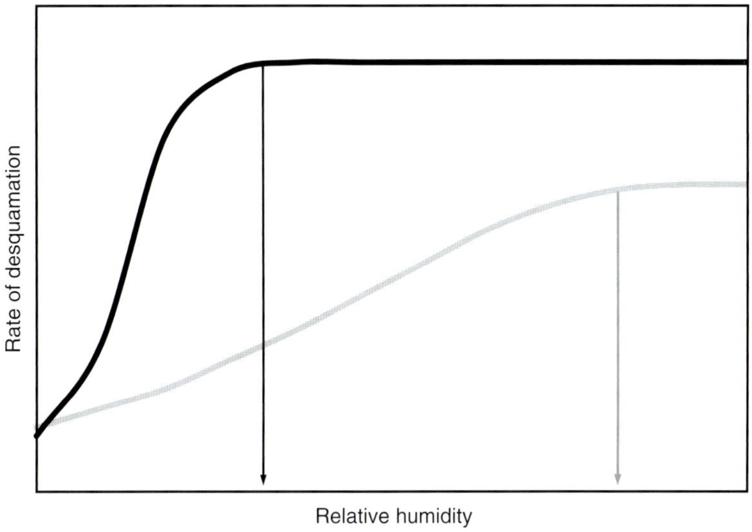

Fig. 11.9 The rate of desquamation depends on relative humidity. Skin with a reduced water-holding capacity (*gray line*) may be more sensitive to low relative humidity conditions than normal hydrated skin (*black line*) (Modified from [140])

abdomen, back, thigh) [76]. Unfortunately the authors did not evaluate facial skin which has been shown to have elevated protease activity on SC extract (cf. posterior chapter) [138].

11.8.1.2 Influence of Relative Humidity on Desquamation

Exposure to a dry environment leads to depletion of water from the outermost SC layers in a process dependent on the relative humidity (RH) and the water-holding capacity of the tissue. Desmosomal degradation was shown by Rawlings et al. to be a humidity-dependent event, being significantly reduced at low RH [43]. Moreover, Watkinson et al. demonstrated that by modulating the water content in the surface layers of the SC, RH effects the rate of desquamation by modulating the activity of desquamatory enzymes, specifically KLK7 [24]. Below 80% RH, corneocyte release was decreased, and KLK7 activity was significantly higher at 100% than at 44% RH. Furthermore increases in KLK7 activity was induced by applying a 10% glycerol solution. KLK7 showed a small tolerance to water restriction, which may be an adaptation to maintain enzyme activity even within the water-depleted SC intercellular space. In a study on mice, Sato et al. found that dry SC (10% RH) contains the same activity of trypsin-like protease as the control in an aqueous based assay but more undegraded desmosomal protein [139]. This suggests that deficiency of water in the SC may suppress desquamation through reduction of protease activities. Skin with a low water-holding capacity may be more sensitive to dry skin conditions and show more scaliness in dry season (Fig. 11.9) [140].

Skin chronically exposed to a hot, dry environment exhibits strong skin barrier functions and low basal transepidermal water loss (TEWL). The amount of active KLK7 was found to be higher in the skin of subjects exposed to low RH, suggesting that upregulation of the amount of active proteases may be part of an adaptation response to ensure proper desquamation at low humidity. Interestingly, human skin can adapt to a low humidity environment by increasing epidermal barrier function and modulating desquamation [141].

11.8.1.3 Depth Profiling of Desquamatory and Inflammatory Serine Protease Activities in the SC on Different Body Sites

In a study with healthy Caucasian subjects in winter season, we compared SC cohesion, SC hydration, and TEWL with depth profiles of enzymatic activities of desquamatory serine proteases (trypsin-like and chymotrypsin-like kallikreins) and inflammatory serine proteases (plasmin-, uPA-, and SC tryptase-like proteases) on SC extracts of ventral

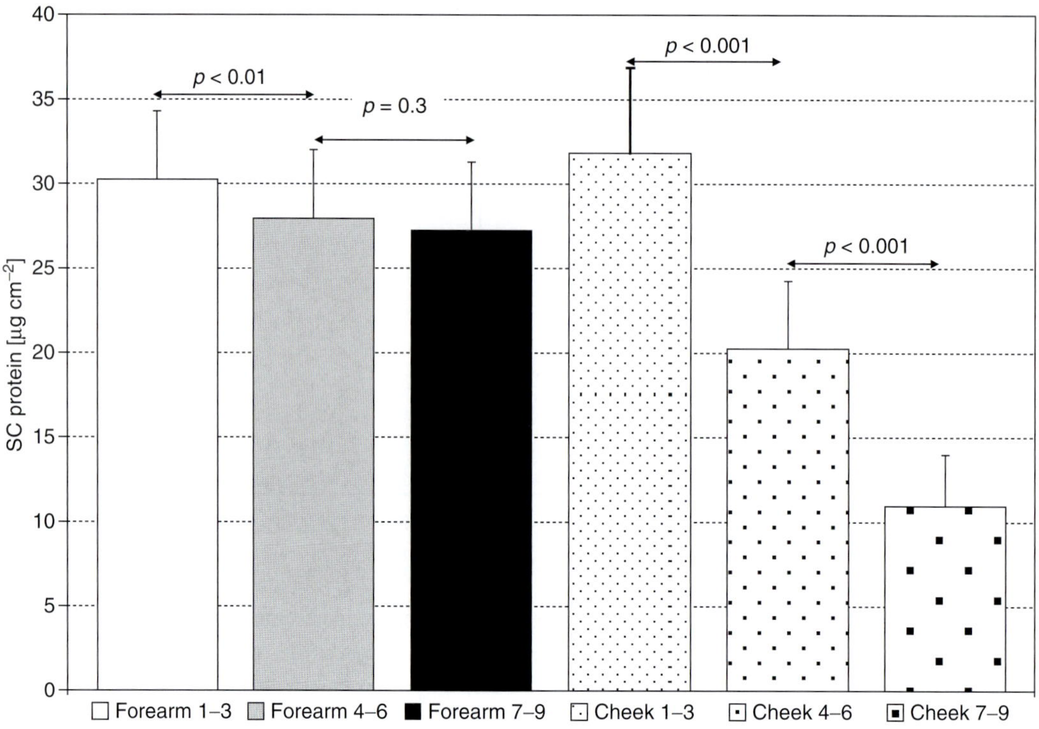

Fig. 11.10 Cohesion of healthy forearm and cheek SC. Protein content (mean per tape ± SEM, $n = 14$ subjects) on tape stripping pools (tapes 1–3, 4–6, 7–9) of forearm and of cheek (Modified from [138])

Table 11.3 (a) Biometric data of the subjects and (b) SC serine protease activities on 9 consecutive tape stripping extracts of healthy forearm and facial skin (mean ± SEM; $n = 14$ per group)

(a)			
Biometric data	Forearm	Cheek	
Skin surface pH	4.75 ± 0.08	4.93 ± 0.04	
SC hydration (DPM)	104 ± 4	110 ± 3	
TEWL ($g \cdot m^{-2} h^{-1}$)	13.5 ± 0.9	28.6 ± 2.8**	
SC cohesion (μg protein cm^{-2}), 9 tape strippings	28.5 ± 4.0	21.0 ± 4.0**	
(b)	Protease activity (μU/mg SC protein)		
Serine protease	Forearm (F)	Cheek (C)	Factor C/F
Trypsin-like kallikreins	3.20 ± 0.47	12.05 ± 1.57**	3.8
Chymotrypsin-like kallikreins	1.45 ± 0.35	3.77 ± 0.48**	2.6
SC tryptase-like	1.62 ± 0.58	13.44 ± 1.50**	8.3
Plasmin-like	1.39 ± 0.29	9.91 ± 1.25**	7.1
Urokinase-like	0.92 ± 0.16	6.99 ± 1.31**	7.6

Modified from [138]
*$p < 0.05$; **$p < 0.01$ for cheek vs. forearm

forearm and facial tape strippings [138]. There was no difference in SC hydration, whereas SC cohesion, determined via IR densitometry (Fig. 11.10) [142], TEWL, and protease activities were increased on the cheek (Tables 11.3a, b). Inflammatory enzymes showed 7–8 times and desquamatory

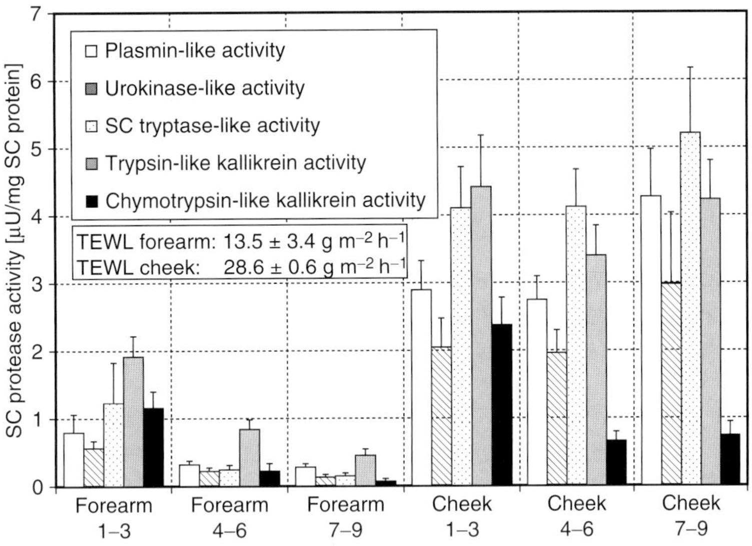

Fig. 11.11 Depth profiling of serine protease activity (mean ± SEM, $n = 14$ subjects) on tape stripping pools (tapes 1–3, 4–6, 7–9) of healthy forearm and cheek SC. The TEWL of the cheek is twice as much the one of the forearm, indicating an impaired barrier (Modified from [138])

enzymes 2.5–4 times greater activities. Except the chymotrypsin-like kallikreins, all tested protease activities positively correlated with TEWL and negatively with SC hydration [143]. On the forearm, all serine proteases showed a distinct gradient with highest activity in the outermost layers of the SC (Fig. 11.11), whereas on the cheek area, the activity gradients were less distinct except for chymotrypsin-like kallikrein activity which, like the samples from the forearm, showed increased activation toward the surface layers of the SC. There was a greater trypsin-like kallikrein than a chymotrypsin-like kallikrein activity on both body sites.

Many authors [27, 73] describe that processing of kallikreins probably occurs within early SC development. Conversely, using a sensitive approach, we have established that both trypsin- and chymotrypsin-like kallikreins show increased activities toward the surface layers of the SC on samples from the forearm skin. Like we, Chang-Yi et al. have found higher chymotrypsin- and trypsin-like protease activities in the outer part of the SC [134]. Presumably, the processing of these enzymes is occurring much later than assumed by others. Similar activation processes can be observed for chymotrypsin-like kallikreins on samples from the face, but on this body site, trypsin-like kallikreins seem to be activated consistently throughout the inner and outer SC. Differences in the control mechanisms of activation of these enzymes may occur on these two different skin areas.

Mohammed et al. found similar results [144]; moreover, they report decreased corneocyte maturity and surface area with increasing number of tape strippings similar to Hirao [145] and Harding et al. [146].

Although the subjects of our study had clinically normally looking facial skin, TEWL values were clearly above the values of the forearm (29 vs. 14 $g{\cdot}m^{-2}{\cdot}h^{-1}$) indicating a barrier disturbance (Table 11.3a). Thus, the elevated serine protease activities on the face may be due to a subclinical microinflammatory or preinflammatory condition induced, e.g., by environmental influences. Serine proteases might represent key markers for underlying and sometimes nonobservable skin abnormalities.

Reduced SC thickness, corneocyte size [147, 148] and maturity, elevated SC cohesion, and TEWL indicate that facial SC disjunctum is not existing probably due increased proteolytic activity leading to premature corneodesmosomal degradation. Facial skin is the most exposed skin of the body and is submitted to numerous environmental attacks for long periods each day as it is not protected by clothing. Paradoxically, facial skin is particularly sensitive because it possesses a thin epidermis and a thin SC [149].

11.8.1.4 Desquamation in Dry Skin, Winter Xerosis, and Soap-Induced Xerotic Skin

In xerotic skin, the degradation of corneodesmosomes is perturbed, and the proteolysis of their components is impaired [44]. This is also the case in psoriatic scales [41]. As demonstrated by Rawlings et al. and Simon et al., the persistence of DSG1 is a characteristic of hyperkeratosis [41, 42]. DSC1 proteolysis is reduced in dry skin [41, 146], and degradation of the DSG1, DSC1, and CDSN is reduced in winter and soap-induced xerotic skin [42–44].

Harding et al. and van Overloop et al. observed a chronic decrease in KLK5 and KLK7 and a diminished protease activity that may contribute to the induction of a scaly dry skin. Inverse correlation between skin scaliness and KLK5 and KLK7 activities [150] and reduced expression of KLK5 and KLK7 has been shown in the outer layers of the SC in dry skin [31, 150].

Interestingly surfactants lead to contrary effects. While soap decreases the activity of KLK7 [31] and SLES the activity of KLK5 [135], SLS increases the activities of KLK 5 and KLK7 [54] after topical application. The differences are due to the application regimes. Single application of surfactants leads to irritation in the epidermis and the up regulation of gene synthesis. Chronic application, as in the examples with soap washing, leads to lipid lamellae disruption and either leaching or denaturing of the SC proteases.

Alternatively there may be changes to the LEKTI inhibition system as there is after UV irradiation. Reduced expression of LEKTI-1 and increased expression of KLK5 and KLK7 in human epidermal keratinocytes after UVB irradiation may contribute to desquamation of the SC [151].

Disturbances to the plasminogen system have also been described in dry skin. Kitamura et al. [152] demonstrated that plasminogen that was only located at the basal layer in healthy subjects was expressed in all epidermal cell layers in dry skin. Moreover, Kawai et al. [153] reported that uPA was also present in the SC especially in experimentally induced dry skin on back skin of individuals. They further demonstrated that increased extractable uPA activity was present in SC samples from the cheek in subjects with visibly dry skin and subjects with TEWL levels above $16\,g{\cdot}m^{-2}{\cdot}h^{-1}$. In subjects with normal appearing skin and a TEWL below $16\,g{\cdot}m^{-2}{\cdot}h^{-1}$, no activity was found.

11.8.2 Psoriasis and Ichthyosis

In several hyperkeratotic disorders, such as psoriasis and ichthyosis, corneodesmosome retention is elevated and corneocyte cohesion increased [16, 154]. Psoriasis is a chronic inflammatory skin disease. It is characterized by hyperproliferation and altered differentiation of keratinocytes leading to red, scaly skin, abnormal desquamation, and a defective epidermal barrier. Currently, psoriasis is considered a T-cell-mediated inflammatory disease [155].

KLK7 has been proposed to be a candidate marker for psoriasis as increased amount of the zymogen and the activated protease in lesional psoriatic skin have been shown [35, 156]. On the other hand, there has no significant genetic association been found between psoriasis and KLK7. These findings suggest that KLK7 is unlikely to be involved in psoriasis and that the overexpression of KLK7 observed in lesional psoriatic skin could be the consequence of an unspecific response to epidermal hyperproliferation and inflammation [157].

The SC of lesional psoriatic skin was immunochemically shown by Komatsu et al. to contain significantly higher amounts of all SC kallikreins, including KLK7, as compared with normal SC [34, 36]. Enzymatic assays showed that the plasmin-like, furin-like, and overall trypsin-like kallikrein activities were significantly elevated in lesional psoriatic SC, whereas the chymotrypsin-like kallikrein activity was only slightly elevated. Such an increased expression of proteases in the psoriatic scales is apparently contradictory to a reduced proteolysis of corneodesmosomes. However, overexpression does not obligatorily mean higher activity in situ, as protease activity in the SC is controlled by protease inhibitors, such as the LEKTIs, and by physicochemical properties, such as SC pH or water content [32, 49, 158].

Also the intercellular lipids are altered in the SC of psoriatic skin, especially the level and nature of ceramides [159, 160]. As the corneodesmosomes directly interact with the lipid lamellae and the kallikreins are present within the lipids, the physical properties of these lipids probably influence the enzyme activity and the corneodesmosome degradation. One may speculate that, in psoriasis, KLK7, even present in large amounts in the SC, is inhibited or may not be able to cleave corneodesmosome components. As a feedback mechanism, other kallikreins are overexpressed. However, because they are not able to degrade corneodesmosomes for similar reasons, they do not permit the defect to be overcome. Finally, other proteases potentially involved in desquamation, e.g., cathepsins, may be downregulated in psoriatic skin. As a whole, this results in reduced desquamation and scale retention [41].

11.8.3 Atopic Dermatitis

Atopic dermatitis (AD) is a chronic inflammatory disease associated with changes in SC structure and function. The breakdown of epidermal barrier function in AD is associated with changes in corneocyte size and maturation, desquamation, lipid profiles, and some protease activities. Changes in the expression and activity of serine proteases in skin have been reported in epidermal samples taken from subjects with AD [37, 38, 161–163].

11.8.3.1 Serine Protease Profiling in Atopic Xerosis

Komatsu et al. compared SC mass levels of all the eight SC kallikreins together with the trypsin-like kallikrein, chymotrypsin-like kallikrein, and plasmin-like and furin-like enzyme activities on the outermost SC of the forearms from AD patients having very mild lichenification with skin from healthy subjects [37]. In the SC of AD skin, the mass levels of all kallikreins, except for KLK11, were found to be elevated. The increase of the mass level of chymotrypsin-like KLK7 was predominant compared with the trypsin-like kallikreins. Therefore, Komatsu et al. hypothesize that KLK7 could be a key enzyme in AD skin lesions. However, trypsin-like and chymotrypsin-like kallikrein activities were not increased, in marked contrast to the plasmin-like and furin-like enzyme activities.

11.8.3.2 Serine Protease Profiling in Acute Eczematous Atopic Skin

We compared physiological changes in acute eczematous lesional skin of AD patients, with nonlesional AD skin and skin of healthy subjects on ventral forearms, and determined protease mass levels (KLK5, KLK7, KLK11, KLK14, plasmin, and uPA) and enzyme activities on 15 consecutive tape strippings [38, 163].

TEWL levels were elevated before and after tape stripping in lesional skin compared with nonlesional and healthy skin. Conversely, the amount of SC removed by sequential tape stripping was decreased in L skin, indicating increased intracorneocyte cohesion. By correlating reciprocal TEWL values and the amount of SC removed [164], we estimated a significantly thinner SC in lesional skin compared with both nonlesional and healthy skin (Table 11.4a).

There were no differences in the mass levels of KLK5, KLK14, and uPA between healthy, nonlesional, and lesional skin. KLK5 mass levels were large, whereas KLK14 and uPA levels were very low and close or even at detection limit. However, there was a trend of increasing KLK7 levels (3x), and the levels of KLK11 (4x) and plasmin (83x) were significantly elevated in lesional skin (Table 11.4b). Although mass levels of serine proteases tended to be higher in the deeper SC layers for lesional skin, there was no change in the mass levels of any enzyme measured with increasing depth from either nonlesional or healthy skin (data not shown). Unfortunately we did not succeed to establish useful antibody constructs for leukocyte elastase, tryptase, and KLK8. KLK8 has been of interest as it has been suggested to be involved in pathogenesis of inflammatory skin diseases [77].

In contrast to protease mass levels, the enzyme activities of all the tested SC serine proteases were elevated in lesional skin (11.4c). The order compared to healthy skin was plasmin (69x), SC

Table 11.4 (a) Biometric data of the subjects, (b) SC serine protease mass, and (c) activities on 15 consecutive tape stripping extracts of healthy (H), nonlesional (NL), and lesional (L) atopic dermatitis skin (mean ± SEM; *n* = 6 per group)

(a)			
Biometric data	Healthy	Nonlesional	Lesional
Local SCORAD	0.0 ± 0.0	0.2 ± 0.4	7.0 ± 1.2
Irritation score	0.0 ± 0.0	0.0 ± 0.0	5.8 ± 1.8
Mexameter data	203 ± 60	162 ± 30	323 ± 73*
Skin surface pH	6.1 ± 0.7	6.4 ± 0.7	6.0 ± 0.4
SC hydration (AU)	29.6 ± 3.2	26.9 ± 5.0	13.4 ± 1.5*
TEWL ($g \cdot m^{-2} h^{-1}$) before tape stripping	8.2 ± 1.9	12.5 ± 3.4	41.8 ± 9.5*
TEWL ($g \cdot m^{-2} h^{-1}$) after 20 tape strippings	34.9 ± 5.5	27.3 ± 6.9	81.3 ± 7.1
SC thickness [μm]	17 ±1.13	20 ±2.84	10 ±1.80*
SC cohesion (μg protein cm^{-2}), 20 tape strippings	20.8 ± 1.4	17.8 ± 2.6	7.2 ± 1.7

(b)	Protease mass (ng protease/mg SC protein)				
Serine protease	Healthy	Nonlesional	Lesional	Factor L/H	Factor L/NL
KLK5 (trypsin-like)	234 ± 69	151 ± 34	190 ± 75	0.8	1.3
KLK7 (chymotrypsin-like)	21.9 ± 5.2	18.3 ± 3.9	62.0 ± 26.0	2.8	3.4
KLK11 (trypsin-like)	7.18 ± 0.80	7.20 ± 1.07	29.0 ± 9.7**	4.0	4.0
KLK14 (trypsin- and chymotrypsin-like)	0.26 ± 0.11	0.28 ± 0.12	0.21 ± 0.09	0.7	0.8
Plasmin	0.54 ± 0.14	1.09 ± 0.41	45.0 ± 10.7**	83	41
Urokinase	0.036 ± 0.007	0.040 ± 0.010	0.052 ± 0.018	1.4	1.3
(c)	Protease activity (μU/mg SC protein)				
Serine protease	Healthy	Nonlesional	Lesional	Factor L/H	Factor L/NL
Trypsin-like kallikreins	1.40 ± 0.27	1.26 ± 0.25	7.29 ± 1.48**	5.2	5.8
Chymotrypsin-like kallikreins	0.84 ± 0.18	0.42 ± 0.09	1.62 ± 0.28*	1.9	3.8
SC tryptase-like	0.71 ± 0.29	0.87 ± 0.32	39.4 ± 10.8*	55	45
Plasmin-like	0.53 ± 0.11	1.22 ± 0.34	36.4 ± 10.4*	69	30
Urokinase-like	0.40 ± 0.13	0.46 ± 0.12	3.25 ± 0.75*	8.1	7.1
Leukocyte elastase-like	0.01 ± 0.01	0.16 ± 0.16	3.13 ± 1.45*	n.a.	n.a.

Modified from [38, 163]
*p <0.05; **p <0.01 for L vs. H

tryptase-like enzyme (55x), uPA (8x), trypsin-like kallikreins (5x), and chymotrypsin-like kallikreins (2x). Leukocyte elastase showed considerable activity in lesional skin indicating an infiltration of neutrophils, whereas in the SC samples from nonlesional and healthy skin, no activity was found. Analyzing these enzymes with depth showed increased extractable protease activity toward the surface of the SC in nonlesional and healthy skin. Conversely, the activities of inflammatory proteases were elevated in the deeper layers of lesional SC, whereas the desquamatory proteases showed no obvious gradient (data not shown).

The mass levels of KLK14 in lesional skin were very low and not elevated compared with nonlesional or healthy skin. These results would suggest that the increases in SC chymotrypsin-like kallikrein activity we observed are probably due to the increased mass levels of KLK7, although KLK14 exerts a high catalytic efficiency (Tables 11.4b, c) [73, 74]. As we did not measure the mass levels of all SC trypsin-like kallikreins but did not observe increased KLK5 mass levels in lesional skin, other trypsin-like kallikrein activities are probably contributing to the increased SC trypsin-like kallikrein activity. KLK11 would appear to be a candidate but not KLK14.

For the first time we report massively increased mass levels and activity of plasmin in SC extracts from atopic patients with acute eczema; the correlation between mass levels and activity was statistically highly significant ($R^2 = 0.822$, $p = 10^{-5}$). uPA, the major plasminogen activator, is present at very low concentration within the studied SC layers, although uPA-like activity levels were increased in lesional skin. This fact raises the question: is plasminogen activated at the basal layer only by uPA/uPAR or are there other plasminogen activators than uPA within the SC such as KLK5 [79]? Not much is known about the interaction of desquamatory kallikreins and proteases of the thrombostasis axis. Yoon et al. [78] demonstrated the potential for important regulatory interactions between these two major protease families. It might be hypothesized that activation of proKLK7 and/or proKLK11 by plasmin in AD and vice versa may occur and that these KLKs may play a role in the inflammatory cascade in AD.

There exists a discrepancy between protease mass levels and the corresponding enzyme activities that could be explained by the facts (1) that antibodies do not differentiate between inactive zymogen, active protease, and inactive protease/inhibitor complex and (2) that enzyme substrates may exhibit a certain unspecificity.

The reason for the increased protease mass levels and activities in AD is not known. The study results imply that there is insufficient amount of LEKTIs, or any other inhibitor, to inhibit the elevated protease activity in chronic lesions [165]. Increased expression may occur due to kallikrein gene polymorphisms such as those reported for KLK7 by Vasilopoulous et al. who suggest that this enzyme could have an important role in the development of AD [157]. Barrier perturbation also leads to increased inflammatory protease levels, e.g., uPA after tape stripping the SC of a mouse model of AD [166]. We have shown SC protease activities are also increased in barrier-compromised conditions even in nondiseased skin [138, 143]. However, we did not observe any impaired barrier function or increased serine protease activity in nonlesional skin sites, implying that the impairment of barrier function is not intrinsic in subjects with AD, as reported by Kikuchi et al. [167].

The question remains, do these elevated protease levels impair SC or epidermal functioning? Statistically significantly increased irritation, increased TEWL, and decreased hydration levels were found in lesional skin. It is highly likely that the elevated levels of serine proteases in patients with active lesions were contributing to their apparently thinner SC. The increased cohesion in the remaining SC probably indicates that the desquamation is occurring above the stratum compactum and not at the stratum compactum/SG interface.

While Komatsu et al. [37] found increased mass levels of all kallikreins in lesional skin except KLK11, we only observed increased mass levels of KLK11 but not of KLK5 or KLK14 but with a tendency of KLK7 to be increased. We also observed greater quantities of KLK5 but similar quantities of KLK7, KLK11, and KLK14. Moreover, in contrast to our study, Komatsu et al. did not measure increased trypsin-like and chymotrypsin-like kallikrein activities in lesional skin.

The differences in protease mass and activity levels to the Komatsu et al. study [37] may be related to the differences in the skin condition of the AD patients as well as to different sampling procedures and assays having been used. We examined subjects with active lesions having an exacerbated inflammatory condition, whereas the subjects of the Komatsu et al. study showed very mild lichenification only, a condition with retention hyperkeratosis and not premature desquamation. Komatsu et al. collected uppermost corneocytes only, whereas we did 15 subsequent tape strippings, allowing depth profiling. Perhaps one of the major reasons for the differing results between the two studies is the corticosteroid medication of the AD patients in the Komatsu et al. study. It has been shown that the application of clobetasol propionate to normal human skin induces the expression of the mRNA for KLK7 [168, 169]. Obviously the results of the two studies cannot be directly compared.

11.8.4 Effect of Topically Applied Protease Inhibitors on SC Barrier Function and Dry Skin

Several topically applied trypsin-like serine protease inhibitors have been shown by Denda et al., Kitamura et al., and Hachem et al. to accelerate barrier recovery in experimentally damaged (sodium lauryl sulfate, acetone, tape stripping) mouse and human skin models [58, 89, 152]. Inhibitors for chymotrypsin-like serine proteases, aspartic proteases, cysteine proteases, and matrix metalloproteases had no beneficial effects on barrier recovery. The uPA and plasmin inhibitor trans-4-(aminomethyl) cyclohexane carboxylic acid (t-AMCHA) and the dual tryptic/chymotryptic inhibitor aprotinin showed accelerated barrier recovery, paralleled by decreased serine protease activity and improved hydration on damaged skin.

Interestingly, neither lipid synthesis nor lipid processing was altered by serine protease inhibitors. Instead, serine protease inhibitor treatment accelerated LB secretion. These observations suggest that serine proteases suppress the LB secretory responses to acute barrier perturbations (Fig. 11.8) [58].

Take Home Messages

- Corneodesmosomes, modified desmosomes, are the primary mediator of intercorneocyte cohesion between corneocytes. Their transmembranal, intercellular components are composed of desmogleins, desmocollins, and corneodesmosin. Desquamation is mediated by their degradation.
- Epidermal proteases control desquamation, corneocyte maturity, and the number of cell layers in the SC. Excess of protease activity can lead to SC thinning, while reduced protease activity can lead to SC thickening.
- In healthy skin, serine protease activity in the SC varies on skin areas. Compared to other body sites, facial skin shows higher proteolytic activity resulting in premature corneodesmosomal degradation. This indicates that facial SC disjunctum is probably not present. The elevated serine protease activities on the face may be due to a subclinical microinflammatory or preinflammatory condition induced, e.g., by environmental impacts.
- Delayed desquamation is the accumulation of corneocytes on the surface of the SC that leads ultimately to the cosmetic condition commonly termed as "dry skin" and which has been described best as a cyclical model [158]. Much more is known about body dry skin rather than dry facial skin. The latter tends to become rough rather than flaky. The biology of skin moisturization, of which hydration is only one benefit, is highly complex. We are convinced that the future of all new moisturizers lies in the fully understanding of the control and impairment of desquamation [170].
- Changes in the proteolytic balance of the skin can result in inflammation, which leads to the typical clinical signs of redness, scaling, and itching. Increased serine protease activity occurs in most, if not all, inflammatory dermatoses, ranging from genetic disorders, such as Netherton syndrome, psoriasis, and AD, to subclinical barrier abnormalities induced, e.g., by alkaline soaps or by environmental influences. Serine proteases might represent key markers for underlying and sometimes nonobservable skin abnormalities.
- Better understanding of the multistep proteolytic events and of the regulatory

mechanisms involved in desquamation should enable the design of new treatments for the skin disorders associated with disturbance in the SC turnover. This will be the ultimate approach to corneocare.

- A vast number of data and hypothesis have been generated on SC proteases and their influences to the skin. Some of them are contradictory due to the chosen variable conditions; most of them are fragmentary making it difficult to assemble the complete puzzle with pieces that do not fit exactly. To get a holistic view of the picture, a broad scientific collaboration is needed mutually discussing and investigating the profiling of proteases and other enzymes, inhibitors, as well as desmosomal and CE proteins to fully understand the maturation and desquamation of the SC in healthy and diseased skin. An open and informal scientific desquamation community should regularly meet to discuss the mechanisms of human desquamation. Perhaps through a workshop in association with the Stratum Corneum Conference series.

Abbreviations and Synonyms

A2ML1	α2-macroglobulin-like 1
AD	atopic dermatitis
CE	cornified envelope
CDSN	corneodesmosin
CTSD	cathepsin D
CTSL2	cathepsin L2 = cathepsin V = stratum corneum thiol protease= SCTP
CTSL-like	cathepsin L-like
DSC	desmocollin
DSG	desmoglein
Elafin	skin-derived antileukoprotease = SKALP
KLK	kallikrein
KLK5	stratum corneum trypsin-like enzyme = SCTE
KLK7	stratum corneum chymotrypsin-like enzyme = SCCE
LB	lamellar bodies = lamellar granules = Odland bodies = keratinosomes
LEKTI-1	lymphoepithelial Kazal-type 5 serine protease inhibitor
LEKTI-2	lymphoepithelial Kazal-type 9 serine protease inhibitor
LEKTI-3	lymphoepithelial Kazal-type 6 serine protease inhibitor
PAI-2	plasminogen activator inhibitor-2 = SERPINB2
PAR	protease-activated receptor
RH	relative humidity
SC	stratum corneum
SG	stratum granulosum
SLPI	secretory leukocyte protease inhibitor = antileukoprotease (ALP)
SPINK5	serine protease inhibitor Kazal-type 5 gene
SPINK6	serine protease inhibitor Kazal-type 6 gene
SPINK9	serine protease inhibitor Kazal-type 9 gene
t-AMCHA	trans-4-(aminomethyl) cyclohexane carboxylic acid
TEWL	transepidermal water loss
TJ	tight junction
UPA	urokinase = urokinase-type plasminogen activator
UPAR	urokinase-type plasminogen activator receptor

References

1. Kligman AM (2011) Corneobiology and corneotherapy – a final chapter. Int J Cosmet Sci 33(3):197–209
2. Elias PM (2005) Stratum corneum defensive functions: an integrated view. J Invest Dermatol 125(2):183–200
3. Chaturvedi V et al (2006) Defining the caspase-containing apoptotic machinery contributing to cornification in human epidermal equivalents. Exp Dermatol 15(1):14–22
4. Egelrud T (1993) Purification and preliminary characterization of stratum corneum chymotryptic enzyme: a proteinase that may be involved in desquamation. J Invest Dermatol 101(2):200–204

5. Haftek M, Simon M, Serre G (2006) Corneodesmosomes: Pivotal Actors in the Stratum Corneum Cohesion and Desquamation. In: Elias PM, Feingold KR (eds) Skin barrier. Taylor & Francis, New York, pp 171–189
6. Marks R (2004) The stratum corneum barrier: the final frontier. J Nutr 134(8 Suppl):2017S–2021S
7. Jonca N et al (2002) Corneodesmosin, a component of epidermal corneocyte desmosomes, displays homophilic adhesive properties. J Biol Chem 277(7):5024–5029
8. Michaels AS, Chandrasekaran SK, Shaw JE (1975) Drug permeation through human skin: Theory and invitro experimental measurement. AIChE J 21(5):985–996
9. Elias PM (1983) Epidermal lipids, barrier function, and desquamation. J Invest Dermatol 80(Suppl):44s–49s
10. Wepf R et al (2007) Multimodal imaging of skin structures: imagining imaging of the skin. In: Wilhelm K-P et al (eds) Bioengineering of the skin: skin imaging and analysis. Informa Healthcare, New York
11. Cork MJ et al (2009) Epidermal barrier dysfunction in atopic dermatitis. J Invest Dermatol 129(8):1892–1908
12. Serre G et al (1991) Identification of late differentiation antigens of human cornified epithelia, expressed in re-organized desmosomes and bound to cross-linked envelope. J Invest Dermatol 97(6):1061–1072
13. Lundström A et al (1994) Evidence for a role of corneodesmosin, a protein which may serve to modify desmosomes during cornification, in stratum corneum cell cohesion and desquamation. Arch Dermatol Res 286(7):369–375
14. Brandner JM, Haftek M, Niessen CM (2010) Adherens junctions, desmosomes and tight junctions in epidermal barrier function. Open Dermatol J 4:14–20
15. Egelrud T (1999) Desquamation. In: Loden M, Maibach H (eds) Dry skin and moisturizers. CRC Press, Boca Raton, pp 109–117
16. Chapman SJ, Walsh A (1990) Desmosomes, corneosomes and desquamation. An ultrastructural study of adult pig epidermis. Arch Dermatol Res 282(5):304–310
17. Fartasch M, Bassukas ID, Diepgen TL (1993) Structural relationship between epidermal lipid lamellae, lamellar bodies and desmosomes in human epidermis: an ultrastructural study. Br J Dermatol 128(1):1–9
18. Neubert RHH, Wepf R (2008) Das stratum corneum – struktur und morphologie einer hoch effizienten barriere. Medicos 4:21–28
19. Stokes DL (2007) Desmosomes from a structural perspective. Curr Opin Cell Biol 19(5):565–571
20. Green KJ, Simpson CL (2007) Desmosomes: new perspectives on a classic. J Invest Dermatol 127(11):2499–2515
21. Green KJ, Gaudry CA (2000) Are desmosomes more than tethers for intermediate filaments? Nat Rev Mol Cell Biol 1(3):208–216
22. Kottke MD, Delva E, Kowalczyk AP (2006) The desmosome: cell science lessons from human diseases. J Cell Sci 119(5):797–806
23. Garrod D, Chidgey M, North A (1996) Desmosomes: differentiation, development, dynamics and disease. Curr Opin Cell Biol 8(5):670–678
24. Watkinson A et al (2001) Water modulation of stratum corneum chymotryptic enzyme activity and desquamation. Arch Dermatol Res 293(9):470–476
25. Naoe Y et al (2010) Bidimensional analysis of desmoglein 1 distribution on the outermost corneocytes provides the structural and functional information of the stratum corneum. J Dermatol Sci 57(3):192–198
26. Horikoshi T et al (1999) Role of endogenous cathepsin D-like and chymotrypsin-like proteolysis in human epidermal desquamation. Br J Dermatol 141(3):453–459
27. Ekholm IE, Brattsand M, Egelrud T (2000) Stratum corneum tryptic enzyme in normal epidermis: a missing link in the desquamation process? J Invest Dermatol 114(1):56–63
28. Watkinson A (1999) Stratum corneum thiol protease (SCTP): a novel cysteine protease of late epidermal differentiation. Arch Dermatol Res 291(5):260–268
29. Skerrow CJ, Clelland DG, Skerrow D (1989) Changes to desmosomal antigens and lectin-binding sites during differentiation in normal human epidermis: a quantitative ultrastructural study. J Cell Sci 92(4):667–677
30. Chapman SJ et al (1991) Lipids, proteins and corneocyte adhesion. Arch Dermatol Res 283(3):167–173
31. Harding CR et al (2000) Dry skin, moisturization and corneodesmolysis. Int J Cosmet Sci 22(1):21–52
32. Caubet C et al (2004) Degradation of corneodesmosome proteins by two serine proteases of the kallikrein family, SCTE//KLK5//hK5 and SCCE//KLK7//hK7. J Invest Dermatol 122(5):1235–1244
33. Öhman H, Vahlquist A (1998) The pH gradient over the stratum corneum differs in X-linked recessive and autosomal dominant ichthyosis: a clue to the molecular origin of the "acid skin mantle"? J Invest Dermatol 111(4):674–677
34. Komatsu N et al (2007) Aberrant human tissue kallikrein levels in the stratum corneum and serum of patients with psoriasis: dependence on phenotype, severity and therapy. Br J Dermatol 156(5):875–883
35. Simon M et al (2002) Abnormal proteolysis of corneodesmosin in psoriatic skin. Br J Dermatol 147(5):1053
36. Komatsu N et al (2005) Multiple tissue kallikrein mRNA and protein expression in normal skin and skin diseases. Br J Dermatol 153(2):274–281
37. Komatsu N et al (2007) Human tissue kallikrein expression in the stratum corneum and serum of atopic dermatitis patients. Exp Dermatol 16(6):513–519
38. Voegeli R et al (2009) Increased stratum corneum serine protease activity in acute eczematous atopic skin. Br J Dermatol 161:70–77
39. Cork MJ et al (2006) New perspectives on epidermal barrier dysfunction in atopic dermatitis: gene-environment interactions. J Allergy Clin Immunol 118(1):3–21, quiz 22–3
40. Haftek M et al (1997) Expression of corneodesmosin in the granular layer and stratum corneum of normal and diseased epidermis. Br J Dermatol 137(6):864–873

41. Simon M et al (2008) Alterations in the desquamation-related proteolytic cleavage of corneodesmosin and other corneodesmosomal proteins in psoriatic lesional epidermis. Br J Dermatol 159(1):77–85
42. Rawlings AV et al (1994) Abnormalities in stratum corneum structure, lipid composition, and desmosome degradation in soap-induced winter xerosis. J Soc Cosmet Chem 45:203–220
43. Rawlings AV et al (1995) The effect of glycerol and humidity on desmosome degradation in stratum corneum. Arch Dermatol Res 287(5):457–464
44. Simon M et al (2001) Persistence of both peripheral and non-peripheral corneodesmosomes in the upper stratum corneum of winter xerosis skin versus only peripheral in normal skin. J Invest Dermatol 116(1): 23–30
45. Brandner JM (2009) Tight junctions and tight junction proteins in mammalian epidermis. Eur J Pharm Biopharm 72(2):289–294
46. Schlüter H et al (2004) Sealing the live part of the skin: the integrated meshwork of desmosomes, tight junctions and curvilinear ridge structures in the cells of the uppermost granular layer of the human epidermis. Eur J Cell Biol 83(11–12):655–665
47. Haftek M et al (2011) Compartmentalization of the human stratum corneum by persistent tight junction-like structures. Exp Dermatol 20(8):617–621
48. Igawa S et al (2011) Tight junctions in the stratum corneum explain spatial differences in corneodesmosome degradation. Exp Dermatol 20(1):53–57
49. Hachem JP et al (2005) Sustained serine proteases activity by prolonged increase in pH leads to degradation of lipid processing enzymes and profound alterations of barrier function and stratum corneum integrity. J Invest Dermatol 125(3):510–520
50. Parra JL, Paye M (2003) EEMCO guidance for the in vivo assessment of skin surface pH. Skin Pharmacol Appl Skin Physiol 16(3):188–202
51. Öhman H, Vahlquist A (1994) In vivo studies concerning a pH gradient in human stratum corneum and upper epidermis. Acta Derm Venereol 74(5):375–379
52. Behne MJ et al (2002) NHE1 regulates the stratum corneum permeability barrier homeostasis. Microenvironment acidification assessed with fluorescence lifetime imaging. J Biol Chem 277(49): 47399–47406
53. Behne MJ et al (2003) Neonatal development of the stratum corneum pH gradient: localization and mechanisms leading to emergence of optimal barrier function. J Invest Dermatol 120(6):998–1006
54. Suzuki Y et al (1993) Detection and characterization of endogenous protease associated with desquamation of stratum corneum. Arch Dermatol Res 285(6):372–377
55. Ovaere P et al (2009) The emerging roles of serine protease cascades in the epidermis. Trends Biochem Sci 34(9):453–463
56. Morizane S et al (2010) Kallikrein expression and cathelicidin processing are independently controlled in keratinocytes by calcium, vitamin D(3), and retinoic acid. J Invest Dermatol 130(5):1297–1306
57. Menon GK et al (1992) Localization of calcium in murine epidermis following disruption and repair of the permeability barrier. Cell Tissue Res 270(3):503–512
58. Hachem J-P et al (2006) Serine protease signaling of epidermal permeability barrier homeostasis. J Invest Dermatol 126(9):2074–2086
59. Demerjian M et al (2008) Acute modulations in permeability barrier function regulate epidermal cornification. Role of caspase-14 and the protease-activated receptor type 2. Am J Pathol 172(1):86–97
60. Sexsmith E, Petersen WF (1918) Skin ferments. J Exp Med 27(2):273–282
61. Di Cera E (2009) Serine proteases. IUBMB Life 61(5):510–515
62. Emami N, Diamandis EP (2007) Human tissue kallikreins: a road under construction. Clin Chim Acta 381(1):78–84
63. Bissett DL, McBride JF, Patrick LF (1987) Role of protein and calcium in stratum corneum cell cohesion. Arch Dermatol Res 279(3):184–189
64. Egelrud T, Hofer PA, Lundstrom A (1988) Proteolytic degradation of desmosomes in plantar stratum corneum leads to cell dissociation in vitro. Acta Derm Venereol 68(2):93–97
65. Lundström A, Egelrud T (1988) Cell shedding from human plantar skin in vitro: evidence of its dependence on endogenous proteolysis. J Invest Dermatol 91(4):340–343
66. Egelrud T, Lundstrom A (1990) The dependence of detergent-induced cell dissociation in non-palmoplantar stratum corneum on endogenous proteolysis. J Invest Dermatol 95(4):456–459
67. Lundström A, Egelrud T (1990) Evidence that cell shedding from plantar stratum corneum in vitro involves endogenous proteolysis of the desmosomal protein desmoglein I. J Invest Dermatol 94(2):216–220
68. Lundström A, Egelrud T (1990) Cell shedding from human plantar skin in vitro: evidence that two different types of protein structures are degraded by a chymotrypsin-like enzyme. Arch Dermatol Res 282(4):234–237
69. Egelrud T, Lundström A (1991) A chymotrypsin-like proteinase that may be involved in desquamation in plantar stratum corneum. Arch Dermatol Res 283(2):108–112
70. Lundström A, Egelrud T (1991) Stratum corneum chymotryptic enzyme: a proteinase which may be generally present in the stratum corneum and with a possible involvement in desquamation. Acta Derm Venereol 71(6):471–474
71. Paliouras M, Diamandis EP (2006) The kallikrein world: an update on the human tissue kallikreins. Biol Chem 387(6):643–652
72. Clements JA et al (2004) The tissue kallikrein family of serine proteases: functional roles in human disease and potential as clinical biomarkers. Crit Rev Clin Lab Sci 41(3):265–312
73. Brattsand M et al (2005) A proteolytic cascade of kallikreins in the stratum corneum. J Invest Dermatol 124(1):198–203

74. Stefansson K et al (2006) Kallikrein-related peptidase 14 may be a major contributor to trypsin-like proteolytic activity in human stratum corneum. Biol Chem 387(6):761–768
75. Komatsu N et al (2005) Quantification of human tissue kallikreins in the stratum corneum: dependence on age and gender. J Invest Dermatol 125(6):1182–1189
76. Komatsu N et al (2006) Quantification of eight tissue kallikreins in the stratum corneum and sweat. J Invest Dermatol 126(4):927–931
77. Kishibe M et al (2007) Kallikrein 8 is involved in skin desquamation in cooperation with other kallikreins. J Biol Chem 282(8):5834–5841
78. Yoon H et al (2008) Activation profiles of human kallikrein-related peptidases by proteases of the thrombostasis axis. Protein Sci 17:1998–2007
79. Debela M et al (2008) Structures and specificity of the human kallikrein-related peptidases KLK 4, 5, 6, and 7. Biol Chem 389(6):623
80. Alfano D et al (2005) The urokinase plasminogen activator and its receptor: role in cell growth and apoptosis. Thromb Haemost 93(2):205–211
81. Rockway TW, Nienaber V, Giranda VL (2002) Inhibitors of the protease domain of urokinase-type plasminogen activator. Curr Pharm Des 8(28): 2541–2558
82. Mondino A, Resnati M, Blasi F (1999) Structure and function of the urokinase receptor. Thromb Haemost 82(Suppl 1):19–22
83. Ogura Y et al (2008) Plasmin induces degradation and dysfunction of laminin 332 (laminin 5) and impaired assembly of basement membrane at the dermal-epidermal junction. Br J Dermatol 159(1):49–60
84. Rosenberg S (2001) New developments in the urokinase-type plasminogen activator system. Expert Opin Ther Targets 5(6):711–722
85. Schaefer BM et al (1995) Differential expression of urokinase-type plasminogen activator (uPA), its receptor (uPA-R), and inhibitor type-2 (PAI-2) during differentiation of keratinocytes in an organotypic coculture system. Exp Cell Res 220(2):415–423
86. Jensen PJ, Lavker RM (1999) Urokinase is a positive regulator of epidermal proliferation in vivo. J Invest Dermatol 112(2):240–244
87. Spiers EM, Lazarus GS, Lyons-Giordano B (1994) Expression of plasminogen activator enzymes in psoriatic epidermis. J Invest Dermatol 102(3): 333–338
88. Katsuta Y et al (2003) Urokinase-type plasminogen activator is activated in stratum corneum after barrier disruption. J Dermatol Sci 32(1):55–57
89. Denda M et al (1997) trans-4-(aminomethyl)cyclohexane carboxylic acid (T-AMCHA), an anti-fibrinolytic agent, accelerates barrier recovery and prevents the epidermal hyperplasia induced by epidermal injury in hairless mice and humans. J Invest Dermatol 109(1):84–90
90. Marschall C et al (1999) UVB increases urokinase-type plasminogen activator receptor (uPAR) expression. J Invest Dermatol 113(1):69–76
91. Miralles F et al (1998) UV irradiation induces the murine urokinase-type plasminogen activator gene via the c-Jun N-terminal kinase signaling pathway: requirement of an AP1 enhancer element. Mol Cell Biol 18(8):4537–4547
92. Oxholm A et al (1988) Immunohistological detection of interleukin I-like molecules and tumour necrosis factor in human epidermis before and after UVB-irradiation in vivo. Br J Dermatol 118(3): 369–376
93. Sales KU et al (2010) Matriptase initiates activation of epidermal pro-kallikrein and disease onset in a mouse model of Netherton syndrome. Nat Genet 42(8):676–683
94. List K et al (2002) Matriptase/MT-SP1 is required for postnatal survival, epidermal barrier function, hair follicle development, and thymic homeostasis. Oncogene 21(23):3765–3779
95. List K et al (2003) Loss of proteolytically processed filaggrin caused by epidermal deletion of Matriptase/MT-SP1. J Cell Biol 163(4):901–910
96. List K et al (2006) Delineation of matriptase protein expression by enzymatic gene trapping suggests diverging roles in barrier function, hair formation, and squamous cell carcinogenesis. Am J Pathol 168(5):1513–1525
97. Deraison C et al (2007) LEKTI fragments specifically inhibit KLK5, KLK7, and KLK14 and control desquamation through a pH-dependent interaction. Mol Biol Cell 18(9):3607–3619
98. Zeeuwen PL et al (2007) Colocalization of cystatin M/E and cathepsin V in lamellar granules and corneodesmosomes suggests a functional role in epidermal differentiation. J Invest Dermatol 127(1):120–128
99. Igarashi S et al (2004) Cathepsin D, but not cathepsin E, degrades desmosomes during epidermal desquamation. Br J Dermatol 151(2):355–361
100. Meyer-Hoffert U (2009) Reddish, scaly, and itchy: how proteases and their inhibitors contribute to inflammatory skin diseases. Arch Immunol Ther Exp (Warsz) 57(5):345–354
101. Bernard D et al (2001) Purification and characterization of the endoglycosidase heparanase 1 from human plantar stratum corneum: a key enzyme in epidermal physiology? J Invest Dermatol 117(5): 1266–1273
102. Goettig P, Magdolen V, Brandstetter H (2010) Natural and synthetic inhibitors of kallikrein-related peptidases (KLKs). Biochimie 92(11):1546–1567
103. Borgono CA et al (2007) Expression and functional characterization of the cancer-related serine protease, human tissue kallikrein 14. J Biol Chem 282(4):2405–2422
104. Debela M et al (2007) Structural basis of the zinc inhibition of human tissue kallikrein 5. J Mol Biol 373(4):1017–1031
105. Debela M et al (2007) Chymotryptic specificity determinants in the 1.0 A structure of the zinc-inhibited human tissue kallikrein 7. Proc Natl Acad Sci USA 104(41):16086–16091

106. Sato J et al (1998) Cholesterol sulfate inhibits proteases that are involved in desquamation of stratum corneum. J Invest Dermatol 111(2):189–193
107. Ishida-Yamamoto A et al (2005) LEKTI is localized in lamellar granules, separated from KLK5 and KLK7, and is secreted in the extracellular spaces of the superficial stratum granulosum. J Invest Dermatol 124(2):360–366
108. Roelandt T et al (2009) LEKTI-1 in sickness and in health. Int J Cosmet Sci 31(4):247–254
109. Borgono CA et al (2007) A potential role for multiple tissue kallikrein serine proteases in epidermal desquamation. J Biol Chem 282(6):3640–3652
110. Egelrud T et al (2005) hK5 and hK7, two serine proteinases abundant in human skin, are inhibited by LEKTI domain 6. Br J Dermatol 153(6):1200–1203
111. Schechter NM et al (2005) Inhibition of human kallikreins 5 and 7 by the serine protease inhibitor lympho-epithelial Kazal-type inhibitor (LEKTI). Biol Chem 386(11):1173–1184
112. Meyer-Hoffert U, Wu Z, Schroder JM (2009) Identification of lympho-epithelial Kazal-type inhibitor 2 in human skin as a kallikrein-related peptidase 5-specific protease inhibitor. PLoS One 4(2):e4372
113. Brattsand M et al (2009) SPINK9: a selective, skin-specific Kazal-type serine protease inhibitor. J Invest Dermatol 129(7):1656–1665
114. Meyer-Hoffert U et al (2010) Isolation of SPINK6 in human skin: selective inhibitor of kallikrein-related peptidases. J Biol Chem 285(42):32174–32181
115. Franzke C-W et al (1996) Antileukoprotease inhibits stratum corneum chymotryptic enzyme. Evidence for a regulative function in desquamation. J Biol Chem 271(36):21886–21890
116. Tian X et al (2004) Expression of human kallikrein 7 (hK7/SCCE) and its inhibitor antileukoprotease (ALP/SLPI) in uterine endocervical glands and in cervical adenocarcinomas. Oncol Rep 12:1001–1006
117. Molhuizen HO et al (1993) SKALP/elafin: an elastase inhibitor from cultured human keratinocytes. Purification, cDNA sequence, and evidence for transglutaminase cross-linking. J Biol Chem 268(16):12028–12032
118. Taggart CC et al (2001) Cathepsin B, L, and S cleave and inactivate secretory leucoprotease inhibitor. J Biol Chem 276(36):33345–33352
119. Galliano MF et al (2006) A novel protease inhibitor of the alpha2-macroglobulin family expressed in the human epidermis. J Biol Chem 281(9):5780–5789
120. Oji V et al (2006) Plasminogen activator inhibitor-2 is expressed in different types of congenital ichthyosis: in vivo evidence for its cross-linking into the cornified cell envelope by transglutaminase-1. Br J Dermatol 154(5):860–867
121. Hibino T et al (1999) Suppression of keratinocyte proliferation by plasminogen activator inhibitor-2. J Invest Dermatol 112(1):85–90
122. Lian X, Yang T (2004) Plasminogen activator inhibitor 2: expression and role in differentiation of epidermal keratinocyte. Biol Cell 96(2):109–116
123. Chavanas S et al (2000) Mutations in SPINK5, encoding a serine protease inhibitor, cause Netherton syndrome. Nat Genet 25(2):141–142
124. Hachem J-P et al (2006) Serine protease activity and residual LEKTI expression determine phenotype in Netherton syndrome. J Invest Dermatol 126(7): 1609–1621
125. Komatsu N et al (2002) Elevated stratum corneum hydrolytic activity in Netherton syndrome suggests an inhibitory regulation of desquamation by SPINK5-derived peptides. J Invest Dermatol 118(3):436–443
126. Sevilla LM et al (2007) Mice deficient in involucrin, envoplakin, and periplakin have a defective epidermal barrier. J Cell Biol 179(7):1599–1612
127. Eissa A, Diamandis EP (2008) Human tissue kallikreins as promiscuous modulators of homeostatic skin barrier functions. Biol Chem 389(6):669–680
128. Yoon H et al (2007) Activation profiles and regulatory cascades of the human kallikrein-related peptidases. J Biol Chem 282(44):31852–31864
129. Simon M et al (2001) Refined characterization of corneodesmosin proteolysis during terminal differentiation of human epidermis and its relationship to desquamation. J Biol Chem 276(23):20292–20299
130. Bernard D et al (2003) Analysis of proteins with caseinolytic activity in a human stratum corneum extract revealed a yet unidentified cysteine protease and identified the so-called "stratum corneum thiol protease" as cathepsin L2. J Invest Dermatol 120(4):592–600
131. Stefansson K et al (2008) Activation of proteinase-activated receptor-2 by human kallikrein-related peptidases. J Invest Dermatol 128(1):18–25
132. Oikonomopoulou K et al (2006) Proteinase-activated receptors. Targets for kallikrein signaling. J Biol Chem 281(43):32095–32112
133. Egberts F et al (2004) Cathepsin D is involved in the regulation of transglutaminase 1 and epidermal differentiation. J Cell Sci 117(11):2295–2307
134. Chang-Yi C, Takahashi M, Tezuka T (1997) 30-kDa trypsin-like proteases in the plantar stratum corneum. J Dermatol 24(8):504–509
135. Schepky AG et al (2004) Influence of cleansing on stratum corneum tryptic enzyme in human skin. Int J Cosmet Sci 26(5):245–253
136. Hansson L et al (2002) Epidermal overexpression of stratum corneum chymotryptic enzyme in mice: a model for chronic itchy dermatitis. J Invest Dermatol 118(3):444–449
137. Koyama J et al (1996) The mechanism of desquamation in the stratum corneum and its relevance to skin care. In: Proceedings of the 19th IFSCC congress, Sydney, 1996
138. Voegeli R et al (2007) Profiling of serine protease activities in human stratum corneum and detection of a stratum corneum tryptase-like enzyme. Int J Cosmet Sci 29(3):191–200
139. Sato J et al (1998) Dry condition affects desquamation of stratum corneum in vivo. J Dermatol Sci 18(3):163–169

140. Sato J (2002) Desquamation and the Role of Stratum Corneum Enzymes. In: Leyden JJ, Rawlings AV (eds) Skin moisturization. Marcel Dekker, New York, pp 81–94
141. Declercq L et al (2002) Adaptation response in human skin barrier to a hot and dry environment. J Invest Dermatol 119(3):716
142. Voegeli R et al (2007) Efficient and simple quantification of stratum corneum proteins on tape strippings by infrared densitometry. Skin Res Technol 13(3):242–251
143. Voegeli R et al (2008) Increased basal transepidermal water loss leads to elevation of some but not all stratum corneum serine proteases. Int J Cosmet Sci 30(6):435–442
144. Mohammed D et al (2011) Depth profiling of stratum corneum biophysical and molecular properties. Br J Dermatol 164(5):957–965
145. Hirao T (2003) Involvement of transglutaminase in ex vivo maturation of cornified envelopes in the stratum corneum. Int J Cosmet Sci 25(5):245–257
146. Harding CR et al (2003) The cornified cell envelope: an important marker of stratum corneum maturation in healthy and dry skin. Int J Cosmet Sci 25(4): 157–167
147. Hadgraft J, Lane ME (2009) Transepidermal water loss and skin site: a hypothesis. Int J Pharm 373(1–2):1–3
148. Machado M, Hadgraft J, Lane ME (2010) Assessment of the variation of skin barrier function with anatomic site, age, gender and ethnicity. Int J Cosmet Sci 32:397–409
149. Proksch E (2008) Protection against dryness of facial skin: a rational approach. Skin Pharmacol Physiol 22(1):3–7
150. Van Overloop L, Declercq L, Maes D (2001) Visual scaliness of human skin correlates to decreased ceramide levels and decreased stratum corneum protease activity. J Dermatol 117(3):811
151. Nina M et al (2009) Dichotomous effect of ultraviolet B on the expression of corneodesmosomal enzymes in human epidermal keratinocytes. J Dermatol Sci 54(1):17–24
152. Kitamura K (2002) Advances in dry skin care technology extend beyond the category of cosmetic products. IFSCC Mag 5(3):177–187
153. Kawai E et al (2002) Can inorganic powders provide any biological benefit in stratum corneum, while residing on skin surface. IFSCC Mag 5(4):269–275
154. Suzuki Y et al (1996) The role of two endogenous proteases of the stratum corneum in degradation of desmoglein-1 and their reduced activity in the skin of ichthyotic patients. Br J Dermatol 134(3):460–464
155. Bowcock AM, Krueger JG (2005) Getting under the skin: the immunogenetics of psoriasis. Nat Rev Immunol 5(9):699–711
156. Ekholm E, Egelrud T (1999) Stratum corneum chymotryptic enzyme in psoriasis. Arch Dermatol Res 291(4):195–200
157. Vasilopoulos Y et al (2004) Genetic association between an AACC insertion in the 3′UTR of the stratum corneum chymotryptic enzyme gene and atopic dermatitis. J Invest Dermatol 123(1):62–66
158. Rawlings AV, Matts PJ (2005) Stratum corneum moisturization at the molecular level: an update in relation to the dry skin cycle. J Invest Dermatol 124(6):1099–1110
159. Choi MJ, Maibach HI (2005) Role of ceramides in barrier function of healthy and diseased skin. Am J Clin Dermatol 6(4):215–223
160. Holleran WM, Takagi Y, Uchida Y (2006) Epidermal sphingolipids: metabolism, function, and roles in skin disorders. FEBS Lett 580(23):5456–5466
161. Redoules D et al (1999) Characterisation and assay of five enzymatic activities in the stratum corneum using tape-strippings. Skin Pharmacol Appl Skin Physiol 12(4):182–192
162. Tarroux R et al (2002) Variability of enzyme markers during clinical regression of atopic dermatitis. Skin Pharmacol Appl Skin Physiol 15:55–62
163. Voegeli R et al (2011) Increased mass levels of serine proteases in the stratum corneum in acute eczematous atopic skin. Int J Cosmet Sci 33(6):560–565
164. Kalia YN et al (2001) Assessment of topical bioavailability in vivo: the importance of stratum corneum thickness. Skin Pharmacol Appl Skin Physiol 14(suppl 1):82–86
165. Roedl D et al (2009) Serine protease inhibitor lymphoepithelial Kazal type-related inhibitor tends to be decreased in atopic dermatitis. J Eur Acad Dermatol Venereol 23(11):1263–1266
166. Descargues P et al (2006) Corneodesmosomal cadherins are preferential targets of stratum corneum trypsin- and chymotrypsin-like hyperactivity in Netherton syndrome. J Invest Dermatol 126(7): 1622–1632
167. Kikuchi K et al (2006) Impairment of skin barrier function is not inherent in atopic dermatitis patients: a prospective study conducted in newborns. Pediatr Dermatol 23(2):109–113
168. Cork MJ et al (2006) Interaction of topical corticosteroids and pimecrolimus with the skin barrier: Implications for efficacy and safety of treatment for atopic dermatitis. J Am Acad Dermatol 54(suppl S):AB3 P10
169. Sugarman JL (2008) The epidermal barrier in atopic dermatitis. Semin Cutan Med Surg 27(2):108–114
170. Rawlings AV (2009) 50 years of stratum corneum and moisturization research. IFSCC Mag 12(3):169–172
171. Jonca N et al (2009) Corneodesmosomal Proteins. In: Rawlings AV, Leyden JJ (eds) Skin moisturization. Informa Healthcare, New York, pp 99–123

Endogenous Retroviral-Like Aspartic Protease, SASPase as a Key Modulator of Skin Moisturization

12

Takeshi Matsui

12.1 Introduction

About 360 million years ago (the late Devonian period), the first terrestrial vertebrate amphibian emerged from water and adapted to life on land. These animals evolved their skin epidermis into a keratinized stratified squamous epithelium, baring the stratum corneum (SC) as the outermost layer, to prevent water loss and as protection from sunlight [1, 67]. Genomic analysis of various vertebrate species reveals that dynamic changes in epithelia are correlated with the integration of new stratified epithelia-specific genes (Fig. 12.1). Therefore, identification and deletion of these genes in mammals such as mice may help us to understand the molecular mechanisms of adaptive evolution of epithelium, termed "epithelial evolution."

Skin is composed of three layers: the epidermis, dermis, and hypodermis. The epidermis is a keratinized stratified squamous epithelium and forms an effective barrier between the organism and the environment that is indispensable for the prevention of the invasion of microorganisms, chemical compounds, and allergens [50, 66]. This layer is also crucial in the maintenance of moisture levels of the skin. It composed of the stratum basale (SB), stratum spinosum (SS), stratum granulosum (SG), and stratum corneum (SC). Epidermal differentiation consists of a multiple-step process accompanied by various gene expression and concomitant morphological changes [18, 19, 68, 77] Keratinocytes proliferate and differentiate as they move upward from the SB. Gene expression is finished in the "living" SG by maturation of intra/extracellular processes. Intracellular changes consist of the formation of a protein-rich envelope and an outer lipid membrane that provides flexibility to the SC [11, 72]. At the extracellular level, the extrusion of lamellar granules occurs to produce waterproof barrier lipids by secreting membrane-coating granules. At the "dead" SC, corneocytes and intracellular lipids form a functional barrier between the organism and the environment, i.e. "air-liquid interface," which is indispensable for the physiology of the skin [11]. At the SG-to-SC transition stage, keratinocytes dramatically transform themselves from living cells to flat-shaped dead cells with loss of intracellular organelles and contain keratin bundles and lipids to constitute the SC [39]. During this dynamic terminal differentiation with cell death, keratinocytes still express various proteins, such as keratins, profilaggrin/filaggrin, involucrin, small proline-rich proteins, loricrin, cystatin A, and elafin, which participate in forming the cornified

T. Matsui, Ph.D.
Hiiragi Laboratory, Institute for Integrated Cell – Material Sciences (iCeMS), Kyoto University, iCeMS Complex2, Yoshida-Honmachi, Sakyo-ku, Kyoto 606-8501, Japan
e-mail: tmatsui@icems.kyoto-u.ac.jp

M. Lodén, H.I. Maibach (eds.), *Treatment of Dry Skin Syndrome*,
DOI 10.1007/978-3-642-27606-4_12, © Springer-Verlag Berlin Heidelberg 2012

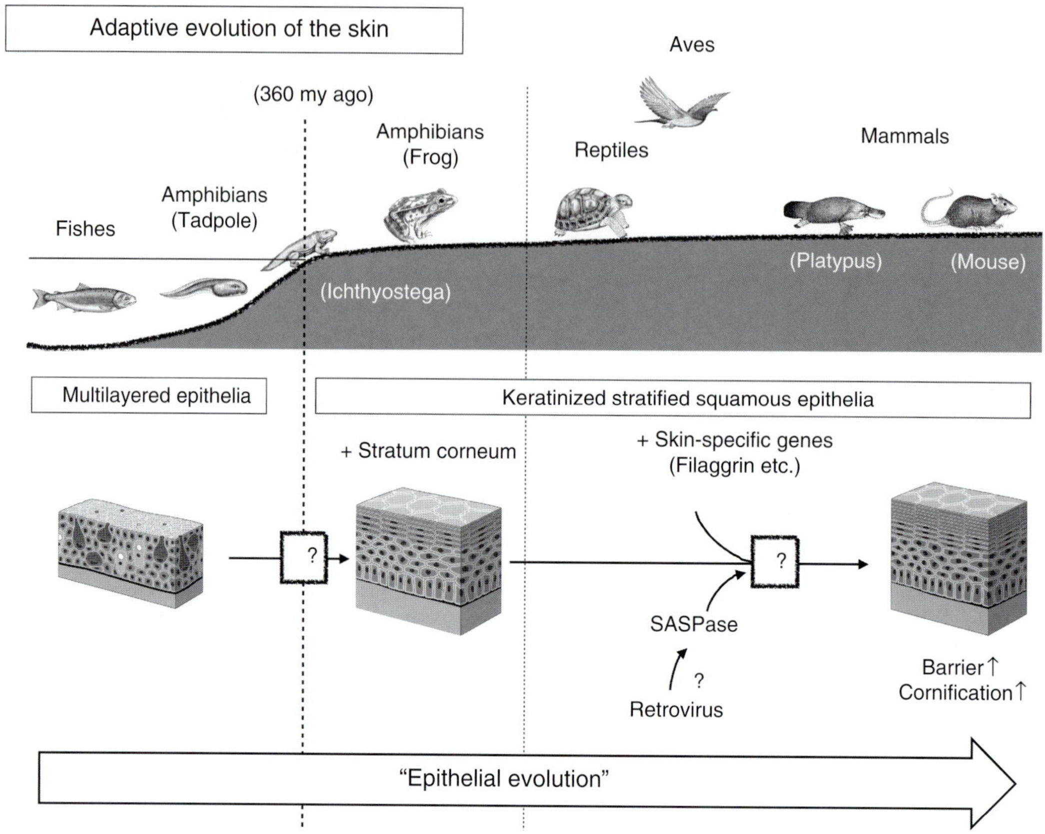

Fig. 12.1 Adaptive evolution of the skin. About 360 million years ago (the late Devonian period, *360 my ago*), the first terrestrial vertebrate amphibian (e.g., *Ichthyostega*) emerged from the water and adapted to life on land. They evolved their surface epithelium from multilayered epithelia into keratinized stratified squamous epithelia, baring the stratum corneum to prevent water loss and for protection from sunlight. Genomic analysis of various terrestrial vertebrate species reveals that new stratified epithelia-specific genes including filaggrin and SASPase were integrated into their genome. SASPase may have derived from an ancient retroviral infection. Therefore, the identification of skin-specific genes and generation of knockout mice may aid our understanding of the molecular mechanisms of "epithelial evolution"

envelope of mature corneocytes [11]. Therefore, "the SG-expressing genes/proteins" serve important roles in the final stage of epidermal differentiation, cornification, and barrier function.

12.2 The Skin-Specific and SG-Specific Protein, Filaggrin

Filaggrin is known as a skin-specific protein that is expressed from the SG as a phosphorylated profilaggrin of >400 kDa in humans and is a major component of keratohyalin granules in the SG of the epidermis [15, 49]. Profilaggrin is linked to 10–12 tandem filaggrin monomer repeats [15, 25, 37]. At the SG-to-SC transition, each filaggrin repeat is cleaved by a particular protease(s) to generate the filaggrin monomer (37 and 28 kDa in humans and mice, respectively). The cleaved filaggrin monomer strongly binds to keratin, and the resulting keratin bundles are thought to contribute to the production of functional SC [13, 24]. Regions of the filaggrin-keratin complex are cross-linked by transglutaminase to build the skin barrier [11, 12, 25, 69]. Keratin-bound filaggrin is citrullinated and degraded into amino acids, which constitutes the major part of the natural moisturizing factor (NMF) in the upper SC [8, 17, 28–30, 38,

41, 54, 74]. Therefore, at the SG-to-SC transitional stage, the processing from profilaggrin to filaggrin is the rate-limiting step for the profilaggrin processing cascade.

Several proteases are reported to be involved in the profilaggrin-to-filaggrin processing [44, 62, 10]. Calpain I and profilaggrin endopeptidase I (PEP-I) are reported to cleave the linker peptides of profilaggrin in vitro [56–59, 79]; furin or convertase has been demonstrated to be involved in the cleavage of the N-terminus from profilaggrin [47]; and matriptase/MT-SP1- and prostasin (CAP1/Prss8)-deficient mice show aberrant processing of profilaggrin to filaggrin [32, 33]. The possible linker cleavage sites of mouse, rat, and human profilaggrin have been determined from endogenous filaggrin [57–59, 75, 76]. It remains to be elucidated that the corresponding linker sequences of profilaggrin are cleaved by matriptase or prostasin in vitro.

Historically, the existence of a certain heritable component for the development of atopic dermatitis (AD) has long been known [3, 9, 40]. Filaggrin was reported to have nonsense mutations in ichthyosis vulgaris (IV) patients and is the major predisposing factor for atopic eczema, asthma, and allergies [45, 62, 63, 10]. It was indicated that the early onset of AD is caused by outside-to-inside paradigms, namely a primary barrier abnormality [20]. Filaggrin null mutations showed population specificity [10]. For instance, filaggrin nonsense mutations are carried by ~9% of the Irish population. Such filaggrin mutations are found in ~50% and 20% of Irish and Japanese AD patients, respectively [2, 42, 62, 63]. The remaining patients with AD who have normal filaggrin alleles are likely to be affected by other predisposing factors [22, 46, 71].

12.3 Skin-Specific and SG-Specific Protease, SASPase

Proteases play an important role in many physiological processes [5]. Proteases are classified into five distinct classes: aspartic, metallo, cysteine, serine, and threonine proteases. Aspartic proteases are expressed in various species such as vertebrates, invertebrates, fungi, plants, and retroviruses [52, 73]. Eukaryotic aspartic proteases are ~330 residues and are monomeric enzymes that consist of two homologous domains (the structure is analogous to a pair of scissors connected by a rope). Each domain contains an active site centered on a catalytically essential aspartic acid residue. On the other hand, retroviral aspartic proteases are encoded in the retroviral genome and are expressed as part of a large polyprotein precursor that undergoes autoprocessing in viral particles to produce an active enzyme that exists as a homodimer (like a pair of scissors) (See Fig.12. 9). These proteases are essential for maturation and assembly of infectious virus particles [53].

A number of retroviral protease sequences with retroviral elements are integrated in every eukaryotic genome as endogenous retroviruses [51]. Most of these human endogenous retroviruses have been acquired 10–100 million years ago [34]. Krylov and Koonin have described new subfamilies of predicted retroviral-like aspartic proteases that were not embedded within endogenous retroviral elements throughout the eukaryotic and prokaryotic genomes [31].

Bernard et al. have identified a novel retroviral-like aspartic protease, SASPase (skin aspartic protease; Asprv1) from total protein extracts of the human reconstructed epidermis [4]. Using high-throughput in situ hybridization screening, we have also identified a mouse homolog of SASPase [35] as an SG-expressing gene. This protease has also been cloned as a 12-O-tetradecanoylphorbol-13-acetate (TPA)-induced gene (Taps) from cDNA of mouse back skin epidermis [60]. Human and mouse SASPase/Asprv1/Taps were primarily expressed in skin and exclusively expressed in the SG of the epidermis (Fig. 12.2). This retroviral-like aspartic protease was only found in mammals. Immunoblotting of human and mouse epidermal extracts revealed the expression of two forms of the enzyme: the 28 and 14 kDa forms in human and the 32 and 15 kDa forms in mouse. Although there are putative transmembrane domains in human and mouse SASPase, the full-length protein was not detected in epidermal lysates of human and mouse. It has also been demonstrated that mouse SASPase is found in the medium when the full-length protein was expressed in the HeLa

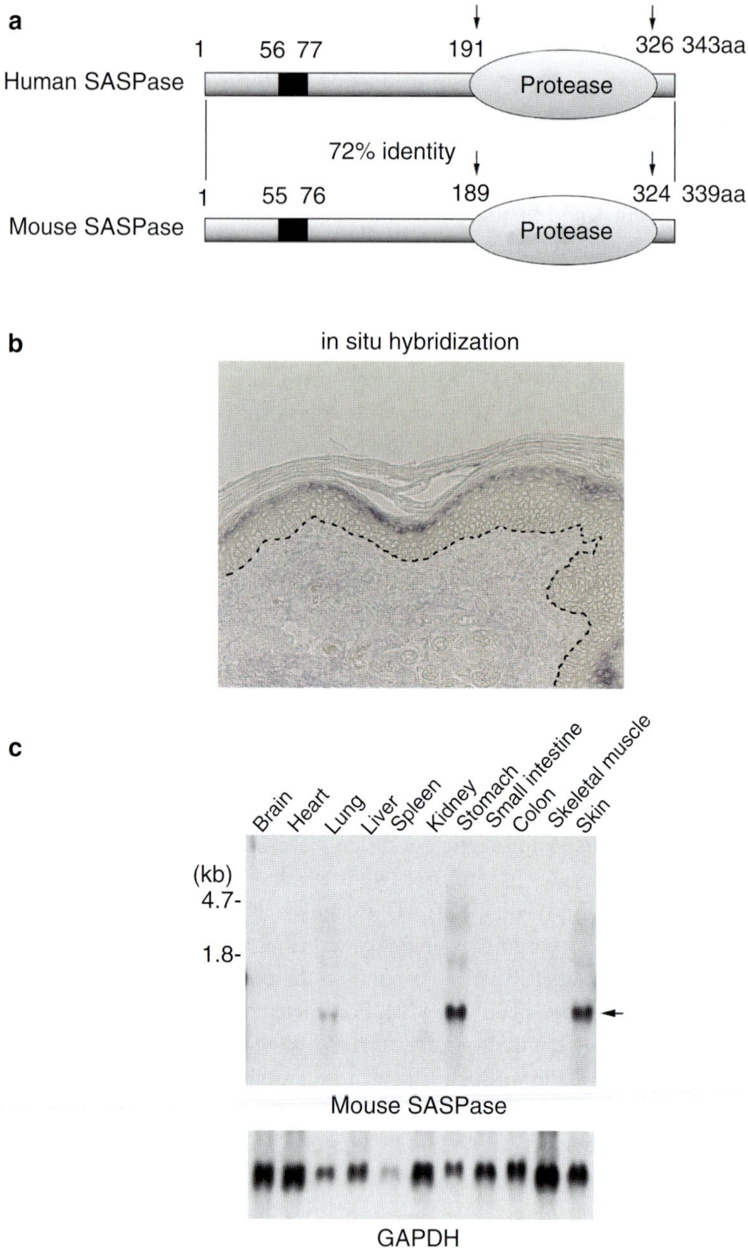

Fig. 12.2 Retroviral-like aspartic protease, SASPase. (**a**) Schematic representation of human and mouse SASPase. At the amino acid sequence level, human and mouse SASPase show 72% identity. The putative transmembrane domain is denoted as a *black square*. *Arrows* indicate the autoprocessing sites. (**b**) In situ hybridization signals obtained with the mouse SASPase antisense probe in sections of adult mouse foot pad epidermis. The SASPase probe gives an intense signal in the granular layer of the epidermis. A *dashed line* represents the border between the epidermis and dermis. (**c**) The expression of mouse SASPase mRNA in various tissues in northern blotting. SASPase was expressed in the stomach, skin, and weakly in the lung (*arrow*). The control-GAPDH probe was also hybridized (This was reproduced and modified from Matsui et al. [35]. Reprinted with permission. © 2006 The American Society for Biochemistry and Molecular Biology. All rights reserved)

cell line [60]. Thus, the function of the transmembrane domain of SASPase remains to be elucidated. Similar to other retroviral proteases such as the HIV protease, recombinant human 28 kDa and mouse 32 kDa SASPase forms undergo autoactivation processing in vitro, and this cleavage event generates a 14-kDa (human)/15-kDa (mouse) derived protease domain [4, 35]. We also demonstrated that the optimum pH of the active form of mouse SASPase is 5.77, which is similar to the optimum pH for HIV protease activity. Interestingly, this pH corresponds to the pH of the upper surface of the epidermis. Recently, aberrant SASPase expression in transgenic mice was reported to cause impaired skin regeneration and remodeling after cutaneous injury and chemically induced hyperplasia, suggesting that when expressed in skin, SASPase cleaves particular substrates involved in these processes [27].

12.4 The Phenotype of SASPase-Deficient "Hairless" Mice

To understand the physiological role of evolutionally conserved SASPase in mammals, we have generated SASPase-deficient mice. These mice were found to show fine wrinkles that ran parallel on the lateral trunk at 5 weeks of age (Fig. 12.3; [35]). This phenotype indicated that SASPase is involved in the prevention of fine wrinkle formation. As SASPase is an SG-expressing gene, these fine wrinkles of SASPase-deficient mice were hypothesized to be derived from the aberrant functions of the SG and/or SC. To further analyze the phenotype on the epidermal surface physiology of SASPase-deficient mice, we transferred the ablated allele to a Hos:HR-1 hairless background [36].

As shown in Fig. 12.4, $SASP^{-/-}$ hairless mice had more fine wrinkles and drier, rougher skin than their $SASP^{+/+}$ and $SASP^{+/-}$ counterparts [36]. Electron microscopic analysis of $SASP^{-/-}$ hairless mice showed that the epidermis had more tightly and electron densely compacted cornified cells. Moreover, the number of layers was found to have increased when compared with $SASP^{+/+}$ mice (Fig. 12.5) [36].

Physiological characterization of the epidermal surface of the $SASP^{-/-}$ hairless mice revealed a marked decrease in SC hydration without alteration to the barrier function (TEWL: trans-epidermal water loss) (Fig. 12.6) [36]. Decreased SC hydration is found in several diseases, such as AD, eczema, or psoriasis [26]. Consistent with our results, although the TEWL is an important hallmark for skin barrier function, TEWL has been

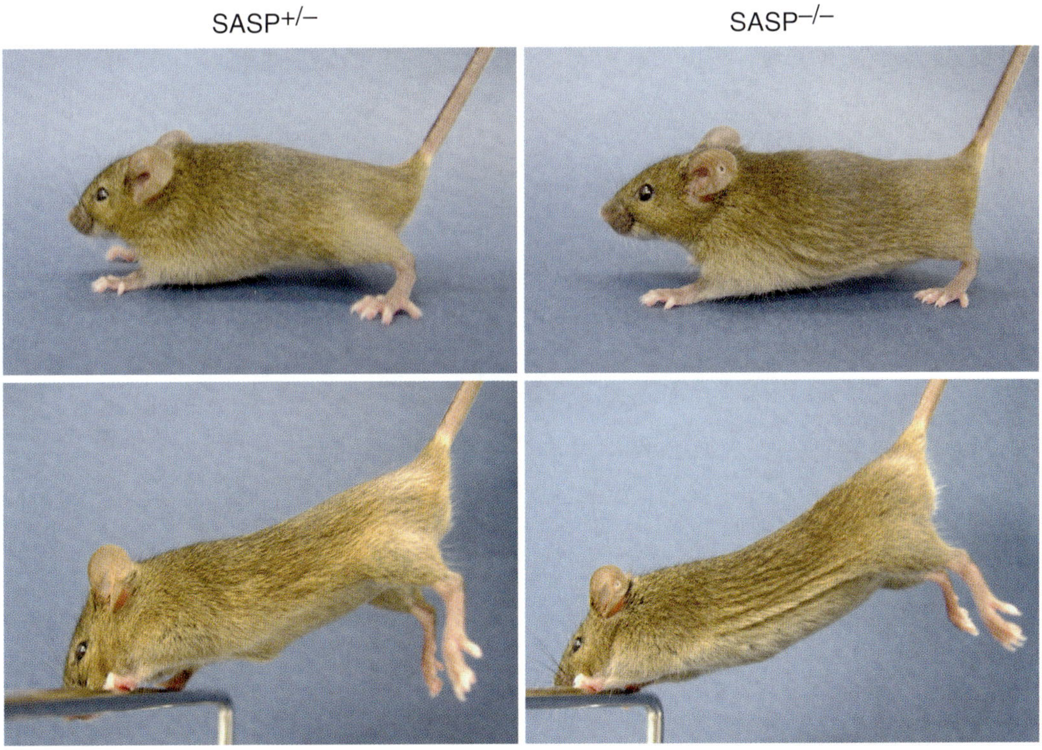

Fig. 12.3 Wrinkle formation in SASPase-deficient mice. A lined appearance on the skin surface of the lateral trunk of SASPase-deficient mice is observed. Static state of 14-week-old female heterogenic (*$SASP^{+/-}$*) and homogenic (*$SASP^{-/-}$*) mice (*upper panel*). In $SASP^{-/-}$ mice, lined grooves appear parallel to the body axis. These grooves were more enhanced by stretching the hind legs backward (*lower panel*) (This was reproduced and modified from Matsui et al. [35]. Reprinted with permission. © 2006 The American Society for Biochemistry and Molecular Biology. All rights reserved)

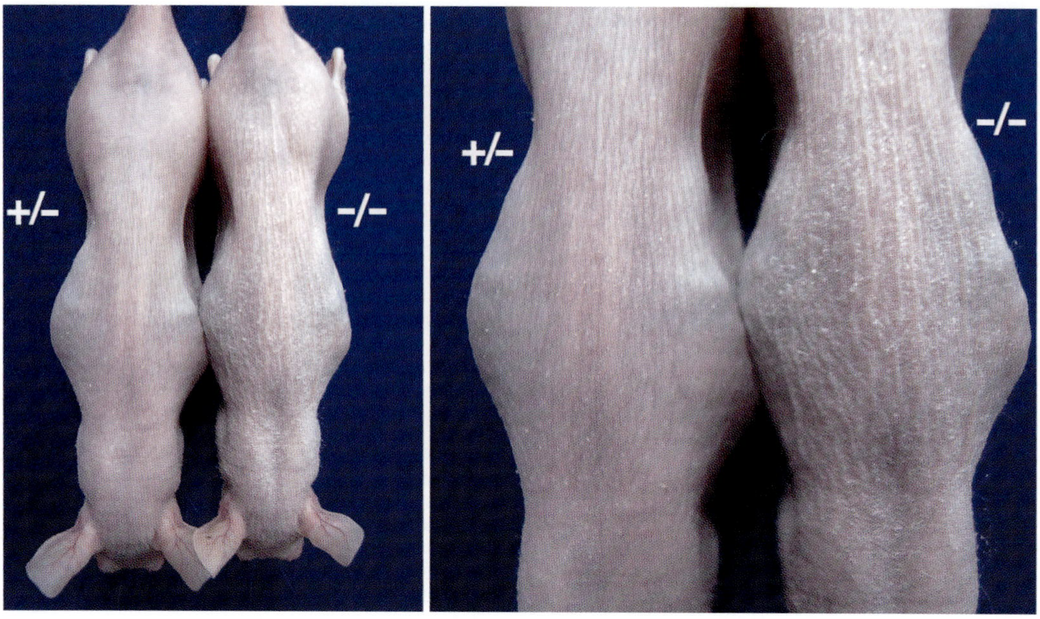

Fig. 12.4 Dry skin-like phenotype in hung SASP$^{-/-}$ hairless mice. When hung by the tail, more wrinkles appeared on the surface of the back skin in SASP$^{-/-}$ hairless mice when compared with SASP$^{+/-}$ hairless mice (Copyright 2011 Wiley. Used with permission from Mastui et al. [36])

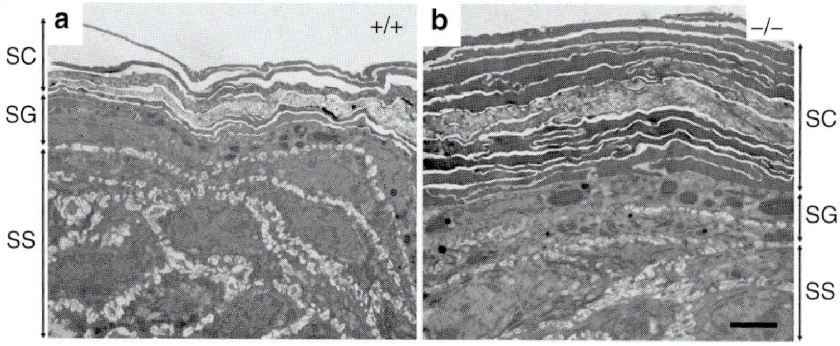

Fig. 12.5 *S*ASP$^{-/-}$ hairless mouse epidermis shows an increase in the number of layers in the aberrant SC. Sections of SASP$^{+/+}$ (**a**) and SASP$^{-/-}$ (**b**) epidermis examined by electron microscopy are shown. Transmission electron microscopic analysis of SASP$^{+/+}$ and SASP$^{-/-}$ epidermis showed an increase in the number of electron dense layers in the SC of SASP$^{-/-}$ mice compared with SASP$^{+/+}$ mice. *Scale bars*: 4 μm. *SC* stratum corneum, *SG* stratum granulosum, *SS* stratum spinosum (Copyright 2011 Wiley. Used with permission from Mastui et al. [36])

reported to be sometimes not correlated with human dry skin [6, 21, 78].

12.5 SASPase as a Profilaggrin Processing Enzyme

The expression of several epidermal differentiation markers (keratin 14, keratin 10, involucrin, loricrin) revealed normal expression and localization in SASP$^{-/-}$ hairless mice, whereas staining with an antifilaggrin antibody revealed the accumulation of aberrant dimeric and trimeric filaggrin, i.e., premature profilaggrin processing (Fig. 12.7) [36]. We also showed that recombinant human SASPase (14 kDa form) directly cleaves the human profilaggrin linker sequence in vitro. Considering that the processing of mouse profilaggrin occurs in a two-step process via two types of profilaggrin linker sequences (with or without FYPV), aberrant accumulation of dimeric- and trimeric-like

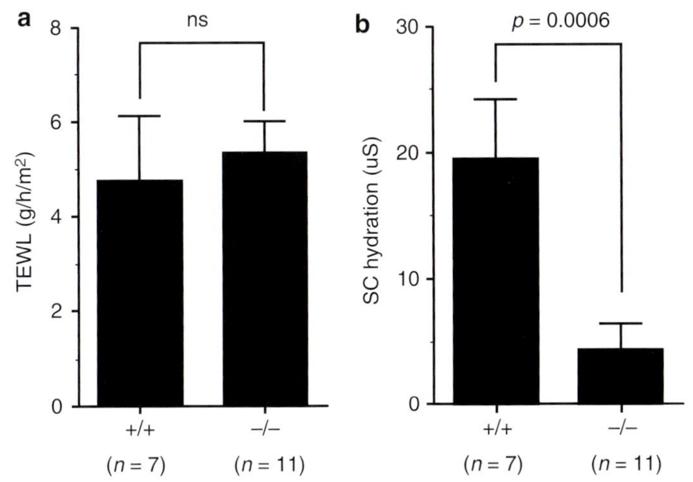

Fig. 12.6 Trans-epidermal water loss (TEWL) (**a**) and SC hydration levels (**b**) of $SASP^{+/+}$ and $SASP^{-/-}$ hairless mice were measured, respectively. The numbers of animals tested were: $SASP^{+/+}$, $n=7$ and $SASP^{-/-}$, $n=11$. Each p value is indicated above the bar (Mann Whitney test on mean values ± SD). The SC hydration of SASP. The SC hairless mice hydration levels were significantly lower than the $SASP^{+/+}$ and $SASP^{+/-}$ hairless mice hydration levels (Copyright 2011 Wiley. Used with permission from Mastui et al. [36])

profilaggrin in the mouse $SASP^{-/-}$ SC suggests that SASPase may be involved in either processing steps in mouse [56, 59].

As described in Sect. 12.2, filaggrin is thought to have two major functions in the SC: the formation of keratin microfibrils in the lower SC and the production of NMFs in the upper SC [54]. It is widely believed that SC hydration is closely linked and dependent on the three-dimensional keratin structural organization. Accumulation of aberrant profilaggrin in the lower SC may affect the cubic-like, rod-packing symmetry of keratin filaments at the lower SC, resulting in the alteration of the hydration level and the texture of SCin the $SASP^{-/-}$ epidermis [43]. In support of this concept, on the contrary to $SASP^{-/-}$ hairless mice, it was reported that the SC of flaky tail mice, in which filaggrin is absent, showed normal SC hydration and numbers of SC layers [23, 48, 64]. It is possible that in addition to profilaggrin, SASPase may also cleave other substrates and effect SC hydration via, for instance, abnormalities in the intercellular lamellar lipids barrier formation, the diffusion path length, and/or the composition of nonfilaggrin-derived NMFs [54, 55]. These possibilities will be clarified by crossing $SASP^{-/-}$ mice with filaggrin-deficient mice. Future detailed analysis of $SASP^{-/-}$ hairless mice SC will provide additional molecular mechanism that is important in the maintenance of the moisturization levels of the skin.

12.6 Human Mutations of SASPase

We have performed a mutation search on the human SASPase gene against a Japanese cohort. Two types of missense mutations (D232Y and V243A: 3.5% [1/28]) in the 28 control subjects, four types of missense mutations (A54S: 0.5% [1/196], I186T: 0.5% [1/196], V187I: 1.5% [3/196], R311C: 0.5% [1/196]), and three types of silent mutations (F101F: 0.5% [1/196], P206P: 3.1% [6/196], N276N: 1.5% [3/196]) in the 196 AD patients were identified (Fig. 12.8) [36]. All mutations were identified as heterozygous. V187I was the most frequently identified (three AD patients). Biochemical analysis has shown that among these, the V243A mutation abolished protease activity in vitro, whereas the V187I mutation was observed to induce a marked decrease in protease activity. In the future, it will be necessary to perform a large-scale cohort analysis to clarify the clinicopathological significance of these heterogenic loss-of-function mutations of SASPase and whether they affect human skin physiology (See

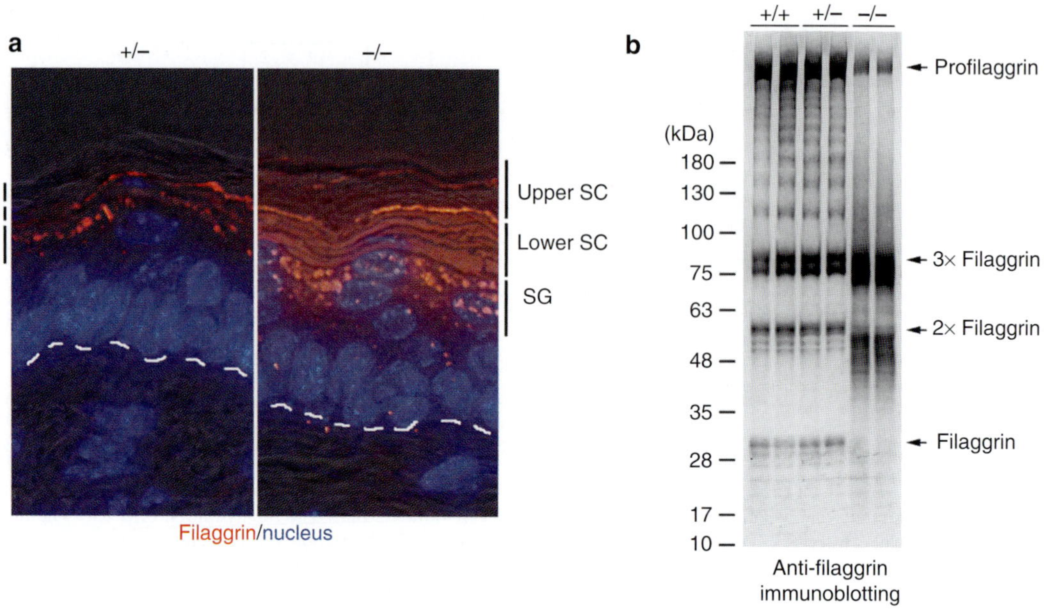

Fig. 12.7 Aberrant expression of filaggrin in SASP$^{-/-}$ hairless mice. (**a**) Immunofluorescence staining of frozen sections of the back skin of SASP$^{+/-}$ and SASP$^{-/-}$ mice stained with an antifilaggrin antibody (*red*). Nuclei were counterstained with bisbenzimide (*blue*). The SASP$^{-/-}$ epidermis showed an increase in the amount of filaggrin-positive staining in the lower SC. *Dashed lines* represent the border between the epidermis and dermis. *SC* stratum corneum, *SG* stratum granulosum. (**b**) Equivalent amounts of tape-stripped extracts (10 times, 5 μg) from SASP$^{+/+}$ ($n=2$), SASP$^{+/-}$ ($n=2$), and SASP$^{-/-}$ ($n=2$) mice were immunoblotted with antifilaggrin antibodies, demonstrating that an accumulation of aberrant filaggrin degradation products (dimer and trimer sizes) was detected (2× *filaggrin* and 3× *filaggrin*), whereas mature filaggrin (*filaggrin*) was rarely detected. As equivalent amounts of SC extracts were loaded, the intensity of the profilaggrin band (*profilaggrin*) had decreased in SASP$^{-/-}$, possibly due to an increase in the concentrations of other smear proteins (Copyright 2011 Wiley. Used with permission from Mastui et al. [36])

also Sect. 12.7). We also performed mutation searches against South African and Irish atopic eczema cases and Scottish dry skin cases. However, we failed to find an association between SASPase mutations and atopic eczema or clinically dry skin in the European populations, suggesting the possibility that these mutations are likely to be specific to the Japanese population [65]. Due to complex disorders, like AD, it is particularly difficult to establish a direct role of these sequence variants in the pathogenesis of known disease states.

Of note, there are various human epidermal diseases with aberrant expression and processing of profilaggrin to filaggrin (reviewed in [14]). Bernard et al. have also shown high expression of active SASPase in the SC of psoriasis patients by immunoblotting and immunofluorescence [4].

Therefore, it is possible that patients who do not have a nonsense mutation of filaggrin, but who exhibit xerosis or AD, may have an aberrant profilaggrin processing pattern. The involvement of SASPase in the progression of these diseases from the viewpoint of the profilaggrin processing pathway should be examined. The profilaggrin degradation pattern may prove useful in the diagnosis of xerosis and the early onset of AD.

12.7 Possible Physiological Role of SASPase

Our findings of the analysis of SASPase-deficient hairless mice are summarized in Fig. 12.9 (Modified from [36]). In normal mice and human epidermis, phosphorylated profilaggrin is

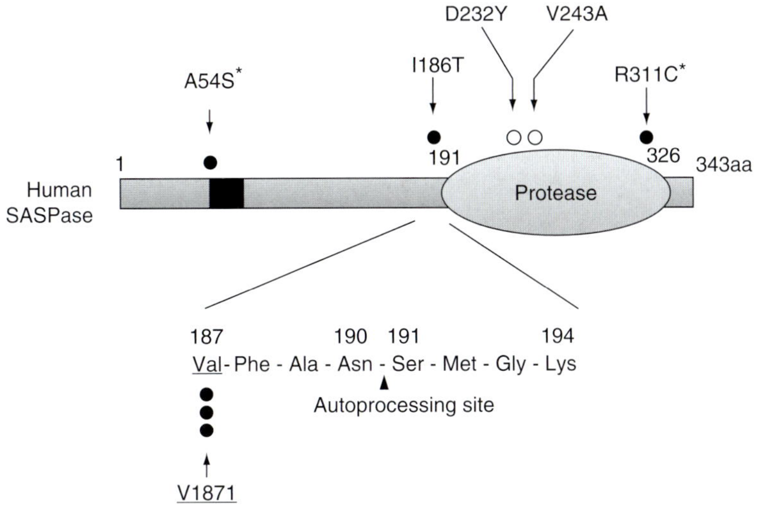

Fig. 12.8 Schematic representation of human mutations identified in Japanese AD patients (*n*=196; *closed circles*) and case controls (*n*=28; *open circles*). The amino acid sequence of the autoprocessing site (between Asn[190] and Ser[191]) is indicated. *Asterisks* of A54S and R311C indicate that these mutations were found in the same patient and in the same allele. The V243A mutation abolished protease activity, whereas the V187I mutation induced a marked decrease in protease activity in vitro (underlined). (Copyright 2011 Wiley. Used with permission from Mastui et al. [36])

dephosphorylated and processed into filaggrin monomers and bundle keratin filaments at the "lower SC." They are subsequently further degraded to free amino acids that constitute most of the NMFs in the "upper SC." SASPase deficiency causes incomplete linker cleavage of profilaggrin resulting in the accumulation of trimeric and dimeric profilaggrins in the "lower SC." Such aberrant profilaggrin may bind to keratin filaments and then degrade into a normal composition of free amino acids in the "upper SC." Overall, the SC of the SASP$^{-/-}$ epidermis has an increase in the number of layers and produces a wrinkled, dry, rough skin. SASPase, as a retroviral aspartic protease, must undergo homodimeric formation for its protease activity (Fig. 12.9, [4, 35]). In the case of the human epidermis with a heterogenic mutation of SASPase (such as V187I or V243A), the dominant negative effects would expect to lead to one functional domain of the SASPase (Fig. 12.9, see the picture of the scissors). This postulate is consistent with the HIV protease, where a subunit exchange reaction of the protease with a catalytically inactive mutation results in 50% inhibition of enzymatic activity [16].

12.8 Origin of SASPase and Adaptation to Life on Land

Collectively, these results indicate that the activity of SASPase plays a key role in determining the texture of the SC by modulating SC hydration, as well as profilaggrin-to-filaggrin processing. Moreover, these results, in combination with clinicopathological investigations of epidermal diseases derived from the aberrant processing of profilaggrin by mutation or decreased activity of SASPase should provide valuable data that enable researchers to dissect the complex mechanisms of percutaneous antigen priming in atopic diseases.

SASP$^{-/-}$ hairless mice have provided the first evidence that one of the genome-integrated retroviral-like aspartic protease family members is functionally important in mammalian tissue architecture. Interestingly, the SASPase gene is only found in the mammalian genome. Although it has not been proven that the SASPase gene in mammals is derived from an ancient retroviral infection into the germline, this molecular mechanism would be the first example of a virus-related element that has contributed to the evolution of

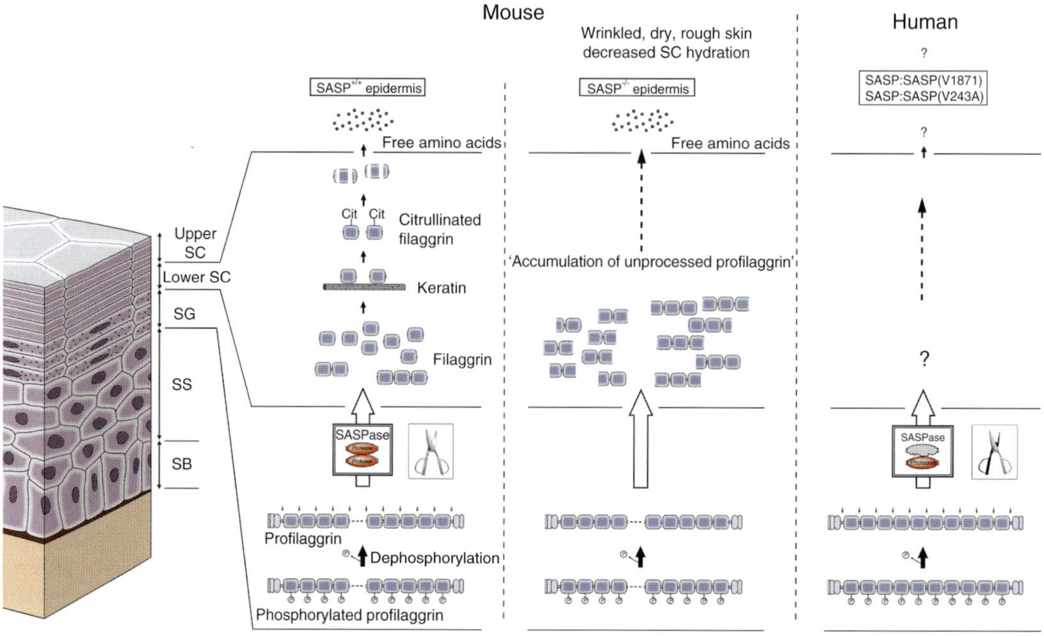

Fig. 12.9 Schematic representation of the possible profilaggrin processing pathway observed in the SASP$^{+/+}$ and SASP$^{-/-}$ epidermis. In the mouse SASP$^{+/+}$ epidermis, highly phosphorylated profilaggrin expressed in the SG is dephosphorylated in the uppermost SG. The linker sequence that connects each filaggrin monomer is then cleaved by SASPase at the SG-to-SC transition. Monomeric filaggrin strongly binds to keratin filaments in the lower SC to form bundled keratin filaments. After citrullination, filaggrin is released from keratin and further degraded to form free amino acids, which constitute most of the NMFs in the upper SC. In the mouse SASP$^{-/-}$ epidermis, trimeric and dimeric profilaggrins are slightly degraded from either N- or C-terminal ends and accumulate because of incomplete linker sequence cleavage. Aberrantly processed profilaggrin binds to keratin filaments and degrades into free amino acids without the production of monomeric filaggrin. Finally, aberrant SC causes wrinkled, dry, rough skin with decreased SC hydration. In the case of the human epidermis which has heterogenic mutations of SASPase (such as V187I or V243A), dominant negative effects would be expected to be observed because one side of the scissors is dysfunctional. The clinicopathological significance of these heterogenic loss-of-function mutations of SASPase has not been fully determined. *SC* stratum corneum, *SG* stratum granulosum, *SS* stratum spinosum, *SB* stratum basale (Copyright 2011 Wiley. Used with permission from Mastui et al. [36])

vertebrate skin [7, 70]. Therefore, the study of the SASPase physiological function should provide valuable clues that reveal the role of the SC in mammals and how they adapted to life on land.

Take Home Messages

- SASPase is a retroviral-like aspartic protease that is expressed primarily in the skin and exclusively in the stratum granulosum.
- SASPase-deficient hairless mice show drier and more wrinkled skin.
- SASPase activity is indispensable for SC hydration.
- SASPase activity is indispensable for profilaggrin processing.
- SASPase directly cleaves the profilaggrin linker peptide in vitro.
- Loss-of-function mutations of SASPase in the human genome have been identified.

Acknowledgments I thank Itsumi Ohmori and Sayaka Katahira-Tayama for their technical assistance. I thank Keiko Mizuno and Kaoru Orihashi for critical reading of the manuscript. I thank Drs. Masayuki Amagai, Akiharu Kubo, Jun Kudoh and Kenichi Miyamoto (Keio University) and Dr. Johji Inazawa (Tokyo Medical and Dental University) for supporting this project and Mr. Yoshihiko Tsuda (Davinci Medical Illustration Office) for illustration of figures. I also thank KAN Research Insitute Inc. for provising materials. This work was supported by a Grant-in-Aid for Scientific Research to Takeshi Matsui, "Program for Improvement of Research Environment for Young Researchers" from the Ministry of Education, Culture, Sports, Science and Technology (MEXT) of Japan to Takeshi Matsui, research grants from the Nakatomi Foundation, the Cosmetology Research Foundation, and the Naito Foundation to Takeshi Matsui, and Health and Labour Sciences Research Grants for Research on Allergic Diseases and Immunology from the Ministry of Health, Labour, and Welfare.

References

1. Alibardi L (2003) Adaptation to the land: the skin of reptiles in comparison to that of amphibians and endotherm amniotes. J Exp Zool B Mol Dev Evol 298(1):12–41. doi:10.1002/jez.b.24
2. Barker JN, Palmer CN, Zhao Y et al (2007) Null mutations in the filaggrin gene (FLG) determine major susceptibility to early-onset atopic dermatitis that persists into adulthood. J Invest Dermatol 127:564–567
3. Barnes KC (2010) An update on the genetics of atopic dermatitis: scratching the surface in 2009. J Allergy Clin Immunol 125(1):16–29 e11–11; quiz 30–11. doi:S0091-6749(09)01722-9 [pii] 10.1016/j.jaci.2009.11.008
4. Bernard D, Mehul B, Thomas-Collignon A, Delattre C, Donovan M, Schmidt R (2005) Identification and characterization of a novel retroviral-like aspartic protease specifically expressed in human epidermis. J Invest Dermatol 125(2):278–287. doi:JID23816 [pii] 10.1111/j.0022-202X.2005.23816.x
5. Barret AJ, Rawlings ND, Woessner JF (eds) (1998) Handbook of proteolytic enzymes. Academic, San Diego
6. Berry N, Charmeil C, Goujon C, Silvy A, Girard P, Corcuff P, Montastier C (1999) A clinical, biometrological and ultrastructural study of xerotic skin. Int J Cosmet Sci 21(4):241–252. doi:ICS196570 [pii] 10.1046/j.1467-2494.1999.196570.x
7. Blikstad V, Benachenhou F, Sperber GO, Blomberg J (2008) Evolution of human endogenous retroviral sequences: a conceptual account. Cell Mol Life Sci 65(21):3348–3365. doi:10.1007/s00018-008-8495-2
8. Bonnart C, Deraison C, Lacroix M, Uchida Y, Besson C, Robin A, Briot A, Gonthier M, Lamant L, Dubus P, Monsarrat B, Hovnanian A (2010) Elastase 2 is expressed in human and mouse epidermis and impairs skin barrier function in netherton syndrome through filaggrin and lipid misprocessing. J Clin Invest 120(3):871–882. doi:41440 [pii] 10.1172/JCI41440
9. Brown SJ, McLean WH (2009) Eczema genetics: current state of knowledge and future goals. J Invest Dermatol 129:543–552
10. Brown SJ, McLean WH (2012) One remarkable molecule: filaggrin. J Invest Dermatol 132(3 Pt 2):751–762
11. Candi E, Schmidt R, Melino G (2005) The cornified envelope: a model of cell death in the skin. Nat Rev Mol Cell Biol 6(4):328–340. doi:nrm1619 [pii] 10.1038/nrm1619
12. Candi E, Tarcsa E, Digiovanna JJ, Compton JG, Elias PM, Marekov LN, Steinert PM (1998) A highly conserved lysine residue on the head domain of type II keratins is essential for the attachment of keratin intermediate filaments to the cornified cell envelope through isopeptide crosslinking by transglutaminases. Proc Natl Acad Sci USA 95(5):2067–2072
13. Dale BA, Holbrook KA, Steinert PM (1978) Assembly of stratum corneum basic protein and keratin filaments in macrofibrils. Nature 276(5689):729–731
14. Dale BA, Resing KA, Haydock PV (1990) Filaggrins. In: Goldman RD, Steinert PM (eds) Cellular and molecular biology of intermediate filaments, 1st edn. Plenum Press, New York, London, pp 393–412
15. Dale BA, Resing KA, Lonsdale-Eccles JD (1985) Filaggrin: a keratin filament associated protein. Ann N Y Acad Sci 455:330–342
16. Darke PL (1994) Stability of dimeric retroviral proteases. Methods Enzymol 241:104–127
17. Denecker G, Hoste E, Gilbert B, Hochepied T, Ovaere P, Lippens S, Van den Broecke C, Van Damme P, D'Herde K, Hachem JP, Borgonie G, Presland RB, Schoonjans L, Libert C, Vandekerckhove J, Gevaert K, Vandenabeele P, Declercq W (2007) Caspase-14 protects against epidermal UVB photodamage and water loss. Nat Cell Biol 9(6):666–674. doi:ncb1597 [pii] 10.1038/ncb1597
18. Eckert RL (1989) Structure, function, and differentiation of the keratinocyte. Physiol Rev 69(4):1316–1346
19. Eckert RL, Crish JF, Robinson NA (1997) The epidermal keratinocyte as a model for the study of gene regulation and cell differentiation. Physiol Rev 77(2): 397–424
20. Elias PM, Steinhoff M (2008) "Outside-to-inside" (and now back to "outside") pathogenic mechanisms in atopic dermatitis. J Invest Dermatol 128:1067–1070
21. Engelke M, Jensen JM, Ekanayake-Mudiyanselage S, Proksch E (1997) Effects of xerosis and ageing on epidermal proliferation and differentiation. Br J Dermatol 137(2):219–225
22. Esparza-Gordillo J, Weidinger S, Folster-Holst R et al (2009) A common variant on chromosome 11q13 is associated with atopic dermatitis. Nat Genet 41: 596–601
23. Fallon PG, Sasaki T, Sandilands A, Campbell LE, Saunders SP, Mangan NE, Callanan JJ, Kawasaki H, Shiohama A, Kubo A, Sundberg JP, Presland RB,

Fleckman P, Shimizu N, Kudoh J, Irvine AD, Amagai M, McLean WH (2009) A homozygous frameshift mutation in the mouse Flg gene facilitates enhanced percutaneous allergen priming. Nat Genet 41(5):602–608. doi:ng.358 [pii] 10.1038/ng.358
24. Gruber R, Elias PM, Crumrine D et al (2011) Filaggrin genotype in ichthyosis vulgaris predicts abnormalities in epidermal structure and function. Am J Pathol 178:2252–2263
25. Harding CR, Scott IR (1983) Histidine-rich proteins (filaggrins): structural and functional heterogeneity during epidermal differentiation. J Mol Biol 170(3):651–673
26. Harding CR, Watkinson A, Rawlings AV, Scott IR (2000) Dry skin, moisturization and corneodesmolysis. Int J Cosmet Sci 22:21–52
27. Hildenbrand M, Rhiemeier V, Hartenstein B, Lahrmann B, Grabe N, Angel P, Hess J (2010) Impaired skin regeneration and remodeling after cutaneous injury and chemically induced hyperplasia in taps-transgenic mice. J Invest Dermatol 130(7):1922–1930. doi:jid201054 [pii] 10.1038/jid.2010.54
28. Hoste E, Kemperman P, Devos M, Denecker G, Kezic S, Yau N, Gilbert B, Lippens S, De Groote P, Roelandt R, Van Damme P, Gevaert K, Presland RB, Takahara H, Puppels G, Caspers P, Vandenabeele P, Declercq W (2011) Caspase-14 is required for filaggrin degradation to natural moisturizing factors in the skin. J Invest Dermatol 131(11):2233–2241. doi:jid2011153 [pii] 10.1038/jid.2011.153
29. Ishida-Yamamoto A, Senshu T, Eady RA, Takahashi H, Shimizu H, Akiyama M, Iizuka H (2002) Sequential reorganization of cornified cell keratin filaments involving filaggrin-mediated compaction and keratin 1 deimination. J Invest Dermatol 118(2):282–287. doi:1671 [pii] 10.1046/j.0022-202x.2001.01671.x
30. Kamata Y, Taniguchi A, Yamamoto M, Nomura J, Ishihara K, Takahara H, Hibino T, Takeda A (2009) Neutral cysteine protease bleomycin hydrolase is essential for the breakdown of deiminated filaggrin into amino acids. J Biol Chem 284(19):12829–12836. doi:M807908200 [pii] 10.1074/jbc.M807908200
31. Krylov DM, Koonin EV (2001) A novel family of predicted retroviral-like aspartyl proteases with a possible key role in eukaryotic cell cycle control. Curr Biol 11(15):R584–R587. doi:S0960-9822(01), 00357-8 [pii]
32. Leyvraz C, Charles RP, Rubera I, Guitard M, Rotman S, Breiden B, Sandhoff K, Hummler E (2005) The epidermal barrier function is dependent on the serine protease CAP1/Prss8. J Cell Biol 170(3):487–496. doi:jcb.200501038 [pii] 10.1083/jcb.200501038
33. List K, Szabo R, Wertz PW, Segre J, Haudenschild CC, Kim SY, Bugge TH (2003) Loss of proteolytically processed filaggrin caused by epidermal deletion of matriptase/MT-SP1. J Cell Biol 163(4):901–910. doi:10.1083/jcb.200304161 jcb.200304161 [pii]
34. Lower R, Lower J, Kurth R (1996) The viruses in all of us: characteristics and biological significance of human endogenous retrovirus sequences. Proc Natl Acad Sci USA 93(11):5177–5184
35. Matsui T, Kinoshita-Ida Y, Hayashi-Kisumi F, Hata M, Matsubara K, Chiba M, Katahira-Tayama S, Morita K, Miyachi Y, Tsukita S (2006) Mouse homologue of skin-specific retroviral-like aspartic protease involved in wrinkle formation. J Biol Chem 281(37):27512–27525. doi:M603559200 [pii] 10.1074/jbc.M603559200
36. Matsui T, Miyamoto K, Kubo A et al (2011) SASPase regulates stratum corneum hydration through profilaggrin-to-filaggrin processing. EMBO Mol Med 3:320–333
37. McGrath JA, Uitto J (2008) The filaggrin story: novel insights into skin-barrier function and disease. Trends Mol Med 14(1):20–27. doi:S1471-4914(07), 00221-3 [pii] 10.1016/j.molmed.2007.10.006
38. Mechin MC, Enji M, Nachat R, Chavanas S, Charveron M, Ishida-Yamamoto A, Serre G, Takahara H, Simon M (2005) The peptidylarginine deiminases expressed in human epidermis differ in their substrate specificities and subcellular locations. Cell Mol Life Sci 62(17):1984–1995. doi:10.1007/s00018-005-5196-y
39. Montagna W, Parakkal PF (1974) The structure and function of skin. Academic Press, Orlando
40. Morar N, Willis-Owen SA, Moffatt MF, Cookson WO (2006) The genetics of atopic dermatitis. J Allergy Clin Immunol 118:24–34; quiz 35–36
41. Nachat R, Mechin MC, Takahara H, Chavanas S, Charveron M, Serre G, Simon M (2005) Peptidylarginine deiminase isoforms 1–3 are expressed in the epidermis and involved in the deimination of K1 and filaggrin. J Invest Dermatol 124(2):384–393. doi:JID23568 [pii] 10.1111/j.0022-202X.2004.23568.x
42. Nomura T, Akiyama M, Sandilands A, Nemoto-Hasebe I, Sakai K, Nagasaki A, Ota M, Hata H, Evans AT, Palmer CN, Shimizu H, McLean WH (2008) Specific filaggrin mutations cause ichthyosis vulgaris and are significantly associated with atopic dermatitis in Japan. J Invest Dermatol 128(6):1436–1441. doi:5701205 [pii] 10.1038/sj.jid.5701205
43. Norlen L, Al-Amoudi A (2004) Stratum corneum keratin structure, function, and formation: the cubic rod-packing and membrane templating model. J Invest Dermatol 123(4):715–732.doi:10.1111/j.0022-202X.2004.23213.x JID23213 [pii]
44. Ovaere P, Lippens S, Vandenabeele P, Declercq W (2009) The emerging roles of serine protease cascades in the epidermis. Trends Biochem Sci 34(9):453–463. doi:S0968-0004(09), 00136-4 [pii] 10.1016/j.tibs.2009.08.001
45. Palmer CN, Irvine AD, Terron-Kwiatkowski A, et al. (2006) Common loss-of-function variants of the epidermal barrier protein filaggrin are a major predisposing factor for atopic dermatitis. Nat Genet 38, 441–446
46. Paternoster L, Standl M, Chen CM et al (2011) Meta-analysis of genome-wide association studies identifies three new risk loci for atopic dermatitis. Nat Genet 44:187–192
47. Pearton DJ, Nirunsuksiri W, Rehemtulla A, Lewis SP, Presland RB, Dale BA (2001) Proprotein convertase expression and localization in epidermis: evidence for multiple roles and substrates. Exp Dermatol 10(3):193–203. doi:exd100307 [pii]

48. Presland RB, Boggess D, Lewis SP, Hull C, Fleckman P, Sundberg JP (2000) Loss of normal profilaggrin and filaggrin in flaky tail (ft/ft) mice: an animal model for the filaggrin-deficient skin disease ichthyosis vulgaris. J Invest Dermatol 115(6):1072–1081. doi:jid178 [pii] 10.1046/j.1523-1747.2000.00178.x
49. Presland RB, Rothnagel JA, Lawrence OT (2006) Profilaggrin and the fused S100 family of calcium-binding proteins. In: Elias PM, Feingold KR (eds) Skin barrier. Taylor & Francis, New York, pp 111–140
50. Proksch E, Brandner JM, Jensen JM (2008) The skin: an indispensable barrier. Exp Dermatol 17(12):1063–1072
51. Puente XS, Sanchez LM, Overall CM, Lopez-Otin C (2003) Human and mouse proteases: a comparative genomic approach. Nat Rev Genet 4(7):544–558. doi:10.1038/nrg1111 nrg1111 [pii]
52. Rao JK, Erickson JW, Wlodawer A (1991) Structural and evolutionary relationships between retroviral and eucaryotic aspartic proteinases. Biochemistry 30(19): 4663–4671
53. Ratner L, Haseltine W, Patarca R, Livak KJ, Starcich B, Josephs SF, Doran ER, Rafalski JA, Whitehorn EA, Baumeister K et al (1985) Complete nucleotide sequence of the AIDS virus, HTLV-III. Nature 313(6000):277–284
54. Rawlings AV, Harding CR (2004) Moisturization and skin barrier function. Dermatol Ther 17(Suppl 1):43–48. doi:04S1005 [pii]
55. Rawlings AV, Matts PJ (2005) Stratum corneum moisturization at the molecular level: an update in relation to the dry skin cycle. J Invest Dermatol 124:1099–1110
56. Resing KA, al-Alawi N, Blomquist C, Fleckman P, Dale BA (1993) Independent regulation of two cytoplasmic processing stages of the intermediate filament-associated protein filaggrin and role of Ca2+ in the second stage. J Biol Chem 268(33):25139–25145
57. Resing KA, Johnson RS, Walsh KA (1993) Characterization of protease processing sites during conversion of rat profilaggrin to filaggrin. Biochemistry 32(38):10036–10045
58. Resing KA, Thulin C, Whiting K, al-Alawi N, Mostad S (1995) Characterization of profilaggrin endoproteinase 1. A regulated cytoplasmic endoproteinase of epidermis. J Biol Chem 270(47):28193–28198
59. Resing KA, Walsh KA, Haugen-Scofield J, Dale BA (1989) Identification of proteolytic cleavage sites in the conversion of profilaggrin to filaggrin in mammalian epidermis. J Biol Chem 264(3):1837–1845
60. Rhiemeier V, Breitenbach U, Richter KH, Gebhardt C, Vogt I, Hartenstein B, Furstenberger G, Mauch C, Hess J, Angel P (2006) A novel aspartic proteinase-like gene expressed in stratified epithelia and squamous cell carcinoma of the skin. Am J Pathol 168(4):1354–1364. doi:168/4/1354 [pii]
61. Rodriguez E, Baurecht H, Herberich E et al (2009) Meta-analysis of filaggrin polymorphisms in eczema and asthma: robust risk factors in atopic disease. J Allergy Clin Immunol 123:1361–70 e7
62. Sandilands A, Sutherland C, Irvine AD, McLean WH (2009) Filaggrin in the frontline: role in skin barrier function and disease. J Cell Sci 122(Pt 9):1285–1294. doi:122/9/1285 [pii] 10.1242/jcs.033969
63. Sandilands A, Terron-Kwiatkowski A, Hull PR, O'Regan GM, Clayton TH, Watson RM, Carrick T, Evans AT, Liao H, Zhao Y, Campbell LE, Schmuth M, Gruber R, Janecke AR, Elias PM, van Steensel MA, Nagtzaam I, van Geel M, Steijlen PM, Munro CS, Bradley DG, Palmer CN, Smith FJ, McLean WH, Irvine AD (2007) Comprehensive analysis of the gene encoding filaggrin uncovers prevalent and rare mutations in ichthyosis vulgaris and atopic eczema. Nat Genet 39(5):650–654. doi:ng2020 [pii] 10.1038/ng2020
64. Scharschmidt TC, Man MQ, Hatano Y, Crumrine D, Gunathilake R, Sundberg JP, Silva KA, Mauro TM, Hupe M, Cho S, Wu Y, Celli A, Schmuth M, Feingold KR, Elias PM (2009) Filaggrin deficiency confers a paracellular barrier abnormality that reduces inflammatory thresholds to irritants and haptens. J Allergy Clin Immunol 124(3):496–506, 506 e491–496. doi:S0091–6749(09)01012–4 [pii] 10.1016/j.jaci.2009.06.046
65. Sandilands A, Brown SJ, Goh CS et al (2012) Mutations in the SASPase gene (ASPRV1) are not associated with atopic eczema or clinically dry skin. J Invest Dermatol. doi:10.1038/jid.2011.479
66. Schauber J, Gallo RL (2009) Antimicrobial peptides and the skin immune defense system. J Allergy Clin Immunol 124(3Suppl2):R13–R18.doi:S0091-6749(09), 01124-5 [pii] 10.1016/j.jaci.2009.07.014 http://books.google.co.uk/books/about/Cellular_and_molecular_biology_of_interm.html?id =uYXwAAAAMAAJ&redir_esc=y
67. Schempp C, Emde M, Wolfle U (2009) Dermatology in the Darwin anniversary. Part 1: evolution of the integument. J Dtsch Dermatol Ges 7(9):750–757. doi:DDG7193 [pii] 10.1111/j.1610–0387.2009.07193.x
68. Simpson CL, Patel DM, Green KJ (2011) Deconstructing the skin: cytoarchitectural determinants of epidermal morphogenesis. Nat Rev Mol Cell Biol 12:565–580
69. Steinert PM, Marekov LN (1995) The proteins elafin, filaggrin, keratin intermediate filaments, loricrin, and small proline-rich proteins 1 and 2 are isodipeptide cross-linked components of the human epidermal cornified cell envelope. J Biol Chem 270(30): 17702–17711
70. Stocking C, Kozak CA (2008) Murine endogenous retroviruses. Cell Mol Life Sci 65(21):3383–3398. doi:10.1007/s00018-008-8497-0
71. Sun LD, Xiao FL, Li Y et al (2011) Genome-wide association study identifies two new susceptibility loci for atopic dermatitis in the Chinese Han population. Nat Genet 43:690–694
72. Swartzendruber DC, Wertz PW, Madison KC, Downing DT (1987) Evidence that the corneocyte has a chemically bound lipid envelope. J Invest Dermatol 88(6):709–713
73. Tang J, Wong RN (1987) Evolution in the structure and function of aspartic proteases. J Cell Biochem 33(1):53–63. doi:10.1002/jcb.240330106

74. Tarcsa E, Marekov LN, Mei G, Melino G, Lee SC, Steinert PM (1996) Protein unfolding by peptidylarginine deiminase. Substrate specificity and structural relationships of the natural substrates trichohyalin and filaggrin. J Biol Chem 271(48):30709–30716
75. Thulin CD, Taylor JA, Walsh KA (1996) Microheterogeneity of human filaggrin: analysis of a complex peptide mixture using mass spectrometry. Protein Sci 5(6):1157–1164. doi:10.1002/pro.5560050618
76. Thulin CD, Walsh KA (1995) Identification of the amino terminus of human filaggrin using differential LC/MS techniques: implications for profilaggrin processing. Biochemistry 34(27):8687–8692
77. Watt FM (1989) Terminal differentiation of epidermal keratinocytes. Curr Opin Cell Biol 1(6):1107–1115
78. Wilhelm KP, Cua AB, Maibach HI (1991) Skin aging. Effect on transepidermal water loss, stratum corneum hydration, skin surface pH, and casual sebum content. Arch Dermatol 127(12):1806–1809
79. Yamazaki M, Ishidoh K, Suga Y, Saido TC, Kawashima S, Suzuki K, Kominami E, Ogawa H (1997) Cytoplasmic processing of human profilaggrin by active mu-calpain. Biochem Biophys Res Commun 235(3):652–656. doi:S0006-291X(97), 96809-1 [pii] 10.1006/bbrc.1997.6809

13 Vernix Caseosa and Its Substitutes: Lipid Composition and Physicochemical Properties

Marty O. Visscher and Steven B. Hoath

13.1 Introduction

Appropriate moisturization is essential for optimum stratum corneum (SC) function [1, 2]. Among the multiple functions of the skin affected by SC water content are desquamation and self-renewal, restoration of barrier integrity after wounding, acid mantle formation, microbial colonization, tactile discrimination, infection control, immunosurveillance, and protection against ultraviolet light and environmental irritants [3]. Operationally, "appropriate" hydration may be defined as: that amount of SC water which optimizes local SC biomechanics while facilitating terminal differentiation, programmed cell death, and orderly corneocyte incorporation into the inner SC with balanced pH-dependent desquamation of the outer SC. Overhydration can cause maceration, disruption of the intercellular lipid bilayers, degradation of desmosomes and creation of amorphous regions, corneocyte swelling, and enhanced molecular transport with increased permeability [4–6], as well as inflammation, irritation, and urticaria [7–12]. Low hydration can cause visible dryness/scaling, aberrant desquamation via reduced enzyme activity, cracking, reduced flexibility, tightness, and itching. On balance, the SC water-handling properties must be sufficiently robust to respond to local, potentially disruptive forces, for example, friction, heat, humidity, bathing, clothing, secretions, and topical product applications [13].

Throughout life, the SC must adapt quickly to sudden changes in hydration imposed by open arid environments, topical occlusion, and immersion in water of varying salinities. In humans, birth marks a sudden transition from a controlled aqueous environment to a dry extrauterine state. A mature, flexible, relatively impermeable SC is essential to life after birth, and, yet, this structure develops in utero under aqueous conditions in the amniotic fluid. Recent evidence supports the notion that epidermal barrier maturation in utero is a function of the direction of nutrient delivery, i.e., from "bottom to top" [14]. Structures which influence nutrient and water gradients in utero, therefore, may be important modifiers of fetal skin maturation under submerged conditions.

M.O. Visscher, Ph.D.
Skin Sciences Program, Cincinnati Children's Hospital Medical Center, Cincinnati, OH, USA

Division of Plastic Surgery, College of Medicine, University of Cincinnati,Cincinnati, OH, USA
e-mail: marty.visscher@cchmc.org

S.B. Hoath, M.D. (✉)
Skin Sciences Program, Cincinnati Children's Hospital Medical Center, Cincinnati, OH, USA

Perinatal Institute, Cincinnati Children's Hospital, Medical Center, Cincinnati, OH, USA

Department of Pediatrics, College of Medicine, University of Cincinnati, Cincinnati, OH, USA
e-mail: steven.hoath@cchmc.org

M. Lodén, H.I. Maibach (eds.), *Treatment of Dry Skin Syndrome*,
DOI 10.1007/978-3-642-27606-4_13, © Springer-Verlag Berlin Heidelberg 2012

Vernix caseosa, from the Greek word for "varnish" and the Latin word for "cheese," is defined as "a grayish-white cheese-like substance, consisting of sebaceous gland secretions, lanugo, and desquamated epithelial cells, that covers the skin of the fetus and newborn" [15]. This chapter addresses the lipid composition and physicochemical properties of vernix caseosa and its substitutes. Within the theme of skin moisturization, specific vernix constituents and functions are closely related to epidermal barrier development in utero and adaptation after birth. The potential applications of vernix and synthetic analogs for the treatment of compromised skin for neonatal, pediatric, and adult populations are discussed.

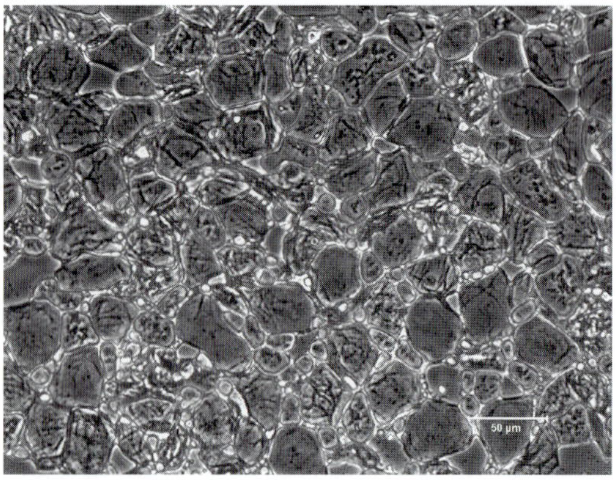

Fig. 13.1 Phase contrast image of native vernix showing dense packing of fetal corneocytes surrounded by a thin lipid matrix. The cells are heterogenous in size and structure. Many nuclear ghosts are evident. Scale bar is shown in the figure

13.2 Vernix Composition, Formation, and Impact on Cornification

Vernix is a complex mixture of 80% water, 10% protein, and 10% lipid fractions, consisting primarily of cornified cells embedded in an amorphous lipid matrix [16–18]. The remarkably high water content is associated with, i.e., "packaged" within, the cellular component. The densely packed, flattened cells are differentiated corneocytes with cell envelopes approximately 1–2 μm thick which lack distinct nuclei and have lower keratin levels than fully mature stratum corneum cells (Fig. 13.1) [17]. There is no evidence of corneodesmosomes or distinct cellular organization. Ultrastructural evaluation shows the individual cells in vernix to be variable with respect to the stage of keratinization [19].

An understanding of the potential roles of vernix in neonatal development begins with consideration of fetal skin formation. In an elegant electron microscopy investigation, Holbrook and Odland showed eight distinct stages of fetal epidermal differentiation from approximately 5–26 weeks gestation occurring under the influence of the periderm (Fig. 13.2) [20]. The periderm appears to protect the developing epidermis from amniotic fluid and to manage secretory processes such as the uptake of glucose. By 20 weeks (stage 7), keratin-containing squames and follicular regions appear within the interfollicular space as well as discrete waxy material [20]. Keratinized cells are present along the hair follicle and the interfollicular spaces around week 23.5, and the periderm disappears around this time [20]. During fetal (human and animal) development, the barrier forms around the hair follicle beginning at 18–19 gestational weeks and along the hair canal by week 21 [21]. Interfollicular development occurs in a programmatic fashion, initially at week 23 on the head and week 25 on the abdomen. This folliculocentric pattern of organized intrauterine epidermal maturation supports an important role for the hair follicle in barrier formation.

Of note, vernix can be observed around the eyebrows as early as gestational week 17. During the last trimester, vernix begins to coat the fetal skin surface from head to toe and back to front, presumably under hormonal control. In one form of this working hypothesis, corticotropin-releasing factors (CRF) from either the placenta or hypothalamus initiate adrenocorticotropic hormone (ACTH) release from the pituitary gland. ACTH adrenal gland stimulation promotes synthesis and release of androgenic steroids (e.g., dehydroepiandrosterone) which are converted to active androgens within the sebaceous gland. More recent data support the hypothesis of a local hypothalamic-pituitary-adrenal-like axis in the hair follicle itself [22]. Concordant with this hypothesis, vernix lipids include types produced

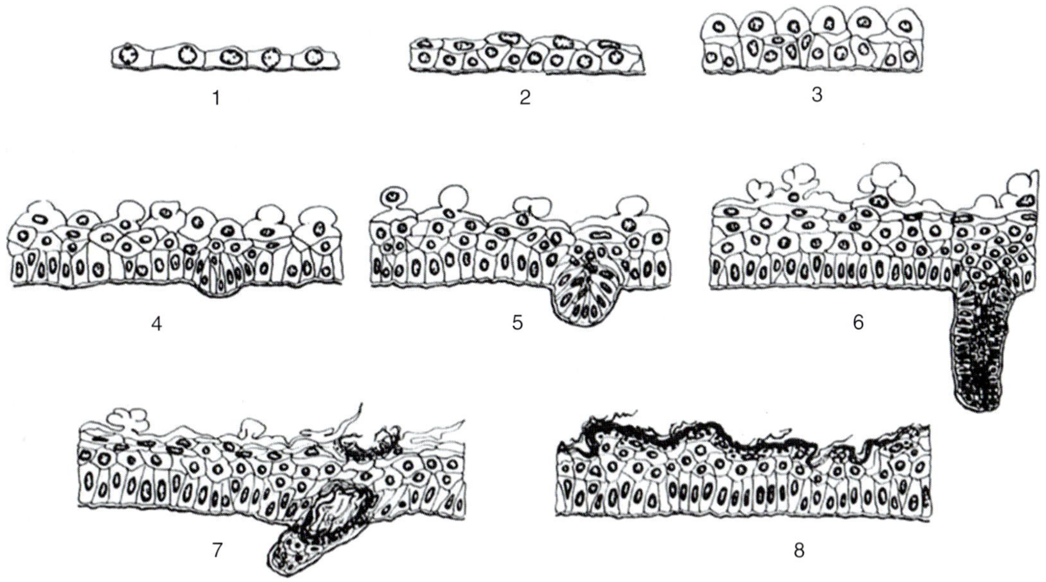

Fig. 13.2 Schematic diagram of the eight stages of periderm development and epidermal differentiation. Corresponding estimated gestation ages for each stage are (1) <36 days, (2) 35–55 days, (3) 55–75 days, (4) 65–95 days, (5) 85–110 days, (6) 95–120 days, (7) 110–160 days, and (8) >160 days. Vernix production corresponds to the loss of periderm and the transition from stage 7 to stage 8 (Modified from Holbrook and Odland [20])

by the sebaceous glands [18, 23], and the cornified fetal cells may originate from the hair follicles, analogous to the production of terminally differentiated infundibular keratinocytes in acne [24]. In this scenario, vernix is "extruded" or squeezed out through the hair shaft and onto the interfollicular epidermis, eventually spreading over the entire surface as production continues throughout gestation [25]. The superficial vernix film is hydrophobic due to the lipids which coat the hydrated cells [26]. During gestation, vernix presumably protects the underlying epidermis from exposure to water [26]. Normal stratum corneum has a water gradient with higher levels in the lower layers and reduced hydration toward the surface [27–29]. Repair of superficial SC wounds is regulated by the transepidermal water gradient via increased synthesis of DNA and lipids [30–33]. Vernix films are semipermeable to water vapor transport ex utero [34]. Presumably, fetal epidermis has a high water flux potential driven by osmotic gradients since cornification is not complete. Therefore, vernix may impose a semiregulated barrier and/or physiological gradient for transepidermal water and nutrients in utero, thereby facilitating cornification via mechanisms involving increased DNA and lipid synthesis. The asymmetric submerged culture model of Thakoersing et al. is consistent with this hypothesis [14].

13.3 Vernix Lipid Composition and Structural Organization

Vernix contains both free lipids and lipids bound to corneocytes. The components of free lipids include sterol esters, wax esters, dihydroxy wax esters, squalene, triglycerides, diacylglycerol, monoacylglycerol, phospholipids, cholesterol, fatty acids, and ceramides [18, 35]. The bound lipids in vernix include ω-hydroxy acids (bound to corneocyte envelope), fatty acids, ω-hydroxyceramides CerA (sphingosine), and CerB (6-hydroxysphingosine) [18].

Early work on vernix lipid composition focused on the free lipid component containing both squalene and triglycerides [23, 36–38], supporting the conjecture that vernix was, in part, of sebaceous origin. Rissmann et al. analyzed the free lipid fraction from vernix samples derived from term infants by high-performance thin-layer

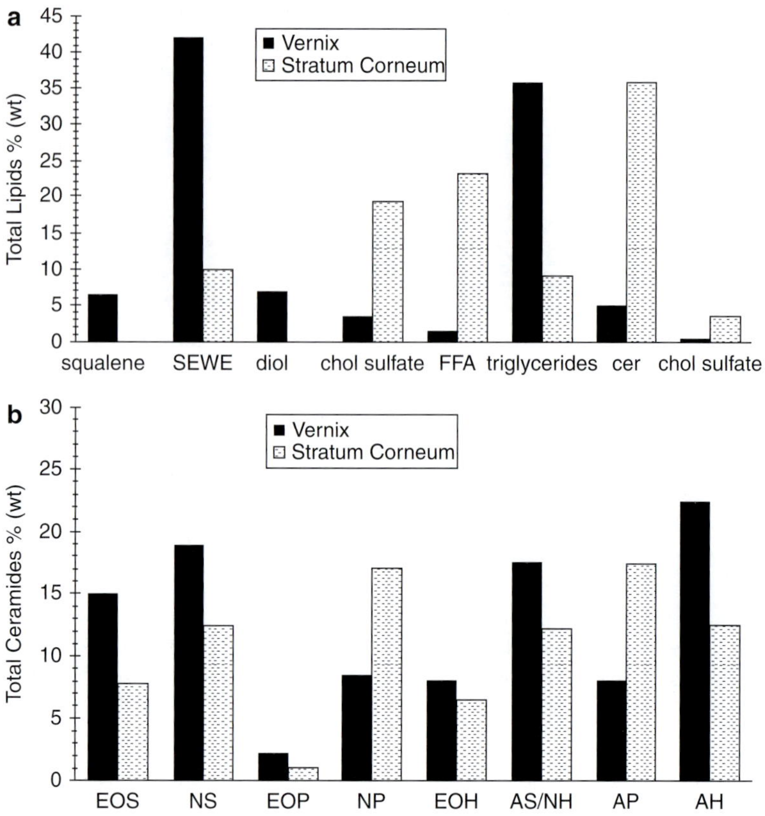

Fig. 13.3 (**a**) Comparison of total lipids in vernix caseosa and stratum corneum (Adapted from Rissmann et al. [18]). (**b**) Comparison of different classes of ceramides in vernix caseosa and stratum corneum (Adapted from Rissmann et al. [18])

chromatography (Fig. 13.3) [18]. Approximately 11% of the total weight of vernix is comprised of lipids with nonpolar lipids predominating. As opposed to native SC wherein barrier lipids such as cholesterol, free fatty acids, and ceramides constitute 80% of total lipids, these lipid classes represent only 10% of total lipids in vernix. Nonpolar lipids are the major components of vernix.

More recent analyses have shed light on the highly complex lipid species present in vernix including branched-chain fatty acids and lipids bound to the cornified cell envelope [16, 18, 35, 39, 40]. The free fatty acid component of vernix is particularly complex and includes oleic, linoleic, long-chain species between 14 and 32 carbons long, and branched-chain types (Tables 13.1 and 13.2) [18, 40]. The FFA profile is dominated by saturated chain lengths C16:0 (14%) and C24:0 (24.5%). The predominant monounsaturated fatty acid is C18:1n-9 (6.4%), and the predominant polyunsaturated fatty acid is C18:2n-6 (9.6%) [35]. Branched-chains account for 29% of the fatty acids and include 30 different chain lengths, from 11 to 26 carbons (Fig. 13.4) [40]. In contrast, SC fatty acids are straight-chained and generally 22 or 24 carbons [41]. Ran-Ressler et al. investigated branched-chain fatty acids (BCFA) in vernix in relation to meconium in the fetal gut [40]. They found a reduction of BCFA in meconium and speculated that BCFA in vernix, swallowed by the fetus, was absorbed or modified within the healthy term gastrointestinal tract, thus playing a putative nutritional, adaptive, or anti-infective role. BCFA are known membrane constituents of many commensal bacteria, including lactobacilli, which are considered probiotic candidates promoting colonization of the GI tract [42, 43]. Tollin et al. observed that free fatty acids in vernix exhibit antibacterial activity [35].

Both vernix and stratum corneum exhibit structures consisting of hydrophilic corneocytes

Table 13.1 Composition of free fatty acids in vernix caseosa [35]

Species	%, weight/weight
Saturated fatty acids	*50.1*
C14:0	2.0
C15:0	1.0
C16:0	14.0
C17:0	0.4
C18:0	2.0
C20:0	0.8
C22:0	5.4
C24:0	24.5
Monounsaturated fatty acids	*11.4*
C16:ln-9	2.0
C16:ln-7	1.3
C18:ln-9	6.4
C18:ln-7	1.7
Polyunsaturated fatty acids	*15.0*
C18:2n-6	9.6
C20:2n-6	1.3
C22:4n-6	4.1
Unidentified fatty acids	*23.0*

Table 13.2 Profile of total fatty acid classes in vernix caseosa from term infants

Species	%, weight/weight
Saturated fatty acids	34.0
Monounsaturated fatty acids	31.0
Polyunsaturated fatty acids	3.9
Branched-chain fatty acids	29.1

Data adapted from Ran-Ressler et al. [40]

embedded in a hydrophobic lipid matrix; there are important architectural differences. Vernix is a malleable cream which can be spread manually over the skin surface or detached in bulk into the amniotic fluid [44]. In SC, the free lipids consist primarily of cholesterol, free fatty acids, and ceramides which form a tightly organized lamellar pattern with repeat distances of 6 and 13 nm [45, 46]. Presumably, these alternative structures reflect important physiological differences. Rissmann et al. have proposed that the lower levels of ceramides with long fatty acid chains in vernix coupled with the high proportion of unsaturated or branched fatty acids may lead to the more fluid, nonlamellar organization seen in vernix [18]. They note that the majority of lipids in SC have straight unsaturated fatty acid chains.

A major difference between vernix and SC is the lack of corneodesmosal linkages in the former. Corneocytes in vernix are therefore amenable to shear force application and can be spread on a flat surface (Fig. 13.1). Despite the lack of desmosomes, vernix does contain bound lipids covalently linked to the cornified envelope. After saponification and extraction, these lipids constitute approximately 1% of the total vernix weight [18]. In general, vernix-bound lipids are the same as those found in the SC, i.e., fatty acids, ω-hydroxy acids, ω-hydroxyceramides CerA (sphingosine), and CerB (6-hydroxysphingosine) [47]. Compared to SC, however, vernix has higher levels of ω-hydroxyeicosanoic acid and nearly absent levels of ω-hydroxyacid with 30 C-atoms [18].

13.4 Comparison: Epidermal Lipids and Vernix Lipids

During fetal development, the epidermal lipid composition is relatively constant from gestational week 8 through 16 [48]. By week 19, the fraction of sterol esters and wax esters is substantially higher with an increase in epidermal triglycerides. Interestingly, sterol esters/wax esters (SEWE) are the largest fraction of vernix lipids, followed by triglycerides [18]. The presence of epidermal SEWE is an indicator of fetal cornification [48, 49]. An examination of the epidermal lipids from fetal samples of 14–17 and 20–28 weeks gestation compared with samples from full terms ($n=1$) and adults showed a marked difference in the sterol ester/wax ester fraction between the 14–17- and 20–28-week groups [50]. Additionally, fatty acids were lower and ceramides increased, although the comparison is limited by only one sample from a 38-week infant. Interestingly, the triglyceride level was much higher in vernix than any other epidermal or SC sample. The high triglyceride and SEWE fractions in vernix likely reflect the contribution of sebaceous lipids which are dominated by triglyceride (41%) and SEWE (27%) [51]. Cholesterol levels were much higher in fetal and infant epidermis compared to adults and vernix

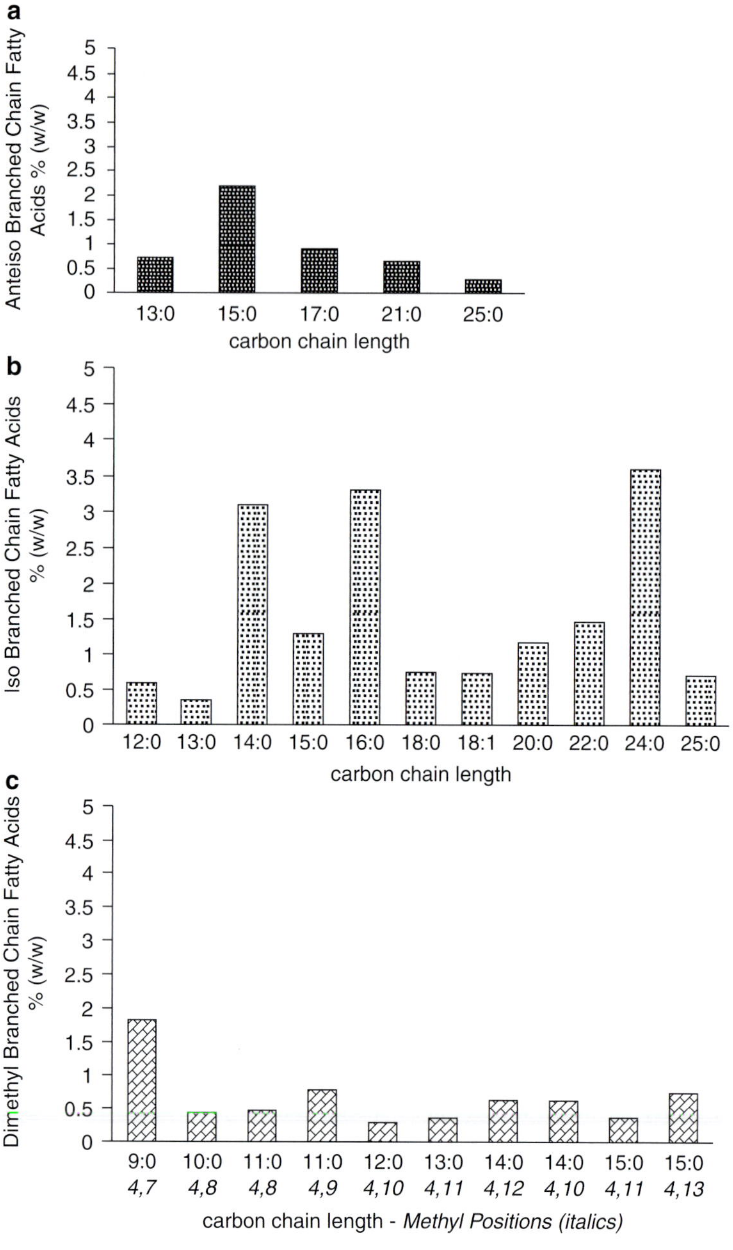

Fig. 13.4 Branched-chain fatty acids in vernix caseosa (Adapted from RanRessler et al. [40]). (**a**) Anteiso branched-chain fatty acids. (**b**) Iso branched-chain fatty acids. (**c**). Dimethyl branched-chain fatty acids

[18]. Free fatty acid levels were considerably higher in all fetal, neonatal, and infant samples compared to vernix.

Given that the composition of epidermal lipids changes during gestation, it is possible that the composition of vernix also changes throughout the last trimester as the infant prepares to transition to the dry environment. To date, there is one report on the vernix lipid composition as a function of gestational age among infants of 31–40 weeks gestation [52]. The cholesterol/squalene ratio decreases around 36 weeks GA, i.e., it is higher for premature infants and lower at term. This change reflected an increase in squalene content relative to other vernix lipids, indicating a possible surge in fetal sebaceous gland function near the time of delivery.

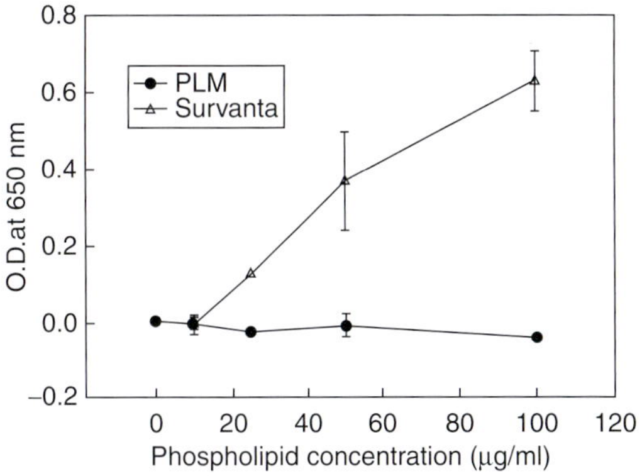

Fig. 13.5 Increase in solution turbidity arising from vernix-coated microfuge tubes following incubation overnight with increasing concentrations of the bovine pulmonary surfactant Survanta® [53]. Incubation with an equimolar phospholipid mixture not containing surfactant proteins had no effect. This in vitro experiment is consistent with an effect of pulmonary surfactant to induce vernix detachment from the fetal skin surface, thereby giving rise to amniotic fluid turbidity seen in the last trimester of human pregnancy [53]

13.5 Vernix: Physical Properties

The lipid-coated, high-water-containing cellular architecture of vernix gives rise to interesting physical and water-handling properties. Rheological measurements indicate a much higher shear rate (flow) at body temperature than at ambient (room temperature) conditions, consistent with vernix spreading and coating the fetal skin surface in utero, while becoming increasingly viscous and immobile following birth [53]. The addition of native, protein-containing pulmonary surfactant to vernix increases its flow and ability to spread, an effect which does not occur with phospholipids alone [53] (Fig. 13.5). As the fetal lungs mature, increasing amounts of pulmonary surfactant are secreted into the amniotic fluid. Hypothetically, as term approaches, the quantity is sufficient to detach vernix from the skin surface thereby increasing the turbidity of the amniotic fluid (which is used as an indirect indicator of lung maturity) (Fig. 13.4). Surface tension measurements indicate that vernix has a critical surface tension of 39 dyne/cm which is comparable to that of petrolatum (100% lipid) and much lower than water, despite its high water content [26]. Surface free

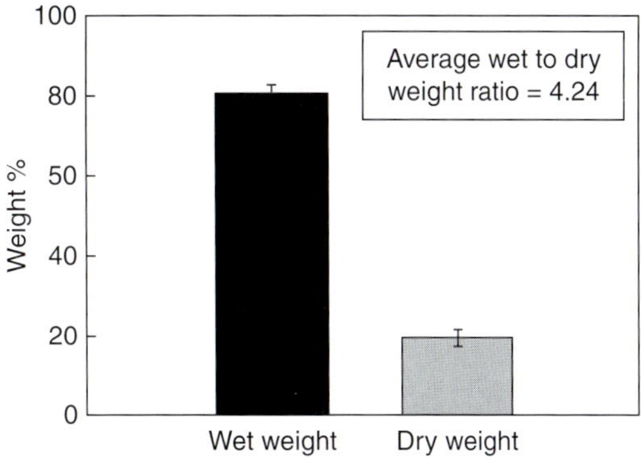

Fig. 13.6 Wet weight and dry weight of fresh native vernix caseosa prior to dehydration postnatally. The ratio of the average wet-to-dry weight dose is shown [54]

energy measurements show vernix to be unwettable, suggesting that it forms a hydrophobic coating for the developing infant with "water-proofing" effects to exogenous water and materials of high critical surface tension [26].

13.5.1 Water Content

Vernix specimens have a remarkably high and consistent water content of approximately 80.7±2.2% [54]. In determining the water content of vernix, care must be taken to prevent condensation of water on the inner surface of the storage container. Ex utero studies of isolated vernix corneocytes demonstrate that these cells can swell and contract as a function of a hypoosmotic or hyperosmotic environment [55], supporting a potential role for vernix in osmoregulation intra-amniotically. Of theoretical interest, the wet to dry weight ratio of vernix, i.e., 4.24 (Fig. 13.6), is indistinguishable from the cube of the golden section ratio (phi), i.e., 1.6180^3 [55]. Bulienkov has postulated that "water structures" found in self-organizing biological systems are a power function of phi [56]. Based on empirical data, phi proportionality figures prominently into the cellular organization of the human epidermis [57]. The proposition that synthetic vernix-based analogs and skin creams based on phi-proportional water structures might synergize particularly well with human epidermis has not been rigorously tested.

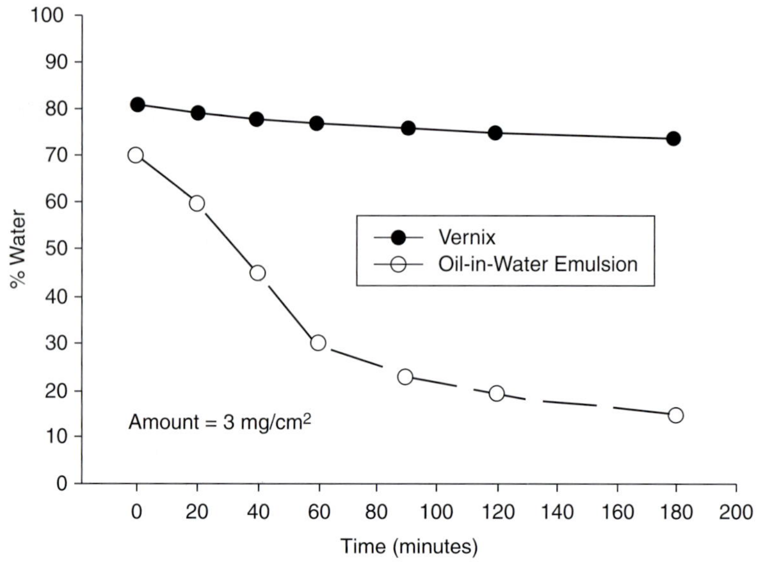

Fig. 13.7 Dehydration kinetics of vernix caseosa compared to a typical oil-in-water emulsion over 3 h [17, 59]

Whereas most of the water content in vernix is localized to the intracorneocyte region, several studies have noted apparent hydrated domains in the nonlamellar lipid matrix [17, 18]. Thus, cryo-SEM shows small round structures within the lipid domains which may represent water droplets. The origin and function of these structures remain unclear, but they may represent a pool of rapidly releasable extracorneocyte water [54]. Larger, hydrated inclusion bodies containing antimicrobial peptides such as lysozyme and lactoferrin have been described by Akinbi et al. [58]. The larger size of the inclusions in the latter study may result from process-induced coalescence. The presence of a quick release pool of soluble antimicrobials would be a major benefit for the fetus faced with chorioamnionitis or other intrauterine infection. This physicochemical hypothesis has not yet been tested.

13.5.2 Water Binding

Despite a high (80%) water content, vernix films lose water slowly compared to standard water-in-oil emulsions and display first order kinetics consistent with a biphasic release process (Fig. 13.7) [17, 59, 60]. Complete water loss may take days, depending upon environmental conditions. The rate of water loss depends upon the thickness of the vernix films and thicker films lose water more slowly [60]. The water behavior of native vernix and isolated vernix corneocytes (lipid removed) has been quantified by measuring the water sorption and desorption over varying (high to low) water activities [54]. At equilibrium, the vernix water content decreases with decreasing water activity (relative humidity) and regains water as the humidity is increased again. This behavior suggests the presence of an internal, structured microenvironment responsible for the water-binding properties. The behavior of vernix at low humidity is comparable to that of native stratum corneum indicating a small, constant amount of bound water [54]. As humidity increases, the cells swell to expose more water-binding sites, thereby increasing the water content. When the lipid fraction was removed, the water sorption/desorption profile differed from that of native vernix especially between water activities of 0.64 and 0.75, i.e., before the normal inflection point for water binding, suggesting that the lipid component is important for the normative sorption–desorption behavior of vernix (Fig. 13.8) [54].

13.5.3 Water Vapor Transport

Water vapor transport (WVT) of vernix films in vitro was measured quantitatively by application of

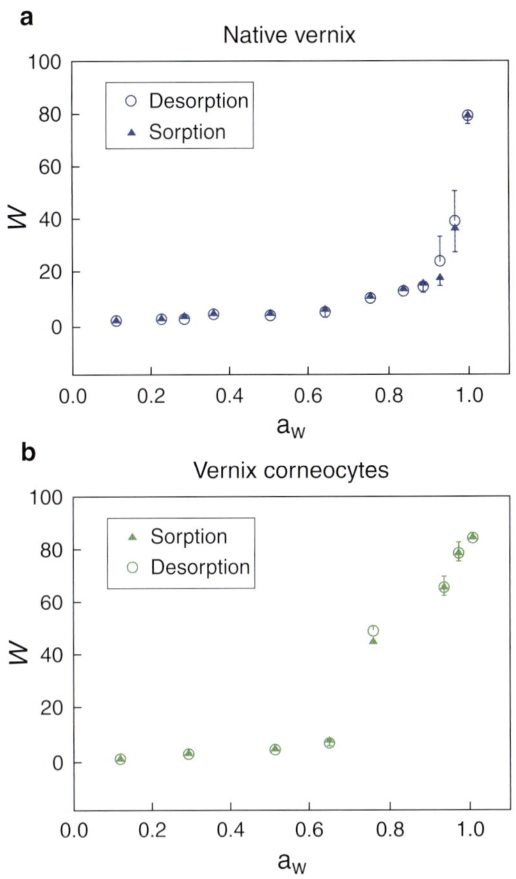

Fig. 13.8 Equilibrium water sorption–desorption behavior from Tansirikongkol et al. [54]. (**a**) Native vernix ($n = 4$) and (**b**) isolated vernix corneocytes ($n = 6$) expressed as weight % water in the tissue (mean ± SD) versus water activity. Key: (▲) Sorption experiment, (○) Desorption experiment. Equilibrium water content within all test materials is water activity dependent

vernix to a highly porous membrane over water with equilibration at room temperature. Gravimetric measurements were made at multiple intervals to derive the rate of water loss. Water vapor transport measurements indicate that vernix films are semipermeable, with transmission rates of 19–70 g/m^2/h, depending upon thickness (19 for 5 mg/cm^2 and 70 for 0.5 mg/cm^2) [59, 60]. Petrolatum-based films have low water vapor transport, i.e., 1.5 g/m^2/h for films of 2 mg/cm^2, indicating that they are almost fully occlusive compared with vernix films (at 2 mg/cm^2) that have a WVT of 45 g/m^2/h [61]. Treatment of superficial SC damage with semipermeable films results in more rapid barrier recovery than damaged skin treated with either complete occlusion (no water vapor transport) or no occlusion [62]. The water vapor transport results suggest that vernix films may promote the formation of the stratum corneum in premature infants and the barrier repair process in damaged skin.

13.5.4 Skin Cleansing

The effectiveness of native vernix as a skin cleanser was evaluated following application of a simulated soil (uniform carbon particles) to adult volar forearm skin [63]. Vernix was comparable to or superior to standard skin cleansers. Visualization of the skin dermatoglyphics in high-resolution images suggests that vernix intercolates or penetrates into skin furrows, pores, and around the hair shaft to remove the soil. This effect is most likely due to the compatability of vernix with cutaneous lipids and an expected tropism to follicular pores [21, 64]. These results are consistent with vernix as both a naturally occurring emollient (moisturizer) and a skin cleanser.

13.6 Vernix: Biochemical Properties

Multiple other biological functions have been demonstrated or proposed for vernix [55]. They are discussed in the following sections.

13.6.1 Antimicrobial/Anti-infective Agents

Vernix contains antimicrobial agents, including proteins and lipids, and exhibits a range of bioactivity against common fungal and bacterial pathogens [35, 58, 65, 66]. The protein human cathelicidin (hCAP18) is part of the cutaneous innate immune system with antimicrobial properties and protection against keratinocyte apoptosis attributed to the 37 amino acids in the C-terminal portion, known as LL-37 [67]. Vernix from full-term infants contains lysozyme and LL-37, the latter of which had antimicrobial activity against *B. megaterium* Bm11 (gram-positive) [65]. A second study on vernix and amniotic fluid from healthy infants showed activity to Bm11 and to *C. albicans* [66]. The antimicrobial proteins α-defensins (HNP1–3), lysozyme, and LL-37 were identified. Two other peptides, ubiquitin and psoriasin, were in the lysozyme-containing fraction, so their antimicrobial activity could not be differentiated. A series of proteonomic and fractionation experiments identified five additional proteins of the innate immune system, i.e., calgranulin A, B, and C; cystatin A; and UGRP-1 [35]. The antimicrobial efficacy of 88 vernix samples against *B. megaterium*, group B *Streptococcus*, *C. albicans*, and *E. coli* was greatest for *B. megaterium* and group *B. Streptococcus* [35]. All of the vernix samples inhibited *B. megaterium* and *C. albicans*; 78% inhibited group *B strep*; and 31% were active against *E. coli*. Combinations of vernix lipids and LL-37 in ratios of 3:1 and 7:1 displayed greater antimicrobial inhibition than LL-37 alone, indicating synergetic innate immunity for the mixtures. In another study, the antimicrobial proteins lactoferrin, lysozyme, secretory leukocyte protease inhibitor, and human neutrophil peptides 1–3 were found in vernix from healthy full-term births [58]. Vernix samples had muramidase activity and were active against the growth of group B *Streptococcus*, *L. monocytogenes*, and *K. pneumoniae*. However, these samples did not contain detectable levels of human beta defensin-2, lactoperoxidase, or LL-37. Ceramides, sterols, and fatty acids on the SC surface inhibit attachment of C. albicans in vitro [68]. These lipid components of vernix left on the skin surface after birth may also serve the same function.

13.6.2 Skin Hydration/Moisturization

The high water content, the slow water release from the cellular component, and the resorption of water suggest that vernix might function as an ideal skin moisturizer, i.e., to promote hydration for optimum stratum corneum function. Application of native vernix to adult volar forearm skin (2.5 mg/cm^2) significantly increased the water-holding capacity (WHC) versus an untreated control ($p<0.05$) [69]. In contrast, treatment with a water-in-oil cream (Eucerin©), an anhydrous barrier (petrolatum), and a low-water cream (Aquaphor©) did not differ in WHC from untreated skin. The water-binding capacity (peak sorption following application of exogenous water) of vernix-treated skin was significantly higher than the untreated control, while values for Eucerin, petrolatum, and aquaphor were significantly lower. Along with baseline hydration and moisture accumulation rate, these measures show a unique temporal change in skin hydration which is different from common topical treatments.

The provision of skin hydration for the newborn infant is of interest. Within minutes to hours after birth, newborn skin hydration varies with body site (chest, back, forehead) and time under the radiant warmer [70]. Hydration decreases rapidly in the first day and then increases during the first 2 weeks, in contrast to mother's skin where hydration is relatively constant. Water-binding capacity increases over this period as well, suggesting adaptive changes to the postnatal environment [71]. Newborn skin is significantly drier than the skin of their mothers and older infants (1, 2, and 6 months) [72]. In various settings worldwide, vernix is removed immediately after birth. Visscher et al. examined the effect of vernix retention at birth by comparing parallel groups of healthy full-term newborns. In one group, vernix was wiped off immediately at delivery following common local hospital practices at the time. In the second group, vernix was retained on the skin and allowed to rub in naturally. Vernix retention led to significantly higher skin hydration at birth and 24 h later ($p<0.05$) [73]. Vernix-treated skin was significantly less erythematous versus skin for which vernix removed. In another study among healthy full-term newborn infants, vernix was removed at delivery and saved. Following delivery, a small area on the chest was treated with alcohol to remove residual vernix. A sample of vernix was then reapplied to one side of the chest. The alcohol-treated contralateral site was used as the control. The water-handling behavior was evaluated 24 h later, and no additional treatments (e.g., bathing, lotions) were applied. The vernix-treated site had a significantly higher water-holding capacity than the control site.

To further probe the cause of low skin hydration at birth, the levels of free amino acids (FAA) were determined [74]. Free amino acids are water-binding moieties that constitute about 40% of natural moisturizing factor in the upper SC. In the absence of vernix, FAA levels were extremely low at birth, increased over the first month but remained markedly lower than typical adult quantities [74]. The FAA levels in newborn skin were also examined as a function of vernix treatment with the hypothesis that FAA would be higher following vernix retention after birth. Vernix itself contains FAA at levels corresponding to about 0.3 μmol/cm^2 which may account in part for the slow water release and water resorption. The relative amounts of histidine and glutamic acid in vernix were higher than expected from filaggrin proteolysis alone, indicating that vernix may contain other sources of soluble amino acids [74]. Vernix retention led to higher levels of FAA 24 h after birth ($p<0.05$). The three most abundant FAAs, i.e., glycine, serine, and glutaminic acid ($p<0.005$), as well as arginine ($p=0.05$) and citrulline ($p=0.03$), were significantly higher for VC-retained samples. FAAs at 24 h paralleled the higher SC hydration. The results suggest another adaptive function of vernix, namely to provide water-binding FAAs to plasticize the skin before the longer-term adaptive epidermal changes and subsequent increased SC hydration have occurred [71, 74].

13.6.3 Skin Surface Acidity

In a study of the effect of vernix retention versus removal at birth, the skin surface acidity was significantly lower in the vernix-retained group at birth and 24 h later, suggesting that vernix assists in the development of the acid mantle [73]. An acid surface is necessary for the effective functioning of enzymes in SC formation and integrity, i.e., lipid metabolism, bilayer structure, ceramide synthesis, and desquamation [75, 76], as well as bacterial homeostasis, skin colonization, and inhibition of pathogenic bacteria [77–79]. At birth, the pH of full-term skin following vernix removal is relatively neutral, decreases significantly during the first 1–4 days, and continues to drop during the first 3 months as the enzymes needed to generate acidic components are activated [71, 80, 81]. Topical treatment of the SC with PPARα activators increases the rate of skin pH lowering after birth in neonatal animals, demonstrating that the adaptive mechanisms can be influenced with exogenous materials [82]. Acidification of the SC enhances its integrity and cohesion, in part by improving lipid processing and decreasing corneodesmosomal degradation [83] as well as improving SC barrier homeostasis in neonatal and aged skin [84]. The application of acidic treatments has been proposed as a method for treating inflammation and normalizing SC structure and function [83].

13.6.4 Lipids and SC Barrier

The lipid components of vernix may facilitate SC barrier development in utero or as a topical treatment for underdeveloped skin, for example, premature infants. Fatty acids, particularly linoleic acid, activate peroxisome proliferator-activated receptor-α (PPARα) which increases the rate of barrier formation [85]. Linoleic acid has anti-inflammatory properties [86]. The postnatal application of linoleic-containing sunflower seed oil to the skin of premature infants less than 33 weeks gestational age reduced the incidence of nosocomial blood infections by 41% [87]. Treatment of tape-stripped skin with SC lipids increases the barrier repair rate [88]. The ceramide component of the treatment, i.e., the type and ratio of ceramides to other lipid classes, influences the barrier properties in SC model systems [89]. A mixture of physiological barrier lipids, viz., cholesterol, ceramide, palmitate, and linoleate (ratio 3:1:1:1), is optimum for barrier repair [90]. Future studies on the effects and fate of vernix components for premature SC maturation are warranted.

13.6.4.1 Physical Barrier

The juxtaposition of vernix between the fetal skin surface and the amniotic fluid suggests that it functions as a physical barrier and perhaps regulates the transport of in utero "agents" either by keeping them away from the developing skin, filtering desirable substances to the skin surface, or by sequestering epidermal products from loss in the amniotic fluid. Exposure of the nascent stratum corneum to chymotrypsin enzyme and other protease or lipase agents in amniotic fluid, for example, could have deleterious effects on the skin. Meconium (fetal stool) is commonly passed prenatally and is particularly noxious if aspirated by the fetus. Neutralization or binding of meconium by vernix would be advantageous. Tansirikongkol et al. evaluated the effect of vernix in vitro on the penetration of exogenous chymotrypsin. Films of vernix provided a protective barrier impeding the penetration of the exogenous chymotrypsin [91]. This effect was due to mechanical obstruction and not to enzyme inhibition. Hypothetically, vernix in vivo protects against penetration of exogenous proteolytic enzymes while facilitating production and/or localization of endogenous materials involved in normal cornification and desquamation. Vernix may also act as a sump mechanism clearing the amniotic fluid of unwanted hydrophilic or hydrophobic agents passed in the fetal urine. Vernix has been reported to bind bile pigments and bilirubin in vitro [92].

13.6.5 Skin Barrier Maturation, SC Compromise, Wound Healing

13.6.5.1 Significance

Premature infants have an incompetent SC barrier, leading to problems with fluid balance, temperature control, infection, and skin damage [93, 94]. The premature SC is functionally compromised for several weeks after birth [95], and estimates of the time to complete barrier maturation vary from 2 to 9 postnatal weeks [96–99]. Attempts to improve barrier function with topical treatments have had limited success [100–102]. Neonates <28 weeks gestation lack significant vernix caseosa. The potential effects of vernix on skin barrier maturation for restoration of SC compromise in premature infants and for epidermal wound healing are of interest. The relevance for premature infants can be determined by investigating the effects using animal models, for example, removal of SC to simulate premature skin possessing only a few cornified layers, and using tape-stripped human adult skin to replicate superficial wounds. Lower extremity wounds improved following treatment with vernix [103]. Vernix may also serve as a natural wound healing agent for the maternal perineum at birth [55].

13.6.5.2 Animal and Human Studies

In the hairless mouse model, one application of vernix (5 mg/cm^2) increased the rate of barrier relative to no treatment following complete removal of the SC via tape stripping [104]. A petrolatum-based treatment also accelerated barrier repair, but the skin was more erythematous, and the epidermis was thickened compared to vernix-treated skin (Fig. 13.9a, b). In the murine tape-stripped model, native vernix elicits epidermal cornification within 2–6 h, suggesting that the effects of vernix on epidermal cornification may be very rapid [104].

In the Yorkshire hybrid minipig, minor epidermal wounds were made with a dual-mode erbium:YAG laser at nominal depths of 20 and 25 μm. Five sites at each level were treated twice a day with 2.5 mg/cm^2 of vernix caseosa or a petrolatum-based cream (Aquaphor®, Beiersdorf AG, Hamburg, Germany). Untreated (no occlusion) sites served as controls [105]. TEWL values after wounding and prior to treatment ranged from 29 to 50 g/m^2/h, comparable to values for infants <30 weeks gestation [106]. Vernix and the petrolatum-based treatment produced significantly greater barrier repair than the untreated, no occlusion site for both ablation levels.

In a human trial, tape-stripped maternal volar forearm skin (a common model for premature skin) was used to compare the effects of vernix, a petrolatum-based cream (Aquaphor®), and an oil-in-water cream (Hand Medic®, GOJO Industries, Inc., Akron, OH, USA) on the rate of

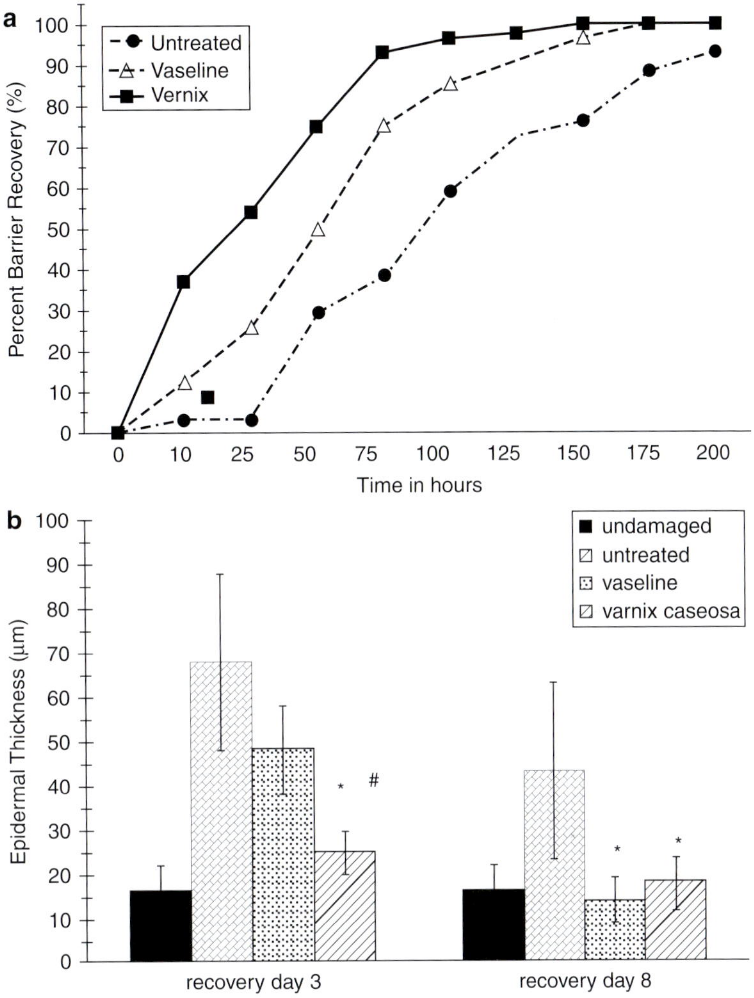

Fig. 13.9 (**a**). Rapid recovery of barrier function measured as return of transepidermal water loss to baseline levels following epidermal damage due to tape stripping. Vernix treatment was superior to Vaseline (petrolatum) compared to control results. (**b**). Increase in epidermal thickening observed in untreated epidermis and following Vaseline application in the tape-stripped murine mouse model. * Indicates significant difference versus untreated skin ($p<0.05$), # indicates significant difference versus Vaseline treatment ($p<0.05$) (Data modified and adapted from Oudshoorn et al. [112])

SC barrier repair, skin hydration, erythema, and dryness [105]. Vernix and the creams were applied twice daily at 2.5 mg/cm^2. The vernix was from each mother's own infant to address potential safety issues posed by human-derived materials. Additional stripped sites were treated with full occlusion (FO, impermeable to water vapor); a semipermeable film (SP) and no occlusion (NO) were controls for comparison with previous work [62, 107]. The semipermeable film produced more rapid barrier recovery than FO and NO, consistent with previous findings. Barrier recovery was greater for vernix than FO and similar for the petrolatum-based cream, the oil-in-water cream, and no occlusion. The moisture accumulation rate tended to be higher for vernix than the oil-in-water cream. The initial hydration for vernix-treated skin was directionally higher than NO. These findings suggest that the SC recovering with vernix may be more hydrated than with the oil-in-water cream or no occlusion. Skin dryness was higher for the petrolatum treatment than no occlusion and directionally higher for the petrolatum treatment compared to vernix and the oil-in-water cream, suggesting a difference in desquamation and/or hyperproliferation among them. Overall, the findings suggest that vernix-based topical creams may be effective for the treatment of epidermal wounds and show promise to augment SC repair and maturation in infants [105, 108, 109].

13.7 Vernix Substitutes: Synthetic Analogs

It is not feasible to topically apply vernix from one infant to another or to anyone other than the infant's mother due to the limitations on the use of human-derived materials. Therefore, there is a need to formulate topical creams based on native vernix caseosa as a prototype. Formulation of high-water-phase emulsions with lipid mixtures resulted in several stable creams with high water content and slow water release [34]. Preparations with vernix-like lipids demonstrated water release profiles closer to the native vernix benchmark than those with conventional lipids. In addition, the water vapor transport rates were in the range to facilitate barrier repair [34].

Lipid mixtures, based on the composition of native vernix lipids, were formulated and evaluated for their effects on stratum corneum barrier formation in the tape-stripped hairless mouse model [110]. Triglycerides, cholesterol, fatty acids, ceramides, and squalene were combined with sterol esters and wax esters isolated from lanolin in order to include the branched-chain component of the native vernix lipid matrix [110]. The formulas that matched the thermal and structural properties of native vernix were evaluated for effect on barrier repair. The synthetic lipid mixtures were comparable to native vernix and provided increased barrier repair versus a petrolatum treatment [110].

Synthetic vernix formulations were made with microgels of hyperbranched polyglycerol glycidyl methacrylate to simulate the water-containing cells in vernix [111]. In some formulations, the hydrated particles were coated with lipids to more closely simulate the native vernix structure. The lipid fraction was constituted as shown in Table 13.3. The formula with lipid-coated microgel particles in a ratio of 2:1 particles/lipid had an experimental water level of 57% and most closely resembled the water release profile of native vernix [111].

Table 13.3 Lipid mixture used to formulate synthetic vernix [111]

Lipid	Amount (%)
Sterol ester/wax ester	48.0
Triglycerides	
Trinervonin	11.9
Tripalmitolein	11.9
Triolein	11.9
Cholesterol	3.5
Fatty acids	
Palmitic	0.8
Palmitoleic	0.3
Steric	0.1
Oleic	0.3
Ceramides	
EOS	0.7
NS	1.0
NP (C24)	0.4
NP (C16)	0.4
AS	0.8
AP	1.6
Squalene	6.4

In further work, Oudshoorn et al. examined the following effects of synthetic formulations on SC barrier recovery in the hairless mouse: hydrated particle/lipid ratio (2:1 and 5:1), presence of lipid particle coating (with, without), vernix lipids only (no particles), and vernix lipids (no hydrated component) minus barrier lipids (i.e., sterol esters/wax esters, squalene, triglycerides) (Table 13.4) [112]. The synthetic versions were compared to native vernix, a petrolatum cream (Vaseline), and a water-in-oil emulsion (Eucerin©) at a single application dose of 5 mg/cm^2. Their efficacy for SC barrier repair was evaluated with multiple measures including evaluation of barrier recovery rate (measured as TEWL) at specific time points, epidermal thickness, and erythema and crust formation (measures of quality of recovering SC). The findings are summarized as follows (Table 13.5) [112]. Overall, the formula (B1) with microgel particles, 50% initial water content, a particle-to-lipid ratio of 2:1, and a lipid mixture based on vernix (i.e., including barrier lipids) resulted in SC barrier repair comparable to that of native vernix [112]. This formulation produced no erythema or crust formation early in the recovery period and did not cause epidermal thickening. In contrast, formulas with a higher microgel particle-to-lipid ratio (5:1) resulted in a thickened epidermis at

Table 13.4 Synthetic vernix formulations used in evaluation of SC barrier recovery [112]

Code	Lipids	Particle/lipid ratio	Lipid coated	Formulated water level (%)	Initial water release profile
L1	Lipid mixture only (Table 13.3)	n/a	n/a	n/a	n/a
L2	Lipids without barrier lipids (cholesterol, fatty acid, ceramide)	n/a	n/a	n/a	n/a
B1	L1	2:1	n/a	50	
B1c	L1	2:1	Coated	50	
B2c	L1	2:1	Coated	80	
B4	L1	5:1	n/a	80	Greater than B1, B1c, B2

day 3 and intermediate erythema and crust formation over time. The formulas containing only the lipid component (L1) showed comparable SC repair to B1, and therefore native vernix, except for a markedly thickened SC at 3 h. The lipid formulation without cholesterol, fatty acids, and ceramides was not as effective for SC repair. Results of treatment with a higher dose, 15 mg/cm^2, for B1 were comparable to those of the lower dose. Both formula B1 and the vernix-lipid-only treatment resulted in faster SC repair than petrolatum (Vaseline) from 8 h after initial application. Barrier repair was slower than with native vernix and was complete 150 h after treatment with the water-in-oil system (Eucerin©). For SC barrier repair, the permeable lipid-based systems, i.e., synthetic formulations with hydrated moieties, the physiological lipid mixture (L1), and native vernix, were more effective than occlusive treatments (i.e., petrolatum) [112].

13.8 Summary

Vernix caseosa has multiple physical and biological functions [55]. It contains lysozyme, lactoferrin, and other microbials with demonstrated anti-infective properties [35, 58, 65, 66]. Films of vernix in vitro impede penetration of the exogenous enzyme chymotrypsin (found in meconium) [91] and, hypothetically, serves to establish epidermal-amniotic fluid gradients of water, nutrients, and electrolytes necessary for normal "inside/outside" architecture and barrier formation [14]. Vernix has been implicated in the establishment of the high electrical resistance of fetal skin during the last trimester of pregnancy [113]. In animals with barrier compromise (via tape stripping), vernix enhances SC formation without increasing epidermal thickness [104]. Vernix functions as a natural moisturizing agent [54, 69] and as a skin cleanser [63], although it is often viewed as a soil itself [63]. In vitro measurements indicate a low surface energy for vernix, suggesting that it creates a protective hydrophobic layer around the fetus [26]. Vernix contains multiple cytokines such as IL1α, IL1β, TNFα, IL-6, IL-8, and MCP1 [44]. The role of these cytokines is the subject of future investigations, but the association of specific antimicrobials with hydrated granules within vernix supports a mechanism for "quick release" in the presence of chorioamnionitis [58]. Vernix contains cholesterol, ceramides, and a number of fatty acids (including oleic, linoleic, and long-chain species) [18, 35]. Fatty acids, particularly linoleic, activate peroxisome proliferator-activated receptor-α (PPARα) which increases the rate of barrier formation [85]. Linoleic acid has anti-inflammatory properties [86]. Overall, vernix facilitates development of the stratum corneum protective barrier in the normal, full-term infant through a variety of protective and adaptive mechanisms. These functions, coupled with its anti-infective properties, are essential for a premature infant who may not have exposure to vernix in utero. The findings provide support for the practice of vernix retention (rather than removal) at birth. The World Health Organization

Table 13.5 Effects of synthetic vernix formulations on SC barrier repair and histological properties [112]

	Erythema and crust		Epidermal thickness		Stratum corneum barrier recovery[a]			
Code (Table 13.4)	Initial	Over time	Day 3	Day 8	Initial <3 h	3–75 h	100 h	150 h
B1	None	Slight	Normal skin, no thickening, similar to native VC	Normal skin, no thickening	Similar to native VC	Similar to native VC	Faster than native VC, complete	
B1c	Slight	Slight			Similar to native VC	Slower than native VC	Same as native VC	
B2c	Slight	Slight	Thicker by 4× vs. untreated skin	Normal skin, no thickening	Similar to native VC	Slower than native VC	Same as native VC, complete	
B4	Slight	Intermediate	Thicker by 4× vs. untreated skin	Normal skin, no thickening	More rapid than B1, B2			Complete
L1	None	Slight	Very thickened SC	Normal skin, no thickening	Similar to B1c, B2c	Similar to B1, vernix		
L2	Slight	Slight	Thickened vs. L1 Very thin SC	Normal skin, no thickening	Delayed vs. L2, B1	Delayed vs. L2	B1	Complete
Petrolatum (Vaseline)	Slight	Slight	Thicker by 2.5× vs. untreated skin	Similar to damaged, untreated skin	Low TEWL (3 g/m^2/h) due to occlusion	Delayed vs. native VC TEWL ~ pre-treatment at 4 h	Delayed vs. native VC	Complete
Water in oil (Eucerin[b])	Slight	Slight	Thicker by 2.5× vs. untreated skin	Similar to damaged, untreated skin	Delayed vs. native VC	Delayed vs. native VC	Delayed vs. native VC	Complete

[a]Tape-stripped, untreated skin required 200 h for complete SC recovery
[b]Water content ~50%

recommends that vernix be left in place and that caregivers wait for at least 6 h prior to bathing newborn infants [114].

Take Home Messages

- Vernix caseosa is a naturally occurring, uniquely human fetal skin cream which exhibits multiple positive physical and biological functions during the last trimester of gestation. In conjunction with pulmonary surfactant, vernix detaches from the skin surface and is swallowed by the fetus. Vernix retained on the skin surface aides in the transition to a dry, microbe-laden environment after birth.
- Vernix is a complex mixture of proteins and lipids with a highly conserved water content present primarily within fetal corneocytes surrounded by an amorphous lipid matrix. The composition and structure of vernix confer water handling and rheological properties that differ from typical oil-in-water or water-in-oil topical skin creams.
- Vernix is putatively produced under hormonal control by "coextrusion" of sebaceous secretions and cells from the hair follicle onto the fetal skin surface first around the hair shaft and then spreading onto the interfollicular areas.
- Vernix contains antimicrobial agents, including proteins and lipids, and exhibits a range of bioactivity against common fungal and bacterial pathogens.
- The moisturization effects of vernix on normal skin, both adults and infants after birth, may be due to its slow water release and the presence of the free amino acid component of natural moisturizing factor.
- Vernix-based topical treatments may be effective for the treatment of epidermal wounds, for the repair of SC compromise, and to facilitate maturation of an effective SC barrier in premature infants.
- The very premature infant is deprived of the benefits of vernix in utero, and treatments based on vernix biology may protect them from vulnerabilities including delayed barrier maturation, delayed acid mantle formation, infection, and water loss.
- The demonstrated properties of vernix caseosa support retention at birth. The World Health Organization recommends retention and delay of bathing for at least 6 h after birth.
- Vernix substitutes have been successfully formulated with stratum corneum barrier repair rates and water release profiles comparable to native vernix. The effects of some of these formulations on SC barrier repair have been demonstrated. An important next step is to evaluate these systems in trials in premature infants to determine effects on SC barrier maturation and infection control and in pediatric and adult patients with SC barrier compromise, epidermal wounds, and dry skin.

References

1. Blank IH (1952) Factors which influence the water content of the stratum corneum. J Invest Dermatol 18:433–440
2. Gloor M, Bettinger J, Gehring W (1998) Modification of stratum corneum quality by glycerin-containing external ointments. Hautarzt 49(1):6–9
3. Rawlings AK, Leyden JJ (eds) (2009) Skin moisturization, 2nd edn. Informa Healthcare, New York
4. Warner RR et al (1999) Water disrupts stratum corneum lipid lamellae: damage is similar to surfactants. J Invest Dermatol 113(6):960–966
5. Warner RR, Stone KJ, Boissy YL (2003) Hydration disrupts human stratum corneum ultrastructure. J Invest Dermatol 120(2):275–284
6. Zimmerer RE, Lawson KD, Calvert CJ (1986) The effects of wearing diapers on skin. Pediatr Dermatol 3(2):95–101
7. Halkier-Sorensen, Petersen BH, Thestrup-Pedersen K (1995) Epidemiology of occupational skin diseases in Denmark: notification, recognition and compensation. In: Van der Valk PGM, Maibach HI (eds) The irritant

contact dermatitis syndrome. CRC Press, Boca Raton, pp 23–52
8. Hurkmans JF, Bodde HE, Van Driel LM, Van Doorne H, Junginger HE (1985) Skin irritation caused by transdermal drug delivery systems during long-term (5 days) application. Br J Dermatol 112(4):461–467
9. Kligman AM (1996) Hydration injury to human skin. In: van der Valk P, Maibach H (eds) The irritant contact dermatitis syndrome. CRC Press, Boca Raton, pp 187–194
10. Medeiros M Jr (1996) Aquagenic urticaria. J Investig Allergol Clin Immunol 6(1):63–64
11. Rustemeyer T, Frosch PJ (1996) Occupational skin diseases in dental laboratory technicians. (I). Clinical picture and causative factors. Contact Dermatitis 34(2):125–133
12. Willis I (1973) The effects of prolonged water exposure on human skin. J Invest Dermatol 60:166–171
13. Visscher MO, Chatterjee R, Ebel JP, LaRuffa AA, Hoath SB (2002) Biomedical assessment and instrumental evaluation of healthy infant skin. Pediatr Dermatol 19(6):473–481
14. Thakoersing VS, Ponec M, Bouwstra JA (2010) Generation of human skin equivalents under submerged conditions-mimicking the in utero environment. Tissue Eng Part A 16(4):1433–1441
15. Anonymous (2009) Mosby's medical dictionary. Elsevier, Amsterdam, Netherlands
16. Hoeger PH et al (2002) Epidermal barrier lipids in human vernix caseosa: corresponding ceramide pattern in vernix and fetal skin. Br J Dermatol 146(2): 194–201
17. Pickens WL, Warner RR, Boissy YL, Boissy RE, Hoath SB (2000) Characterization of vernix caseosa: water content, morphology, and elemental analysis. J Invest Dermatol 115(5):875–881
18. Rissmann R et al (2006) New insights into ultrastructure, lipid composition and organization of vernix caseosa. J Invest Dermatol 126(8):1823–1833
19. Agorastos T, Hollweg G, Grussendorf EI, Papaloucas A (1988) Features of vernix caseosa cells. Am J Perinatol 5(3):253–259
20. Holbrook KA, Odland GF (1975) The fine structure of developing human epidermis: light, scanning, and transmission electron microscopy of the periderm. J Invest Dermatol 65(1):16–38
21. Hardman MJ, Moore L, Ferguson MW, Byrne C (1999) Barrier formation in the human fetus is patterned. J Invest Dermatol 113(6):1106–1113
22. Ito N et al (2005) Human hair follicles display a functional equivalent of the hypothalamic-pituitary-adrenal axis and synthesize cortisol. FASEB J 19(10): 1332–1334
23. Nicolaides N, Fu HC, Ansari MN, Rice GR (1972) The fatty acids of wax esters and sterol esters from vernix caseosa and from human skin surface lipid. Lipids 7(8):506–517
24. Kurokawa I et al (2009) New developments in our understanding of acne pathogenesis and treatment. Exp Dermatol 18(10):821–832
25. Hardman MJ, Sisi P, Banbury DN, Byrne C (1998) Patterned acquisition of skin barrier function during development. Development 125(8):1541–1552
26. Youssef W, Wickett RR, Hoath SB (2001) Surface free energy characterization of vernix caseosa. Potential role in waterproofing the newborn infant. Skin Res Technol 7(1):10–17
27. Caspers PJ, Lucassen GW, Puppels GJ (2003) Combined in vivo confocal Raman spectroscopy and confocal microscopy of human skin. Biophys J 85(1):572–580
28. Verdier-Sevrain S, Bonte F (2007) Skin hydration: a review on its molecular mechanisms. J Cosmet Dermatol 6(2):75–82
29. Warner RR, Myers MC, Taylor DA (1988) Electron probe analysis of human skin: determination of the water concentration profile. J Invest Dermatol 90(2):218–224
30. Denda M et al (1998) Exposure to a dry environment enhances epidermal permeability barrier function. J Invest Dermatol 111(5):858–863
31. Denda M, Sato J, Tsuchiya T, Elias PM, Feingold KR (1998) Low humidity stimulates epidermal DNA synthesis and amplifies the hyperproliferative response to barrier disruption: implication for seasonal exacerbations of inflammatory dermatoses. J Invest Dermatol 111(5):873–878
32. Fluhr JW, Lazzerini S, Distante F, Gloor M, Berardesca E (1999) Effects of prolonged occlusion on stratum corneum barrier function and water holding capacity. Skin Pharmacol Appl Skin Physiol 12(4):193–198
33. Proksch E, Feingold KR, Man MQ, Elias PM (1991) Barrier function regulates epidermal DNA synthesis. J Clin Invest 87(5):1668–1673
34. Tansirikongkol A, Visscher MO, Wickett RR (2007) Water-handling properties of vernix caseosa and a synthetic analogue. J Cosmet Sci 58(6):651–662
35. Tollin M et al (2005) Vernix caseosa as a multi-component defence system based on polypeptides, lipids and their interactions. Cell Mol Life Sci 62(19–20): 2390–2399
36. Fu HC, Nicolaides N (1969) The structure of alkane diols of diesters in vernix caseosa lipids. Lipids 4(2):170–175
37. Haahti E, Nikkari T, Salmi AM, Laaksonen AL (1961) Fatty acids of vernix caseosa. Scand J Clin Lab Invest 13:70–73
38. Kaerkkaeinen J, Nikkari T, Ruponen S, Haahti E (1965) Lipids of vernix caseosa. J Invest Dermatol 44:333–338
39. Hauff S, Vetter W (2010) Exploring the fatty acids of vernix caseosa in form of their methyl esters by off-line coupling of non-aqueous reversed phase high performance liquid chromatography and gas chromatography coupled to mass spectrometry. J Chromatogr A 1217(52):8270–8278
40. Ran-Ressler RR, Devapatla S, Lawrence P, Brenna JT (2008) Branched chain fatty acids are constituents of the normal healthy newborn gastrointestinal tract. Pediatr Res 64(6):605–609

41. Wertz PW (2006) Biochemistry of human stratum corneum lipids. In: Elias P, Feingold K (eds) Skin barrier. Taylor & Francis, New York, pp 33–42
42. Huang HY et al (2007) Basic characteristics of sporolactobacillus inulinus BCRC 14647 for potential probiotic properties. Curr Microbiol 54(5):396–404
43. Veerkamp JH (1971) Fatty acid composition of bifidobacterium and lactobacillus strains. J Bacteriol 108(2):861–867
44. Narendran V, Visscher MO, Abril I, Hendrix SW, Hoath SB (2010) Biomarkers of epidermal innate immunity in premature and full-term infants. Pediatr Res 67(4):382–386
45. Bouwstra JA et al (1996) Phase behavior of isolated skin lipids. J Lipid Res 37(5):999–1011
46. Bouwstra JA et al (1991) Structural investigations of human stratum corneum by small-angle X-ray scattering: phase behavior of isolated skin lipids. J Invest Dermatol 97(6):1005–1012
47. Swartzendruber DC, Wertz PW, Madison KC, Downing DT (1987) Evidence that the corneocyte has a chemically bound lipid envelope. J Invest Dermatol 88(6):709–713
48. Williams ML, Hincenbergs M, Holbrook KA (1988) Skin lipid content during early fetal development. J Invest Dermatol 91(3):263–268
49. Freinkel RK, Fiedler-Weiss V (1974) Esterification of sterols during differentiation and cornification of developing rat epidermis. J Invest Dermatol 62(4):458–462
50. Tachi M, Iwamori M (2008) Mass spectrometric characterization of cholesterol esters and wax esters in epidermis of fetal, adult and keloidal human skin. Exp Dermatol 17(4):318–323
51. Downing DT, Strauss JS, Pochi PE (1969) Variability in the chemical composition of human skin surface lipids. J Invest Dermatol 53(5):322–327
52. Wysocki SJ, Grauaug A, O'Neill G, Hahnel R (1981) Lipids in forehead vernix from newborn infants. Biol Neonate 39(5–6):300–304
53. Narendran V, Pickens W, Wickett R, Hoath S (2000) Interaction between pulmonary surfactant and vernix: a potential mechanism for induction of amniotic fluid turbidity. Pediatr Res 48(1):120–124
54. Tansirikongkol A, Hoath SB, Pickens WL, Visscher MO, Wickett RR (2008) Equilibrium water content in native vernix and its cellular component. J Pharm Sci 97(2):985–994
55. Hoath SB, Pickens WL, Visscher MO (2006) The biology of vernix caseosa. Int J Cosmet Sci 28(5): 319–333
56. Bulienkov NA (2003) The role of system-forming modular water structures in self-organization of biological systems. J Mol Liquids 106(2–3):257–275
57. Hoath SB, Leahy DG (2003) The organization of human epidermis: functional epidermal units and phi proportionality. J Invest Dermatol 121(6):1440–1446
58. Akinbi HT, Narendran V, Pass AK, Markart P, Hoath SB (2004) Host defense proteins in vernix caseosa and amniotic fluid. Am J Obstet Gynecol 191(6):2090–2096
59. Gunt H (2002) Water handling properties of vernix caseosa. University of Cincinnati, Cincinnati
60. Tansirikongkol A (2006) Development of a synthetic vernix equivalent, and its water handling and barrier protective properties in comparison with vernix caseosa. PhD, University of Cincinnati, Cincinnati
61. Visscher M, Narendran V, Joseph W, Gunt H, Hoath S (2002) Development of topical eqidermal barriers for preterm infant skin: comparison of aquaphor and vernix caseosa. Pediatric Academic Society Annual Meeting, May 4-7, Baltimore, MD, USA
62. Visscher M, Hoath SB, Conroy E, Wickett RR (2001) Effect of semipermeable membranes on skin barrier repair following tape stripping. Arch Dermatol Res 293(10):491–499
63. Moraille R, Pickens WL, Visscher MO, Hoath SB (2005) A novel role for vernix caseosa as a skin cleanser. Biol Neonate 87(1):8–14
64. Hashimoto K (1970) The ultrastructure of the skin of human embryos. IX. Formation of the hair cone and intraepidermal hair canal. Arch Klin Exp Dermatol 238(4):333–345
65. Marchini G et al (2002) The newborn infant is protected by an innate antimicrobial barrier: peptide antibiotics are present in the skin and vernix caseosa. Br J Dermatol 147(6):1127–1134
66. Yoshio H et al (2003) Antimicrobial polypeptides of human vernix caseosa and amniotic fluid: implications for newborn innate defense. Pediatr Res 53(2): 211–216
67. Bouzari N, Kim N, Kirsner RS (2009) Defense of the skin with LL-37. J Invest Dermatol 129:814
68. Law S, Fotos PG, Wertz PW (1997) Skin surface lipids inhibit adherence of candida albicans to stratum corneum. Dermatology 195(3):220–223
69. Bautista MI, Wickett RR, Visscher MO, Pickens WL, Hoath SB (2000) Characterization of vernix caseosa as a natural biofilm: comparison to standard oil-based ointments. Pediatr Dermatol 17(4):253–260
70. Visscher M, Maganti S, Munson KA, Bare DE, Hoath SB (1999) Early adaptation of human skin following birth: a biophysical assessment. Skin Res Technol 5:213–220
71. Visscher MO, Chatterjee R, Munson KA, Pickens WL, Hoath SB (2000) Changes in diapered and nondiapered infant skin over the first month of life. Pediatr Dermatol 17(1):45–51
72. Nikolovski J, Stamatas GN, Kollias N, Wiegand BC (2008) Barrier function and water-holding and transport properties of infant stratum corneum are different from adult and continue to develop through the first year of life. J Invest Dermatol 128(7):1728–1736
73. Visscher MO et al (2005) Vernix caseosa in neonatal adaptation. J Perinatol 25(7):440–446
74. Visscher MO et al (2011) Neonatal skin maturation-vernix caseosa and free amino acids. Pediatr Dermatol 28(2):122–132
75. Schmid-Wendtner MH, Korting HC (2006) The pH of the skin surface and its impact on the barrier function. Skin Pharmacol Physiol 19(6):296–302

76. Rippke F, Schreiner V, Schwanitz HJ (2002) The acidic milieu of the horny layer: new findings on the physiology and pathophysiology of skin pH. Am J Clin Dermatol 3(4):261–272
77. Aly R, Shirley C, Cunico B, Maibach HI (1978) Effect of prolonged occlusion on the microbial flora, pH, carbon dioxide and transepidermal water loss on human skin. J Invest Dermatol 71(6):378–381
78. Puhvel SM, Reisner RM, Amirian DA (1975) Quantification of bacteria in isolated pilosebaceous follicles in normal skin. J Invest Dermatol 65(6):525–531
79. Fluhr JW et al (2001) Generation of free fatty acids from phospholipids regulates stratum corneum acidification and integrity. J Invest Dermatol 117(1):44–51
80. Hoeger PH, Enzmann CC (2002) Skin physiology of the neonate and young infant: a prospective study of functional skin parameters during early infancy. Pediatr Dermatol 19(3):256–262
81. Yosipovitch G, Maayan-Metzger A, Merlob P, Sirota L (2000) Skin barrier properties in different body areas in neonates. Pediatrics 106(1 Pt 1):105–108
82. Fluhr JW et al (2009) Topical peroxisome proliferator activated receptor activators accelerate postnatal stratum corneum acidification. J Invest Dermatol 129:365–374, Epub 2008 Aug 14
83. Hachem JP et al (2010) Acute acidification of stratum corneum membrane domains using polyhydroxyl acids improves lipid processing and inhibits degradation of corneodesmosomes. J Invest Dermatol 130(2):500–510
84. Hatano Y et al (2009) Maintenance of an acidic stratum corneum prevents emergence of murine atopic dermatitis. J Invest Dermatol 129(7):1824–1835
85. Darmstadt GL et al (2002) Impact of topical oils on the skin barrier: possible implications for neonatal health in developing countries. Acta Paediatr 91(5):546–554
86. Schurer NY (2002) Implementation of fatty acid carriers to skin irritation and the epidermal barrier. Contact Dermatitis 47(4):199–205
87. Darmstadt GL et al (2005) Effect of topical treatment with skin barrier-enhancing emollients on nosocomial infections in preterm infants in Bangladesh: a randomised controlled trial. Lancet 365(9464):1039–1045
88. Yang L, Mao-Qiang M, Taljebini M, Elias PM, Feingold KR (1995) Topical stratum corneum lipids accelerate barrier repair after tape stripping, solvent treatment and some but not all types of detergent treatment. Br J Dermatol 133(5):679–685
89. Kessner D, Ruettinger A, Kiselev MA, Wartewig S, Neubert RH (2008) Properties of ceramides and their impact on the stratum corneum structure. Part 2: Stratum corneum lipid model systems. Skin Pharmacol Physiol 21(2):58–74
90. Elias PM, Mao-Qiang M, Thornfeldt CR, Feingold KR (1999) The epidermal permeability barrier: effects of physiologic and non-physiologic lipids. In: Hoppe U (ed) The lanolin book. Beiersdorf AG, Hamburg, pp 253–279
91. Tansirikongkol A, Wickett RR, Visscher MO, Hoath SB (2007) Effect of vernix caseosa on the penetration of chymotryptic enzyme: potential role in epidermal barrier development. Pediatr Res 62(1):49–53
92. Narendran V, Pickens WL, Visscher MO, Alla SK, Hoath SB (2010) Binding of unconjugated bilirubin to human epidermis and vernix caseosa: the physiological basis of jaundice. Society for Pediatric Research, May 1-4, Vancouver, Canada
93. Hoath S, Narendran V (2000) Adhesives and emollients in newborn care. Semin Neonatol 5(289–296)
94. Rutter N (1996) The immature skin. Eur J Pediatr 155(Suppl 2):S18–S20
95. Darmstadt GL, Dinulos JG (2000) Neonatal skin care. Pediatr Clin North Am 47(4):757–782
96. Agren J, Sjors G, Sedin G (1998) Transepidermal water loss in infants born at 24 and 25 weeks of gestation. Acta Paediatr 87(11):1185–1190
97. Harpin VA, Rutter N (1983) Barrier properties of the newborn infant's skin. J Pediatr 102(3):419–425
98. Kalia YN, Nonato LB, Lund CH, Guy RH (1998) Development of skin barrier function in premature infants. J Invest Dermatol 111(2):320–326
99. Nonato LB, Lund CH, Kalia YN, Guy RH (2000) Transepidermal water loss in 24 and 25 weeks gestational age infants. Acta Paediatr 89(6):747–748
100. Edwards WH, Conner JM, Soll RF (2004) The effect of prophylactic ointment therapy on nosocomial sepsis rates and skin integrity in infants with birth weights of 501 to 1000 g. Pediatrics 113(5):1195–1203
101. Nopper AJ et al (1996) Topical ointment therapy benefits premature infants. J Pediatr 128(5 Pt 1): 660–669
102. Pabst RC, Starr KP, Qaiyumi S, Schwalbe RS, Gewolb IH (1999) The effect of application of aquaphor on skin condition, fluid requirements, and bacterial colonization in very low birth weight infants. J Perinatol 19(4):278–283
103. Zhukov BN, Neverova EI, Nikitin KE, Kostiaev VE, Myshentsev PN (1992) A comparative evaluation of the use of vernix caseosa and solcoseryl in treating patients with trophic ulcers of the lower extremities. Vestn Khir Im I I Grek 148(6):339–341
104. Oudshoorn MH et al (2009) Development of a murine model to evaluate the effect of vernix caseosa on skin barrier recovery. Exp Dermatol 18(2):178–184
105. Visscher MO, Barai N, LaRuffa AA, Pickens WL, Narendran V, Hoath SB (2011) Epidermal barrier treatments based on vernix caseosa. Skin Pharmacol Physiol 24:322–329
106. Sedin G, Hammarlund K, Stromberg B (1983) Transepidermal water loss in full-term and pre-term infants. Acta Paediatr Scand Suppl 305:27–31
107. Visscher M, Robinson M, Wickett R (2011) Stratum corneum free amino acids following barrier perturbation and repair. Int J Cosmet Sci 33(1):80–89
108. Barai N (2005) Effect of vernix caseosa on epidermal barrier maturation and repair: implications in wound healing. PhD, University of Cincinnati, Cincinnati

109. Oudshoorn MH et al (2009) Development of a murine model to evaluate the effect of vernix caseosa on skin barrier recovery. Exp Dermatol 18(2): 178–184
110. Rissmann R et al (2008) Lanolin-derived lipid mixtures mimic closely the lipid composition and organization of vernix caseosa lipids. Biochim Biophys Acta 1778(10):2350–2360
111. Rissmann R et al (2009) Mimicking vernix caseosa – preparation and characterization of synthetic biofilms. Int J Pharm 372(1–2):59–65
112. Oudshoorn MH et al (2009) Effect of synthetic vernix biofilms on barrier recovery of damaged mouse skin. Exp Dermatol 18:695–703
113. Wakai R, Lengle J, Leuthold A (2000) Transmission of electric and magnetic foetal cardiac signals in a case of ectopia cordis: the dominant role of the vernix caseosa. Phys Med Biol 45(7):1989–1995
114. Anonymous (2009) Newborn care until the first week of life. World Health Organization, Geneva, Switzerland

14 The Role of Tight Junctions and Aquaporins in Skin Dryness

J.M. Brandner

14.1 Introduction

The water content of the *stratum corneum* (SC) and the viable layers of the epidermis have a major influence on physical properties and appearance of the skin. Adequate water supply is necessary for enzymatic processes which are, e.g. required for normal desquamation and barrier formation/maintenance. Further, SC hydration also seems to fulfil a biosensor function, as it appears to be directly linked to epidermal hyperplasia and inflammation [20, 71]. To obtain optimal water content, water uptake into the epidermis, water (and solute) transport through the epidermis, water binding in the SC and the transepidermal water loss (TEWL) have to be orchestrated. Imbalance results in roughness, scaling, flaking and dryness of the skin. Reduced SC hydration is found in several skin diseases, including psoriasis, atopic dermatitis, eczema, hereditary ichthyosis as well as in senile xerosis and UV-exposed skin (for review see [110]).

J.M. Brandner
Department of Dermatology and Venerology, University-Hospital Hamburg-Eppendorf, Martinistrasse 52, Hamburg, 20246, Germany
e-mail: brandner@uke.de

The concentration profile of water in the epidermis is very characteristic. While water content in the viable epidermis is high (up to 70%), it distinctly decreases at the border between *stratum granulosum* (SG) and SC (15–35% water) (for review see [110]). Water transport through the epidermis can occur transcellular, i.e. through the cells, e.g. via aquaporins (AQPs), and paracellular, i.e. through the extracellular space, which is controlled by tight junctions (TJs) (Figs. 14.1 and 14.2). Of note, AQPs are only present in the living cell layers with a (slight) decrease of the main AQP, AQP3, in the SG, and barrier-forming TJs are only found in the SG. This hints for a role of these proteins/structures in formation of the water gradient and therefore of skin hydration. Several experimental data strengthen this hypothesis as will be shown in the following sections.

14.2 Aquaporins

AQPs are six-membrane spanning transmembrane proteins with a molecular weight of ca. 30 kDa. They are thought to form tetramers in the membrane with independently functioning pores [28, 109]. In mammalian, the family of aquaporins comprises 13 members (AQP0–12). All of them transport water in response to osmotic gradients, but a subgroup, the so-called aquaglyceroporins (AQP3, 7, 9, 10), also transports glycerol and (possibly) other small molecules (for reviews see [2, 9, 111, 122]).

M. Lodén, H.I. Maibach (eds.), *Treatment of Dry Skin Syndrome*,
DOI 10.1007/978-3-642-27606-4_14,

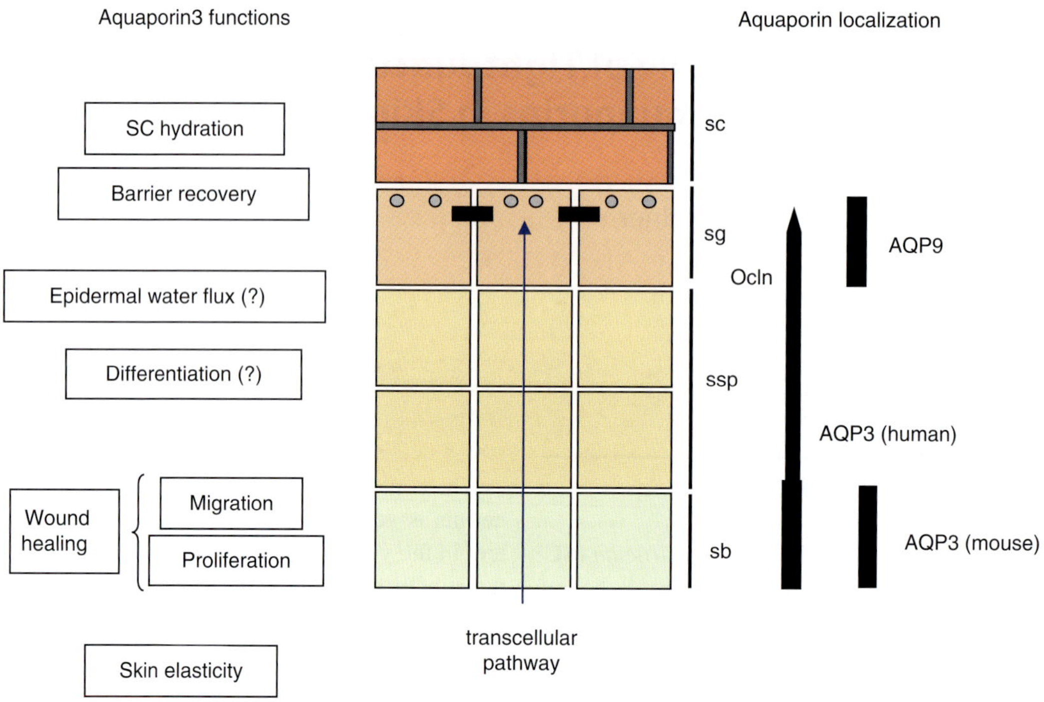

Fig. 14.1 Schematic drawing of the localization of aquaporins in human and mouse epidermis and the (putative) functions of AQPs. mRNA coding for AQP10 has also been demonstrated in human keratinocytes, but its localization has not been shown as yet. *SC* stratum corneum, *SG* stratum granulosum, *SSP* stratum spinosum, *SB* stratum basale. *Grey circles*: lamellar bodies; (?): function proposed and experimentally supported but not as yet unambiguously shown. *Blue arrow*: AQPs facilitate the transcellular pathway of water and glycerol

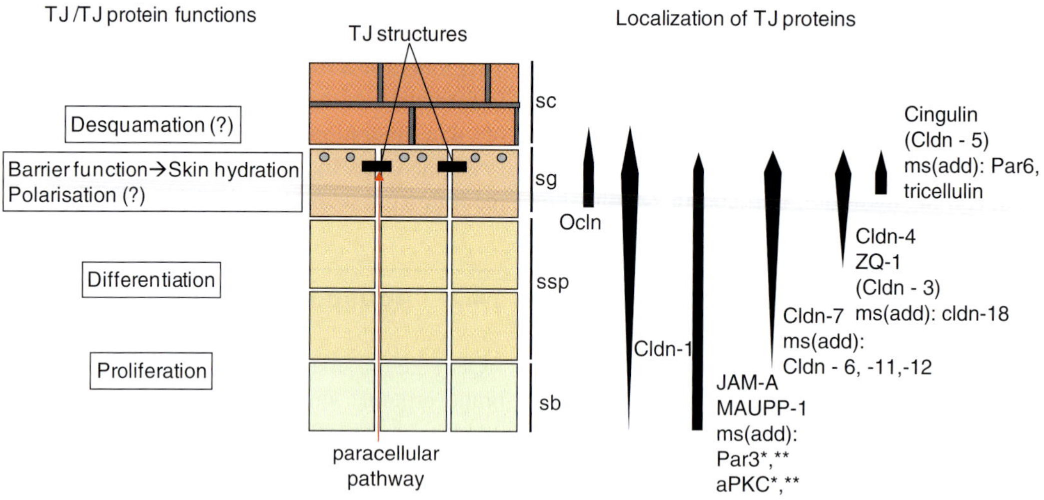

Fig. 14.2 Schematic drawing of the localization of TJ structures and TJ proteins in human and mouse epidermis and the (putative) functions of TJs and TJ proteins. mRNAs coding for Cldn-8 (human and mouse) and Cldn-2, -11, -12, -15, 17 and 23 (human) have also been detected in keratinocytes, but their localization has not been shown as yet. *SC* stratum corneum, *SG* stratum granulosum, *SSP* stratum spinosum, *SB* stratum basale. *Grey circles*: lamellar bodies. *: different isoforms show different localization; **: membrane and cytoplasmic localization; (): very faint staining; (?): function proposed and experimentally supported but not as yet unambiguously shown. *Red arrow*: TJ are barriers for the paracellular pathway of solutes

Mammalian AQPs are found in simple epithelial and endothelial cells involved in fluid transport (e.g. kidney), in brain glial cells, in the epidermis and in adipocytes. Their functions – often demonstrated by knockout mice and by the rare patients with loss of AQP subtypes – are as manifold as their localizations. For example, they are involved in the urinary-concentrating function (AQP1–4, kidney), glandular fluid secretion (e.g. AQP5, AQP1 salivary and airway submucosal glands, choroid plexus and ciliary epithelium), brain water balance (AQP4), cell migration (e.g. AQP1, AQP3; brain astroglial cells, corneal epithelial cells, skin cells and tumour cells), cell proliferation (e.g. AQP3), epidermal hydration (AQP3) and adipocyte function (AQP7) (for review see [112]).

14.2.1 Aquaporins in the Skin

Several aquaporins have been identified in the skin: AQP1 was found by immunostaining in capillary endothelial cells [81] as well as by RT-PCR in cultured melanocytes [12]. AQP3 was demonstrated in keratinocytes (e.g. [41, 68, 72, 97, 100]) and fibroblasts [16] as well as Langerhans cells and dermal dendritic cells [70]. In addition, it was found in hair follicles and sebaceous glands [3]. Interestingly, while AQP3 was described to be mainly restricted to the basal cell layer of adult mouse skin (e.g. [12, 40, 41, 68]), it was detected in several layers of human skin with a (slightly) more intense staining in the basal cell layer. It is absent in the (uppermost) granular layer(s) and in the SC (Fig. 14.1) ([8, 12, 40, 51, 65, 97], slight differences of stainings are seen between different publications). AQP5 is present in sweat glands and was shown to play a role in sweat secretion [81]. AQP7 was found in adipocytes and seems to be important for glycerol release into the plasma [37]. AQP9 was described in the SG of mouse epidermis [89]; its presence was also confirmed in differentiated cultured human keratinocytes [100] and human skin [99]. mRNA coding for AQP10 was identified in (undifferentiated) human keratinocytes [12, 100]. Its localization is still unknown.

14.2.2 Functions of Epidermal Aquaporins

Because skin hydration mainly depends on epidermal AQP function, this chapter will concentrate on aquaporins present in keratinocytes, i.e. AQP3, 9 and 10, even though it cannot be excluded that AQPs of, e.g. sebaceous glands, may be involved in skin hydration [27].

14.2.2.1 AQP3

AQP3 is an aquaglyceroporin, i.e. it transports water and glycerol. Also a permeability for urea is discussed [48]. In keratinocytes, AQP3 colocalizes with phospholipase D2 in caveolin-rich membrane microdomains (lipid rafts) and might transport glycerol to phospholipase D2 which synthesizes phophatidylglycerol, a bioactive lipid involved in keratinocyte function [126]. In addition, a colocalization with E-cadherin was described [51], a protein important for the formation of cell-cell contacts.

Mice deficient of AQP3 exhibit impaired *SC hydration*, reduced *skin elasticity* and delayed recovery of *barrier function* after removal of the SC. In addition, slowed *wound healing* was observed [38, 41, 42, 68]. Epidermal cells of AQP3 KO mice showed more than fourfold reduced osmotic water permeability and more than twofold reduced glycerol permeability [68]. The authors demonstrated a significantly reduced *glycerol content* in SC and epidermis while there was no difference in SC structure and its content of ions and small solutes as well as lipids and free amino acids [41, 42]. Further investigations showed that the reduced levels of glycerol in skin were responsible for the decreased SC hydration as well as delayed barrier recovery and reduced skin elasticity because these deficiencies could be corrected by supplementation with glycerol (topical, oral and intraperitoneal), but not by occlusion or high humidity [42]. However, because oral and i.p. supplementation improved epidermal and SC glycerol content as well as SC hydration and barrier recovery in wild-type and in AQP3-deficient mice, there have to be AQP-3-independent pathways for the uptake of glycerol into the epidermis. One possibility could be glycerol provided from sebaceous glands [26].

Boury-Jamot (2006) demonstrated that after consecutive tape stripping in wild-type (wt) as well as AQP3-deficient mice, hyperplasia was observed. In wild-type mice, AQP3 was localized in all hyperplastic layers. Interestingly, in knock-out (KO) mice, intercellular oedema was present in the hyperplastic layers. This hints for a role of AQP3 in *water movement* especially in 'thicker' epidermis which might therefore also apply especially for human skin. This is supported by Agren et al. [3] who described in rat embryonic skin – which has increased transepidermal water loss (TEWL) – an elevated expression of AQP3 and a localization of the proteins in more layers compared to adult skin.

Delayed wound healing in AQP3-deficient mice was shown to be a consequence of impaired *migration* as well as decreased *proliferation* of keratinocytes [38]. Knockdown of AQP3 in human and mouse keratinocytes results in decreased lamellipodia formation at the leading edge of the cells, impaired migration in a chemotactic driven transwell assay and delayed wound healing in a cell scratch assay. Because the migration defect can be rescued by transfection with AQP3 as well as AQP1 – the latter being an exclusive water channel – the involvement of water flux in migration is likely. Further, KO mice as well as AQP3-siRNA-treated human keratinocytes show decreased numbers of proliferative cells at the wound margins, a mechanism which seems to involve p38 (and JNK). The impaired proliferation can be rescued by oral glycerol supplementation in mice, and AQP3, but not AQP1, transfection in cultured keratinocytes, hinting for a major effect of glycerol in proliferation [38]. Glycerol may play an important role for the generation of energy in form of ATP which, in turn, is necessary to drive the cellular processes of proliferation. Decreased levels of ATP were detected in mouse AQP3 KO keratinocytes as well as human AQP3-siRNA-treated keratinocytes and a positive correlation between glycerol content, ATP content and proliferation of the cells was observed. Addition of glycerol-3-phosphate, an important intermediate for glycerol-driven ATP generation, restores the ATP levels in AQP3-deficient cells [39]. Of note, wound healing cannot be completely restored by addition of glycerol, emphasizing the important role of water movement for migration and therefore wound healing [38].

The importance of AQP3 for cell *migration* and wound healing is also confirmed by further data. Epidermal growth factor (EGF) increases cell migration and wound healing in human fibroblasts and HaCaT keratinocytes [16]. This is accompanied by a time- and dose-dependent increase of AQP3. EGF-induced cell migration is reduced by inhibitors of water and glycerol transport through AQPs and by a knockdown of AQP3. EGF receptor, ERK and PI3K are likely to play a role in the AQP3-mediated cell migration [16].

The role of AQP3 in cell *proliferation* is supported by findings that overexpression of AQP3 in human keratinocytes results in increased [79] decrease of AQP3 in decreased cell counts [51], even though the authors did not specifically look for proliferation in their experiments. Straseski et al. [98] have shown that hypoxia results in a downregulation of APQ3, and this is accompanied by a decrease of basal keratinocyte proliferation in human skin equivalents. Further, treatment with retinoic acid resulted in a less increase of proliferative cells in the epidermis of AQP3 KO mice than in wild-type mice [40]. And finally, mice which are deficient for 3β-hydroxysterol-Δ24-reductase, an enzyme converting desmosterol to cholesterol, exhibit increased proliferation as well as elevated levels of AQP3 and increased water and glycerol content in the epidermis. This hints for a correlation of AQP3 levels and proliferation, even though the epidermis also shows further alterations, e.g. decreased levels of cholesterol and impaired differentiation which also may play a role in altered proliferation [74, 75]. Summarizing all these data, proliferation of keratinocytes clearly seems to be associated with AQP3 levels.

The role of AQP3 in *differentiation* of keratinocytes is a matter of debate. Zheng and Bollinger-Bollag [126] described that the induction of differentiation by 1,25 dihydroxyvitamin D_3 or high concentrations of extracellular calcium result in a downregulation of AQP3 in murine keratinocytes [126]. In addition, this group showed that overexpression of AQP3 decreased the promoter activity of keratin 5 and increased that of keratin 10 [10], again hinting for an inhibiting effect of AQP3 on differentiation. In line with these results, Kim and Lee [51] observed a decrease of the differentiation markers K10, involucrin and loricrin in AQP3-deficient human keratinocytes, even though they did not find an alteration for K14 (which is coexpressed with K5 in undifferentiated keratinocytes). However, the group of Hara-Chikuma did not observe a difference of K5, K14, K10, involucrin or loricrin in low or high Ca conditions or in the course of differentiation induced by VD3 in knockdown experiments of human and mouse keratinocytes [40], and overexpression of AQP3 resulted in increased mRNA levels of K5 and K14 while there was no alteration for K1 and K10 [79]. The causes for these discrepancies are not clear at the moment; different experimental systems may play a role.

Interestingly, Roudier et al. [90] described two AQP3-deficient patients who were identified during the screening of individuals producing alloantibodies against so far unidentified high-frequency antigens on red blood cells. These patients did not show any obvious clinical symptoms. However, the same is true for AQP1-deficient patients, but they show defects in stress conditions [52]. Therefore, future investigations are necessary to clarify the phenotype of AQP3-deficient patients in 'non-normal' conditions.

14.2.2.2 AQP9 and 10

AQP9 and 10 are also aquaglyceroporins. Up to now, their roles in the epidermis are unknown. AQP9 localization is found in more layers in hypertrophic skin after wounding compared to normal mouse skin. However, AQP9-deficient mice do neither show a wound healing defect nor any other obvious skin phenotype [89]. Of note, AQP9 is downregulated in psoriatic lesions (see below).

14.2.3 AQPs in Skin Diseases and Skin Ageing

Several skin diseases, as well as aged skin, are characterized by dry skin and therefore have deficits in skin hydration. Therefore, it is of special interest to investigate the role of AQPs in these diseases.

In *atopic dermatitis* (*AD*), an *upregulation* of AQP3 was observed on mRNA and protein level, and immunostaining revealed increased staining intensity especially in the *stratum spinosum* (SSP). Also in non-lesional skin, a mild alteration of AQP3 staining was observed [84]. The authors suggest that increased AQP3 expression results in enhanced water transport to the SC and might, together with the impaired water holding capacity in skin of patients with atopic dermatitis, result in increased loss of water and dry skin. The upregulation of AQP3 in AD, especially in suprabasal layers, was confirmed by Nakahigashi et al. [79]. They further investigated AQP3 in an AD mouse model where they also found an upregulation of AQP3. CCL17, which is highly expressed in AD skin, induces upregulation of AQP3 and leads to an AQP3-dependent increase of proliferation in HaCaT keratinocytes. Consequently, when inducing AD in AQP3-deficient mice, they observed decreased hyperplasia and decreased numbers of proliferative cells [79]. These data suggest that AQP3 not only plays a role in increased TEWL but also in hyperproliferation in AD.

In a study investigating three patients suffering from *eczema*, with or without intercellular *oedema*, AQP3 was *absent* in cases with oedema. This might hint for a relationship between the loss of AQP3 and intercellular oedema, i.e. defect in water movement, and supports data found in AQP3-deficient mice after consecutive tape stripping (see also above; [12]).

In 8 out of 10 patients with *psoriasis*, *cytoplasmic* instead of cell border staining of *AQP3* was observed [114]. A comparison of mRNA levels of lesional versus non-lesional skin before and 12 weeks after etanercept – a TNFα and TNFβ binding protein – treatment showed a *downregulation* of *AQP9* in lesional skin which is not completely reversed by etanercept [99]. As AQP3 is not mentioned in this manuscript, its expression does not seem to be significantly different between lesional and non-lesional skin.

In depigmented areas of *vitiligo* patients – which exhibit reduced SC hydration but no alteration of

TEWL [66] – *decreased* levels of AQP3 were observed. A downregulation of AQP3 via RNAi in human primary keratinocytes results in decreased levels of phospho-PI3K, E-cadherin, β-catenin and γ-catenin, molecules known to be downregulated in vitiligo [51]. In addition, it results in reduced cell counts (see above). The authors suggest that the decreased amount of keratinocytes results in decreased levels of growth factors and therefore demise of melanocytes.

A decrease of AQP3 expression was also described during *skin ageing* [21, 65]. Of note, the loss of AQP3 was mainly found in the suprabasal layers [65].

The role of AQP3 in *skin cancer* is a matter of debate. The group of Verkman showed that AQP3-deficient mice develop less papilloma in a two-step skin carcinoma model, mainly due to decreased susceptibility to tumour promoter (TPA)-induced proliferation. In addition, they described strong expression of AQP3 in 40 cases of squamous cell carcinoma (SSC) [39] and suggest therefore a *tumour-promoting* potential of AQP3. Unfortunately, it was not shown whether the expression of AQP3 in SSC compared to normal skin is up- or downregulated (or not changed at all). Voss et al. [114] demonstrated a downregulation of AQP3 in basal cell carcinoma compared to normal skin and a patchy staining in SCC with decreased staining intensity in highly proliferative areas and suggest therefore that *downregulation* of AQP3 may be a marker for tumourigenic potential, but the number of cases investigated was quite small (13 BCC, 5 SCC). Horie and colleagues [46] demonstrated the presence of AQP3 in the cutaneous squamous cell carcinoma cell line DJM-1, Nakakoshi et al. [80] in one out of three keratocarcinoma cell lines. Further investigations using a larger number of SCC but also precursor lesions, e.g. actinic keratosis and Bowen's disease, and comparison of the stainings with healthy skin as well as correlating them with different grades of SCC and its precursors may help to elucidate the role of AQP3 in skin cancer. However, as long as there are doubts about the impact of upregulation of AQP3 on skin carcinogenesis, this should be carefully observed.

14.2.4 Alteration of AQPs by External Stimuli

UV irradiation of HaCaT keratinocytes results in a dose- and time-dependent *downregulation* of AQP3 by a signalling pathway which involves MEK/ERK, but not p38 and JNK. It might be mediated by reactive oxygen species [17]. This is accompanied by decreased water permeability of the HaCaT cells [50]. A slight decrease of AQP3 expression was also described in a group of 10 Asian women in *sun-exposed skin*. Of note, this decrease is only observed in females more than 40 years of age [22].

Hypoxia leads to a reversible *decrease* of AQP3, especially in the granular cell layer, of human skin equivalents (HSEs). In addition, filaggrin, E-cadherin and β-catenin are downregulated, and the transcription factor slug is upregulated. The HSEs further exhibit reduced proliferation of basal keratinocytes and swelling in the stratum granulosum [98].

H_2O_2 leads to a time- and dose-dependent *downregulation* of AQP3 in HaCaT cells [17].

Tape stripping results in an *upregulation* of AQP3 in human skin explants [22, 31]. Dumas et al. suggest that the upregulation of AQP3 ensures that the cells have the necessary water-rich environment to rebuild skin barrier. More detailed investigation of AQP3 after barrier disruption will surely be interesting. Consecutive tape stripping of mouse skin results in hyperplasia and a localization of AQP3 in all living layers, comparable to human skin [12].

Osmotic stress by various molecules results in an *upregulation* of AQP3 mRNA [31, 100].

14.2.5 Influence of Cytokines and Growth Factors on AQP3

TNFα – a cytokine often increased in inflammatory dermatoses characterized by dry skin – *decreases* AQP3 protein expression levels and water permeability in the cutaneous squamous cell carcinoma line DMJ1. The mechanism involves TNF receptor 1 as well as p38 and ERK, but not NFκB [46].

EGF induces an *upregulation* of AQP3 in a time- and dose-dependent manner in cultured human fibroblasts and HaCaT keratinocytes. EGFR, PI3K and ERK are involved in this upregulation which is accompanied by accelerated migration of the cells [16].

14.2.6 Influence of External Applied Substances on AQP3

All-trans retinoic acid (ATRA), a substance often used in dermatology, results in an *upregulation* of mRNA and protein levels of AQP3 in human primary keratinocytes and HaCaT cells, in topically treated human skin explants and in mouse skin [8, 17, 40]. The upregulation is likely (among others) to be mediated by transactivation of EGFR and ERK signalling because their inhibition abolishes the effect of ATRA on AQP3 in HaCaT cells [17, 96]. Upregulation of AQP3 is accompanied by an upregulation of K5 and K14 as well as an increase of BrdU-labelled cells which are absent/reduced in AQP3 KO mice [40]. Pre-treatment of cells with ATRA attenuates UV (and H_2O_2)-induced downregulation of AQP3 in HaCaT cells [17]. On the other hand, pre-treatment of cells with *nicotinamide* attenuates the effect of ATRA on AQP3, even though nicotinamide itself only decreases AQP3 expression at very high concentrations [96]. This is of special interest as topical treatment of skin with ATRA improves the clinical and histological appearance of photo-damaged skin [25] but frequently shows skin dryness as a side effect. Topical nicotinamide application on dry human skin seems to improve epidermal barrier function, and myristyl nicotinate provides tolerability of retinoic acid [49, 101].

An *extract from Ajuga turkestanica*, a plant from Central Asia, was described to *increase* AQP3 in human-reconstructed epidermis. In in vivo studies, the extract resulted in decreased TEWL after 21 days of treatment in tape-stripped skin, but a direct correlation of AQP3 and this effect was not investigated in the volunteers [22].

A *hydroglycolic extract of Piptadenia colubrina (HEPC)*, a tree from the South American rain forest, *increases* the mRNA levels of AQP3 in human keratinocytes in a dose- and time-dependent manner. In addition, also the levels of filaggrin and involucrin are increased. Investigation of volunteers treated with HEPC or placebo showed an increased glycerol content and increased skin capacitance in the HEPC group, but the authors did not specifically investigate the levels of AQP3 (and filaggrin and involucrin) n these volunteers [86]. The same group also described an *upregulating* effect of *green Coffea Arabica L. seed oil* (GCO) on AQP3 in keratinocytes (as well as collagen, elastin, glycosaminoglycan, TGF-β1 and GM-CSF) [108].

Trans-zeatin, a cytokinin plant growth factor derived from Zea Mays, *induces* AQP3 expression and reduces UV-induced loss of AQP3 and activation of MEK/ERK. In addition, it attenuates UV-induced decreased water permeability and wound healing delay in HaCaT keratinocytes [50].

A purified *Ceratonia siliqua (carob) seed extract* which is rich in amino acids and peptides corresponding to conserved motifs in the pore channel of aquaporins also results in an *increased* staining intensity of AQP3 in human keratinocytes. It also further increases the osmotic stress (sorbitol) or tape-stripping-induced upregulation of AQP3 in keratinocytes/skin. Of note, the upregulation of AQP3 seems to protect keratinocytes from cold stress. Treatment of volunteers with dry skin with the carob seed extract result in 'healthier appearance'; a correlation to AQP3 levels was not investigated [31].

A diet for 4 weeks with 4.5% *Bakkokinanjinto (BKN)*, a herbal medicine which reduces diuresis, thirst and pruritus in patients with diabetes mellitus results in an *increase* of AQP2 in kidney and AQP3 in the skin in KKAy mice, a model system for diabetes type 2. The authors suggest that the upregulation of AQP may contribute to the reduction of pruritus in skin which is in turn caused by dry skin [1]. It is not known whether KKAy mice show reduced levels of AQP3 in skin compared to wild-type mice of the same background which would be a very interesting information concerning the role of AQP3 in pruritus in diabetes.

14.2.7 Specific Modulation of AQPs

An up- or downregulation of AQP3, dependent on skin condition and additional external influences, might be beneficial to restore normal AQP levels in the skin and therefore improve skin dryness and clinical symptoms. For example, in atopic dermatitis or ATRA-pre-treated skin which show increased AQP3 levels, a downregulation might be advantageous, while in UV-irradiated or aged skin, which show decreased levels, an upregulation may be favourable. The putative influence of AQP3 levels on skin carcinogenesis should be kept in mind.

For an optimized modulation of AQPs, specific inhibitors or activators are desirable. However, even though several AQP inhibitors exist, e.g. sulfhydryl-reactive mercurials, they are non-selective between the various AQPs and toxic. The development of subtype specific inhibitors, which also have access to the appropriate organs (e.g. inhibitors for AQP4 will have to cross the blood–brain barrier), will be a challenge for the future. The same is true for AQP enhancers. Because AQPs may already have maximal per channel function, an increase of function can only be achieved on expression level. Substances used so far to upregulate AQP3 also influence other proteins. Therefore, the development of AQP-selective transcriptional upregulators will be necessary.

14.3 Tight Junctions

Tight junctions (TJs) are cell-cell junctions localized at the apical part of the lateral plasma membranes of cells. They are composed of transmembrane proteins, e.g. the family of claudins (Cldns), occludin (Ocln), tricellulin and the family of junctional adhesion molecules (JAMs), as well as cytoplasmic plaque proteins, e.g. zonula occludens (ZO) proteins, MUPP-1, cingulin, symplekin and the cell polarity complex proteins aPKC, Par3 and Par6. The particular composition of TJs depends on the cell type, differentiation of the cells and physiologic and non-physiologic stimuli. In transmission electron microscopy, TJs are identified as sites of close membrane contact ('kissing points'); in freeze fracture electron microscopy, networks of TJ strands are typical for simple epithelia. TJs were identified in simple and multilayered epithelia as well as endothelia. TJ proteins are also found in additional cell types, e.g. neutrophils or dendritic cells. TJs and TJ proteins are involved in (1) barrier function for the paracellular pathway of ions, water, small molecules and inflammatory cells, (2) the formation of a barrier between the apical and the basolateral plasma membrane domains of the cells to prevent intramembrane diffusion of lipids and proteins ('fence function') which is important for cell polarity, (3) the regulation of gene expression on transcriptional and translational level, (4) cell proliferation, (5) cell differentiation and (6) vesicle transport (for reviews see: [4, 7, 23, 30, 55, 57, 93, 107]).

14.3.1 TJs and TJ Proteins in the Skin

A variety of TJ transmembrane proteins, i.e. several Cldns, Ocln, tricellulin and JAM-A as well as TJ plaque proteins, e.g. the TJ scaffolding/adaptor proteins ZO-1, ZO-2 and MUPP-1 and the cell polarity proteins aPKC, Par3 and Par6, have been identified in mammalian epidermis (Fig. 14.2; for reviews see: [15, 82]). Further, several TJ proteins were identified in hair follicles and sweat glands in human and murine skin [14, 61, 76, 118] as well as in dermal blood vessels [67, 77].

The localization patterns of TJ proteins in the epidermis are very complex. For example, Cldn-1 is found in all epidermal layers, while Ocln is restricted to the *stratum granulosum* (SG) and Cldn-4 is found in the upper layers of the epidermis. All TJ proteins colocalize in the SG, and in horizontal sections, it could be shown that the TJ proteins encircle the cells entirely in this layer [13, 58]. In addition, typical TJ structures were found at the lateral plasma membranes of SG cells by transmission electron microscopy [13, 29, 55, 87, 123]. However, typical extended networks of TJ strands known from freeze-fracture experiments of simple epithelia remain to be shown in the SG, even though TJ-like structures have been demonstrated at the border between SG and SC [92].

14.3.2 Functions of TJs and TJ Proteins in the Epidermis

The skin provides an important barrier for the body. It prevents the uncontrolled loss of water and solutes and protects the body from external assaults (e.g. invasion of pathogens, penetration of harmful substances and UV irradiation). Besides the very well-established contribution of the SC, TJs have also been shown to be involved in *barrier function* of the skin. The function of TJs as a barrier for dermal supplied tracers was first suggested in human skin by electron microscopical investigations using lanthanum [43] and was later confirmed in mouse and men for the first time on light microscopic level by using a biotinylation reagent which biotinylate proteins extracellular and is stopped at TJs [29, 55]. Several authors have confirmed these experiments (e.g. [64, 95, 105, 125]). The importance of the TJ barrier for skin barrier function is demonstrated by Cldn-1 KO mice which exhibit leaky TJs for the biotinylation reagent and which die at the first day of birth due to a tremendous TEWL [29]. The same is true for epidermal E-cadherin-deficient mice which also exhibit a loss of Cldn-1 in the SG [105]. In human, the loss of Cldn-1 is apparently not lethal but results in the NISCH syndrome (neonatal ichthyosis sclerosing cholangitis; [24, 34]; OMIM # 607626) which comprises a severe skin disease with dry skin. However, one cannot completely exclude lethality in human, because up to now, only very few cases of Cldn-1-deficient patients have been identified, which might be due to high lethality during development without diagnosis. On the other hand, the period of embryonic development is much longer in human than in men; therefore, compensation mechanism might take effect in human which are not present in mice, preventing the death of the patients. Of note, skin from Cldn-1-deficient mice transplanted onto nude mice is characterized by epidermal thickening [29], hinting for compensation. Interestingly, a leaky TJ barrier does not necessarily result in increased TEWL. TRPV4 channel-deficient mice show permeable TJs but exhibit no difference in TEWL. Only after additional alteration of the SC barrier by acetone TEWL is profoundly increased in KO mice compared to WT mice [95]. Therefore, it will be of great interest to elucidate the molecular link between leaky TJ and TEWL/impaired barrier function of the skin. Putatively, not the loss of the TJ barrier is the primary cause for the water loss, but it results in a change of ion gradients or cell polarity which leads to an alteration of the SC. Indeed, an alteration of SC structure was observed in Cldn-1-deficient mice [29]. In addition, the impairment of TJs by sodium caprate results in an alteration of Ca^{2+} gradient in epidermis equivalents [59]. However, because sodium caprate targets phospholipase C and results in increased intracellular IP3, DAG and Ca^{2+} levels which lead to several cellular alterations including an opening of TJ [44], it remains to be shown whether this is indeed a TJ-specific effect.

The establishment of barrier-forming TJs in keratinocyte cultures depends on Ca^{2+} concentration. Ca^{2+} induces a continuous localization of TJ proteins at the cell-cell borders [13, 45, 73, 87, 124] and subsequently leads to the generation of a transepithelial resistance (TER), a measure for ion permeability of TJs, and reduced paracellular permeability for larger molecules [45, 73, 124]. For the establishment of a TER, the cell polarity complex Par3/Par6/aPKC is necessary [45]. Tiam1 (T-lymphoma invasion and metastasis), an exchange factor for the small GTPase Rac, is involved through the activation of Rac and aPKC [73]. One putative target molecule of aPKC in TJs of keratinocytes is Cldn-4 which was shown to be phosphorylated during TJ formation in HaCaT cells [5].

Downregulation of Cldn-1 in human keratinocytes results in decreased transepithelial resistance (TER) and increased paracellular permeability for larger molecules, e.g. FITC albumin [19, 120]. Also the downregulation of Ocln by RNAi was shown to decrease TJ barrier function in cultured keratinocytes [120]. However, Ocln-deficient mice do not show any obvious defect in skin barrier [91], again hinting for a compensation mechanism.

In addition to play a pivotal role in TJ barrier function, Cldn-1 was also shown to play a role in *proliferation* and *differentiation*. Downregulation of Cldn-1 results in increase of proliferation in human [19] and a downregulation of the differentiation markers filaggrin and loricrin in mouse keratinocytes [56]. Also the overexpression of Cldn-6, as well as specific deletion mutants of this molecule, results in increased proliferation of keratinocytes and dysregulated epidermal and hair follicle differentiation [102–104, 106].

TJs/TJ proteins are also known to participate in the *paracellular migration of inflammatory cells* through endothelia and simple epithelia (for reviews see [4, 93, 116]). This might also be true for the skin. TJ proteins are downregulated in psoriasis near specific subgroups of inflammatory cells, particularly neutrophils [54], and one could suggest that neutrophils migrate through the skin by downregulation of TJ proteins. In mouse skin, it was shown that dendrites of activated Langerhans cells (LHC) are positive for Cldn-1 and ZO-1 and that functional bicellular and tricellular TJs form between Langerhans cells and keratinocytes [58]. This may preserve TJ integrity during external antigen uptake by Langerhans cells. Also in human skin, Cldn-1, as well as JAM-A, is present in LHC [53, 127, 128].

For the formation of a functional SC, it is necessary that cells of the SG secrete their lamellar bodies only to the apical site but not to the basolateral sites of the cells. Therefore, *cell polarity* with directed vesicle transport has to be established in SG cells. Because TJs are known to be involved in cell polarity in simple epithelia and are localized in the SG, it is tempting to speculate that they are involved in this mechanism. Indeed, Kuroda et al. [60] observed that treatment of human skin equivalents and cultured keratinocytes with sodium caprate results in altered intracellular localization of a fluorescent ceramide (BODIPY) and decreases the secretion of this ceramide as well as of the lymphoepithelial Kazal-type-related inhibitor LEKTI. However, as mentioned above, due to the fact that sodium caprate increases the levels of several second messengers which also influence other molecules than TJ proteins, it is not sure whether this effect is TJ specific. CD44-deficient keratinocytes show prominent decreased levels of TJ proteins and impaired cell polarity formation in cultured cells, as well as lost polarity of lamellar body localization in the SG of KO mice during embryonic development [56]. This also strongly suggests for a role of TJs in cell polarity. However, again, also the absence of CD44 influences other proteins in addition to TJs; therefore, it cannot be excluded that other molecules might also be involved in perturbed polarity. Nonetheless, both findings clearly suggest the involvement of TJs in keratinocyte polarity which should be further clarified in future experiments.

Lastly, Cldn-1 and Ocln, as well as TJ-related structures, were also found in the lower layers of SC and were suggested to play a role in protection of corneodesmosomes at the lateral plasma membranes from precocious degradation, therefore contributing to orchestrated *desquamation* [35, 47, 36].

14.3.3 TJs and TJ Proteins in Skin Diseases

Alterations of TJ proteins have been observed in several skin diseases with dry skin. They are often characterized by impaired skin barrier function, altered proliferation/differentiation of the epidermis and/or infiltration of inflammatory cells.

In *psoriasis*, a broader expression of TJ proteins which are normally restricted to the SG/SSP, i.e. Ocln, ZO-1 and Cldn-4, and a (restricted to the uppermost and lowermost layers) downregulation of proteins, which are normally found in all layers, i.e. Cldn-1 and Cldn-7, were observed [53, 54, 87, 115, 123]. Even though these alterations are already observed in early stage psoriasis [53], there is no obvious alteration in non-lesional skin, and the alterations are widely reversed in healed psoriatic plaques [85]. The alteration of localization of TJ proteins results in a relocation of their colocalization from the SG to the upper spinous cell layers which is reflected by a relocation of TJ structures in electron microscopy [123] and a relocation of the TJ barrier function for the biotinylation reagent [54]. The biological meaning of this relocated TJ barrier function is not clear yet. It might be a rescue mechanism to compensate for the impaired SC barrier already in deeper layers. Suarez-Farinas et al. [99] found in their comparison of mRNA levels of lesional versus non-lesional skin before and 12 weeks after etanercept treatment (see also AQP section) also a downregulation of Cldn-8 and Cldn-10 which is not completely reversed by etanercept. In addition, they confirmed the upregulation of Ocln and ZO-1 and showed that it is normalized after etanercept treatment. As Cldn-1 is not mentioned in this manuscript, its expression might not have been investigated or does not seem to be significantly different between lesional and non-lesional skin.

In *non-lesional skin* of *atopic dermatitis (AD)* patients, a downregulation of Cldn-1 and Cldn-23 was observed in the epidermis [19]. The authors further describe a negative correlation between Cldn-1 expression and total serum IgE and eosinophils. Skin barrier function of suction blisters was impaired, as shown by Ussing chamber experiments, but TJ-specific barrier experiments in the skin were not performed. Of note, the authors found preliminary results hinting for a correlation of specific CLDN-1 SNPs with AD [19]. It is tempting to speculate that the impairment of both barriers, SC and TJs, results in increased uptake of antigens leading in turn to increased skin inflammation. Yang et al. [121] described that the downregulation of FGF receptor 1 and 2 in mice results in a downregulation of TJ proteins, including Cldn-1, and a loss of sebaceous glands and, subsequently, in the development of an inflammatory skin disease. Unfortunately, assays for in vivo TJ permeability, i.e. penetration of the biotinylation reagent could not be performed in these mice because the method is only established for newborn/embryonic mice but the phenotype of these mice only developed later.

In *ichthyosis vulgaris* patients with filaggrin mutation, a downregulation of Ocln and ZO-1 was described. Of note, the downregulation was more pronounced in homozygous compared to heterozygous filaggrin carriers [32]. On the other hand, as already described before, Cldn-1-deficient patients suffer from the NISCH syndrome which shows an ichthyosis skin phenotype [24, 34].

Skin infection (impetigo contagiosa) leads to a downregulation of all TJ proteins in the areas of acute invasion, while there is an upregulation of Ocln and ZO-1 in areas with colonization of bacteria [83].

Alterations of TJ protein expression and localization have also been described in *keratinocytic skin carcinomas, Merkel cell carcinomas and melanomas* [18, 33, 62, 63, 78, 94, 117]. In a two-step mouse carcinogenesis model, Arabzadeh and coworkers [6] noted a downregulation of Cldn-1 in the basal cell layer and of Cldn-1, 6,-11, -12 and −18 in the lower suprabasal epidermal layers. The impact of these alterations on tumourigenesis still has to be elucidated, but the fact that in psoriasis, non-lesional skin from AD patients and squamous cell carcinoma (SSC), which are all characterized by hyperproliferation and altered differentiation, a (limited) downregulation of Cldn-1 is found ([6, 19, 53, 62, 78, 115], submitted) and an influence of Cldn-1 on proliferation/differentiation was shown in knockdown experiments [19, 56] hints for an involvement of Cldn-1 in proliferation/differentiation of the tumours.

14.3.4 Influence of External Stimuli on TJs/TJ Proteins

UV exposure of mouse and human keratinocytes, as well as skin explants and skin equivalents, results in a decreased TJ barrier function. Chronic UV exposure as found in sun-exposed skin results in a downregulation of Cldn-1 in the lowermost layers and a broader expression of Ocln, ZO-1 and Cldn-4 (Rachow et al.).

Tape stripping of mouse skin results in an upregulation of Cldn-4 mRNA 1 and 3 h after tape stripping, while there was no significant change for Ocln and Cldn-1 [56]. Malminen et al. [69] also did not observe an effect of tape stripping on Ocln (and ZO-1) in human skin 24 h, 2d, 3d and 5d after tape stripping. They did not investigate Cldn-4.

Transient receptor potential vanilloid 4 (TRPV4) channel is a physiological sensor for hypo-osmolarity, mechanical deformation and warm temperature. TRPV4-deficient mice show leaky TJ and the absence of typical TJ structures while there is no obvious change in protein levels of Cldn-1 and Ocln [95]. Up to now, nothing is known about changes in TJ function as a result of physiologic stimulation of TRPV4, but due to the knockout results, an influence can be expected.

14.3.5 Influence of Extracellular Signalling Molecules on Epidermal TJs

The proinflammatory cytokines *IL-1*β and *TNF*α lead to an upregulation of Ocln and ZO-1 in ex vivo skin models. In addition, they increase and decrease TER in a time- and dose-dependent manner in primary keratinocytes [53]. IL-1β also results in a downregulation of Cldn-1 in human primary [53] and HaCat [112] keratinocytes and reduces Cldn-1 immunostaining after injection in human volunteers [115].

IL-4 and *IL-13* result in an upregulation of Cldn-1 levels in primary human keratinocytes, while there is no change of Ocln and ZO-1. In addition, IL-4 results in an increase of TER. These data render it unlikely that the decreased level of Cldn-1 in non-lesional skin from patients with AD is just a simple result of increased levels of IL-4 and IL-13 [19].

TGF-β1 decreases the levels of ZO-1 (and E-cadherin), markers for epithelial-mesenchymal transition, in HaCaT cell subtypes of various malignancy [88].

FGF7 increases Cldn-1 and Cldn-3 levels on mRNA and protein levels in cultured mouse keratinocytes [121].

Somatostatin (SST) increases TER in cultured human keratinocytes via the SST receptor 3. This is accompanied by an upregulation of Cldn-4 on mRNA and protein level [113].

CD44-deficient keratinocytes show alterations of TJ protein composition in the course of barrier formation during embryonic development, after tape stripping and in cell culture. In addition, they show delayed TJ barrier formation in cell culture and impaired skin barrier formation in embryonic and adult mice [56]. The main ligand of CD44 is *hyaluronic acid* (*HA*), but the large-size form of HA, which is known to influence differentiation as well as lamellar body formation and secretion in keratinocytes [11], does not influence TJ barrier function [56]. Therefore, the appropriate ligand to influence TJs via CD44, which might be HA of a different size or other glycosaminoglycans, still has to be identified.

14.3.6 Influence of External Substances on Epidermal TJs

Soybean-derived phospholipids modified with phospholipase A2 and C (lysophospholipids; *LPL*) stimulate the expression of Cldn-1 and Ocln (in addition to profilaggrin and serine palmitoyltransferase) in human keratinocytes. Treatment of human volunteers for 6 weeks with LPL resulted in increased SC hydration, but no direct correlation to TJ proteins was investigated [118].

14.3.7 Specific Modulation of TJs

Regarding the observations in mouse models and human diseases, an upregulation of Cldn-1 in diseased skin might be beneficial, also to improve skin dryness. However, as seen for Cldn-6, not only downregulation but also overexpression of a Cldn can disturb TJ barrier homeostasis. Therefore, the effect of Cldn-1 overexpression (and other TJ proteins) should be clarified first to evaluate the benefit of upregulation of TJ proteins.

In addition, as already mentioned for AQPs, specific upregulation of genes on transcriptional level is not easily achieved and will be a challenging task for the future.

Conclusion

Aquaporins and tight junctions are both involved in skin hydration. In addition, they are involved in various other functions. Their expression patterns are characteristically changed in skin diseases associated with dry skin and are influenced by cytokines and external stimuli known to change skin hydration. Knockout models of key epidermal aquaporins (AQP3) and TJ proteins (Cldn-1) result in dry skin/increased TEWL. Approaches to modify AQPs as well as the various proteins of TJs to improve skin dryness may therefore be reasonable but have to take into account the particular skin condition to which treatment is applied and other functions of AQPs/TJs which also might be influenced.

Take Home Messages

- Aquaglyceroporins are pore-forming transmembrane proteins. They transport water and glycerol into or out of the cells. In keratinocytes, AQP3, 9 and 10 are present.
- The major aquaglyceroporin in skin, AQP3, is (putatively) involved in skin hydration, proliferation (differentiation), migration, wound healing, barrier recovery, skin elasticity (and skin carcinogenesis).
- An up- or downregulation of AQP3 might be beneficial to improve skin moisturization depending on the skin condition and additional external influences.
- Tight junctions are complex cell-cell junctions that control the paracellular pathway of molecules in the stratum granulosum. TJ proteins are found in various expression patterns in several layers of the epidermis.
- TJs and TJ proteins are (putatively) involved in skin hydration, proliferation, differentiation, (stratum granulosum polarization) and (desquamation).
- An upregulation of Cldn-1, a major TJ protein, might be beneficial for skin moisturization, as its downregulation is observed in several skin diseases characterized by dry skin, but the consequence of a putative Cldn-1 overexpression is not clarified yet.

Abbreviations

AQP	Aquaporin
Cldn	Claudin
Ocln	Occludin
SC	Stratum corneum
SG	Stratum granulosum
TJ	Tight junctions

References

1. Aburada T, Ikarashi N, Kagami M, Ichikawa Y, Sugitani M, Maniwa A, Ueda H, Toda T, Ito K, Ochiai W, Matsushita R, Miyamoto K, Sugiyama K (2011) Byakkokaninjinto prevents body water loss by increasing the expression of kidney aquaporin-2 and skin aquaporin-3 in KKAy mice. Phytother Res 25:897–903
2. Agre P (2006) The aquaporin water channels. Proc Am Thorac Soc 3:5–13
3. Agren J, Zelenin S, Hakansson M, Eklof AC, Aperia A, Nejsum LN, Nielsen S, Sedin G (2003) Transepidermal water loss in developing rats: role of aquaporins in the immature skin. Pediatr Res 53:558–565
4. Aijaz S, Balda MS, Matter K (2006) Tight junctions: molecular architecture and function. Int Rev Cytol 248:261–298
5. Aono S, Hirai Y (2008) Phosphorylation of claudin-4 is required for tight junction formation in a human keratinocyte cell line. Exp Cell Res 314:3326–3339
6. Arabzadeh A, Troy TC, Turksen K (2007) Changes in the distribution pattern of Claudin tight junction proteins during the progression of mouse skin tumorigenesis. BMC Cancer 7:196
7. Balda MS, Matter K (2009) Tight junctions and the regulation of gene expression. Biochim Biophys Acta 1788:761–767
8. Bellemere G, Von Stetten O, Oddos T (2008) Retinoic acid increases aquaporin 3 expression in normal human skin. J Invest Dermatol 128:542–548
9. Benga G (2009) Water channel proteins (later called aquaporins) and relatives: past, present, and future. IUBMB Life 61:112–133
10. Bollag WB, Xie D, Zheng X, Zhong X (2007) A potential role for the phospholipase D2-aquaporin-3 signaling module in early keratinocyte differentiation: production of a phosphatidylglycerol signaling lipid. J Invest Dermatol 127:2823–2831
11. Bourguignon LY, Ramez M, Gilad E, Singleton PA, Man MQ, Crumrine DA, Elias PM, Feingold KR (2006) Hyaluronan-CD44 interaction stimulates keratinocyte differentiation, lamellar body formation/secretion, and permeability barrier homeostasis. J Invest Dermatol 126:1356–1365
12. Boury-Jamot M, Sougrat R, Tailhardat M, Le Varlet B, Bonte F, Dumas M, Verbavatz JM (2006) Expression and function of aquaporins in human skin:

Is aquaporin-3 just a glycerol transporter? Biochim Biophys Acta 1758:1034–1043
13. Brandner JM, Kief S, Grund C, Rendl M, Houdek P, Kuhn C, Tschachler E, Franke WW, Moll I (2002) Organization and formation of the tight junction system in human epidermis and cultured keratinocytes. Eur J Cell Biol 81:253–263
14. Brandner JM, McIntyre M, Kief S, Wladykowski E, Moll I (2003) Expression and localization of tight junction-associated proteins in human hair follicles. Arch Dermatol Res 295:211–221
15. Brandner JM (2009) Tight junctions and tight junction proteins in mammalian epidermis. Eur J Pharm Biopharm 72:289–294
16. Cao C, Sun Y, Healey S, Bi Z, Hu G, Wan S, Kouttab N, Chu W, Wan Y (2006) EGFR-mediated expression of aquaporin-3 is involved in human skin fibroblast migration. Biochem J 400:225–234
17. Cao C, Wan S, Jiang Q, Amaral A, Lu S, Hu G, Bi Z, Kouttab N, Chu W, Wan Y (2008) All-trans retinoic acid attenuates ultraviolet radiation-induced down-regulation of aquaporin-3 and water permeability in human keratinocytes. J Cell Physiol 215: 506–516
18. Cohn ML, Goncharuk VN, Diwan AH, Zhang PS, Shen SS, Prieto VG (2005) Loss of claudin-1 expression in tumor-associated vessels correlates with acquisition of metastatic phenotype in melanocytic neoplasms. J Cutan Pathol 32:533–536
19. De Benedetto A, Rafaels NM, McGirt LY, Ivanov AI, Georas SN, Cheadle C, Berger AE, Zhang K, Vidyasagar S, Yoshida T, Boguniewicz M, Hata T, Schneider LC, Hanifin JM, Gallo RL, Novak N, Weidinger S, Beaty TH, Leung DY, Barnes KC, Beck LA (2011) Tight junction defects in patients with atopic dermatitis. J Allergy Clin Immunol 127(773–86):e1–e7
20. Denda M, Sato J, Tsuchiya T, Elias PM, Feingold KR (1998) Low humidity stimulates epidermal DNA synthesis and amplifies the hyperproliferative response to barrier disruption: implication for seasonal exacerbations of inflammatory dermatoses. J Invest Dermatol 111:873–878
21. Dumas M, Langle S, Noblesse E, Bonnet-Duquennoy M, Pelle de Queral D, Tadokoro T, Bonte F (2005) Histological variation of Japanese skin with aging. Int J Cosmet Sci 27:47–50
22. Dumas M, Sadick NS, Noblesse E, Juan M, Lachmann-Weber N, Boury-Jamot M, Sougrat R, Verbavatz JM, Schnebert S, Bonte F (2007) Hydrating skin by stimulating biosynthesis of aquaporins. J Drugs Dermatol 6:s20–s24
23. Ebnet K, Suzuki A, Ohno S, Vestweber D (2004) Junctional adhesion molecules (JAMs): more molecules with dual functions? J Cell Sci 117:19–29
24. Feldmeyer L, Huber M, Fellmann F, Beckmann JS, Frenk E, Hohl D (2006) Confirmation of the origin of NISCH syndrome. Hum Mutat 27:408–410
25. Fisher GJ, Voorhees JJ (1998) Molecular mechanisms of photoaging and its prevention by retinoic acid: ultraviolet irradiation induces MAP kinase signal transduction cascades that induce Ap-1-regulated matrix metalloproteinases that degrade human skin in vivo. J Investig Dermatol Symp Proc 3:61–68
26. Fluhr JW, Mao-Qiang M, Brown BE, Wertz PW, Crumrine D, Sundberg JP, Feingold KR, Elias PM (2003) Glycerol regulates stratum corneum hydration in sebaceous gland deficient (asebia) mice. J Invest Dermatol 120:728–737
27. Fluhr JW, Darlenski R, Surber C (2008) Glycerol and the skin: holistic approach to its origin and functions. Br J Dermatol 159:23–34
28. Fujiyoshi Y, Mitsuoka K, de Groot BL, Philippsen A, Grubmuller H, Agre P, Engel A (2002) Structure and function of water channels. Curr Opin Struct Biol 12:509–515
29. Furuse M, Hata M, Furuse K, Yoshida Y, Haratake A, Sugitani Y, Noda T, Kubo A, Tsukita S (2002) Claudin-based tight junctions are crucial for the mammalian epidermal barrier: a lesson from claudin-1-deficient mice. Journal of Cell Biology 156:1099–1111
30. Furuse M, Tsukita S (2006) Claudins in occluding junctions of humans and flies. Trends Cell Biol 16: 181–188
31. Garcia N, Gondran C, Menon G, Mur L, Oberto G, Guerif Y, Dal Farra C, Domloge N (2011) Impact of AQP3 inducer treatment on cultured human keratinocytes, ex vivo human skin and volunteers. Int J Cosmet Sci 33:432–442
32. Gruber R, Elias PM, Crumrine D, Lin TK, Brandner JM, Hachem JP, Presland RB, Fleckman P, Janecke AR, Sandilands A, McLean WH, Fritsch PO, Mildner M, Tschachler E, Schmuth M (2011) Filaggrin genotype in ichthyosis vulgaris predicts abnormalities in epidermal structure and function. Am J Pathol 178:2252–63
33. Haass NK, Houdek P, Wladykowski E, Moll I, Brandner JM (2003) Expression patterns of tight junction proteins in Merkel cell carcinoma. In: Baumann KI, Halata Z, Moll I (eds) The Merkel Cell. Springer, Berlin, Heidelberg
34. Hadj-Rabia S, Baala L, Vabres P, Hamel-Teillac D, Jacquemin E, Fabre M, Lyonnet S, De Prost Y, Munnich A, Hadchouel M, Smahi A (2004) Claudin-1 gene mutations in neonatal sclerosing cholangitis associated with ichthyosis: a tight junction disease. Gastroenterology 127:1386–1390
35. Haftek M (2009) Tight junction-like structures contribute to the lateral contacts between corneocytes and protect corneodesmosomes from premature degradation. J Invest Dermatol 129:S65
36. Haftek M, Callejon S, Sandjeu Y, Padois K, Falson F, Pirot F, Portes P, Demarne F, Jannin V (2011) Compartmentalization of the human stratum corneum by persistent tight junction-like structures. Experimental Dermatology 20:617–621
37. Hara-Chikuma M, Sohara E, Rai T, Ikawa M, Okabe M, Sasaki S, Uchida S, Verkman AS (2005) Progressive adipocyte hypertrophy in aquaporin-7-deficient mice: adipocyte glycerol permeability as a novel regulator of fat accumulation. J Biol Chem 280: 15493–15496

38. Hara-Chikuma M, Verkman AS (2008) Aquaporin-3 facilitates epidermal cell migration and proliferation during wound healing. J Mol Med 86:221–231
39. Hara-Chikuma M, Verkman AS (2008) Prevention of skin tumorigenesis and impairment of epidermal cell proliferation by targeted aquaporin-3 gene disruption. Mol Cell Biol 28:326–332
40. Hara-Chikuma M, Takahashi K, Chikuma S, Verkman AS, Miyachi Y (2009) The expression of differentiation markers in aquaporin-3 deficient epidermis. Arch Dermatol Res 301:245–252
41. Hara M, Ma T, Verkman AS (2002) Selectively reduced glycerol in skin of aquaporin-3-deficient mice may account for impaired skin hydration, elasticity, and barrier recovery. J Biol Chem 277: 46616–46621
42. Hara M, Verkman AS (2003) Glycerol replacement corrects defective skin hydration, elasticity, and barrier function in aquaporin-3-deficient mice. Proc Natl Acad Sci U S A 100:7360–7365
43. Hashimoto K (1971) Intercellular spaces of the human epidermis as demonstrated with lanthanum. Journal of Investigative Dermatology 57:17–31
44. Hayashi M, Sakai T, Hasegawa Y, Nishikawahara T, Tomioka H, Iida A, Shimizu N, Tomita M, Awazu S (1999) Physiological mechanism for enhancement of paracellular drug transport. J Control Release 62:141–148
45. Helfrich I, Schmitz A, Zigrino P, Michels C, Haase I, le Bivic A, Leitges M, Niessen CM (2007) Role of aPKC isoforms and their binding partners Par3 and Par6 in epidermal barrier formation. J Invest Dermatol 127:782–791
46. Horie I, Maeda M, Yokoyama S, Hisatsune A, Katsuki H, Miyata T, Isohama Y (2009) Tumor necrosis factor-alpha decreases aquaporin-3 expression in DJM-1 keratinocytes. Biochem Biophys Res Commun 387: 564–568
47. Igawa S, Kishibe M, Murakami M, Honma M, Takahashi H, Iizuka H, Ishida-Yamamoto A (2011) Tight junctions in the stratum corneum explain spatial differences in corneodesmosome degradation. Exp Dermatol 20:53–57
48. Ishibashi K, Sasaki S, Fushimi K, Uchida S, Kuwahara M, Saito H, Furukawa T, Nakajima K, Yamaguchi Y, Gojobori T et al (1994) Molecular cloning and expression of a member of the aquaporin family with permeability to glycerol and urea in addition to water expressed at the basolateral membrane of kidney collecting duct cells. Proc Natl Acad Sci U S A 91:6269–6273
49. Jacobson EL, Kim H, Kim M, Williams JD, Coyle DL, Coyle WR, Grove G, Rizer RL, Stratton MS, Jacobson MK (2007) A topical lipophilic niacin derivative increases NAD, epidermal differentiation and barrier function in photodamaged skin. Exp Dermatol 16:490–499
50. Ji C, Yang Y, Yang B, Xia J, Sun W, Su Z, Yu L, Shan S, He S, Cheng L, Wan Y, Bi Z (2011) Trans-Zeatin attenuates ultraviolet induced down-regulation of aquaporin-3 in cultured human skin keratinocytes. Int J Mol Med 26:257–263
51. Kim NH, Lee AY (2011) Reduced aquaporin3 expression and survival of keratinocytes in the depigmented epidermis of vitiligo. J Invest Dermatol 130:2231–2239
52. King LS, Choi M, Fernandez PC, Cartron JP, Agre P (2001) Defective urinary-concentrating ability due to a complete deficiency of aquaporin-1. N Engl J Med 345:175–179
53. Kirschner N, Poetzl C, von den Driesch P, Wladykowski E, Moll I, Behne MJ, Brandner JM (2009) Alteration of tight junction proteins is an early event in psoriasis: putative involvement of proinflammatory cytokines. Am J Pathol 175:1095–1106
54. Kirschner N, Houdek P, Fromm M, Moll I, Brandner JM (2010) Tight junctions form a barrier in human epidermis. Eur J Cell Biol 89:839–842
55. Kirschner N, Bohner C, Rachow S, Brandner JM (2010) Tight junctions: is there a role in dermatology? Arch Dermatol Res 302:483–493
56. Kirschner N, Haftek M, Niessen CM, Behne MJ, Furuse M, Moll I, Brandner JM (2011) CD44 regulates tight-junction assembly and barrier function. J Invest Dermatol 131:932–943
57. Kohler K, Zahraoui A (2005) Tight junction: a co-ordinator of cell signalling and membrane trafficking. Biol Cell 97:659–665
58. Kubo A, Nagao K, Yokouchi M, Sasaki H, Amagai M (2009) External antigen uptake by Langerhans cells with reorganization of epidermal tight junction barriers. J Exp Med 206:2937–2946
59. Kurasawa M, Maeda T, Oba A, Yamamoto T, Sasaki H (2011) Tight junction regulates epidermal calcium ion gradient and differentiation. Biochem Biophys Res Commun 406:506–511
60. Kuroda S, Kurasawa M, Mizukoshi K, Maeda T, Yamamoto T, Oba A, Kishibe M, Ishida-Yamamoto A (2010) Perturbation of lamellar granule secretion by sodium caprate implicates epidermal tight junctions in lamellar granule function. J Dermatol Sci 59:107–114
61. Langbein L, Grund C, Kuhn C, Praetzel S, Kartenbeck J, Brandner JM, Moll I, Franke WW (2002) Tight junctions and compositionally related junctional structures in mammalian stratified epithelia and cell cultures derived therefrom. Eur J Cell Biol 81:419–435
62. Langbein L, Pape U-F, Grund C, Kuhn C, Praetzel S, Moll I, Moll R, Franke WW (2003) Tight junction-related structures in the absence of a lumen: Occludin claudins and tight junction plaque proteins in densely packed cell formations of stratified epithelia and squamous cell carcinomas. European Journal of Cell Biology 82:385–400
63. Leotlela PD, Wade MS, Duray PH, Rhode MJ, Brown HF, Rosenthal DT, Dissanayake SK, Earley R, Indig FE, Nickoloff BJ, Taub DD, Kallioniemi OP, Meltzer P, Morin PJ, Weeraratna AT (2007) Claudin-1 overexpression in melanoma is regulated by PKC and contributes to melanoma cell motility. Oncogene 26:3846–3856
64. Leyvraz C, Charles RP, Rubera I, Guitard M, Rotman S, Breiden B, Sandhoff K, Hummler E (2005) The epidermal barrier function is dependent on the serine protease CAP1/Prss8. J Cell Biol 170:487–496

65. Li J, Tang H, Hu X, Chen M, Xie H (2011) Aquaporin-3 gene and protein expression in sun-protected human skin decreases with skin ageing. Australas J Dermatol 51:106–112
66. Liu J, Man WY, Lv CZ, Song SP, Shi YJ, Elias PM, Man MQ (2010) Epidermal permeability barrier recovery is delayed in vitiligo-involved sites. Skin Pharmacol Physiol 23:193–200
67. Ludwig RJ, Zollner TM, Santoso S, Hardt K, Gille J, Baatz H, Johann PS, Pfeffer J, Radeke HH, Schon MP, Kaufmann R, Boehncke WH, Podda M (2005) Junctional adhesion molecules (JAM)-B and -C contribute to leukocyte extravasation to the skin and mediate cutaneous inflammation. J Invest Dermatol 125:969–976
68. Ma T, Hara M, Sougrat R, Verbavatz JM, Verkman AS (2002) Impaired stratum corneum hydration in mice lacking epidermal water channel aquaporin-3. J Biol Chem 277:17147–17153
69. Malminen M, Koivukangas V, Peltonen J, Karvonen SL, Oikarinen A, Peltonen S (2003) Immunohistological distribution of the tight junction components ZO-1 and occludin in regenerating human epidermis. Br J Dermatol 149:255–260
70. Marchini G, Stabi B, Kankes K, Lonne-Rahm S, Ostergaard M, Nielsen S (2003) AQP1 and AQP3, psoriasin, and nitric oxide synthases 1–3 are inflammatory mediators in erythema toxicum neonatorum. Pediatr Dermatol 20:377–384
71. Matsuki M, Yamashita F, Ishida-Yamamoto A, Yamada K, Kinoshita C, Fushiki S, Ueda E, Morishima Y, Tabata K, Yasuno H, Hashida M, Iizuka H, Ikawa M, Okabe M, Kondoh G, Kinoshita T, Takeda J, Yamanishi K (1998) Defective stratum corneum and early neonatal death in mice lacking the gene for transglutaminase 1 (keratinocyte transglutaminase). Proc Natl Acad Sci U S A 95:1044–1049
72. Matsuzaki T, Suzuki T, Koyama H, Tanaka S, Takata K (1999) Water channel protein AQP3 is present in epithelia exposed to the environment of possible water loss. J Histochem Cytochem 47:1275–1286
73. Mertens AE, Rygiel TP, Olivo C, van der Kammen R, Collard JG (2005) The Rac activator Tiam1 controls tight junction biogenesis in keratinocytes through binding to and activation of the Par polarity complex. J Cell Biol 170:1029–1037
74. Mirza R, Hayasaka S, Takagishi Y, Kambe F, Ohmori S, Maki K, Yamamoto M, Murakami K, Kaji T, Zadworny D, Murata Y, Seo H (2006) DHCR24 gene knockout mice demonstrate lethal dermopathy with differentiation and maturation defects in the epidermis. J Invest Dermatol 126:638–647
75. Mirza R, Hayasaka S, Kambe F, Maki K, Kaji T, Murata Y, Seo H (2008) Increased expression of aquaporin-3 in the epidermis of DHCR24 knockout mice. Br J Dermatol 158:679–684
76. Morita K, Itoh M, Saitou M, Ando-Akatsuka Y, Furuse M, Yoneda K, Imamura S, Fujimoto K, Tsukita S (1998) Subcellular distribution of tight junction-associated proteins (occludin, ZO-1, ZO-2) in rodent skin. Journal of Investigative Dermatology 110: 862–866
77. Morita K, Sasaki H, Furuse K, Furuse M, Tsukita S, Miyachi Y (2003) Expression of claudin-5 in dermal vascular endothelia. Exp Dermatol 12:289–295
78. Morita K, Tsukita S, Miyachi Y (2004) Tight junction-associated proteins (occludin, ZO-1, claudin-1, claudin-4) in squamous cell carcinoma and Bowen's disease. Br J Dermatol 151:328–334
79. Nakahigashi K, Kabashima K, Ikoma A, Verkman AS, Miyachi Y, Hara-Chikuma M (2011) Upregulation of aquaporin-3 is involved in keratinocyte proliferation and epidermal hyperplasia. J Invest Dermatol 131: 865–873
80. Nakakoshi M, Morishita Y, Usui K, Ohtsuki M, Ishibashi K (2006) Identification of a keratinocarcinoma cell line expressing AQP3. Biol Cell 98:95–100
81. Nejsum LN, Kwon TH, Jensen UB, Fumagalli O, Frokiaer J, Krane CM, Menon AG, King LS, Agre PC, Nielsen S (2002) Functional requirement of aquaporin-5 in plasma membranes of sweat glands. Proc Natl Acad Sci U S A 99:511–516
82. Niessen CM (2007) Tight junctions/adherens junctions: basic structure and function. J Invest Dermatol 127:2525–2532
83. Ohnemus U, Kohrmeyer K, Houdek P, Rohde H, Wladykowski E, Vidal S, Horstkotte MA, Aepfelbacher M, Kirschner N, Behne MJ, Moll I, Brandner JM (2008). Regulation of epidermal tight-junctions (TJ) during infection with exfoliative toxin-negative Staphylococcus strains. J Invest Dermatol 128:906–16
84. Olsson M, Broberg A, Jernas M, Carlsson L, Rudemo M, Suurkula M, Svensson PA, Benson M (2006) Increased expression of aquaporin 3 in atopic eczema. Allergy 61:1132–1137
85. Peltonen S, Riehokainen J, Pummi K, Peltonen J (2007) Tight junction components occludin, ZO-1, and claudin-1, -4 and –5 in active and healing psoriasis. Br J Dermatol 156:466–472
86. Pereda Mdel C, Dieamant Gde C, Eberlin S, Werka RM, Colombi D, Queiroz ML, Di Stasi LC (2010) Expression of differential genes involved in the maintenance of water balance in human skin by Piptadenia colubrina extract. J Cosmet Dermatol 9:35–43
87. Pummi K, Malminen M, Aho H, Karvonen S-L, Peltonen J, Peltonen S (2001) Epidermal tight junctions: ZO-1 and occludin are expressed in mature, developing, and affected skin and in vitro differentiating keratinocytes. Journal of Investigative Dermatology 117:1050–1058
88. Rasanen K, Vaheri A (2011) TGF-beta1 causes epithelial-mesenchymal transition in HaCaT derivatives, but induces expression of COX-2 and migration only in benign, not in malignant keratinocytes. J Dermatol Sci 58:97–104
89. Rojek AM, Skowronski MT, Fuchtbauer EM, Fuchtbauer AC, Fenton RA, Agre P, Frokiaer J, Nielsen S (2007) Defective glycerol metabolism in aquaporin 9 (AQP9) knockout mice. Proc Natl Acad Sci U S A 104:3609–3614

90. Roudier N, Ripoche P, Gane P, Le Pennec PY, Daniels G, Cartron JP, Bailly P (2002) AQP3 deficiency in humans and the molecular basis of a novel blood group system, GIL. J Biol Chem 277:45854–45859
91. Saitou M, Furuse M, Sasaki H, Schulzke J-D, Fromm M, Takano H, Noda T, Tsukita S (2000) Complex phenotype of mice lacking occludin, a component of tight junction strands. Mol Biol Cell 11:4131–4142
92. Schlüter H, Wepf R, Moll I, Franke WW (2004) Sealing the live part of the skin: the integrated meshwork of desmosomes, tight junctions and curvilinear ridge structures in the cells of the uppermost granular layer of the human epidermis. Eur J Cell Biol 83:655–665
93. Schneeberger EE, Lynch RD (2004) The tight junction: a multifunctional complex. Am J Physiol Cell Physiol 286:C1213–C1228
94. Smalley KS, Brafford P, Haass NK, Brandner JM, Brown E, Herlyn M (2005) Up-regulated expression of zonula occludens protein-1 in human melanoma associates with N-cadherin and contributes to invasion and adhesion. Am J Pathol 166:1541–1554
95. Sokabe T, Fukumi-Tominaga T, Yonemura S, Mizuno A, Tominaga M (2011) The TRPV4 channel contributes to intercellular junction formation in keratinocytes. J Biol Chem 285:18749–18758
96. Song X, Xu A, Pan W, Wallin B, Kivlin R, Lu S, Cao C, Bi Z, Wan Y (2008) Nicotinamide attenuates aquaporin 3 overexpression induced by retinoic acid through inhibition of EGFR/ERK in cultured human skin keratinocytes. Int J Mol Med 22: 229–236
97. Sougrat R, Morand M, Gondran C, Barre P, Gobin R, Bonte F, Dumas M, Verbavatz JM (2002) Functional expression of AQP3 in human skin epidermis and reconstructed epidermis. J Invest Dermatol 118: 678–685
98. Straseski JA, Gibson AL, Thomas-Virnig CL, Allen-Hoffmann BL (2009) Oxygen deprivation inhibits basal keratinocyte proliferation in a model of human skin and induces regio-specific changes in the distribution of epidermal adherens junction proteins, aquaporin-3, and glycogen. Wound Repair Regen 17:606–616
99. Suarez-Farinas M, Fuentes-Duculan J, Lowes MA, Krueger JG (2011) Resolved psoriasis lesions retain expression of a subset of disease-related genes. J Invest Dermatol 131:391–400
100. Sugiyama Y, Ota Y, Hara M, Inoue S (2001) Osmotic stress up-regulates aquaporin-3 gene expression in cultured human keratinocytes. Biochim Biophys Acta 1522:82–88
101. Tanno O, Ota Y, Kitamura N, Katsube T, Inoue S (2000) Nicotinamide increases biosynthesis of ceramides as well as other stratum corneum lipids to improve the epidermal permeability barrier. Br J Dermatol 143:524–531
102. Troy TC, Rahbar R, Arabzadeh A, Cheung RM, Turksen K (2005) Delayed epidermal permeability barrier formation and hair follicle aberrations in Inv-Cldn6 mice. Mech Dev 122:805–819
103. Troy TC, Turksen K (2007) The targeted overexpression of a Claudin mutant in the epidermis of transgenic mice elicits striking epidermal and hair follicle abnormalities. Mol Biotechnol 36:166–174
104. Troy TC, Arabzadeh A, Lariviere NM, Enikanolaiye A, Turksen K (2009) Dermatitis and aging-related barrier dysfunction in transgenic mice overexpressing an epidermal-targeted claudin 6 tail deletion mutant. PLoS One 4:e7814
105. Tunggal JA, Helfrich I, Schmitz A, Schwarz H, Gunzel D, Fromm M, Kemler R, Krieg T, Niessen CM (2005) E-cadherin is essential for in vivo epidermal barrier function by regulating tight junctions. Embo J 24:1146–1156
106. Turksen K, Troy TC (2002) Permeability barrier dysfunction in transgenic mice overexpressing claudin 6. Development 129:1775–1784
107. Van Itallie CM, Anderson JM (2006) Claudins and epithelial paracellular transport. Annu Rev Physiol 68:403–429
108. Velazquez Pereda Mdel C, Dieamant Gde C, Eberlin S, Nogueira C, Colombi D, Di Stasi LC, de Souza Queiroz ML (2009) Effect of green Coffea arabica L. seed oil on extracellular matrix components and water-channel expression in in vitro and ex vivo human skin models. J Cosmet Dermatol 8:56–62
109. Verbavatz JM, Brown D, Sabolic I, Valenti G, Ausiello DA, Van Hoek AN, Ma T, Verkman AS (1993) Tetrameric assembly of CHIP28 water channels in liposomes and cell membranes: a freeze-fracture study. J Cell Biol 123:605–618
110. Verdier-Sevrain S, Bonte F (2007) Skin hydration: a review on its molecular mechanisms. J Cosmet Dermatol 6:75–82
111. Verkman AS (2005) More than just water channels: unexpected cellular roles of aquaporins. J Cell Sci 118:3225–3232
112. Verkman AS (2009) Aquaporins: translating bench research to human disease. J Exp Biol 212: 1707–1715
113. Vockel M, Breitenbach U, Kreienkamp HJ, Brandner JM (2010) Somatostatin regulates tight junction function and composition in human keratinocytes. Exp Dermatol 19:888–894
114. Voss KE, Bollag RJ, Fussell N, By C, Sheehan DJ, Bollag WB (2011) Abnormal aquaporin-3 protein expression in hyperproliferative skin disorders. Arch Dermatol Res 303:591–600
115. Watson RE, Poddar R, Walker JM, McGuill I, Hoare LM, Griffiths CE, O'Neill CA (2007) Altered claudin expression is a feature of chronic plaque psoriasis. J Pathol 212:450–458
116. Weber C, Fraemohs L, Dejana E (2007) The role of junctional adhesion molecules in vascular inflammation. Nat Rev Immunol 7:467–477
117. Werling AM, Doerflinger Y, Brandner JM, Fuchs F, Becker JC, Schrama D, Kurzen H, Goerdt S, Peitsch WK (2011) Homo- and heterotypic cell-cell contacts

in Merkel cells and Merkel cell carcinomas: heterogeneity and indications for cadherin switching. Histopathology 58:286–303
118. Wilke K, Wepf R, Keil FJ, Wittern KP, Wenck H, Biel SS (2006) Are sweat glands an alternate penetration pathway? Understanding the morphological complexity of the axillary sweat gland apparatus. Skin Pharmacol Physiol 19:38–49
119. Yahagi S, Koike M, Okano Y, Masaki H (2011) Lysophospholipids improve skin moisturization by modulating of calcium-dependent cell differentiation pathway. Int J Cosmet Sci 33:251–256
120. Yamamoto T, Saeki Y, Kurasawa M, Kuroda S, Arase S, Sasaki H (2008) Effect of RNA interference of tight junction-related molecules on intercellular barrier function in cultured human keratinocytes. Arch Dermatol Res 300:517–524
121. Yang J, Meyer M, Muller AK, Bohm F, Grose R, Dauwalder T, Verrey F, Kopf M, Partanen J, Bloch W, Ornitz DM, Werner S (2010) Fibroblast growth factor receptors 1 and 2 in keratinocytes control the epidermal barrier and cutaneous homeostasis. J Cell Biol 188:935–952
122. Yasui M (2004) Molecular mechanisms and drug development in aquaporin water channel diseases: structure and function of aquaporins. J Pharmacol Sci 96:260–263
123. Yoshida Y, Morita K, Mizoguchi A, Ide C, Miyachi Y (2001) Altered expression of occludin and tight junction formation in psoriasis. Archives of Dermatological Research 293:239–244
124. Yuki T, Haratake A, Koishikawa H, Morita K, Miyachi Y, Inoue S (2007) Tight junction proteins in keratinocytes: localization and contribution to barrier function. Exp Dermatol 16:324–330
125. Yuki T, Hachiya A, Kusaka A, Sriwiriyanont P, Visscher MO, Morita K, Muto M, Miyachi Y, Sugiyama Y, Inoue S (2011) Characterization of tight junctions and their disruption by UVB in human epidermis and cultured keratinocytes. J Invest Dermatol 131:744–752
126. Zheng X, Bollinger-Bollag W (2003) Aquaporin 3 colocates with phospholipase d2 in caveolin-rich membrane microdomains and is downregulated upon keratinocyte differentiation. J Invest Dermatol 121: 1487–1495
127. Zimmerli SC, Hauser C (2007) Langerhans cells and lymph node dendritic cells express the tight junction component claudin-1. J Invest Dermatol 127:2381–2390
128. Zimmerli SC, Kerl K, Hadj-Rabia S, Hohl D, Hauser C (2008) Human epidermal Langerhans cells express the tight junction protein claudin-1 and are present in human genetic claudin-1 deficiency (NISCH syndrome). Exp Dermatol 17:20–23

Biomechanics of the Barrier Function of Human Stratum Corneum

15

Kemal Levi and Reinhold H. Dauskardt

15.1 Introduction

The outermost layer of skin, the stratum corneum (SC), provides mechanical protection and a controlled permeable barrier to the external environment. It is subject to highly variable conditions including changing temperature, humidity, mechanical and abrasive contact. In addition, the SC must withstand daily application of topical cleaning agents and potentially damaging acute and chronic chemical exposure. The mechanical properties of the SC are crucial not only for its mechanical and biophysical function [1], but are also a vital factor in the cosmetic aspects of skin appearance, "feel" and "firmness." In addition, they play a central role in skin chapping and cracking associated with dry skin conditions [2].

Mechanical behavior of the SC is also important for wound healing, adhesive dressings, and emerging biosensor and drug delivery technologies which must all have a reliable mechanical interface with skin. Residual stress in the SC affects the growth and healing of skin. Fibrosis, scar formation, and various tissue responses including inflammation and expression of growth factors may be affected by mechanical loading [3–7]. As the outermost layer of skin, the SC, acts as the principal mechanical interface between the epidermal and dermal layers and the exterior environment and thus plays a crucial role in determining the stress state in skin. Surprisingly, the connection to the mechanical properties and stresses in the skin remain elusive due in part to a paucity of mechanical properties of the skin layers as a function of tissue condition and treatment.

15.2 Drying Stress and Relationship to Tissue Damage

Daily exposures to variable temperature and moisture conditions, together with application of cleansing agents, lead to skin "dryness" and "tightness." If left untreated, dry skin conditions can lead to tissue damage in the form of chapping and cracking, which is directly related to intercellular delamination and fracture of the SC layer. Such damage can ultimately lead to tissue responses including inflammation, scarring, and abnormal desquamation and further exacerbate the effects of skin disorders such as atopic dermatitis, ichthyosis vulgaris, and chronic xerosis [2–8]. Skin tightness is likely related to changes in the stiffness of the SC layer and the buildup of tensile biaxial SC drying stresses in the plane of the SC layer [9–11]. The presence of these

K. Levi • R.H. Dauskardt (✉)
Department of Materials Science and Engineering, Stanford University,
496 Lomita Mall, Durand Bldg., Rm 121, Stanford, CA 94305, USA
e-mail: levik@stanford.edu; dauskardt@stanford.edu

M. Lodén, H.I. Maibach (eds.), *Treatment of Dry Skin Syndrome*,
DOI 10.1007/978-3-642-27606-4_15, © Springer-Verlag Berlin Heidelberg 2012

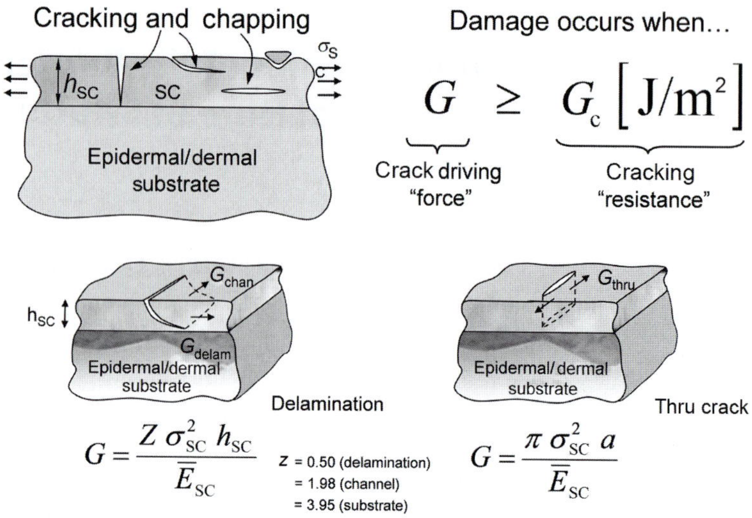

Fig. 15.1 A schematic illustration showing typical dry skin cracking and chapping processes that result from the development of drying stresses in SC. The driving force for these damage processes, G, can be quantified in terms of the SC stress, elastic properties and thickness. The parameter Z is determined by the cracking configuration only. The resistance to SC damage is given in terms of the intercellular delamination energy, G_c. Damage occurs when $G \geq G_c$ as indicated

stresses and their potential role in skin damage processes have been well cited, and connections have been suggested to water loss during drying of treated tissue [9, 10, 12–14]. However, quantitative methods to characterize these stresses have been still lacking until very recently, and little understanding existed regarding the effects of drying environment, chemical exposures, and moisturizing treatments.

From a mechanics viewpoint, the SC drying stress, σ_{SC}, provides a mechanical "driving force" for dry skin damage such as cracking and chapping of the SC as shown in Fig. 15.1. The stressed SC layer can then be treated as a thin (15–30 μm) stiff film on a thick (1–3 mm) substrate consisting of the epidermal and dermal layers. The driving force for crack propagation for the cracking configurations shown in Fig. 15.1 can be quantified in terms of the strain energy release rate, G, [15]:

$$G = \frac{Z\sigma_{SC}^2 h_{SC}}{\bar{E}_{SC}} \qquad (15.1)$$

G depends on the SC stress squared divided by the SC biaxial elastic modulus, $\bar{E}_{SC}$, which provides a measure of the elastic strain energy density stored in the film, the SC thickness, h_{SC}, and a nondimensional parameter Z which provides information about the specific cracking type (peeling, channel cracking, delamination, etc.). Note that the mechanics presented here assumes that the SC is a linear elastic thin film on an elastic substrate and has been shown to be accurate for the low strains, hydration conditions, and time scales important for dry skin damage processes [16]. Cracking and chapping will develop in the SC during drying when the value of G exceeds the intercellular delamination energy, G_c, which is a property of the tissue and provides a measure of tissue resistance to cracking [17–19]. Then, the ratio between G and G_c, G/G_c, can then be used to infer the propensity of cracking in the tissue following its exposure to a certain condition or treatment.

15.3 Measurement of Drying Stress

15.3.1 Microtension

It is well known that isolated SC exhibits significant shrinkage when dried from a hydrated condition. If the SC is constrained from shrinking, then stresses develop as it dries and attempts to contract. (Note that, in vivo, the constraint results from the underlying skin layers which resist SC shrinking in the plane of the SC). The development of uniaxial drying stresses in isolated SC

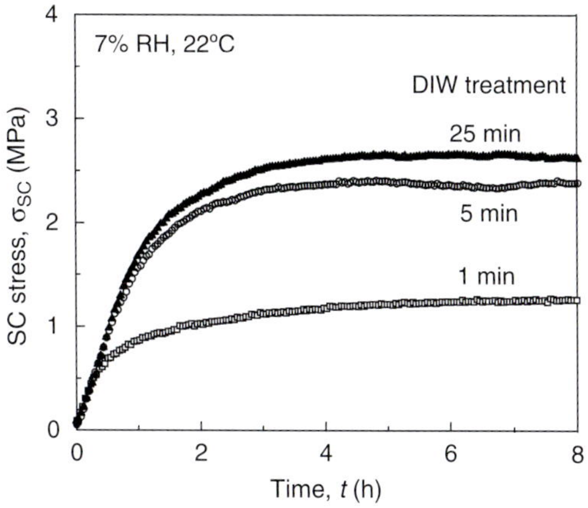

Fig. 15.2 The uniaxial σ_{SC} for tissue initially treated with distilled water (DIW) for 1, 5, and 25 min and then exposed to 7% RH and 25°C air

can be shown with microtension experiments where following treatment or conditioning the wet tissue is clamped between two fixed grips of a tensile testing unit and exposed to a certain drying environment [16, 20]. The σ_{SC} values are then determined using the measured loads and the SC thickness.

The microtension technique can be used to detect sensitivity of SC to changes in hydration [16, 20]. The reported σ_{SC} for tissue initially treated with distilled water (DIW) for 1, 5, and 25 min and then exposed to 7% RH and 25°C air is shown in Fig. 15.2. The σ_{SC} values for all specimens rise immediately after exposure to dry air and begin to stabilize after ~2 h. Note that the final σ_{SC} values increase with increasing exposure to hydration due to greater water loss during drying.

The microtension technique provides a quick method to measure the SC drying stress. However, microtension experiments are challenging since the SC is mechanically fragile and difficult to handle after isolation and treatment. The transfer of the wet tissue to the grips of the tensile testing unit, particularly after exposure to damaging treatments (e.g., sodium dodecyl sulfate, acetone), is quite difficult. Often, wet tissue has been observed to curl or fold onto itself after being clamped between the two fixed grips of a tensile testing unit. This may result in inaccurate thickness and stress measurements. Also, the microtension technique simulates neither the in vivo drying conditions where moisture can only escape from the outer SC surface nor the roughly equal in vivo biaxial stress state of SC.

15.3.2 Substrate Curvature

The substrate curvature technique is widely used in thin-film materials science to quantify the stresses of thin films on elastic substrates [21–24], and was recently adapted to measure SC drying stresses from the curvature of an elastic substrate onto which the SC adhered [16]. Briefly, inplane tensile or compressive stresses that develop in a film adhered to an elastic substrate result in a concave or convex elastic curvature of the substrate, respectively. This elastic curvature, K, can be measured using optical, interferometric or capacitative methods [23–25]. In recent studies, a scanning laser substrate curvature instrument was used to measure the substrate angle of deflection, α, in terms of the dimensions L_y and L_z, as a function of position, y as defined in Fig. 15.3. K was subsequently calculated from a linear regression analysis of α versus position data [16].

Using this technique, the biaxial SC film stress, σ_{SC}, adhered to an elastic substrate can be determined from K using the Stoney's equation [16, 26]:

$$\sigma_{SC} = \left(\frac{E_{sub}}{1 - \nu_{sub}}\right)\frac{h^2_{sub}}{6h_{SC}}K, \tag{15.2}$$

where E_{sub}, ν_{sub}, h_{sub} and h_{SC} are the Young's modulus, Poisson's ratio, and thickness of the substrate and SC specimen thickness, respectively. This relationship is based on the "thin-film" assumption that generally requires the product of the film biaxial modulus and thickness to be ≤1/80 of the equivalent product for the substrate to ensure an error less than ~5% in the resulting film stress. An important advantage of this assumption and Stoney's equation is that the film elastic properties are not required to calculate the film stress, making the SC stress analysis

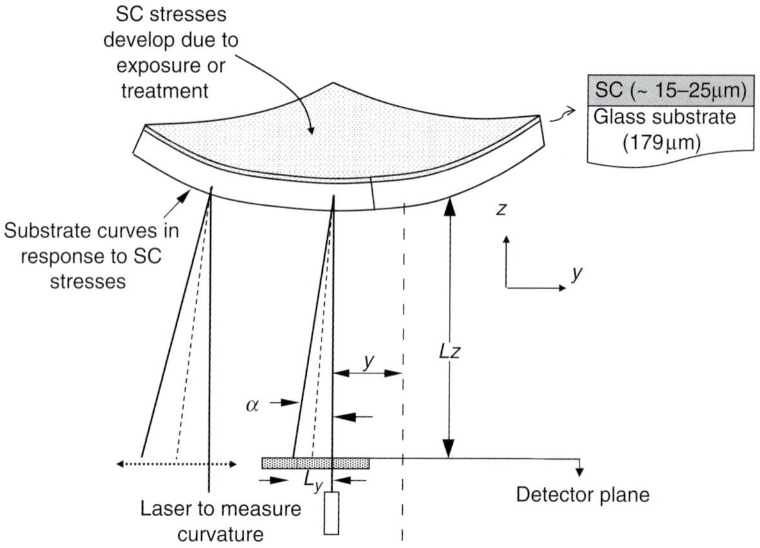

Fig. 15.3 The experimental arrangement for the substrate curvature technique showing the SC mounted on a glass substrate. A scanning laser equipped with detector measures the angle of deflection, α, versus position, y, on the substrate. The average curvature is calculated from a linear regression of the deflection angle

particularly straightforward in terms of the measured elastic curvature of the substrate using Stoney's equation. Nevertheless, as the SC film thickness is quite large compared to the substrate thickness, a more complete "thick-film" analysis has been undertaken to validate the thin-film approach, and σ_{SC} values have been reported to be insensitive to E_{SC} and ν_{SC} as anticipated by the thin-film assumption [16].

As discussed, in vivo wet SC is constrained from shrinking in-plane by the underlying epidermal and dermal skin layers as it dries and attempts to contract. The out-of-plane SC dimension is not constrained and free to contract without any through-thickness stress buildup. The substrate curvature technique provides the same type of biaxial constraint with an artificial substrate. There are two important requirements for the accuracy of this method. First, the mechanical properties of the substrate must be elastic for the range of strains experienced during drying of the SC. Second, the tissue must be well adhered to the substrate. An epoxy can certainly be used to adhere the tissue to the substrate. However, this can further complicate the method, as the curvature of the added epoxy layer will also have to be taken into account for stress measurements with the possibility of epoxy impregnation into the SC layer. As such, the SC has been shown to naturally adhere well to clean glass surface without the use of an epoxy. Furthermore, digital image correlation studies have shown there are no net displacement of strains in the SC while drying [16], proving that an adhesive is not required for accurate substrate curvature measurements on SC.

The reported σ_{SC} for DIW-treated tissue measured using the substrate curvature technique as a function of drying time in 15% RH and 25°C air is shown in Fig. 15.4 [16]. The σ_{SC} of the wet tissue is ~0 MPa and does not change for a period of 2 h. The σ_{SC} then rapidly increases and stabilizes after ~4 h to a final value of ~2.5 MPa at 8 h. The uniaxial drying stress measured using the microtension technique under identical drying conditions is included in the figure for comparison. By contrast, the uniaxial σ_{SC} values rise immediately after exposure to the drying air and stabilize after ~4 h to a final value of ~1.48 MPa at 8 h. However, the time after which the drying stress stabilizes is similar in both cases following the onset of the first drying stresses.

The immediate development of drying stresses in the microtension test is attributed to the fact that both sides of the SC specimen are exposed to the drying environment, thus allowing faster water loss [16]. In the substrate curvature test, water can only escape from the original outer surface of the SC. Although the final σ_{SC} value measured using substrate curvature is significantly

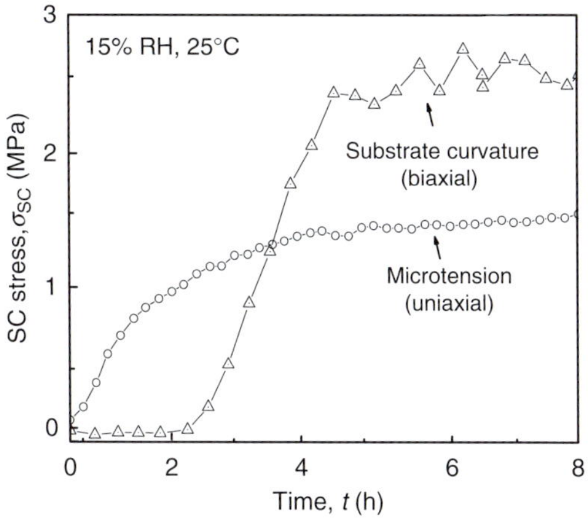

Fig. 15.4 The biaxial and uniaxial SC drying stress as a function of drying time for DIW-treated tissue exposed to 15% RH and 25°C air

higher than the microtension value, they are entirely consistent with simple elastic predictions for films that are constrained under biaxial and uniaxial conditions, while undergoing a transformation (drying) strain. Using Hooke's laws for linear elastic films, the relationship between the biaxial and uniaxial σ_{SC} is given by:

$$\frac{\sigma_{SC}^{\text{biaxial}}}{\sigma_{SC}^{\text{uniaxial}}} = \frac{1}{1-\nu_{SC}}. \quad (15.3)$$

Using $\nu_{SC} \sim 0.4$ for dried SC, the expected ratio of 1.8 from Eq. 15.3 is close to the measured stress ratio of 1.7. This means that the biaxial constraint of the SC in the substrate curvature method results in stresses that are consistent with the uniaxial microtension results.

The measured biaxial SC stresses in substrate curvature measurements more closely approximate the biaxial in vivo stress state of SC compared to uniaxial stresses measured in a uniaxial tension test. Furthermore, water loss occurs only through the outer SC surface, again more closely approximating in vivo drying conditions. The substrate curvature technique also has experimental advantages compared with tensile testing. SC can be more easily transferred to the substrate, particularly when it is mechanically fragile after treatment. The tissue is positioned on the substrate while it is still inside the treatment solution. As the solution is removed, SC settles onto the substrate. This prevents SC from curling or folding onto itself as experienced in tensile testing. In addition, if SC mechanical properties and thickness compared to those of the substrate employed for curvature measurements satisfy the "thin-film" assumption, SC mechanical properties are not required to determine the SC stresses. This simplifies the stress analysis significantly compared to other methods.

15.4 Effect of Environmental Conditions and Chemical Treatment on Drying Stress

15.4.1 Overview of Water Effects on Tissue Structure and Its Mechanical Properties

The hydration characteristics of SC have been extensively investigated using methods such as gravimetry [27–29] and spectroscopic techniques including infrared [30], Raman [31], and nuclear magnetic resonance spectroscopy [32, 33]. These studies have shown that the water content of the tissue and its microstructure is very sensitive to the RH and temperature of the environment it is conditioned at. In dry environments (<20% RH), SC has a dense, semicrystalline structure. There is a strong interaction between the keratin chains due to hydrogen bonding between the polar-side groups of the keratin chains [34, 35]. The intercellular lipids are closely packed and rigid. As the tissue hydrates, the primary hydration sites, such as the strong polar groups of keratin chains in corneocytes, covalently bound lipids of the cellular protein envelope and intercellular lipids, become saturated and then additional water binds to the secondary hydration binding sites, namely, tightly bound water and dipolar sites on the protein [36]. This reduces the interaction between the keratin chains [37]. In the case of the lipids, increasing water presence reduces the intermolecular forces between the intercellular lipids and loosens their packing [38]. As the tissue continues to hydrate, secondary hydration binding sites become saturated and water can no longer be sorbed locally. Consequently, water condenses as unbound water [36]. The unbound water disrupts the hydrogen bonding between the keratin chains allowing them to be less constrained and move more easily relative to each other while being strained [34, 39]. Meanwhile, the intercellular lipids of the hydrated tissue are less tightly packed and more fluid and permeable.

SC can be further hydrated if conditioned at very moist environments (>90% RH) or soaked in water. Increasing unbound water in the tissue has been reported to have damaging effects on SC depending on the length of exposure to hydration. While short exposures to water (<1 h), even with repetitive applications during a day or over many days, have no damaging effect on SC intercellular lipids [40, 41], long exposures (>1 h) cause significant swelling in the corneocytes followed by formation of amorphous-appearing material and pooling of water in the intercellular lipids [41, 42]. The dilation of the lipids due to pooling of water has been shown to disrupt SC lamellar lipid ultrastructure and produce corneocyte separations [41]. Furthermore, degradation of corneodesmosomes between corneocytes has been associated with increased hydration content [43, 44].

The hydration state of SC has direct implications on its mechanical properties and propensity for cracking. With respect to elastic behavior, tissue modulus has been reported to decrease from ~265 to 14 MPa with increasing humidity [16]. This is associated with the effect of water on molecular mobility in the SC. With increasing water content, the interaction between keratin chains is progressively weakened as discussed above. This involves substitution of existing protein–protein hydrogen bonds with water-mediated bonding to facilitate greater chain mobility [34, 45, 46]. Similar trends have been observed with nanoindentation measurements to obtain the compression modulus of porcine SC, and the SC modulus has been measured to decrease from ~120 to 26 MPa with increasing humidity [47]. Interestingly, the effect of hydration on the SC in-plane and out-of-plane fracture properties is different. The in-plane fracture (tearing) energy of the tissue has been shown to increase from 580 to 1,390 J/m^2 with increasing RH from 35% to 85% [48]. This trend is not observed for out-of-plane fracture properties due to constrained plasticity [17]. The intercellular delamination energy of the tissue has been shown to decrease from ~4 to ~1 J/m^2 with increasing RH from 40% to 100%. This decrease has been associated with the separation of interfaces in the presence of water in the intercellular space [18].

15.4.2 Water Effects

SC drying stresses have been shown to be strongly dependent on the hydration level of the drying environment [16]. The reported σ_{SC} values for DIW-treated tissue as a function of drying time in 15%, 30%, 45%, and 100% RH and 25°C air are shown in Fig. 15.5a. As moisture increases in the drying environment, both the drying stress rate (the increase in σ_{SC} with time following treatment and exposure to air), $d\sigma_{SC}/dt$, and the plateau σ_{SC} values significantly decrease. No drying stresses are observed for SC exposed to the 100% RH air as the tissue remains fully hydrated in a 100% RH environment. The σ_{SC} also changes rapidly in response to changes in the hydration level of the drying environment as shown in Fig. 15.5b. This is not surprising considering that SC is a biosensor which communicates outside changes to the underlying skin layers. The σ_{SC} values alternate between ~2.1 to 2.8 MPa and ~0 MPa as the tissue is cycled between 15% and 100% RH over 2-h periods after an initial drying period in 15% RH air.

The sensitivity of σ_{SC} values to the hydration level of the drying environment is strongly linked to the moisture content of the tissue, which is determined by how much water SC loses based on the chemical potential of water, μ_w, in the environment [16]. μ_w is a function of both RH and temperature and is defined by:

$$\mu_w = \mu_0 + RT\ln(a_{H_2O}), \qquad (15.4)$$

where μ_0 is the standard chemical potential, R the universal gas constant, T the temperature in Kelvin, and a_{H2O} the activity of water in the drying

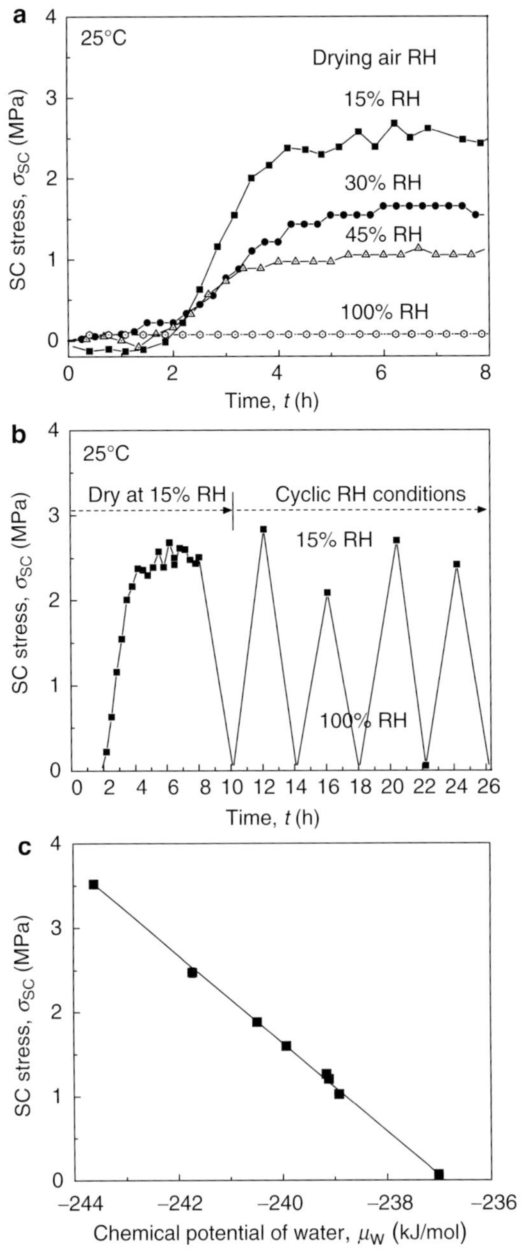

Fig. 15.5 (**a**) SC drying stress as a function of drying time for DIW-treated tissue exposed to 15%, 30%, 45%, and 100% RH air at 25°C for up to 8 h. (**b**) SC drying stress as a function of drying time for specimen exposed to 15% RH and 25°C drying environment for ~8 h and then cycled between 100% RH and 15% RH at 2-h intervals. (**c**) SC final drying stress as a function of chemical potential of water in the drying environment. The linear fit shows a strong correlation between the drying stress and the chemical potential of water ($R^2 = -0.999$)

environment given by [49]. The strong linear relationship apparent between σ_{SC} and μ_w values shown in Fig. 15.5c for conditions listed in further proves that desorption of water from SC during drying is the main driving force for evolution of drying stresses in the tissue.

15.4.3 Modeling Water Effects

A thin-film mechanics model that predicts the amount of water loss from the SC during drying from measured values of SC drying stress, elastic modulus, and SC thickness has recently been reported [16]. Using this model, the shrinkage of the tissue during drying, Δ^{dry}, can now be written in terms of measured quantities:

$$\Delta^{dry} = -2\left(\frac{1-\nu_{SC}}{E_{SC}}\right)\sigma_{SC} + \left(\frac{h_f - h_0}{h_0} + \frac{2\nu_{SC}}{E_{SC}^{\perp}}\sigma_{SC}\right), \quad (15.5)$$

where E_{SC}, $E_{SC}^{\perp}$, h_0 and h_f are the in-plane and out-of-plane Young's modulus of the SC and initial and final tissue thickness, respectively. Then, the mass of water lost during drying of the SC that accounts for the drying stress can be obtained from:

$$m_w = \rho_w V_{wet} \Delta^{dry}, \quad (15.6)$$

where ρ_w is the density of water, and V_{wet} is the volume of the wet tissue.

From the measured drying stress, modulus, and SC thickness measurements, the predicted water loss is compared to the measured water loss in Fig. 15.6. The calculated water loss only slightly exceeds the measured values by up to ~16% for the SC dried in 45% RH air. The strong linear relationship between the predicted and measured water loss suggests that the SC drying stress is mainly related to the reduction of the volume occupied by water, regardless of the bound states of water that were discussed. This result also suggests that that the reorientation of proteins and lipids which have commonly been thought to provide a significant

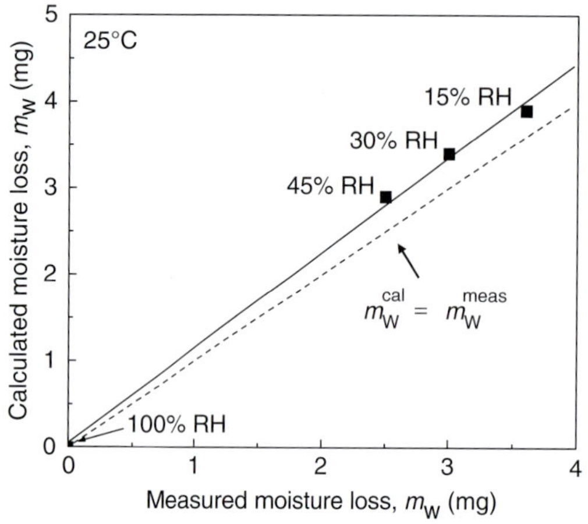

Fig. 15.6 The predicted moisture loss as a function of the measured moisture loss. The linear fit shows a strong correlation between the two ($R^2=0.998$)

contribution to the drying strains and stresses may in fact be quite small. Based on this result, the relationship between the drying stresses and the water loss can be used to understand how a certain treatment affects the water retention in the tissue. We will use this relationship later in the chapter.

15.4.4 Chemical Treatment Effects

The substrate curvature technique has also been used to characterize SC drying stresses following exposure to different treatments [16]. The reported final σ_{SC} values of SC initially treated with surfactant sodium dodecyl sulfate (SDS), moisturizing glycerin (GLY), and DIW (control) for 25 min and then dried for 8 h in 15% RH and 25°C or 27% RH and 32°C air are plotted as a function of the chemical potential of water, μ_w, in the drying environment in Fig. 15.7. For both drying conditions, the σ_{SC} of the tissue treated with the harsh cleanser surfactant, SDS, is significantly higher than that of the control-treated tissue. SDS treatment is known to have damaging effects on all SC components and is widely used to study surfactant-induced dry scaly skin [50, 51]. It disrupts the barrier properties of the intercellular lipids increasing their fluidity and permeability [52]. As a result, more water can penetrate into the tissue during treatment. SDS also binds to SC proteins resulting in conformational changes in their structure leading to transient swelling and hyperhydration of corneocytes [9, 14, 53, 54]. Thus, the water content of the tissue during exposure to SDS is much higher compared to that of the tissue exposed to DIW. Additionally, following exposure to SDS, SC has been reported to return to a lower hydration state compared to that of the tissue exposed to DIW because surfactant binding reduces the ability of SC proteins to bind and hold water [9].

The increased σ_{SC} values of SDS-treated tissue compared to DIW-treated tissue has been mainly linked to the increased volume of water lost during drying which is anticipated from our model in the previous section [16]. The other possible causes of high SC drying stress values may be conformational changes in the keratin chains following SDS binding and contraction of lipids due to extraction of a fraction of the intercellular lipids or changes in the lipid composition and content. The σ_{SC} of the SDS-treated tissue is significantly reduced when the availability of water in the drying environment increases suggesting that the damage caused by SDS may be suppressed when the tissue is conditioned at moist environments.

In contrast to the harsh SDS treatment, the σ_{SC} of the tissue treated with GLY is significantly lower than that of the control-treated tissue for both drying conditions. This trend is expected considering that the GLY is a well-known moisturizing treatment which increases water-holding capacity of SC and accelerates the recovery of its barrier function after exposure to damaging treatments [55, 56]. Following exposure to GLY, corneocytes and SC intercellular spaces have been observed to expand, and the tissue has been reported to be at a higher hydration state compared to that of the tissue exposed to DIW [57]. Additionally, after exposure to GLY, SC in-plane modulus significantly decreases with respect to that of the DIW-treated tissue and the extensibility of SC significantly increases [43].

The reported effects of GLY above on SC hydration and mechanical properties suggest that the decreased σ_{SC} values of GLY-treated tissue

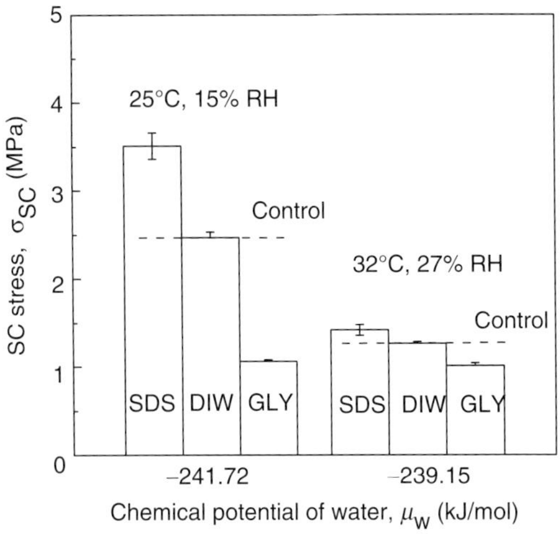

Fig. 15.7 SC final drying stress as a function of chemical potential of water for specimens treated with GLY, SDS and DIW (control) and exposed to either 15% RH and 25°C or 27% RH and 32°C air

compared to DIW-treated tissue may be due to the decreased volume of water lost during drying and the decreased SC modulus. The other possible cause of low drying stress may be expansion of lipids due to GLY increasing their fluidity. The effects of corneodesmosome degradation are not considered since it is reported to occur when the tissue is conditioned at moist environments (>80% RH) [43]. Note that the σ_{SC} of the GLY-treated tissue remained the same at different drying conditions. This means that the tissue maintains a certain level of hydration independent of the availability of water in the drying environment after being treated with GLY. Altogether, the data in Fig. 15.7 suggests that the substrate curvature technique can be used to easily detect and distinguish the σ_{SC} of SC treated with different chemicals.

15.5 Extension of the Substrate Curvature Method to Assess the Effect of Topical Coatings on Stratum Corneum

Topical coatings are extensively used in medical and cosmetic formulations [58]. Despite their extensive use, little is understood of their effects on the perception of skin "dryness" and "tightness." It also remains unclear whether these perceptions are related to the drying of the coating itself or the interaction of the coating with the underlying SC. For example, the coating may affect the water content of the SC or may contain molecules that diffuse into the SC and change its mechanical properties and stress state. In addition, the coating may itself develop drying stresses that may be perceived as skin tightness. This section first describes the application of the substrate curvature technique to characterize stresses in drying and nondrying occlusive topical coatings and then extensions of the technique to measure the effects of the coating applied to the SC where the overall drying stresses may have contributions from the coating, the SC, and the interaction of the coating with the SC. This section also discusses how these separate contributions in the coating and SC layers can be differentiated.

15.5.1 Substrate Curvature Technique for Multiple Layers

The theory behind the substrate curvature method and the relationship between the SC stresses and curvature have been described in detail in Sect. 15.3.2. The extension of the substrate curvature technique to characterize the effects of topical coatings on SC stresses requires taking the contribution of the coating to the overall curvature of the specimen into account. If the treatment involves a coating applied to the SC that develops stresses after application, the total substrate curvature, K_T, will be given by [59–61]:

$$K_T = K_{SC} + K_{coat}, \tag{15.7}$$

where K_{coat} is the curvature associated with the stress developed in the treatment coating, and K_{SC} is the curvature associated with the drying stress of the underlying SC. If the coating does not develop any stresses, then $K_{coat} = 0$ and the curvature measured is related to the stress in the SC, σ_{SC}, only. On the other hand, if the treatment coating hardens and develops stresses of its own, σ_{coat}, then these will add to the curvature measured.

If the multiple films together satisfy the thin-film assumption, then Stoney's equation can be applied to relate the contribution of individual film stresses to the substrate curvature. Any significant changes in the SC and coating thickness, h_{coat}, during the experiment must be taken into account in Stoney's equation (Eq. 15.2). Note that the overall substrate curvature is measured, and the individual SC and coating stresses cannot be deconvoluted without additional information. For example, if the coating stresses are separately measured, then their contribution to the substrate curvature can be determined and subtracted from the total curvature using Eq. 15.7 to obtain the curvature related to the SC stresses provided that the presence of the SC under the coating does not change the coating stresses.

15.5.2 Effects of Topical Coatings on Stratum Corneum

Stresses that develop in topical coatings can be measured by applying the topical coating directly to a glass substrate. Characterizing the stresses in topical coatings helps to isolate their effect on the SC. Since when they are applied to the SC, the overall drying stresses have contributions from the coating, the SC, and the interaction of the coating with the SC. This section reviews the effects of nondrying and drying occlusive barriers (NDO and DO) on SC.

The reported coating stress and associated substrate curvature for a drying occlusive barrier (DO) and a nondrying occlusive barrier (NDO) applied directly to a glass substrate and exposed to the 26% RH and 26°C drying environment are shown as a function of time in Fig. 15.8a. The DO coating hardens in the drying environment, and a positive curvature develops in the substrate as a result of the presence of tensile drying stresses in the coating. These stresses have been linked to the loss of water bound to the humectant molecules in the DO coating or contractions as a result of cross-linking of emollient molecules in the coating when exposed to air.

The NDO coating does not harden in the drying environment, and no substrate curvature is detected, indicating zero coating stress. This also suggests that there is no moisture diffusing out of the coating.

Prior to the application of coatings on the SC, the curvature and σ_{SC} of isolated SC should be measured as control in the same drying environment as shown in Figs. 15.8b and c. Both NDO and DO are then applied to the SC, and the substrate curvature is measured as a function of time (Fig. 15.8b).

The NDO coating does not harden, and the results shown in Fig. 15.8a show that no coating stresses develop. The curvature measured is therefore associated with stresses in the SC only which are calculated using Stoney's equation (Eq. 15.2) and shown in Fig. 15.8c. In the presence of NDO, the plateau σ_{SC} is significantly lower than that of the control.

For the DO-coated specimen, it is assumed that the coating hardens and develops the same stresses as it does when applied directly to the substrate. Using Eq. 15.7, the curvature associated with the DO coating stresses (Fig. 15.8a) can be subtracted from the total curvature (Fig. 15.8b) to obtain just the curvature associated with stresses in the SC. The σ_{SC} value can then be determined using Stoney's equation (Eq. 15.2) as shown in Fig. 15.8c. Interestingly, the σ_{SC} values stabilize for the DO-coated SC at values almost identical to those of the SC with the NDO coating.

The principal effect of the occlusive coatings on the SC is to maintain higher moisture content in the SC when exposed to the drying environment. For the NDO- and DO-coated tissue, the final drying stresses are observed to be the same despite the initial difference in the stress profiles following application of the coatings (Fig. 15.8c). This observation demonstrates that both coatings are equally effective at maintaining higher moisture content in SC. To better understand the effect of occlusive barriers in maintaining higher moisture content in SC, the relationship between the SC drying stresses and the chemical potential of water in the drying environment (Fig. 15.5c) shown in Sect. 15.4.2 can be used. The decreased σ_{SC} values observed in the presence of the occlusive barriers are equivalent to SC stresses that would be observed in a 49% RH, 26°C drying environment without any

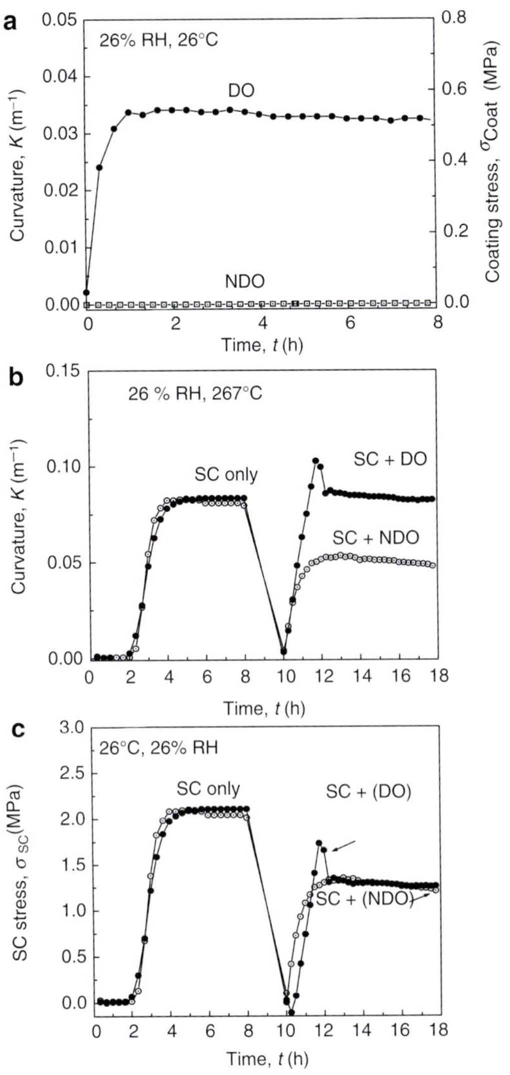

Fig. 15.8 (**a**) The curvature and stress values as a function of drying time for drying occlusive (*DO*) and nondrying occlusive (*NDO*) coatings exposed to 26% RH and 26°C air. (**b**) The total curvature values as a function of drying time for stratum corneum (*SC*) treated with DO and NDO coatings and exposed to 26% RH and 26°C air. (**c**) SC drying stress as a function of drying time for SC treated with DO and NDO coatings and exposed to 26% RH and 26°C air

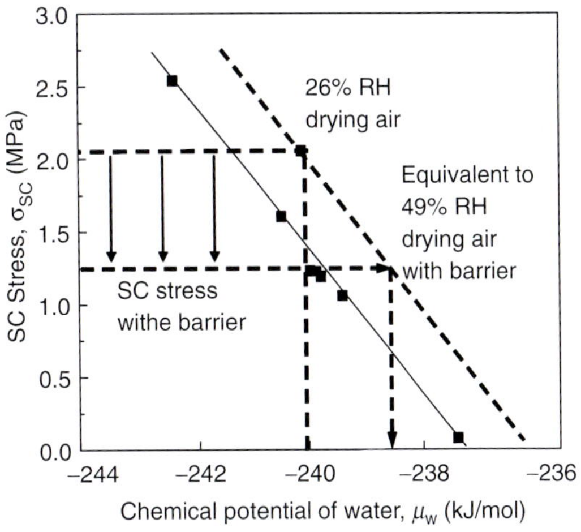

Fig. 15.9 SC final drying stress as a function of chemical potential of water in the drying environment. The decreased SC stresses observed in the presence of the occlusive barriers are equivalent to SC stresses that would be observed in a 49% RH, 26°C drying environment without any occlusive barrier

occlusive barrier as shown in Fig. 15.9. This suggests that the SC retains some water in the presence of the occlusive barriers.

For the DO-treated SC, the stress relaxation following initial stress increase to a peak stress value may be the diffusion of moisturizing molecules such as emollients in the coating into the SC and softening the tissue. This behavior is similar to the behavior observed in other studies where diffusion of emollient molecules in the occlusive coating into the intercellular boundaries of SC causes significant softening of the tissue within minutes of application [60, 61].

The methodology presented in this study provides direct opportunities for studying the effects of moisturizing treatments and occlusive barrier films used to control water loss on SC and alleviate the propensity for dry skin damage. This will be discussed in the next section.

15.6 Assessing Moisturizer Efficacy with the Substrate Curvature Method

Topical moisturizer products are formulated based on their molecular, biochemical, and moisture occlusive properties to improve skin sensory properties and alleviate dry skin [1, 9–11]. Control of transepidermal water loss (TEWL), effects on skin components including lipid organization, irritation potential, optical spectroscopy, and imaging together with consumer product

Table 15.1 The treatments used in this study, their compositions, their physical states, and their mechanism of action to moisturize skin are listed

Treatment	Composition	Physical state	Type
GLY	10%, 30%, and 100% (v/v) in DIW	Liquid	Humectant
GLY-A	40–50% (v/v) Glycerin 40–50% (v/v) Water 1–5% (v/v) Glyceryl polyacrylate	Solid (gel)	Humectant
GLY-B	40% Glycerin (v/v),cetearyl alcohol, stearic acid, sodium cetearyl sulfate, methylparaben, propylparaben, dilauryl thiodipropionate, sodium sulfate	Solid (cream)	Oil/lamellar gel/ water emulsion
AL	C12–C15 Alkyl esters (lactic acid, lauryl and myristyl alcohol)	Liquid	Emollient
DA	Diisopropyl adipate (adipic acid, isopropyl alcohol)	Liquid	Emollient
EP	Ethylhexyl palmitate (palmitic acid, 2-ethylhexanol)	Liquid	Emollient
IN	Isostearyl neopentanoate (neopentanoic acid, isostearyl alcohol)	Liquid	Emollient
ISS	Isocetyl steaoryl stearate (stearic acid, isocetyl alcohol)	Liquid	Emollient
OSS	Octyldodecyl stearoyl stearate (atearic acid, octyldodecanol)	Liquid	Emollient
PET	100% White petrolatum USP	Solid (gel)	Occlusive

For the emollients, the main component of the composition is listed first. The remaining ingredients of the composition which were used to construct the emollient molecule are in parenthesis

perceptions are used to assess efficacy [62]. However, these do not measure the effects of moisturizing treatments on skin biomechanical function, which affect not only the perception of dry skin stiffness and tightness but also underlie the biomechanical component for dry skin damage [16, 59].

This section discusses the application of the substrate curvature technique to measure the efficacy of selected moisturizers commonly used in topical moisturizing products using the methodology presented in Sect. 15.5 [60, 61]. SC is shown to have distinct drying stress profiles after application of various moisturizers. The section also discusses how these moisturizers reduce σ_{SC} and alleviate the propensity for mechanically induced dry skin damage. The effect of the moisturizers on the SC drying stresses is explained in terms of SC water loss and the chemical state of the SC components.

The moisturizers discussed in this section are listed in Table 15.1 and classified according to their mechanism of action to moisturize skin. These moisturizers include the purified mixture of hydrocarbons taken from petroleum, petrolatum (PET), long considered as the "gold standard" occlusive treatment in cosmetic science; various concentrations and different formulations of the nonvolatile trihydroxylated humectant, glycerin (GLY), widely used as a hydrating agent in personal care products; and a range of undiluted ester-based emollients with diverse physicochemical properties including alkyl lactate (AL), diisopropyl adipate (DA), ethylhexyl palmitate (EP), isostearyl neopentanoate (IN), isocetyl stearoyl stearate (ISS), and octyldodecyl stearoyl stearate (OSS).

15.6.1 Petrolatum

PET is regarded as one of the most effective occlusive emollients for skin care, and its topical application is used as a standard to achieve reduced TEWL following insults to the SC barrier [63–65]. This section reviews drying stress measurements on PET-coated SC and demonstrates how the principal effect of the occlusive PET coating on the SC stresses is achieved through control of the SC water content.

The reported σ_{SC} of PET-coated SC exposed to 7% RH and 22°C air is shown as a function of drying time in Fig. 15.10a [61]. Note that these σ_{SC} values are determined by taking the contribution

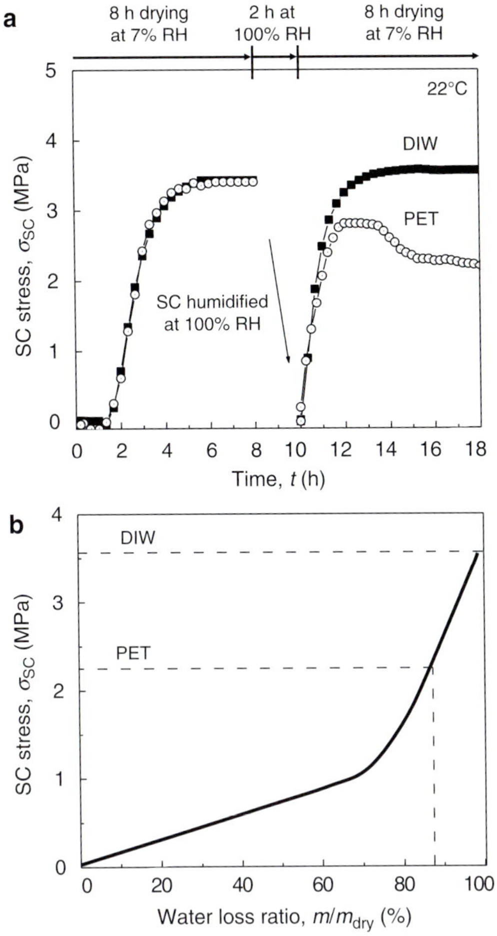

Fig. 15.10 (**a**) SC drying stress as a function of drying time for SC treated with the occlusive PET coating and exposed to 7% RH and 22°C air. (**b**) SC drying stress as a function of % water loss. The final stress value of PET-coated SC and the corresponding percentage water loss value is plotted with *dashed lines*

of the coating to the overall substrate curvature into account as described in Sect. 15.5.2. The σ_{SC} values of PET-coated SC rise rapidly to a peak σ_{SC} value, remain relatively constant for ~2 h, and then slowly relax to a final σ_{SC} value of ~2.3 MPa, ~37% lower than the DIW (control)-treated tissue.

The contribution of reduced water loss to the reduced final σ_{SC} values following PET treatment can be determined using the mechanics model presented in Sect. 15.4.3 assuming that the stress is generated only by the strain change associated with the volume of water lost to the drying environment. The predicted reduction in water lost compared to DIW (control) is ~13% as shown in Fig. 15.10b. As expected, a small reduction in the water lost is enough to fully account for the reduced drying stresses, given the sensitivity of SC drying stresses to SC water content. The retention of water in the SC in the presence of occlusive PET coating is also consistent with reported reduced TEWL following insults to the SC barrier [63–65].

The other possible reason for lower σ_{SC} values following PET treatment may be related to increased intercellular lipid fluidity reported using attenuated total reflectance Fourier transform infrared spectroscopy (ATR – FTIR) as a function of tissue depth [61]. This would act to reduce the drying stresses by viscous flow allowing some corneocyte movement in the plane of the SC, particularly in the outer SC layers where there are few corneodesmosomes connecting corneocytes. The relaxation in SC stresses after ~4 h in the drying environment strengthens this argument [61].

15.6.2 Glycerin-Based Humectants

Glycerin-based humectants have a significant proclivity to bind with water and attract water from the viable skin layers to the SC and from the environment if the ambient RH exceeds 70% [66]. This section reviews reported drying stress measurements on SC following application of humectant GLY coatings listed in Table 15.1 and the contribution of reduced water loss to the resulting decrease in σ_{SC} values.

Following application of GLY coatings, the reported σ_{SC} values are observed to rapidly increase and stabilize after ~2 h in the drying environment where they remain relatively constant as shown in Fig. 15.11a [61]. Since no stresses develop in the humectant coatings when applied directly on the glass substrate, the σ_{SC} values are determined from the overall substrate curvature as described for NDO coatings in Sect. 15.5.2.

With increasing GLY concentration, the drying stress rate and the final σ_{SC} values are observed to decrease compared to DIW (control). This decrease, along with observed penetration of

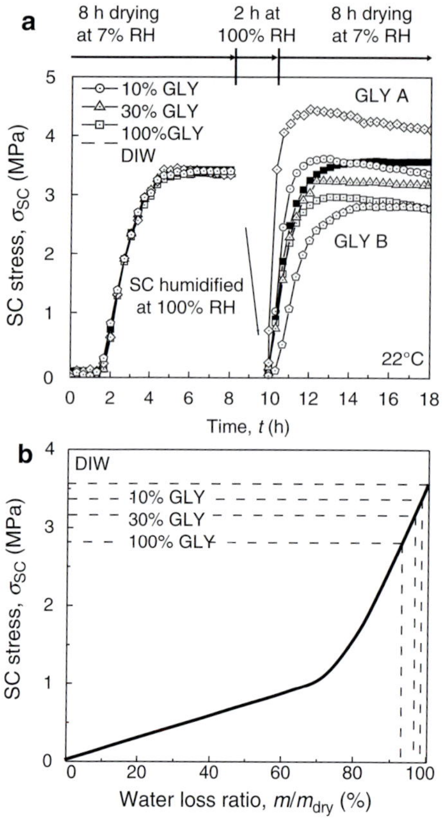

Fig. 15.11 (**a**) SC drying stress as a function of drying time for SC treated with the humectant coatings and exposed to 7% RH and 22°C air. (**b**) SC drying stress as a function of % water loss. The final stress values of GLY-treated specimens and the corresponding % water loss values are plotted with *dashed lines*

GLY into the SC, suggests that GLY reduces water loss from the SC due to its proclivity to bind with water. The penetration of GLY coatings into the SC has been measured with ATR-FTIR measurements as a function of tissue depth using a delamination technique [61]. Additionally, in reported substrate curvature measurements, the humectant GLY coatings are applied to the SC adhered to a glass substrate. These coatings can neither attract water from the underlying glass substrate as they will in vivo nor can they draw from the external dry (7% RH) environment. Therefore, the resulting drying stresses can be explained solely in terms of the effect of humectant coatings on SC water loss and the SC components themselves.

The contribution of water loss to the reduced final σ_{SC} values following GLY application can be determined from the relationship between measured σ_{SC} values and water loss ratio [61]. Using this relationship, the predicted reduction in water loss compared to the control is ~2%, 4%, and 8% after 10%, 30%, and 100% GLY application, respectively (Fig. 15.11b). So again, given the sensitivity of SC drying stresses to SC water content, only a small reduction in the water lost due to the treatment may fully account for the reduced drying stresses. The observed retention of water in the SC in the presence of GLY is consistent with reported corneocyte and SC intercellular space expansion together with higher hydration states reported for GLY-treated SC [57].

The other possible reason for lower σ_{SC} values with increasing glycerin concentration may be the reported increase in intercellular lipid fluidity after application of the GLY coatings [61]. In addition, when GLY is added to SC lipids in vitro, it has been reported to interact with the intercellular lipids and maintain the intercellular lipid matrix in a fluid, liquid crystalline phase [55, 67]. Considering that the SC lipids alone account for ~5–30 vol.% of the total tissue volume, their expansion could act to reduce drying stresses by viscous flow and increased movement of the corneocytes. The extent to which the observed drying stress reductions are related to such viscous flow associated with increased lipid fluidity is not currently known. Also, although the final σ_{SC} values are lower for GLY-coated SC compared to control, the σ_{SC} values stabilize after ~2 h in the drying environment, and there is no evidence of further relaxation that would be expected in the case of viscous flow. Note that viscous intercellular boundary sliding could be arrested by stretching of the corneodesmosomes to establish force equilibrium after a predetermined amount of sliding. Such mechanisms for drying stress reduction are currently speculative and await further study.

While different concentrations of GLY in DIW have been observed to reduce SC stresses, the efficacy of other GLY-containing formulations in reducing these stresses has been shown to vary. The reported σ_{SC} values following application of two different formulations, GLY-A and GLY-B, containing 40–50% (v/v) glycerin are shown in Fig. 15.11a. σ_{SC} values of GLY-A-coated specimens increase rapidly to a peak and then decrease to a final σ_{SC} value higher than that of the control. In contrast, the σ_{SC} values of specimens coated with GLY-B increase and stabilize at σ_{SC} values lower than that of the control after ~2 h in the drying environment.

These drastically different stress profiles following application of two formulations containing similar amounts of GLY have been discussed in terms of the effect of these coatings on SC water loss and its components [61]. The significantly higher final σ_{SC} and $d\sigma_{SC}/dt$ values for specimens coated with GLY-A suggest that SC is more sensitive to water loss following exposure to this treatment despite the high GLY content and humectancy of GLY-A. This nondrying gel with a simple chemical composition consisting of GLY and glyceryl polyacrylate does not readily release the water contained within its molecular structure even under severe drying conditions due to its clathrate (group of molecules that form a cage-like matrix) structure. Water molecules are held within the glyceryl polyacrylate clathrate matrix and released when disrupted by the salt content, pH and surface temperature of skin [68].

The increased σ_{SC} and $d\sigma_{SC}/dt$ values following application of GLY-A has been associated with the poor diffusion of the gel ingredients into the SC and the strong affinity of both glycerin and glyceryl polyacrylate in the gel to absorb water from the humid SC in the meantime. Finally, the significantly larger stress relaxation observed for GLY-A compared to GLY coatings has been linked to increased lipid fluidity due to penetration of glyceryl polyacrylate into the SC [61].

The final σ_{SC} values of GLY-B-coated SC is similar to the σ_{SC} values observed for tissue coated with 100% (v/v) GLY although the formulation contains only 40–50% (v/v) GLY. The lower σ_{SC} values observed with GLY-B have been associated with the increased GLY penetration in the presence of the emulsifiers used in the treatment [61]. The formulation also contains an oil/lamellar gel-/water-type emulsion that forms a hydrophobic film on SC that further reduce water loss.

These reported results show that the effective delivery of GLY into the SC is crucial for it to reduce water loss from the tissue. Otherwise, the presence of a humectant coating on SC can actually increase water loss from the tissue for the isolated SC experimental model discussed in this section.

15.6.3 Ester-Based Emollients with Partially Occlusive Behavior

Emollients are used as key ingredients in moisturizing and cleansing formulations to improve skin sensory properties and alleviate dry skin. They provide an oily partially occlusive film over the surface of the skin which fills in the interstices between the desquamating corneocytes abundant in dry skin conditions, smoothing the rough SC surface and increasing the ability of the skin to hold water [66, 69]. Their occlusivity depends in part on their molecular weight, viscosity, and spreading characteristics on SC. If the emollient molecules penetrate into the SC, they may interact with the intercellular lipids or corneocytes depending on their hydrophilicity/lipophilicity, and in vivo, they may eventually be metabolized and modify lipid secretory mechanisms [70–72]. This section discusses reported effects of emollient molecules listed in Table 15.1 on SC drying stresses in terms of their direct effects on the components of the SC and moisture exchange with the environment.

The molecular structure of these emollients together with their calculated partition coefficient, log *P*, used to measure the hydrophilic/lipophilic balance, and other salient physical characteristics (molecular weight (MW), viscosity and spreading characteristics) are listed in Table 15.2. Among these treatments, DA is the least lipophilic (log $P \sim 2.8$) and likely to diffuse rapidly into the SC and partition well between its hydrophilic and lipophilic lipid domains [73]. The other emollients are unlikely to partition into the hydrophilic domains of the SC with log *P* values increasing above 5. Rather, they are expected to partition into the skin lipids and have extreme difficulty partitioning out of the SC [74].

Table 15.2 The molecular structure of the emollient coatings, their corresponding calculated log *P* values and other salient physical characteristics (molecular weight (MW), viscosity and spreading characteristics) are listed

Treatment	Molecular structure	log *P*	MW (g)	Viscosity (Pa·s)	Spreading
DA	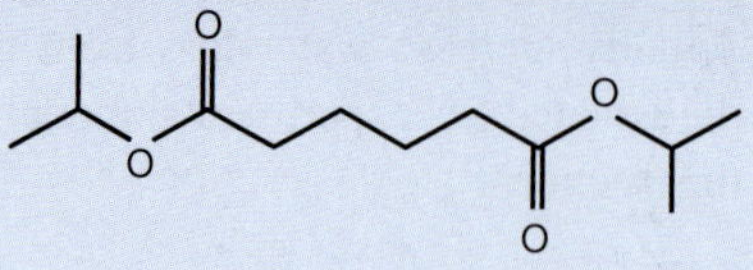	2.79	230.2	0.004	High
AL	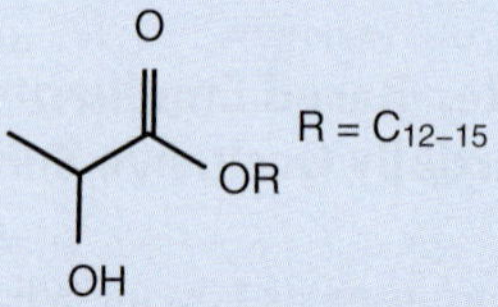	5.92	286.5	0.018	High
IN	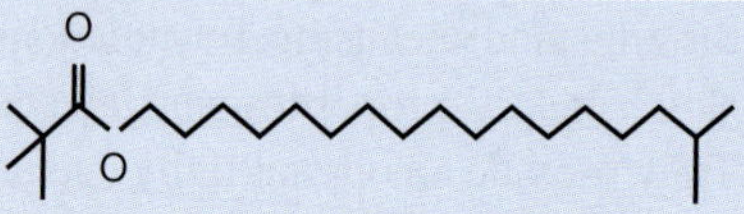	10.25	354.4	0.015	Medium
EP	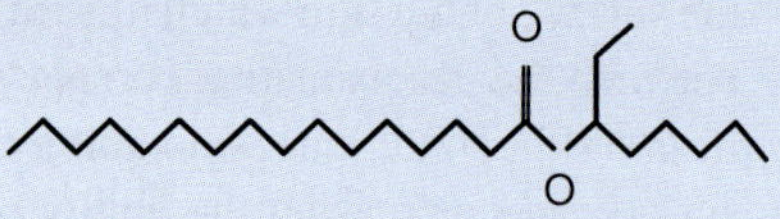	11.15	368.4	0.014	Medium
ISS	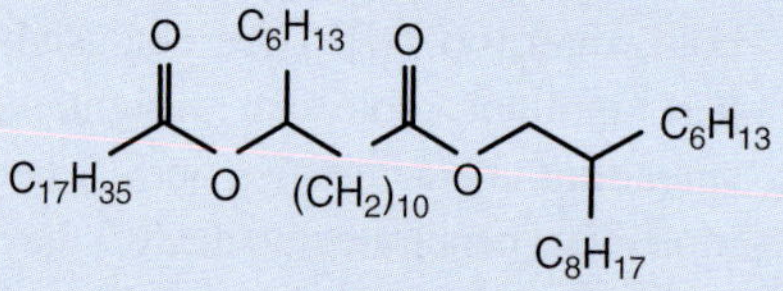	20.02	791.4	0.090	Low
OSS	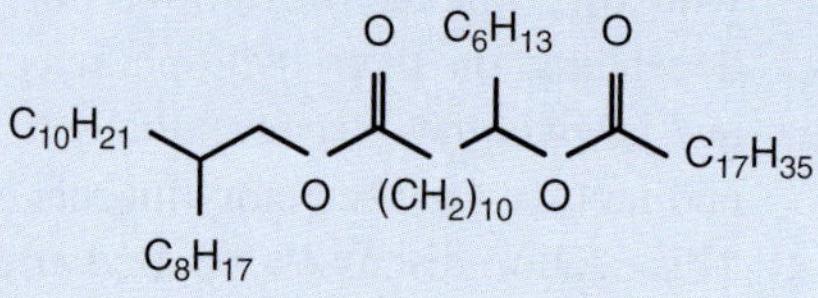	26.92	846.9	0.083	Low

Following application of emollient coatings on SC, the reported σ_{SC} values are nonzero; they increase rapidly to initial peak values in <1 h and relax to final values that are significantly lower than DIW (control)-treated tissue as shown in Fig. 15.12 [60]. Since no stresses develop in the emollient coatings when applied directly on the glass substrate, the σ_{SC} values are determined from the overall substrate curvature as described for NDO coatings in Sect. 15.5.2.

The complex drying stress profiles for emollient-coated SC have been associated with the effects of emollient molecules on lipid extraction and fluidity together with their effects on control of SC water content [60]. The initial nonzero σ_{SC} values have been linked to contraction of SC lipids due to extraction of a fraction of intercellular lipids immediately following application of the

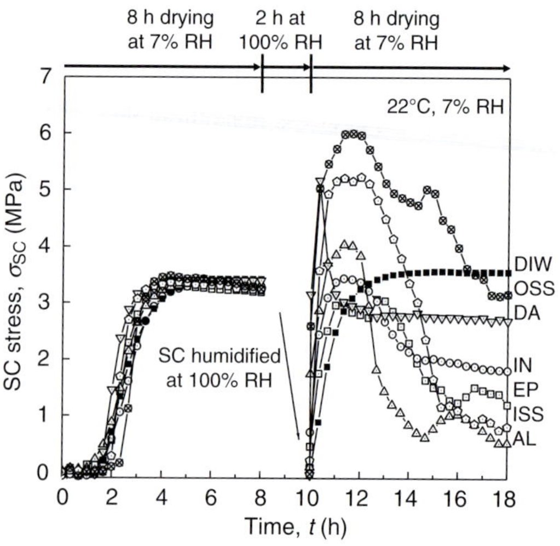

Fig. 15.12 SC drying stress as a function of drying time for SC treated with the emollient coatings (DA, AL, IN, EP, ISS, OSS) and exposed to 7% RH and 22°C air

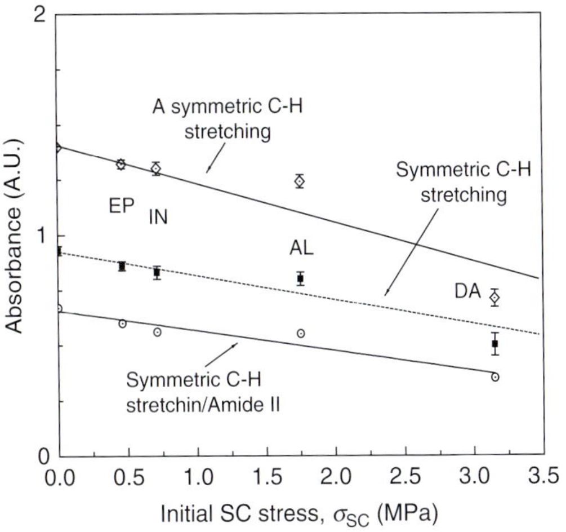

Fig. 15.13 The first stress values following application of emollient coatings as a function of the height of asymmetric and symmetric C–H bond stretching peak and the ratio of the height of symmetric C–H stretching peak to the height of the amide II peak. The linear fits show a strong correlation between the drying stress and the height of the asymmetric and symmetric C–H bond stretching peaks and the ratio of the height of symmetric C–H stretching peak to the height of the amide II peak

emollient molecules. The extraction of SC lipids has been measured with ATR-FTIR by monitoring changes in the height of the symmetric and anti-symmetric C–H stretching peaks and the ratio of the height of symmetric C–H stretching peak to the height of the amide II peak [60]. These peaks and ratios are indicators of lipid extraction. For the emollients that resulted in lipid extraction, the initial σ_{SC} values have been observed to correlate well with the height of the symmetric and assymetric C–H stretching peaks and the ratio of the height of the symmetric C–H stretching peak to the height of the amide II peak as shown in Fig. 15.13.

The reported high $d\sigma_{SC}/dt$ and peak σ_{SC} values following application of the emollient coatings have been associated with the humectancy of the emollient coating on the SC, the extraction of a fraction of intercellular lipids with emollient penetration into the SC, or the increased water loss from the tissue as the emollients fluidize the SC lipids [60]. The high initial and peak σ_{SC} values following exposure to DA and AL (low-MW emollients with low lipophilicity) have been attributed to the ability of these coatings to extract moisture out of SC due to their significant proclivity to bind with water and the perturbation of the SC barrier properties due to extraction of a fraction of SC lipids with emollient penetration into the tissue as confirmed by spectroscopy results. Additionally, the possibility of the DA treatment to dissolve and remove the natural moisturizing factor components of SC has been suggested. This can reduce the natural humectancy of the tissue as DA can penetrate into both the hydrophilic and lipophilic domains of the tissue (based on its calculated log *P* value). On the other hand, the high peak σ_{SC} values observed following exposure to ISS and OSS (high-MW emollients with high lipophilicity) have been attributed to two contributing effects. First, the emollients act to fluidize the lipids and in doing so they free bound water, which can escape from the SC. This is consistent with a reported increase in water loss from the SC with increasing lipid fluidity as measured by the increase in lipid symmetric stretching frequency [75]. The second is related to the inability of these emollients to form a continuous occlusive coating and their subsequent failure to prevent water loss from the tissue, which includes the previously bound water.

Finally, the relaxation of SC stresses from a peak σ_{SC} value to a final σ_{SC} value has been linked to changes in the lipid fluidity of the tissue due to penetration of emollients into the SC. The penetration of GLY coatings into the SC has been measured with ATR-FTIR measurements as a function of tissue depth using a delamination technique [60]. For the low-MW emollients, the sudden rapid decrease in SC stresses has been attributed to the increase in lipid rigidity. On the other hand, the gradual stress relaxation for medium and high-MW emollients has been attributed to the ability of the corneocytes to move somewhat due to increased fluidity of the lipid matrix and gradual softening of the tissue due to increased penetration of the emollients.

We conclude by noting that the drying stress profiles of the emollient-treated SC are more complex than those observed for DIW-treated specimens or after application of humectant or occlusive treatments where the major contribution to the drying stresses is primarily due to the volume of water lost as discussed in Sects. 15.6.1 and 15.6.2. The drying stress profiles following application of humectant or occlusive treatments does not exhibit the peaks and significant relaxation exhibited after the emollient treatments where both lipid extraction and changes in lipid fluidity contributed to the drying stresses in addition to the volume of water lost. For the emollients discussed in this section, the effects of other SC components on the resulting drying stresses are not expected to be significant because these emollients (excluding DA) are likely to strongly partition into the SC lipids based on their high partition coefficient value. However, we note that the extraction of the lipids and changes in lipid fluidity may be encountered by reorientation of the covalently linked protein scaffolding constituted by the cornified SC envelope and stretching of corneodesmosomes to establish force equilibrium. This can especially play a role to arrest viscous intercellular boundary sliding or movement of corneocytes due to increased fluidity of the lipid matrix. The effect of such mechanisms on the SC drying stresses is currently speculative and awaits further study.

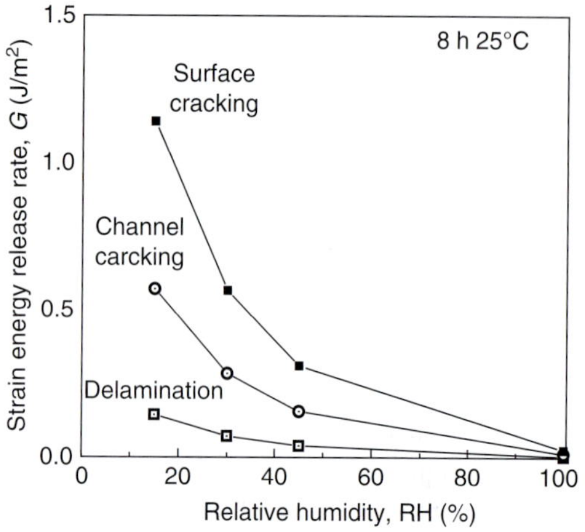

Fig. 15.14 Crack driving force, *G*, values that result from the SC drying stresses for surface cracking, channel cracking and delamination as a function of the RH of the drying environment for DIW-treated tissue exposed to air at 15%, 30%, 45%, and 100% RH and 25°C for 8 h

15.6.4 Implications for Damage

We now consider the biomechanics model described in Sect. 15.2 to infer the propensity for dry skin damage by computing the strain energy release rate, *G*, from the reported values of σ_{SC} and E_{SC} and comparing them to the SC resistance to cracking, G_c. *G* values of DIW-treated SC for the cracking configurations shown in Fig. 15.1 are shown as a function of the RH of the drying environment in Fig. 15.14 [16]. It is clear from the figure that *G* values increase with decreasing RH of the drying environment. We note that the mechanical driving force for skin damage is particularly sensitive to the SC stress since *G* scales with the square of σ_{SC}. On the other hand, the reported increasing stiffness of the SC with decreasing RH of the drying environment would act to decrease *G* values since E_{SC} appears on the denominator of Eq. 15.1. However, the SC stress dominates and the values of *G* increase markedly with decreasing RH suggesting that the driving force for dry skin cracking and chapping damage increases as the skin is exposed to increasingly dry environments.

The *G* values determined must exceed the SC resistance to cracking, G_c, in order for such skin damage processes to occur. G_c values reported in the literature range from ~0.5 to 8 J/m^2 for human SC treated in different drying environments [17–19]. The *G* values estimated clearly equal or exceed G_c values in the lower part of the range that we have previously reported (they are likely to be higher due to the epidermal/dermal viscoelastic relaxation processes mentioned in the introduction). Taken together, the results for the value of *G* and the associated G_c values for dry skin strongly suggest that the drying stress in SC provides the principal mechanical driving force for the formation and propagation of dry skin damage. The results shown in Fig. 15.14 also suggest that the driving force for surface cracking which involves the propagation of a through thickness SC crack into the underlying epidermal layers has the largest value of *G* making this the most prevalent form of skin damage. These results are suggested from the mechanical models for the different possible SC cracking configurations but are clearly consistent with clinical observations of severe dry skin damage. The surface cracking configuration provides a direct path for environmental species to penetrate the SC barrier and enter the underlying skin layers.

Using the biomechanics model, it is also possible to predict the effect of chemical and moisturizing treatments discussed in this chapter on skin damage processes. By observing the ratio of

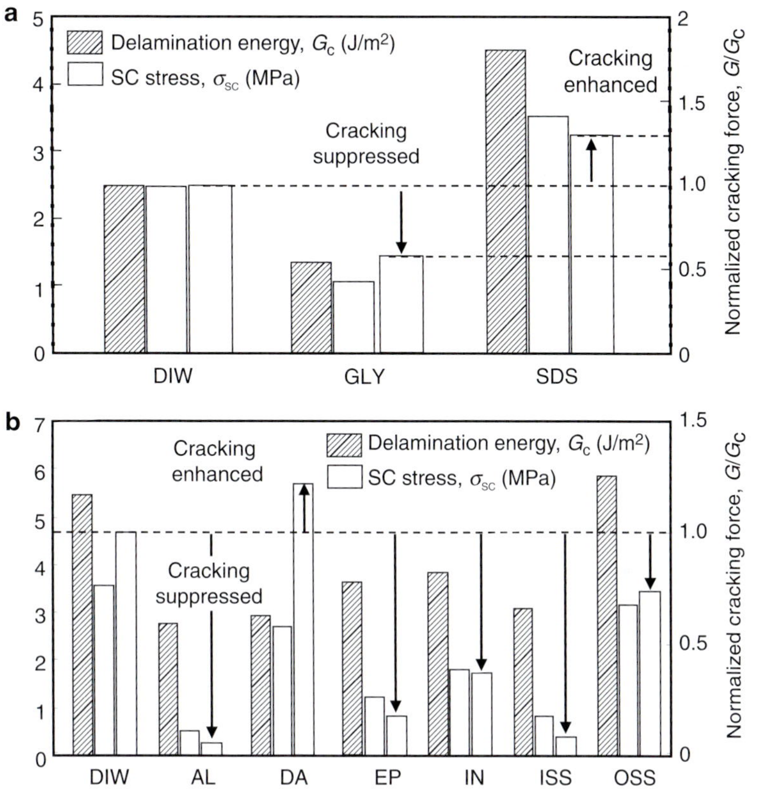

Fig. 15.15 (**a**) SC drying stress, σ_{SC}, intercellular delamination energy, G_c, and the normalized crack driving force, G/G_c, shown as a function of chemical treatment (SDS, DIW and GLY) for SC exposed to 15% RH air at 25°C. The cracking potential is significantly increased after the SC is damaged by the SDS treatment, and the cracking potential is markedly reduced after moisturizing with GLY. (**b**) SC drying stress, σ_{SC}, intercellular delamination energy, G_c, and the normalized crack driving force, G/G_c, shown as a function of emollient coatings

G/G_c and using the values for DIW-treated tissue exposed to a drying environment as a control, the propensity for SC cracking for SDS- and GLY-treated tissue exposed to the same 15% RH and 25°C drying environment can immediately be observed (Fig. 15.15a). The normalized cracking ratio for SDS-treated tissue increased significantly with the higher drying stresses compared to the DIW-treated control, suggesting that the harsh SDS treatment enhances the propensity for cracking. In contrast, the normalized cracking ratio for the GLY-treated tissue with the lower drying stresses is significantly reduced compared to the control, indicating the beneficial effects of moisturizing treatments on reducing dry skin damage.

The same model can also be used to show the efficacy of emollient coatings discussed in this chapter as shown in Fig. 15.15b. The propensity for cracking is significantly reduced for SC treated with the emollient coatings (excluding DA) indicating again the beneficial effects of moisturizing treatments on reducing dry skin damage. On the other hand, the propensity for cracking for DA-coated SC is higher compared to control suggesting that this treatment may cause damage to the tissue. Our visual observations of a dry SC surface with evidence of cracking and flaking following exposure to this treatment and the drying environment strengthen this argument.

Conclusion

The research described in this chapter involves synergistic experimental and mechanics modeling efforts to provide a fundamental scientific and clinically relevant basis from which skin damage processes associated with dry skin conditions in isolated human SC can be quantitatively characterized and understood. This research also provides the basis from which biomechanical models can be employed to evaluate the efficacy of treatments on the propensity for dry skin damage. Thin-film mechanics techniques currently used to characterize skin stresses are reviewed. The relationship of these stresses to tissue components and moisture content is discussed by using environmental, damaging and moisturizing chemical treatments to systematically manipulate and influence components of the SC tissue including intercellular lipids, corneodesmosomes, and intracellular keratin. Finally, a mechanics framework is used to evaluate the efficacy of moisturizing treatments in alleviating the potential for dry skin damage. Taken together, this chapter discusses new and unique approaches to characterize and model the fundamental biomechanics of human SC and skin damage processes.

Take Home Messages

- We review the application of the substrate curvature technique to characterize drying stresses in human stratum corneum (SC) following environmental preconditioning, chemical and moisturizing treatment in a range of drying environments.
- We describe a biomechanical model that explains how these stresses provide the propensity for dry skin damage such as cracking and chapping.
- We review extensions of the substrate curvature technique to measure the efficacy of topical coatings applied to SC where the overall drying stresses may have contributions from the coating, the SC, and the interaction of the coating with the SC.
- We elucidate the effects of occlusive, humectant, and emollient moisturizers on the mechanical properties and drying stresses in SC.
- We explain how moisturizers affect the water content and structural components of the tissue and how these subsequently determine the stress state in the tissue.
- Using the biomechanical model reviewed in the chapter, we demonstrate how damaging treatments enhance and moisturizing treatments alleviate the propensity for dry skin damage.

References

1. Harding CR (2004) The stratum corneum: structure and function in health and disease. Dermatol Ther 17:6–15
2. Harding CR, Long S, Richardson J, Rogers J, Zhang Z, Rawlings AV (2003) The cornified envelope: an important marker of stratum corneum in healthy and dry skin. J Cosmet Sci 25:157–163
3. Mustoe TA, Cooter RD, Gold MH, Hobbs FD, Ramelet AA, Shakespeare PG et al (2002) International clinical recommendations on scar management. Plast Reconstr Surg 110:560–571
4. Longacre JJ, Berry HK, Basom CR, Townsend SF (1976) The effects of Z plasty on hypertrophic scars. Scand J Plast Reconstr Surg 10:113–128
5. Scars BM (1998) Can they be minimised? Aust Fam Physician 27:275–278
6. Edlich RF, Carl BA (1998) Predicting scar formation: from ritual practice (Langer's lines) to scientific discipline (static and dynamic skin tensions). J Emerg Med 16:759–760
7. Atkinson JM, Barnett AG, McGrath DJ, Rudd M (2005) A randomized controlled trial to determine the efficacy of paper tape in preventing hypertrophic scar formation. Plast Reconstr Surg 116:1648–1656
8. Gaul LE, Underwood GB (1952) Relation of dew point and barometric pressure to chapping of normal skin. J Invest Dermatol 19(1):9–19
9. Ananthapadmanabhan KP, Moore DJ, Subramanyan K, Misra M, Meyer F (2004) Cleansing without compromise: the impact of cleansers on the skin barrier and the technology of mild cleansing. Dermatol Ther 17(Suppl 1):16–25
10. Subramanyan KF (2007) Advances in the materials science of skin: a composite structure with multiple functions. MRS Bull 32(10):770
11. Rudikoff D (1998) The effect of dryness on skin. Clin Dermatol 16:99–107
12. Rawlings AV, Matts PJ (2005) Stratum corneum moisturization at the molecular level: an update in relation to the dry skin cycle. J Invest Dermatol 124:1099–1110
13. Harding CR, Watkinson A, Rawlings AV, Scott IR (2000) Dry skin, moisturization and corneodesmolysis. Int J Cosmet Sci 1:21–52
14. Rhein L, Robbins C, Fernee K, Cantore R (1986) Surfactant structure effects on swelling of isolated human stratum corneum. J Soc Cosmet Chem 37:125–139
15. Hutchinson JW, Suo Z (1992) Mixed mode cracking in layered materials. Adv Appl Mech 29:63–191
16. Levi K, Weber RJ, Do JQ, Dauskardt RH (2009) Drying stress and damage processes in human stratum corneum. Int J Cosmet Sci 32(4):276–293
17. Wu KS, Van Osdol WW, Dauskardt RH (2005) Mechanical properties of human stratum corneum: effects of temperature, hydration, and chemical treatment. Biomaterials 27(5):785–795
18. Wu KS, Li J, Ananthapadmanabhan KP, Dauskardt RH (2006) Time-dependent intercellular delamination of human stratum corneum. J Mater Sci 42(21):8986

19. Wu KS, Stefik MM, Ananthapadmanabhan KP, Dauskardt RH (2006) Graded delamination behavior of human stratum corneum. Biomaterials 27: 5861–5870
20. Mukherjee S, Richardson J, Margosiak M, Lei X (1999) Understanding dry rough skin: a physical basis for the effects of dry environment and surfactant treatment on corneum fracture. In: Lal M, Lillford PJ, Naik VM, Prakash V (eds) Supramolecular and colloidal structures in biomaterials and biosubstrates – Proceedings of the fifth royal society-Unilever Indo-UK forum in materials science and engineering, held in Mysore, India, on January 10–14, 1999. World Scientific Publishing Company, Singapore, pp 306–324
21. Flinn PA, Gardner DS, Nix WD (1987) Measurements and interpretation of stress in aluminum-based metallization as a function of thermal history. IEEE Trans Electron Dev ED-34(3):689–699
22. Gardner DS, Flinn PA (1988) Mechanical stress as a function of temperature in aluminum films. IEEE Trans Electron Dev 35(12):2160–2169
23. Moske M, Samwer K (1988) New UHV dilatometer for precise measurement of internal stresses in thin binary-alloy films from 20–750K. Rev Sci Instrum 59:2012
24. Bader S, Kalaugher EM, Arzt E (1995) Comparison of mechanical properties and microstructure of Al (1 wt. % Si) and Al (1 wt. % Si, 0.5 wt. % Cu) thin films. Thin Solid Films 262:175–184
25. Keller RM, Baker SP, Arzt E (1998) Quantitative analysis of strengthening mechanisms in thin cu films: effects of film thickness, grain size, and passivation. J Mater Res 13(5):1307–1317
26. Stoney GG (1909) The tension of metallic films deposited by electrolysis. Proc R Soc Lond B Biol 82(553):172
27. Anderson RL, Cassidy JM, Hansen JR, Yellin W (1973) Hydration of stratum corneum. Biopolymers 12(12):2789–2802
28. Liron Z, Wright RL, McDougal JN (1994) Water diffusivity in porcine stratum corneum measured by a thermal gravimetric analysis technique. J Pharm Sci 83(4):457–462
29. Kasting GB, Barai ND (2003) Equilibrium water sorption in human stratum corneum. J Pharm Sci 92(8):1624–1631
30. Potts RO, Guzek DB, Harriss RR, McKie JE (1985) A non invasive, in vivo, technique to quantitatively measure water concentration of the stratum corneum using attenuated total-reflectance infrared spectroscopy. Arch Dermatol Res 277:489–495
31. Caspers PJ, Lucassen GW, Wolthuis R, Bruining HA, Puppels GJ (1998) In vitro and in vivo Raman spectroscopy of human skin. Biospectroscopy 4(5 Suppl):9
32. Hansen JR, Yellin W (1972) NMR and infrared spectroscopic studies of stratum corneum hydration. Plenum Press, New York
33. Gilard V (1998) Measurement of total water and bound water contents in human stratum corneum by in vitro proton nuclear magnetic resonance spectroscopy. Int J Cosmet Sci 20(2):117
34. Takahashi M, Kawasaki K, Tanaka M, Ohta S, Tsuda Y (1981) The mechanism of stratum corneum plasticization with water. In: Marks RM, Payne PA (eds) Bioengineering and the skin. MTP Press Ltd, Lancaster, pp 67–73
35. Jokura Y, Ishikawa S, Tokuda H, Imokawa G (1995) Molecular analysis of elastic properties of the stratum corneum by solid-state 13C-nuclear magnetic resonance spectroscopy. J Invest Dermatol 104(5):806–812
36. Guo X, Imhof RE, Rigal J (2001) Spectroscopic study of water-keratin interactions in stratum corneum. Anal Sci 17:s342
37. Leveque JL (2004) Bioengineering of the skin: water and the stratum corneum. CRC Press, Boca Raton
38. Barry BW (1988) Action of skin penetration enhancers-the lipid protein partitioning theory. Int J Cosmet Sci 10(6):281
39. Wu KS (2006) Mechanical behavior of human stratum corneum: relationship to tissue structure and condition. Stanford University, Stanford
40. Ramsing DW (1997) Effect of water on experimentally irritated human skin. Br J Dermatol 136(3):364
41. Warner RR, Boissy YL, Lilly NA, Spears MJ, McKillop K, Marshall JL et al (1999) Water disrupts stratum corneum lipid lamellae: damage is similar to surfactants. J Invest Dermatol 113(6):960–966
42. Van Hal DA, Jeremiasse E, Junginger HE, Spies F, Bouwstra JA (1996) Structure of fully hydrated human stratum corneum: a freeze-fracture electron microscopy study. J Invest Dermatol 106(1):89–95
43. Rawlings A, Harding C, Watkinson A, Banks J, Ackerman C, Sabin R (1995) The effect of glycerol and humidity on desmosome degradation in stratum corneum. Arch Dermatol Res 287(5):457–464
44. Bouwstra JA, de Graaff A, Gooris GS, Nijsse J, Wiechers JW, van Aelst AC (2003) Water distribution and related morphology in human stratum corneum at different hydration levels. J Invest Dermatol 120(5):750–758
45. Wilkes GL, Wildnauer RH (1973) Structure–property relationships of the stratum corneum of human and neonatal rat. II. Dynamic mechanical studies. Biochim Biophys Acta 304(2):276–289
46. Wilkes GL, Nguyen AL, Wildnauer R (1973) Structure–property relations of human and neonatal rat stratum corneum. I. Thermal stability of the crystalline lipid structure as studied by X-ray diffraction and differential thermal analysis. Biochim Biophys Acta 304(2):265–275
47. Yuan Y, Verma R (2006) Measuring microelastic properties of stratum corneum. Colloids Surf B 48(1):6
48. Nicolopoulos CS, Giannoudis PV, Glaros KD, Barbenel JC (1998) In vitro study of the failure of skin surface after influence of hydration and preconditioning. Arch Dermatol Res 290(11):638–640
49. Murray FW (1967) On the computation of saturation vapor pressure. J Appl Meteorol 6:203–204

50. Imokawa G, Akasaki S, Minematsu Y, Kawai M (1989) Importance of intercellular lipids in water-retention properties of the stratum corneum: induction and recovery study of surfactant dry skin. Arch Dermatol Res 281(1):45–51
51. Fulmer AW, Kramer GJ (1986) Stratum corneum lipid abnormalities in surfactant-induced dry scaly skin. J Invest Dermatol 86(5):598–602
52. Downing DT, Abraham W, Wegner BK, Wilman KW, Marshall JL (1993) Partition of sodium dodecyl sulfate into stratum corneum lipid liposomes. Arch Dermatol Res 285(3):151
53. Ananthapadmanabhan KP, Lips A, Vincent C, Meyer F, Caso S, Johnson A et al (2003) pH-induced alterations in stratum corneum properties. Int J Cosmet Sci 25(3):103
54. Putterman GJ, Wolsejsza NF, Wolfram MA, Laden K (1977) The effect of detergents on swelling of stratum corneum. J Soc Cosmet Chem 28:521–532
55. Froebe CL, Simion FA, Ohlmeyer H, Rhein LD, Mattai J, Cagan RH (1990) Prevention of stratum corneum lipid phase transitions in vitro by glycerol – an alternative mechanism for skin moisturization. J Soc Cosmet Chem 41:51
56. Fluhr JW, Gloor M, Lehmann L, Lazzerini S, Distante F, Berardesca E (1999) Glycerol accelerates recovery of barrier function in vivo. Acta Derm Venereol 79(6):418–421
57. Orth DS, Appa Y (1999) Glycerine: a natural ingredient for moisturizing skin. In: Loden M, Maibach HI (eds) Dry skin and moisturizers. CRC Press, Boca Raton
58. Loden M (2003) Role of topical emollients and moisturizers in the treatment of dry skin barrier disorders. Am J Clin Dermatol 4(11):771–788
59. Levi K, Dauskardt RH (2010) Application of substrate curvature method to differentiate drying stresses in topical coatings and human stratum corneum. Int J Cosmet Sci 32(4):294–298
60. Levi K, Kwan A, Rhines AS, Gorcea M, Moore DJ, Dauskardt RH (2010) Emollient molecule effects on the drying stresses in human stratum corneum. Br J Dermatol 163(4):695–703
61. Levi K, Kwan A, Rhines AS, Gorcea M, Moore DJ, Dauskardt RH (2011) Effect of glycerin on drying stresses in human stratum corneum. J Dermatol Sci 61(2):129–131
62. Hannon W, Maibach HI (1998) Efficacy of moisturizers assessed through bioengineering techniques. In: Baran R, Maibach HI (eds) Textbook cosmetic dermatology. Taylor & Francis Group, Boca Raton
63. Loden M (1992) The increase in skin hydration after application of emollients with different amounts of lipids. Acta Derm Venereol 72:327–330
64. Ghadially R, Halkier-Sorensen L, Elias PM (1992) Effects of petrolatum on stratum corneum structure and function. J Am Acad Dermatol 26(3 Pt 2): 387–396
65. O'Goshi KI, Tabata N, Sato Y, Tagami H (2000) Comparative study of the efficacy of various moisturizers on the skin of the ASR miniature swine. Skin Pharmacol Appl Skin Physiol 13(2):120–127
66. Draelos ZD (2000) Therapeutic moisturizers. Dermatol Clin 18(4):597–607
67. Hara M, Verkman AS (2003) Glycerol replacement corrects defective skin hydration, elasticity, and barrier function in aquaporin-3-deficient mice. Proc Natl Acad Sci USA 100(12):7360
68. Greff, D. (2000). Cosmetic, dermopharmaceutical or veterinary compositions for disinfecting human or animal skin. U.S. Patent 6,123,953, filed February 20, 1997, and issued September 26, 2000
69. Cork MJ (1997) The importance of skin barrier function. J Dermatolog Treat 8:7
70. Kucharekova M, Van de Kerkhof PCM, Van der Valk PGM (2003) A randomized comparison of an emollient containing skin-related lipids with a petrolatum-based emollient as adjunct in the treatment of chronic hand dermatitis. Contact Dermatitis 48(6):293–299
71. Wertz PW, Downing DT (1990) Metabolism of topically applied fatty acid methyl esters in BALB/C mouse epidermis. J Dermatol Sci 1(1):33
72. Mao-Qiang M, Brown BE, Wu-Pong S, Feingold KR, Elias PM (1995) Exogenous nonphysiologic vs physiologic lipids: divergent mechanisms for correction of permeability barrier dysfunction. Arch Dermatol 131:809–816
73. Hadgraft J (2001) Skin, the final frontier. Int J Pharm 224(1–2):1
74. Hadgraft J, Finnin BC (2006) Fundamentals of retarding penetration. In: Smith EW, Maibach HI (eds) Percutaneous penetration enhancers. CRC Press, Boca Raton
75. Potts RO, Francoeur ML (1990) Lipid biophysics of water loss through the skin. Proc Natl Acad Sci USA 87:3871–3873

Part III

Dry Skin Disorders and Treatments

Update on Atopic Eczema with Special Focus on Dryness and the Impact of Moisturizers

16

Eric Simpson

16.1 Clinical Presentation

Atopic dermatitis (AD) is the most common skin disease of childhood and is characterized by erythematous papules and papulovesicles during its initial presentation, followed by subacute lesions that are crusted, weeping, scaling, and excoriated. Chronic lesions show skin thickening, xerosis, and exaggerated skin markings (lichenification) that are the skin's response to rubbing (Fig. 16.1). Sites of predilection are the face and extensor extremities in infancy, with more frequent involvement of the flexural areas after age 1 [27]. Skin lesions are accompanied by intractable pruritus, the primary symptom leading to the reduced quality of life observed in these children.

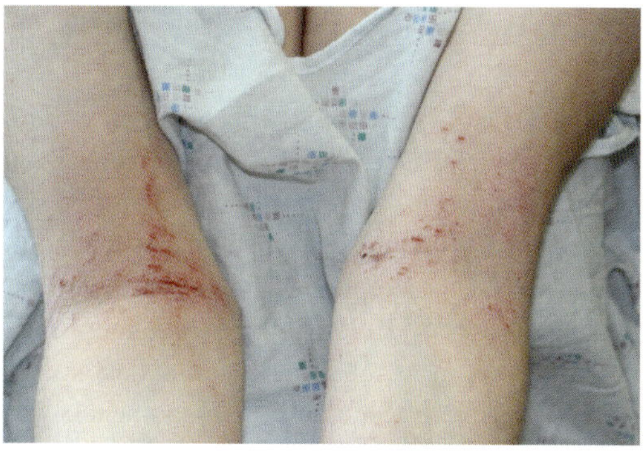

Fig. 16.1 Erythematous papules, crusting, and lichenified plaques on the flexural ankles typical of atopic dermatitis in a pediatric patient with moderate disease

16.2 Impact on Quality of Life

Children with AD display measurable emotional and behavioral differences compared to their peers without AD [10]. Recent data show that the sleep loss associated with AD increases the prevalence of attention deficit hyperactivity disorder [55]. Several other neuropsychiatric conditions have recently been reported to be associated with AD including anxiety, depression, and autism [83]. These associations display a dose-dependent response based on AD severity. A child's AD often affects an entire family as well. Caring for a child with AD impacts a family to a greater degree than caring for a child with type I diabetes [70].

16.3 Nomenclature

Historically, the terms prurigo of Besnier, neurodermatitis, and allergic eczema all represented what we now know as AD. Even today, there are many attempts to rename AD based on whether the disease is accompanied by IgE sensitization or not. The role of IgE in AD has been a controversial

E. Simpson, MD, M.C.R
Department of Dermatology, Oregon Health & Science University, Center for Health and Healing,
3303 SW Bond Ave, MC: CH16D, Portland, OR 97239, USA
e-mail: simpsone@ohsu.edu

M. Lodén, H.I. Maibach (eds.), *Treatment of Dry Skin Syndrome*,
DOI 10.1007/978-3-642-27606-4_16, © Springer-Verlag Berlin Heidelberg 2012

subject for many years, but several studies have shown that the IgE need not be present to make a diagnosis. Flohr found no association between IgE sensitization and flexural eczema in rural environments [23]. We recommend and continue to use the term atopic dermatitis for all children who meet standard criteria for the disease [28]. Documenting the presence or absence of IgE may be of use when managing concomitant type I allergic diseases or performing genetic studies but should not be an essential component to establishing the diagnosis of AD or to influence the treatment of the skin.

16.4 Diagnostic Criteria

In 1980, Hanifin and Rajka proposed their criteria for diagnosing AD after input from experts from around the world during the first International Symposium of Atopic Dermatitis in Stockholm [29]. These criteria represent the gold standard for the diagnosis of AD, although the large number of minor criteria makes it somewhat cumbersome to use in the clinic. Similar to AD nomenclature, numerous criteria for the diagnosis of AD have been proposed. Most sets of criteria have not undergone formal validation studies. The criteria that have been most extensively validated are the UK Working Party criteria, a systematic distillation of the Hanifin-Rajka criteria designed for epidemiological studies. The millennium criteria have been recently validated [59]. While being a more concise instrument than the Hanifin-Rajka criteria, the millennium criteria contain the requirement that IgE sensitization be present in order to establish a diagnosis of AD. As discussed previously, the significance of IgE for AD diagnosis and therapy has not been established. The American Academy of Dermatology Consensus criteria may serve as a more practical guide to AD diagnosis in the clinical setting, although they have not yet been validated [15].

16.5 Prevalence

There is significant worldwide variation in the prevalence of AD [51]. A higher disease prevalence exists in more industrialized countries, with a 1-year period prevalence ranging between 10% and 18% in the United States [62] and 20% in Northern Europe [51]. Similar to asthma and food allergy, the prevalence of AD has increased over the past 50 years and continues to increase in developing countries [60] for unclear reasons [81]. Environmental factors associated with industrialization likely play a role [51]. In high prevalence areas of Europe and Asia, this increase appears to be stabilizing at approximately 20% [81, 85].

16.6 Allergic Comorbidity

Between 60% and 80% of patients with AD have specific IgE sensitization, although the strength of this association varies by disease severity, the age of the patient, and geographical location. The etiologic basis of IgE sensitization in AD is not clear and is likely multifactorial. IgE sensitization may occur before or after AD development [44], so the cause-and-effect relationship between AD and IgE is unclear. In theory, children may be born with a genetic predisposition to the development of IgE, and genetic polymorphisms in Th2 cytokine pathways that could be responsible for this predisposition have been found in AD. On the other hand, several lines of evidence suggest elevated IgE levels may develop secondarily from a genetically disrupted skin barrier [20, 58]. Mouse models reveal that a disrupted skin barrier leads to significant IgE production targeted to skin-applied protein antigens [33, 68]. Lack and colleagues first provided clinical evidence of epicutaneous sensitization when his group showed that the strongest predictor of peanut allergy was the previous use of peanut oil on the skin [40]. Most recently, genetic defects in the gene encoding the skin barrier protein filaggrin have been shown to be associated with peanut allergy independent of eczema development, suggesting early peanut exposure to a disrupted skin barrier may promote type I peanut allergy [7]. As a consequence of IgE sensitization, patients with AD are at increased risk for developing asthma, allergic rhinitis, and food allergy. The prevalence of asthma in patients with AD varies depending upon AD severity and ranges between 14.2% and 52.7% according to a systematic review of cohort studies [78]. Children with eczema prior to the age of 4 had a greater than twofold odds increased risk of asthma at age 6.

16.7 Pathogenesis Overview

Twin studies reveal that AD has a strong genetic basis, although the inheritance pattern is non-Mendelian, suggesting that multiple genes and/or external factors contribute to its development [75]. While most experts agree that the disease is characterized by immune hyperactivity and skin barrier dysfunction, there has been significant disagreement regarding what constitutes the most important driving force for expression of the disease. There are those who propose the underlying and most influential defect in AD lies within the epidermis (outside-in hypothesis), and there are those who propose that the initiating event lies within a dysregulated immune system (inside-out hypothesis) [16]. In recent years, it is becoming clear that there is a complex relationship between the epidermis and the immune system in this disorder and that the disease may develop from contributions from both defects in the structural components of the skin barrier and from aberrant immune responses, with environmental factors modifying this relationship [17] (Fig. 16.2).

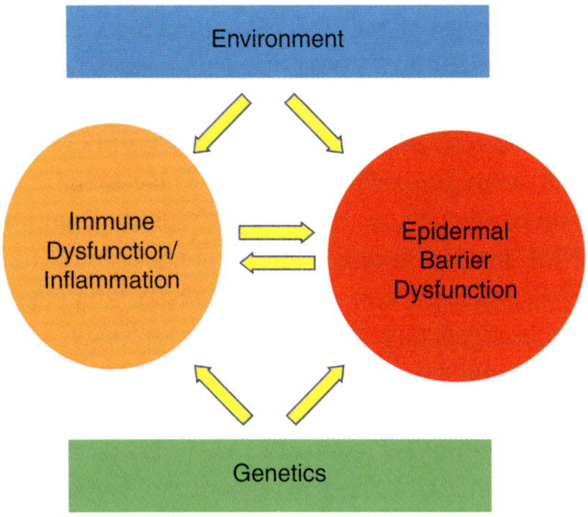

Fig. 16.2 The pathogenesis of atopic dermatitis involves the interplay between genetic defects in the skin barrier, hyperactive immune responses, skin barrier abnormalities that are not genetically determined, and environmental factors

16.8 Genetic Factors

While over 20 genes have been associated with atopic dermatitis, defects in the skin barrier gene filaggrin (FLG) have emerged as the most replicated and most important to date [2]. Candidate gene studies have found polymorphisms in several components of various immune pathways, but, unlike FLG studies, most have failed study replication [2]. Over 30 papers examining populations primarily in Asia and Europe have confirmed the importance of FLG mutations in AD [1]. Over 40 mutations have been described, all leading to an absence of protein expression through nonsense or frame-shift mutations [1]. Both mouse and human studies suggest the mechanism by which FLG deficiency leads to AD is through impaired barrier function. Filaggrin deficiency leads to a dry and impaired skin barrier through reduced NMF levels (see Sect. 16.11), a paracellular lipid defect, and an elevated stratum corneum pH. An elevated pH may have multiple negative downstream effects on barrier function such as a reduction in lamellar body secretion and activation of serine proteases [18]. Mouse models of filaggrin deficiency reveal this skin barrier defect alone leads to increased transepidermal water loss, cutaneous inflammation, the development of Th2-dominant inflammation, and IgE sensitization to topically applied allergens [20]. A meta-analysis of FLG associations reveals that people with AD and FLG mutations have earlier onset disease, more severe disease, more IgE sensitization, and asthma than AD controls without an FLG defect [77]. The mechanisms underlying the relationship between an epidermal FLG defect and the increased risk of IgE sensitization and asthma are not yet known, but mouse models confirm that protein exposed to the filaggrin-deficient epidermis leads to epicutaneous sensitization and markedly elevated IgE [20, 58]. More research is needed regarding the full downstream molecular effects of FLG deficiency.

While filaggrin mutations have been the strongest risk factor ever found for this disease, in population-based studies of children with more mild disease, the percent of the total AD burden that may be explained by FLG mutations may be as low as 13% (attributable risk) [80]. This fact and the increase in disease prevalence over time suggest environmental factors play a role in AD expression.

16.9 Environmental Factors

Environmental factors likely play a role in AD given the significant geographic variability found in the disease [51, 62] and the changes in disease prevalence over time. Children who immigrate to a new country adopt the AD risk of the destination country, strongly suggesting environmental factors play a role [41]. Observational studies have shown factors such as urban living and proximity to pollution may modify one's risk of developing AD [48, 62]. Exposure to hard water had been associated with a higher prevalence of AD, but a recent randomized controlled trial failed to find utility in water softeners as an adjunct to AD therapy [74]. Repeated skin exposure to water and detergents during infancy has also been proposed as a cause of the increasing prevalence of AD [53]. We recently showed a large proportion of parents use fragranced lotions on a regular basis on their infants, supporting this hypothesis [54]. Most recently, the complex interactions between FLG mutations and environmental factors are being elucidated; for example, the combination of an FLG mutation plus cat ownership increased the risk of AD development in two studies [4, 61]. Deciphering these complex gene-environmental interactions is the first step toward the development of comprehensive prevention strategies.

16.10 Immunological and Proinflammatory Factors

In some cases of AD, a genetically determined predisposition toward immune dysregulation could primarily drive the disease. Examples of this are seen with common variable immunodeficiency or autosomal recessive hyper-IgE syndrome: Both are primarily immune disorders that have AD as an associated feature. In addition, many epidermal defects in AD may be explained by the effects of Th2 inflammation on epidermal function. Th2 cytokines have been shown to downregulate filaggrin expression, ceramide synthesis, and antimicrobial production [35, 36]. Recently, Suárez-Fariñas and colleagues showed that nonlesional skin in atopic dermatitis has a significantly altered epidermal differentiation program, suggesting systemic inflammation plays a role in epidermal dysfunction in AD [71]. Treatment of lesional skin with topical steroids or topical pimecrolimus upregulates multiple terminal differentiation markers in the lesional skin of AD [38]. In addition, intermittent anti-inflammatory treatment, even of normal-appearing skin, can have beneficial effects on AD [52].

16.11 Etiology of Atopic Dry Skin

Virtually all children with atopic dermatitis have xerosis [6]. Xerosis has been reported in both lesional and nonlesional skin in AD, and the degree of xerosis often corresponds to the overall severity of the disease [73]. The etiology of xerosis in AD is multifactorial, but reduced NMF levels play a major role. A reduction of NMF is likely a global feature of atopic dermatitis and can be caused by either filaggrin deficiency or inflammation. Kezic and colleagues recently found the primary determinant of reduced NMF levels in AD was filaggrin genotype [39]. Filaggrin is normally proteolytically processed into the primary components of NMF-polycarboxylic acids and hygroscopic amino acids [57]. NMF levels as measured by Raman spectroscopy accurately correlate to FLG genotype [50]; however, Kezic's study also found that filaggrin genotype is not the only determinant of NMF levels. Disease severity, independent of the FLG genotype, also correlated directly with NMF levels, suggesting the inflammatory process may further influence NMF levels possibly by altering FLG expression as discussed earlier.

In addition to reduced levels of NMF, alterations in lipid composition and organization contribute to the xerosis seen in AD by increasing water permeability. Several studies have found reduced levels of ceramide species in the lesional skin of patients with AD [5, 14, 37, 84]. Imokawa found reduced levels of ceramide in both lesional and nonlesional skin, suggesting a ceramide deficiency may be a primary defect in AD. Farwanah, however, was unable to confirm these results in nonlesional skin [21]. Altered sphingomyelin metabolism likely explains the lipid abnormalities in lesional skin [49]. Hatano showed that the Th2 cytokine, IL-4, downregulates ceramide synthesis probably by reducing the expression of sphingomyelinase and glucocerebrosidase [31]. Mouse models of FLG deficiency reveal a paracellular permeability defect due to disorganized lamellar lipid sheets [58] that has recently been confirmed in human subjects with genetically confirmed filaggrin deficiency [25]. Abnormal lamellar body loading and unloading of lipids likely underlies the lipid disorganization caused by filaggrin deficiency. Tight junctions and corneodesmosome numbers were also reduced in FLG deficient patients, likely contributing to the permeability barrier defect.

16.12 Therapeutic Overview

The overall strategy for control of atopic dermatitis can be divided into the three following phases: clearance, maintenance, and rescue of flares [64]. The clearance phase usually involves the application of a medium potency topical steroid in an ointment base to all affected surfaces after twice daily bathing. A bland emollient is used on nonaffected skin. Application should be 7–14 days, and, if the proper strength of topical steroid is used, this should lead to significant clearing in nearly all patients in 1–2 weeks.

The maintenance phase of therapy then begins and consists of primarily emollient therapy on a daily basis for patients with mild to moderate disease as the topical steroids are tapered. The use of a bland petrolatum-based emollient can drastically improve disease control and reduce topical steroid use [11, 72]. Petrolatum incorporates into the interstitial space of the stratum corneum and improves skin barrier function, likely explaining its efficacy in atopic dermatitis [24]. The optimal emollient formulation for AD management is not known.

For eczema that quickly recurs despite proper emollient use, topical steroids may be used twice weekly to recurrent disease. Topical calcineurin inhibitors may also be initiated to early disease recurrence twice daily to reduce steroid use [79]. In patients with moderate to severe disease, treatment of normal skin frequent flare sites represents a new paradigm of anti-inflammatory use. Intermittent topical steroids or calcineurin inhibitors, when applied to normal skin frequent flare sites, dramatically increase the number of days without flare [3, 52].

Even with the best maintenance program, flares of AD will occur. This phase is treated by identifying and correcting flare factors such as a cutaneous infection or xerosis and reinstituting the induction phase therapy for 3–4 days. Patients with moderate to severe disease failing this aggressive topical approach often need phototherapy or systemic therapy with cyclosporine, azathioprine, methotrexate, or mycophenolate mofetil.

Lastly, effective patient and parental education regarding the risks and benefits of topical steroids, proper application of topical therapies, proper bathing, and clarifying the role of food allergy are all essential to achieving successful outcomes in this disease. Studies of nurse educators in AD illustrate the importance of education in achieving successful outcomes in AD [11]. A discussion of factors that worsen itch is also important and patients should be instructed to avoid contact with wool, irritating over-the-counter products, and low-humidity environments. Attempting to improve adherence to the treatment regimen is also important. One study found frequent follow-up visits may be one potentially useful strategy [56].

16.13 Emollients in AD

16.13.1 Overview

Despite the fact that emollients are considered first-line treatment for AD in several published guidelines [15, 19, 30], there is a paucity of data examining the optimal emollient for this condition. Most oil-in-water emollients improve skin barrier function, which likely explains their clinical benefit; however, some emollient formulations may have detrimental effects on the skin barrier. Held and colleagues showed a slight increase in irritant response in normal skin after treatment with an oil-in-water emollient but no negative effect on TEWL was seen [32]. Buraczewska and colleagues showed pretreatment of normal skin with an emollient containing canola oil and urea worsened the skin barrier function after challenge with a skin irritant [8]. Mustard oil, commonly used on infant skin in India, negatively affected skin barrier recovery kinetics in a mouse model in contrast to petrolatum [12]. Water itself has also been shown to be a skin irritant making emollients high in water content (e.g., lotions) less appealing for AD therapy [26, 76].

16.13.2 Simple Oil-in-Water Emollients

Petrolatum-based emollients have been the workhorse for flare prevention in AD. The lipids found in petrolatum permeate the interstitial compartment of the stratum corneum and enhance the lipid barrier [24]. The other advantage of plain petrolatum is that it does not need preservatives or fragrances, two potential sources of contact sensitization. Most simple emollients improve barrier function and improve long-term control of the disease while reducing topical steroid use [45, 72]. A study of nurse education in AD illustrates the power of simple petrolatum-based emollients in AD therapy. Patients randomized to a nurse education program experienced significant improvements in disease severity, with a concomitant decrease in topical steroid use. The authors attributed this effect to an 800% increase in emollient use [11].

16.13.3 Emollients Specially Designed for AD

As advances in the laboratory shed light on the various epidermal defects in AD, new emollient formulations are arriving in the marketplace that attempt to tailor their effects to AD skin. Emollients containing niacinamide, urea, vitamin B12, ceramides, and natural moisturizing factor components have all been shown to improve skin barrier function in AD skin and in some cases to improve clinical outcomes [42, 67, 69, 82]. The most commonly added ingredients in moisturizers designed to address the skin of AD patients are ceramides. A recent study revealed a ceramide-containing moisturizer led to improvements in transepidermal water loss and skin hydration [66]. The question remains whether any of the new moisturizers with AD-specific ingredients perform better than simple and less expensive petrolatum-based moisturizers on clinical outcomes such as flare prevention or reductions in topical steroid use. Few comparative studies have been performed to date. A ceramide-rich emollient was shown to be more effective in improving TEWL levels and clinical disease scores than routine emollients in one poorly controlled study [9]. In contrast, a study by Loden and colleagues did not see a benefit of skin-identical lipids over pure petrolatum in repairing the skin barrier after experimental perturbation [43]. Most recently, a study found a petrolatum-based emollient to yield similar or better outcomes than a ceramide-dominant cream while being considerably more cost effective [47].

16.13.4 Emollients for Primary Prevention of AD

While emollients represent the gold standard for secondary prevention of AD (flare prevention), their use as a potential primary prevention strategy is just now being realized. The dramatic rise of AD prevalence over the past 50 years and associated comorbidity makes AD prevention an important goal. Hoare's Health Technology Assessment from 2000 listed AD prevention as an "urgent call" for research [34]. Atopic dermatitis prevention strategies have primarily focused on allergen avoidance such as maternal allergen avoidance and child dietary manipulation, although no allergy-based strategy has been consistently effective [63]. Most recently, probiotic supplementation and hydrolyzed formula feeding have had some positive results, although studies have been conflicting. These disappointing results coupled with new data implicating the skin barrier to be central to initiating AD make emollient intervention from birth an intriguing new AD prevention strategy.

Several lines of evidence suggest that emollient therapy from birth may delay the onset or prevent the development of AD. Topical petrolatum or sunflower oil improved the skin barrier function of premature infants and can prevent skin inflammation in several studies [13]. A case-control study from Kenya found the early use of petrolatum to be protective from AD development in neonates [46]. Finally, Flohr was able to detect altered TEWL readings prior to the onset of inflammatory lesions [22], suggesting early correction of an altered barrier can prevent the development of inflammation. We previously showed that applying a simple moisturizer starting near birth is both safe and feasible in a small cohort of infants [65]. Controlled studies from various groups, including our own, are currently ongoing.

Take Home Messages

- Atopic dermatitis is a common skin disorder affecting children on a worldwide scale.
- Asthma, skin infections, and mental health disorders are important comorbidities found in atopic dermatitis.
- The pathogenesis of atopic dermatitis involves a combination of dysfunctional immune responses, abnormal skin barrier function, genetic factors, and environmental influences.
- Functional mutations in the gene encoding the skin barrier protein filaggrin represent the strongest risk factors for atopic dermatitis development identified to date.
- Filaggrin gene mutations and inflammation both contribute to reduced natural moisturizing factor in the stratum corneum in atopic dermatitis leading to a dry barrier.
- Emollients correct skin barrier dysfunction in atopic dermatitis, reduce the need for topical steroid, and their use leads to improved outcomes.
- New information regarding the defective skin barrier in atopic dermatitis is driving the development of disease-specific emollients, but comparative effectiveness studies are needed.

Conclusions

Atopic dermatitis represents a complex disorder whose expression is modified by both genetic and environmental factors. Skin barrier dysfunction is a hallmark of the disease, making moisturizer therapy integral to the management of AD. Recent genetic discoveries have refocused interest on the epidermal barrier, spurring new developments in moisturizer technology. Further studies are needed to clarify the comparative effectiveness of specially designed moisturizers, and more data regarding moisturizers as a primary prevention strategy are eagerly awaited.

References

1. Akiyama M (2010) FLG mutations in ichthyosis vulgaris and atopic eczema: spectrum of mutations and population genetics. Br J Dermatol 162(3):472–477
2. Barnes KC (2010) An update on the genetics of atopic dermatitis: scratching the surface in 2009. J Allergy Clin Immunol 125(1):16–29
3. Berth-Jones J, Damstra RJ, Golsch S, Livden JK, Van Hooteghem O, Allegra F, Parker CA, Group MS (2003) Twice weekly fluticasone propionate added to emollient maintenance treatment to reduce risk of relapse in atopic dermatitis: randomised, double blind, parallel group study. Br Med J 326(7403):1367
4. Bisgaard H, Simpson A, Palmer CN, Bønnelykke K, McLean I, Mukhopadhyay S, Pipper CB, Halkjaer LB, Lipworth B, Hankinson J, Woodcock A, Custovic A (2008) Gene-environment interaction in the onset of eczema in infancy: filaggrin loss-of-function mutations enhanced by neonatal cat exposure. PLoS Med 5(6):e131
5. Bleck O, Abeck D, Ring J, Hoppe U, Vietzke JP, Wolber R, Brandt O, Schreiner V (1999) Two ceramide subfractions detectable in Cer(AS) position by

HPTLC in skin surface lipids of non-lesional skin of atopic eczema. J Invest Dermatol 113(6):894–900
6. Böhme M, Svensson A, Kull I, Wahlgren CF (2000) Hanifin's and Rajka's minor criteria for atopic dermatitis: which do 2-year-olds exhibit? J Am Acad Dermatol 43(5 Pt 1):785–792
7. Brown SJ, Asai Y, Cordell HJ, Campbell LE, Zhao Y, Liao H, Northstone K, Henderson J, Alizadehfar R, Ben-Shoshan M, Morgan K, Roberts G, Masthoff LJ, Pasmans SG, van den Akker PC, Wijmenga C, Hourihane JO, Palmer CN, Lack G, Clarke A, Hull PR, Irvine AD, McLean WH (2011) Loss-of-function variants in the filaggrin gene are a significant risk factor for peanut allergy. J Allergy Clin Immunol 127(3): 661–667
8. Buraczewska I, Berne B, Lindberg M, Torma H, Loden M (2007) Changes in skin barrier function following long-term treatment with moisturizers, a randomized controlled trial. Br J Dermatol 156(3):492–498
9. Chamlin SL, Kao J, Frieden IJ, Sheu MY, Fowler AJ, Fluhr JW, Williams ML, Elias PM (2002) Ceramide-dominant barrier repair lipids alleviate childhood atopic dermatitis: changes in barrier function provide a sensitive indicator of disease activity. J Am Acad Dermatol 47:198–208
10. Chamlin SL (2006) The psychosocial burden of childhood atopic dermatitis. Dermatol Ther 19(2): 104–107
11. Cork MJ et al (2003) Comparison of parent knowledge, therapy utilization and severity of atopic eczema before and after explanation and demonstration of topical therapies by a specialist dermatology nurse. Br J Dermatol 149:582–589
12. Darmstadt GL, Mao-Qiang M, Chi E, Saha SK, Ziboh VA, Black RE, Santosham M, Elias PM (2002) Impact of topical oils on the skin barrier: possible implications for neonatal health in developing countries. Acta Paediatr 91(5):546–554
13. Darmstadt GL, Saha SK, Ahmed AS, Ahmed S, Chowdhury MA, Law PA, Rosenberg RE, Black RE, Santosham M (2008) Effect of skin barrier therapy on neonatal rates in preterm infants in Bangladesh: a randomized, controlled, clinical trial. Pediatrics 121(3): 522–529
14. Di Nardo A, Wertz P, Giannetti A, Seidenari S (1998) Ceramide and cholesterol composition of the skin of patients with atopic dermatitis. Acta Derm Venereol 78(1):27–30
15. Eichenfield LF, Hanifin JM, Luger TA, Stevens SR, Pride HB (2003) Consensus conference on pediatric atopic dermatitis. J Am Acad Dermatol 49(6): 1088–1095
16. Elias PM, Feingold KR (2001) Does the tail wag the dog? Role of the barrier in the pathogenesis of inflammatory dermatoses and therapeutic implications. Arch Dermatol 137(8):1079–1081
17. Elias PM, Steinhoff M (2008) "Outside-to-inside" (and now back to "outside") pathogenic mechanisms in atopic dermatitis. J Invest Dermatol 128(5): 1067–1070
18. Elias PM (2010) Therapeutic implications of a barrier-based pathogenesis of atopic dermatitis. Ann Dermatol 22(3):245–254
19. Ellis C et al (2003) International Consensus Conference on Atopic Dermatitis II (ICCAD II): clinical update and current treatment strategies. Br J Dermatol 148(Suppl 63):3–10
20. Fallon PG, Sasaki T, Sandilands A, Campbell LE, Saunders SP, Mangan NE, Callanan JJ, Kawasaki H, Shiohama A, Kubo A, Sundberg JP, Presland RB, Fleckman P, Shimizu N, Kudoh J, Irvine AD, Amagai M, McLean WH (2009) A homozygous frameshift mutation in the mouse FLG gene facilitates enhanced percutaneous allergen priming. Nat Genet 41(5): 602–608
21. Farwanah H, Raith K, Neubert RH, Wohlrab J (2005) Ceramide profiles of the uninvolved skin in atopic dermatitis and psoriasis are comparable to those of healthy skin. Arch Dermatol Res 296(11):514–521
22. Flohr C, England K, Radulovic S, McLean WH, Campbel LE, Barker J, Perkin M, Lack G (2010) Filaggrin loss-of-function mutations are associated with early-onset eczema, eczema severity and transepidermal water loss at 3 months of age. Br J Dermatol 163(6):1333–1336
23. Flohr C, Weiland SK, Weinmayr G, Bjorksten B, Braback L, Brunekreef B et al (2008) The role of atopic sensitization in flexural eczema: findings from the International Study of Asthma and Allergies in Childhood Phase Two. J Allergy Clin Immunol 121(1):141–147
24. Ghadially R, Halkier-Sorensen L, Elias PM (1992) Effects of petrolatum on stratum corneum structure and function. J Am Acad Dermatol 26(3 Pt 2): 387–396
25. Gruber R, Elias PM, Crumrine D, Lin TK, Brandner JM, Hachem JP, Presland RB, Fleckman P, Janecke AR, Sandilands A, McLean WH, Fritsch PO, Mildner M, Tschachler E, Schmuth M (2011) Filaggrin genotype in ichthyosis vulgaris predicts abnormalities in epidermal structure and function. Am J Pathol 178(5): 2252–2263
26. Grunewald AM et al (1995) Damage to the skin by repetitive washing. Contact Dermatitis 32(4):225–232
27. Halkjaer LB, Loland L, Buchvald FF, Agner T, Skov L, Strand M, Bisgaard H (2006) Development of atopic dermatitis during the first 3 years of life: the Copenhagen prospective study on asthma in childhood cohort study in high-risk children. Danish Pediatric Asthma Centre, Department of Pediatrics, Copenhagen University Hospital. Arch Dermatol 142(5):561–566
28. Hanifin JM (2002) Atopiform dermatitis: do we need another confusing name for atopic dermatitis? Br J Dermatol 147(3):430–432
29. Hanifin JM, Rajka G (1980) Diagnostic features of atopic dermatitis. Acta Dermatovener (Suppl) 92:44–47
30. Hanifin JM et al (2004) Guidelines of care for atopic dermatitis, developed in accordance with the American Academy of Dermatology (AAD)/American Academy

of Dermatology Association "Administrative Regulations for Evidence-Based Clinical Practice Guidelines". J Am Acad Dermatol 50(3):391–404
31. Hatano Y, Katagiri K, Arakawa S, Fujiwara S (2007) Interleukin-4 depresses levels of transcripts for acid-sphingomyelinase and glucocerebrosidase and the amount of ceramide in acetone-wounded epidermis, as demonstrated in a living skin equivalent. J Dermatol Sci 47(1):45–47
32. Held E, Sveinsdottir S, Agner T (1999) Effect of long-term use of moisturizer on skin hydration, barrier function and susceptibility to irritants. Acta Derm Venereol 79(1):49–51
33. Herrick CA et al (2000) Th2 responses induced by epicutaneous or inhalational protein exposure are differentially dependent on IL-4. J Clin Invest 105: 765–775
34. Hoare C, Li Wan Po A, Williams H (2000) Systematic review of treatments for atopic eczema. Health Technol Assess 4(37):1–191
35. Howell MD, Novak N, Bieber T, Pastore S, Girolomoni G, Boguniewicz M, Streib J, Wong C, Gallo RL, Leung DY (2005) Interleukin-10 downregulates anti-microbial peptide expression in atopic dermatitis. J Invest Dermatol 125(4):738–745 (Erratum in: J Invest Dermatol (2005) 125(6):1320)
36. Howell MD, Kim BE, Gao P, Grant AV, Boguniewicz M, Debenedetto A, Schneider L, Beck LA, Barnes KC, Leung DY (2007) Cytokine modulation of atopic dermatitis filaggrin skin expression. J Allergy Clin Immunol 120(1):150–155
37. Imokawa G, Abe A, Jin K, Higaki Y, Kawashima M, Hidano A (1991) Decreased level of ceramides in stratum corneum of atopic dermatitis: an etiologic factor in atopic dry skin? J Invest Dermatol 96(4): 523–526
38. Jensen JM, Pfeiffer S, Witt M, Bräutigam M, Neumann C, Weichenthal M, Schwarz T, Fölster-Holst R, Proksch E (2009) Different effects of pimecrolimus and betamethasone on the skin barrier in patients with atopic dermatitis. J Allergy Clin Immunol 124(3 Suppl 2):R19–R28
39. Kezic S, O'Regan GM, Yau N, Sandilands A, Chen H, Campbell LE, Kroboth K, Watson R, Rowland M, Irwin McLean WH, Irvine AD (2011) Levels of filaggrin degradation products are influenced by both filaggrin genotype and atopic dermatitis severity. Allergy 66(7):934–940
40. Lack G, Fox D, Northstone K, Golding J (2003) Avon Longitudinal Study of Parents and Children Study Team. Factors associated with the development of peanut allergy in childhood. N Engl J Med 348(11): 977–985
41. Leung R (1994) Asthma, allergy and atopy in South-east Asian immigrants in Australia. Aust N Z J Med 24(3):255–257
42. Loden M, Andersson AC, Lindberg M (1999) Improvement in skin barrier function in patients with atopic dermatitis after treatment with a moisturizing cream (Canoderm). Br J Dermatol 140:264–267
43. Loden M, Barany E (2000) Skin-identical lipids versus petrolatum in the treatment of tape-stripped and detergent-perturbed human skin. Acta Derm Venereol 80(6):412–415
44. Lowe AJ, Abrahamson MJ, Hosking CS, Carlin JB, Bennett CM, Dharmage SC, Hill DJ (2007) The temporal sequence of allergic sensitization and onset of infantile eczema. Clin Exp Allergy 37:536–542
45. Lucky AW, Leach AD, Laskarzewski P, Wenck H (1997) Use of an emollient as a steroid-sparing agent in the treatment of mild to moderate atopic dermatitis in children. Pediatr Dermatol 14:321–324
46. Macharia WM, Anabwani GM, Owili DM (1991) Effects of skin contactants on evolution of atopic dermatitis in children: a case control study. Trop Doct 21(3):104–106
47. Miller DW, Koch SB, Yentzer BA, Clark AR, O'Neill JR, Fountain J, Weber TM, Fleischer AB Jr (2011) An over-the-counter moisturizer is as clinically effective as, and more cost-effective than, prescription barrier creams in the treatment of children with mild-to-moderate atopic dermatitis: a randomized, controlled trial. J Drugs Dermatol 10(5):531–537
48. Morgenstern V, Zutavern A, Cyrys J, Brockow I, Koletzko S, Krämer U, Behrendt H, Herbarth O, Von Berg A, Bauer CP, Wichmann HE, Heinrich J, GINI Study Group, LISA Study Group (2008) Atopic diseases, allergic sensitization, and exposure to traffic-related air pollution in children. Am J Respir Crit Care Med 177(12):1331–1337
49. Murata Y, Ogata J, Higaki Y, Kawashima M, Yada Y, Higuchi K, Tsuchiya T, Kawainami S, Imokawa G (1996) Abnormal expression of sphingomyelin acylase in atopic dermatitis: an etiologic factor for ceramide deficiency? J Invest Dermatol 106(6):1242–1249
50. O'Regan GM, Kemperman PM, Sandilands A, Chen H, Campbell LE, Kroboth K, Watson R, Rowland M, Puppels GJ, McLean WH, Caspers PJ, Irvine AD (2010) Raman profiles of the stratum corneum define 3 filaggrin genotype-determined atopic dermatitis endophenotypes. J Allergy Clin Immunol 126(3): 574–580
51. Odhiambo JA, Williams HC, Clayton TO, Robertson CF, Asher MI (2009) Global variations in prevalence of eczema symptoms in children from ISAAC phase three. J Allergy Clin Immunol 124(6):1251–1258
52. Paller AS, Eichenfield LF, Kirsner RS, Shull T, Jaracz E, Simpson EL, US Tacrolimus Ointment Study Group (2008) Three times weekly tacrolimus ointment reduces relapse in stabilized atopic dermatitis: a new paradigm for use. Pediatrics 122(6):e1210–e1218
53. Proksch E, Elias PM (2002) Epidermal barrier in atopic dermatitis. In: Bieber T, Leung DYM (eds) Atopic dermatitis. Marcel Dekker, Inc, New York
54. Rendell ME, Baig-Lewis SF, Berry TM, Denny ME, Simpson BM, Brown PA, Simpson EL (2011) Do early skin care practices alter the risk of atopic dermatitis? A case-control study. Ped Dermatol 28(5):593–595
55. Romanos M, Gerlach M, Warnke A, Schmitt J (2010) Association of attention-deficit/hyperactivity disorder

and atopic eczema modified by sleep disturbance in a large population-based sample. J Epidemiol Community Health 64(3):269–273
56. Sagransky MJ, Yentzer BA, Williams LL, Clark AR, Taylor SL, Feldman SR (2010) A randomized controlled pilot study of the effects of an extra office visit on adherence and outcomes in atopic dermatitis. Arch Dermatol 146(12):1428–1430
57. Sandilands A, Sutherland C, Irvine AD, McLean WH (2009) Filaggrin in the frontline: role in skin barrier function and disease. J Cell Sci 122(Pt 9):1285–1294
58. Scharschmidt TC, Man MQ, Hatano Y, Crumrine D, Gunathilake R, Sundberg JP, Silva KA, Mauro TM, Hupe M, Cho S, Wu Y, Celli A, Schmuth M, Feingold KR, Elias PM (2009) Filaggrin deficiency confers a paracellular barrier abnormality that reduces inflammatory thresholds to irritants and haptens. J Allergy Clin Immunol 124(3):496–506
59. Schram ME, Leeflang MM, DEN Ottolander JP, Spuls PI, Bos JD (2011) Validation and refinement of the millennium criteria for atopic dermatitis. J Dermatol [epub ahead of print]
60. Schultz Larsen F, Hanifin JM (1992) Secular change in the occurrence of atopic dermatitis. Acta Derm Venereol (Stockh) 176(Suppl):7–12
61. Schuttelaar ML, Kerkhof M, Jonkman MF, Koppelman GH, Brunekreef B, de Jongste JC, Wijga A, McLean WH, Postma DS (2009) Filaggrin mutations in the onset of eczema, sensitization, asthma, hay fever and the interaction with cat exposure. Allergy 64(12): 1758–1765
62. Shaw TE, Currie GP, Koudelka C, Simpson EL (2010) Eczema prevalence in the United States: data from the 2003 National Survey of Children's Health. J Invest Dermatol 131(1):67–73
63. Simpson EL (2006) Atopic dermatitis prevention. Dermatol Ther 19(2):108–117
64. Simpson EL (2010) Atopic dermatitis – a review of topical treatment options. Curr Med Res Opin 26(3):633–640
65. Simpson EL, Berry TM, Brown PA, Hanifin JM (2010) A pilot study of emollient therapy for the primary prevention of atopic dermatitis. J Am Acad Dermatol 63(4):587–593
66. Simpson EL, Dutronc Y (2011) A new body moisturizer increases skin hydration and improves atopic dermatitis symptoms among children and adults. J Drugs Dermatol 10(7):744–749
67. Soma Y, Kashima M, Imaizumi A, Takahama H, Kawakami T, Mizoguchi M (2005) Moisturizing effects of topical nicotinamide on atopic dry skin. Int J Dermatol 44(3):197–202
68. Spergel JM, Mizoguchi E, Brewer JP, Martin TR, Bhan AK, Geha RS (1998) Epicutaneous sensitization with protein antigen induces localized allergic dermatitis and hyperresponsiveness to methacholine after single exposure to aerosolized antigen in mice. J Clin Invest 101:1614–1622
69. Stücker M, Pieck C, Stoerb C, Niedner R, Hartung J, Altmeyer P (2004) Topical vitamin B12 – a new therapeutic approach in atopic dermatitis – evaluation of efficacy and tolerability in a randomized placebo-controlled multicentre clinical trial. Br J Dermatol 150(5):977–983
70. Su JC, Kemp AS, Varigos GA, Nolan TM (1997) Atopic eczema: its impact on the family and financial cost. Arch Dis Child 76(2):159–162
71. Suárez-Fariñas M, Tintle SJ, Shemer A, Chiricozzi A, Nograles K, Cardinale I, Duan S, Bowcock AM, Krueger JG, Guttman-Yassky E (2011) Nonlesional atopic dermatitis skin is characterized by broad terminal differentiation defects and variable immune abnormalities. J Allergy Clin Immunol 127(4):954–964
72. Szczepanowska J, Reich A, Szepietowski JC (2008) Emollients improve treatment results with topical corticosteroids in childhood atopic dermatitis: a randomized comparative study. Pediatr Allergy Immunol 19(7):614–618
73. Tagami H, Kobayashi H, O'goshi K, Kikuchi K (2006) Atopic xerosis: employment of noninvasive biophysical instrumentation for the functional analyses of the mildly abnormal stratum corneum and for the efficacy assessment of skin care products. J Cosmet Dermatol 5(2):140–149
74. Thomas KS, Dean T, O'Leary C, Sach TH, Koller K, Frost A, Williams HC (2011) SWET Trial Team. A randomised controlled trial of ion-exchange water softeners for the treatment of eczema in children. PLoS Med 8(2):e1000395
75. Thomsen SF, Ulrik CS, Kyvik KO, Hjelmborg JB, Skadhauge LR, Steffensen I, Backer V (2007) Importance of genetic factors in the etiology of atopic dermatitis: a twin study. Allergy Asthma Proc 28(5):535–539
76. Tsai TF, Maibach HI (1999) How irritant is water? An overview. Contact Dermatitis 41(6):311–314
77. van den Oord RA, Sheikh A (2009) Filaggrin gene defects and risk of developing allergic sensitisation and allergic disorders: systematic review and meta-analysis. Br Med J 339:b2433. doi: 10.1136/bmj.b2433
78. van der Hulst AE, Klip H, Brand PL (2007) Risk of developing asthma in young children with atopic eczema: a systematic review. J Allergy Clin Immunol 120(3):565–569
79. Wahn U, Bos JD, Goodfield M, Caputo R, Papp K, Manjra A, Dobozy A, Paul C, Molloy S, Hultsch T, Graeber M, Cherill R, de Prost Y (2002) Flare Reduction in Eczema with Elidel (Children) Multicenter Investigator Study Group. Efficacy and safety of pimecrolimus cream in the long-term management of atopic dermatitis in children. Pediatrics 110(1 Pt 1):e2
80. Weidinger S, O'Sullivan M, Illig T, Baurecht H, Depner M, Rodriguez E, Ruether A, Klopp N, Vogelberg C, Weiland SK, McLean WH, von Mutius E, Irvine AD, Kabesch MJ (2008) Filaggrin mutations, atopic eczema, hay fever, and asthma in children. J Allergy Clin Immunol 121(5):1203–1209
81. Williams H, Stewart A, von Mutius E, Cookson W, Anderson HR (2008) Is eczema really on the increase

worldwide? J Allergy Clin Immunol 121(4): 947–954
82. Woods MT, Brown PA, Baig-Lewis SF, Simpson EL (2011) Effects of a novel formulation of fluocinonide 0.1% cream on skin barrier function in atopic dermatitis. J Drugs Dermatol 10((2):171–176
83. Yaghmaie P, Koudelka CW, Simpson EL (2011) Psychiatric comorbidity in pediatric eczema. J Invest Dermatol 131(Suppl 1):41 (Abstract #246)
84. Yamamoto A, Serizawa S, Ito M, Sato Y (1991) Stratum corneum lipid abnormalities in atopic dermatitis. Arch Dermatol Res 283(4):219–223
85. Yura A, Kouda K, Iki M, Shimizu T (2011) Trends of allergic symptoms in school children: large-scale long-term consecutive cross-sectional studies in Osaka Prefecture, Japan. Pediatr Allergy Immunol 5. doi:10.1111/j.1399-3038.2011.01159.x [Epub ahead of print]

Update on Hand Eczema with Special Focus on the Impact of Moisturisers

17

Christina Williams and Mark Wilkinson

17.1 Hand Eczema

The hands are a common site of dermatitis as they are often exposed to irritants and allergens in the home and work environments. Contact irritants are the most common exogenous cause of hand eczema, but chronic hand eczema is usually due to a combination of various interacting factors that cannot be viewed in isolation. The effects of these factors may be cumulative and exacerbated by water, humidity, dryness, friction and cold.

17.1.1 Epidemiology

According to a review of studies performed between 1964 and 2007, the point prevalence of hand eczema in the general population is around 4%, the one year prevalence nearly 10% and the lifetime prevalence almost 15% [1]. The median incidence rate is 5.5 cases/1,000 person-years with a high incidence rate associated with female sex, contact allergy especially nickel allergy, wet work or frictional irritancy and atopic dermatitis [2]. The prevalence of hand eczema in adults reporting moderate and severe atopic dermatitis in childhood has been reported as 25% and 41%, respectively [3]. Atopic dermatitis associated with null mutations within the gene encoding the key epidermal protein filaggrin is particularly associated with an earlier onset and higher persistence of hand eczema [4]. Other endogenous risk factors include psoriasis and subclinical barrier deficiency. Hand eczema has a relapsing course and variable disease duration [5]. Approximately half of cases develop into a chronic disease, and symptoms may persist for many years or may recur after disease-free intervals [5, 6].

17.1.2 Diagnosis

An accurate diagnosis of hand eczema leads to better management, but no single classification of hand eczema has been satisfactory. The morphology can often change in an individual case, and one morphology can have several different causes; hence, a new classification of hand eczema has recently been proposed for use in clinical practice and research applications [7]. Based on an analysis of patients attending European patch-testing centres, it defines seven subgroups according to demographics, medical history and lesion morphology. The most common subgroups are irritant (27%), allergic (19%) and combined irritant and allergic hand eczema (19%). Atopic hand eczema and atopic in combination with irritant hand

C. Williams (✉) • M. Wilkinson
Department of Dermatology, Leeds General Infirmary, Great George Street, Leeds, LS1 3EX, UK
e-mail: tinawilliams@doctors.org.uk

M. Lodén, H.I. Maibach (eds.), *Treatment of Dry Skin Syndrome*,
DOI 10.1007/978-3-642-27606-4_17, © Springer-Verlag Berlin Heidelberg 2012

eczema constitute 18%, with other endogenous forms constituting only a minor group.

The differential diagnosis of a dermatological dermatosis affecting the hand includes psoriasis/pustulosis, fungal infection, keratoderma, lichen planus, granuloma annulare and infection/infestation. The pattern of skin lesions may suggest the diagnosis, but patch testing, considered in the context of the patient's history, is essential for patients with chronic hand eczema. Patch testing with a standard series of allergens will often identify substances to which the patient is allergic, and avoidance can lead to an improvement in their hand eczema.

17.1.3 Quality of Life

Hand dermatitis accounts for up to 90% of all occupational skin diseases [8, 9], with important issues regarding the use of medical resources, productivity loss, disability and litigation [1, 10]. The burden of hand dermatitis is therefore high for individual patients and for society.

Chronic hand eczema has been shown to adversely affect quality of life. A survey in the USA found that people with chronic hand eczema report worse quality of life and impaired activity and work performance compared with those without hand eczema [11]. A study of 416 patients with hand eczema recruited from European patch test clinics found that quality of life (measured by the DLQI) correlated with disease severity (measured by the Hand Eczema Severity Index) [12], but the validity of this finding is not supported by the fact that there was no difference in quality of life between men and women, although disease severity was significantly worse in men.

US national statistics suggest that 15% of people with contact dermatitis have limitation of activity due to hand involvement. In Denmark, follow-up after 10 years in a cohort of 274 people with hand eczema found that 12.4% had taken sick leave and 8.5% had changed jobs [13]. The prognosis for moderately severe hand dermatitis is poor. A UK-reporting scheme (EPIDERM) found that 20% of reported cases led to the individual requiring time off work and 16% did not improve at repeat assessment [5]. In a 15-year follow-up of a Swedish general population sample, the majority of patients with hand eczema had ongoing symptoms, about a third needed ongoing medical treatment, and 5% experienced long periods of sickness absence, loss or change of job and ill-health retirement [5]. The 12-year prognosis of hand dermatitis in a study of Finnish farmers was equally poor, with 26% of men and 21% of women reporting current symptoms at follow-up [14]. It seems that hand dermatitis tends to persist with exposure to wet work, irritants or allergens, and a high proportion of workers change job as a result. This productivity loss and sick leave can result in high costs [8]. In the Netherlands, annual costs of medical care, absenteeism and disability pensions attributable to occupational skin disease in employees are estimated to be 98.1 million € [9].

17.2 Prevention

The management of patients with chronic hand eczema can often be unsatisfactory [15]. For this reason, primary and secondary prevention is potentially an important strategy, especially in professions known to have an increased risk of hand dermatitis. A systematic review of the literature by van Gils et al. [16] assessed the effectiveness of prevention programmes for hand dermatitis. They found that there is moderate evidence for the effect of prevention programmes, including skin care education, on lowering occurrence and improving adherence to preventive measures, and low evidence for the effect on improving clinical outcomes and self-reported outcomes. No studies reporting on the cost-effectiveness of prevention however were found.

Primary prevention aims to reduce the incidence of hand eczema by targeting the healthy population. The regulation of exposure to allergens either by legislation on threshold values or regulations on precautions in the handling of allergenic products reduces allergen exposure and subsequently reduces the frequency of allergic contact dermatitis [17]. Exposure to wet work is a particular risk factor for the development of hand eczema, and the use of gloves in wet work has generally been recommended and accepted as an important preventive measure, particularly when combined with other preventative measures. Compliance with this recommendation is good in some but not all occupations [18]. However, gloves may also sometimes be the cause of hand eczema, since protective rubber gloves may cause irritant dermatitis from heat and sweating, or allergic contact dermatitis from contact sensitisation to rubber additives or contact urticaria caused by immediate allergy to natural rubber latex [19–21].

Secondary prevention strategies are recommended when skin manifestations are apparent on the hands. The objective of secondary prevention is to spot early skin changes in order to rapidly implement corrective measures. Outpatient skin-protection seminars have been suggested for those in wet work occupations such as health-care workers, hairdressers, cooks, caterers and other food handlers and cleaners [22–24]. These provide theoretical background knowledge and training in the selection and use of adequate skin-protection strategies. They are aimed at helping people keep working in their occupation and to motivate people to use adequate skin protection. Although this area still needs more research, the results are very promising.

Lifestyle change is therefore recommended for all patients, particularly those involved in wet work or high-risk occupations. This involves avoidance of relevant allergens and irritants, substituting alternatives where possible, use of hand protection such as occlusive gloves and/or barrier creams and avoidance of wet work and mechanical irritation. A skin-protection programme should be tailored to individual need, and this should include education about hand eczema with the aim of giving the patient realistic expectations of treatment outcomes [25]. Working organisations should play an active role in providing opportunities for prevention and making protection measures available [14].

17.3 Treatment

17.3.1 Soap Substitutes

Careful hand washing to remove irritants and allergens is an important part of skin care in any high-risk occupation. However, the mechanical trauma of repeated washing and drying and the detergents themselves can give rise to skin irritation, particularly in the finger web spaces. Emollient soap substitutes containing nonionic surface active agents may be beneficial in these circumstances. In an attempt to improve compliance with infection control procedures in the health-care setting, the introduction of alcohol-based gels for hand decontamination as a substitute for hand washing with conventional soaps and disinfectants when the hands are not visibly soiled has been advocated by the World Health Organization, the Centres for Disease Control in the USA, and the National Patient Safety Agency and Infection Prevention Society (formerly Infection Control Nurses Association) in the UK. Most of the studies that evaluate different hand hygiene regimens are focused on their effectiveness at reducing skin colonisation [26]. In a recent study by Loffler et al., it was suggested that alcohol hand rubs cause less skin irritation than hand washing with detergents/soaps and should therefore be preferred from the dermatological viewpoint. They went on to state that alcohol hand rubs may even decrease rather than increase skin irritation after a hand wash due to a partial mechanical elimination of the detergent [27]. It is still not clear however, whether different hand hygiene regimens have an important impact on the prevention or management of dermatitis in health-care workers.

17.3.2 Pre-work Creams

Pre-work creams are designed for application at the start of work or after rest breaks. Many pre-work creams have oily formulations and therefore have emollient properties. They also make it easier to wash off contaminants, allowing milder cleansing agents to be used. Therefore, they can play a useful role in an overall skin management programme.

They are sometimes referred to as barrier creams. However, this term can be misleading, giving rise to a perception that these agents form a physical barrier to protect skin and are a substitute for wearing gloves or other protective equipment. In fact, evidence from animal studies indicates that they are very limited in forming a true barrier [28, 29].

A systematic review revealed that there is mixed evidence for the effectiveness of pre-work creams [30]. Limitations of pre-work creams include a well-recognised failure of users to apply them properly [31], uncertainty about penetration or permeation rates for many substances [29] and difficulty for workers in recognising when the creams wear off during a shift. While some are effective in preventing irritant contact dermatitis or allergic contact dermatitis for specific allergens, there are limitations in the extent to which this finding can be generalised. Three studies explored the use of prework creams as a preventative measure against specific agents (epoxy resins, glass fibres, sodium lauryl sulphate and toluene) and found that they offered no or very limited protection [32–34]. A randomised controlled trial of workers in the building and timber trades found no clinical evidence that pre-work creams alone prevent dermatitis, although such creams in combination with cleansing and after-work creams were effective in improving skin condition, measured by trans-epidermal water loss [35]. A systematic review of latex allergy concluded that prior use of protective hand creams cannot be recommended for people who wear latex gloves and found some indication that such creams may favour the uptake of allergens from gloves [36].

17.3.3 Moisturisers

Emollients or moisturisers are preparations that increase skin hydration and replace depleted skin lipids that form an important part of the barrier function of normal healthy skin. Most are oil-in-water preparations with a variable fat content (commonly petrolatum, paraffins, glycerides or lanolin). The development of topical agents that improve skin barrier function is a promising approach for the prevention and management of hand dermatitis. A good skin barrier helps to avoid the penetration of both allergens and irritants. Well-selected moisturisers that maintain and support skin barrier function are therefore considered useful treatment adjuncts for hand eczema [37, 38]. However, more rigorous data on the preventive effectiveness of moisturisers are required [39], as moisturisers have different effects on the skin and some formulations may deteriorate skin barrier function and increase susceptibility to irritants, with possible negative consequences for the eczema [40–43].

Earlier studies suggested that moisturisers help to re-establish normal skin physiology in various diseases characterised by abnormal barrier function, with those containing humectants, for example, urea or glycerine, being typically more efficacious than those without humectants [44], and that they may be effective in the prevention of contact and occupational irritant dermatitis. One field study indicated a positive effect on skin hydration from the use of moisturisers in 55 cleaners and kitchen assistants exposed to water and detergents [45], and another study found that moisturisers prevented cumulative irritant contact dermatitis and speeded healing [46]. Hannuksela and Kinnunen asked their subjects to wash their upper arms with a liquid detergent and applied eight moisturisers after each wash in the first week to one upper arm and twice daily without wash in the second week. Evaluation of skin blood flow and TEWL concluded that the regular use of emollients prevented irritant dermatitis from this detergent. In a single-blinded study, Loden reported that urea-containing moisturiser speeds healing and decreases susceptibility to sodium lauryl sulphate SLS [47]. TEWL and skin capacitance of surfactant-damaged skin and normal skin were measured at baseline and after 14 days of treatment with the moisturiser. The authors found that barrier recovery and influence of irritant stimuli in skin treated with a moisturising cream were significantly more favourable than untreated skin.

Other reports further support the role of moisturisers in preventing irritant contact dermatitis. Ramsing and Agner [38], using the hand-immersion test, studied the effect of a moisturiser on experimentally irritated human skin using SLS and found that moisturiser was not only effective in preventing the development of irritant contact dermatitis but also significantly accelerated skin barrier repair, judged by measurement of TEWL and electrical capacitance, and it improved the clinical signs, which were observed on the control hand. Held and Agner also reported that moisturiser speeds healing in hand-immersion and SLS-patch tests [48]. Goh et al. showed that an after-work moisturiser appeared to reduce the incidence of irritant dermatitis, and reduced TEWL increase from cutting oil, among metal workers [49]. A recent study modelling an almost real work situation assessed the effect of the regular use of detergents and emollients in a wash test [50]. This double-blind, randomised study examined whether the regular use of a moisturising product after repeated washing of the hands over a 2-week period in healthy adult volunteers would maintain skin barrier function compared to a soap-only control group not exposed to moisturiser over the same time period. Objective subclinical assessment of the skin barrier function using TEWL and epidermal hydration showed that three of the five moisturisers tested were more effective in increasing epidermal hydration and one moisturiser out of five led to a significant reduction in TEWL. These results supported the findings of previous studies that the regular application of moisturisers to normal skin does offer a protective effect against repeated exposure to irritants.

In contrast, however, Held et al. in 1999 and 2001 reported that moisturisers, which improve stratum corneum hydration, may increase skin susceptibility to contact irritants [48, 51]. In these studies, a 4-week treatment of normal skin with moisturiser three times a day increased susceptibility to SLS as demonstrated by a statistically significant higher TEWL on the treated forearm compared with the other untreated forearm. The results suggest that long-term treatment with moisturisers on normal skin may not necessarily offer any protection against irritant trauma caused by a detergent. On the contrary, daily use of moisturizers under these conditions may increase skin susceptibility to irritants. The authors suggested that increasing the hydration level of the stratum corneum progressively may reduce its barrier efficiency and allow the permeation of noxious substances into the skin with greater ease.

In summary, it would appear that most studies support the 'protective' effects of moisturisers against skin irritants. However, the protective effects of moisturisers may not be broad spectrum, and different moisturisers with different constituents may be specifically more effective against different skin irritants and in different individuals. A number of practical factors might also limit clinical efficacy in the workplace, including compliance, availability, interaction with other substances and removal by repeated washing. Further field studies, however, are therefore required to evaluate skin care programmes in a practical workplace environment.

17.3.4 Types of Moisturisers

Lipid content and natural moisturising factors such as urea have been suggested to be the most important constituents of emollients. Emollients with high lipid content accelerate the healing after experimental damage to the skin [52]. Humectants may sometimes improve barrier function, mainly by increasing the hydration of the stratum corneum and for some humectants also by anti-irritant capacity [53]. Efforts to improve the efficacy of moisturisers have included using skin-related lipids (e.g. ceramides) in formulations. However, no superiority of an emollient containing ceramide used twice daily over an ordinary petrolatum emollient used twice daily was observed in patients with chronic hand dermatitis [54]. A similar result was seen in experimentally irritated skin [55], where two models for barrier deterioration were used. One reflected irritant contact dermatitis, caused by exposure to an aqueous solution of a surfactant and in the other model, TEWL was increased by mechanical removal of the outer layers of the stratum corneum by stripping the skin with adhesive tape.

Repairing the barrier or preventing barrier dysfunction are important strategies for reducing the risks for eczema. Elias et al. suggested that pathogenesis-based therapy with an ideal ratio of lipid to ceramide, directed at the lipid biochemical abnormality that is responsible for the barrier defect in atopic dermatitis, could be an effective treatment model [56]. One 5% urea-containing moisturiser has repeatedly been shown to improve skin barrier function in dry atopic skin [57, 58]. In a single blinded study, Loden et al. [58] showed that the susceptibility to irritation by SLS decreased, as measured by skin blood flow and TEWL, and skin capacitance was significantly increased in cream-treated skin, indicating increased hydration. Similar findings were also reported by Buraczewska et al. in normal skin [40]. Maintenance treatment with this urea-containing moisturiser was recently found to reduce the relapse of flares of eczema on corticosteroid-healed sites in atopic dermatitis patients to approximately one-third of that of patients with no such maintenance treatment [59]. In a study by Loden et al. [60], the time to relapse of eczema during treatment with a barrier strengthening moisturiser (5% urea) was compared with no treatment (no medical or non-medicated preparations) in 53 randomised patients with successfully treated hand eczema. The median time to relapse was 20 days in the moisturiser group compared with 2 days in the no-treatment group ($p=0.04$). Eczema relapsed in 90% of the patients within 26 weeks. No difference in severity was noted between the groups at relapse. Dermatology Life Quality Index (DLQI) increased significantly in both groups, from 4.7 to 7.1 in the moisturiser group and from 4.1 to 7.8 in the no treatment group ($p<0.01$) at the time of relapse. Hence, the application of moisturisers seems to prolong the disease-free interval in patients with controlled hand eczema.

17.3.5 Other Topical Therapies

After barrier creams, soap substitutes and emollients, the topical treatment of choice is a topical steroid. These agents are very effective in the short term, but they inhibit repair of the stratum corneum and may interfere with recovery in the long term. There is some evidence for long-term intermittent treatment of chronic hand eczema with mometasone furoate cream [61]. The adverse effects of topical steroids include cutaneous atrophy, tachyphylaxis and adrenal suppression after systemic absorption.

Two topical calcineurin inhibitors are licensed for the treatment of atopic dermatitis when topical steroids have failed or not been tolerated: tacrolimus for moderate to severe disease and pimecrolimus for mild to moderate disease. Tacrolimus has been shown to be as effective as mometasone furoate [62] whereas pimecrolimus appears to be equivalent to a mildly potent topical steroid [63]. Adverse effects include transient stinging, flushing with alcohol and skin infection. There has been no short- or intermediate-term evidence of systemic immunosuppression or an increased risk for malignancy, although long-term data collection is ongoing. Other topical agents include the retinoid bexarotene, which is licensed in a gel formulation in the USA for the treatment of lymphoma. This has been shown to improve severe chronic hand eczema. Adverse effects include irritation, stinging or burning and flare of dermatitis [64]. Other treatments include superficial X-ray and particularly Grenz rays [65], botulinum toxin [66] and iontophoresis [67].

17.3.6 Phototherapy

Small trials have shown that ultraviolet (UV) B may improve chronic hand eczema over a period of 10 weeks, but topical psoralen UVA (PUVA) is superior [68]. Most dermatologists would use topical PUVA rather than systemic PUVA as it likely to be safer. UVA1 may also be effective, although provision of this in the UK is very limited [69].

17.3.7 Systemic Therapies

The systemic therapies most widely used in the treatment of chronic hand eczema include corticosteroids, azathioprine, cyclosporine, methotrexate and acitretin. The only systemic agent licensed for treatment of hand eczema is the oral retinoid alitretinoin, which is specifically approved for the treatment of adults with hand eczema unresponsive to topical steroids, and is supported by evidence from a large randomised trial [70].

17.3.7.1 Systemic Corticosteroids

Systemic corticosteroids can be used briefly to treat acute severe hand eczema (generally 0.5–1 mg/kg body weight per day prednisolone equivalent, for a maximum period of 3 weeks). Systemic corticosteroids are not appropriate for use in the chronic phases of chronic hand eczema, as they are associated with long-term side effects such as osteoporosis, glaucoma, cataracts, hypothalamic-pituitary-adrenal axis suppression, hyperglycaemia, hypertension and immunosuppression

17.3.7.2 Azathioprine

Azathioprine has been reported to improve atopic eczema and pompholyx [71]. Patients on azathioprine require regular blood monitoring, as it can cause a reduction of the white blood cell count. Measurement of blood levels of thiopurine methyltransferase (TPMT) before initiating therapy is helpful to find the suitable dose for each individual patient.

17.3.7.3 Cyclosporine

In a double-blind study of 41 patients with severe chronic hand eczema randomised to either oral cyclosporine (3 mg/kg/day) or 0.05% betamethasone dipropionate cream, disease activity decreased by 50%, compared to 32% in the steroid group, which was not statistically significantly different. The relapse rate for both groups was 50% after 2 weeks of follow-up [72]. In a second, open-label study, 75 patients treated for 6 weeks with oral cyclosporine 3 mg/kg/day showed 1-year success rates of 79% and 74% for atopic and chronic hand eczema, respectively [73]. A recent meta-analysis suggested the efficacy of cyclosporine after 6–8 weeks of treatment was 55% in atopic eczema [74].

The use of cyclosporine also requires careful monitoring, as it can be associated with potentially serious adverse events including nephrotoxicity, risk of malignancy, increased blood pressure and increased risk of infection. In general, therapy with cyclosporine is recommended for a maximum of 6 months at the lowest therapeutic dose, followed by a dose reduction over a period of 3 months.

17.3.7.4 Methotrexate

Case reports have shown that low doses of methotrexate led to improvement or clearing of hand dermatitis, together with a decreased need for concomitant systemic corticosteroids [75]. Long-term use of methotrexate is associated with significant potential for side effects including hepatitis, liver cirrhosis, pancytopenia, pulmonary fibrosis and teratogenicity, but these can be minimised if it is appropriately dosed, and patients are selected and monitored carefully.

17.3.7.5 Acitretin

Acitretin is currently not licensed for the treatment of hand dermatitis. There are limited data on its efficacy, but a small, open-label study of 29 patients with hyperkeratotic dermatitis of the palms, 30 mg daily for 4 weeks was associated with a 51% reduction of all symptoms, compared to only 9% in a placebo control group. No further improvement was seen with 4 additional weeks of treatment [76]. Being a retinoid, acitretin is teratogenic, and therefore, pregnancy prevention measures are indicated during treatment and for at least 2–3 years after discontinuation. Additionally, in combination with alcohol, acitretin has been associated with the formation of etretinate, which increases the duration of teratogenic potential for female patients.

17.3.7.6 Alitretinoin (9-Cis Retinoic Acid)

Alitretinoin is approved for use in treating severe, chronic hand eczema that does not respond, or responds inadequately, to topical corticosteroids. Alitretinoin is an agonist of both vitamin A acid receptors. Its main mechanism of action is immunomodulatory and anti-inflammatory (and, in contrast to retinoids, it has a minimal drying effect). Treatment should be stopped if no effect has occurred after 3 months. In 1,032 patients with severe refractory HE, 48% of randomised patients treated with alitretinoin were clear (Physician Global Assessment) or almost clear within 12–24 weeks compared with 17% assigned to placebo [70]. The commonest adverse effect was headache, reported by 11% and 20% of patients at doses of 10 and 30 mg daily compared with 6% with placebo. The response was more marked in patients with hyperkeratotic hand eczema (49% at 30 mg daily, 28% at 10 mg daily) than in those with vesicular disease (33% and 23%, respectively). Alitretinoin is associated with an increase in plasma cholesterol, thyroid function and triglyceride levels, and these should be monitored during therapy. Like all retinoic acid derivatives, alitretinoin is teratogenic. Pregnancy prevention 1 month before, during and for 1 month after cessation of treatment is therefore required in women of childbearing potential.

Take Home Messages

- Initial management should include a full history, exclusion of infection and advice on a skin-protection programme.
- Skin barrier function should be maintained and supported by preventive measures, for example, emollients, barriers and soap substitutes, if avoidance of contact factors is not possible.
- Moisturisers differ in composition and in their influence on skin properties. Further field studies are required to investigate this objectively.
- Initial treatment should include a trial of treatment with a topical steroid.
- Systemic therapies include cyclosporine and azathioprine. Alitretinoin is a new option licensed for severe chronic hand eczema and showing good clearance rates in a clinical trial that included patients with all forms of hand eczema
- PUVA and/or acitretin may be considered first for hyperkeratotic hand eczema.
- Oral steroids can be considered when rapid control is needed.
- Options after other systemic therapies have failed include methotrexate and mycophenolate mofetil.

References

1. Thyssen JP, Johansen JD, Linneberg A, Menne T (2010) The epidemiology of hand eczema in the general population – prevalence and main findings. Contact Dermatitis 62:75–87
2. Meding B (1990) Epidemiology of hand eczema in an industrial city. Acta Derm Venereol Suppl (Stockh) 153:1–43
3. Rystedt I (1985) Long term follow-up in atopic dermatitis. Acta Derm Venereol Suppl (Stockh) 114: 117–120
4. Thyssen JP, Carlsen BC, Menne T et al (2010) Filaggrin null mutations increase the risk and persistence of hand eczema in subjects with atopic dermatitis: results from a general population study. Br J Dermatol 163:115–120
5. Meding B, Wrangsjo K, Jarvholm B (2005) Fifteen-year follow-up of hand eczema: persistence and consequences. Br J Dermatol 152:975–980
6. Halkier-Sorensen L (1996) Occupational skin diseases. Contact Dermatitis 35(Suppl 1):1–120
7. Diepgen TL, Andersen KE, Brandao FM et al (2009) Hand eczema classification: a cross-sectional, multicentre study of the aetiology and morphology of hand eczema. Br J Dermatol 160:353–358
8. Koch P (2001) Occupational contact dermatitis. Recognition and management. Am J Clin Dermatol 2:353–365
9. Dickel H, Kuss O, Blesius CR, Schmidt A, Diepgen TL (2001) Occupational skin diseases in Northern Bavaria between 1990 and 1999: a population-based study. Br J Dermatol 145:453–462
10. Cvetkovski RS, Rothman KJ, Olsen J, Mathiesen B, Iversen L, Johansen JD, Agner T (2005) Relation between diagnoses on severity, sick leave and loss of job among patients with occupational hand eczema. Br J Dermatol 152:93–98
11. Fowler JF, Ghosh A, Sung J et al (2006) Impact of chronic hand dermatitis on quality of life, work productivity, activity impairment, and medical costs. J Am Acad Dermatol 54:448–457
12. Agner T, Andersen KE, Brandao FM et al (2008) Hand eczema severity and quality of life: a cross-sectional, multicentre study of hand eczema patients. Contact Dermatitis 59:43–47
13. Lerbaek A, Kyvik KO, Ravn H et al (2008) Clinical characteristics and consequences of hand eczema – an 8-year follow-up study of a population-based twin cohort. Contact Dermatitis 58:210–216
14. Susitaival P, Hannuksela M (1995) The 12-year prognosis of hand dermatosis in 896 Finnish farmers. Contact Dermatitis 32(4):233–237
15. Diepgen TL, Agner T, Aberer W, Berth-Jones J, Cambazard F, Elsner P, McFadden J, Coenraads PJ (2007) Management of chronic hand eczema. Contact Dermatitis 57:203–210
16. van Gils RF, Boot CRL, van Gils PF et al (2011) Effectiveness of prevention programmes for hand

dermatitis: a systematic review of the literature. Contact Dermatitis 64:63–72
17. Nielsen NH, Linneberg A, Menné T, Madsen F, Frolund L, Dirksen A, Jørgensen T (2002) The association between contact allergy and hand eczema in two cross-sectional surveys 8 years apart. Contact Dermatitis 47:71–77
18. Wrangsjo K, Wallenhammar LM, Ortengren U, Barregard L, Andreasson H, Bjorkner B, Karlsson S, Meding B (2001) Protective gloves in Swedish dentistry: use and side effects. Br J Dermatol 145:32–37
19. Ramsing DW, Agner T (1996) Effect of glove occlusion on human skin. (I). Short-term experimental exposure. Contact Dermatitis 34(1):1–5
20. Ramsing DW, Agner T (1996) Effect of glove occlusion on human skin (II). Long-term experimental exposure. Contact Dermatitis 34(4):258–262
21. Strauss RM, Gawkrodger DJ (2001) Occupational contact dermatitis in nurses with hand eczema. Contact Dermatitis 44:293–296
22. Schürer NY, Klippel U et al (2005) Secondary individual prevention of hand dermatitis in geriatric nurses. Int Arch Occup Environ Health 78:149–157
23. Schwanitz HJ, Riehl U et al (2003) Skin care management: educational aspects. Int Arch Occup Environ Health 76(5):374–381
24. Weisshaar E, Radulescu M et al (2007) Secondary individual prevention of occupational skin diseases in health care workers, cleaners and kitchen employees: aims, experiences and descriptive results. Int Arch Occup Environ Health 80(6):477–484
25. English J, Aldridge R, Gawkrodger DJ, Kownacki S, Statham B, White JM et al (2009) Consensus statement on the management of chronic hand eczema. Clin Exp Dermatol 34:761–769
26. Boyce JM, Pittet D, Healthcare Infection Control Practices Advisory Committee et al (2000) Guideline for Hand Hygiene in Health-Care Settings. Recommendations of the Healthcare Infection Control Practices Advisory Committee and the HICPAC/SHEA/APIC/IDSA Hand Hygiene Task Force. Society for Healthcare Epidemiology of America/Association for Professionals in Infection Control/Infectious Diseases Society of America. MMWR Morb Mortal Wkly Rep 51(RR-16):1–45
27. Loffler H, Kampf G, Schermund D, Maibach HI (2007) How irritant is alcohol? Br J Dermatol 157:74–81
28. Frosch PJ, SchulzeDirk A, Hoffmann M et al (1993) Efficacy of skin barrier creams. (I). The repetitive irritation test (RIT) in the guinea pig. Contact Dermatitis 28(2):94–100
29. Kresken J, Klotz A (2003) Occupational skin-protection products – a review. Int Arch Occup Environ Health 76(5):355–358
30. Saary J, Qureshi R, Palda V, DeKoven J, Pratt M, Skotnicki-Grant S et al (2005) A systematic review of contact dermatitis treatment and prevention. J Am Acad Dermatol 53:845–855
31. Kelterer D, Fluhr JW, Elsner P (2003) Application of protective creams: use of a fluorescence-based training system decreases unprotected areas on the hands. Contact Dermatitis 49(3):159–160
32. Bendsoe N, Bjornberg A, Lowhagen GB, Tengberg JE (1987) Glass fibre irritation and protective creams. Contact Dermatitis 17:69–72
33. Elsner P (2007) Skin protection in the prevention of skin diseases. Curr Probl Dermatol 34:1–10
34. Krajewska D, Rudzki E (1976) Sensitivity to epoxy resins and triethylenetetramine. Contact Dermatitis 2:135–138
35. Winker R, Salameh B, Stolkovich S, Nikl M, Barth A, Ponocny E et al (2009) Effectiveness of skin protection creams in the prevention of occupational dermatitis: results of a randomized, controlled trial. Int Arch Occup Environ Health 82:653–662
36. (NHS Plus 2008) NHS Plus/Royal College of Physicians (2008) Latex allergy: occupational health aspects of management: a national guideline. Royal College of Physicians, London
37. Loden M, Andersson AC (1996) Effects of topically applied lipids on surfactant irritated skin. Br J Dermatol 134:215–220
38. Ramsing DW, Agner T (1997) Preventive and therapeutic effects of a moisturizer. Acta Derm Venereol 77:335–337
39. Hoare C, Li Wan Po A, Williams H (2000) Systematic review of treatments for atopic eczema. Health Technol Assess 4:1–191
40. Buraczewska I, Berne B, Lindberg M, Torma H, Loden M (2007) Changes in skin barrier function following long-term treatment with moisturizers, a randomized controlled trial. Br J Dermatol 156:492–498
41. Held E, Sveinsdottir S, Agner T (1999) Effect of long-term use of moisturizer on skin hydration, barrier function and susceptibility to irritants. Acta Derm Venereol 79:49–51
42. Zachariae C, Held E, Johansen JD, Menne T, Agner T (2003) Effect of a moisturizer on skin susceptibility to $NiCl_2$. Acta Derm Venereol 83:93–97
43. Vilaplana J, Coll J, Trullás C, Axón A, Pelejero C (1992) Clinical and non-invasive evaluation of 12% ammonium lactate emulsion for the treatment of dry skin in atopic and non-atopic subjects. Acta Derm Venereol 72:28–33
44. Loden M (2005) The clinical benefit of moisturizers. J Eur Acad Dermatol Venereol 19:672–688
45. Halkier-Sorensen L, Thestrup-Pedersen K (1993) The efficacy of a moisturizer (Locobase) among cleaners and kitchen assistants during everyday exposure to water and detergents. Contact Dermatitis 29:1–6
46. Hannuksela A, Kinnunen T (1992) Moisturizers prevent irritant dermatitis. Acta Derm Veneroel (Stockh) 72:42–44
47. Loden M (1997) Barrier recovery and influence of irritant stimuli in skin treated with a moisturizing cream. Contact Dermatitis 36:256–260
48. Held E, Agner T (1999) Comparison between 2 test models in evaluating the effect of a moisturizer on irritated human skin. Contact Dermatitis 40:261–268

49. Goh CL, Gan SL (1994) Efficacies of a barrier cream and an afterwork emollient cream against cutting fluid dermatitis in metalworkers: a prospective study. Contact Dermatitis 31:176–180
50. Williams C, Wilkinson SM, McShane P et al (2010) A double-blind, randomized study to assess the effectiveness of different moisturizers in preventing dermatitis induced by hand washing to simulate healthcare use. Br J Dermatol 162(5):1088–1092
51. Held E (2001) So moisturizers may cause trouble! Int J Dermatol 40:12–13
52. Held E, Lund H, Agner T (2001) Effect of different moisturizers on SLS-irritated human skin. Contact Dermatitis 44:229–234
53. Loden M (2004) Do moisturizers work? J Cosmet Dermatol 2:141–149
54. Kucharekova M, Van De Kerkhof PC, Van Der Valk PG (2003) A randomized comparison of an emollient containing skin related lipids with a petrolatum-based emollient as adjunct in the treatment of chronic hand dermatitis. Contact Dermatitis 48:293–299
55. Lodén M, Barany E (2000) Skin-identical lipids versus petrolatum in the treatment of tape-stripped and detergent-perturbed human skin. Acta Derm Venereol 80:412–415
56. Elias PM, Hatano Y, Williams ML (2008) Basis for the barrier abnormality in atopic dermatitis: outside-inside-outside pathogenic mechanisms. J Allergy Clin Immunol 121:1337–1343
57. Andersson A-C, Lindberg M, Lodén M (1999) The effect of two urea-containing creams on dry, eczematous skin in atopic patients. I. Expert, patient and instrumental evaluation. J Dermatol Treat 10:165–169
58. Lodén M, Andersson A-C, Lindberg M (1999) Improvement in skin barrier function in patients with atopic dermatitis after treatment with a moisturizing cream (Canoderm®). Br J Dermatol 140:264–267
59. Wirén K, Nohlgård C, Nyberg F, Holm L, Svensson M, Johannesson A et al (2009) Treatment with a barrier-strengthening moisturizing cream delays relapse of atopic dermatitis: a prospective and randomized controlled clinical trial. J Eur Acad Dermatol Venereol 23:1267–1272
60. Loden M, Wiren K, Smerud K et al (2010) Treatment with a barrier-strengthening moisturizer prevents relapse of hand eczema: an open, randomized, prospective, parallel group study. Acta Derm Venereol 90:602–606
61. Veien NK, Olholm Larsen P, Thestrup-Pedersen K et al (1999) Long-term, intermittent treatment of chronic hand eczema with mometasone furoate. Br J Dermatol 140:882–886
62. Schnopp C, Remling R, Möhrenschlager M et al (2002) Topical tacrolimus (FK506) and mometasone furoate in treatment of dyshidrotic palmar eczema: a randomized, observer-blinded trial. J Am Acad Dermatol 46:73–77
63. El-Batawy MM, Bosseilo MA, Marshaly HM et al (2009) Topical calcineurin inhibitors in atopic dermatitis: a systematic review and meta-analysis. J Dermatol Sci 54:76–87
64. Hanifin JM, Stevens V, Sheth P et al (2004) Novel treatment of chronic severe hand dermatitis with bexarotene gel. Br J Dermatol 150:545–553
65. Lindelof B, Wrangsjo K, Liden S (1987) A double-blind study of Grenz ray therapy in chronic eczema of the hands. Br J Dermatol 117:77–80
66. Wollina U, Karamfilov T (2002) Adjuvant botulinum toxin A in dyshidrotic hand eczema: a controlled prospective pilot study with left-right comparison. J Eur Acad Dermatol Venereol 16:40–42
67. Odia S, Vocks E, Rakoski J, Ring J (1996) Successful treatment of dyshidrotic hand eczema using tap water iontophoresis with pulsed direct current. Acta Derm Venereol 76:472–474
68. Rosen K, Mobacken H, Swanbeck G (1987) Chronic eczematous dermatitis of the hands. A comparison of PUVA and UVB treatment. Acta Derm Venereol 67:48–54
69. Schmidt T, Abeck D, Boeck K et al (1998) UVA1 irradiation is effective in treatment of chronic vesicular dyshidrotic hand eczema. Acta Derm Venereol 78:318–319
70. Ruzicka T, Lynde CW, Jemec GB et al (2008) Efficacy and safety of oral alitretinoin (9-cis retinoic acid) in patients with severe chronic hand eczema refractory to topical corticosteroids: results of a randomized, double-blind, placebo-controlled, multicentre trial. Br J Dermatol 158:808–817
71. Scerri L (1999) Azathioprine in dermatological practice. An overview with special emphasis on its use in non-bullous inflammatory dermatoses. Adv Exp Med Biol 455:343–348
72. Granlund H, Erkko P, Eriksson E et al (1996) Comparison of cyclosporine and topical betamethasone-17,21-dipropionate in the treatment of severe chronic hand eczema. Acta Derm Venereol 76:371–376
73. Granlund H, Erkko P, Reitamo S (1998) Long-term follow-up of eczema patients treated with cyclosporine. Acta Derm Venereol 78:40–43
74. Schmitt J, Schmitt N, Meurer M (2007) Cyclosporin in the treatment of patients with atopic eczema – a systematic review and meta-analysis. J Eur Acad Dermatol Venereol 21(5):606–619
75. Egan CA, Rallis TM, Meadows KP, Krueger GC (1999) Low-dose oral methotrexate treatment for recalcitrant palmoplantar pompholyx. J Am Acad Dermatol 40:612–614
76. Thestrup-Pedersen K, Andersen KE, Menné T et al (2001) Treatment of hyperkeratotic dermatitis of the palms (eczema keratoticum) with oral acitretin. A single-blind placebo-controlled study. Acta Derm Venereol 81:353–355

18 Update on Ichthyosis with Special Emphasis on Dryness and the Impact of Moisturizers

Johannes Wohlrab

18.1 Introduction

Patients with ichthyoses typically suffer their whole life under the hereditary keratosis of the skin organ. Depending on heredity, genetic characteristics and clinical expression patterns, retention hyperkeratosis or alternatively proliferation hyperkeratosis [25] result. This causes functional damage to the layers of the stratum corneum, which causes the typical clinical phenotype, i.e. raw, dry skin. Some ichthyoses are frequent genodermatoses. In particular, the autosomal dominant form of ichthyosis vulgaris with 1:300 is the most frequently occurring within genetically conditioned skin disorders [25].

The historical systematics of ichthyoses describes two main types:

1. Common ichthyoses (without concomitant inflammation)
2. Congenital lamellar ichthyoses (with concomitant inflammation)

Both types have numerous genetic and phenotypic variants and occur as isolated disorders, but they can rarely also display additional symptoms in extracutaneous organ systems as ichthyosis syndromes with many clinical variants. The molecular etiopathogenesis and the genetic defect are not known for all forms and are also heterogenous in most types. However, the ichthyoses have a more or less functionally effective microstructural alteration of the physicochemically complex milieu of the stratum corneum and its microcompartments. Since state-of-the-art molecular and genetic methods have allowed ever deeper insights into the etiopathogenetic contexts of disorders of cornification (DOC), but are not available for area-covering routine diagnostics, an international expert commission worked out a new systematics and nomenclature in 2009, which is more strongly oriented toward clinical criteria and includes the molecular and pathogenetic relationships if known [14]. The historically characterized concept of the 'ichthyoses', which is oriented to the phenotypical picture, particularly of the lamellar ichthyoses, and refers to the appearance of fish skin, is ultimately inapplicable and has therefore faded into the background in the new pathophysiologically oriented nomenclature (Fig. 18.1). Nevertheless, in analogy to historical systematics, two main groups are differentiated: non-syndromal ichthyoses (exclusively cutaneous manifestations) and syndromal ichthyoses (cutaneous manifestation in combination with participation of other organs) [14]. For the much more frequent and thus also more practically relevant non-syndromal forms, five pathogenetic patterns have been defined (Fig. 18.1) [14]. To understand this systematics, the processes of the keratinocyte differentiation as well as the functional structure of the stratum corneum (bricks-and-mortar model) are an essential foundation [3].

J. Wohlrab, M.D., Ph.D.
Department of Dermatology and Venereology, Martin Luther University Halle-Wittenberg, Ernst-Grube-Straße 40, D-06097 Halle (Saale), Germany
e-mail: johannes.wohlrab@medizin.uni-halle.de

M. Lodén, H.I. Maibach (eds.), *Treatment of Dry Skin Syndrome*,
DOI 10.1007/978-3-642-27606-4_18, © Springer-Verlag Berlin Heidelberg 2012

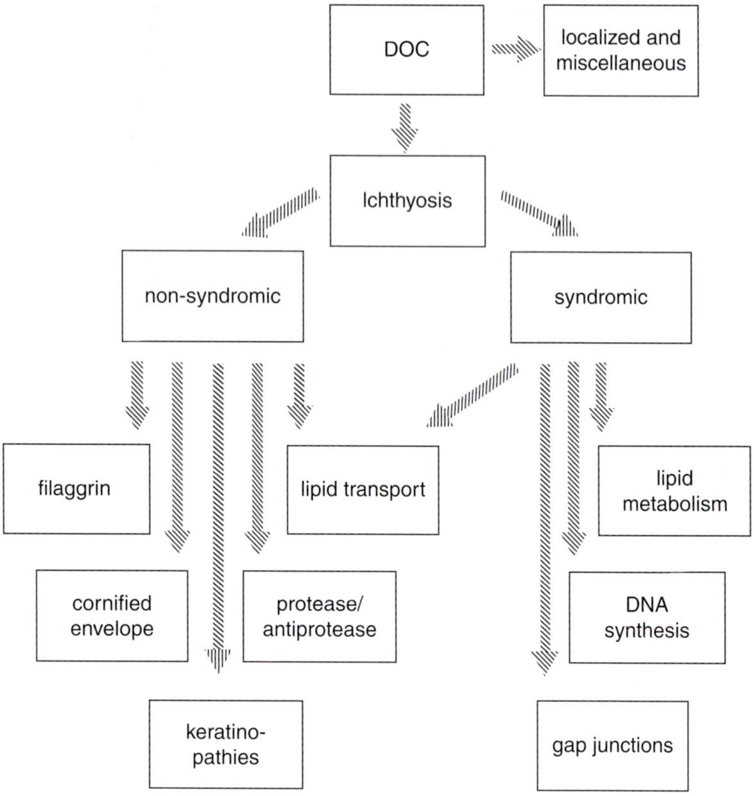

Fig. 18.1 Overview of the disorders of cornification (DOC) (adapted from Oji et al. [14])

18.2 Defects of the Corneocyte Proteins

The defined group of keratinopathic ichthyoses (KPI) subsumes all subtypes of the epidermolytic ichthyoses (EI) [14]. Spontaneous mutations in genes that code for keratins (in particular K1, K2 or K10) [18, 19] are typical. The functional deficits frequently clinically result, even prenatally or perinatally, in blister formation and exfoliation without syndromal phenotype. However, defects can also first manifest themselves postnatally as a consequence of the functional decomposition of the epidermal barrier [25]. In this context, the barrier damage is primarily due to the fragility of the upper nucleated cell layers.

Disorders of the corneocyte envelope, particularly in the form of ichthyosis vulgaris (IV), are frequent [23]. A clinical differentiation to atopical dermatitis or xerosis, respectively, can be difficult, particularly since the type IV ichthyosis typically establishes itself only in the first few months of life. Either insertion or deletion mutations in the filaggrin gene (FLG) is recognized as being the causal factor as heterozygotic form they are usually mild and as homozygotic form they express the full phenotype. In this case, overlaps to atopic dermatitis exist for which mutations in the FLG gene are known [2]. Pro-FLG, the translation product of the FLG gene, is located in the keratohyalin granules in the granular layer, which is reduced or absent in cases involving existing mutation or mutations. The filaggrin defect results in a reduction in the intracorneocytic amino acid concentration produced by proteolysis and thus reduces the hygroscopic binding capacity of the stratum corneum. The altered swelling behaviour of corneocytes then effects a retention of the stratum corneum and a reduced acidification and forms the basis for a scaling abnormality [21].

More rarely, loss-of-function mutations of the transglutaminase 1 (TGM1) gene occur under the clinical phenotype of an autosomal recessive congenital ichthyosis (ARCI) [1, 20]. Moreover, clinically variable, erythrodermic pictures are observed, which are subsumed under the phenotype of an ichthyosis en confetti (IEC) [14].

18.3 Defects of Keratinocyte Lipid Transport

Disturbances of the exocytosis-like processes of secretion of the lipid fractions, which are synthesized in the keratinocytes, from the lamellar bodies are functionally more severe [26]. The lysosome-like lamellar bodies additionally contain a series of enzymatically active substances, which belong to the group of the lipid hydrolases, proteases or anti-proteases, respectively. Additionally, apolipoproteins, anti-microbial peptides (β-defensin hBD2, cathelicidin LL-37) and additional functional peptides are separated with the lipid fractions which contribute to the particular organizational structure of the intercellular lipid matrix. To achieve this, the organelles must migrate centrifugally to the cell membrane, which is regulated by special proteins. The motor and non-motor proteins (e.g. CLIP-170, Cdc42, Arf, Rab7, Rab 11) are very significant, and functional deficits of this system result in severe phenotypes of the disease (e.g. harlequin ichthyosis), mostly even as syndromal form (e.g. CEDNIK Syndrome, MEDNIK Syndrome) [8, 17].

18.4 Protease/Anti-protease Defects

The process of desquamation is enzymatically controlled and thus represents a biochemically active process. The interaction of proteases and anti-proteases is to be understood as a type of equilibrium process. An enzyme that regulates the activity of serine proteases is LEKTI-1, which is encoded by the SPINK5 gene and, as is well known, exhibits mutations in the Netherton syndrome or in the peeling skin syndrome [14]. In the meantime, it has become additionally clear that LEKTI-1 also participates in inducing and maintaining an inflammatory response [6]: For this reason, parallels are also drawn to the pathogenetic concept of atopic dermatitis [2].

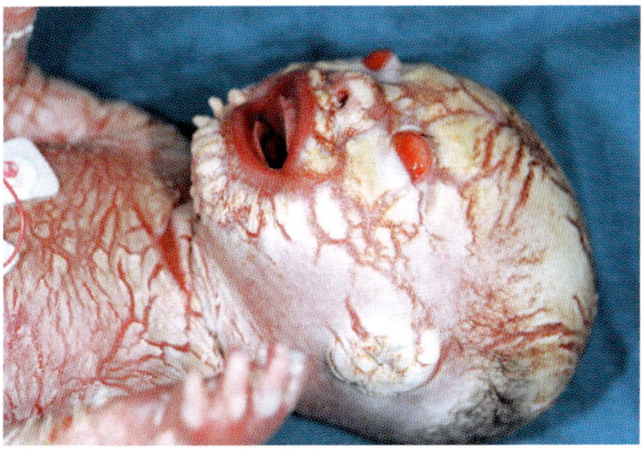

Fig. 18.2 A 2-day-old girl with harlequin ichthyosis

18.5 Defects of the Keratinocyte Lipid Metabolism

The broad spectrum of lipids and their functional significance in the particular organizational structure of the lamellar and extralamellar phases of the stratum corneum are only partially known to date. Nevertheless, defined defects of lipid metabolism clearly illustrate which effects the lack or the functional failure of certain fatty acids can have non-syndromally (e.g. autosomal recessive congenital ichthyoses, ARCI) or syndromally (e.g. Chanarin-Dorfman syndrome, Sjögren-Larsson syndrome, Morbus Refsum). In addition, disorders of the cholesterol (e.g. CHILD syndrome, Conradi-Hünermann-Happle syndrome) or sphingolipid metabolism (e.g. Gaucher disease) have syndromal phenotypes [14].

18.6 Therapeutic Options

Because of the multifarious pathological concepts of the DOC, it is clear that ichthyoses do not represent a uniform entity and therefore no uniform therapy approach can be propagated [11]. From a clinical point of view, however, depending on the ichthyosis (DOC) type and manifestation pattern, the following significant aspects can be considered in therapeutic management after meticulous consideration of the individual benefit-risk ratio:

- Barrier substitution (moisturizer) [4, 12, 22]
- Anti-proliferative therapy (retinoids (Figs. 18.2, 18.3), Vitamin D analogues) [7, 9, 13]

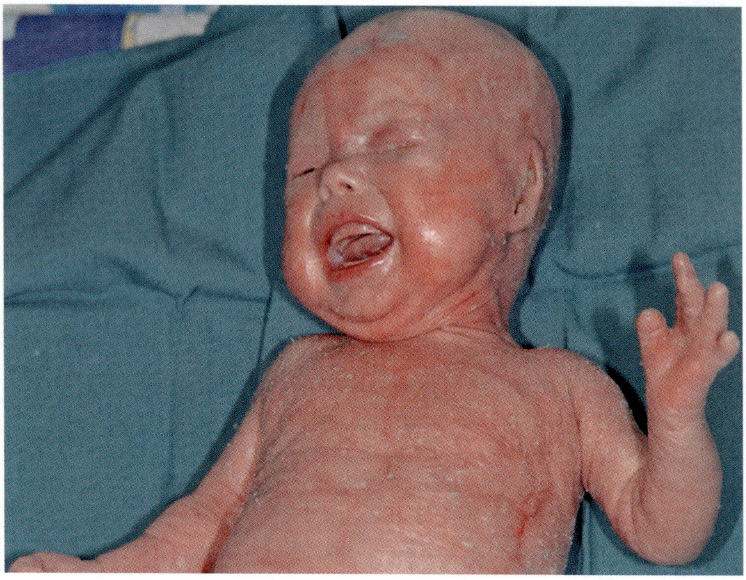

Fig. 18.3 The girl of Fig. 18.2 after perinatal 6 month of oral 1 mg/kg body weight/day acitretin in combination with 5% urea, 5% glycerol, 20% water in cold cream TID

- Anti-septic measures (triclosan, octenidine, polyhexanide, chlorhexidine)
- Anti-inflammatory therapy (glucocorticoids, calcineurin inhibitors)
- Anti-pruritic therapy (polidocanol)
- Keratolytic/keratoplastic therapy (2–10% urea, 10–25% propylene glycol, α-hydroxy acids, e.g. 5–15% lactic acid, salicylic acid, bath additive of approximately 20–50 g/bath sodium hydrogen carbonate) [5, 10–12]
- Nutritional counselling (elevated basal metabolism) [11]
- Measures for anhidrosis (e.g. cooling)
- Psychosocial counselling

The criteria for evidence-based medicine can only be conditionally applied because of the rarity of most ichthyoses and the lack of prospective, controlled therapy studies according to GCP standard. Fundamentally, the active-substance–specific risks of the individual therapy options and the special resorption conditions of the pathologically altered skin as well as the extent of the affected skin area are to be considered. The compliance of those affected and their social environment are of great importance, and judging from my own experience can only be maintained by an empathic and patient informative guidance by a competent and experienced therapist. Depending on the extent of the disease's clinical relevance and the individual impairment of quality of life, the affected person should be given individually selected, barrier-effective and optionally pharmaceutical therapy options so that an individualized, symptom-oriented therapy for the patient is enabled.

18.7 Significance of Moisturizers

A great significance is frequently ascribed to the application of moisturizers in the management of ichthyoses. However, depending on the individual circumstances and the disease type, a critical assessment of the individual therapy options should be performed. As is well known, the application of false or falsely concentrated moisturizer can also result in irritations or toxicologically relevant side effects [16]. Hence, a generalized recommendation is not advisable and also not professional. Similarly to the management of atopic dermatitis, adherence of the affected person to the therapy regime is of decisive importance in the middle- and long-term. Not only the optimized composition of the therapeutic concept, but – above all – the regular and consequent application is decisive for the effect [22]. Therefore, the acceptance of the therapeutic preparations is so important; this can only be achieved when the appropriate moisturizer mixtures are selected and tested in a dynamic process, quasi-empirically, in cooperation with the patient. In this context, the patient's expectations, which are normally shaped by a generally defined ideal (i.e. ideal of beauty), are also to be taken into consideration to ensure therapeutic success. The definition of a realistic therapeutic objective is particularly relevant for the orientation of the patient and the trust-based physician-patient relationship. Additionally, there are slightly different experiences in the use of moisturizers in individual countries. In Germany (and as far as the author knows, also in other European countries), urea (2–10%) alone and in combination with glycerol (5%) are frequently recommended. However, in the USA, α-hydroxy acids and propylene glycol (up to 20%) are preferred. Basically, combination preparations of at least two, better three, moisturizers is to be preferred to a monotherapy. The use of moisturizers is an essential component of basic therapeutic management for the majority of ichthyoses [12, 16, 22].

Take Home Messages

- Since 2009, there is a revised pathophysiologically oriented nomenclature and classification of inherited ichthyoses.
- Two main groups, non-syndromal and syndromal ichthyoses, are differentiated.
- The classification is oriented at (1) defects of the corneocyte proteins, (2) defects of keratinocyte lipid transport, (3) protease/anti-protease defects and (4) defects of the keratinocyte lipid metabolism.
- The use of moisturizers and the basis of therapeutic management are established.
- There are different experiences in the use of moisturizers in individual countries.
- Urea, glycerol, α-hydroxy acids and propylene glycol alone or in combination are frequently recommended.
- Therapeutic options are the topical and/or systemic administration of anti-proliferative (retinoids, Vitamin D analogues), anti-inflammatory (glucocorticoids, calcineurin inhibitors), anti-septic (triclosan, octenidine, polyhexanide, chlorhexidine) and/or anti-pruritic (polidocanol) active substances.
- Nutritional counselling, measures for anhidrosis and psychosocial counselling can be important.

References

1. Akiyama M, Takizawa Y, Kokaji T (2001) Novel mutations of TGM1 in a child with congenital ichthyosiform erythroderma. Br J Dermatol 144:401–407
2. Elias PM, Hatano Y, Williams ML (2008) Basis for the barrier abnormality in atopic dermatitis: outside-inside-outside pathogenic mechanisms. J Allergy Clin Immunol 121:1337–1343
3. Elias PM, Schmuth M, Uchida Y, Rice RH, Behne M, Crumrine D, Feingold KR, Holleran WM, Pharm D (2002) Basis for the permeability barrier abnormality in lamellar ichthyosis. Exp Dermatol 11:248–256
4. Ganemo A, Virtanen M, Vahlquist A (1999) Improved topical treatment of lamellar ichthyosis: a double-blind study of four different cream formulations. Br J Dermatol 141:1027–1032
5. Goldsmith LA, Baden HP (1972) Propylene glycol with occlusion for treatment of ichthyosis. JAMA 220:579–580
6. Hachem JP, Wagberg F, Schmuth M, Crumrine D, Lissens W, Jayakumar A, Houben E, Mauro TM, Leonardsson G, Brattsand M, Egelrud T, Roseeuw D, Clayman GL, Feingold KR, Williams ML, Elias PM (2006) Serine protease activity and residual LEKTI expression determine phenotype in Netherton syndrome. J Invest Dermatol 126:1609–1621
7. Hofmann B, Stege H, Ruzicka T, Lehmann O (1999) Effect of topical tazarotene in the treatment of congenital ichthyoses. Br J Dermatol 141:642–646
8. Ishida-Yamamoto A, Kishibe M, Takahashi H, Iizuka H (2007) Rab11 is associated with epidermal lamellar granules. J Invest Dermatol 127:2166–2170
9. Kragballe K, Steijlen PM, Ibsen HH, Van de Kerkhof PC, Esmann J, Sorensen LH, Axelsen MB (1995) Efficacy, tolerability, and safety of calcipotriol ointment in disorders of keratinization. Results of a randomized, double-blind, vehicle-controlled, right/left comparative study. Arch Dermatol 131:556–560
10. Küster W, Bohnsack K, Rippke F, Upmeyer HJ, Groll S, Traupe H (1998) Efficacy of urea therapy in children

with ichthyosis. A multicenter randomized, placebo-controlled, double-blind, semilateral study. Dermatology 196:217–222
11. Küster W (2006) Ichthyosen: Vorschläge für eine verbesserte therapie. Dt Ärzteblatt 103:A1684–A1689
12. Lodén M (2003) Role of topical emollients and moisturizers in the treatment of dry skin barrier disorders. Am J Clin Dermatol 4:771–788
13. Nikhar B, Atherton DJ, Harper JI (1996) An appraisal of acitretin therapy in children with inherited disorders of keratinisation. Br J Dermatol 134:1023–1029
14. Oji V, Tadini G, Akiyama M, Blanchet Bardon C, Bodemer C, Bourrat E, Coudiere P, DiGiovanna JJ, Elias P, Fischer J, Fleckman P, Gina M, Harper J, Hashimoto T, Hausser I, Hennies HC, Hohl D, Hovnanian A, Ishida-Yamamoto A, Jacyk WK, Leachman S, Leigh I, Mazereeuw-Hautier J, Milstone L, Morice-Picard F, Paller AS, Richard G, Schmuth M, Shimizu H, Sprecher E, Van Steensel M, Taïeb A, Toro JR, Vabres P, Vahlquist A, Williams M, Traupe H (2010) Revised nomenclature and classification of inherited ichthyoses: results of the first ichthyosis consensus conference in Sorèze 2009. J Am Acad Dermatol 63:607–641
15. Oren A, Ganz T, Liu M, Meerloo T (2003) In human epidermis, beta-defensin 2 is packaged in lamellar bodies. Exp Mol Pathol 74:180–182
16. Rawlings AV, Scott IR, Harding CR, Bowser PA (1994) Stratum corneum moisturization at the molecular level. J Invest Dermatol 103:731–741
17. Raymond AA, de Gonzalez de Peredo A, Stella A, Ishida-Yamamoto A, Bouyssie D, Serre G, Monsarrat B, Simon M (2008) Lamellar bodies of human epidermis: proteomics characterization by high throughput mass spectrometry and possible involvement of CLIP-170 in their trafficking/secretion. Mol Cell Proteomics 7:2151–2175
18. Rothnagel JA, Dominey AM, Dempsey LD, Longley MA, Greenhalgh DA, Gagne TA, Huber M, Frenk E, Hohl D, Roop DR (1992) Mutations in the rod domains of keratins 1 and 10 in epidermolytic hyperkeratosis. Science 257:1128–1130
19. Rothnagel JA, Wojcik S, Liefer KM, Dominey AM, Huber M, Hohl D, Roop DR (1995) Mutations in the 1A domain of keratin 9 in patients with epidermolytic palmoplantar keratoderma. J Invest Dermatol 104:430–433
20. Russell LJ, DiGiovanna JJ, Rogers GR, Steinert PM, Hashem N, Compton JG, Bale SJ (1995) Mutations in the gene for transglutaminase 1 in autosomal recessive lamellar ichthyosis. Nat Genet 9:279–283
21. Scott IR, Harding CR (1986) Filaggrin breakdown to water binding compounds during development of the rat stratum corneum is controlled by the water activity of the environment. Dev Biol 115:84–92
22. Simion FA, Abrutyn ES, Draelos ZD (2005) Ability of moisturizers to reduce dry skin and irritation and to prevent their return. J Cosmet Sci 56:427–444
23. Steinert PM, Marekov LN (1999) Initiation of assembly of the cell envelope barrier structure of stratified squamous epithelia. Mol Biol Cell 10:4247–4261
24. Sybert VP, Dale BA, Holbrook KA (1985) Ichthyosis vulgaris: identification of a defect in synthesis of filaggrin correlated with an absence of keratohyaline granules. J Invest Dermatol 84:191–194
25. Traupe H (1989) The ichthyoses: a guide to clinical diagnosis, genetic counselling, and therapy. Springer, New York, p. 253ff
26. Williams ML, Coleman RA, Placezk D, Grunfeld C (1991) Neutral lipid storage disease: a possible functional defect in phospholipids-linked triacylglycerol metabolism. Biochim Biophys Acta 1096:162–169
27. Zeeuwen PL (2004) Epidermal differentiation: the role of proteases and their inhibitors. Eur J Cell Biol 83:761–773

Psoriasis and Dry Skin: The Impact of Moisturizers

19

Joachim W. Fluhr, Enzo Berardesca, and Razvigor Darlenski

19.1 Introduction

Psoriasis is a chronic, systemic, inflammatory disorder with predominant affection of the skin. It affects around 2% of the general population [1]. The disease has a serious impact on the quality of life of the patients [2]. Psoriasis is clinically heterogeneous disease, characterized by variable clinical features, with plaque type being the most common clinical form [3].

The pathophysiological mechanisms include epidermal hyperproliferation and inflammatory reactions of the dermis and epidermis [4]. Psoriasis is characterized by an elevated turnover rate of keratinocytes and a shortened cell cycle. Furthermore, the desquamation process is altered. Inflammation is characterized by the release of cytokines in psoriatic lesions of the affected patients. Scaling marks the clinical feature associated with hyperkeratosis, pruritus, inflammation and SC dryness. Today, psoriasis is accepted as a disease characterized by chronic systemic inflammation and enhanced secretion of proinflammatory cytokines that are capable of inducing pathological skin changes [5].

The chronic-relapsing course of psoriasis requires lifelong management in most of the patients. To date, only disease control or immune suppressive therapy is possible [6]. The available treatments are intended to minimize the development of new skin lesions and the associated symptoms [1, 7]. The aim of any treatment is the decrease or remission of inflammation, scaling, subjective symptoms and skin dryness. The classical topical treatment includes dithranol (anthralin), vitamin D analogues, topical glucocorticosteroids, vitamin A derivates, coal tar, keratolytic agents and emollients. Photochemotherapy with systemic PUVA, bath PUVA and cream PUVA, and phototherapy with UVB light have shown to be effective. Methotrexate, cyclosporine, etretinate, fumaric acid and recently biologicals (ustekinumab, alefacept, etanercept, infliximab, adalimumab) have shown their efficacy upon systemic administration [8].

19.2 Topical Therapy of Psoriasis: The Place of Moisturizers

Topical therapies are adequate in patients with limited plaque psoriasis or less than 20% involved body surface area. The variables to be considered

J.W. Fluhr M.D. (✉)
Department of Dermatology, Venereology and Allergology, Charité - Universitätsmedizin Berlin, Chariteplatz 1, Berlin 10117, Germany
e-mail: joachim.fluhr@charite.de

E. Berardesca, M.D.
San Gallicano Dermatological Institute, Rome, Italy
e-mail: berardesca@berardesca.it

R. Darlenski, M.D., Ph.D.
Department of Dermatology and Venereology, Tokuda Hospital Sofia, Sofia, Bulgaria
e-mail: darlenski@abv.bg

M. Lodén, H.I. Maibach (eds.), *Treatment of Dry Skin Syndrome*,
DOI 10.1007/978-3-642-27606-4_19, © Springer-Verlag Berlin Heidelberg 2012

when choosing topical agents include patient's age, skin type, affected anatomical site, patient's preference (in order to increase the treatment adherence), cost of medication, likelihood of remission and possible side effects. In some cases, a combination therapy with more than one medication may be indicated [7]. The aim of the present chapter is to summarize the knowledge and clinical value on moisturizing agents and emollients in the topical treatment of psoriasis. The most important indications of emollients and moisturizing agents are as an adjuvant therapy of classical psoriasis treatment modalities and the supportive treatment in remission phases.

For topical therapy, Greaves and Weinstein [9] scored emollients lowest taking into account relapse rate, side effects, cosmetic acceptance and efficacy, followed by keratolytic agents, coal tar, dithranol and corticosteroids. For the adjuvant therapy of mild cases of psoriasis, a low risk rate (side effects, cosmetic problems) and no necessity for a strong and rapid efficacy is required. These requirements are met by emollients, moisturizing and keratolytic agents reducing scaling, itch and subjective discomfort and inducing an increased hydration of dry SC and barrier repair. Altered structure and function of the skin measured by increased transepidermal water loss, dysfunction of skin lipid barrier, augmented skin permeability and increased skin roughness can be improved, relieving clinical symptoms and decreasing relapses [10]. Regular application of moisturizers helps to maintain hydration and overall integrity of the SC [11].

A second indication for keratolytic and some moisturizing agents (e.g. urea), when co-applied, is the penetration enhancement of other topical antipsoriatic drugs. A frequently used compound is salicylic acid in dithranol, coal tar or glucocorticosteroid treatment modalities. This may result in an economical benefit by reducing the required amount of topical drug and decreased side effects with a better adherence to the therapeutic regimen [10]. One has to be aware of the potential induction of toxic effects when large surface areas are treated with salicylic acid (salicylism) [12].

19.3 Moisturizers and Emollients in Psoriasis

Emollients are agents designed to soften the SC corneum and to render the skin more supple by increasing its hydration and by reducing superficial scales. They are the most frequently used products in dermatology [13]. A study found that the application of emollients took in average 25 h/year for psoriasis patients [14]. More than 76% of patients had to cover a part or the entire cost of these products.

Emollients induce an occlusive film that limits evaporation of water from deeper parts of the skin and allows the SC to be rehydrated by endogenous supply of water. Furthermore, by including natural moisturizing factors, they induce an increase in water-binding capacity of the SC. Regular use over a sufficiently long period of emollients and/or moisturizers is important. Several products are available today, e.g. moisturizing creams and ointments, as well as bath oils. Creams or ointments are preferable to lotions. They tend to be thicker, more occlusive and therefore more effective in the induction of occlusion and rehydrating the SC [7]. Emollients do not work as a monotherapy in an already fully developed psoriasis. They should be used in combination with other therapies. For chronic plaque psoriasis, it has been reported that water-in-oil emollients are useful as steroid-sparing agent [15]. The use of an emollient limited relapses after the end of therapy with topical steroids and maintained the improvement obtained after 1-month corticotherapy [1]. The hydration of the SC leads to an enhanced delivery of topical glucocorticosteroids. The replacement of one of the twice daily application of betamethasone dipropionate treatment by a water-in-oil emollient showed the same efficacy. A paper summarizing topical therapies in psoriasis found that vehicle (or placebo) was efficient in a broad range from 15% to almost 50% of cases [16]. These results confirm the positive response to an emollient-only treatment.

In an early study, it could be demonstrated that white soft paraffin may inhibit the development of Koebner response in psoriasis [17]. Finlay reported of an effective cream therapy adjunct to dithranol for the treatment of chronic plaque psoriasis [18]. Nola showed that the electrical properties of the SC change after application of an emollient and that there is also an anti-inflammatory activity of these substances [13]. Witman proposed that patients with psoriasis should be encouraged to take a daily bath in warm water followed by generalized application of cream or ointment containing moisturizers [7]. A second or third application of a moisturizer during the day should exert an additional benefit [7]. A study on palmoplantar psoriasis showed that adding an emollient to the topical corticosteroid therapy significantly reduced the desquamation, affected surface area and subjective symptoms at week 4 [19].

Tanghetti performed an observational study evaluating the treatment of plaque psoriasis with tazarotene gels alone and an emollient and/or corticosteroid to investigate whether the efficacy and tolerability of tazarotene treatment can be optimized through the additional use of an emollient and/or a topical corticosteroid [20]. The use of an emollient and/or a corticosteroid enhanced the efficacy of tazarotene treatment and increased the percentage of patients who were satisfied with their treatment [20].

Two randomized controlled studies revealed controversial results on the efficacy of aloe vera gel containing topical cream, with one study showing superiority of the product over placebo [21] and the other one no difference between both [22].

Emollients can cause a few side effects, such as irritant dermatitis, allergic contact dermatitis, fragrance allergy or allergy to other constituents, stinging, cosmetic acne and pigmentary disorders [13]. However, some reports indicate a potentially negative effect of emollients on the susceptibility of the SC to irritants after long-term use [23, 24].

Additionally, regular full-body baths should be performed in order to reduce the scale load and to increase the SC hydration. Two forms of bath formulations are available: dispersion bath oils and spreading bath oils, with the latter being more effective in SC hydration and barrier repair [25]. Furthermore, a shampoo with compounds enhancing desquamation should be used. After hair washing, lotions with keratolytic agents should be applied into the dry hair, especially onto the scalp. Polidocanol-containing formulations might relieve the symptoms of itch. At current, phytoproducts should be avoided since UV therapy is a central part of the treatment, and undesired side effects like allergic contact dermatitis are frequent with the combination of phytoproducts and extended UV exposure. Rim et al. could show a good correlation between skin capacitance and TEWL with the visual assessment of skin dryness. Both TEWL and capacitance values improved in psoriatic lesions in a 6 weeks trial [26].

An emollient-based mild psoriasis treatment induced normalization of several proliferation and differentiation markers, while the clinical response hardly showed any changes after 2 weeks [27]. A point of discussion was raised on the blocking effect of petrolatum pretreatment in phototherapy. While petrolatum was recommended before UVB 311–313 nm phototherapy by one group [28], a petrolatum and salicylic acid in petrolatum treatment just before PUVA therapy was not recommended due to their blocking effects in another publication [29]. The latter group also showed a blocking effect for petrolatum and salicylic acid formulated in petrolatum in the UVB treatment of plaque psoriasis [30].

The patient acceptance of emollients is generally excellent. An additional advantage of emollient therapies is the fact that they are relatively inexpensive (for the health care system). However, in many countries, no reimbursement is available for emollients in psoriasis. More controlled, randomized trials with a high evidence level might help to change the lack of reimbursement since these patients might use, in severe SC dryness, more than 250 g of emollients per day.

A moisturizing cream was studied in participants with mild to moderate plaque psoriasis who were not treated or had discontinued the use of all topical psoriasis medications and all other moisturizers. The use of the product resulted in improvement of skin hydration and desquamation and no further increase in the skin barrier damage [31].

Table 19.1 Critical points in moisturizer therapy of psoriasis

How often to apply a moisturizer	1–3 times/day
How much to apply	Use fingertip units if applicable; if not – enough to create a smooth film over the entire skin surface
Where to apply	Entire skin, not just the affected sites
Which moisturizer to choose	Individual, depends on the patient preference, financial status, cosmetic properties of the product
Contraindications	Uncommon and rare, most often- irritation, contact allergy, cosmetic acne
Pregnancy/nursing	Considered safe
Use in children (paediatric patients)	Generally safe

A guideline from the American Academy of Dermatology summarized the current view on the application of moisturizers on psoriasis [16]. Table 19.1 is reviewing the critical points in moisturizer therapy of psoriasis.

19.4 Effects of Moisturizer and Keratolytic Agents in Psoriasis

19.4.1 Salicylic Acid

Since the beginning of the twentieth century, salicylic acid is known to exert a specific effect on the SC. Salicylic acid is widely used as a keratolytic (facilitating the desquamation process) agent in the treatment of hyperkeratotic dermatoses, e.g. psoriasis [32]. It is mainly used in concentrations of 0.5–60% in almost any vehicle. As mechanism of action for topical salicylic acid corneocyte intercellular bonding, corneocyte desquamation, SC hydration, corneocyte swelling and SC softening has been proposed [32]. Salicylic acid is most beneficial in thick or scaly psoriatic plaques [7]. It is the most effective of the known keratolytic compounds. Several over-the-counter medicated shampoos and scalp solutions aimed for treatment of the scaly scalp contain salicylic acid. Furthermore, compounded ointments with salicylic acid are helpful for localized psoriasis [32]. Moncorps reported as early as 1929 about different penetration properties of salicylic acid from different vehicles [33]. The delivered concentration does not only depend on the original concentration within the vehicle but also on the type of ointment [33]. The resorption rate of salicylic acid on psoriatic lesions is higher, with a faster and longer resorption than on skin of healthy subjects [34]. The resorption rate also depends on the severity of the inflammation [34]. However, the liberation of salicylic acid from different formulations did not correlate with the penetration rate into the skin [35]. An additional study of the same group showed a dose-dependent percutaneous absorption of salicylic acid in vivo [36]. In contrast to the antihyperplastic properties of salicylic acid on pathological hyperproliferation of the epidermis, a promotion of the epidermopoiesis in normal guinea pig skin has been shown with a 1% salicylic acid-acetone-ethanol solution [37]. The mitotic index was increased by 17%, epidermis thickness by 40% and the thickness of the deep epidermis by 19% [37]. Pullman et al. reported an increase of the proliferation rate of psoriatic epidermal cells in humans in an autoradiographic study [38]. Roberts et al. could show a reduction of SC cell layers after 3 weeks [39]. The keratolytic effect was visualized with the surfometry and scanning electron microscopy by Davies and Marks [40]. Huber and Christophers could show for a 50% salicylic acid solution that corneocytes did not change their morphology while the intercellular structure was altered [41]. This treatment resulted in desquamation of the corneocytes. In vivo, with the silver nitrate staining technique, Nook could provide evidence for a keratolytic effect for the combination of a water-soluble ointment containing 5% salicylic acid and 10% urea in comparison to 5% and 10% salicylic acid alone in petrolatum [42]. The combination therapy was as effective as 10% salicylic acid and significantly more effective than a 5% salicylic acid formulation. The keratolytic effect of salicylic acid 6% in an isopropyl solution has been shown with the cantharidin blister method [43]. Going et al. reported the successful treatment of scalp psoriasis with a salicylic acid gel with a negligible systemic absorption of salicylic acid [44].

The negative interaction of dithranol and zinc oxide in pastes could be partly inhibited by combining them with salicylic acid [45]. The addition of salicylic acid to dithranol formulations improves the clinical efficacy of dithranol due to the antioxidant properties of salicylic acid [46].

Salicylic acid can be helpful as a monotherapy. Witman reported an enhanced penetration of glucocorticosteroids. Concentration of salicylic acid used for this purpose is 2–10% [7]. Such combinations require compounding by a pharmacist and carry the risk of imprecise formulations that are potentially unstable, unsafe or ineffective [7].

The major problem in the topical treatment of psoriasis with salicylic acid is the potential chronic and/or acute systemic intoxication (called salicylism), with the symptoms of burning of oral mucosa, frontal headache, CNS symptoms, pH deviation (metabolic acidosis), tinnitus, nausea, vomiting and gastric symptoms [47–49]. These symptoms may occur in topical treatment of large body surfaces, especially in children [50–52]. Even lethal cases are reported [53, 54]. Therefore, a concentration higher than 10%, and an application on larger body surface areas, especially in children, is not recommended. Salicylic acid should not be applied to more than 20% of the body surface area [32]. If larger surfaces need salicylic acid treatment, e.g. for initial keratolysis with an important hyperkeratosis, a sequential treatment is useful (e.g. affected areas in the upper part of the body at night time and the lower part in the morning). Careful clinical monitoring helps to avoid salicylic acid intoxication. It should be noted that some topical treatments of psoriasis such as calcipotriol are inactivated by salicylic acid [55]. It has been shown that salicylic acid exerts a more superficial keratolytic effect compared to benzoyl peroxide and retinoic acid in a test model using chromameter measurements and sequential tape stripping [56]. Bashir et al. used a comparable model with squamometry, protein measurements after sequential tape stripping to assess the scaliness and desquamation for different formulations of salicylic acid [57]. Local irritation but not the clinical efficacy was increased by an acidic pH of the preparation. A constant drug penetration rate was measured for salicylic acid using microdialysis techniques [58, 59].

19.4.2 Urea

The moisturizing effect of urea in dry and scaly skin conditions is widely studied and accepted [60–63]. Urea is known to exert a proteolytical, mild keratolytic, hydrating, hygroscopical, penetration-enhancing, epidermis thinning and antipruritic effect [64]. An increased water-binding capacity could be shown under a treatment with w/o-emulsions containing 10% urea [65]. An increased hydration comparing 10% urea to 5% was not detectable in both o/w- and w/o-emulsions [66]. This indicates that 5% urea is sufficient for a good hydration effect in the SC.

In vitro and in vivo data showed a decreased DNA synthesis index, with a thinning of the epidermis and a reduction of epidermal cells [67]. The mechanisms of urea on epidermal function result in an epidermal thinning (~ −20%). Furthermore, a reduction of the cells in the DNA synthesis in basal layers (~ −45%) and a prolongation of the generation time of postmitotic epidermal cells were detectable [68]. There is data suggesting that lipid biosynthesis may be increased by topical application of high concentration of urea [60].

An improved drug liberation of steroids with ointments containing urea has been reported [69]. Furthermore, penetration enhancement for glucocorticosteroids by urea is well studied [70–76]. Such a penetration enhancement leads to a steroid-sparing effect and an increased clinical efficacy of steroid ointments containing urea. The maximum of the steroid penetration is within psoriatic lesions. But it has still not been studied whether the penetration enhancement improves the clinical outcome in psoriasis.

Dithranol in combination with urea is a standard combination used in psoriasis to improve the clinical efficacy. This effect minimizes the dithranol concentration and shortens the contact time. Furthermore, a better hydration of the SC and a decreased proliferation rate of the keratinocytes can be achieved. Gabard and Bieli showed an increased keratolytic effect of salicylic acid by adding 10% urea [77]. Hagemann and Proksch [78] showed with a 10% urea ointment in 10 psoriasis patients an increased SC hydration and a small decrease in TEWL, a reduction in epidermal thickness (−29%) and a decreased epidermal proliferation (−51%). The altered expression of involucrin and cytokeratins as marker for epidermal proliferation was partially reversed [78]. Sasaki et al. showed for topically applied 10% urea ointment an improvement of SC hydration, water-binding capacity and TEWL in patients with psoriasis vulgaris [79].

Shemer reported a treatment of scalp seborrheic dermatitis and psoriasis with a 40% urea-1% bifonazole ointment [80]. This study showed a benefit of the combination of urea and bifonazole over bifonazole alone by enhancing the bifonazole penetration. These authors reported that urea reduces the plaque thickness [80]. Gloor et al. showed a significant keratolytic activity of five different salicylic acid and high-dose urea compounded formulations from the German pharmacopoeia (NRF) in an in vivo study [81].

19.4.3 Alpha Hydroxy Acids

Alpha hydroxy acids(AHA), such as glycolic acid or lactic acid, are organic acids present in natural sources (e.g. fruits, wine and milk). They exert specific benefits on structure and function of the skin [82]. AHA have been proposed as therapeutic options against hyperkeratotic skin conditions. They penetrate the epidermis, inducing an increased SC turnover. The precise mechanism by which AHA regulate desquamation is not fully understood [82]. AHA appear to decrease cohesion of the corneocytes [83]. Kostarelos revealed synergistic effects between AHA and betamethasone lotions in the topical treatment of scalp psoriasis [84]. Moreover, the therapeutic synergy between AHA and topical glucocorticosteroids was evident without systemic or topical side effects in this clinical trial.

Berardesca et al., in a controlled study, treated 12 psoriasis patients with a glycolic acid lotion 15% versus a 0.05% betamethasone valerate cream [85]. TEWL, blood perfusion (laser Doppler) and skin colour (chromametry) were assessed on psoriatic lesions. The TEWL values decreased significantly. Betamethasone valerate exerted no significant better TEWL improvement compared to glycolic acid. Redness (chromametry a* values) decreased significantly during the treatment without significant differences between glycolic acid- and betamethasone valerate-treated lesions. Laser Doppler values decreased significantly during the study, with lower values in the steroid treated site induced by the known vasoconstrictive activity of glucocorticosteroids. The measurement results were clinically confirmed with a reduction of hyperkeratosis and erythema induced by both treatment modalities. The study shows that AHA are useful not only in the control of hyperkeratosis but also in the modulation of keratinocyte proliferation.

19.4.4 Omega (ω)-Fatty Acids

Oral or topical supplementation of eicosapentaenoic acid (EPA) and/or ω-3 derivatives can decrease not only skin dryness and scaling but also the severity of inflammatory skin diseases such as psoriasis [86, 87]. Omega (ω)-3 derivatives can be incorporated into cell membranes. They are utilized as substrate for phospholipase activity. This may lead to an increase of free EPA, which can be used as substrate for cyclooxygenase and lipooxygenase activities resulting in an increased production of anti-inflammatory leukotrienes LTB5 and PG3 [88]. Abnormal serum fatty acid profiles in Darier's disease, ichthyosis vulgaris, psoriasis and Sjögren-Larsson syndrome have been reported [89]. Berardesca et al. tested topical corticosteroids in combination with 5% linoleic acid. An improvement of epidermal barrier function was reported. Formulations containing omega-3 and omega-6 fatty acids may help in the restoration of barrier properties. Higher efficacy of these products may be achieved by combining different classes of SC lipids [90]. However, in a double-blind, placebo-controlled multicentre study with highly purified omega-3-polyunsaturated fatty acids for topical treatment in psoriasis, no statistical or clinical differences between the omega-3-polyunsaturated fatty acid and the placebo-treated lesions were found [91]. Escobar et al. [86] showed a clinical improvement of scaling and plaque thickness for topical fish oil compared to the base-treated site in a 4-week treatment.

Conclusion

Moisturizers and emollients have a central role in topical treatment modalities of psoriasis. They are adjuvants for classical treatments and help to reduce the scale load of the individual patient. The major role for emollients and moisturizers is to support the improvement in dermal hyperproliferation, differentiation and apoptosis. The anti-inflammatory effect and the stabilization of epidermal barrier function reduce the induction of Köbner phenomena. Co-administration of moisturizers and emollients to the specific antipsoriatic agents improves the course of psoriasis and is a helpful tool in the hands of the dermatologist.

Take Home Messages

- Psoriatic skin is characterized by increased dryness and impeded epidermal barrier function.
- Moisturizers and emollients are indivisible and integral part of the topical psoriasis therapy.
- Moisturizers pursue the classical and novel treatment modalities for the life-long therapy of psoriasis.
- The major effects of moisturizers are based on their adjuvant role in reducing the scaling, supporting the normalizing of hyperproliferation and differentiation as well as on exerting anti-inflammatory effects.
- Moisturizers increase skin hydration and improve the epidermal barrier function thus reducing the risk for the development of Köbner phenomenon.

References

1. Seite S, Khemis A, Rougier A et al (2009) Emollient for maintenance therapy after topical corticotherapy in mild psoriasis. Exp Dermatol 18:1076–1078
2. Murphy G, Reich K (2011) In touch with psoriasis: topical treatments and current guidelines. J Eur Acad Dermatol Venereol 25(Suppl 4):3–8
3. Christopheres E, Mrowietz U (2003) Psoriasis. In: Freedberg IR, Eisen AZ, Wolff K et al (eds) Fitzpatrick's dermatology in general medicine, McGraw-Hill Professional, New York City, USA, vol, 6th edn, pp 407–427
4. Zeichner JA, Lebwohl MG, Menter A et al (2010) Optimizing topical therapies for treating psoriasis: a consensus conference. Cutis 86:5–31; quiz 2
5. Guttman-Yassky E, Krueger JG (2007) Psoriasis: evolution of pathogenic concepts and new therapies through phases of translational research. Br J Dermatol 157:1103–1115
6. Wippel-Slupetzky K, Stingl G (2009) Future perspectives in the treatment of psoriasis. Curr Probl Dermatol 38:172–189
7. Witman PM (2001) Topical therapies for localized psoriasis. Mayo Clin Proc 76:943–949
8. Garcia-Valladares I, Cuchacovich R, Espinoza LR (2011) Comparative assessment of biologics in treatment of psoriasis: drug design and clinical effectiveness of ustekinumab. Drug Des Devel Ther 5:41–49
9. Greaves MW, Weinstein GD (1995) Treatment of psoriasis. N Engl J Med 332:581–588
10. Schopf E, Mueller JM, Ostermann T (1995) Value of adjuvant basic therapy in chronic recurrent skin diseases. Neurodermatitis atopica/psoriasis vulgaris. Hautarzt 46:451–454
11. Bikowski J (2001) The use of therapeutic moisturizers in various dermatologic disorders. Cutis 68:3–11
12. Brubacher JR, Hoffman RS (1996) Salicylism from topical salicylates: review of the literature. J Toxicol Clin Toxicol 34:431–436
13. Nola I, Kostovic K, Kotrulja L et al (2003) The use of emollients as sophisticated therapy in dermatology. Acta Dermatovenerol Croat 11:80–87
14. Meyer N, Paul C, Feneron D et al (2010) Psoriasis: an epidemiological evaluation of disease burden in 590 patients. J Eur Acad Dermatol Venereol 24: 1075–1082
15. Watsky KL, Freije L, Leneveu MC et al (1992) Water-in-oil emollients as steroid-sparing adjunctive therapy in the treatment of psoriasis. Cutis 50:383–386
16. Menter A, Korman NJ, Elmets CA et al (2009) Guidelines of care for the management of psoriasis and psoriatic arthritis. Section 3. Guidelines of care for the management and treatment of psoriasis with topical therapies. J Am Acad Dermatol 60:643–659
17. Comaish JS, Greener JS (1976) The inhibiting effect of soft paraffin on the Kobner response in psoriasis. Br J Dermatol 94:195–200
18. Finlay AY (1997) Emollients as adjuvant therapy for psoriasis. J Dermatolog Treat 8(Suppl 1):S25–S27
19. Cassano N, Mantegazza R, Battaglini S et al (2010) Adjuvant role of a new emollient cream in patients with palmar and/or plantar psoriasis: a pilot randomized open-label study. G Ital Dermatol Venereol 145:789–792
20. Tanghetti EA (2000) An observation study evaluating the treatment of plaque psoriasis with tazarotene gels, alone and with an emollient and/or corticosteroid. Cutis 66:4–11
21. Syed TA, Ahmad SA, Holt AH et al (1996) Management of psoriasis with Aloe vera extract in a hydrophilic cream: a placebo-controlled, double-blind study. Trop Med Int Health 1:505–509

22. Paulsen E, Korsholm L, Brandrup F (2005) A double-blind, placebo-controlled study of a commercial Aloe vera gel in the treatment of slight to moderate psoriasis vulgaris. J Eur Acad Dermatol Venereol 19: 326–331
23. Held E, Sveinsdottir S, Agner T (1999) Effect of long-term use of moisturizer on skin hydration, barrier function and susceptibility to irritants. Acta Derm Venereol 79:49–51
24. Gloor M, Hauth A, Gehring W (2003) O/W emulsions compromise the stratum corneum barrier and improve drug penetration. Pharmazie 58:709–715
25. Fluhr JW, Gloor M, Bettinger J et al (1998) On the influence of bath oils with different solvent characteristics and different amounts of a non-ionic tenside on the hydration and barrier function of the stratum corneum. J Cosmet Sci 49:343–350
26. Rim JH, Jo SJ, Park JY et al (2005) Electrical measurement of moisturizing effect on skin hydration and barrier function in psoriasis patients. Clin Exp Dermatol 30:409–413
27. van Duijnhoven MW, Hagenberg R, Pasch MC et al (2005) Novel quantitative immunofluorescent technique reveals improvements in epidermal cell populations after mild treatment of psoriasis. Acta Derm Venereol 85:311–317
28. Penven K, Leroy D, Verneuil L et al (2005) Evaluation of Vaseline oil applied prior to UVB TL01 phototherapy in the treatment of psoriasis. Photodermatol Photoimmunol Photomed 21:138–141
29. Birgin B, Fetil E, Ilknur T et al (2005) Effects of topical petrolatum and salicylic acid upon skin photoreaction to UVA. Eur J Dermatol 15:156–158
30. Fetil E, Ozka S, Soyal MC et al (2002) Effects of topical petrolatum and salicylic acid on the erythemogenicity of UVB. Eur J Dermatol 12:154–156
31. Draelos ZD (2008) Moisturizing cream ameliorates dryness and desquamation in participants not receiving topical psoriasis treatment. Cutis 82:211–216
32. Lebwohl M (1999) The role of salicylic acid in the treatment of psoriasis. Int J Dermatol 38:16–24
33. Moncorps C (1929) Untersuchungen über die Pharmakologie und Pharmakodynamik von Salben und salbeninkorporierten Medikamenten II. Mitteilung: Über die Resorption und Pharmakodynamik der salbeninkorporiereten Salizylsäure. Arch Exp Path Pharm 155 (1–2): 51–69
34. Arnold W, Trinnes F, Schroeder I (1979) Skin resorption of salicylic acid in psoriasis patients and persons with healthy skin. Beitr Gerichtl Med 37:325–328
35. Gabard B, Treffel P, Schwarb F, Surber C, Bieli E, Lüdi S (1997) Salicylic acid release from topical formulations does not predict in vitro skin absorption. Dermatology 195:37–43
36. Schwarb F, Gabard B, Jost G, Rufli Th, Surber C (1997) Percutaneous absorption of salicylic acid in man following topical administration of different formulations. Dermatology 195
37. Weirich EG, Longauer JK, Kirkwood AH (1978) Effect of topical salicylic acid on animal epidermopoiesis. Dermatologica 156:89–96
38. Pullmann H, Lennartz KJ, Steigleder GK (1975) The effect of salicylic acid on epidermal cell proliferation kinetics in psoriasis. Autoradiographic in vitro-investigations(author's transl). Arch Dermatol Forsch 251:271–275
39. Roberts DL, Marshall R, Marks R (1980) Detection of the action of salicylic acid on the normal stratum corneum. Br J Dermatol 103:191–196
40. Davies M, Marks R (1976) Studies on the effect of salicylic acid on normal skin. Br J Dermatol 95:187–192
41. Huber C, Christophers E (1977) "Keratolytic" effect of salicylic acid. Arch Dermatol Res 257:293–297
42. Nook TH (1987) In vivo measurement of the keratolytic effect of salicylic acid in three ointment formulations. Br J Dermatol 117:243–245
43. Gloor M, Beier B (1984) Keratoplastic effect of salicyclic acid, sulfur and a tensio-active mixture. Z Hautkr 59:1657–1660
44. Going SM, Guyer BM, Jarvie DR et al (1986) Salicylic acid gel for scalp psoriasis. Clin Exp Dermatol 11:260–262
45. Hulsebosch HJ, Ponec-Waelsch M (1972) The interaction of anthralin, salicylic acid and zinc oxide in pastes. Dermatologica 144:287–293
46. Runne U (1974) Anthralin-salicylic acid therapy of psoriasis. Cignolin-salicylic acid-vaseline treatment and Lasan paste in a right-left comparison. Hautarzt 25:199–200
47. Diem E, Fritsch P (1973) Salicylate poisoning by percutaneous resorption. Hautarzt 24:552–555
48. Zesch A (1986) Short and long-term risks of topical drugs. Br J Dermatol 115(Suppl 31):63–70
49. Chapman BJ, Proudfoot AT (1989) Adult salicylate poisoning: deaths and outcome in patients with high plasma salicylate concentrations. Q J Med 72: 699–707
50. Pec J, Strmenova M, Palencarova E et al (1992) Salicylate intoxication after use of topical salicylic acid ointment by a patient with psoriasis. Cutis 50: 307–309
51. Luderschmidt C, Plewig G (1975) Chronic percutaneous salicylic acid poisoning. Hautarzt 26:643–646
52. Germann R, Schindera I, Kuch M et al (1996) Life threatening salicylate poisoning caused by percutaneous absorption in severe ichthyosis vulgaris. Hautarzt 47:624–627
53. Vonweiss JF, Lever WF (1964) Percutaneous salicylic acid intoxication in psoriasis. Arch Dermatol 90: 614–619
54. Taylor JR, Halprin KM (1975) Percutaneous absorption of salicylic acid. Arch Dermatol 111:740–743
55. van de Kerkhof PC, Vissers WH (2003) The topical treatment of psoriasis. Skin Pharmacol Appl Skin Physiol 16:69–83
56. Waller JM, Dreher F, Behnam S et al (2006) 'Keratolytic' properties of benzoyl peroxide and retinoic acid resemble salicylic acid in man. Skin Pharmacol Physiol 19:283–289
57. Bashir SJ, Dreher F, Chew AL et al (2005) Cutaneous bioassay of salicylic acid as a keratolytic. Int J Pharm 292:187–194

58. Klimowicz A, Farfal S, Bielecka-Grzela S (2007) Evaluation of skin penetration of topically applied drugs in humans by cutaneous microdialysis: acyclovir vs. salicylic acid. J Clin Pharm Ther 32:143–148
59. Klimowicz A, Bielecka-Grzela S, Groth L et al (2004) Use of an intraluminal guide wire in linear microdialysis probes: effect on recovery? Skin Res Technol 10:104–108
60. Loden M (1996) Urea-containing moisturizers influence barrier properties of normal skin. Arch Dermatol Res 288:103–107
61. Loden M (1997) Barrier recovery and influence of irritant stimuli in skin treated with a moisturizing cream. Contact Dermatitis 36:256–260
62. Treffel P, Gabard B (1995) Stratum corneum dynamic function measurements after moisturizer or irritant application. Arch Dermatol Res 287:474–479
63. Bettinger J, Gloor M, Gehring W, Wolf W (1995) Influence of emulsions with and without urea an water-binding capacity of the stratum corneum. J Soc Cosmet Chem 46:247–254
64. Muller KH, Pflugshaupt C (1989) Urea in dermatology I. Hautarzt 40(Suppl 9):1–12
65. Wohlrab W (1988) Effect of urea on the water binding capacity of the human stratum corneum. Dermatol Monatsschr 174:622–627
66. Fluhr JW, Vrzak G, Gloor M (1998) Hydratisierende und die Steroidpenetration verbessernder Effekt von Harnstoff und Glycerin in Abhänigkeit von der verwendeten Grundlage. Z Hautkr 73:55–59
67. Wohlrab W, Schiemann S (1976) Investigations on the mechanism of the activity of urea upon the epidermis (author's transl). Arch Dermatol Res 255:23–30
68. Wohlrab W (1992) Harnstoff-ein bewährter Wirkstoff in der Dermatologie und Kosmetik. P Z 33:2483–2489
69. Wohlrab W (1986) Recovery rate of externally administered glucocorticoids on the skin surface. Dermatol Monatsschr 172:615–619
70. Feldmann RJ, Maibach HI (1974) Percutaneous penetration of hydrocortisone with urea. Arch Dermatol 109:58–59
71. Wohlrab W (1984) The influence of urea on the penetration kinetics of topically applied corticosteroids. Acta Derm Venereol 64:233–238
72. Stuttgen G (1989) Promoting penetration of locally applied substances by urea. Hautarzt 40(Suppl 9): 27–31
73. Gloor M, Lindemann J (1980) The influence of ceratolytics and moisturizers on the bio-availability of triamcinolone acetonide following topical application (author's transl). Dermatol Monatsschr 166:102–106
74. Kalbitz J, Neubert R, Wohlrab W (1996) Modulation of drug penetration in the skin. Pharmazie 51:619–637
75. Fluhr JW, Gloor M, Gehring W (2000) Physiology of Skin cleaning and functional mechanism of bath oils. In: Berardesca E, Picardo M, Pigatto P (eds) Irritant contact dermatitis – proceedings of the 3 rd International Symposium (ISICD). Medical Publishing & New Media, Milano, pp 291–307
76. Müller KH, Pflugshaupt Ch (1979) Harnstoff in der Dermatologie. Zbl Haut 1:14–15
77. Gabard B, Bieli E (1989) Salicylic acid and urea–possible modification of the keratolytic effect of salicylic acid by urea. Hautarzt 40(Suppl 9):71–73
78. Hagemann I, Proksch E (1996) Topical treatment by urea reduces epidermal hyperproliferation and induces differentiation in psoriasis. Acta Derm Venereol 76:353–356
79. Sasaki Y, Tadaki T, Tagami H (1989) The effects of a topical application of urea cream on the function of pathological stratum corneum. Acta Dermatol – Kyoto 84:31
80. Shemer A, Nathansohn N, Kaplan B et al (2000) Treatment of scalp seborrheic dermatitis and psoriasis with an ointment of 40% urea and 1% bifonazole. Int J Dermatol 39:532–534
81. Gloor M, Fluhr J, Wasik B et al (2001) Clinical effect of salicylic acid and high dose urea applied according to the standardized New German Formulary. Pharmazie 56:810–814
82. Hardening CR, Watkinson A, Rawlings AV, Scott IR (2000) Dry skin, moisturization and corneodesmolysis. Int J Cosmet Sci 22:21–52
83. Lynde CW (2001) Moisturizers: what they are and how they work. Skin Therapy Lett 6:3–5
84. Kostarelos K, Teknetzis A, Lefaki I et al (2000) Double-blind clinical study reveals synergistic action between alpha-hydroxy acid and betamethasone lotions towards topical treatment of scalp psoriasis. J Eur Acad Dermatol Venereol 14:5–9
85. Berardesca E, Piero Vignoli G, Distante E (1998) Effects of glycolic acid on psoriasis. Clin Exp Dermatol 23:190–191
86. Escobar SO, Achenbach R, Iannantuono R et al (1992) Topical fish oil in psoriasis – a controlled and blind study. Clin Exp Dermatol 17:159–162
87. Dewsbury CE, Graham P, Darley CR (1989) Topical eicosapentaenoic acid (EPA) in the treatment of psoriasis. Br J Dermatol 120:581
88. Kragballe K, Voorhees P, Darley CR, Goetzl EJ (1985) Leukotriene B5 derived from eicosapentaenoic acid does not stimulate DNA synthesis of cultured human keratinocytes but inhibits the stimulation induced by leukotriene B4. J Invest Dermatol 84:349
89. Williams ML (1991) Lipids in normal and pathological desquamation. Adv Lipid Res 24:211–262
90. Berardesca E, Borroni G (1998) Oral and topical supplementation of linoleic acid and skin disease. Medecine, Biologie, Environnement 26(2):159–163
91. Henneicke-von Zepelin HH, Mrowietz U, Farber L et al (1993) Highly purified omega-3-polyunsaturated fatty acids for topical treatment of psoriasis. Results of a double-blind, placebo-controlled multicentre study. Br J Dermatol 129:713–717

Update on Infant Skin with Special Focus on Dryness and the Impact of Moisturizers

20

Georgios N. Stamatas and Neena K. Tierney

20.1 Introduction

Healthy skin is a reflection of its integrity as physical barrier against, among others, external mechanical, microbial, and oxidative insults and loss of moisture and nutrients. This barrier is mostly provided by the superficial layers of the epidermis, the *stratum corneum* (SC), and is sustained by a constant process of cell proliferation, differentiation, and shedding that involves a specialized form of programmed cell death [1]. The basal layer (*stratum basale*) of the epidermis is mostly comprised of keratinocytes, rapidly replicating cells, part of which migrate toward the skin surface and differentiating into flat, nonnucleated cells (squames) [2]. In the basal layer, keratinocytes are connected to each other via protein-rich desmosomes. During the differentiation process, keratin and lamellar bodies are synthesized in the *stratum spinosum* and *stratum granulosum*, respectively, and cell organelles including the nucleus are degraded through nonapoptotic programmed cell death. The lamellar bodies are precursors of the intercellular lipid matrix and are discharged into the extracellular space where they organize into stacks of bilayers that predominantly contain ceramides, fatty acids, and cholesterol [3]. Differentiated keratinocytes (corneocytes) are encapsuled in the cornified envelope (CE) which consists of highly linked, insoluble proteins, mostly loricrin, small proline-rich proteins, and involucrin [4], that are cross-linked to the cytoplasmic keratin filaments and to the lipid matrix [5]. Ten to 15 layers of corneocytes embedded in the lipid matrix make up the SC, the end point of the differentiation process. In the SC, the CE and the corneodesmosomes (specialized desmosomes of the SC) confer the mechanical strength and the intercellular lipid matrix providing the structural foundation for its permeability properties [6]. Before the corneocytes are shed from the skin surface in the desquamation process, the corneodesmosomes are degraded mainly by serine proteases [7].

Keratinization starts around 23 weeks of gestation with ongoing expression of CE precursor proteins and lamellar granule-associated proteins. At this point, the ultrastructure of the keratinocyte cell membrane resembles that of the CE in the adult epidermis with about 15 nm thickness [8]. Histologically, a well-defined SC emerges at 34 weeks of gestation in the developing fetus, and babies born at full term have a developed epidermis several layers thick [9].

Yet, the skin of babies is markedly distinct from adults with regard to its structural, compositional, and functional properties [10–12]. Among the prominent differences are a thinner epidermis and smaller cells [11]. Together with the relatively higher surface area to body weight, this implies

G.N. Stamatas, Ph.D. (✉)
Research and Development, Johnson & Johnson Santé Beauté France, 1, rue Camille Desmoulins, Issy-les-Moulineaux 92787, France
e-mail: gstamata@its.jnj.com

N.K. Tierney, Ph.D
Research and Development, Johnson & Johnson Consumer Companies Inc, Skillman, NJ, USA

M. Lodén, H.I. Maibach (eds.), *Treatment of Dry Skin Syndrome*,
DOI 10.1007/978-3-642-27606-4_20, © Springer-Verlag Berlin Heidelberg 2012

the possibility of a more readily percutaneous absorption of substances through infant skin. Infant skin is more hydrated than that of adults [10, 13]; nevertheless, atopic dermatitis, an inflammatory skin condition marked by extreme skin dryness, is a common affliction at young age [14]. The "acid mantle" of the skin is not yet developed in newborns [13], and the high skin pH and hydration levels in part contribute to frequent damage to diapered skin [15, 16]. Furthermore, sebaceous glands and eccrine sweat glands are not functioning maturely yet [17, 18]. High pH and reduced or lacking sebum and sweat production imply that the antimicrobial properties of the skin are not fully developed. Baby skin provides less protection against the damaging effect of UV radiation because of limited skin pigmentation [19]. Accordingly, skin water barrier function is not fully mature early on in life [10].

Nowadays, we possess numerous and complementary methods that are suitable to study epidermal barrier physiology in infants in vivo. This allows us to document the uniqueness of infant skin and to study the conditions that relate to dry skin in infants. We discuss particular issues of infant skin health and how moisturizers can help to keep baby skin healthy. We will limit this review to healthy babies from 0 to 36 months of life. The SC barrier and hydration needs of preterm infants are out of scope of the present work.

20.2 Skin Barrier Function and How It Is Assessed

20.2.1 Physiological Aspects of Skin Barrier Function

A series of intrinsic and extrinsic factors regulate epidermal barrier function. An important regulatory role is attributed to the hydration status of the skin. The SC with its layers of corneocytes embedded in the intercellular lipid matrix provides an efficient protective barrier that, among others, prevents uncontrolled transcutaneous loss of water [20]. Barrier function and the hydration status of the skin are interdependent factors. The latter is largely influenced by the organization and composition of the intercellular lipid matrix [21], the natural moisturization factors (NMF) which are comprised of hygroscopic components and exclusively found in the SC [22], and by the permeation path length through the SC [23]. On the other hand, the water content of the skin influences barrier function by regulating hydrolytic enzyme activities involved in SC maturation and desquamation of corneocytes [24].

NMF components are highly concentrated in the corneocytes and make up 20–30% of the SC dry weight [25]. Due to their hygroscopic properties, they bind and retain water in the corneocytes, which contain most of the water in the SC [26], thereby keeping the SC hydrated. Proteolytic activity degrades the epidermal protein filaggrin to produce the free amino acids that make up the major components of the NMF [27, 28]. Filaggrin proteolysis is regulated by the water activity in the tissue, with too humid or too dry conditions inhibiting the process [27]. Another component of the NMF is glycerol, which is derived endogenously either from hydrolysis of sebum triglycerides by lipases within the SC or taken up from the circulation into the epidermis by aquaporin channels [29]. This explains why skin rich in sebaceous glands has higher SC hydration than skin with few such glands and is supported by the correlation of hydration levels and SC glycerol content [29, 30]. It was suggested that components of the NMF, including lactate, amino acids, and potassium [31], also contribute to skin pH regulation.

The perpetual sloughing off of corneocytes from the outermost SC through desquamation is required to maintain epidermal homeostasis. The process whereby corneodesmosomes are digested is regulated by a combination of proteases (predominantly by the serine proteases SC chymotryptic and tryptic enzymes) and their inhibitors [32]. Environmental humidity influences desquamation, such that dry conditions have an inhibitory effect on the desquamation process [24] and high humidity stimulates protease activity [33], suggesting that the water content of the SC has an important role in desquamation by regulating protease activity. The desquamatory proteases are contained in lamellar bodies and secreted into the SC intercellular space together with lipids. One

Table 20.1 Methods for the assessment of skin hydration and epidermal barrier function used on infants

Skin hydration		
Microscopy	Skin surface appearance	In vivo microscopy D-squames CLSM
Electrical measurements	SC water content (indirect)	Capacitance Impedance Conductance
Spectroscopy	SC water content (direct)	Raman confocal microspectroscopy FTIR
Epidermal barrier function		
TEWL	Inside-out water barrier	Open chamber Simple closed chamber Closed ventilated chamber Closed condenser chamber
Sorption–desorption	Water barrier (both directions)	One of the electrical methods above

of the components of the lipid matrix, cholesterol sulfate, also acts as regulator of the desquamation process and inhibits serine protease activity [34].

Barrier homeostasis and SC integrity are also controlled by skin pH and calcium concentration. The proteases and their inhibitors involved in desquamation each have their own optimal pH [35, 36], and shifts in pH induce abnormal desquamation [37]. In addition, aberrations in the skin pH also affect lipid processing and maturation of lamellar membranes through the pH-sensitive enzyme beta-glucocerebrosidase [38]. Enhanced protease activity and decreased synthesis of the lipid lamellae lead to exacerbated breakdown of the epidermal barrier when elevated pH is sustained. Keratinocyte differentiation processes, including lamellar body secretion [39], and the processing of CE precursors [40] are also regulated by calcium. Calcium concentration in the epidermis follows a vertical gradient with a low concentration in the basal layers and a progressively higher concentration to reach a maximum concentration in the stratum granulosum and a subsequent decline in the SC [41]. It was found that the formation of the calcium gradient is regulated by the epidermal barrier function and that the gradient disappears upon epidermal barrier disruption [42].

It is thus evident that different homeostatic mechanisms regulate skin hydration and barrier function and that these processes are mutually dependent.

20.2.2 Assessment of Skin Barrier Structure and Function

A series of noninvasive techniques is at the disposal of researchers to quantitatively study the biophysical properties, including barrier function and hydration of human skin, in vivo under physiological, pathological, and experimental conditions. Since these techniques are noninvasive in nature and measurements can mostly be taken in a matter of seconds and by simply holding a small probe against the skin surface, they are suitable for the use in infants (Table 20.1).

Superficial structures of the SC can be visualized with in vivo microscopy [43]. Topographical features include the microrelief lines (crisscrossing the skin surface), the SC island structures between the lines, skin pores, hair follicles, etc. The dryness of the surface correlates with the size of shed corneocytes. Well-hydrated skin sheds individual corneocytes, whereas dry skin with disrupted desquamation sheds scales consisting of partly cross-linked corneocytes. These can be collected with adhesive tape strips (D-squames) and the desquamation rate estimated as a function of the area covered by corneocytes in conjunction with video microscopy [44]. This method also provides information about corneocyte size.

Features within the skin can be revealed by in vivo confocal laser scanning microscopy

(CLSM). This method creates images composed of serial optical sections in the horizontal plain and allows to section tissue at different depths and to gain information of the whole epidermis, underlying dermal papillae (undulating structures at the interface between dermis and epidermis), and dermal structures [45]. Analysis of confocal images provides information on microrelief line depth, the projected area of cells in different epidermal layers, the thickness of the layers, structure and distribution of dermal papillae, etc. [11].

As emphasized above, skin water content is a decisive factor in skin barrier homeostasis; measuring the hydration status can thus give important insights into skin pathophysiology. The ease of flow of electrons in the skin depends on the water content of the SC and increases with increasing hydration. Skin hydration can thus be indirectly assessed with methods that measure the electrical properties of the skin, including skin capacitance, impedance, and conductance [46]. Depending on the chosen method, these measurements permit the assessment of the hydration status of superficial SC layers or much deeper layers including parts of the viable epidermis [46, 47]. A small probe is brought into contact with the skin, and measurements are taken in a matter of seconds, which allows repetitive measurements. Environmental parameters such as ambient temperature and relative humidity influence the readings. It is thus important to control and record these parameters and to let study participants acclimate to the given conditions.

In addition to these indirect measurements, the concentration of water and other substances in the skin can be directly measured with spectroscopic techniques, such as Raman confocal microspectroscopy [48, 49]. The physical principle of this method is the inelastic scattering of laser light (Raman scattering) that results from the interaction between the light and the vibrations of chemical bonds of the molecules in the sample. Based on the shift in the energy of the laser photons, information about the identity and concentration of the molecules present is obtained. The sampling penetration depth in the skin for this technique is up to about 120 μm [48], which encompasses the SC and the viable epidermis and reaches into the papillary dermis. This method allows also measuring the concentration of NMF and other skin components with characteristic Raman signals.

Attenuated total reflectance Fourier transform infrared (ATR-FTIR) spectroscopy is another means to measure the molecular composition of the skin in vivo. This method collects reflection spectra in the mid-IR region of molecules with characteristic vibrational modes and distinct IR absorbance bands. The SC surface water content and lipid types, concentration, and ordering in the SC can be recorded [50].

A widely accepted surrogate marker for SC barrier function is the assessment of transepidermal water loss (TEWL). TEWL measurements register water vapor loss other than through sweating [51]. The rate of water loss is indirectly proportional to the integrity of the water barrier function. At least four distinct methods exist to measure TEWL: the simple closed chamber, the closed ventilated chamber, the closed condenser chamber, and the open chamber method [52, 53]. The simple closed chamber approach measures the relative humidity inside a chamber. Its rapid response makes it suitable for measurements on infant skin. In the closed ventilated method, a carrier gas is used to eliminate water, but this may influence evaporation if the gas is too dry. In the condenser chamber method, the carrier gas mechanism is replaced by water condensation at the top of the chamber. Both the ventilated and the closed condenser chamber method may be forcing water evaporation beyond the nominal state. When performed properly, the open chamber method appears to be more accurate but takes long and can be impractical in certain cases, such as measuring infants. Ambient temperature, humidity, air movement, and direct light are environmental factors that influence TEWL measurements in addition to subject-specific parameters such as sweating, stress, etc. [52, 54].

The capacity of the skin to absorb and retain water can be assessed with sorption–desorption tests that consist of repeated electromeasurements (conductance or capacitance) before and after application of water on the skin surface [55]. The rates of sorption and desorption are inversely related to the water barrier function of the skin area tested, and the time for desorption relates to the water-holding capacity of the SC.

Other methods used to assess skin barrier function rely on measurement of skin reaction (erythema) following the uptake of specific molecules, such as the methyl nicotinate, into the SC or measurement of the concentration of a dye after a defined time following topical application. Due to skin permeation concerns, these methods are not used on infants.

20.3 Baby Skin Properties Differ Compared to Those of Adult Skin

20.3.1 Infant Skin Maturation

The skin of newborns is markedly distinct from adults in structure, function, and composition and remains different throughout infancy while skin maturation continues [19]. At birth, the skin is covered with a protective layer with high water content, the vernix caseosa, composed of corneocytes and lipids similar to SC but with a distinct architecture [56]. As part of the developing epidermal barrier, the vernix provides numerous functions to fetal and newborn skin, including waterproofing in the womb and anti-infectious, moisturizing, and cleansing properties, as well as promotion of the acid mantle development in newborns.

The surface structure of infant skin is characterized by a denser network of the microrelief lines and smaller and less flat island structures compared to adult skin, as analyzed by in vivo video microscopy [11]. CLSM showed that the islands are matched in a one-to-one ratio to the underlying dermal papillae, which is not seen in adults. Furthermore, the dermal papillae are of more homogenous distribution, size, and density than in adult skin. The SC and the suprapapillary epidermis are on average 30% and 20% thinner, respectively. Both corneocytes and keratinocytes are smaller in infants compared to adults. The smaller cell size and higher cell density observed in this age group may be explained by the higher cell proliferation rate observed using fluorescence microscopy in young infants which decreases with age. Structural differences are also observed in the dermis with less dense bundling of collagen fibers [57].

Considerable differences between infants and adults are also manifested in skin composition as indicated by the electrical measurements mentioned above. Skin hydration goes through significant changes during infancy. At birth, the SC of babies is drier compared to older infants, children, and adults [58–60]. The difference between infants and adults is reversed through a significant increase in skin hydration during the first month of life [58, 61] that leads to higher skin hydration in older infants (3–24 months) compared to adults [10, 13]. Together with increasing hydration, the initially relatively rough skin smoothens during the first month [58]. Raman spectroscopy indicated that compared to adults, infants have a higher total water concentration and a steeper water gradient in the SC [10].

Despite the high moisture content of infant skin, the NMF is significantly lower compared to adult skin as measured by Raman spectroscopy [10]. The surface of infant skin is also less rich in sebaceous lipids [17]. This seemingly paradoxical observation of a high water content in spite of relatively low NMF and lipid levels and an apparently shorter pathway for water molecules to evaporate from skin as suggested by the smaller cell size and thinner SC [11] indicates that there are regulatory mechanisms at work that control skin hydration in infants that are different from those of adults.

A thin, highly hydrated SC as is the case in infants [10, 11, 13] presumably causes reduced light scattering. This, together with lower levels of photoprotective melanin compared to adults [62], may increase the probability of UV-induced damage in childhood and could explain the increased risk for malignant skin tumors through sunburns incurred in childhood [63, 64].

After birth, the surface of infant skin undergoes rapid bacterial colonization [65]. In parallel to the ongoing changes in skin structure and function, the composition of the cutaneous microflora evolves over the first year of life [66]. While adult skin is mostly colonized by the phyla Proteobacteria, Actinobacteria, and Firmicutes [67–70], infant skin is colonized predominantly by Firmicutes (predominantly *Staphylococci*), followed by Actinobacteria, Proteobacteria, and Bacteroidetes. Originally dominated by *Staphylococci*, the relative abundance of the genera present grows more even during the first year. Similar to adults, the composition of infant skin microflora appears to be site specific. Cutaneous bacteria modulate the innate immune response [71] and may be involved in the maturation of other skin barrier functions.

The structural differences together with the distinct composition of infant skin probably explain the functional differences in barrier function and water-handling properties compared to adult skin. In analogy to a brick wall, where the corneocytes represent the bricks and the intercellular lipids the mortar [72], smaller cell size and less abundant lipids in infants may account for an immature barrier.

As mentioned above, the barrier function of the SC is commonly indirectly assessed by measuring TEWL. Although contradictory data exist [13, 59, 60] (possibly due to the susceptibility of the method to external and subject specific parameters), we and others found a significantly higher TEWL rate in infants compared to adults [10, 60] together with a large interperson variability [10], which is indicative of an immature barrier function. Furthermore, the water-holding capacity of infant skin is reduced as suggested by its water sorption and desorption properties [10]. Infant skin absorbs larger amounts of water which is then lost more quickly than in adults. A possible explanation for the high desorption rate in infants is the relative scarcity of water-retaining NMF [10] or a larger surface area due to higher density of the microrelief structures [10].

Compared to the acidic skin of adults with a pH in the range of 4.5–6.7 [60, 73, 74], the skin pH of newborns is close to neutral, with values ranging from 6.6 to 7.5, depending on the body site [13, 58, 60, 61]. Skin acidification commences rapidly after birth, causing a drop in pH within a few days [60] that continues to decrease during the first month [58]. Nevertheless, skin pH remains significantly higher throughout infancy compared to adults [13]. This relatively high pH most likely influences skin barrier function, as a number of process in the skin that are crucial for maturation or maintenance of the epidermal barrier are pH sensitive, such as bacterial proliferation on the skin [75, 76], processing of intercellular lipids [36, 77], and desquamation [35]. The diapered area with pH values even higher than other regions is in particular prone to skin irritation (diaper rash) that is accompanied by a broken barrier [16].

A further difference with adult skin is the immature activity of sebaceous and sweat glands in babies. Maternal hormones stimulate sebum production in the uterus, and the residual presence of these hormones is thought to induce high sebum production in newborns [78]; however, sebum levels diminish during the first year [17], and the sebum glands remain quiescent until puberty. Eccrine sweat glands are fully developed in utero. Eccrine glands of palms and soles of the feet are functioning at birth, and their activity is related to the emotional state [79]. However, the thermoregulatory function of sweat glands is minimal in babies [80].

20.3.2 Infant Skin Reaction to Environmental Factors

Exposure to the elements (hot or cold climate, sun, wind) can leave skin red, dry, and scaly. Infants are at a particular risk to react to environmental factors due to the immature protective function of their skin, such as the abovementioned scarcity of melanin [81]. In addition to the temporary discomfort or pain, accumulating damage through repeated sunburns in childhood can have long-term consequences, such as premature aging and skin cancer [82].

Clinical features of skin reactivity of the face and body show a seasonal dependence as demonstrated in a study on infants conducted in Beijing [83]. The stark difference in climatic characteristics between summer (hot and humid summers and dry, cold, and windy winters) correlated with significantly more cases with skin dryness and erythema in winter compared to summer, with erythema being most prominent on cheeks and the chin (Fig. 20.1, Table 20.2). The exact physiological mechanism that underlies the susceptibility to seasonal differences has not been studied in infants. We know however from studies in adults that ceramides and total SC lipids get depleted in winter [84]. Furthermore, the concentration of lactate and potassium (both components of the NMF) diminishes in winter, and this correlates with decreased skin hydration, increased stiffness, and increased pH [31]. It remains to be tested if this is also the case in infants.

Skin reactivity can be measured by assessing the ratio of the concentration of the cytokine interleukin-1 receptor antagonist (IL-1RA) to that of interleukin-1α (IL-1α) in the SC. These concentrations are measured by collecting tape strips from the SC and analyzing the obtained soluble fraction by enzyme-linked immunosorbent assays (ELISA) [85]. It was suggested that IL-1RA modulates inflammatory responses of the skin, as the IL-1RA/IL-1α ratio is increased in UV-exposed areas as opposed to protected areas of healthy skin and in lesions of inflammatory diseases including psoriasis and atopic dermatitis in adults [85, 86] as well as in infant skin exhibiting diaper dermatitis, heat rash, or erythema [87]. Thus, assessing the IL-1RA/IL-1α ratio as a nonspecific indicator of skin reactivity and in the absence of any particular stressors, we found that healthy infant skin is significantly more reactive to the external environment than adult skin [88] (Fig. 20.2).

20.4 Specific Dry Skin Problems in Infants

Dry scaly skin is very common in newborns [59] but can appear at any stage of development resulting from environmentally induced hydration loss of the SC (low humidity, wind, cold). However, the need of protection and moisturization may not always be recognized. In a recent study, 90% of the mothers surveyed believed that their child's skin was not dry, although according to clinical evaluation, only 37% of the children had nondry skin, while the rest had clinical signs of low to moderately dry skin (unpublished results).

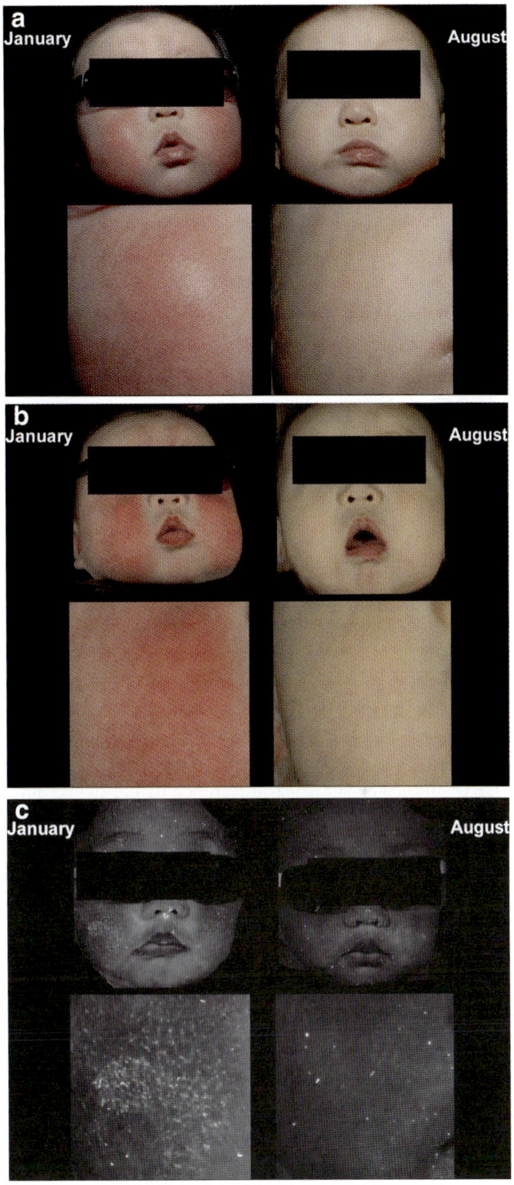

Fig. 20.1 Skin dryness and erythema are evident during winter but not during summer in infants in Beijing. Skin reactions are documented by high-resolution digital imaging at different imaging modalities (**a** regular visible photo, **b** orthogonal polarization imaging, **c** UV-excitation fluorescence imaging). Orthogonal polarization imaging minimizes surface glare and is used to document skin erythema in winter: blood vessels and uneven erythema are visible on the cheek. UV-excitation fluorescence imaging is used to document skin dryness as dry corneocytes show as white flakes under this modality. The images below the full face pictures are magnified areas of the left cheek

Table 20.2 Percentage of infant subjects (aged 3–36 months) with clinical signs of dryness or erythema in Beijing

	Winter (%)	Summer (%)
Dryness (face)	49.6	1.6
Dryness (body)	50.4	0.0
Erythema (face)	68.1	1.6
Erythema (body)	16.0	0.0

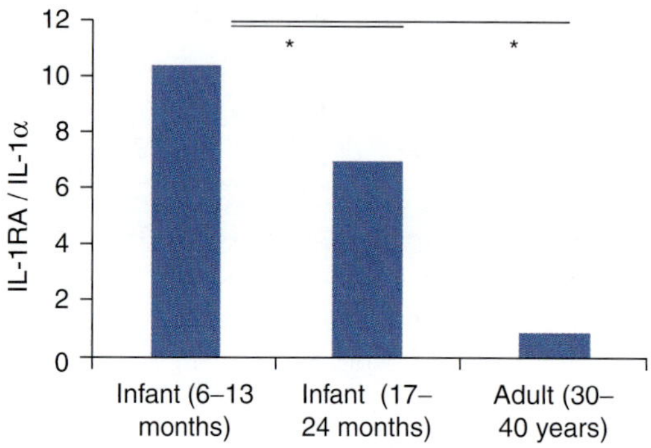

Fig. 20.2 Infants appear to have more reactive skin than adults. The ratio of IL-1RA/IL-1α is calculated from the normalized values of IL-1RA and IL-1α from tapes sampled from the volar forearms of infants and adults. The *star* (*) indicates statistical difference of the two groups joined by the line on top at the level of $p<0.05$

20.4.1 Allergic and Irritant Contact Dermatitis

Cutaneous disturbances are frequent in childhood and include allergic and irritant types of dermatitis. Atopic dermatitis (AD) is an allergic inflammatory skin condition that features as key characteristic extremely dry and scaly skin. The opposite of dry skin, excessive skin hydration, is at the core of another inflammatory skin condition, irritant diaper dermatitis or diaper dermatitis (DD).

DD is among the leading issues in infant skin health. More than half of the infant population has at least one episode during the diaper-wearing phase [89, 90]. This condition afflicts the buttocks, perianal region, inner thighs, and abdomen and presents with redness and scaling of the skin and in severe cases with papules and edema [91]. Diapering creates an environment with distinct characteristics that comprise skin occlusion and friction [92], fecal enzyme activity [93], excessive hydration, and increased pH [16, 94]. All these factors weaken the barrier function and contribute to the risk of developing diaper dermatitis. Prevention or treatment of mild cases involve frequent diaper changes, use of gentle cleansers to remove fat-containing feces, keeping the skin as dry as possible, and application of a barrier cream [92, 95–97], while severe cases that involve secondary yeast or bacterial infections require medical treatment in addition [98].

AD concerns around 20% of children [99–101]. In 60% of those afflicted, the onset occurs before the first birthday [101]. The clinical features of AD vary with age: infants usually have extremely pruritic erythematous papules and vesicles on the cheeks, forehead, or scalp, while chronic disease characteristics in children involve lichenified papules and plaques [14]. The etiology of this disease is not yet fully elucidated; however, a combination of environmental and genetic factors appears implicated [102]. Genetic predisposition involves mutations in structural proteins, epidermal proteases, and protease inhibitors. The most significant genetic factors predisposing to AD appear to be loss-of-function mutations in the filaggrin-encoding gene [102]. Among the environmental risk factors are sensitization to food allergens and aeroallergens [14]. AD that arises in childhood is frequently a precursor of allergic asthma and allergic rhinitis acquisition [103]. One study found that in a population of children with AD, 43% developed asthma and 45% allergic rhinitis [104]. When asthma coexists with AD, it is more severe and persistent than without it [105].

TEWL and pH are higher [106] and the lipid content is reduced in skin with AD lesions [30]. However, a defective skin barrier function in AD is not limited to lesional skin only. Even unaffected skin appears frequently dry. Moreover, TEWL and pH values of noninvolved skin in children with AD are different from that in healthy children [106]. Possibly related to the obvious barrier dysfunction is the risk of microbial infection in children with AD [107].

The following scenario may explain how AD predisposes to allergenic airway diseases: barrier dysfunction may constitute the primary event in the disease development [102] and subsequently enable the penetration of allergens and irritants through the skin. As a consequence of this allergen sensitization, a systemic allergic response may be provoked, characterized by elevated levels of serum IgE antibodies, eosinophils, macrophages, and T cells, which are biological markers of leukocyte activation [108]. It was suggested that the systematic sensitization may facilitate the infiltration of respiratory mucosa with primed T cells, eosinophils, and macrophages after allergen infiltration [108]. This is supported by the evidence that avoidance of food- and air-derived allergens can reduce the development of AD and allergic disease [109].

Besides airborne and food-borne allergens, irritants such as clothing, soaps, hot water, microorganisms, and stress may act as triggers for AD or worsen existing conditions. Special care has to be taken not to exacerbate skin barrier dysfunction in AD through inadequate skin care practices (discussed below).

20.4.2 Baby Skin Moisturization and Barrier Function Protection

Moisturizers are hydrating agents that increase the water content of the SC and result in skin that feels and looks smoother. Key ingredients are emollients (lipids of mineral, animal, or vegetal origin, such as mineral oils, waxes, triglycerides, lanolin, etc.), emulsifiers (which blend the moisturizer ingredients and prevent them from separating), and humectants (e.g., alpha-hydroxy acids, urea, glycerin) [110]. Fats such as petrolatum ("petroleum jelly") have an occlusive effect and increase skin hydration by preventing water from escaping. More than just creating a water-impermeable layer, petrolatum penetrates the SC and aids in epidermal barrier repair [111]. Humectants, including glycerol, increase skin hydration by binding and holding water. Glycerol provides also other benefits for dry skin. It acts as occlusive agent (although to a lesser degree than petrolatum), it may reduce water loss by preventing lipid crystal-phase transitions, and it enhances corneodesmolysis [112]. Emulsifiers are surfactants (surface active agents) that also affect the phase behavior of lipids and facilitate desquamation.

Depending on their water content, moisturizers are either lotions (with high water content), creams (with less water and more oils or occlusive agents), or ointments (oil-based compounds with little or no water in the product).

The increased reactivity and reduced barrier function of infant skin as well as conditions of inflammatory skin disease have implications for skin care in this age group. Specific guidelines developed by dermatologists, pediatricians, and midwives and based on scientific evidence give advice on topics such as the first bath, routine bathing, vernix care, dry skin care, and management of AD and DD in babies [97, 113]. Infant bathing, including that of newborns, is considered a safe practice when performed for a few minutes, not more than 2–3 times per week at 37–40°C and preferably with a gentle, pH-neutral cleanser. A comparative study between cloth washing and bathing in newborns found no clinical harm elicited by either method [114]. Nevertheless, bathing is considered preferable to cloth washing [97] based on evidence that it may better protect barrier function (with lower TEWL and higher SC hydration in some body areas [114]) and thermal stability [115, 116].

To soothe dry and flaking skin, emollients may be applied after bathing [97]. Emollient formulations can be either oil-in-water emulsions (creams) or water-in-oil emulsions (ointments). Current guidelines on AD treatment consider emollients as effective first-line agents in the management of this skin condition [14, 117]. It is recommended to bath children with AD using a moisturizing cleanser and to use emollients after bathing either alone or in combination with topical medication. Repeated application is advised, even in the absence of obvious skin lesions.

20.4.3 Improvement of Baby Skin Barrier Function and Hydration with Moisturizers

The benefit of application of a topical cream after bathing was shown in a study that evaluated the effect of twice weekly bathing with water alone or with a pH 5.5 wash gel with or without

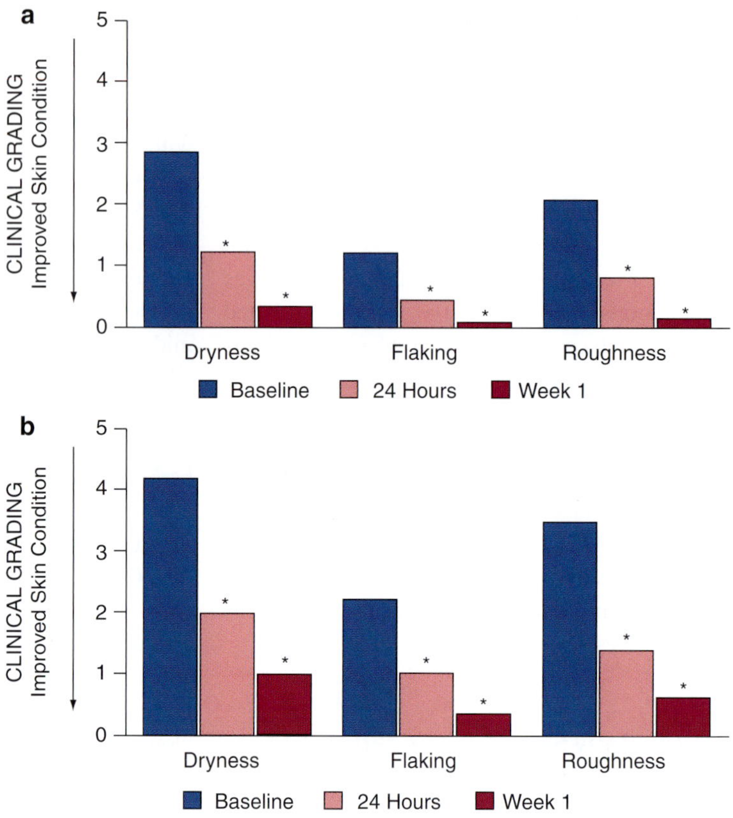

Fig. 20.3 Significant improvement in the skin condition of infants with dry skin and extradry patches 24 h after a single application of a moisturizer and after 1 week of following a regimen consisting of use of a mild cleanser combined with the same moisturizer. The effect of the regimen on the skin condition was evaluated in a blinded, 1-week clinical study under the supervision of a pediatrician. Parents bathed their infants daily using the moisturizing wash and applied the lotion twice daily, with one application being immediately after the bath. The skin condition was assessed using clinical grading of dryness, flaking, and tactile roughness. (**a**) Improvements of dry skin and (**b**) improvements of extradry patches. The *star* (*) indicates statistical difference from baseline at the level of $p<0.05$

cream application for 2 months in newborns [118]. Babies bathed with or without the wash gel and treated with cream had higher SC hydration and lower TEWL than those that were bathed only.

Moisturizers can exert their beneficial effect on skin properties after a single application. In a study, we tested a daily regimen using a gentle, moisture-rich cleanser with twice daily application of a nourishing moisturizer on 6–36-month-old infants with mild to moderate dry and chapped facial skin. The skin condition showed significant improvement 24 h after the first application of the moisturizer [119]. After 1 week of using this regimen, skin conditions remained significantly improved according to both clinical evaluation (Fig. 20.3) and assessment by the parents. We obtained similar results on dryness, erythema, and roughness with the daily use of a moisturizing balm used without any specifically defined washing regimen (Fig. 20.4) [120].

20.4.4 Water Alone Does Not Moisturize Skin: The Complete Skin Care Regimen Is Important

Excessive exposure to water damages skin by disrupting the intercellular lipid lamellae in the SC accompanied with the appearance of large water pools in the intercellular space [121]. It is thus somewhat counterintuitive that washing with water alone does not increase skin hydration. When 3–12-month-old babies underwent a regimen of twice daily washing for 2 weeks, their skin water barrier function showed a small but significant decrease, as indicated by TEWL (authors' unpublished results). At the same time, neither a positive nor negative effect on barrier function was observed for the adults who participated in this study. However, another study that evaluated the effect of twice weekly bathing with water alone or with a pH 5.5 wash gel for 2 months in newborns did not find any nonphysiological values for SC hydration and TEWL despite the

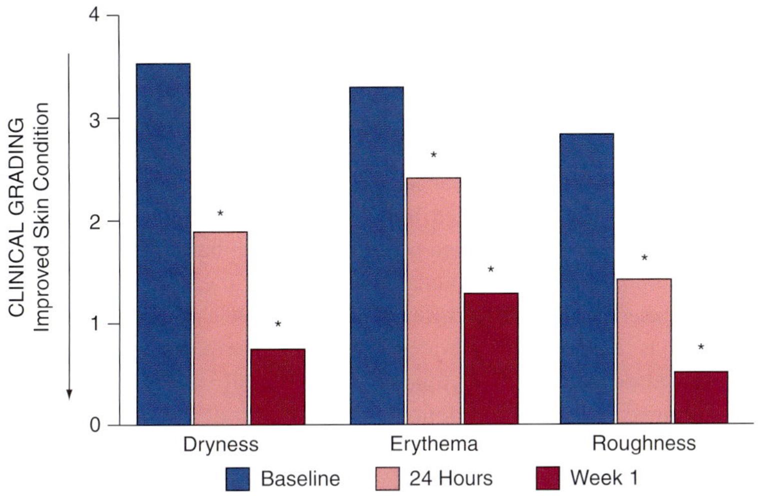

Fig. 20.4 Significant improvement in the skin condition of mild to moderate dry/chapped facial infant skin 24 h after a single application of a balm and after 1 week of twice daily application. The effect of the balm on the skin condition was evaluated in a blinded, 1-week clinical study under the supervision of a pediatrician. Parents were instructed to use the balm on their baby's face daily and to apply to other body areas as needed. The skin condition was assessed using clinical grading of dryness, flaking, and tactile roughness. The *star* (*) indicates statistical difference from baseline at the level of $p<0.05$

observation that bathing with or without the wash gel and application of cream resulted in lower TEWL rates and higher SC hydration than bathing alone [118]. It is conceivable that the observed divergence in results depends on the physical properties of the water used, in particular its hardness (i.e., its calcium content). Hard water can increase the irritant potential of harsh surfactants [122] and was found to correlate with the prevalence of AD in children [123].

20.4.5 Infant Moisturizers Need to be Safe and Effective

Naturally, skin care products, including moisturizers, intended for the use in infants as well as in adults should in no way negatively affect skin function. They should be clinically tested for safety and tolerance and for their efficacy to provide moisture and maintain barrier function. Sometimes even skin care products that are claimed to be in particular suited for sensitive skin may have irritant potential as shown in a comparative study on commercial shower and bath oils designed for dry skin in adults [124]. Some of these products had a damaging effect on skin as evidenced by erythema and increased TEWL after patch testing and left skin reaction-inducing residues after washing. The composition of the formulations is necessarily decisive for their effect on skin barrier function. It remains to be demonstrated which ingredients in particular or combinations thereof have an enhancing or weakening effect. In a study conducted in adults, twice daily application for 7 weeks of moisturizers with simplified (40% lipids of mineral or vegetable origin) or complex (20% lipids of mineral and vegetable origin) creams demonstrated increased TEWL rates and increased susceptibility to sodium lauryl sulfate with the simplified creams, while the opposite was true for the complex cream [125].

We found that neonatal skin does not show any clinical signs of irritation or erythema after 6 weeks of washing with a mild baby cleanser in combination with the application of an appropriately formulated baby lotion (unpublished results). In accordance with this, a previous study on 3–6-month-old infants bathed with a liquid cleanser found no negative effect on barrier function measured with TEWL 15 min after the bath [126].

We observed differences in efficacy of different formulation when assessing the impact of regular moisturizer utilization on skin barrier function and hydration in 3–12-month-old babies. After twice daily lotion application during a period of 6 weeks, we found significant changes in barrier function compared to baseline as indicated by TEWL. The nature of the changes depended on the chemical composition of the test products used (authors' unpublished results). Two different oil-in-water lotions resulted in elevated TEWL and thus decreased water barrier function, which was sustained after the daily lotion applications were terminated. In contrast, a third oil-in-water lotion with silicon, glycerol, and petrolatum improved the skin water barrier function (reduced TEWL) even after application cessation. Among the test products, only the third lotion increased skin hydration and improved the water-holding capacity of the skin during the entire application period.

This data suggest that the choice of a suitable moisturizing product is crucial to support baby skin moisturization.

Conclusion

The skin barrier of infants continues to develop during the first years of life, which reaffirms that infant skin is different than adult skin and remains so for an extended period of childhood. Moisturizers for infants should have clinically proven safety, tolerance, and suitability for the use on infant skin, as well as efficacy in maintaining barrier integrity and providing moisture.

Take Home Messages

- Infant skin displays a developing barrier function and water-handling properties that are distinct from those in adults.
- The unique characteristics of infant skin in structure and composition suggest the presence of distinct mechanisms that regulate water handling and may explain the immature barrier function.
- Atopic dermatitis has higher frequency in infants compared to adults.
- In atopic dermatitis, inhibiting the entry of allergens and other irritants by keeping the barrier function intact may possibly prevent disease progression to allergic airway disease.
- Moisturizers alleviate dry skin due to their occlusive and/or humectant properties.
- Water alone does not provide moisturization and may even dry skin.
- Appropriate formulation is key for the efficacy of a moisturizer.

Abbreviations

AD	Atopic dermatitis
ATR-FTIR	Attenuated total reflectance Fourier transform infrared spectroscopy
CE	Cornified envelope
CLSM	Confocal laser scanning microscopy
DD	Diaper dermatitis
ELISA	Enzyme-linked immunosorbent assays
IL-1α	Interleukin-1α
IL-1RA	Interleukin-1 receptor antagonist
IR	Infrared
NMF	Natural moisturizing factor
SC	Stratum corneum
TEWL	Transepidermal water loss
UV	Ultraviolet

Acknowledgement The authors would like to thank Dr. Beate Gerstbrein of Ascopharm for editorial assistance.

References

1. Lippens S, Hoste E, Vandenabeele P, Agostinis P, Declercq W (2009) Cell death in the skin. Apoptosis 14:549–569
2. Williams AC (2003) Structure and function of human skin. Transdermal and topical drug delivery. Pharmaceutical Press, London

3. Elias PM (1991) Epidermal barrier function: intercellular lamellar lipid structures, origin, composition and metabolism. J Control Release 15:199–208
4. Candi E, Oddi S, Terrinoni A, Paradisi A, Ranalli M et al (2001) Transglutaminase 5 cross-links loricrin, involucrin, and small proline-rich proteins in vitro. J Biol Chem 276:35014–35023
5. Pillai S, Cornell M, Oresajo C (2010) Epidermal barrier. In: Draelos ZD (ed) Cosmetic dermatology. Wiley-Blackwell, Chichester, pp 3–12
6. Wertz PW (2000) Lipids and barrier function of the skin. Acta Derm Venereol Suppl (Stockh) 208:7–11
7. Suzuki Y, Nomura J, Koyama J, Horii I (1994) The role of proteases in stratum corneum: involvement in stratum corneum desquamation. Arch Dermatol Res 286:249–253
8. Akiyama M, Smith LT, Yoneda K, Holbrook KA, Hohl D et al (1999) Periderm cells form cornified cell envelope in their regression process during human epidermal development. J Invest Dermatol 112:903–909
9. Evans NJ, Rutter N (1986) Development of the epidermis in the newborn. Biol Neonate 49:74–80
10. Nikolovski J, Stamatas GN, Kollias N, Wiegand BC (2008) Barrier function and water-holding and transport properties of infant stratum corneum are different from adult and continue to develop through the first year of life. J Invest Dermatol 128:1728–1736
11. Stamatas GN, Nikolovski J, Luedtke MA, Kollias N, Wiegand BC (2010) Infant skin microstructure assessed in vivo differs from adult skin in organization and at the cellular level. Pediatr Dermatol 27:125–131
12. Chiou YB, Blume-Peytavi U (2004) Stratum corneum maturation. A review of neonatal skin function. Skin Pharmacol Physiol 17:57–66
13. Giusti F, Martella A, Bertoni L, Seidenari S (2001) Skin barrier, hydration, and pH of the skin of infants under 2 years of age. Pediatr Dermatol 18:93–96
14. Akdis CA, Akdis M, Bieber T, Bindslev-Jensen C, Boguniewicz M et al (2006) Diagnosis and treatment of atopic dermatitis in children and adults: European Academy of Allergology and Clinical Immunology/American Academy of Allergy, Asthma and Immunology/PRACTALL Consensus Report. J Allergy Clin Immunol 118:152–169
15. Berg RW, Milligan MC, Sarbaugh FC (1994) Association of skin wetness and pH with diaper dermatitis. Pediatr Dermatol 11:18–20
16. Stamatas GN, Zerweck C, Grove G, Martin KM (2011) Documentation of impaired epidermal barrier in mild and moderate diaper dermatitis in vivo using noninvasive methods. Pediatr Dermatol 28:99–107
17. Agache P, Blanc D, Barrand C, Laurent R (1980) Sebum levels during the first year of life. Br J Dermatol 103:643–649
18. Behrendt H, Green M (1969) Drug-induced localized sweating in full-size and low-birth-weight neonates. Am J Dis Child 117:299–306
19. Stamatas GN, Nikolovski J, Mack MC, Kollias N (2011) Infant skin physiology and development during the first years of life: a review of recent findings based on in vivo studies. Int J Cosmet Sci 33:17–24
20. Lee SH, Jeong SK, Ahn SK (2006) An update of the defensive barrier function of skin. Yonsei Med J 47:293–306
21. Rawlings AV (2003) Trends in stratum corneum research and the management of dry skin conditions. Int J Cosmet Sci 25:63–95
22. Rawlings AV, Scott IR, Harding CR, Bowser PA (1994) Stratum corneum moisturization at the molecular level. J Invest Dermatol 103:731–741
23. Machado M, Salgado TM, Hadgraft J, Lane ME (2010) The relationship between transepidermal water loss and skin permeability. Int J Pharm 384:73–77
24. Rawlings A, Harding C, Watkinson A, Banks J, Ackerman C et al (1995) The effect of glycerol and humidity on desmosome degradation in stratum corneum. Arch Dermatol Res 287:457–464
25. Rawlings AV, Harding CR (2004) Moisturization and skin barrier function. Dermatol Ther 17(Suppl 1): 43–48
26. Wertz PW (2004) Stratum corneum lipids and water. Exog Dermatol 3:53–56
27. Scott IR, Harding CR (1986) Filaggrin breakdown to water binding compounds during development of the rat stratum corneum is controlled by the water activity of the environment. Dev Biol 115:84–92
28. Bouwstra JA, Groenink HW, Kempenaar JA, Romeijn SG, Ponec M (2008) Water distribution and natural moisturizer factor content in human skin equivalents are regulated by environmental relative humidity. J Invest Dermatol 128:378–388
29. Choi EH, Man MQ, Wang F, Zhang X, Brown BE et al (2005) Is endogenous glycerol a determinant of stratum corneum hydration in humans? J Invest Dermatol 125:288–293
30. Sator PG, Schmidt JB, Honigsmann H (2003) Comparison of epidermal hydration and skin surface lipids in healthy individuals and in patients with atopic dermatitis. J Am Acad Dermatol 48:352–358
31. Nakagawa N, Sakai S, Matsumoto M, Yamada K, Nagano M et al (2004) Relationship between NMF (lactate and potassium) content and the physical properties of the stratum corneum in healthy subjects. J Invest Dermatol 122:755–763
32. Sato J (2002) Desquamation and the role of stratum corneum enzymes. In: Leyden JJ, Rawlings AV (eds) Skin moisturization. Marcel Dekker Inc, New York, pp 79–92
33. Watkinson A, Harding C, Moore A, Coan P (2001) Water modulation of stratum corneum chymotryptic enzyme activity and desquamation. Arch Dermatol Res 293:470–476
34. Sato J, Denda M, Nakanishi J, Nomura J, Koyama J (1998) Cholesterol sulfate inhibits proteases that are involved in desquamation of stratum corneum. J Invest Dermatol 111:189–193
35. Deraison C, Bonnart C, Lopez F, Besson C, Robinson R et al (2007) LEKTI fragments specifically inhibit KLK5, KLK7, and KLK14 and control desquamation

through a pH-dependent interaction. Mol Biol Cell 18:3607–3619
36. Hachem JP, Man MQ, Crumrine D, Uchida Y, Brown BE et al (2005) Sustained serine proteases activity by prolonged increase in pH leads to degradation of lipid processing enzymes and profound alterations of barrier function and stratum corneum integrity. J Invest Dermatol 125:510–520
37. Hachem JP, Crumrine D, Fluhr J, Brown BE, Feingold KR et al (2003) pH directly regulates epidermal permeability barrier homeostasis, and stratum corneum integrity/cohesion. J Invest Dermatol 121:345–353
38. Choi EH, Man MQ, Xu P, Xin S, Liu Z et al (2007) Stratum corneum acidification is impaired in moderately aged human and murine skin. J Invest Dermatol 127:2847–2856
39. Menon GK, Price LF, Bommannan B, Elias PM, Feingold KR (1994) Selective obliteration of the epidermal calcium gradient leads to enhanced lamellar body secretion. J Invest Dermatol 102:789–795
40. Hitomi K (2005) Transglutaminases in skin epidermis. Eur J Dermatol 15:313–319
41. Menon GK, Grayson S, Elias PM (1985) Ionic calcium reservoirs in mammalian epidermis: ultrastructural localization by ion-capture cytochemistry. J Invest Dermatol 84:508–512
42. Elias P, Ahn S, Brown B, Crumrine D, Feingold KR (2002) Origin of the epidermal calcium gradient: regulation by barrier status and role of active vs passive mechanisms. J Invest Dermatol 119: 1269–1274
43. Chu M, Kollias N (2011) Documentation of normal stratum corneum scaling in an average population: features of differences among age, ethnicity and body site. Br J Dermatol 164:497–507
44. Schatz H, Altmeyer PJ, Kligman AM (1995) Dry skin and scaling evaluated by D-squames and image analysis. In: Serup J, Jemec GBE (eds) Handbook of non-invasive methods and the skin. CRC Press, Boca Raton, pp 377–384
45. Corcuff P (2004) In vivo confocal microscopy. In: Agache P, Humbert P (eds) Measuring the skin. Springer, Berlin/Heidelberg/New York, pp 183–193
46. Berardesca E (1997) EEMCO guidance for the assessment of stratum corneum hydration: electrical methods. Skin Res Technol 3:126–132
47. Blichmann CW, Serup J (1988) Assessment of skin moisture. Measurement of electrical conductance, capacitance and transepidermal water loss. Acta Derm Venereol 68:284–290
48. Caspers PJ, Lucassen GW, Bruining HA, Puppels GJ (2000) Automated depth-scanning confocal Raman microspectrometer for rapid *in vivo* determination of water concentration profiles in human skin. J Raman Spectrosc 31:813–818
49. Caspers PJ, Lucassen GW, Carter EA, Bruining HA, Puppels GJ (2001) In vivo confocal Raman microspectroscopy of the skin: noninvasive determination of molecular concentration profiles. J Invest Dermatol 116:434–442
50. Brancaleon L, Bamberg MP, Sakamaki T, Kollias N (2001) Attenuated total reflection-Fourier transform infrared spectroscopy as a possible method to investigate biophysical parameters of stratum corneum in vivo. J Invest Dermatol 116:380–386
51. Levin J, Maibach H (2005) The correlation between transepidermal water loss and percutaneous absorption: an overview. J Control Release 103:291–299
52. Distante F, Berardesca E (1995) Transepidermal water loss. In: Berardesca E, Elsner P, Wilhelm K-P, Maibach HI (eds) Bioengineering of the skin: methods and instrumentation. CRC Press, Boca Raton/New York/London/Tokyo, pp 1–4
53. Imhof RE, De Jesus ME, Xiao P, Ciortea LI, Berg EP (2009) Closed-chamber transepidermal water loss measurement: microclimate, calibration and performance. Int J Cosmet Sci 31:97–118
54. Pinnagoda J, Tupker RA (1995) Measurement of the transepidermal water loss. In: Serup J, Jemec BE (eds) Handbook of non-invasive methods and the skin. CRC Press, Boca Raton/Ann Arbor/London/Tokyo, pp 173–178
55. Tagami H, Kanamaru Y, Inoue K, Suehisa S, Inoue F et al (1982) Water sorption–desorption test of the skin in vivo for functional assessment of the stratum corneum. J Invest Dermatol 78:425–428
56. Hoath SB, Pickens WL, Visscher MO (2006) The biology of vernix caseosa. Int J Cosmet Sci 28:319–333
57. Vitellaro-Zuccarello L, Cappelletti S, Dal Pozzo Rossi V, Sari-Gorla M (1994) Stereological analysis of collagen and elastic fibers in the normal human dermis: variability with age, sex, and body region. Anat Rec 238:153–162
58. Hoeger PH, Enzmann CC (2002) Skin physiology of the neonate and young infant: a prospective study of functional skin parameters during early infancy. Pediatr Dermatol 19:256–262
59. Saijo S, Tagami H (1991) Dry skin of newborn infants: functional analysis of the stratum corneum. Pediatr Dermatol 8:155–159
60. Yosipovitch G, Maayan-Metzger A, Merlob P, Sirota L (2000) Skin barrier properties in different body areas in neonates. Pediatrics 106:105–108
61. Visscher MO, Chatterjee R, Munson KA, Pickens WL, Hoath SB (2000) Changes in diapered and non-diapered infant skin over the first month of life. Pediatr Dermatol 17:45–51
62. Mack MC, Tierney NK, Ruvolo E Jr, Stamatas GN, Martin KM et al (2010) Development of solar UVR-related pigmentation begins as early as the first summer of life. J Invest Dermatol 130:2335–2338
63. Gallagher RP, Hill GB, Bajdik CD, Fincham S, Coldman AJ et al (1995) Sunlight exposure, pigmentary factors, and risk of nonmelanocytic skin cancer. I. Basal cell carcinoma. Arch Dermatol 131:157–163
64. Mills O, Messina JL (2009) Pediatric melanoma: a review. Cancer Control 16:225–233
65. Dominguez-Bello MG, Costello EK, Contreras M, Magris M, Hidalgo G et al (2010) Delivery mode

shapes the acquisition and structure of the initial microbiota across multiple body habitats in newborns. Proc Natl Acad Sci U S A 107:11971–11975
66. Capone K, Dowd SE, Stamatas GN, Nikolovski J (2010) Survey of bacterial diversity on infant skin over the first year of life (abstract 744). J Invest Dermatol 130(S1):S124
67. Costello EK, Lauber CL, Hamady M, Fierer N, Gordon JI et al (2009) Bacterial community variation in human body habitats across space and time. Science 326:1694–1697
68. Gao Z, Tseng CH, Pei Z, Blaser MJ (2007) Molecular analysis of human forearm superficial skin bacterial biota. Proc Natl Acad Sci U S A 104:2927–2932
69. Grice EA, Kong HH, Conlan S, Deming CB, Davis J et al (2009) Topographical and temporal diversity of the human skin microbiome. Science 324:1190–1192
70. Grice EA, Kong HH, Renaud G, Young AC, Bouffard GG et al (2008) A diversity profile of the human skin microbiota. Genome Res 18:1043–1050
71. Wanke I, Steffen H, Christ C, Krismer B, Gotz F et al (2011) Skin commensals amplify the innate immune response to pathogens by activation of distinct signaling pathways. J Invest Dermatol 131:382–390
72. Elias PM (1983) Epidermal lipids, barrier function, and desquamation. J Invest Dermatol 80(Suppl):44s–49s
73. Braun-Falco O, Korting HC (1986) Normal pH value of human skin. Hautarzt 37:126–129
74. Fluhr JW, Pfisterer S, Gloor M (2000) Direct comparison of skin physiology in children and adults with bioengineering methods. Pediatr Dermatol 17:436–439
75. Matousek JL, Campbell KL (2002) A comparative review of cutaneous pH. Vet Dermatol 13:293–300
76. Korting HC, Hubner K, Greiner K, Hamm G, Braun-Falco O (1990) Differences in the skin surface pH and bacterial microflora due to the long-term application of synthetic detergent preparations of pH 5.5 and pH 7.0. Results of a crossover trial in healthy volunteers. Acta Derm Venereol 70:429–431
77. Mauro T, Holleran WM, Grayson S, Gao WN, Man MQ et al (1998) Barrier recovery is impeded at neutral pH, independent of ionic effects: implications for extracellular lipid processing. Arch Dermatol Res 290:215–222
78. Henderson CA, Taylor J, Cunliffe WJ (2000) Sebum excretion rates in mothers and neonates. Br J Dermatol 142:110–111
79. Harpin VA, Rutter N (1982) Development of emotional sweating in the newborn infant. Arch Dis Child 57:691–695
80. Rutter N (2003) Eccrine sweating in the newborn. In: Hoath SB, Maibach HI (eds) Neonatal skin structure and function. Marcel Dekker, New York
81. Brenner M, Hearing VJ (2008) The protective role of melanin against UV damage in human skin. Photochem Photobiol 84:539–549
82. Berneburg M, Surber C (2009) Children and sun protection. Br J Dermatol 161(Suppl 3):33–39
83. Chu M, Tierney N, Ruvolo E, Stamatas GN, Kollias N et al (2010) Infant skin is similar in New Jersey and Mumbai and markedly different in Beijing in winter (abstract 253). J Invest Dermatol 130(S1):S43
84. Rogers J, Harding C, Mayo A, Banks J, Rawlings A (1996) Stratum corneum lipids: the effect of ageing and the seasons. Arch Dermatol Res 288:765–770
85. Hirao T, Aoki H, Yoshida T, Sato Y, Kamoda H (1996) Elevation of interleukin 1 receptor antagonist in the stratum corneum of sun-exposed and ultraviolet B-irradiated human skin. J Invest Dermatol 106: 1102–1107
86. Terui T, Hirao T, Sato Y, Uesugi T, Honda M et al (1998) An increased ratio of interleukin-1 receptor antagonist to interleukin-1alpha in inflammatory skin diseases. Exp Dermatol 7:327–334
87. Perkins MA, Osterhues MA, Farage MA, Robinson MK (2001) A noninvasive method to assess skin irritation and compromised skin conditions using simple tape adsorption of molecular markers of inflammation. Skin Res Technol 7:227–237
88. Tierney NK, Kothari PD, Martin KM (2010) Investigation into skin reactivity as a function of age: a focus on children less than 2 years of age. International Pediatric Association 26th International Congress of Pediatrics. Johannesburg, South Africa
89. Adalat S, Wall D, Goodyear H (2007) Diaper dermatitis-frequency and contributory factors in hospital attending children. Pediatr Dermatol 24:483–488
90. Jordan WE, Lawson KD, Berg RW, Franxman JJ, Marrer AM (1986) Diaper dermatitis: frequency and severity among a general infant population. Pediatr Dermatol 3:198–207
91. Visscher MO, Chatterjee R, Munson KA, Bare DE, Hoath SB (2000) Development of diaper rash in the newborn. Pediatr Dermatol 17:52–57
92. Atherton DJ (2001) The aetiology and management of irritant diaper dermatitis. J Eur Acad Dermatol Venereol 15(Suppl 1):1–4
93. Buckingham KW, Berg RW (1986) Etiologic factors in diaper dermatitis: the role of feces. Pediatr Dermatol 3:107–112
94. Berg RW, Buckingham KW, Stewart RL (1986) Etiologic factors in diaper dermatitis: the role of urine. Pediatr Dermatol 3:102–106
95. Benjamin L (1987) Clinical correlates with diaper dermatitis. Pediatrician 14(Suppl 1):21–26
96. Atherton D, Mills K (2004) What can be done to keep babies' skin healthy? RCM Midwives 7:288–290
97. Blume-Peytavi U, Cork MJ, Faergemann J, Szczapa J, Vanaclocha F et al (2009) Bathing and cleansing in newborns from day 1 to first year of life: recommendations from a European round table meeting. J Eur Acad Dermatol Venereol 23:751–759
98. Gupta AK, Skinner AR (2004) Management of diaper dermatitis. Int J Dermatol 43:830–834
99. Laughter D, Istvan JA, Tofte SJ, Hanifin JM (2000) The prevalence of atopic dermatitis in Oregon schoolchildren. J Am Acad Dermatol 43:649–655
100. Schultz Larsen F, Diepgen T, Svensson A (1996) The occurrence of atopic dermatitis in north Europe:

an international questionnaire study. J Am Acad Dermatol 34:760–764
101. Kay J, Gawkrodger DJ, Mortimer MJ, Jaron AG (1994) The prevalence of childhood atopic eczema in a general population. J Am Acad Dermatol 30:35–39
102. Cork MJ, Danby SG, Vasilopoulos Y, Hadgraft J, Lane ME et al (2009) Epidermal barrier dysfunction in atopic dermatitis. J Invest Dermatol 129:1892–1908
103. Spergel JM, Paller AS (2003) Atopic dermatitis and the atopic march. J Allergy Clin Immunol 112: S118–S127
104. Gustafsson D, Sjoberg O, Foucard T (2000) Development of allergies and asthma in infants and young children with atopic dermatitis – a prospective follow-up to 7 years of age. Allergy 55: 240–245
105. Eichenfield LF, Hanifin JM, Beck LA, Lemanske RF Jr, Sampson HA et al (2003) Atopic dermatitis and asthma: parallels in the evolution of treatment. Pediatrics 111:608–616
106. Seidenari S, Giusti G (1995) Objective assessment of the skin of children affected by atopic dermatitis: a study of pH, capacitance and TEWL in eczematous and clinically uninvolved skin. Acta Derm Venereol 75:429–433
107. Krakowski AC, Eichenfield LF, Dohil MA (2008) Management of atopic dermatitis in the pediatric population. Pediatrics 122:812–824
108. Beck LA, Leung DY (2000) Allergen sensitization through the skin induces systemic allergic responses. J Allergy Clin Immunol 106:S258–S263
109. Arshad SH, Bateman B, Sadeghnejad A, Gant C, Matthews SM (2007) Prevention of allergic disease during childhood by allergen avoidance: the Isle of Wight prevention study. J Allergy Clin Immunol 119:307–313
110. Loden M (2003) Role of topical emollients and moisturizers in the treatment of dry skin barrier disorders. Am J Clin Dermatol 4:771–788
111. Stamatas GN, de Sterke J, Hauser M, von Stetten O, van der Pol A (2008) Lipid uptake and skin occlusion following topical application of oils on adult and infant skin. J Dermatol Sci 50:135–142
112. Harding CR, Watkinson A, Rawlings AV, Scott IR (2000) Dry skin, moisturization and corneodesmolysis. Int J Cosmet Sci 22:21–52
113. Lund CH, Kuller J, Raines DA, Ecklund S, Archambault ME et al (2007) Neonatal skin care – evidence-based clinical practice guideline. Association of Women's Health, Obstetric and Neonatal Nurses and the National Association of Neonatal Nurses, Washington
114. Garcia Bartels N, Mleczko A, Schink T, Proquitte H, Wauer RR et al (2009) Influence of bathing or washing on skin barrier function in newborns during the first four weeks of life. Skin Pharmacol Physiol 22:248–257
115. Bryanton J, Walsh D, Barrett M, Gaudet D (2004) Tub bathing versus traditional sponge bathing for the newborn. J Obstet Gynecol Neonatal Nurs 33:704–712
116. Henningsson A, Nystrom B, Tunnell R (1981) Bathing or washing babies after birth? Lancet 2:1401–1403
117. Eichenfield LF, Hanifin JM, Luger TA, Stevens SR, Pride HB (2003) Consensus conference on pediatric atopic dermatitis. J Am Acad Dermatol 49: 1088–1095
118. Garcia Bartels N, Scheufele R, Prosch F, Schink T, Proquitte H et al (2010) Effect of standardized skin care regimens on neonatal skin barrier function in different body areas. Pediatr Dermatol 27:1–8
119. Telofski LS, Niciporciukas C, Kurtz ES (2007) Regimen of a moisturizing cleanser and gentle moisturizer provides soothing relief of dry skin and extra-dry patches for infants. International Pediatric Association 25th International Congress of Pediatrics. Athens, Greece
120. Telofski LS, Niciporciukas C, Kurtz ES (2007) Evaluation of tolerance and efficacy of an infant facial balm on mild to moderate dry/chapped facial skin. International Pediatric Association 25th International Congress of Pediatrics. Athens, Greece
121. Warner RR, Stone KJ, Boissy YL (2003) Hydration disrupts human stratum corneum ultrastructure. J Invest Dermatol 120:275–284
122. Warren R, Ertel KD, Bartolo RG, Levine MJ, Bryant PB et al (1996) The influence of hard water (calcium) and surfactants on irritant contact dermatitis. Contact Dermatitis 35:337–343
123. McNally NJ, Williams HC, Phillips DR, Smallman-Raynor M, Lewis S et al (1998) Atopic eczema and domestic water hardness. Lancet 352:527–531
124. Loden M, Buraczewska I, Edlund F (2004) Irritation potential of bath and shower oils before and after use: a double-blind randomized study. Br J Dermatol 150:1142–1147
125. Buraczewska I, Berne B, Lindberg M, Torma H, Loden M (2007) Changes in skin barrier function following long-term treatment with moisturizers, a randomized controlled trial. Br J Dermatol 156: 492–498
126. Visscher MO, Chatterjee R, Ebel JP, LaRuffa AA, Hoath SB (2002) Biomedical assessment and instrumental evaluation of healthy infant skin. Pediatr Dermatol 19:473–481

Part IV

Ingredients and Treatment Effects

The Composition and Development of Moisturizers

21

Steve Barton

21.1 Overview

"Moisturizer" is such a commonplace term undoubtedly meaning many things to different people. So while the common feature of skin needing moisturization is a loss of the natural stratum corneum moisture content, the quantitative and qualitative extent will vary. According to Marie Lodén, moisturizers "should be tailored with respect to the dermatological abnormality" [1]. Defining "the dermatological abnormality" may help understand the consumer need, but acceptance by the end user, whether patient or cosmetic user, may be driven by other factors. Individuals with a "xerosis" arising from pathology – e.g. ichthyosis or eczema – may have similar needs to someone with senile xerosis, but the intensity, persistence and cosmetic properties of the treatment may vary, as may the appropriate ingredients. Likewise, there may be subtle differences between the needs of those who seek improvement in "skin moisturization" as a result of environmental challenges such as surfactant drying, short-term sun exposure and ageing. The concept of the "dry-skin cycle" has shifted thinking on the "dermatological abnormality" from a "dry versus moisturised" state to a dynamic model [2, 3]. This helps explain why moisturization remains the top unmet consumer skin needs, a constant point of reference in this chapter and further defined in Sect. 21.2.

Given this background, it is no surprise that while the fundamental principles will be similar, there exist a number of strategies to "moisturize" the skin. As discussed by Lodén, terms such as "moisturizers" and "emollients" are often used interchangeably, highlighting the focus on the mode of action (adding moisture) and the benefit (skin softening). Over time, and with advances in understanding dry skin, such terms have become imprecise, with a recognition that "moisturising ingredients" have a number of benefits. Hydrophilic systems deliver water and humectants providing optimum conditions for desquamation. Lipophilic materials (emollients) reduce water loss, trap existing moisture into the skin and improve skin softness and flexibility. Section 21.3 develops these ideas.

Between the hydrophilic and lipophilic extremes, there exist emulsions – offering the "best of both worlds." Whether the moisturizer is designed to reduce skin roughness or improve skin flexibility, this end point should be delivered at least in part on first application. If any long-term effect is to be achieved, it needs to be perceived. This is where emulsions come into their own, with many aesthetic possibilities. The focus of Sect. 21.4 will be the characteristics of emulsions and the

S. Barton
Skincare and Claim Support,
Oriflame Research and Development Ltd,
Bray Business Park, Kilruddery, Bray,
Co.Wicklow, Ireland
e-mail: steve.barton@oriflame.com

M. Lodén, H.I. Maibach (eds.), *Treatment of Dry Skin Syndrome*,
DOI 10.1007/978-3-642-27606-4_21, © Springer-Verlag Berlin Heidelberg 2012

implications of efficacy, sensory characteristics, format, etc. on their composition and development.

The most important constraint of using thermodynamically unstable systems in emulsion moisturizers – stability – will be covered in Sect. 21.5. Together with other influences on the choice of ingredient – regulatory compliance, quality, manufacture – this section will further emphasise that moisturizers are multi-phase products, whose ingredients contribute more than one function. Ingredients contributing to stability can also contribute to aesthetics and physiologically.

The foregoing hopefully explains the number of ingredients used in a moisturizer product. Whilst some examples and variants will be referenced, this chapter will not be a formulary. There are many such sources [4–9]. The composition and development of moisturizers is not only a technological process. Moisturizers compounded in a pharmacist's dispensary for specific dermatological needs or manufactured on a large scale for mass consumption will have different commercial constraints. This will impact on choice of ingredients and production methods – what is deemed commercially acceptable for one application may find no place in others.

21.2 Consumers' Skin Needs

There are many levels of consumer need. The subjective level that the consumer directly experiences – scaling, stiffness, tightness, irritation, reactivity, sensitivity, dullness, softness, smoothness and powdery appearance are amongst these. At another level, functional need is "the dermatological abnormality" referred to by Lodén – correction of a biological or physiological process that can be measured in some way. Such measurement should preferably relate to the consumer perception; this may not always be possible (see Sect. 21.3.1).

The "dry-skin cycle" [3] view of skin moisturization focuses the product developer on the potential to interrupt at any stage of this cycle and thus helps skin recover its inherent self-preserving moisturising systems. The dry-skin cycle view emphasises increasing severity of the skin changes as an important consumer need especially "time to improve" – different skin needs may not be satisfied at the same rate. As referenced earlier, this gives rise to the need for "early perception of benefit" so that any longer-term strategy is given a chance to work. This is where the developer has to consider carefully the aesthetic characteristics that influence positive perception (see Sect. 21.4). Targeting one, some or all of these and their different levels of severity will raise different considerations from a formulation development and ingredient standpoint. Figure 21.1 outlines how these two different needs can be brought together to help define the compositional needs of a moisturizer under development.

Further considerations of consumer need will be driven by demographics – motivation, age, ethnicity and geographical location. Motivation will differ between those in search of therapeutic relief from serious pathological condition and those who believe their skin is losing its youthful appearance. The latter "beauty moisturizer" users in general may have less to provide them with early evidence of benefit and thus more likely to cease use if dissatisfied (and more alternatives to try until their needs are met). By contrast, a "medicinal moisturizer" user may tolerate poorer cosmetic properties if the product is being applied for them or healthcare professionals underwrite the relief of the more serious skin symptoms. Self-application of medicinal moisturizers may have driven different acceptability parameters [10].

Age and ethnicity carry with them similar considerations [11] – what constitutes "moisturized skin" varies with age and ethnicity. The geographical and climatic factors influencing dry skin and its successful treatment are covered elsewhere in this book.

21.3 Correcting the Dermatological Abnormality

21.3.1 Just Add Water and Test?

Blank described the need for a minimal level of water within the stratum corneum if plasticity was to be retained [12] and the role of low levels of humidity in decreased stratum corneum flexibility. Although water is the principal plasticiser

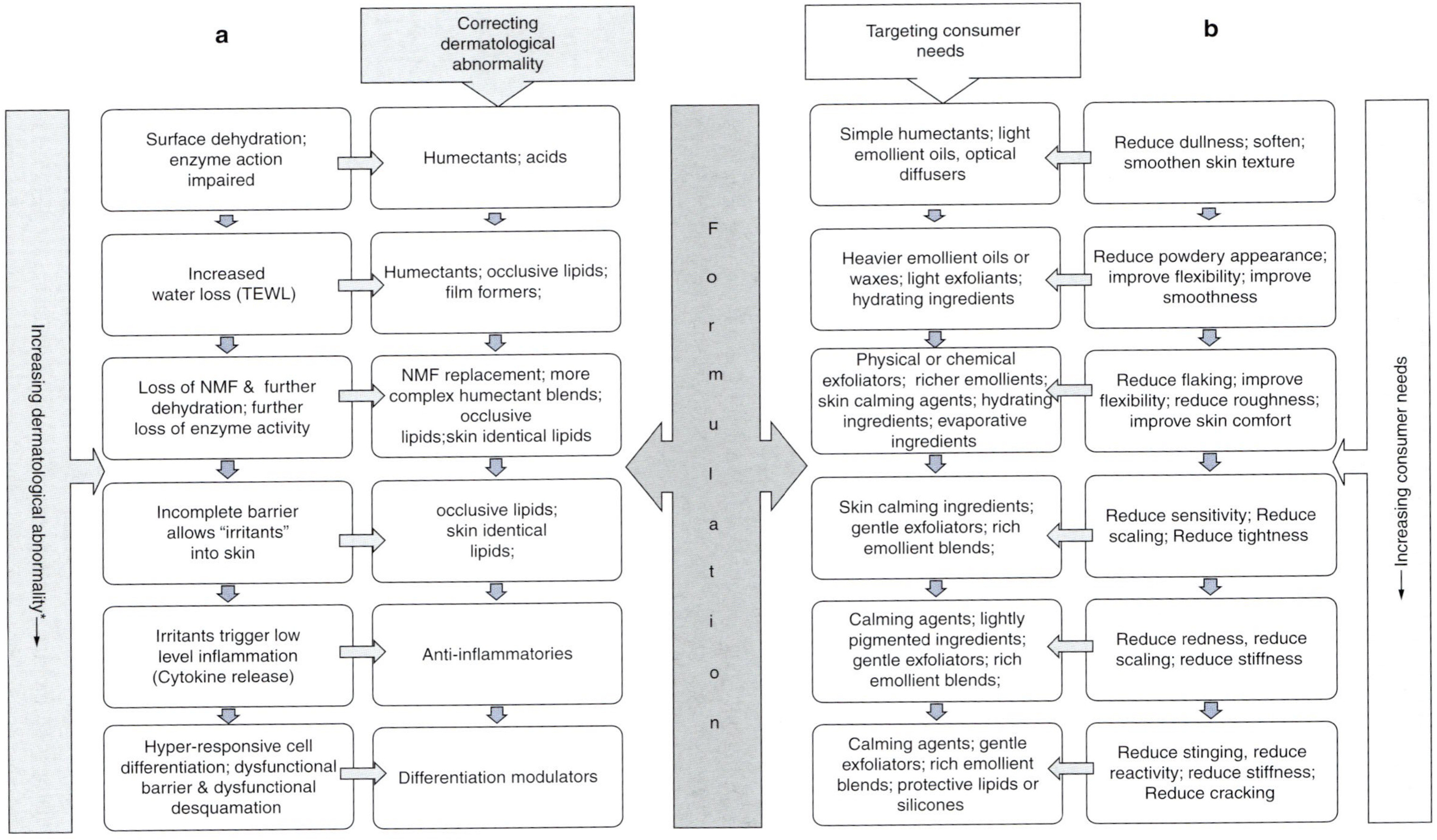

Fig. 21.1 Formulation strategy drivers. Formulation of moisturiser requires bringing together the functional and aesthetic needs. The dermatological abnormality can be increasingly severe (block **a**). A number of ingredient options exist to help correct these dermatological abnormalities. These are discussed in Sect. 21.3. Consumer needs may or may not be consistent with a dermatological abnormality but also can be described in terms of increasing severity (block **b**). Targeting these consumer needs gives rise to a number of ingredient options. These are discussed in Sect. 21.4. There may be some commonality across these ingredients, and the composition and development of a moisturiser involve balancing these factors along with others discussed in Sect. 21.5 (Modified after Rawlings and Matts [3])

of the stratum corneum, the water within a moisturizer delivers only transient effectiveness when assessed by skin extensibility [13]. Indeed, water alone may have deleterious effects on stratum corneum lipid-phase structure [14]. The development and composition of moisturizers focus on maintaining an optimally hydrated state within the stratum corneum.

Hydration can be assessed in a number of ways – see [15], Chaps. 35, 36, 37 and 40. Stratum corneum electrical properties, barrier properties (TEWL) and flexibility offer indirect ways of assessing skin hydration. More direct spectroscopic methods (e.g. Raman spectroscopy) have become more practical [16, 17].These methods can be applied to normal or clinically dry skin. Alternatively, they can be used to assess the recovery on stratum corneum compromised with soap, SLS or tape stripping. Whether these represent the true picture of dry-skin cycle or are predictive of efficacy in all cases of dry skin is debatable.

From the 1970s onward, these techniques provided an array of insights into skin hydration and thus means of assessing moisturizer development. Unfortunately, in addition to the shortcomings of the methods themselves, at a more fundamental level, a direct relationship between any given measurement of hydration and an end-user perception of "moisturization" is challenging given the variety of expectations. The clinical improvement of dry skin – reduced skin roughness, improved skin flexibility, decreased scaling and reduced sensitivity – as well as beauty benefits – decreased dullness, a more youthful complexion and plumped surface micro-relief – can be related to hydration, but for greater consumer effectiveness, additional measures of end-user satisfaction are required.

This factor was highlighted in studies showing that, though water is the principle plasticizer in stratum corneum, plasticization also correlated with product greasiness [18]. In addition, the suggestion that moisturization and elasticity originate from different mechanisms [19] confirm the empirical knowledge that a good moisturizer needs to combine water with other materials that help maintain the functions of hydrated stratum corneum.

21.3.2 Skin Biology as a Guide to Developing Moisturizers

Stratum corneum biology, with its hydrophilic and lipophilic domains, suggests that combinations of such constituents offer a good approach to dealing with the biological problems underlying dry skin. Whilst some products use a single lipid or aqueous phase to deliver moisturization, the majority comprise different combinations and levels of hydrophilic ingredients (salts, amino acids, humectants, etc.) together with lipophilic materials (oils, waxes, etc.) – properties not dissimilar to stratum corneum chemistry.

For simplicity, here the two physico-chemical domains will be used to describe the types of ingredients and their role.

21.3.3 Hydrophilic Materials

These ensure that the hydrophilic domain(s) within the skin are optimally hydrated and/or that some of the components responsible for this in the skin (but have been depleted for some reason) are replaced in fact or by action.

Many of the hydrophilic materials used for this purpose may have little direct sensory impact. Whilst water itself only adds temporary benefit, from a commercial standpoint, it adds to cost-effectiveness of the final formulation. Its solvent capabilities provide the means of adding benefits via other materials. The most important materials, humectants, work by physico-chemical covalent binding of water into the desiccated stratum corneum. The most important class of these materials is polyols and especially glycols.

Glycerol appears to be a special case, backed up the fact that skin generates its own endogenous glycerol [20]. Its performance, better than its humectant properties would suggest, may be due to its small molecular size in proportion to its covalent binding. A comparison of several glycols, their in vitro water uptake and their in vivo water binding found that glycerol, though having the lowest humectancy in vitro, had better in vivo moisturizing effects than other glycols with better in vitro performance [21]. Similar conclusions were made by Takahashi et al. [22] comparing stratum corneum water-binding capacity in the presence of several humectants, including glycerol, pyrrolidone carboxylic acid (PCA) and sodium lactate.

Humectancy ensures some important stratum corneum properties are enhanced. Glycerol provides more rapid induction of hysteresis (creep), but not distensibility, compared to water alone [23], thus enhancing mechanical flexibility. Glycerol has barrier stabilization properties and thus important for skin homeostasis [24]. Stratum corneum extensibility improvements were confirmed by Rawlings et al. [25] after 7 days use of lotions containing 5% or 10% glycerol. Their observations also suggested that glycerol exerted its effects via insertion into the lipid lamellae, a mechanism proposed by Batt et al. [26] to explain the persistence of glycerol's effectiveness after product use stopped.

The role of glycerol in controlling desquamation has been further defined – in particular providing the correct water content for the enzymes responsible for breakdown of desmosomes in the superficial layers of xerotic stratum corneum [27, 28]. Moisturizers containing glycerol are superior in this regard [29]. Glycol humectants have other attributes associated with their humectancy and solvent characteristics – enhanced percutaneous penetration [30] and as a vehicle for antimicrobial materials also influence its use. There are stability considerations from this as glycols can interfere with emulsion structure and rheological behavior. Polyols also improve measures of stratum corneum hydration and barrier – e.g. panthenol [31] – and are common components of moisturizers.

Stratum corneum hydration is naturally maintained via a number of processes. The term natural moisturizing factor (coined by Jacobi [32] and often termed NMF) describes the mixture of amino acids, organic acids, urea and inorganic ions found to make up about 10% of the dry weight of the stratum corneum. These materials have found use in skincare products for many years.

Special prominence was given to the NMF resulting from the breakdown of the histidine-rich protein filaggrin – including sodium lactate, urea and PCA – within the stratum corneum during keratinisation [33]. Generating NMF has been proposed as one of the many functions of stratum corneum [34] providing an essential role in maintaining hydration and maturation of stratum corneum. The trigger for filaggrin breakdown is water gradient found in stratum corneum; effective moisturization thus has a potential role in the "natural moisturization process" in the epidermis. Dry-skin conditions have been found lacking in NMF, correlated with the state of hydration, and moisturizer use can improve stratum corneum amino acid content [35]. Recent findings show loss of function mutations in filaggrin, and this takes the idea of diversity of end-user need to a new level, and NMF quality [36] may influence future moisturizer formulation strategy. "NMF replacement" is a common strategy – prolonged application of a lotion containing PCA has been more effective than a placebo [37].

Urea is a common ingredient used in therapeutic moisturizers; its influence and action are dealt with elsewhere in this book. The choice between this and glycerol tends to be driven by regional market expectations. Comparative performance has been studied showing superior clinical effectiveness in atopic dermatitis patients using a moisturizer containing urea [38]. However, the study used a level of glycerol far higher than usual, and a different result was obtained in soap-dried winter xerosis [39]. Like glycerol, urea improves barrier, the latter producing improved resistance to an SLS challenge [40]. Unlike glycerol, its charged nature can give rise to poor formulation stability (including formation of ammonia) and skin tolerance; thus, pH and concentration are important considerations. Levels of use vary – one study showed 10% and 3% urea similar for subjectively assessed efficacy, though 10% proved better by objective measures of barrier improvement [41]. Urea formulated at 10% was effective in both water-in-oil (W/O) and oil-in-water (O/W) emulsions [42] and withstands the influence of other charged aqueous components – sodium chloride [43], ammonium lactate or urea combinations in O/W or W/O emulsions [44] showed similar improvements in hydration. Studies on short-term benefit of urea have been shown to be predictive of longer-term benefit [45].

Other charged "NMF ingredients" are the organic acids. The alpha hydroxy acids (AHA) in particular showed powerful therapeutic action in several common xerotic dermatoses [46]. Like urea, despite formulation and tolerability factors, AHA have become useful ingredients in cosmetic skincare. Hyperacidification of stratum corneum has recently been proposed as a means of improving stratum corneum integrity and cohesion [47].

Lactic acid enhances the pliability of stratum corneum [48] independently of the hydrating effect of lactate in cosmetic moisturizers. A further study clearly demonstrated the pH dependencies of AHA action [49]. Both pH and concentration are critical in the lactic acid effect. At a fixed lactic acid concentration, the desquamative effect was highly pH dependent. At a fixed pH, the turnover rate of skin was concentration dependent. Though chain length is important, glycolic, lactic, tartaric and gluconolactone formulated at 8% in a common base [50] all improved skin barrier. The early site of action of AHA appears to be the outer layers (stratum disjunctum) [51] emphasizing their role as exfoliants in moisturizers.

Further specificity of the effects of AHA has been demonstrated; the L isomer acid (rather than the D isomer) of lactic or glycolic acid were the most effective, primarily on the basis of their greater consumer tolerability [52]. The L isomers also have a role in stimulating ceramide biosynthesis, hence improving barrier function [53].

AHA are used in cosmetics at up to 8% but at higher concentrations [54] increase skin thickness, peel significant layers of stratum corneum and epidermis, and improvements in the histological signs of photoageing were noted without any signs of inflammation. Even citric acid, which is relatively ineffective at low concentrations, has been shown to have effects similar to other more effective AHA [55].

There has been concern about the safety in the use of AHA in daily skincare products. Studies showing an increased sensitivity to UV after use of AHA [56] brought about a practice advising sun protection whilst using AHA-based products.

Consumer tolerability is a key determinant when formulating with AHA – free acid, counter-ion, chain length and formulation vehicle are all important [57]. Commercially available AHA have been produced to help the formulator create better, and a number of strategies exist to allow successful benefits with reduced irritation [58]. Similar management of the benefit/tolerability paradox has been achieved for salicylic acid [59], a beta hydroxy acid with an exfoliating action.

Other common hydrophilic materials in moisturizers include osmoprotectants extracted from plants. Aloe vera, possibly the best known, comprising polysaccharides, glycoproteins and minerals, has benefits beyond simple moisturization [60]. Soothing components may help deliver this requirement sought as a desirable consumer end point. There are many grades available including freeze-dried powders, reconstituted concentrates and native juices. Aloe vera gel can be used alone or as the major component of an aqueous moisturising gel designed for use in conditions such as sunburn. Incorporation into emulsions is common, and the potential interactions with other ingredients are an important stability consideration.

Similarities can be found in extracts of certain seaweed species. Both plants survive long periods of water deprivation and have adapted their own ways of resisting desiccation. Like aloe vera, the benefits of seaweed may go beyond simple moisturization [61]. Water-holding properties of the complex polysaccharides that comprise the alginates and carrageenans may account for their "moisturizing" properties, but like aloe, these gels also modify the sensory perception on the skin. Enhancing the sensory properties, stability and rheological properties of the formulation adds to the reasons for their use. This highlights again the multi-functional properties of moisturizing ingredients (a theme reiterated throughout this chapter). Trehalose is another material that absorbs and retains water in biological systems, and this too finds use in moisturizers.

Oats provide another source of material with use in dry-skin conditions – colloidal preparations contain starch and beta-glucans with water-binding properties as well as avenanthramides that may help skin barrier recovery properties [62, 63]. The husk of oats also finds use as an exfoliating agent.

These large molecules with water-binding capability, and others such as hyaluronic acid, unlike glycerol are too large to insert into the stratum corneum. Their moisturizing action, apart from sensorial, probably derives from coating the skin with a hydrated "buffer" at the skin surface. Smaller-molecular-size fractions of hyaluronic acid may have greater penetration into stratum corneum and thus have greater effectiveness.

Two per cent nicotinamide in a moisturizer has been shown to improve atopic dry skin over an 8-week period [64]. Nicotinamide reduced TEWL whereas petrolatum did not, and whilst both treatments improved measures of hydration, nicotinamide was superior. Together with vitamin B3, it also improved skin barrier function [16].

21.3.4 Lipophilic Materials

Whilst glycerol may soften the skin as an undiluted material, this is not a universal effect of hydrophilic moisturizer ingredients at normal use levels. Lipophilic materials by contrast will possess emollient properties – slip, glide and lubricity – forming a soft layer on the skin surface. They also change the optical properties of the skin. As such, they address many of the consumer needs required to correct dry skin (thus "moisturising"). Many lipophilic materials will have "occlusive" effects on the skin, thereby reducing water loss, further enhancing their "moisturization" capabilities.

The chemistry of emollients can be roughly broken down into different classes – hydrocarbons, fatty alcohols, fatty acids, esters, ethers, glycerides and complex mixtures. Selection of particular materials depends on a number of criteria – all of which are driven by consumer need – spreading characteristics, sensory impact, stability, solubilising properties and skin compatibility. In turn, these performance characteristics evolve from a number of chemical properties – molecular structure (straight chain versus branched; saturation), molecular species (alkane versus alcohol versus aldehyde versus acid versus amide) and molecular size. Examples of some commonly used emollient materials together with their characteristics can be found in the Table 21.1 (see also Chap. 27).

Hydrocarbon oils and waxes have been useful ingredients in formulations, and Kligman's definitive study [65] showed petrolatum to gradually and temporarily improve the signs of skin dryness in vivo using clinical grading. The various grades of solid and liquid paraffins in a range of combinations, in W/O or O/W emulsions, can be tailored to reflect sensory requirements. Their limited reactivity provides good stability, and they remain common moisturizer ingredients. As a commodity material, they also have the advantages of low price, though recent cost fluctuations and concerns about the long-term sustainability are just two factors changing patterns of use. A more important factor is the increasing sophistication of consumer needs, driving incorporation of other materials to mitigate the coated and greasy end-feel sensory properties characteristic of paraffins.

Lanolin as a naturally occurring keratin conditioner compensates for many of the deficiencies of petrolatum with similar effectiveness detectable 14 days after ceasing product use. Lanolin is a complex material predominantly comprising sterol esters but also sterols and acids. Its appeal arises from its spreading properties, melting point close to skin temperature and water absorbency. The sterol content also has relevance because of the importance of these materials in skin biology. Lanolin appears to penetrate and integrate itself into the lipid structure within the stratum corneum [66], thus explaining its persistent effects. Lanolin has been used alone as an emollient and also in moisturizer formulations with ingredients of different grades of lanolin alcohols. By analogy, the role of human sebum has similar spreading properties and complexity. Artificial sebum has been proposed comprising 17% fatty acid, 44.7% triglyceride, 25% wax monoester (jojoba oil) and 12.4% squalene [67]. The latter material – a triterpene that is an intermediate of the cholesterol biosynthesis pathway – is a major component of shark oil that used to be a common cosmetic ingredient; more sustainable alternatives include olive oil containing 0.2–0.7% squalene [68].

Vegetable sources of oils easily replace mineral oil in cosmetic moisturizers with parity in their efficacy and safety [69]. Commonly sources are selected on the basis of their sensory properties, but biological activity can influence choice.

Table 21.1 Emollient classes and some characteristics that influence their inclusion in moisturiser formulations

INCI name	Spreading properties	Polarity	Cloud point	HLB value	Viscosity at 20°C (mPas)	Comments
Esters						
Dicaprylyl carbonate	Fast	Weak	<–20°C	–	7	Velvety, dry skin feel, solubilizing capability of UV filters
Isononyl isononanoate	Fast	Weak	<–25°C	12	6	Light emollient with medium to velvety, slippery skin feel; non-greasy with excellent spreadability
Isopropyl myristate	Fast	Medium	<2°C	11.5	5	Good spreading; dry after feel; comedogenic potential
Propylheptyl caprylate	Fast	Medium	<–20°C	–	–	Luxurious – soft; silky; velvety. Hydrolytically stable; supports incorporation of powdery ingredients and UV filters
Cetearyl ethylhexanoate (and) isopropyl myristate	Fast	Weak	<–1°C	8.22	10.4	Forms water repellent films, imparts gloss. Mineral oil alternative
Isopropyl palmitate	Fast	Medium	<15	–	7	Comedogenic potential
Pentaerythrityl tetracaprylate/caprate	Medium		<–2°C	10.59	56	High viscosity; light emollience; high resistance to rub off
Ethylhexyl palmitate	Medium	Low/medium	<2°C	8.5	12	
Pentaerythrityl tetraisostearate	Slow	Strong	<–10°C	7.67	–	Rich, imparts a soft cushiony feel to skin, water repellent, excellent wetting agent
Myristyl myristate	Wax	Medium	41°C	7.52	–	Dry emollient feel, liquefies at body temperature. Improves emulsion stability and texture. Comedogenic potential
Cetyl palmitate	Wax	–	<54°C	–	–	Dry emollient, improves emulsion texture and stability
Ethers						
Dicaprylyl ether	Fast	Weak	<–5°C	–	4	Dry skin feel, hydrolytically stable and particularly suitable for formulations with extreme pH values
PPG-15 stearyl ether	Fast	Strong	<–1°C	7	90 (25°C)	Excellent spreader and lubricant with velvety skin feel. Acts as an excellent solvent for a wide range of actives and component of early liquid crystal emulsions

PPG-3 myristyl ether	Slow	Strong	<–3°C		25	Good spreading, lubricating and co-solvency benefits
Hydrocarbons						
Hydrogenated polyisobutene	Fast	Non-polar	<–55°C	7	15–25 (40°C)	Soft feel, restores skin suppleness
Isohexadecane	Fast	Non-polar	<–70°C (=freezing point)	12	4.1	Light, velvety, dry skin feel, excellent cleansing properties; good alternative to mineral oil
Paraffinum liquidum	Medium/fast	Non-polar	–	–	15.1 (40°C)	
Hydrogenated polydecene	Medium	Non-polar	–	9	16–20 (40°C)	Light, silky, non-oily feel, ideal for dry or damaged skin, replacement for mineral oil
Squalane	Medium	Weak	<0°C	7	–	Emollient with structures similar to those found in the skin
Octyldodecanol	Medium	Medium	<–20°C	–	61	Hydrolytically stable emollient, particularly suitable for formulations with extreme pH values
Glycerides						
Caprylic/capric triglyceride	Medium	Medium	<–5°C	–	30	Good fatting agent and solubiliser
PEG-6 caprylic/capric glycerides	Slow	Strong	<–68°C	13.2	150	Superfatting agent and mildness additive, emollient/solubiliser
Caprylic/capric triglyceride	Medium	Medium	<–10°C	–	30	

Materials are classified by their INCI name – the international standard adopted for pack labelling. The characteristics of importance are spreading properties – speed of response when *spread*; polarity – indicative of *solubilisation* properties for other formulation materials; cloud point – indicative of *stability* at low temperature; HLB – indicative of *stability* requirements in emulsions (see Sect. 21.3.3); viscosity – contributory to *spread* and *sensory* characteristics; comments – on *sensory* and *skin compatibility* factors. *Words in italics are key criteria for selection of a particular emollients* (see Sect. 21.3.2.2)

Virgin coconut oil and virgin olive oil both reduced severity of atopic dermatitis, but the former was superior clinically and resulted in greater reduction of *S. aureus* colonisation [70]. Olive oil has shown effectiveness post-UV challenge [71]. Lanolin/olive oil ointment showed superiority over a commercial moisturizer formulation in managing dermatitis in pre-term infants [72].

The positive health messages about essential fatty acids (EFA) and their profile of stratum corneum lipids have been a justification for inclusion of EFA-rich sources of lipids in moisturizers. Early examples investigated include sunflower seed oil [73], and evening primrose oil or borage oil, following their oral use in the management of atopic eczema [74] – topical efficacy was only demonstrated in W/O emulsion [75]. The role of essential fatty acids may be more fundamental than modification of stratum corneum properties. Effects on cell proliferation [76], wound healing [77] and complementary cancer care [78] whilst outside the remit of this chapter offer potential for future applications of moisturizers.

Natural oils, waxes and natural butters offer greater breadth of sensorial and functional benefit in moisturizers. Shea butter, the non-saponifiable component of the fats and oils derived from the nut of the shea tree (or karite tree, *Butyrospermum parkii*) contains complex mixture of palmitic, stearic, oleic, linoleic and arachidic acid. This material melts at skin temperature thus absorbing well into the skin adding to its sensory appeal in use.

As with other products, sustainability of continued use is an important factor in commercialisation of many natural sources of fats and oils. As with glycols another consideration when using lipophilic materials is potential for enhancing skin penetration [79]. The relationship between emollient action and stratum corneum biomechanics was recently investigated [80] and dealt with elsewhere in this book. Changes in lipid conformation with treatments penetrating into the SC show the potential for emollients to change skin barrier properties, and this needs consideration when selecting ingredients.

The benefit (and the challenge) of using these natural lipids is their complexity. The complex mixtures – with different combinations of branched chain/straight chain, chain length and saturation – provide these materials with their often unique sensory properties. Incorporation of any unsaturated lipid into moisturizers brings stability and efficacy concerns, and in the case of materials like echium oil, odour is a significant disincentive for use. Oxidation of the unsaturated components of a formulation may drive the need for anti-oxidants such as butylated hydroxytoluene (BHT) or those from natural sources. Plant oils comprising both EFA and significant levels of natural anti-oxidants prove useful – e.g. sesame seed oil [81], sea buckthorn oil [82] and many others [83] with anti-oxidant species from tocopherols to anthocyanins and ellagitannins. Thermal and chemical stability of the anti-oxidant itself is important, and the variation in source resulting from processing [84], climate and harvesting [85], and storage [86] are important considerations. In addition to protecting the formulation from oxidation, plant anti-oxidants also protect skin lipids [87] further contributing to the moisturization.

The structural chemistry of the stratum corneum has influenced the choice of lipophilic material in formulations with "skin-identical lipids" (cholesterol, free fatty acids and ceramides) and their contribution to moisturization [88] "correcting the dermatological abnormality" (see Table 21.2). Surfactants selectively reduce cholesterol, cholesterol ester, free fatty acid and sphingolipids from stratum corneum inducing dry skin. Re-incorporation of these molecules via a W/O emulsion resulted in improvement of the dry-skin condition [89]. Their importance in water uptake was demonstrated ex vivo [90] by using de-lipidised corneocytes. However, "skin-identical lipids" in a petrolatum-rich base produced no discernable benefit over placebo over a 14-day period of use [91]. Contrary to this, others showed that an optimal ratio of skin-identical lipids is required to achieve barrier recovery in chronically aged skin [92]. Further studies showed the extent of the ratios and species of "skin-identical lipid" used [93]; a more complete mixture initiating a more rapid barrier recovery [94] but differences in experimental results appear dependent on the type of stratum corneum insult [95, 96].

Table 21.2 Fatty acid chain length of lipophilic species found within the skin[a] and some common moisturiser ingredients[b]

	Palmitic acid C16:0	Palmitoleic acid C16:1	Stearic acid C18:0	Oleic acid C18:1	Linoleic acid C18:2	
Skin	*25*	*22*	*3*	*3*	*0.5*	Additional comments
Butyrospermum parkii (shea butter)	3.5		43	44	6.5	Also contains catechin anti-oxidants
Theobroma cacao (cocoa butter)	26		36	33	3	Contains theobromine, sterols and tocopherol
Olea europaea (olive oil)	13		2.5	71	11	Contains sterols, tocopherols and squalene
Brassica rapa, canola (rapeseed) oil	4		1.5	60	20	Lowered content of erucic acid ensures better tolerability
Oenothera biennis (evening primrose)	8		2	11	69	
Cocos nucifera (coconut oil)	8.5		2.5	7	1.5	Sterols and tocopherols
Gossypium herbaceum (cottonseed oil)	22	0.5	3	17	55	High level of tocopherols and sterols
Sesamum indicum (sesame oil)	9		4	41	45	~10% tocopherols
Glycine max (soybean oil)	10		4	23	54	
Helianthus annuus (sunflower oil)	5.5		4	25	64	Also contains tocopherols and sterols

[a]Common components of stratum corneum and sebaceous lipids from various published sources
[b]*Handbook – Vegetable Oils and Fats*; Pubs Karlshamms AB; first edition 2002

There was some indication of ceramide benefit in a study on the recovery of tape-stripped skin – improved erythema, TEWL and a decrease in numbers of cycling epidermal cells were shown [97]. However, use of a synthetic ceramide showed clear benefits over vehicle control in another study [98].

Other occlusive materials can be introduced to improve the aesthetics and barrier-enhancing properties of a formulation. Silicones are a major class of such materials which partition into the oil phase and have the advantage of being inert and chemically well defined. Volatile silicones – usually cyclomethicones – are preferred where vaporative loss, initial slip and flow in use are required. Non-volatile types, e.g. dimethicones, also confer good skin feel but leave a better film (without shine) and even waterproof the skin. They confer a sensory property of "penetrating" and one study suggested little in the way of interference with the physico-chemical structures important for maintaining hydration of the skin [99].

The choices of hydrophilic and lipophilic composition of a moisturizer outlined above clearly generate a vast number of options. Whilst there are "standard" materials such as glycerol and mineral oil, other materials can be included as a result of previous experience, market or prescriber expectations and cost. Many ingredients will also have supplementary reasons for inclusion – an oil with good levels of self-protection due to anti-oxidant content and a humectant with good solvent properties for other ingredients. There is also the factor of impact on other factors such as aesthetics.

21.4 Targeting Consumer Needs: Aesthetics

Aesthetic factors not only drive success in the beauty moisturizer arena but also contribute to tolerability and acceptability in use for topical therapeutic products. The skin is a sensory organ, and this plays an important role in self-perception of skin quality [100]. From Sect. 21.2, it is clear that unacceptable sensory perception of the skin may be the primary dermatological abnormality to some patients. Many ingredients in moisturizers provide positive aesthetics (or counteract negative characteristics) and improve skin comfort, both during application and for minutes or hours after first use. Aesthetic characteristics also apply to products – ease of application; rub-in period; absorbance into the skin; greasiness and tackiness in use and after use; skin feel (product and skin); product greasiness on the skin; odour. Whilst these factors may not get to the heart of the "dermatological abnormality", they have a great influence in end users' assessment of successful treatment of the abnormality. In practice, it may be difficult to differentiate product and substrate aesthetic.

Perceptions will differ. Depending on the "dermatological abnormality," there will be different levels of initial dryness, roughness and tightness. In addition, there will be individual variation in sensory acuity. As a result, it will prove difficult to satisfy all these needs on an individual basis. The art of formulating a successful moisturizer will be to ensure that the most important sensory requirements are identified and delivered. Understanding which are the most important can be achieved in a number of ways from simple questionnaire analysis and focus groups to more sophisticated pre-development consumer trialling using a number of benchmarks. Having understood these needs, there follows the task of designing a product to deliver the key consumer needs. Sensory evaluation methods of candidate formulations are valuable tools in this respect.

Sensory evaluation is a science in itself, and the reader is referred to other sources for a full explanation [101, 102]. The value is that quantitative and qualitative comparisons can be derived for the formulations aesthetics, textural properties and in-use perception. There are number of ways the product developer can use sensory evaluation to better target these needs. One of the most common is to use trained and validated panels to agree a subjective grading scale with an agreed language to assess the candidate formulations. A benchmark is essential in this model since it allows the language and grading scale to be generated and form a reliable basis for measuring product attributes. The developer can then evaluate the elimination of negative attributes, the retention or improvement of positive attributes and even the introduction of missing attributes.

The major challenge encountered with this useful technique is that it cannot act as anything more than a guide to an experienced formulator. Here, as so often when developing a moisturizer, it is rare that changing one material changes one attribute – e.g. reducing "tackiness" in use could involve introduction of a silicone, reduction or change in a particular wax or oil or all of these. Success is driven by the experience of the formulator and their knowledge of the attributes of the raw materials at their disposal, though mathematical models have been used to optimize formulation characteristics [103].

Having established prototypes, the next step would be to go to end-consumer trialling to qualitatively assess how well the desired aesthetics have been fulfilled and quantitatively assess preference.

It is a generalization to say that for therapeutic products, the balance between aesthetic factors and therapeutic benefit weighs in favour of the therapeutic benefit. However, most commercial development will focus on improving the aesthetics as this has an indirect impact on perception of therapeutic benefit. Creating the correct aesthetic characteristics is central to the art of developing a good moisturizer.

21.4.1 Skin Tolerability as an Aesthetic Need

The safety of topical products is given, and tolerability may be considered a special case of anticipated sensory expectations. This is true of mass market and dermatological products alike, but the target skin need(s) may have an influence on the criteria for any given product. At one extreme, moisturizers designed for the broken and compromised eczema skin will demand far greater skin tolerability than an everyday moisturizer – pharmaceutical regulations are designed to ensure this by way of the permitted ingredients. Replenishment of the lost lipids and NMF will be a key requirement for products designed for damaged or sensitive skin [104]. In some dermatoses, microbial control is important to reduce risk of infection through skin with incomplete barrier whilst reducing risks of sensitization to antimicrobial ingredients.

In the cosmetic arena, there are some product categories where expectations may be higher than the norm. One example would be moisturizers targeted to needs of babies. Whilst these are regulated as cosmetics, there may be a higher expectation on level of safety testing and even higher expectations of ingredients that should or should not be included.

21.4.2 Hydrophilic and Lipophilic Mixtures: Why Emulsions?

Delivering moisturization via an emulsion has many advantages – hydrophilic and lipophilic materials can be mixed to provide the different modes of action and ingredients required to satisfy consumer need and dermatological abnormality. Using infrared spectroscopy, the effects of petrolatum use over 1 week could not be demonstrated whereas an O/W emulsion improved stratum corneum water content 10 h after product application and prolonged 2 days after product use had stopped [105]. One per cent glycerol is ineffective alone but not so in combination with an occlusive material in the formulation – the nature of the lipid influenced the beneficial effects of moisturizers. The combined effect of a bilayer-forming mixture of phospholipids, cholesterol, and fatty acid and glycerol was greater than non-polar petrolatum [106].

Many other studies demonstrate this principle, but this highlights a real issue with moisturizer development – studies on individual ingredients can act as a guide to their inclusion, but ultimately most commercial moisturizers are multi-component systems where almost every ingredient may contribute to at least one of the target end points. Nowhere else is this more true than when creating sensorial properties of the moisturizer. Blending waxes, oils, humectants and water into emulsions offers such a wide range aesthetic possibilities – the cosmetic benefits. Creation of an emulsion adds another variable – the emulsifiers – which, as described later, do more than simply bring the hydrophilic and lipophilic domains together in a relatively stable form. Studying the behaviour of the three phases – lipophilic, hydrophilic and emulsifier – as a function of concentration and plotting this as a triangular graph (ternary diagram) is a practical way to go beyond single ingredient studies. This provides an understanding of the system's properties in terms of emulsion structure, rheology, stability, sensory properties, etc., [107].

21.4.2.1 Emulsifiers

An emulsifier will have a polar species (often referred to as the head group) inserting itself into the water domain whilst the non-polar, the other part (or the tail group) partitions, into the oil phase (see Fig. 21.2). The electrostatic and/or stereochemical repulsion of head and the lipophilicity of the tail will affect the packing and emulsion behaviour. The position of the emulsifier across the interface will determine droplet size, stability and fluidity of this boundary. In practice mixing emulsifiers to create complementary spatial distribution at the interface utilizing the

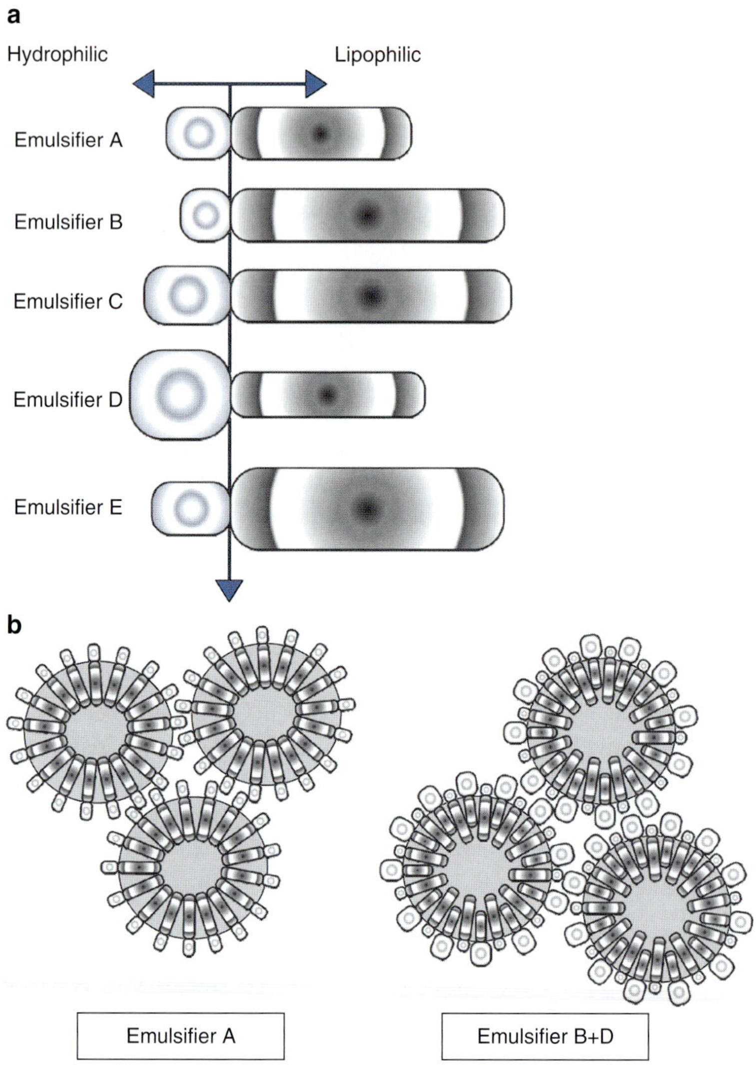

Fig. 21.2 Emulsifiers. (**a**) Emulsifier properties. Emulsifiers act at the interface between the hydrophilic and lipophilic domains to reduce surface tension and allow suspension of one phase in the other. This figure demonstrates some of the factors that influence the behaviour of a particular emulsifier. Hydrophilicity can be the result of larger numbers of hydrophilic sites and/or their stereochemistry. Likewise, lipophilicity increases with increasing molecular size and shape. (**b**) Emulsifier behaviour. The properties described in (**a**) dictate how a particular emulsifier is arranged in an emulsion. Emulsifier A may be effective but due to the stereochemistry may allow droplets closer association with the risk of instability by flocculation or coalescence. By using a combination of two emulsifiers with complementary stereochemistry, the packing may help stabilise the interface and thus provide greater stability

repulsive factors, relative solubility in oil- and water-phase components is central to stabilising complex mixtures of oil and water (rarely do we wish to produce an emulsion of a single oil with pure water).

Emulsifiers can be defined by their chemical nature or by their emulsification behaviour. Chemically, there are amphoteric, anionic, cationic and non-ionic emulsifiers. The most commonly used are the anionic and non-ionic. Examples of cationic emulsifiers are lecithin and some quaternary amines such as stearalkonium chloride. Cationic emulsifiers may be prone to instability at high pH and negative ion concentration. The skin surface has a net negative charge, and cationic emulsifiers may thus bind to the substrate – this can be beneficial in terms of conditioning but can also give rise to irritancy.

The best anionic emulsifier example is soap. Soaps have a charged hydrophilic group and a fatty hydrophobic portion. Heterogeneity in the fatty-acid carbon-chain lengths in starting materials (e.g. coconut oils) calls for careful specification of starting material to ensure predictable performance. Their alkaline pH can be problematic for stability – intolerance to salts in the formulation – and also for skin compatibility. Surface deposits can form leaving the skin looking dull, or irritation develops from the high pH. Sodium lauryl sulphate is a milder and more stable anionic emulsifier choice. However, aqueous cream BP contains emulsifying wax with sodium lauryl sulphate as a component, and this has been implicated in low skin tolerance of aqueous cream [108]. However, another anionic emulsifier – potassium cetyl phosphate – has good skin compatibility, and magnesium stearate is a common emulsifier for basic W/O emulsions.

Overall emulsification behaviour is also dependent on their preference for hydrophilic or lipophilic domain. A means of characterizing this was developed for non-ionic emulsifiers – HLB (hydrophile-lipophile balance) system – a scale between 1 and 50 where 1 shows tendency to far greater lipophilic nature and 50 shows greater hydrophilicity [109]. Cosmetic emulsifiers tend to be between 1 and 20, with HLB 4–6 being useful for W/O and HLB 8–18 for O/W emulsions. As mentioned earlier, the HLB for many emollients can be estimated in simple experimental determinations to determine the HLB requirements of an oil system and emulsifiers selected accordingly. The HLB values are normally published in suppliers' literature and are therefore often readily available. Two conclusions will be provided, one for O/W, the other for W/O systems.

The amphipathic nature of non-ionic emulsifiers derives from their lipophilic long chains species (e.g. fatty alcohols) with the hydrophilic part coming from substitutions with molecules such as ethylene oxide. This process of ethoxylation can be carried out to varying degrees on the same starting material to give a range of different hydrophilic tendencies. Other starting sources are sorbitol and sorbitan esters, again these may be further modified by ethoxylation or esterfication with polyethylene glycol. Other types include polyethylene glycol esters, monoglycerides, and polyglyceride esters. Silicone-based polymers have also become popular as a result of the specific sensory properties that silicones possess. Modification by ethylene glycol or propylene oxide provides the amphipathic nature. Pursuit of more sustainable ingredients (and the availability of natural by-products) has brought the development of natural alternatives to ethoxylated surfactants emulsifiers based on sucrose and glucose and even glycolipids [110]. Glycolipid-based surfactants have also been identified from surprising sources – microorganisms of *Candida* or *Pseudomonas* genus [111]. Lipopeptides have classical structure for an emulsifier – hydrophile-lipophile nature [112].

All these sources can be combined together to provide a variety of emulsifiers, each with their own attributes and cost. See Table 21.3.

Many raw material suppliers combine anionic and non-ionic emulsifiers as a blend for commercial purposes. For many therapeutic applications, this provides a good starting point for formulation and is often self-emulsifying waxes. Choice of emulsifier is not always that straightforward but depends on the consumer needs to be delivered – the sensory properties, the cost and the desired benefits. The reason behind this is that emulsifier type(s), oil loading and rheological properties of the emulsion arise from the emulsion droplet size, oil (including emulsifier) spreading properties, as well as other features. At one extreme, silicone emulsifiers offer very light, quick-break, cooling emulsions; at the other, stearate-based systems generally give long rub-in and heavy feel.

Another important and useful variation is to use a combination of a low and high HLB emulsifier of the same carbon-chain length. This allows for better "packing" of the emulsifiers at the interface. The same principle applies to the use of "co-emulsifiers" – materials with hydrophile-lipophile balance between the continuous phase and emulsifier phase.

Generally, the smaller the particle size, the greater the stability, so mechanical energy can contribute greatly to the overall emulsion stability and aesthetics (Sect. 21.5.5).

Emulsifiers are not inert and have the potential to improve or degrade the moisture-binding capability of the stratum corneum. Gloor suggested that presence of glycerol in O/W emulsions mitigated their drying effects; however, W/O emulsions without glycerine were suitable for atopic dermatitis. Also in stress tests with wash solutions, the damage to the horny layer is reduced by glycerol-containing O/W emulsions. Whereas

Table 21.3 Identity and properties of some ingredients commonly used to create emulsions

INCI name	Type	Comments/properties
Glyceryl stearate	Non-ionic	HLB 3.8
PEG-100 stearate	Non-ionic	HLB 18.8; commercially available as a blend with glyceryl stearate HLB = 11; O/W emulsions; good to build viscosity for sensory and stability benefit
Polyglyceryl-3-oleate	Non-ionic	HLB 5 for W/O but also a co-emulsifier for O/W systems
Cetyl dimethicone copolyol	Non-ionic	W/O and co-emulsifier in O/W systems; adds spreading, waterproofing and cooling effect
Steareth-2	Non-ionic	HLB 4.9 but commonly used in combination with steareth-21 (HLB 15.3) for O/W systems; can form liquid crystals
Cetearyl alcohol	Non-ionic	Co-emulsifier, viscosity enhancer; also adds to the liquid crystalline properties with steareth-2/steareth-21 systems
Polysorbate 20	Non-ionic	HLB 16.7; solubiliser for lipophilic materials in aqueous gel moisturisers
Sorbitan stearate and sucrose cocoate	Non-ionic	HLB 6; O/W emulsion; alternative to ethoxylates steareth-2/steareth-21 for liquid crystalline emulsions
Acrylates/C10–30 alkyl acrylate cross polymer	Polymeric	O/W systems; benefit from electrolyte instability by rapidly breaking on contact with the skin leaving oil phase layer
Stearic acid	Anionic	Sometimes added to anhydrous formulations to enhance dispersion of lipids; co-emulsifier and viscosity enhancer in W/O or O/W systems; neutralisation may be required
Potassium cetyl phosphate	Anionic	Phosphoric acid esters of fatty acids; good pH stability; some similarity in structure to phospholipids

the penetration-promoting effect of O/W emulsions without glycerol is best, only W/O emulsions or glycerol-containing O/W emulsions are suitable for atopic dermatitis. A hydrating effect on the stratum corneum was also found in a propylene glycol ointment [113].

In another study, a range of emulsifiers, in a 50:50 mineral to oil water solution, was tested in normal and SLS-damaged skin [114]. This short-term test showed that some emulsifiers produced significant change in TEWL (but not blood flow) in normal skin, and some had TEWL-reducing effects in SLS-treated skin. The role of the emulsifier cannot therefore be excluded in the design of a moisturizer, and it has been suggested that long-term use of a moisturizer could reduce the skin's barrier [115]. Emulsifier type may be influential, and partition between product and skin lipid phases should be a consideration for selecting emulsifiers for moisturizer formulation.

The potential for an emulsified system to interfere with the stratum corneum lipid domain may also represent a therapeutic opportunity, e.g. enhancing bioavailability of therapeutic materials [116] or getting anti-oxidants deeper into the skin is formulation dependent [117]. Controlling this penetration – targeting the materials to where they are required – is also a theoretical possibility utilizing the relative polarity of the active ingredient, the emulsifier and emollient compared to that of the stratum corneum [118]. Lipid content, emollient and emulsifier, will also influence skin tolerance.

The potential impact of emulsifier on stratum corneum has generated interest in "emulsifier-free" formulations – actually, this means avoidance of the use of classical emulsifiers and reliance on polymeric emulsifiers. Examples include those based on polyacrylic acids – e.g. carbomers. These are synthetic high-molecular-weight polymer of acrylic acid also used to increase stability and improve suspension of added ingredients. They are based on polymers of acrylic acid, cross-linked with an allyl ether pentaerythritol or sucrose or propylene. These polymers distribute themselves along the oil/water interface with side groups of lipophilic and hydrophilic nature inserted into their respectively preferred phase. One of the most widely used applications for such emulsifiers is where "quick-break" properties are required. This can provide a number of sensory and efficacy benefits.

The immediate breakdown or separation of the oil and water phase delivers a cooling effect; it also allows this rapid evaporation to leave a functional oil behind for rapid spreading and drying.

21.4.2.2 Emulsions

There are two fundamental ways of bringing together lipophilic and hydrophilic materials. Lipid droplets dispersed in a hydrophilic continuous phase – O/W emulsions (e.g. milk) – or hydrophilic droplets dispersed in a continuous lipophilic phase – W/O emulsions – as exemplified by butter, also find their application. There are other variants – multiple emulsions where an O/W emulsion is created within an external oil phase (O/W in oil – O/W/O) or vice versa (W/O/W). These and liquid crystalline-structured emulsions are dealt with in Sect. 21.4.2.3.

Consumer need will influence choice of emulsion type, oil/water ratio, efficacy and sensory characteristics and even appearance – conventional emulsion droplet size is large enough to interfere with the pathway of light, hence their "white" appearance. When droplet size falls below the wavelength, not only do these "microemulsions" become clear, the interactions with the substrate change.

Experimental studies have shown that moisturizer effectiveness (targeting the dermatological abnormality) is independent on their penetration profiles into the skin [119]. According to these authors, hydrophilic and lipophilic moisturizers have similar penetration profiles but different effects on SC water distribution in vivo. Three-hour treatment with lipophilic moisturizer did not result in increased water levels in the SC, whereas hydrophilic moisturizers retained water where they are located. O/W emulsions offer a common method of enhancing moisturization using the benefits of water phase (e.g. humectant) and oil phase (e.g. occlusion). Blichmann et al. [120] showed the short-term effects whereas Serup et al. were able to demonstrate cumulative moisturization (cf untreated skin as control) after 2 days of product use and continued enhancement of skin hydration for at least 2 days after product use had ceased [121]. In a separate study, using D-Squame sampling to assess scaling, the same group showed the cumulative effects of a moisturizer against no treatment controls, the benefits were prolonged beyond the cessation of treatment [122].

It is not simply the type of emulsion that can influence the enhancement of skin hydration. Other factors such as droplet size, surfactant organisation and species of lipid are also important [123]. Surfactant organization (micelles, lyotropic liquid crystals) in the emulsion may also affect the cutaneous and percutaneous absorption. This further emphasises the multi-functional mature of moisturising formulations, and the fact that constituents such as emollients and emulsifiers should be selected carefully for optimal efficiency of the formulation.

The short-term effects of product application have been demonstrated. Loden showed that water loss from the skin could not be changed after a 5-min exposure to petrolatum compared to moisturizers with different oil loading (where the loss of water was proportional their aqueous component), whereas after 40 min, the occlusive effects of petrolatum were seen to be superior to these moisturizers [124]. The importance of oil-phase loading is emphasised by these results. W/O emulsions have thus been proposed as more likely to deliver prolonged hydration.

Oil loading, emollient species and emulsifier type affect the emulsion droplet size and viscosity and are all factors that can have an impact on overall efficacy of a moisturizer [125, 126]. Gemec and Wolf [19] compared several commercial moisturizers containing different levels of lipids. Lipid-rich creams (assessed by residual greasiness) conferred greater skin distensibility, whilst moisturizers with lower level of lipid gave higher measures for skin capacitance. The insulating influence of the lipids and short-term nature of the study may account for this conclusion.

21.4.2.3 Advanced Emulsion Systems

For most practical cases, simple emulsions (O/W or W/O) produced by conventional methods (Sect. 21.5.5) will be sufficient to deliver the needs of dry skin. However, there are a number of systems where more complex emulsification creates products with interesting properties. These include liquid crystalline emulsions, multiple emulsions, microemulsions, nano-emulsions and PIT emulsions.

Liquid crystal emulsions are characterized by their macroscopic and microscopic appearance. They tend to have an opalescent rather than bright white appearance to the eye and contain birefringent bodies under polarizing microscopy. The most commonly quoted example is generated in emulsions formed by steareth-2/steareth-21 emulsifiers in the presence of PPG-15 stearyl ether and cetylstearyl alcohol. In these systems, the oil and water phases become distributed as lamellar structures around oil droplets (see Fig. 21.3a). The lamellar phases also surround larger oil droplets and this results in the fluidity and opalescence of such products. The resulting sensory, stability and efficacy from such emulsions has created much interest, as has the homology between these structured emulsions and the organization of the specialized lipids of the inter-corneocyte space [127]. The potential for these emulsions to act as "controlled delivery" of moisturization or of actives in either aqueous or oil phase continues to create interest [128].

Other "multiple emulsions" (see Fig. 21.3b) are formed by adding the third phase and another emulsifier to a two-phase system – oil to an O/W or water to a W/O. The main interest is in their potential to deliver controlled release of moisturization but also to allow incorporation of unstable or incompatible materials within one product – e.g, vitamin C [129]. The complexity and expense of these systems tend to limit their utilization in consumer products.

The smaller droplet size of nano-emulsions offers better spreading and delivery of disperse-phase components. Smaller droplet size can be created using specialised high-pressure homogeniser equipment. Alternative methods utilise the phase inversion temperature – PIT – of the emulsion system, the temperature at which the droplets are at their smallest [130]. PIT is determined by the nature of the oils and the emulsifier concentration (relatively high by comparison to conventional emulsions). W/O PIT emulsions can have higher oil loading whilst remaining more fluid than the conventional systems with high oil.

Nano-emulsions comprising charged lipids phytosphingosine together with ceramide 3, cholesterol and palmitic acid similar to those found in stratum corneum showed enhanced moisturization properties [131].

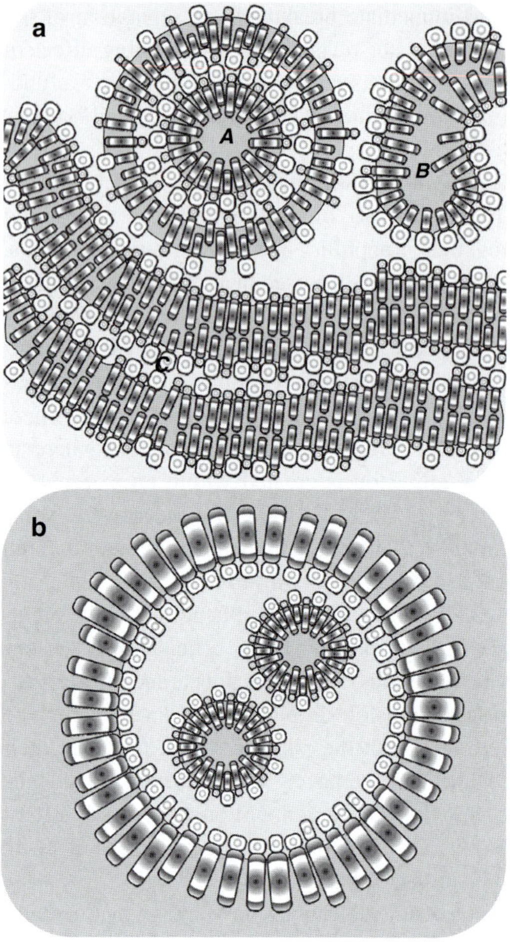

Fig. 21.3 Complex emulsions. (**a**) Liquid crystal emulsions. These emulsions are not simple droplets of disperse phase suspended in a continuous phase. Arrangement of the emulsifiers includes multiple layers around a droplet (*A*), secondary oil droplets (*B*) and formation of sheets (*C*). The layering of hydrophilic phases ( ) and lipophilic phases ( ) is achieved by apposition of hydrophilic and lipophilic domains of the emulsifier trapping lipophilic and hydrophilic materials within these structures. These systems have potential for sustained release of oil- and water-phase ingredients and also reflect organisation of lipids in the inter-corneocyte space. (**b**) Multiple emulsions. An example of an oil-in-water-in-oil (O/W/O) emulsion. Systems such as this also offer potential for sustained release but also the advantage of separating incompatible actives into two compartments

There are applications for micro-emulsions – where the droplet size is so small that it does not interfere with light – and whilst this tends to stem from the novelty of their clarity, they do have other benefits of good thermodynamic stability, high solubilization power and ease of preparation. Again, the cost of bulk – high oil loading; high emulsifier content – is a prime consideration. These systems find use in enhancing skin delivery [132, 133].

Water in silicone emulsions are another variant that could be classed as advanced, finding use in sophisticated cosmetic applications and sunscreens.

21.4.3 Moisturizer: Skin Interaction

The act of rubbing a moisturizer into the skin will begin to disrupt the emulsion structure. It is this interaction that defines consumer perception and influences the successful targeting of the dermatological abnormality. The dynamics and impact of this process will be dependent on rheological factors (see below). The behavior will also depend upon the state of the skin – the level of desiccation, roughness and scaling.

Water will begin to evaporate depending on proportion in the formula, and this can be enhanced by incorporation of ingredients such as alcohols and volatile silicones that evaporate on application. It is difficult to evaluate how the various components of emulsions behave in this initial phase, though studies have been conducted of the microscopic changes seen on evaporation of emulsions on inert models [134]. Gradual evaporation over an hour on an inert substrate showed a linear relationship between water loss and capacitance [135]; however, the role of humectant concentration in this study cannot be discounted since materials with a high dielectric constant may be being measured directly. The persistence of product on the skin surface also highlights the need for care in design and interpretation of instrumental studies [119]. This study showed whilst water evaporated after 15 min, lipids took longer to disappear from the skin (between 2 and 3 h after application). However, hydration remained elevated throughout as assessed by conductance.

An essential part of emulsion use is deposition of an emollient onto the surface of the skin. This has been shown to be influenced by the emollient rather than the emulsifier/co-emulsifier [136]. However, overall hydration is equally important. In studies where the hydration measurements increase early (after one day) moisturizer use and remained higher through the 14-day period, the barrier improved and provided better protection against challenge from SLS [137]. A similar conclusion came from a study using SLS challenge showing a moisturizer conferred both protective and therapeutic effects [138].

The longer-term interactions between skin and moisturizers are dependent on repeated use, though their "cumulative benefit" has been demonstrated [139] and whilst various ingredients such as retinol derivatives may act at a more fundamental level to re-instate the skin's own mechanisms of moisturization, this has not been proven for many other ingredients.

21.4.4 Consistency and Rheology Modifiers

Consistency and "body" of a moisturizer – what makes it a thick cream, a pourable lotion or a sprayable milk – are dictated by many factors including (but not limited to) the type of emulsion system, droplet size, oil loading and the types of oils used. The response of a product to forces – its rheological properties – impacts on manufacturing requirements (e.g. pumping manufactured bulk into pack), the delivery from pack onto the skin and the sensory properties of a moisturizer in use. In addition, the rheological properties can be an important indicator of stability.

The main contributor to these behaviours is the mobility of the disperse (droplet) phase through the continuous phase under forces of shear (short-term breakdown during rub-in) or gravity (long-term separation of phases causing instability). Controlling this mobility can be achieved by thickening the disperse phase, stabilizing the interface between oil and water phases or both [140].

Many natural high-molecular-weight polysaccharides "thicken" the water phase of an O/W emulsion, and their water-binding capacity may also contribute a film of hydration at the skin-air interface. The starting materials include starches, celluloses, alginates and pectins. Industrial processing allows the properties of these naturally occurring materials to be modified for different applications. In the case of xanthan gum, the material is derived from industrial fermentation with *Xanthomonas campestris*, providing a highly reproducible quality material.

Mineral clays are also useful water-phase thickeners – such as those based on montmorillonite clays (bentonite clays). Clays may also have an impact on skin feel and even optical changes to skin surface, another example of multi-functionality for moisturizing ingredients. Other mineral sources can act as oil-phase thickeners – metal stearates and hydroxystearates – and again can modify sensory properties of a product.

Synthetic water-phase thickeners – the carbomers being the most common – provide the advantage of reliability of chemical identity over the natural and naturally derived thickeners. One early disadvantage of these materials, the use of benzene during the processing, has been improved with alternatives using cyclohexane and/or ethyl acetate as solvent. Polyacrylic acids and amides are also common aqueous thickeners in commercial moisturizers.

Carbomers, and other water-phase thickeners, require adequate hydration and swelling to optimize their performance. In the case of carbomers, this requires high shear, adequate neutralization and use of sequestrants such as ethylenediaminetetraacetic acid. Salt tolerance, thermal tolerance and rheological properties of the gels formed by water-phase thickeners are considerations when choosing which thickener(s) to include in the formulation.

Thickening of oil phases can be achieved by including materials that are solid at ambient temperatures – thickeners – waxes are common starting points for this. Again, the quality of the wax can also help provide skin feel and occlusion to the product in use. Other oil-phase thickeners can act as co-emulsifiers and as demonstrated in the case of emulsions comprising a significant proportion of liquid crystals, the rheological properties of a moisturizer are rarely dictated by one ingredient.

Given their physical properties in controlling flow of oil through water (and vice versa), it is no surprise that thickeners have been investigated as alternatives to conventional emulsifiers. Carbomer and clay-based emulsions have been used as the basis "emulsifier-free" products.

21.5 Secondary Consumer Needs: "Hygiene Factors"

Moisturizer users should expect certain properties without question – quality, safety, legality and reliability. Developers respond to this by applying quality standards to aspects during development and production. Since this is not something that can be reverse engineered, it becomes one of the factors influencing ingredient selection. The approaches to this will be guided by local regulations and best practice. Good manufacturing practices adopted by the various national and regional bodies for medicines cover many aspects of product development from training of personnel, documentation control, testing of the product through to ingredient and final product batch traceability. These guidelines also influence how developers and manufacturers of cosmetics conduct their business. The following sections touch on how these indirect consumers' needs impact on ingredient selection and product development.

21.5.1 Microbial and Physical Stability

A successful moisturiser needs to be effective over a period of use. For this, a number of characteristics will need to be assured – at the very least resistance to microbial spoilage and retention of the physical stability. For the latter case, many of the determinants of ingredients have been dealt with in earlier sections – emollient choice, emulsifier choice and rheological modifier.

21.5.1.1 Microbial Stability

There are a number of sources of microbial contamination from raw materials (e.g. natural extracts) through the manufacturing process, packaging, storage and end-user interaction. Where water is a major component of the formulation controlling microbial growth requires preservatives with or without ingredients that reduce water activity. The contribution of product packaging to microbial resistance is also important – pumps and tubes not only reduce entry of microorganisms from atmospheric or direct skin contact, they may, depending on design and material type, also reduce water availability.

Introduction of these materials into emulsions requires careful consideration. Predispersion or solubilisation into glycols or other solvents may be required, and their partitioning into the oil and water domains can change the overall emulsion stability as can preservation aids – materials that reduce water activity in the product or otherwise enhance resistance to microbial contamination.

21.5.1.2 Physical Stability

Whether it is breakdown of lipids in anhydrous ointments or separation of emulsions, physical stability may not just spoil the appearance of the moisturizing preparation – a separated product cannot be guaranteed to deliver the required needs. Any separation of the emulsion can be seen with the naked eye as creaming or sedimentation, but microscopic evaluation provides early warning of this. Microscopy is also useful to check for insolubilities of materials and acts as an essential check that processing has been successful.

Other product stability characteristics are viscosity, pH and odour – each of which is suggestive of change in the physical and chemical nature of the product with implications on the safety, efficacy or tolerability. Rheological assessments are also helpful.

In all cases, testing conditions are designed to accelerate any instability that might occur in normal in-use conditions. Stability protocols therefore include exposing moisturizer formulations to extremes of temperature, cycling between ambient and cool temperature and exposure to light. In some cases, especially medicinal products, it will also be essential to monitor the persistence and activity of active ingredients.

21.5.2 Ingredient Quality

When developing products for markets with different regulations, this can constrain choice in ingredient selection. Whilst these are dealt with more fully elsewhere, they are another factor the consumer unknowingly relies upon the developer to protect them. Ensuring the safety and reliability of performance of a formulation, particularly its stability, requires a comprehensive understanding of the chemical and physico-chemical properties of its ingredients. Working with defined material sources, extraction process and ingredient specifications reduces risks as does implementation of quality assurance procedures.

Ingredients in moisturizers are not only selected on the basis of their effectiveness. Commercial availability is an important consideration. Ingredients for a pharmaceutical product may be prescribed by the appropriate pharmacopoeia and even demand a chemically pure ingredient. This may also be the case for some cosmetic ingredients, but for the most part, there will be a number of commercially available sources. Even "single ingredients", e.g. lanolin, are complex mixtures with many different grades. The detailed specification of two apparently identical materials from different sources may differ, and, as with naturally occurring materials, whilst the minor details of variance may not require recording, logging batch numbers in manufacture provides an essential record for product specification.

From a safety assessor's standpoint, the more complex the material, the more complex will be the safety assessment. Future European regulation (EU Regulation redraft 2013), requiring an additional toxicity end points on all raw materials in cosmetic products, will emphasize the importance of ingredient quality in selection and inclusion into final formulation. Natural, nature-derived or modified natural materials are becoming increasingly sought after by consumers, and their complexity creates a challenge for the safety assessor as well as an impact on an already complex formulation.

As a final comment, once selected, the reliability and consistency of supply are considerations in ingredient selection. The availability of many naturally occurring materials can be subject to variability – seasonal; climate-dependent growth and harvest. Many synthetic materials rely on the availability of a common commodity (e.g. petroleum) and thus subject to market price fluctuations and scarcity of these starting materials.

21.5.3 Cost-Effectiveness

For all consumer products, this factor affects purchase and thus choice of ingredients. At the therapeutic end of the spectrum, the cost and quality of ingredients may have significant commercial impact on the cost of the product hence its viability and sustainability in the market. This is one reason for the resurgence in emollient use in scaling dermatoses [141–144]. The size of the market, the frequency and intensity of use and the acceptability and recommendation by health professionals may all influence commercialization.

Whether the product is aimed at mass market or niche, the overall cost of the product will not only be influenced by cost of ingredients. Market size, frequency of use and area of use also influence the size and frequency of batch production, which in turn influences the minimum order quantities of bulk and special raw materials used in the formulation – all of these influence overall cost.

21.5.4 Manufacturability

Once a successful product has been developed, it has to be reproducibly produced. Processing is a "hidden ingredient". During development, it is important to consider the conditions of manufacture that may influence the quality of the final product. These include, but are not limited to, batch size, shear rate, temperature, order of ingredient addition and cooling rate. The process must also be within the commercial constraints – cost, volume and unit size – dictated by the product and the intended market. Often the grade or format of the particular ingredient is chosen on the basis of enhancing manufacturability – pelletting of waxes, commercial availability of compounded combinations of emulsifiers, may enhance commercial viability of a product. In other cases, it can be that certain conditions need to be placed on inclusion of a particular ingredient because of its lability (e.g. retinol; where packaging is also an essential consideration) or that particular ingredients can only be introduced into certain types of formulation. Finally, the physical conditions of manufacturing may also result in certain ingredients or formulation types being favoured for a given application.

An essential step in developing a moisturizer is transfer from bench formulation to factory scale production. Most new product development will include an interim scaling batch to ensure this transfer is successful, whilst not utilizing large volumes of expensive ingredients and energy.

The normal manufacturing conditions will have oil-phase ingredients heated to above the melting point of the waxes used and water introduced at the same temperature to avoid microcrystallization of waxes. Rheological modifiers are added according to their solubility and temperature stability. Adequate homogenization and mixing are also essential; the whole manufacturing vessel construction should ensure this, and heating/cooling is uniformly achieved. As the emulsion cools, other ingredients can be added as appropriate. For O/W emulsions, the mixture will "invert" from a W/O to O/W, and after this has occurred, other water-phase ingredients can be added as can any heat labile materials provided they are sufficiently solubilised. Choice of ingredient once again has an impact here, and compounded or multi-functional ingredients may offer advantages.

Take Home Messages

- Composition and development of moisturizers is driven by two separate factors – the dermatological abnormality and how the sufferer of this abnormality views successful resolution. There is some common ground between the technological routes to addressing these needs.
- There is a diversity of needs that drives very different formulation strategies for moisturizers designed to address the different aspects of "dry skin" across the spectrum from diseased skin to environmentally compromised skin and on to skin that is perceived to be less beautiful and healthy looking than it should.
- Formulation of moisturizers is the art of balancing functional, sensorial and commercial factors to ensure the needs of the target end user are met.
- Commercial moisturizers are multifunctional systems where one or more end-user needs can be addressed through the same formulation via its different ingredients, and one ingredient can contribute a number of benefits. This makes "placebo" versus "active" studies very challenging for many materials with moisturizing properties.
- The role of stratum corneum as biological sensor to external conditions and the known effects of some moisturizer ingredients on the systems responsible for this demand care in formulating products for dry-skin conditions. There will be continuing focus on delivering the benefits of moisturized skin whilst supporting the skin's own systems for retaining its moisturized state.
- Research into stratum corneum biology will continue to drive new end points and modes of action for moisturizers to address the "dermatological abnormalities".

Acknowledgments I would like to thank my colleagues Adam Muggleton and Mark Hanlon in preparing the figures and tables, Alain Mavon and Aurelie Laloeuf for helpful comments on the text and my wife Julia for assistance in preparing the document.

References

1. Lodén M (2003) Role of topical emollients and moisturizers in the treatment of dry skin barrier disorders. Am J Clin Dermatol 11(4):771–788
2. Lodén M (2003) Do moisturizers work? J Cosmet Dermatol 2(3–4):141–149
3. Rawlings AV, Matts PJ (2005) Stratum corneum moisturization at the molecular level: an update in relation to the dry skin cycle. J Invest Dermatol 124(6):1099–1110
4. de Polo KF (1998) Chapter 8 Cosmetic emulsions. In: A short textbook of cosmetology. Verlag fur Chemische Industrie, H Ziolkowsky GmbH, pp 234–299
5. Hunting ALL (1993) Creams, lotions and milks: a formulary of cosmetic preparations, vol 2. Micelle Press, Dorset, UK
6. http://media.allured.com/documents/CT0801+Formulary.fcx-WEB.pdf
7. http://www.cosmeticsandtoiletries.com/formulating/category/skincare/13041522.html?utm_source=Most+Read&utm_medium=website&utm_campaign=Most+Read
8. http://www.happi.com/formulary/2009/01/
9. Barton S (2002) Formulation of skin moisturizers. In: Leyden JJ, Rawlings AV (eds) Skin moisturization, vol 25, Cosmetic science and technology series. Marcel Dekker, New York, pp 547–584
10. Cork MJ, Britton J, Butler L, Young S, Murphy R, Keohane SG (2003) Comparison of parent knowledge, therapy utilization and severity of atopic eczema before and after explanation and demonstration of topical therapies by a specialist dermatology nurse. Br J Dermatol 149(3):582–589
11. Mahado M, Hadgraft J, Lane ME (2010) Assessment of the variation of skin barrier function with anatomic site, age, gender and ethnicity. Int J Cosmet Sci 323(6):397–409
12. Blank IH (1953) Further observations on factors which influence the water content of the stratum corneum. J Invest Dermatol 21:259–271
13. Auriol F, Vaillant L, Machet L et al (1993) Effects of short-time hydration on skin extensibility. Acta Derm Venereol 73:344–347
14. Warner RR, Boissy YL, Lilly NA, McKillop K, Marshall JL, Stone KJ (1999) Water disrupts stratum corneum lipid lamellae: damage is similar to surfactants. J Invest Dermatol 113(6):960–966
15. Byrne AJ (2010) Bioengineering and subjective approaches to the clinical evaluation of dry skin. Int J Cosmet Sci 32:410–421

16. Crowther JM, Sieg A, Blenkiron P, Marcott C, Matts PJ, Kaczvinsky JR, Rawlings AV (2008) Measuring the effects of topical moisturizers on changes in stratum corneum thickness, water gradients and hydration in vivo. Br J Dermatol 159(3):567–577
17. Förster M, Bolzinger MA, Ach D, Montagnac G, Briançon S (2011) Ingredients tracking of cosmetic formulations in the skin: a confocal Raman microscopy investigation. Pharm Res 28(4):858–872
18. Jemec GB, Wulf HC (1999) Correlation between the greasiness and the plasticizing effect of moisturizers. Acta Derm Venereol 799(2):115–117
19. Wiechers JW, Barlow T (1999) Skin moisturization and elasticity originate from at least two different mechanisms. Int J Cosmet Sci 21:425
20. Choi EH, Man MQ, Wang F et al (2005) Is endogenous glycerol a determinant of stratum corneum hydration in humans? J Invest Dermatol 125(2):288–293
21. Sagiv AE, Marcus Y (2003) The connection between in vitro water uptake and in vivo skin moisturization. Skin Res Technol 9(4):306–311
22. Takahashi M, Yamada M, Machida Y (1984) A new method to evaluate softening effects of cosmetic ingredients on the skin. J Soc Cosmet Chem 35:171–181
23. Pedersen LK, Jemec GB (1999) Plasticising effect of water and glycerin on human skin in vivo. J Dermatol Sci 19(1):8–52
24. Smith W (1999) Stratum corneum barrier integrity controls skin homeostasis. Int J Cosmet Sci 21:99–106
25. Rawlings AV, Watkinson A, Harding CR et al (1995) Changes in stratum corneum lipid and desmosome structure together with water barrier function during mechanical stress. J Soc Cosmet Chem 46:151
26. Batt M et al (1988) Changes in physical properties of stratum corneum following treatment with glycerol. J Soc Cosmet Chem 39:367–381
27. Rawlings AV, Scott IR, Harding CR et al (1994) Stratum corneum moisturization at the molecular level. J Invest Dermatol 103:731–741
28. Rawlings A, Harding C, Watkinson A et al (1995) The effect of glycerol and humidity on desmosome degradation in stratum corneum. Arch Dermatol Res 287:457–464
29. Chander P et al (1996) Superiority of glycerol containing moisturisers on desquamation and desmosome hydrolysis. J Invest Dermatol 106:919
30. Faergemann J, Wahlstrand B, Hedner T, Johnsson J, Neubert RH, Nystrom L, Maibach H (2005) Pentane-1,5-diol as a percutaneous absorption enhancer. Arch Dermatol Res 297(6):261–265
31. Gehring W, Gloor M (2000) Effect of topically applied dexpanthenol on epidermal barrier function and stratum corneum hydration. Results of a human in vivo study. Arzneimittelforschung 50(7):659–663
32. Jacobi O (1959) About the mechanism of moisture regulation in the horny layer of the skin. Proc Sci Sect Toilet Goods Assoc 31:22–26
33. Scott IR, Harding CR (1986) Filaggrin breakdown to water binding compounds during development of the rat stratum corneum is controlled by the water activity of the environment. Dev Biol 115(1):84–92
34. Kligman AM (2011) Corneobiology and corneotherapy – the final chapter. Int J Cosmet Sci 33:197–209
35. Horii I, Nakayama Y, Obata M et al (1989) Stratum corneum hydration and amino acid content in xerotic skin. Br J Dermatol 121:587–592
36. Kezic S, Kemperman PM, Koster ES et al (2008) Loss-of-function mutations in the filaggrin gene lead to reduced level of natural moisturizing factor in the stratum corneum. J Invest Dermatol 128(8):2117–2119
37. Middleton JD, Roberts ME (1978) Effect of a skin cream containing the sodium salt of pyrollidone carboxylic acid on dry and flaky skin. J Soc Cosmet Chem 29(4):201–205
38. Loden M, Andersson AC, Andersson C, Frodin T, Oman H, Lindberg M (2001) Instrumental and dermatologist evaluation of the effect of glycerine and urea on dry skin in atopic dermatitis. Skin Res Technol 7(4):209–213
39. Byrne AJ, Davis M, Laloeuf A, Rawlings AV (2009) Glycerol-containing moisturizers are more effective than urea-containing moisturizers in the relief of soap induced winter xerosis. Poster presentation Stratum Corneum VI, Boston
40. Loden M, Andersson AC, Lindberg M (1999) Improvement in skin barrier function in patients with atopic dermatitis after treatment with a moisturizing cream (Canoderm). Br J Dermatol 140(2):264–267
41. Serup J (1992) A double-blind comparison of two creams containing urea as the active ingredient. Assessment of efficacy and side-effects by non-invasive techniques and a clinical scoring scheme. Acta Derm Venereol Suppl (Stockh) 177:34–43
42. Bettinger JG (1995) Influence of emulsions with and without urea on water- binding capacity of the stratum corneum. J Soc Cosmet Chem 46:247–254
43. Kuzmina N, Hagstromer L, Entestam L (2002) Urea and sodium chloride in moisturisers for skin of the elderly–a comparative, double-blind, randomised study. Skin Pharmacol Appl Skin Physiol 15(3): 166–174
44. Gloor M, Fluhr J, Lehmann L, Gehring W, Thieroff-Ekerdt R (2002) Do urea/ammonium lactate combinations achieve better skin protection and hydration than either component alone? Skin Pharmacol Appl Skin Physiol 15(1):35–43
45. Serup J (1992) A three hour test for rapid comparion of effects of moisturisers and active ingredients (urea). Measurement of hydration, scaling and skin surface lipidisation by noninvasive techniques. Acta Derm Venereol 177(Suppl):29–33
46. Van Scott EJ, Yu RJ (1989) Alpha hydroxy acids: procedures for use in clinical practice. Cutis 43:222–228
47. Hachem JP et al (2010) Acute acidification of stratum corneum membrane domains using polyhydroxyl acids improves lipid processing and inhibits degradation of corneodesmosomes. J Invest Dermatol 130(2): 500–510

48. Takahashi M, Machida Y, Tsuda Y (1985) The influence of hydroxy acids on the rheological properties of stratum corneum. J Soc Cosmet Chem 36:177–187
49. Thueson DO, Chan EK, Oechsli LM et al (1998) The roles of pH and concentration in lactic acid-induced stimulation of epidermal turnover. Dermatol Surg 24:641–645
50. Berardesca E, Distante F, Vignoli GP et al (1997) Alpha hydroxyacids modulate stratum corneum barrier function. Br J Dermatol 137:934–938
51. Fartasch M, Teal J, Menon GK (1997) Mode of action of glycolic acid on stratum corneum: ultrastructural and functional evaluation of the epidermal barrier. Arch Dermatol Res 289:404–409
52. Smith WP (1996) Comparative effectiveness of alpha-hydroxy acids on skin properties. Int J Cosmet Sci 18:75–83
53. Rawlings AV, Davies A, Carlomusto M et al (1996) Effect of lactic acid isomers on keratinocyte ceramide synthesis, stratum corneum lipid levels and stratum corneum barrier function. Arch Dermatol Res 288:383–390
54. Ditre CM, Griffin TD, Murphy GF et al (1996) Effects of alpha-hydroxy acids on photoaged skin: a pilot clinical, histologic, and ultrastructural study. J Am Acad Dermatol 34:187–195
55. Bernstein EF, Underhill CB, Lakkakorpi J et al (1997) Citric acid increases viable epidermal thickness and glycosaminoglycan content of sun-damaged skin. Dermatol Surg 23:689–694
56. Kaidbey K et al (2003) Topical gycolic acid enhances photodamage by ultraviolet light. Photodermatol Photoimmunol Photomed 19(1):21–27
57. Kornhauser A, Coelho SG, Hearing VJ (2010) Applications of hydroxyacids: classification, mechanisms and photoactivity. Clin Cosmet Invest Dermatol 24(3):135–142
58. Green BA, Yu RJ, Van Scott EJ (2009) Clinical and cosmeceutical uses of hydroxyl acids. Clin Dermatol 27(5):495–501
59. Merinville E et al (2010) Three clinical studies showing anti-aging benefits of sodium salicylate in human skin. J Cosmet Dermatol 9(3):174–184
60. Reynolds T, Dweck AC (1999) Aloe vera leaf gel: a review update. J Ethnopharmacol 68(1–3):3–37
61. Fujimura T et al (2002) Treatment of human skin with an extract of Fucus vesiculosus changes its thickness and mechanical properties. J Cosmet Sci 53(1):1–9
62. Kurtz ES (2007) Colloidal oatmeal: history, chemistry and clinical properties. J Drugs Dermatol 6(2):167–170
63. Cerio R et al (2010) Mechanism of action and clinical benefits of colloidal oatmeal for dermatologic practice. J Drugs Dermatol 9(9):1116–1120
64. Soma Y, Kashima M, Imaizumi A, Takahama H, Kawakami T, Mizoguchi M (2005) Moisturizing effects of topical nicotinamide on atopic dry skin. Int J Dermatol 44(3):197–202
65. Kligman A (1978) Regression method for assessing the efficacy of moisturisers. Cosmet Toilet 93:27
66. Clark S (1993) Investigations into biomechanisms of the moisturising function of lanolin. J Soc Cosmet Chem 44:181–195
67. Wertz PW (2009) Human synthetic sebum formulation and stability under conditions of use and storage. Int J Cosmet Sci 31(1):21–25
68. Smith TJ (2000) Squalene: potential chemopreventive agent. Expert Opin Investig Drugs 9(8):1841–1848
69. Agero AL, Verallo-Rowell VM (2004) A randomized double-blind controlled trial comparing extra virgin coconut oil with mineral oil as a moisturizer for mild to moderate xerosis. Dermatitis 159(3):109–116
70. Verallo-Rowell VM, Dillague KM, Syah-Tjundawan BS (2008) Novel antibacterial and emollient effects of coconut and virgin olive oils in adult atopic dermatitis. Dermatitis 19(6):308–315
71. Ichihashi M, Ahmed NU, Budiyanto A, Wu A, Bito T, Ueda M, Osawa T (2000) Preventive effect of antioxidant on ultraviolet-induced skin cancer in mice. J Dermatol Sci 23(Suppl 1):S45–S50
72. Kiechl-Kohlendorfer U, Berger C, Inzinger R (2008) The effect of daily treatment with an olive oil/lanolin emollient on skin integrity in preterm infants: a randomized controlled trial. Pediatr Dermatol 25(2):174–178
73. Prottey C, Hastop PJ, Press M (1975) Correction of the cutaneous manifestations of essential fatty acid deficiency in man by application of sunflower seed oil to the skin. J Invest Dermatol 64:228–234
74. Lovell CR, Burton JL, Horrobin DF (1981) Treatment of atopic eczema with evening primrose oil. Lancet 1(8214):278
75. Gehring W, Bopp R, Rippke F, Gloor M (1999) Effect of topically applied evening primrose oil on epidermal barrier function in atopic dermatitis as a function of vehicle. Arzneimittelforschung 49(7):635–642
76. Morris GM, Hopewell JW, Harold M et al (1997) Modulation of the cell kinetics of pig skin by the topical application of evening primrose oil or lioxasol. Cell Prolif 30:311–323
77. Delair V (1997) The usefulness of topical application of essential fatty acids (EFA) to prevent pressure ulcers. Ostomy Wound Manage 43(5):48–52
78. Haley AC, Calahan C, Gandhi M et al (2011) Skin care management in cancer patients: an evaluation of quality of life and tolerability. Support Care Cancer 19(4):545–554
79. Ibrahim SA, Li S (2010) Efficiency of fatty acids as chemical penetration enhancers: mechanisms and structure enhancement relationship. Pharm Res 27(1):115–125
80. Levi K, Kwan A, Rhines AS, Gorcea M, Moore DJ, Dauskardt RH (2010) Emollient molecule effects on the drying stresses in human stratum corneum. Br J Dermatol 163(4):695–703
81. Nasirullah LRB (2009) Storage stability of sunflower oil with added natural antioxidant concentrate from sesame seed oil. J Oleo Sci 58(9):453–459
82. Yang B, Kallio HP (2001) Fatty acid composition of lipids in sea buckthorn (Hippophae rhamnoides L.)

berries of different origins. J Agric Food Chem 49(4):1939–1947
83. Kahkonen MP, Hopia AI, Heinonen M (2010) Berry phenolics and their antioxidant activity. J Agric Food Chem 49(8):4076–4082
84. Kasparaviciene G, Briedis V, Ivanauskas L (2004) Influence of sea buckthorn oil production technology on its antioxidant activity. [Article in Lithuanian] Medicina (Kaunas) 40(8):753–757
85. Andersson SC, Rumpunen K, Johansson E, Olsson ME (2008) Tocopherols and tocotrienols in sea buckthorn (Hippophae rhamnoides L.) berries during ripening. J Agric Food Chem 56(15):6701–6706
86. Kochhar SP, Henry CJ (2009) Oxidative stability and shelf-life evaluation of selected culinary oils. Int J Food Sci Nutr 60(Suppl 7):289–296
87. Lalouef A (2006) Patent – WO 2006134583 (A1) – cosmetic compositions containing lingonberry (vaccinium vitis idea) extracts
88. Vacata V, Gertchen OB, Ghyczy M (2001) Topical formulations conforming to the structure of the skin. Cosmet Toilet 5(116):67–74
89. Imokawa G, Akasaki S, Minematsu Y et al (1989) Importance of intercellular lipids in water-retention properties of the stratum corneum: induction and recovery study of surfactant dry skin. Arch Dermatol Res 281:45–51
90. Friberg SE, Kayali I, Rhein LD et al (1990) The importance of lipids for water uptake in stratum corneum (L'importance des lipides dans l'absorption d'eau par le stratum corneum). Int J Cosmet Sci 12:5–12
91. Loden M, Barany E (2000) Skin-identical lipids versus petrolatum in the treatment of tape-stripped and detergent-perturbed human skin. Acta Derm Venereol 80(6):412–415
92. Zettersten EM, Ghadially R, Feingold KR et al (1997) Optimal ratios of topical stratum corneum lipids improve barrier recovery in chronologically aged skin. J Am Acad Dermatol 37:403–408
93. Man MQ, Feingold KR, Thornfeldt CR et al (1996) Optimization of physiological lipid mixtures for barrier repair. J Invest Dermatol 106:1096–1101
94. de Paepe K, Roseeuw D, Rogiers V (2002) Repair of acetone- and sodium lauryl sulphate-damaged human skin barrier function using topically applied emulsions containing barrier lipids. J Eur Acad Dermatol Venereol 16(6):587–594
95. Yang L, Mao QM, Taljebini M et al (1995) Topical stratum corneum lipids accelerate barrier repair after tape stripping, solvent treatment and some but not all types of detergent treatment. Br J Dermatol 133:679–685
96. Kucharekova M, van der Kerkhof PC, van der Valk PG (2003) A randomized comparison of an emollient containing skin-related lipids with a petrolatum-based emollient as adjunct in the treatment of chronic hand dermatitis. Contact Dermatitis 48(6):293–299
97. Kucharekova M, Schalkwijk J, van der Kerkhof PC, van der Valk PG (2002) Effect of a lipid-rich emollient containing ceramide 3 in experimentally induced skin barrier dysfunction. Contact Dermatitis 46(6):331–338
98. Lintner K, Mondon P, Girard F et al (1997) The effect of a synthetic ceramide-2 on transepidermal water loss after stripping or sodium lauryl sulfate treatment: an in vivo study. Int J Cosmet Sci 1:15–25
99. Glombitza B, Muller-Goymann CC (2001) Investigation of interactions between silicones and stratum corneum lipids. Int J Cosmet Sci 23:25–34
100. Arbuckle R, Atkinson MJ, Clark M et al (2008) Patient experiences with oily skin: the qualitative development of content for two new patient reported outcome questionnaires. Health Qual Life Outcomes 6:80
101. Meilgaard M, Civille GV, Carr BT (2007) Sensory evaluation techniques, 4th edn. Taylor & Francis, Boca Raton
102. Kemp S, Hollowood T, Hort J (2009) Sensory evaluation: a practical handbook. Wiley-Blackwell, Oxford, UK
103. Balfagon AC et al (2010) Comparative study of neural networks and lest mean square algorithm applied to optimisation of cosmetic formulations. Int J Cosmet Sci 32:376–386
104. Trapp M (2007) Is there room for improvement in the emollients for adjuvant therapy? J Eur Acad Dermatol Venereol 21(Suppl 2):14–18
105. Petersen EN (1991) The hydrating effect of a cream and white petrolatum measured by optothermal infrared spectrometry in vivo. Acta Derm Venereol 71(5):373–376
106. Summers RS, Summers B, Chandar P et al (1996) The effect of lipids, with and without humectant, on skin xerosis. J Soc Cosmet Chem 47:27–39
107. Auguste F, Levy F (2009) Emulsion science and technology. Wiley-VCH Verlag GmbH & Co, KGaA, Weinheim
108. Tsang M, Guy RH (2010) Effect of aqueous cream BP on human stratum corneum in vivo. Br J Dermatol 163(5):954–958
109. Griffin WC (1949) Classification of surface-active agents by 'HLB'. J Soc Cosmet Chem 1:311
110. Faivre V, Rosilio V (2010) Interest of glycolipids in drug delivery: from physicochemical properties to drug targeting. Expert Opin Drug Deliv 7(9):1031–1048
111. Lourith N, Kanlayavattanakul M (2009) Natural surfactants used in cosmetics: glycolipids. Int J Cosmet Sci 31(4):255–261
112. Kanlayavattanakul M, Lourith N (2010) Lipopeptides in cosmetics. Int J Cosmet Sci 32(1):1–8
113. Gloor M (2004) How do dermatological vehicles influence the horny layer. Skin Pharmacol Physiol 17(6):267–273
114. Barany E, Lindberg M, Loden M (2000) Unexpected skin barrier influence from nonionic emulsifiers. Int J Pharm 195(1–2):189–195
115. Held E, Sveinsdottir S, Agner T (1999) Effect of long-term use of moisturizer on skin hydration,

barrier function and susceptibility to irritants. Acta Derm Venereol 79:49–51
116. Wirén K, Frithiof H, Sjöqvist C, Lodén M (2009) Enhancement of bioavailability by lowering of fat content in topical formulations. Br J Dermatol 160(3):552–556
117. Richert S, Schrader A, Schrader K (2003) Transdermal delivery of two antioxidants from different cosmetic formulations. Int J Cosmet Sci 25(1–2):5–13
118. Wiechers JW, Kelly CL, Blease TG, Dederen JC (2004) Formulating for efficacy. Int J Cosmet Sci 26(4):173–182
119. Caussin J, Rozema E, Gooris GS et al (2009) Hydrophilic and lipophilic moisturizers have similar penetration profiles but different effects on SC water distribution in vivo. Exp Dermatol 18(11):954–961
120. Blichmann CW, Serup J, Winther A (1989) Effects of single application of a moisturizer: evaporation of emulsion water, skin surface temperature, electrical conductance, electrical capacitance, and skin surface (emulsion) lipids. Acta Derm Venereol 69:327–330
121. Serup J, Winther A, Blichmann CW (1989) Effects of repeated application of a moisturizer. Acta Derm Venereol 69(5):457–459
122. Serup J, Winther A, Blichmann C (1980) A simple method for the study of scale pattern and effects of a moisturizer–qualitative and quantitative evaluation by D-squame tape compared with parameters of epidermal hydration. Clin Exp Dermatol 14:277–282
123. Otto A, du Plessis J, Wiechers JW (2009) Formulation effects of topical emulsions on transdermal and dermal delivery. Int J Cosmet Sci 31(1):1–19
124. Loden M (1992) The increase in skin hydration after application of emollients with different amounts of lipids. Acta Derm Venereol 72(5):327–330
125. Machado M, Bronze MR, Ribeiro H (2007) New cosmetic emulsions for dry skin. J Cosmet Dermatol 6(4):239–242
126. Dayan N, Sivalenka R, Chase J (2009) Skin moisturization by hydrogenated polyisobutene–quantitative and visual evaluation. J Cosmet Sci 60(1):15–24
127. Friberg SE (1990) Micelles, microemulsions, liquid crystals and the structure of the stratum corneum lipids. J Soc Cosmet Chem 41:155–171
128. Chorillia M, Prestesb PS, Rigonb RB et al (2011) Structural characterization and in vivo evaluation of retinyl palmitate in non-ionic lamellar liquid crystalline system. Colloids Surf B Biointerfaces 85(2): 182–188
129. Farahmand S, Tajerzadeh H, Farboud ES (2006) Formulation and evaluation of a vitamin C multiple emulsion. Pharm Dev Technol 11(2):255–261
130. Shinoda K, Friberg S (1986) Emulsions and solubilisation. Wiley, New York
131. Yilmaz E, Borchert HH (2006) Effect of lipid-containing, positively charged nanoemulsions on skin hydration, elasticity and erythema–an in vivo study. Int J Pharm 307(2):232–238
132. Boonme P (2007) Applications of microemulsions in cosmetics. J Cosmet Dermatol 6(4):223–228
133. Kogan A, Garti N (2006) Microemulsions as transdermal drug delivery vehicles. Adv Colloid Interface Sci 123–126:369–385
134. Bergamaschi MM, Santos OD, Rocha-Filho PA et al (2008) A simple analysis of the changes during evaporation of a commercial emulsion of unknown composition. J Cosmet Sci 59(1):15–32
135. Jemec GB, Na R, Wulf HC (2000) The inherent capacitance of moisturising creams: a source of false positive results? Skin Pharmacol Appl Skin Physiol 13(3–4):182–187
136. Mehling A, Haake H-M, Poly W (2010) Differential deposition of emollients from tripartite formulation systems. Int J Cosmet Sci 32:117–125
137. Loden M (1997) Barrier recovery and influence of irritant stimuli in skin treated with a moisturizing cream. Contact Dermatitis 36(5):256–260
138. Ramsing DW, Agner T (1997) Preventive and therapeutic effects of a moisturizer. An experimental study of human skin. Acta Derm Venereol 77:335–337
139. Nogueira A, Sidou F, Brocard S (2010) Effect of a new moisturizing lotion on immediate and cumulative skin hydration: two randomized, intra-individual, vehicle- and comparator-controlled studies. J Dermatolog Treat. doi:10.3109/09546631003762647
140. Tadros T (2006) Principles of emulsion stabilization with special reference to polymeric surfactants. J Cosmet Sci 57(2):153–169
141. Wirén K, Nohlgård C, Nyberg F et al (2009) Treatment with a barrier-strengthening moisturizing cream delays relapse of atopic dermatitis: a prospective and randomized controlled clinical trial. J Eur Acad Dermatol Venereol 23(11):1267–1272
142. Cork MJ, Danby S (2009) Skin barrier breakdown: a renaissance in emollient therapy. Br J Nurs 18(14): 872–877
143. Hjalte F, Asseburg C, Tennvall GR (2010) Cost-effectiveness of a barrier-strengthening moisturizing cream as maintenance therapy vs. no treatment after an initial steroid course in patients with atopic dermatitis in Sweden – with model applications for Denmark, Norway and Finland. J Eur Acad Dermatol Venereol 24(4):474–480
144. Simpson EL, Berry TM, Brown PA, Hanifin JM (2010) A pilot study of emollient therapy for the primary prevention of atopic dermatitis. J Am Acad Dermatol 63:587–593

22 Ungual Formulations: Topical Treatment of Nail Diseases

Kenneth A. Walters

22.1 Introduction

The human nail can be afflicted by several disease states including paronychia, psoriasis and infections due to bacteria, viruses or fungi. While rarely life threatening, these generate self-consciousness and psychological stress. Approximately 50% of all problems result from fungal infections, onychomycoses, and the prevalence of these may be as high as 27% in Europe [27] and 10% in the USA [15]. Brittle nail syndrome affects approximately 20% of the population, with occurrence in females being twice that of males. Brittle nails can be the result of both internal and external factors, including aging, other nail problems such as psoriasis and fungal infections, exposure to irritants, such as solvents, and excessive water exposure. Although the precise pathogenesis leading to brittle nails is unknown, the involvement of nail coenocytes intercellular adhesion factors seems the most likely explanation [67]. There is certainly evidence to suggest that dry nails are brittle [17], but earlier work indicated that the water content of normal and brittle nails was similar [61]. In the latter work, however, the authors found that nail samples were losing water between clipping and analysis and that the moisture content determinations may not have been indicative of the in vivo situation. Overall, however, the advice of many dermatologists is that the strength and flexibility of brittle nails can be improved using humectant compounds that will increase the water content of the nail plate (see e.g. [31]). For the topical treatment of nail diseases, however, it is a prime requirement that the active ingredient, be it a humectant or an antifungal agent, is capable of penetrating into and diffusing though the nail plate.

Experimental techniques for investigation of the penetration and distribution of chemicals into and through the nail plate have demonstrated that it is possible to deliver drugs to the nail following topical application. This research has led the development of newer more effective topical products and regimens for treatment of onychomycoses and other nail diseases (see examples in: [16, 39, 44, 53, 57, 65]). In this chapter, nail structure and chemical composition will be discussed together with an overview of the permeation of molecules through the nail plate, and this will be followed by a review of selected clinical studies designed to determine the efficacy of topical treatment for nail diseases.

22.2 Nail Structure

The nail plate is composed of layers of flattened keratinized cells fused into a dense but somewhat elastic mass set within periungual grooves (Fig. 22.1). Nail plate cells grow distally from the germinative nail matrix at a rate of about

K.A. Walters, Ph.D.
An-eX Analytical Services Ltd,
14/16 CBTC2, Capital Business Park, Cardiff
CF3 2PX, UK
e-mail: kaw@an-ex.co.uk

M. Lodén, H.I. Maibach (eds.), *Treatment of Dry Skin Syndrome*,
DOI 10.1007/978-3-642-27606-4_22, © Springer-Verlag Berlin Heidelberg 2012

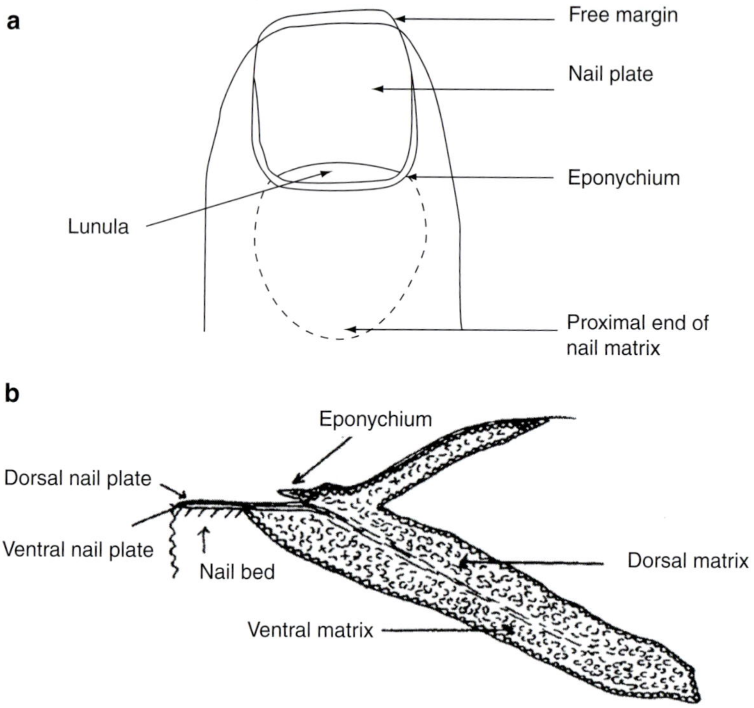

Fig. 22.1 Anatomical features of the human nail plate. (**a**) Top view showing the area of the germinative nail matrix. (**b**) Cross section of the matrix

2–3 mm per month. During keratinization, cells undergo shape and other changes similar to those experienced by the epidermal cells forming the stratum corneum. There are three very tightly knit keratinized layers, a thin outermost dorsal lamina, a thicker intermediate lamina and an innermost ventral layer [54]. Keratins in hair and nail are classified as 'hard' trichocyte keratins.

As a cornified epithelial structure, the chemical composition of the nail plate has many similarities to hair [2]. The major components are hard (80–90%) and soft (10–20%) keratin proteins with small amounts (0.1–1.0%) of lipid, the latter presumably located in the intercellular spaces. In addition, intermediate filament-associated proteins and trichohyalin are also found within the nail [7]. Sulphur content of the nail amounts to about 10% and is mainly present within the cystine disulphide bonds that contribute to nail tensile strength by linking the keratin fibres. The nail contains significant amounts of phospholipid, mainly in the dorsal and intermediate layers, which contribute to its flexibility. Glycolic and stearic acids are also found in the nail. The total lipid content of the nail plate is between 0.1% and 1%, which is considerably different to that of the stratum corneum (~10%). The principal plasticizer of the nail is water, the content of which varies widely dependent on prevailing relative humidity (Table 22.1), but it is normally present at around 18%. When the water content is less than 16%, the nail plate becomes brittle, and when the nail is hydrated to water levels of ~25%, it becomes soft. Minerals are also important constituents of nails. Lack of selenium and magnesium

Table 22.1 Water content of human fingernails as a function of relative humidity (RH). RH was controlled using saturated salt solutions, and nail clippings were positioned above the saturated solutions and exposed for at least 48 h (Data from [17])

RH (%)	Nail water content (%)
0	6
33	9
50	13
65	18
75	25
85	37
100	64

can have a profound effect on the health of the nail plate [4, 35].

22.3 Nail Plate Permeability

Early investigations of nail plate permeability indicated that the nail was significantly more permeable to water than was the stratum corneum [6, 60, 71]. Indeed, when the relative thicknesses were taken into account, water was found to diffuse through the nail plate at approximately 100-fold faster than through the stratum corneum. Given our current knowledge on the role of lipids in the barrier function of the stratum corneum, this is perhaps not surprising. However, at the time the finding that hydrophilic materials could pass through the nail plate with relative ease was viewed with scepticism.

22.3.1 In Vitro Investigations

The first systematic studies on nail plate permeability were carried out in the late 1970s [72–74]. These studies indicated that there were marked differences between the permeability characteristics of the nail plate and stratum corneum. These differences were attributed to the relative amounts of lipid and protein within the structures and possible differences in the physicochemical nature of the respective phases. The nail plate was permeable to dilute aqueous solutions of a series of low molecular weight homologous alcohols, but permeation decreased as a function of increasing alkyl chain length up to octanol (Fig. 22.2). It was suggested that the nail plate possessed a highly 'polar' penetration route that was capable of excluding permeants on the basis of their hydrophobicity. The existence of a minor 'lipid' pathway through the nail plate, which could become rate controlling for hydrophobic solutes, was suggested based on the significant decrease in permeation of hydrophobic *n*-decanol following nail plate delipidization.

In the mid-1990s, Mertin and Lippold [40–42] studied nail and hoof penetration in vitro. Permeability coefficients through both nail plate

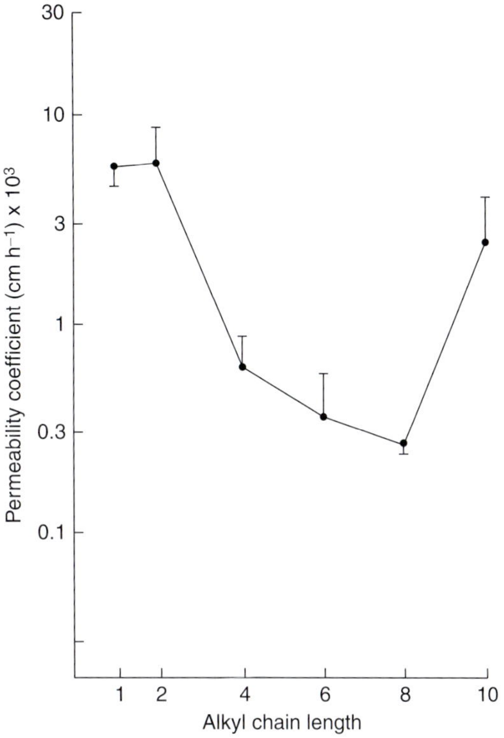

Fig. 22.2 Permeation rates for the *n*-alkanols crossing full-thickness human nail plates mounted in stainless steel side-by-side diffusion chambers in vitro. The alkanols (methanol through decanol) were applied as dilute aqueous solution, and samples taken from the receptor chamber over an 8-h period. Note that the *y*-axis is logarithmic (Data from [72])

and hoof membranes did not increase with increasing oil-water partition coefficient (range 7 to >51,000) or lipophilicity, indicating that these barriers behaved like hydrophilic gel membranes rather than lipophilic partition membranes (as in stratum corneum). Further studies with paracetamol and phenacetin showed that maximum flux was a function of drug solubility in water or in the swollen keratin. Mertin and Lippold were able to predict the maximum flux of ten antimycotics through the nail plate on the basis of their water solubilities and their penetration rates through hoof membrane. Their speculative extrapolation on permeation of amorolfine was in remarkably close agreement to the value obtained by Franz [18] using human nail plate. Bovine hoof membranes were also used by Monti et al.

[44] to evaluate the effect of formulation on the transungual permeation of ciclopirox. Comparison of an experimental water-soluble lacquer (based on hydroxypropyl chitosan) with the marketed water-insoluble lacquer (Penlac) showed that, although steady-state permeation rates were similar, lag times were considerably less for the experimental lacquer. This was tentatively attributed to a strong adhesion between hydroxypropyl chitosan and nail plate keratin. Further work confirmed the validity of using bovine hoof slices as a model for infected human toenails [45, 46]. This group also used bovine hoof membrane to determine penetration of piroctone olamine into keratinous matrices [11]. Although no transmembrane permeation was observed, following 30 h exposure, approximately 11% of the drug penetrated into the hoof.

Measurement of the nail permeation of several model compounds, including a series of *p*-hydroxybenzoic acid esters, indicated that, in broad agreement with earlier work, permeation decreased with increasing hydrophobicity (Table 22.2). It was suggested that molecular size was the principal determinant of the rate and extent of permeation across nail plate [38]. Very importantly, their studies also showed that, for the model permeant 5-fluorouracil, normal nail plate had similar permeation characteristics to infected nail plate, suggesting that normal plates can be used to predict drug distribution in diseased plates.

Table 22.2 Nail permeability coefficients (K_p) and molecular weights (MWt) for several model compounds. Note that for the *p*-hydroxybenzoic acid esters, permeability rates tend to decrease with increasing lipophilicity. Permeation studies were carried out over 5–17 days, and K_p calculated from steady-state regions of cumulative permeation plots (Data from [38])

Model permeant	MWt	K_p ($\times 10^7$ cm/s)
Methyl *p*-hydroxybenzoate	152.2	3.68 ± 0.08
Ethyl *p*-hydroxybenzoate	166.2	2.43 ± 0.48
Propyl *p*-hydroxybenzoate	180.2	2.01 ± 0.35
Butyl *p*-hydroxybenzoate	194.2	2.38 ± 0.32
Amyl *p*-hydroxybenzoate	208.3	2.24 ± 0.39
Hexyl *p*-hydroxybenzoate	222.3	1.24 ± 0.32
Pyridine	79.1	6.36 ± 0.40
Benzoic acid	122.1	12.84 ± 0.05
Sodium benzoate	121.1	0.91 ± 0.14
5-Fluorouracil	130.1	2.08 ± 0.13
Antipyrine	188.2	0.53 ± 0.07
Aminopyrine	232.3	0.09 ± 0.02
Lidocaine	234.3	0.39 ± 0.14
Lidocaine HCl	235.3	0.031 ± 0.003
Procaine HCl	237.3	0.11 ± 0.02
Isosorbide dinitrate	236.1	1.51 ± 0.29
Sodium nicotinate	122.1	0.61 ± 0.20
Barbital sodium	183.2	0.14 ± 0.02
Mexiletine HCl	179.3	0.20 ± 0.06
Isoproterenol HCl	211.2	0.084 ± 0.013
Croconazole HCl	311.8	0.017 ± 0.009

Recognizing the possibility of photodynamic therapy for onychomycosis [32, 59], Donnelly et al. [10] investigated the delivery of 5-aminolevulinic acid (ALA) to the nail from a bioadhesive patch in vitro. After 72 h, approximately 90% of the applied drug had penetrated the nail, with an average flux of 2.54×10^{-4} mg/cm²/s. This was quite a remarkable rate of penetration and, given that ALA is a small highly polar molecule, further confirmation of the hydrophilic nature of the nail barrier.

Hui et al. [30] developed a drilling technique for assessing drug delivery to the inner nail plate in vitro and used it to determine the effect of dimethyl sulfoxide (DMSO) on the penetration of urea, salicylic acid and ketoconazole. Nail plate composition suggests that it would be comparatively insensitive to the effects of stratum corneum penetration enhancers that produce their effects mainly by delipidization or fluidization of intercellular lipids. The nail plate is incapable of absorbing DMSO to any great degree [36], and a decrease in absorption of methanol and hexanol applied with DMSO has been noted [74]. On the other hand, an increase in nail plate content of econazole when applied in a formulation containing DMSO was reported [62], and following pretreatment with DMSO, an increase in the nail absorption of the antifungal amorolfine was demonstrated [18]. Hui et al. [28] determined that DMSO was capable of enhancing the concentration of all three permeants in the ventral region of the nail plate but, paradoxically, reduced the concentration of ketoconazole and salicylic acid in the dorsal regions. The data for the effects of DMSO on the nail, therefore, remain ambiguous.

In later experiments, Hui et al. determined the effects of the lipophilic skin penetration enhancer 2-*n*-nonyl-1,3-dioxolane on the in vitro nail delivery of econazole [29] and evaluated the nail penetration of ciclopirox from three topical formulations [30]. In the first study, lacquer formulations containing econazole with and without the enhancer (18%) were applied twice daily for 14 days to human nail plates. The amounts of econazole in the inner part of the nail plate were 11.1 mg/mg and 1.78 mg/mg nail powder (with and without enhancer, respectively). The amounts of econazole that had permeated through the nail plates with the enhancer were 48 mg and without enhancer 0.2 mg. In a separate study, radiolabelled 2-*n*-nonyl-1,3-dioxolane was found not to significantly penetrate the nail, and the mechanisms of penetration enhancement were presumed to be at the formulation/nail interface. In the subsequent study over 14 days, Penlac lacquer (8% ciclopirox) was evaluated alongside the gels Loprox (0.77% ciclopirox) and an experimental formulation containing 2% ciclopirox. Ciclopirox delivery into and through the nail was greater from the marketed gel than from either the experimental gel or the nail lacquer. The amount of drug that penetrated into and through the nail was also greater from the marketed gel. It was concluded that the delivery of ciclopirox was influenced by the nature of the applied formulation. Notwithstanding the differences in the amount of ciclopirox delivered, all three formulations delivered sufficient drug to generate 'in nail' concentrations far in excess of the minimum inhibitory concentrations (MICs) for most nail invasive dermatophytes and yeasts.

In our laboratory, we have modified the nail drilling technique to allow determination of drug distribution in three layers of the nail plate (dorsal, intermediate and ventral) and successfully adapted the technology as a rapid in vitro formulation-screening tool. More recently, opto-thermal transient emission radiometry (OTTER) has been shown to be capable of monitoring diffusion in nails [77]. The permeation rates of decanol, glycerol and butyl acetate were successfully monitored, and it is interesting to note that the rates of permeation increased with increasing solvent polarity. An advantage of the OTTER technique is that it provides a means of monitoring diffusion into nails in vivo.

The influence of keratolytic agents (papain, urea and salicylic acid) on the permeability of three imidazole antimycotics (miconazole nitrate, ketoconazole and itraconazole) using healthy human nails in vitro has been evaluated [51]. In the absence of any keratolytics, the nail was relatively impermeable to these antimycotics. Furthermore, permeation of these antimycotics was not improved by pretreatment with salicylic acid alone (20% for 10 days) or by application of the drug in a 40% urea solution. The combined effects of papain (15% for 1 day) and salicylic acid (20% for 10 days) were capable of enhancing nail plate permeability.

In contrast, Mohorcic et al. [43], evaluating the use of keratinolytic enzymes to decrease barrier properties, found that keratinase acted on the intercellular regions and caused corneocytes on the dorsal surface to separate. Permeation studies using bovine hoof membranes showed that the enzyme doubled the flux and membrane-vehicle partition coefficient of the model penetrant, metformin, but had little effect on the diffusion coefficient. This suggested that the effect of the enzyme was confined to the outer surface layers of the hoof membrane.

Brown et al. [5] investigated the nail permeability of caffeine, methylparaben and terbinafine and determined the effect of two novel penetration enhancers (thioglycolic acid and urea hydrogen peroxide) on their permeation using human nails in vitro. The penetrants were applied as saturated solutions. In the absence of penetration enhancement, steady-state flux through nails was more dependent on penetrant molecular weight than lipophilicity. While thioglycolic acid increased the flux of caffeine and methylparaben, urea hydrogen peroxide proved ineffective. Interestingly, sequential application of thioglycolic acid followed by urea hydrogen peroxide increased terbinafine flux considerably, but when the

Table 22.3 Flux rates of terbinafine (μg/cm2/h, mean ± SD, $n=3–8$) across nails pretreated with either thioglycolic acid (TA) or urea hydrogen peroxide (UP) or both TA and UP sequentially. Single enhancers were applied (0.5 ml) in solution for 20 h, nails were washed with water, and, if applicable, the second enhancer was applied for a further 20 h. Terbinafine was applied in saturated solution (in 50% ethanol in phosphate-buffered saline), and permeation monitored over about 9 days (Data from [5])

Pretreatment regimen	Terbinafine flux (μg/cm²/h)	ER
None	0.55 ± 0.71	–
5% TA	4.73 ± 1.01	8.6
17.5% UP	0.43 ± 0.29	0.8
5% TA then 17.5% UP	10.22 ± 5.22	18.6
17.5% UP then 5% TA	1.25 ± 0.80	2.3

penetration enhancer application order was reversed, the enhancement effect was considerably reduced (Table 22.3). These findings led to the development and in vitro evaluation of a potential treatment modality for onychomycosis consisting of a pretreatment dose of thioglycolic acid followed by application of a formulation containing urea hydrogen peroxide and the antifungal agent terbinafine [64]. It was clearly demonstrated that this system (MedNail®, MedPharm Ltd) was effective at delivering therapeutic levels of terbinafine to the nail. Furthermore, the enhancer system was also shown to enhance the efficacy of existing antifungal topical formulations. Both thioglycolic acid and urea hydrogen peroxide most likely alter barrier function by disrupting the α-keratin disulfide links. The authors went on to determine how the altering of the reduction/oxidation environment of nail keratin using thioglycolic acid and urea hydrogen peroxide influenced the barrier properties of the nail [34]. The investigation demonstrated that the nail permeability of terbinafine was greatest when relatively low concentrations of the thiolate ion were present in the applied solution and that free radical generation was fundamental in facilitating the redox-mediated keratin disruption of the nail plate.

Hydrophobins are fungal proteins, of about 100 amino acids, that function by self-assembly at hydrophobic-hydrophilic interfaces [9, 76]. They are extremely surface active and form an amphipathic film at interfaces that render hydrophilic surfaces hydrophobic and hydrophobic surfaces hydrophilic. They possess eight cysteine residues that form four disulphide bridges that prevent self-assembly of the hydrophobin in the absence of a hydrophilic-hydrophobic interface. Hydrophobins are subdivided into classes I and II, in which the amino acid sequences diverge considerably. This is reflected in the biophysical properties of these proteins such that assemblages of class I hydrophobins are highly insoluble, while those of class II hydrophobins readily dissolve in a variety of solvents. These proteins have been evaluated as potential enhancers to increase drug delivery to the nail plate. Vejnovic et al. [69] evaluated several nail plate permeation enhancers using caffeine as the model drug. Formulations were prepared in water and 20% (v/v) ethanol/water solutions. The potential enhancers evaluated were urea, DMSO, methanol, *N*-acetyl-*L*-cysteine, sodium docusate, boric acid and hydrophobins. Cadaver nails were used in modified Franz-type diffusion cells. The permeability coefficients of caffeine were increased by *N*-acetyl-*L*-cysteine, but formulations containing methanol generated the highest permeability coefficients for the model drug. The enhancers were classified according to their permeation enhancement. Methanol generated the greatest increase in caffeine permeability over class II hydrophobins. DMSO was more effective than class I hydrophobins and urea. Vejnovic et al. [70] went on to determine the amount of terbinafine that permeated through the human nail plate, from formulations containing hydrophobins at 0.1% (w/v), again using cadaver nails and Franz diffusion cells. Terbinafine remaining in the nail was extracted using 96% ethanol. The hydrophobins tested increased terbinafine permeation after 10 days with a maximum enhancement factor of 13-fold over the reference vehicle (10% terbinafine in a 60% v/v ethanol in water solution). The authors concluded that hydrophobins could be included in the list of potential enhancers for treatment of fungal nail infections.

There is certainly little doubt that effective topical treatment of nail diseases will require

Table 22.4 Enhancement ratios (ER) of terbinafine hydrochloride penetration into nails pretreated with several enhancer candidates (sequential ER) or simultaneous application of drug and enhancer candidate (simultaneous ER) using the TranScreen-NTM method, compared with enhancement ratios obtained for permeation across nails using a simultaneous application in Franz diffusion cells (permeation ER) (Data from [48])

Enhancer candidate	Sequential ER	Simultaneous ER	Permeation ER
Hydrogen peroxide	1.12±0.03	1.41±0.38	1.16±0.11
Salicylic acid	0.87±0.20	0.84±0.02	1.03±0.06
Glycolic acid	0.24±0.07	0.30±0.12	0.83±0.06
Thioglycolic acid	0.89±0.11	0.99±0.09	1.10±0.01
Urea	1.10±0.24	0.84±0.02	1.51±0.09
Thiourea	0.94±0.08	0.92±0.16	1.10±0.02
Cysteine	1.43±0.34	1.29±0.39	1.81±0.08
Sodium lauryl sulphate	2.24±0.03	1.65±0.42	1.76±0.31
Ethanol	1.11±0.04	0.64±0.14	1.00±0.16
Citric acid	1.01±0.11	0.44±0.04	0.60±0.08
Polysorbate 20	0.95±0.01	0.99±0.08	1.10±0.07
Ammonium phosphate	1.25±0.02	9.98±1.44	8.49±0.70
Ammonium carbonate	1.65±0.17	9.31±1.14	9.33±0.85
Potassium phosphate	2.74±0.34	9.98±1.02	8.32±0.64
Sodium phosphate	1.91±0.52	8.85±0.06	6.57±0.33
Sodium carbonate	1.75±0.22	6.90±1.15	4.98±0.20

some form of penetration and/or permeation enhancement to facilitate drug delivery [47]. It is important to note that selecting an effective chemical enhancement system for a given drug and a given formulation is highly critical for therapeutic success. An obvious problem is that there is a large pool of potential enhancers that may be useful for ungual therapy, and a high-throughput method for screening nail permeation enhancers would be a useful investigational tool. Murthy et al. [48] developed a microwell plate method (TranScreen-N) that involved two treatment procedures, simultaneous exposure (drug and enhancer) and sequential exposure (enhancer followed by drug). The drug used was terbinafine hydrochloride. The TranScreen-N method used nail segments, and these were incubated for 24 h at 35°C with drug plus enhancer solutions or with enhancer solutions (24 h exposure) followed by drug solutions (2 h exposure). At the end of the incubation period, the nail segments were washed and dissolved in sodium hydroxide, and the drug content determined. Several chemical enhancers were evaluated and compared with diffusion studies in the Franz diffusion cell in which drug and enhancer solutions were evaluated simultaneously (Table 22.4). Surprisingly, and in contrast to Kobayashi et al. [37] and Khengar et al. [33], the keratolytic enhancer candidates, such as salicylic acid and the thiolytic agents, cysteine and thioglycolic acid, demonstrated no enhancement activity in all of the evaluated scenarios. As the first indication that simple inorganic salts may be useful as nail permeation enhancers, the sodium salts, sodium carbonate, phosphate and citrate provided significant enhancement of terbinafine uptake into and permeation across the nails, as did potassium phosphate and ammonium carbonate. Perhaps unsurprisingly, the simultaneous exposure scenario gave the closest correlation between techniques, which provided validity to the screening method that will undoubtedly prove useful in future studies. The TranScreen-N model was also used to evaluate the effect of chemical etchants, phosphoric acid and lactic acid, on the permeation of terbinafine hydrochloride and 5-fluorouracil into and across human nail [66]. Pretreatment with phosphoric acid was effective in improving drug delivery whereas pretreatment with lactic acid failed to improve drug penetration or permeation.

Other potential nail permeation enhancement strategies that have been evaluated include the use of polyethylene glycols and iontophoresis. The effect of polyethylene glycols (PEGs) on the nail delivery of terbinafine was determined by in vitro permeation studies using passive and iontophoretic (0.5 mA/cm^2) techniques [49] and gel formulations containing different molecular weight PEGs at 30% w/w. There was a moderate enhancement in the permeation using formulations containing low molecular weight PEGs (200 and 400 MW) compared to the control formulation. The effect of low molecular weight PEGs was greater during iontophoresis. High molecular weight PEGs (1,000–3,350 MW) were not effective. The authors suggested that enhancement in drug permeation by low molecular weight PEGs was probably due to their ability to increase hydration of the nail plate. The same group then incorporated polyethylene glycol 400 into a composite nail lacquer comprising an underlying drug-loaded hydrophilic layer and overlying hydrophobic vinyl layer. The hydrophilic drug-containing layer also consists of hydroxypropyl methylcellulose and PEG 400. In vitro permeation studies using Franz diffusion cells indicated that the amount of terbinafine hydrochloride that permeated across the human cadaver nail in 6 days from the bilayer lacquer containing PEG 400 was 1.42 ± 0.53 µg/cm^2, a threefold enhancement over the lacquer without PEG 400. Drug loading within the nail was also enhanced [58].

Early work to determine the feasibility of transungual iontophoresis had been carried out by Li's group at the University of Cincinnati. The initial studies confirmed that hydrated nail plates exhibited electrophoresis-dominant iontophoretic transport [24]. The effects of the chemical enhancers thioglycolic acid (TGA), glycolic acid (GA) and urea (UR) on nail iontophoretic transport of mannitol and tetraethylammonium were subsequently investigated [25]. Nails treated with GA and UR did not show any transport enhancement. Treatment with TGA at 0.5 M enhanced the passive and iontophoretic transport of mannitol, urea and tetraethylammonium. The effect of TGA on the nail plates was irreversible. This group subsequently evaluated the possibilities of enhancing the delivery of ciclopirox across human nail plates and sustaining drug delivery from drug reservoirs in the nail plates with constant voltage iontophoresis [26]. Transungual ciclopirox delivery from Penlac was the control. Iontophoresis increased the flux of ciclopirox across the nail by approximately tenfold compared to passive delivery from the investigational formulation or from Penlac. A significant amount of ciclopirox, estimated to be above the minimum inhibitory concentrations of the drug for dermatophytic moulds, was loaded into the nail. The data suggested that iontophoresis was able to deliver an effective amount of ciclopirox into and across the nails.

The work of Dutet and Delgado-Charro [12–14] further characterized the iontophoretic properties of nail plate transport in vivo. They demonstrated several parameters with regard to cation transport numbers and found nail permselectivity to cations at pH 7 but concluded that electroosmotic flow across the nail may not be easily predictable.

The importance of water to the flexibility of the nail plate has been mentioned previously. Studies using Raman spectroscopy indicated that the water content of the different strata in the nail was variable [75]. Water diffusivity studies showed that there was a non-linear steady-state concentration profile for water [21], and equilibrium sorption studies confirmed that the water was strongly bound to the protein matrix [19]. Gunt and Kasting [20] went on to demonstrate that the penetration of ketoconazole into human nail was enhanced threefold when the nail plate samples were fully hydrated.

22.3.2 In Vivo Investigations

The pharmacokinetics of sertaconazole, an imidazole antifungal drug, following topical application was evaluated in vivo [63]. Sixteen healthy adults were treated with nail patches containing sertaconazole (3.63 mg), which were placed on a thumbnail of each subject. Patches were replaced weekly over 6 weeks. Nail clippings, used

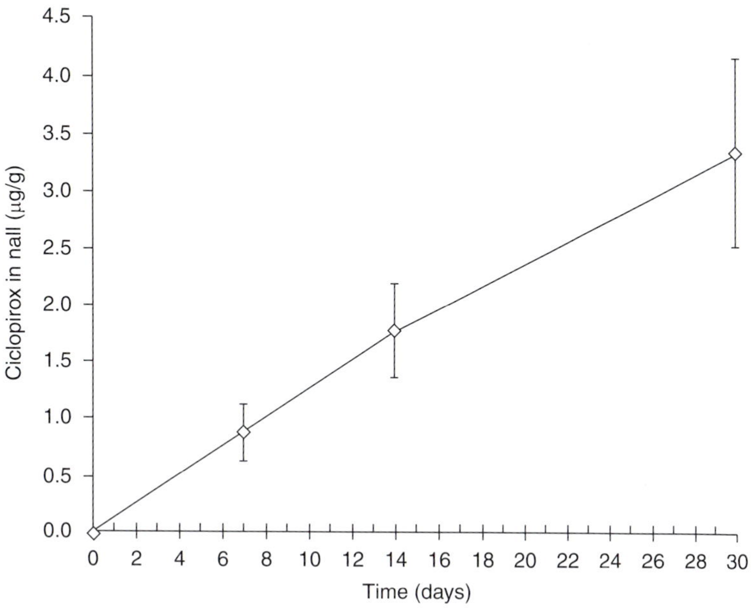

Fig. 22.3 Uptake of ciclopirox into human fingernails in vivo. Ciclopirox (8%) varnish was applied daily to fingernails of nine volunteers. Residual varnish from previous applications was removed prior to application of fresh varnish and prior to sampling. Nail clippings were taken on days 7, 14 and 30. Data shown are mean ± standard error (Data from [8])

nail patches and blood samples were analysed for sertaconazole. Concentrations >100 mg/g, exceeding the MICs for all relevant dermatophytes, were detected in all treated nail samples. Analysis of the residual patches indicated that 16–71% of the drug had penetrated into the nail. No sertaconazole was detected in plasma samples. It was concluded that nail patches should have beneficial therapeutic effects.

Ceschin-Roques et al. [8] assessed the bioavailability of 8% ciclopirox from a lacquer formulation. Nail lacquer was applied to the fingernails of healthy volunteers, and the total amount of ciclopirox in the nail was 3.35 mg/mg following 30 days treatment, and this was considered sufficient to kill the fungal pathogens (Fig. 22.3). Similarly, van Hoogdalem et al. [68] evaluated the in vivo nail penetration of oxiconazole. Six healthy volunteers were treated with 1% w/v oxiconazole lotion applied to the nail twice daily for 6 weeks, and nail clippings were collected every 2 weeks over an 8-week period. Maximum drug levels in the upper 0–50 µm layers varied between 120 and 1420 ng/mg. Total nail uptake was less than 0.2% of the topical dose. Co-delivery with acetylcysteine (15% w/v in the oxiconazole lotion), a compound that will disrupt keratin disulfide bonds, generated a statistically significant prolonged residence time of oxiconazole in the 51–100 µm nail layers. Peak drug levels in the upper 0–50 µm layer increased from 790 ng/mg to 1,570 ng/ml. They concluded that the effect of acetylcysteine was related to increased binding of oxiconazole to nail constituents.

22.4 Clinical Data Supporting Topical Therapy of Nail Diseases

For many years, dermatologists believed that topical treatment for anything other than the most superficial infections of the nail plate was futile. The nail plate was viewed as an impermeable barrier only to be breached via the blood supply to the nail matrix, and prolonged oral dosing with powerful antifungal agents was the order of the day. However, as our knowledge of the nail plate barrier has improved, our ability to rationally develop antifungal and other agents and delivery vehicles specifically for the topical treatment of nail diseases has increased. The dermatologists' armamentarium has been supplemented with nail lacquers and other formulations including those containing tioconazole, amorolfine, ciclopirox, clobetasol-17-propionate, calcipotriol and tazarotene. However, the true test of any therapeutic regimen is efficacy.

The conservative approach is to supplement oral therapy with topical treatment. Nakano et al. [50] performed a pilot study to assess the safety and efficacy of pulse therapy with oral terbinafine in 66 patients with onychomycosis. Each pulse consisted of oral terbinafine (500 mg/day) for 1 week followed by a 3-week interval. Topical 1% terbinafine cream was applied daily. Efficacy was assessed 1 year after treatment initiation. There was a complete cure in 51 patients (approximately 77%), marked improvement in five patients, improvement in five patients and slight improvement in one patient. Four patients showed no change. Although they concluded that terbinafine pulse therapy in combination with topical application of terbinafine cream was safe and effective, it was not possible to determine whether the topical applications improved the outcome. An earlier study [1] using a similar oral treatment regimen but with no supplemental topical therapy reported 74% cure rate, suggesting that topical application was of little additive benefit. However, it is important to appreciate that the application vehicle is a very important determinant for successful delivery of drug to the nail and that the cream used in the Nakano study was probably not optimized in this respect. Furthermore, the highly lipophilic nature of terbinafine suggests that it would not penetrate into the nail to any great extent.

A better indication of the usefulness of supplemental topical therapy can be obtained from the work of Rigopoulos et al. [52] who evaluated the combination of systemic and topical antifungals to improve the cure rates and reduce the duration of systemic treatment for onychomycoses. They used itraconazole pulse therapy combined with amorolfine and compared this with itraconazole alone in the treatment of nail Candida. Ninety patients with Candida fingernail were randomized into two treatment groups of 45. Group 1 received itraconazole pulse therapy for 2 months with amorolfine 5% solution nail lacquer application for 6 months, while group 2 received monotherapy with three pulses of itraconazole. Eighty-five patients, with a mean duration of onychomycosis of 11 months, were analysed. After three months of therapy, mycological cure was seen in 32 (74%) of 43 patients in group 1 and in 25 (60%) of 42 patients in group 2. Following 9 months therapy, a global cure was seen in 40 patients (93%) in group 1 and in 34 patients (81%) in group 2. Compared with oral itraconazole alone, the combination achieved greater mycological cure and increased total cure rate. Although statistical analysis showed no statistically significant difference ($P > 0.1$) between the two treatment groups, the combination of topical amorolfine and oral itraconazole exhibited considerable synergy.

Baran and Coquard [3] treated 13 onychomycotic patients, aged 25–78 years, with a solution of 1% fluconazole and 20% urea in an ethanol-water mixture, applied once daily. There was complete resolution of the condition in four cases, and four patients demonstrated a 90% improvement. Of four patients with onychomycoses in both big toenails, two showed 50% improvement bilaterally, and in the remaining two patients, there was a 90% improvement in one nail and a 50% improvement in the other. Overall the response to local therapy was appreciable.

Gupta et al. [22] reviewed the efficacy and safety of 8% ciclopirox nail lacquer in the treatment of onychomycosis. In one study, 223 patients were randomized to treatment, and in another, 237 subjects were randomized. Both studies were conducted in the USA. The active and placebo formulations were applied daily for 48 weeks, and mycologic evaluation was performed every 12 weeks. Data from these pivotal trials demonstrated that ciclopirox nail lacquer was significantly more effective than placebo in the treatment of onychomycosis. At the end of the treatment period, the mycologic cure rate in the first study was 29% and 11% in the ciclopirox and vehicle groups, respectively, and in the second study, the cure rate was 36% and 9%, respectively. In non-US studies, mycologic cure rates ranged from 47% to 86%, and the lacquer demonstrated a broad spectrum of activity showing efficacy against Candida species and some non-dermatophytes. The authors concluded that the nail lacquer provided a treatment choice with a favourable benefit-to-risk ratio. In subsequent studies, topical ciclopirox efficacy has been confirmed, and more recently, the efficacy of the lacquer in a case of infantile congenital candidal onychomycosis was reported to be excellent [78].

Malay et al. [39] randomly allocated 55 patients to either nail debridement (27 patients) or debridement plus application of a topical antifungal nail lacquer containing 8% ciclopirox (28 patients). After a median follow-up of 10.5 months, patients in the antifungal nail lacquer group showed statistically significantly improvement over those in the debridement-alone group, with an ~77% rate of mycological cure. None of the patients in the debridement-alone group experienced mycological cure.

As previously pointed out, not all nail diseases are fungal or bacterial infections. Psoriasis can affect the entire nail plate and is a common feature in psoriasis patients. A lacquer formulation containing 8% clobetasol-17-propionate was evaluated for the efficacy and safety [55]. Ten patients, with both nail bed and matrix psoriasis, were treated with the nail lacquer applied once daily for 21 days and subsequently twice weekly for 9 months. There was a reduction of all the nail alterations, including nail pain, within 4 weeks of initiating therapy, and response was directly related to the length of treatment. The lacquer was a safe and effective treatment for nail bed and matrix psoriasis.

Tazarotene gel has also been evaluated as a therapy for nail psoriasis. In a double-blind, randomized, vehicle-controlled, parallel-group trial, 31 patients with fingernail psoriasis were randomized to receive tazarotene or vehicle gel, which was applied daily for up to 24 weeks to two target fingernails, one under occlusion and one unoccluded [56]. Tazarotene treatment resulted in a significantly greater reduction in onycholysis (loosening of the nail plate-nail bed connection) in both occluded and non-occluded nails together with a significantly greater reduction in pitting in occluded nails. The gel was well tolerated. Nail psoriasis was also improved following topical application of calcipotriol and betamethasone dipropionate ointment applied once daily for 12 weeks [53].

As noted earlier, brittle nail syndrome is a common problem and refers to nails that exhibit surface roughness, raggedness and peeling. Sherber et al. [57] evaluated the usefulness of tazarotene cream (0.1%) for the treatment of brittle nails. Patients applied tazarotene cream to the nails twice daily for 24 weeks. All participants achieved improvement of the target nails at week 12, and 16 participants (88.9%) at week 24. The study showed that tazarotene was effective at reducing the symptoms of brittle nail syndrome with minimal to no irritation.

22.5 Concluding Remarks

The permeability characteristics of the human nail plate are reasonably well understood, and topical formulations can be designed to optimize drug delivery into the nail. Successful methods of penetration and permeation enhancement are available. For the most part, topical preparations are well tolerated upon prolonged use. Upon clinical examination, the topical formulations have been found to be reasonably effective as either mono- or dual therapies and have been shown to be synergistic with oral therapy. Treatment with topical agents has been described as cost-effective [23]. Further investigation into means to enhance penetration into and permeation across the nail plate will inevitably lead to more effective topical preparations.

Take Home Messages

- Nail structure and morphology: The anatomical and chemical differences between stratum corneum and nail plate are discussed. The properties that make the permeability characteristics of the two structures so different are detailed with an illustration of the importance of water in the nail plate.
- Nail plate permeability in vitro evidence: Given that there is so little lipid in the nail plate, is there any chance that therapeutic molecules can get into and across this tissue? The answer is yes, and this has been shown by in vitro techniques. The potential usefulness of penetration and permeation enhancement strategies is also discussed in this section.
- Nail plate permeability in vivo evidence: If compounds have been shown to get into and through the nail in vitro, will they do the same in vivo? Again the answer is yes.
- Clinical data supporting topical therapy of nail diseases: The fact that therapeutic molecules can penetrate into and permeate across nails in vivo does not necessarily indicate that they will have therapeutic effect. Clinical studies are discussed that illustrate that the topical treatment of nail diseases is partially successful, but there remains much room for improvement.

References

1. Alpsov E, Yilmaz E, Basaran E (1996) Intermittent therapy with terbinafine for dermatophyte toe-onychomycosis: a new approach. J Dermatol 23: 259–262
2. Baden HP, Goldsmith LA, Fleming B (1973) A comparative study of the physicochemical properties of human keratinized tissues. Biochim Biophys Acta 322:269–278
3. Baran R, Coquard F (2005) Combination of fluconazole and urea in a nail lacquer for treating onychomycosis. J Dermatolog Treat 16:52–55
4. Bauer F, Stevens B (1983) Investigations of trace metal content of normal and diseased nails. Australas J Dermatol 24:127–129
5. Brown MB, Khengar RH, Turner RB, Forbes B, Traynor MJ, Evans CRG, Jones SA (2009) Overcoming the nail barrier: a systematic investigation of ungula chemical penetration enhancement. Int J Pharm 370:61–67
6. Burch GE, Winsor T (1946) Diffusion of water through dead plantar, palmar and torsal human skin and through toe nails. Arch Derm Syphilol 53:39–41
7. Cashman MW, Sloan SB (2010) Nutrition and nail disease. Clin Dermatol 28:420–425
8. Ceschin-Roques CG, Hanel H, Pruja-Bougaret SM, Luc J, Vandermander J, Michel G (1991) Ciclopirox nail lacquer 8%: in vivo penetration into and through nails and in vitro effect on pig skin. Skin Pharmacol 4:89–94
9. de Vocht ML, Reviakine I, Wösten HAB, Brisson A, Wessels JGH, Robillard GT (2000) Structural and functional role of the disulfide bridges in the hydrophobin SC3. J Biol Chem 275:28428–28432
10. Donnelly RF, McCarron PA, Lightowler JM, Woolfson AD (2005) Bioadhesive patch-based delivery of 5-aminolevulinic acid to the nail for photodynamic therapy of onychomycosis. J Control Release 103:381–392
11. Dubini F, Bellotti MG, Frangi A, Monti D, Saccomani L (2005) In vitro antimycotic activity and nail permeation models of a piroctone olamine (octopirox) containing transungual water soluble technology. Arzneimittelforschung 55:478–483
12. Dutet J, Delgado-Charro MB (2009) In vivo transungual iontophoresis: effect of DC current application on ionic transport and on transonychial water loss. J Control Release 140:117–125
13. Dutet J, Delgado-Charro MB (2010) Transungual iontophoresis of lithium and sodium: effect of pH and co-ion competition on cationic transport numbers. J Control Release 144:168–174
14. Dutet J, Delgado-Charro MB (2010) Electroosmotic transport of mannitol across human nail during constant current iontophoresis. J Pharm Pharmacol 62: 721–729
15. Elewski E (1998) Onychomycosis: pathogenesis, diagnosis, and management. Clin Microbiol Rev 11:415–429
16. Elkeeb R, AliKhan A, Elkeeb L, Hui X, Maibach HI (2010) Transungual drug delivery: current status. Int J Pharm 384:1–8
17. Farran L, Ennos AR, Eichhorn J (2008) The effect of humidity on the fracture properties of human fingernails. J Exp Biol 211:3677–3681
18. Franz TJ (1992) Absorption of amorolfine through human nail. Dermatology 184(Suppl 1):18–20
19. Gunt HB, Kasting GB (2007) Equilibrium water sorption characteristics of the human nail. J Cosmet Sci 58:1–9
20. Gunt HB, Kasting GB (2007) Effect of hydration on the permeation of ketoconazole through human nail plate in vitro. Eur J Pharm Sci 32:254–260

21. Gunt HB, Miller MA, Kasting GB (2007) Water diffusivity in human nail plate. J Pharm Sci 96:3352–3362
22. Gupta AK, Fleckman P, Baran R (2000) Ciclopirox nail lacquer topical solution 8% in the treatment of toenail onychomycosis. J Am Acad Dermatol 43(4 Suppl):S70–S80
23. Gupta AK, Lynde CW, Barber K (2006) Pharmacoeconomic assessment of ciclopirox topical solution, 8%, oral terbinafine, and oral itraconazole for onychomycosis. J Cutan Med Surg 10(Suppl 2): S54–S62
24. Hao J, Li SK (2008) Transungual iontophoretic transport of polar neutral and positively charged model permeants: effects of electrophoresis and electroosmosis. J Pharm Sci 97:893–905
25. Hao J, Smith KA, Li SK (2008) Chemical method to enhance transungual transport and iontophoresis efficiency. Int J Pharm 357:61–69
26. Hao J, Smith KA, Li SK (2009) Iontophoretically enhanced ciclopirox delivery into and across human nail plate. J Pharm Sci 98:3608–3616
27. Hay R (2005) Literature review. Onychomycosis. J Eur Acad Dermatol Venereol 19(Suppl 1):1–7
28. Hui X, Shainhouse Z, Tanojo H, Anigbogu A, Markus GE, Maibach HI, Wester RC (2002) Enhanced human nail drug delivery: nail inner drug content assayed by new unique method. J Pharm Sci 91:189–195
29. Hui X, Chan TCK, Barbadillo S, Lee C, Maibach HI, Wester RC (2003) Enhanced econazole penetration into human nail by 2-N-nonyl-1,3-dioxolane. J Pharm Sci 92:142–148
30. Hui X, Wester RC, Barbadillo S, Lee C, Patel B, Wortzmman M, Gans EH, Maibach HI (2004) Ciclopirox delivery into the human nail plate. J Pharm Sci 93:2545–2548
31. Hui X, Hornby SB, Wester RC, Barbadillo S, Appa Y, Maibach H (2007) In vitro human nail penetration and kinetics of panthenol. Int J Cosmet Sci 29:277–282
32. Kamp H, Tietz H-J, Lutz M, Piazena H, Sowyrda P, Lademann J, Blume-Peytavi U (2005) Antifungal effect of 5-aminolevulinic acid PDT in *Trichophyton rubrum*. Mycoses 48:101–107
33. Khengar RH, Jones SA, Turner RB, Forbes B, Brown MB (2007) Nail swelling as a pre-formulation screen for the selection and optimisation of ungual penetration enhancers. Pharm Res 24:2207–2212
34. Khengar RH, Brown MB, Turner RB, Traynor MJ, Holt KB, Jones SA (2010) Free radical facilitated damage of ungual keratin. Free Radic Biol Med 49:865–871
35. Kien CL, Ganther HE (1983) Manifestations of chronic selenium deficiency in a child receiving total parenteral nutrition. Am J Clin Nutr 37:319–328
36. Kligman AM (1965) Topical pharmacology and toxicology of dimethylsulfoxide. J Am Med Assoc 193: 796–804
37. Kobayashi Y, Miyamoto M, Sugibayashi K, Morimoto Y (1998) Enhancing effect of N-acetyl-L-cysteine or 2-mercaptoethanol on the in vitro permeation of 5-fluorouracil or tolnaftate through the human nail plate. Chem Pharm Bull 46:1797–1802
38. Kobayashi Y, Komatsu T, Sumi M, Numajiri S, Miyamoto M, Kobayashi D, Sugibayashi K, Morimoto Y (2004) In vitro permeation of several drugs through the human nail plate: relationship between physicochemical properties and nail permeability of drugs. Eur J Pharm Sci 21:471–477
39. Malay DS, Yi SY, Borowsky P, Downey MS, Mlodzienski AJ (2009) Efficacy of debridement alone versus debridement combined with topical antifungal nail lacquer for the treatment of pedal onychomycosis: a randomized, controlled trial. J Foot Ankle Surg 48:294–307
40. Mertin D, Lippold BC (1997) In vitro permeability of the human nail and of a keratin membrane from bovine hooves: influence of the partition coefficient octanol/water and the water solubility of drugs on their permeability and maximum flux. J Pharm Pharmacol 49:30–34
41. Mertin D, Lippold BC (1997) In vitro permeability of the human nail and of a keratin membrane from bovine hooves: penetration of chloramphenicol from lipophilic vehicles and a nail lacquer. J Pharm Pharmacol 49:241–245
42. Mertin D, Lippold BC (1997) In vitro permeability of the human nail and of a keratin membrane from bovine hooves: prediction of the penetration rate of antimycotics through the nail plate and their efficacy. J Pharm Pharmacol 49:866–872
43. Mohorcic M, Torkar A, Friedrich J, Kristl J, Murdan S (2007) An investigation into keratolytic enzymes to enhance ungual drug delivery. Int J Pharm 332:196–201
44. Monti D, Saccomani L, Chetoni P, Burgalassi S, Saetttone MF, Mailland F (2005) In vitro transungual permeation of ciclopirox from a hydroxypropyl chitosan-based, water-soluble nail lacquer. Drug Dev Ind Pharm 31:11–17
45. Monti D, Saccomani L, Chetoni P, Burgalassi S, Senesi S, Ghelardi E, Mailland F (2010) Hydrosoluble medicated nail lacquers: in vitro drug permeation and corresponding antimycotic activity. Br J Dermatol 162:311–317
46. Monti D, Saccomani L, Chetoni P, Burgalassi S, Tampucci S, Mailland F (2011) Validation of bovine hoof slices as model for infected human toenails: in vitro ciclopirox transungual permeation. Br J Dermatol. doi:10.1111/j.1365-2133.2011. 10303.x. [Epub ahead of print]
47. Murdan S (2008) Enhancing the nail plate permeability of topically applied drugs. Expert Opin Drug Deliv 5:1–16
48. Murthy SN, Vaka SRK, Sammeta SM, Nair AB (2009) TransScreen-NTM: method for rapid screening of trans-ungual drug delivery enhancers. J Pharm Sci 98:4264–4271
49. Nair AB, Chakraborty B, Murthy SN (2010) Effect of polyethylene glycols on the trans-ungual delivery of terbinafine. Curr Drug Deliv 7:407–414
50. Nakano N, Hiruma M, Shiraki Y, Chen X, Porgpermdee S, Ikeda S (2006) Combination of pulse therapy with

terbinafine tablets and topical terbinafine cream for the treatment of dermatophyte onychomycosis: a pilot study. J Dermatol 33:753–758

51. Quintanar-Guerrero D, Ganem-Quintanar A, Tapia-Olguin P, Kalia YN, Buri P (1998) The effect of keratolytic agents on the permeability of three imidazole antimycotic drugs through the human nail. Drug Dev Ind Pharm 24:685–690
52. Rigopoulos D, Katoulis AC, Ionnides D, Georgaia S, Kalogeromitros D, Bolbasis I, Karistinou A, Christofidou E, Polydorou D, Balkou P, Fragouli E, Katsambas AD (2003) A randomised trial of amorolfine 5% solution nail lacquer in association with itraconazole pulse therapy compared with itraconazole alone in the treatment of Candida fingernail onychomycosis. Br J Dermatol 149:151–156
53. Rigopoulos D, Gregoriou S, Danielli CR, Belyayeva H, Larios G, Verra P, Stamou C, Kontochristopoulos G, Avgerinou G, Katsambas A (2009) Treatment of nail psoriasis with a two-compound formulation of calcipotriol plus betamethasone dipropionate ointment. Dermatology 218:338–341
54. Runne U, Orfanos CE (1981) The human nail – structure, growth and pathological changes. Curr Probl Dermatol 9:102–149
55. Sanchez Regana M, Martin Ezquerra G, Umbert Millet P, Llambi Mateos F (2005) Treatment of nail psoriasis with 8% clobetasol nail lacquer: positive experience in 10 patients. J Eur Acad Dermatol Venereol 19:573–577
56. Scher RK, Stiller M, Zhu YI, 5 (2001) Tazarotene 0.1% gel in the treatment of fingernail psoriasis: a double-blind, randomised, vehicle-controlled study. Cutis 68:355–358
57. Sherber NS, Hoch AM, Coppola CA, Carter EL, Chang HL, Barsanti FR, Mackay-Wiggan JM (2011) Efficacy and safety study of tazarotene cream 0.1% for the treatment of brittle nail syndrome. Cutis 87:96–103
58. Shivakumar HN, Vaka SR, Madhav NV, Chandra H, Murthy SN (2010) Bilayered nail lacquer of terbinafine hydrochloride for treatment of onychomycosis. J Pharm Sci 99:4267–4276
59. Smijs TGM, Schuitmaker HJ (2003) Photodynamic inactivation of the dermatophyte *Trichophyton rubrum*. Photochem Photobiol 77:556–560
60. Spruit D (1971) Measurement of water vapor loss through human nail in vivo. J Invest Dermatol 56:359–361
61. Stern DK, Diamantis S, Smith E, Wei H, Gordon M, Muigai W, Moshier E, Lebwohl M, Spuls P (2007) Water content and other aspects of brittle versus normal fingernails. J Am Acad Dermatol 57:31–36
62. Stuttgen G, Bauer E (1982) Bioavailability, skin and nail penetration of topically applied antimycotics. Mycosen 25:74–80
63. Susilo R, Korting HC, Greb W, Strauss UP (2006) Nail penetration of sertaconazole with a sertaconazole-containing nail patch formulation. Am J Clin Dermatol 7:259–262
64. Traynor MJ, Turner RB, Evans CR, Khengar RH, Jones SA, Brown MB (2010) Effect of a novel penetration enhancer on the ungula permeation of two antifungal agents. J Pharm Pharmacol 62:730–737
65. Ujiie H, Shibaki A, Akiyama M, Shimizu H (2010) Successful treatment of nail lichen planus with topical tacrolimus. Acta Derm Venereol 90:218–219
66. Vaka SR, Murthy SN, O'Haver JH, Repka MA (2011) A platform for predicting and enhancing model drug delivery across the human nail plate. Drug Dev Ind Pharm 37:72–79
67. van de Kerkhof PC, Pasch MC, Scher RK, Kerscher M, Gieler U, Haneke E, Fleckman P (2005) Brittle nail syndrome: a pathogenesis-based approach with a proposed grading system. J Am Acad Dermatol 53:644–651
68. van Hoogdalem EJ, van den Hoven WE, Terpstra IJ, van Zijtveld J, Verschoor JSC, Visser JN (1997) Nail penetration of the antifungal oxiconazole after repeated topical application in healthy volunteers, and the effect of acetylcysteine. Eur J Pharm Sci 5: 119–127
69. Vejnovic I, Huonder C, Betz G (2010) Permeation studies of novel terbinafine formulations containing hydrophobins through human nails in vitro. Int J Pharm 397:67–76
70. Vejnovic I, Simmler L, Betz G (2010) Investigation of different formulations for drug delivery through the nail plate. Int J Pharm 386:185–194
71. Walters KA, Flynn GL, Marvel JR (1981) Physicochemical characterization of the human nail: I. Pressure sealed apparatus for measuring nail plate permeabilities. J Invest Dermatol 76:76–79
72. Walters KA, Flynn GL, Marvel JR (1983) Physicochemical characterization of the human nail: permeation pattern for water and the homologous alcohols and differences with respect to the stratum corneum. J Pharm Pharmacol 35:28–33
73. Walters KA, Flynn GL, Marvel JR (1985) Penetration of the human nail: the effects of vehicle pH on the permeation of miconazole. J Pharm Pharmacol 37:498–499
74. Walters KA, Flynn GL, Marvel JR (1985) Physicochemical characterization of the human nail: solvent effects on the permeation of homologous alcohols. J Pharm Pharmacol 37:771–775
75. Wessel S, Gniadecka M, Jemec GB, Wulf HC (1999) Hydration of human nails investigated by NIR-FT-Raman spectroscopy. Biochim Biophys Acta 1433:210–216
76. Wösten HA, de Vocht ML (2000) Hydrophobins, the fungal coat unravelled. Biochim Biophys Acta 1469:79–86
77. Xiao P, Zheng X, Imhof RE, Hirata K, McAuley WJ, Mateus R, Hadgraft J, Lane ME (2011) Opto-thermal transient emission radiometry (OTTER) to image diffusion in nails in vivo. Int J Pharm 406:111–113
78. Sardana K, Garg VK, Manchanda V, Rajpal M (2006). Congenital candidal onychomycoses: effective cure with ciclopirox olamine 8% nail lacquer. Br J Dermatol 154:573–575

23 Preservation of Moisturisers

D. Godfrey

23.1 The Consequences of Microbial Growth in Cosmetics

There are several possible adverse effects that may occur in the absence of a sufficiently robust preservation system, and these may be broadly divided into aesthetics and safety issues:

1. Visible growth is one of the more obvious signs of microbial contamination, whether it be a black mould (e.g. *Aspergillus brasiliensis,* formerly *A. niger*) or other discolorations from various different bacteria (e.g. *Pseudomonas aeruginosa* can produce a blue/green, yellow/green or a red/brown colour). The metabolites produced by microbes are often acidic, and the reduction in pH may lead to breakdown of the emulsion. Additionally, the emulsifiers themselves may be used as nutrient source, and this may also lead to phase separation. Microbial growth can also produce unpleasant odours.
2. There are also clear safety issues with microbial contamination. The presence of pathogenic organisms in a product being applied to skin, especially if the skin is damaged, may lead to infection. Staphylococcal infections are particularly easily spread in this manner. Far more seriously but, fortunately, far less common is the possibility of contaminated product entering the eye. For example, sufficient numbers of *Pseudomonas aeruginosa* in the eye will cause blindness [1].

It is essential, therefore, from the dual considerations of product integrity/aesthetics and consumer safety that cosmetic products are sufficiently well-preserved to withstand any possible microbial contamination from reasonably foreseeable conditions of use.

The regulation of cosmetics around the world varies considerably, but no cosmetic product should be unsafe for use, either from a toxicological or a microbiological point of view. It is, therefore, essential that steps be taken to ensure that the product is proven to be adequately preserved.

23.2 Sources of Microbial Contamination

There are three principal sources of microbial contamination in cosmetics:

1. *During the manufacturing process.* Unless the product is manufactured in totally sterile conditions, there will be contamination from the atmosphere and from the skin and clothes of the operators. This is unavoidable, but should be kept to a minimum by using the best manufacturing practise with an emphasis on plant hygiene.

D. Godfrey
Azelis Ltd,
Hertford, UK
e-mail: dene62@hotmail.co.uk

M. Lodén, H.I. Maibach (eds.), *Treatment of Dry Skin Syndrome*,
DOI 10.1007/978-3-642-27606-4_23, © Springer-Verlag Berlin Heidelberg 2012

2. *Raw materials*. Some raw materials may have levels of microbial contamination, especially if they are natural in origin. This should be controlled by the supplier to ensure that any contamination is kept to acceptably low levels.
3. *Consumer use*. This source of contamination is almost entirely unavoidable, as the consumer will inevitably have some contact with the product unless it is supplied in packs designed to eliminate contact, or in single-use packs.

23.3 What Is Preservation?

Preservation may be defined as the art of protecting products against microbial attack during their shelf life.

It should *not* be used to compensate for unhygienic manufacturing conditions, but only to allow for the contamination introduced during consumer use.

23.4 What Is a Preservative?

Any substance used to kill or prevent the growth of microorganisms which, by their growth, will spoil or contaminate a raw material or product.

23.5 Microbial Challenge Testing

The most effective and consistent means of establishing the efficacy of a preservation system is to subject the product to a microbial challenge test. There are many variations on this test but, in its most simple form, the methods prescribed by various pharmacopoeia are a good basis, e.g. United States Pharmacopoeia (USP) and Pharmacopoeia Europa (Ph. Eur.). In the Ph. Eur. method, the product is inoculated with cultures of organisms representative of the four main subgroups of likely contaminants:

1. Gram-negative bacteria – *Pseudomonas aeruginosa*
2. Gram-positive bacteria – *Staphylococcus aureus*
3. Yeasts – *Candida albicans*
4. Moulds – *Aspergillus brasiliensis*

These cultures are inoculated in separate samples and then checked for surviving colonies at specified time points. There are different criteria for success for bacteria than for fungi; both are measured on the degree of logarithmic reduction in colony numbers.

In order to pass the criteria for bacteria, the colony count must be reduced by at least log 2 within 2 days and by at least log 3 within 7 days, with no increase in numbers thereafter (being tested also after 14 and 28 days).

In order to pass the criteria for fungi, the colony count must be reduced by at least log 2 within 7 days, with no increase thereafter, and again, up to 28 days.

The criteria described here, from the Ph. Eur., are the 'A' criteria. There are also 'B' criteria, which are less stringent, but these would not apply to moisturising products.

The USP criteria include the Gram-negative bacterium, *Escherichia coli,* and are less stringent than those of the Ph. Eur., requiring only that there is no increase in the initial numbers of *A. brasiliensis* and *C. albicans* up to 28 days and only a 1 log reduction of bacteria by 7 days and then a 3 log reduction by 14 days, with no increase at 28 days.

23.6 Minimum Inhibitory Concentration Values

When evaluating preservatives and preservative combinations in the development stage of the process, it is common practice to determine the minimum inhibitory concentration (mic) value. This is the lowest concentration at which the test substance prevents further growth of the test organism. This value is specific to both the substance and the organism tested. The concentration required to kill the organism is usually much higher than the mic value. Manufacturers of preservatives usually offer mic data in support of their products, but this information should be treated with a little caution. There is no standard method for the mic test, and the results are subject to wide variability, as there are several factors that have a significant effect on the result. The most important variables are the inoculum count employed and the actual strain of the test organism. The lower the inoculum count, the lower the concentration of test substance required to prevent cells from growing, and it is possible to manipulate the data by using a low inoculum count to produce low mic figures, thereby making the test substance appear unduly active. Microbial cells from all species evolve and adapt to their surroundings, and microbial resistance, or tolerance, can develop in laboratory strains, leading to incorrect mic results. There is also the potential for huge variability in response between the different strains of the same species. (A strain is a subset of a bacterial species differing from other bacteria of that species by some minor, but identifiable difference).

The result of these potential variations within the mic test is that direct comparison of mic data should only be made for the data on one specific substance (i.e. comparing the mic of the substance for all the organisms tested at the same time) and should not be 'read across' to other substances tested separately, other than with a high degree of caution.

For the above reasons, there are no mic data quoted for the preservatives being discussed, only general statements for guidance on the types of organisms against which they are effective.

23.7 Criteria for Preservatives/ Preservation Systems

In order to determine the usefulness of a preservative, or a preservation system, it is important to understand the attributes required for successful preservation of a product.

The most important criterion is broad-spectrum preservation, i.e. the system must be effective against bacteria (normally divided into Gram-negative bacteria and Gram-positive bacteria) and fungi (normally divided into yeasts and moulds). These subdivisions are important, as some preservatives are only effective in one or two of these areas. If the proposed preservation system for any given product is not effective against any of these subgroups, or even just one specific common microorganism, it is not suitable for use without another substance being included that will control the gap in the activity spectrum. For example, *Pseudomonas aeruginosa* is a common Gram-negative bacterium that is relatively difficult to control. If the preservation system controlled all other microorganisms, but allowed *P. aeruginosa* to survive, these bacteria would grow even faster than normal due to the absence of competitive organisms. Partial preservation is barely more effective than the complete absence of preservation. Broad-spectrum antimicrobial protection is the key to a safe and stable product.

The components of the preservation system must be compatible with the other ingredients used in the formulation. Any interaction may result in reduced activity; this would become apparent in the results of the microbial challenge test, unless the interaction develops over a more prolonged period.

The preservation system should be effective at the target pH of the product. Not all preservatives are equally effective across the entire pH range typically seen in moisturisers.

The preservation system should not be prone to discoloration, especially if being considered for use in non-coloured products, and should not impart any detectable/undesirable odour. It may be possible to mask any odour, but this is not ideal.

The preservation system must be appropriate for the intended use of the final product – a substance permitted only in rinse-off products is clearly not suitable for a moisturising lotion.

The preservation system must be as safe as possible. It is inherent amongst biologically active substances to have some potential for skin irritation and, albeit a lower potential, for sensitisation. The choice of preservative is a balance between efficacy and risk of a skin response. As a general rule, the more potent the antimicrobial activity, the higher the risk of a skin response (in relative terms), but this is usually mitigated by the use of lower concentrations – due to the more powerful activity.

23.8 Commonly Used Preservatives

There are 58 entries on Annex VI of the EU Cosmetics Directive (list of permitted preservatives), some covering multiple substances and other antimicrobial substances are also employed in the EU and in other markets. However, the number of commonly used preservatives is relatively low, and the majority of these are discussed here:

23.8.1 Parabens

INCI names:
- Methylparaben
- Ethylparaben
- Propylparaben
- Isopropylparaben
- Butylparaben
- Isobutylparaben

'Parabens' is a contraction of 'esters of *para*-hydroxy*benz*oic acid'. The methyl-, ethyl-, propyl-, isopropyl-, butyl- and isobutyl esters are the ones in general use as preservatives, along with their respective sodium salts (INCI names – sodium methylparaben, etc.).

Parabens have been used as preservatives in personal care products since the late 1920s and have a long and successful history of use, being amongst the preservatives with the lowest rates of irritation and sensitisation, with sensitisation rates amongst dermatological patients as low as 1.2% [2].

The parabens are primarily active against fungi, but they also generally have moderate activity against bacteria.

Methylparaben is the least active of the group, and the antimicrobial activity increases with the increasing carbon chain length of the ester group. The activities of ethylparaben and propylparaben lie between those of methylparaben and butylparaben.

All the parabens have relatively low water solubility, and this decreases with the increasing carbon chain length of the ester group, methylparaben being soluble up to 0.25% in water (25°C) and butylparaben being only 0.02% soluble [3, 4].

Frequently, combinations of parabens are employed in order to maximise the total concentration available in the aqueous phase and also, therefore, the antimicrobial activity. It is relatively unusual to use a single paraben ester in a preservation system. Methylparaben is typically used at 0.1–0.25%, and propylparaben, typically at 0.1–0.15% (as a combination), with the other parabens being mostly used as components of more complex blends, rather than being added as individual ingredients. The typical total parabens concentration is 0.2–0.4%.

In a hot process (c. 80°C), the parabens may be added to either phase prior to emulsification. It is sometimes recommended to split the parabens addition between the two phases, but this is of limited or no value as the parabens will partition between the phases during the emulsification/mixing process.

For cold processes, given the difficulty of dissolving the parabens at low temperatures, the sodium parabens may be used. These are highly water soluble (<50%), but will exert a very high pH, which will require adjustment. A 0.1% aqueous solution of sodium methylparaben is approximately pH 9, so an adjustment is important.

The parabens are compatible with most commonly used cosmetic ingredients, but they may be inactivated by some nonionic species. This effect is strongly concentration dependent, as the paraben ester may be encapsulated within any micelles in the system. Below the critical micelle concentration (CMC), therefore, there is no inactivation, with a progressive reduction in activity above the CMC. There is little effect on the activity of parabens from the pH, within the range pH 4–8.

Parabens are permitted globally for use in personal care products, but with differing maximum permitted concentrations:

European Union
- Methylparaben – 0.4%
- Ethylparaben – 0.4%
- Propylparaben + butylparaben – total 0.19%
- Maximum total parabens concentration – 0.8%

At the time of writing, isopropylparaben and isobutylparaben have been judged to have insufficient data available to assess fully their safety and may be phased out of use.

USA
Safe as used
Japan
Total maximum parabens – 1.0% (Japanese name: parahydroxybenzoate esters)

23.8.2 Imidazolidinyl Urea

Imidazolidinyl urea is primarily an antibacterial preservative, with very little antifungal activity. It has been widely used in many markets since its introduction in the 1980s.

Imidazolidinyl urea is highly water soluble and should be added to the product at temperatures below 40°C to avoid decomposition. It retains its activity over a broad pH range – from pH 3–9. Typical use concentrations are 0.2–0.5%. The potential for imidazolidinyl urea to release very low levels of formaldehyde is perceived by some to be a disadvantage. (See General Note on Formaldehyde Donors below.)

Imidazolidinyl urea is permitted globally, with the following restrictions:
European Union
Maximum 0.6%
USA
Safe as used
Japan
In rinse-off products only, with a maximum of 0.075% (expressed as free formaldehyde) and with special labelling requirements – 'should not be used by infants, or by people who are hypersensitive to formaldehyde'

23.8.3 Diazolidinyl Urea

Diazolidinyl urea is primarily an antibacterial preservative, with activity against moulds, but fairly weak anti-yeast activity. It has been widely used in many markets since its introduction in the 1980s. It is classified as a formaldehyde donor. (See General Note on Formaldehyde Donors below.)

Diazolidinyl urea is highly water soluble and should be added to the product at temperatures below 40°C to avoid decomposition. It retains its activity over a broad pH range – from pH 3–9. Typical use concentrations are 0.1–0.3%.

Diazolidinyl urea is permitted in many territories, with the following restrictions:
European Union
Maximum 0.5%
USA
Maximum 0.5%
Japan
Not permitted

23.8.4 DMDM Hydantoin

DMDM hydantoin is a broad-spectrum preservative, but has better activity against bacteria than against fungi. It is classified as a formaldehyde donor. (See General Note on Formaldehyde Donors below.)

DMDM hydantoin is highly water soluble (it is usually supplied as a 55% aqueous solution) and should be added to the product at temperatures below 40°C to avoid decomposition. It retains its activity over a broad pH range – from pH 3–9. Typical use concentrations are 0.15–0.4%.

DMDM hydantoin is permitted in many territories, with the following restrictions:
European Union
Maximum 0.6%
USA
Safe as used
Japan
In rinse-off products only, with a maximum of 0.075% (expressed as free formaldehyde), with special labelling requirements – 'should not be used by infants, or by people who are hypersensitive to formaldehyde'

23.8.5 Quaternium 15

Quaternium 15 is a broad-spectrum preservative, but has better activity against bacteria than against fungi. It is classified as a formaldehyde donor. (See General Note on Formaldehyde Donors below.) The rate of sensitisation has been reported as high as 10.3% amongst dermatological patients [2], which is higher than most commonly used preservatives. This is still very low in overall terms, given that dermatological patients probably comprise much less than 1% of the general population.

Quaternium 15 is highly water soluble and should be added to the product at temperatures below 40°C to avoid decomposition. It retains its activity over a broad pH range – from pH 3–9. Typical use concentrations are 0.05–0.2%.

Quaternium 15 is permitted in some territories, with the following restrictions:

European Union
  Maximum 0.2%
USA
  Safe as used
Japan
  Not permitted

23.8.6 Sodium Hydroxymethylglycinate

Sodium hydroxymethylglycinate (sodium HMG) is a broad-spectrum preservative, but has slightly better activity against bacteria than against fungi. It is classified as a formaldehyde donor. (See General Note on Formaldehyde Donors below.)

Sodium HMG is highly water soluble and should be added to the product at temperatures below 40°C to avoid decomposition. It retains its activity over a broad pH range – from pH 3–9. Typical use concentrations are 0.4–0.8%.

Sodium HMG is permitted in many territories, with the following restrictions:

European Union
  Maximum 0.5%
USA
  Safe as used
Japan
  Not permitted

General Note on Formaldehyde Donors

Formaldehyde is classified as a category 1 carcinogen (i.e. a proven human carcinogen), and this has led to concerns over the safety of substances having the potential to release formaldehyde. There is no proof, however, that the use of formaldehyde donors in cosmetics results in sufficient exposure to formaldehyde to be of concern. Historically, available formaldehyde levels in cosmetic products have been exaggerated due to a flaw in the standard methods used to detect formaldehyde [5, 6]. In the case of formaldehyde donors, the donor molecule exists in equilibrium with free formaldehyde and the other reaction product. The standard method for determining formaldehyde requires a derivatisation step, which disturbs the equilibrium, thereby producing more free formaldehyde, i.e. formaldehyde that is not actually present in the product prior to the analytical method being performed.

23.8.7 Phenoxyethanol

Phenoxyethanol is one of the most widely used preservatives. It is a broad-spectrum preservative, but it is slightly weaker against Gram-positive bacteria than the other species types.

Phenoxyethanol is slightly water soluble (approximately 2.4%) and is preferably added to the product at temperatures below 40°C to reduce the possibility of evaporative loss, although this is only likely to be an issue should the manufactured batch be held at a high temperature (>80°C) for a prolonged period. It retains its activity over a broad pH range – from pH 3–9. Typical use concentrations are 0.4–1.0%. Phenoxyethanol is more commonly used in combination with other preservatives and is rarely used alone.

Phenoxyethanol is permitted in most territories, with the following restrictions:

European Union
  Maximum 1.0%
USA
  Safe as used
Japan
  Maximum 1.0%

23.8.8 Methylchloroisothiazolinone/Methylisothiazolinone

Methylchloroisothiazolinone/methylisothiazolinone (MCI/MI) is one of the most widely used preservatives. It is a broad-spectrum preservative system, effective at extremely low concentrations.

It is usually supplied as a 1.5% active aqueous solution, stabilised with high concentrations of magnesium salts to prevent degradation of the MCI component.

Methylisothiazolinone (MI) is also available as a single component.

MCI/MI retains its activity over a broad pH range – from pH 3–7.5, but MCI breaks down rapidly above pH 8. MI does not contribute towards any antimicrobial activity in this combination product. Typical use concentrations are 7.5–15 ppm (0.00075–0.0015%) of active MCI/MI.

MI is highly stable and retains its activity from pH 3–9. Typical use concentrations are 0.005–0.01%.

The MCI/MI combination is permitted in most territories, with the following restrictions:

European Union

Maximum 0.0015% (active MCI/MI)

USA

Maximum 0.0015% (active MCI/MI)

Japan

Maximum 0.0015% (active MCI/MI) – rinse-off products only.

Methylisothiazolinone is permitted in most territories, with the following restrictions:

European Union

Maximum 0.01% (active MI)

USA

Maximum 0.01% (active MI)

Japan

Maximum 0.01% (active MI) – rinse-off and leave-on products

23.8.9 Benzyl Alcohol

Benzyl alcohol is a widely used preservative. It is broad spectrum in its range of activity, but it is slightly weak against Gram-positive bacteria.

Benzyl alcohol is slightly water soluble (approximately 2%) and is preferably added to the product at temperatures below 40°C to reduce the possibility of evaporative loss, although this is only likely to be an issue should the manufactured batch be held at a high temperature (>80°C) for a prolonged period. It retains its activity over a broad pH range – from pH 3–8.5. Typical use concentrations are 0.4–1.0%. Benzyl alcohol is more commonly used in combination with other preservatives and is rarely used alone.

Benzyl alcohol is permitted in most territories, with the following restrictions:

European Union

Maximum 1.0%. Benzyl alcohol is one of the 26 designated fragrance allergens, and products containing it must be labelled accordingly.

USA

Safe as used

Japan

Maximum 5.0%

23.8.10 Sorbic Acid/Potassium Sorbate

Sorbic acid/potassium sorbate are food-approved preservatives. They are broad-spectrum preservatives, but they are slightly weak against bacteria.

Sorbic acid is very slightly water soluble, but the potassium salt is highly soluble. They retain their activity over a narrow pH range – from pH 3–6. Typical use concentrations are 0.3–0.5%. (See General Note on Organic Acids below.)

Sorbic acid/potassium sorbate are permitted in most territories, with the following restrictions:

European Union

Maximum 0.6% (as the acid)

USA

Safe as used

Japan

Maximum 0.5%

23.8.11 Benzoic Acid/Sodium Benzoate

Benzoic acid/sodium benzoate are food-approved preservatives. They are broad-spectrum preservatives, but they are slightly weak against bacteria.

Benzoic acid is very slightly water soluble, but the sodium salt is highly soluble. They retain their activity over a narrow pH range – from pH 3–5. Typical use concentrations are 0.2–0.4%. (See General Note on Organic Acids below.)

Benzoic acid/sodium benzoate are permitted in most territories, with the following restrictions:

European Union

Rinse-off products, except oral care products: 2,5 % (as acid)

Oral care products: 1,7 % (as acid)

Leave-on products: 0,5 % (as acid)

USA

Safe as used

Japan

Maximum 0.2%

23.8.12 Dehydroacetic Acid/Sodium Dehydroacetate

Dehydroacetic acid/sodium dehydroacetate are broad-spectrum preservatives, but they are slightly weak against bacteria.

Dehydroacetic acid is very slightly water soluble, but the sodium salt is highly soluble. They retain their activity over a narrow pH range – from pH 3–6.5. Typical use concentrations are 0.3–0.5%. (See General Note on Organic Acids below.)

Dehydroacetic acid/dehydroacetate are permitted in most territories, with the following restrictions:

European Union

Maximum 0.6% (as the acid)

USA

Safe as used

Japan

Maximum 0.5%

General Note on Organic Acids

The organic acids described here are only active in their undissociated form – the ionic species have zero antimicrobial activity; hence the restrictive pH range over which they retain their activity. All three acids are 100% active at pH3 because they are completely undissociated at this pH, but as the pH increases, the concentration of ionic species increases and the activity drops rapidly. For example, benzoic acid is approximately twice as active at pH 5.0 than at pH 5.5. For this reason, it is vital that any finished product being submitted for microbial challenge testing has the pH adjusted to the highest end of the pH specification for that product. This is then testing the worst case scenario, i.e. the pH at which the antimicrobial protection is at its weakest. It the product passes challenge at the highest pH within the specification range, it will pass easily at any other pH within the specification.

23.8.13 Chlorphenesin

Chlorphenesin has broad-spectrum antimicrobial activity against bacteria and fungi, being also effective against *Pseudomonas spp.* and other problematic Gram-negative bacteria.

Chlorphenesin maintains its activity over the range from pH 3.0–8.0 and is compatible with most personal care ingredients. It is only slightly soluble in water (<1%) and may need heating to dissolve in systems with a high water content. Typical use concentrations range from 0.1% to 0.3%.

Chlorphenesin is permitted in most territories, with the following restrictions:

European Union

Maximum 0.3%

USA

Safe as used

Japan

Maximum 0.3% (not permitted for use in product intended to come into contact with mucous membranes)

23.8.14 Iodopropynyl Butylcarbamate

Iodopropynyl butylcarbamate (IPBC) has powerful activity against fungi, but very little antibacterial activity at permitted use concentrations.

IPBC is compatible with most personal care ingredients. It is virtually insoluble in water and may need heating to dissolve in systems with high water content. Typical use concentrations range from 0.01% to 0.02%.

IPBC is permitted in many territories, with the following restrictions:

European Union

Maximum 0.01% in leave-on products (but 0.0075% in deodorants and antiperspirants)

Maximum 0.02% in rinse-off products

Must not be used in lip or oral products, or in products intended for children under 3 years of age, except for bath products, shower gels and shampoo

USA

As for the European Union

Japan

Maximum 0.02% in all product categories

23.8.15 Bronopol

INCI name: 2-bromo-2-nitropropane-1,3-diol

Bronopol has extremely powerful antibacterial activity, but very little antifungal activity at permitted use concentrations. It is especially effective against the Gram-negative bacterium *Pseudomonas aeruginosa*, which, as stated earlier, can cause permanent blindness if sufficient numbers enter the eye.

Bronopol is highly water soluble and compatible with most types of cosmetic ingredients. It should not be used in combination with amines due to the increased potential for nitrosamine formation. It is important to note that bronopol cannot form nitrosamines in the absence of amines.

Typical use concentrations are 0.01–0.04%. Bronopol should be added below 40°C as it is increasingly unstable above this temperature.

European Union
  Maximum 0.1%
USA
  Maximum 0.1%
Japan
  Not permitted

23.9 Preservative Blends

It may be clear from the descriptions of the individual preservatives above that there is no single perfect preservative. Many do not have a complete spectrum of activity, or have weaknesses against certain organisms. In most cases, for good preservation, a broad-spectrum preservation system is essential (unless there is inherent activity against certain organisms from other formulation ingredients). This may be achieved in one of two ways. Either the formulator can make the decision to test various combinations of the individual preservatives or they can test premixed proprietary blends. The use of proprietary blends facilitates ease of handling and accuracy, both on a laboratory scale and in production as it is easier to handle a single preservative blend (they are usually in liquid form) than several individual components, some used in very small quantities. There are also benefits in inventory reduction.

23.10 'Secondary' Preservatives and 'Preservative Free'

In more recent years, there have been an increasing number of adverse reports about some specific preservatives and preservatives in general, mostly based on little or suspect science. Parabens have been especially affected by these recent developments. This is not the forum to discuss these issues in detail, but there is plenty of further reading available for the diligent researcher [7–17].

The result of the pressure, mostly from non-governmental organisations leading to consumer concerns, is that many manufacturers have been looking at alternative ways of preserving their products, simply to avoid having to include a 'dangerous' ingredient on the label. This has paved the way for the fairly recent phenomenon of using secondary preservatives and, in some cases, making overt claims of 'preservative free'.

Within the EU, preservatives are strictly regulated by the EU Cosmetics Directive [18], which must be enacted into law in each member state (to be replaced by the Cosmetics Regulation in 2013, which will apply automatically to all member states). Permitted preservatives are listed in Annex VI of the Directive (which will become Annex V in the Regulation), alongside the various restrictions and maximum permitted concentrations.

There is much less formalised regulation in the USA, and ingredients have their function(s) declared alongside their entry in the International Cosmetic Ingredient Dictionary and Handbook [19]. The Cosmetic Ingredients Review (CIR) Panel assess ingredients along similar lines to the SCCS (see later under Sect. 23.11) in the EU.

The Japanese regulations also include a positive list of permitted preservatives.

In the preamble to Annex VI of the EU Directive, it states:

1. Preservatives are substances which may be added to cosmetic products for the primary purpose of inhibiting the development of microorganisms in such products.
3. Other substances used in the formulation of cosmetic products may also have antimicrobial

properties and thus help in the preservation of the products..... these substances are not included in this Annex.

Therefore, if a substance has antimicrobial activity, but has an alternative (primary?) function in a cosmetic product, it is not officially a preservative. This makes it unclear as to what is *not* a preservative – is it a substance with little or no antimicrobial activity, or is it simply a substance that is not listed on Annex VI of the Cosmetics Directive?

Examples of secondary preservatives are given below, with the approximate concentration required if being used as the sole agent for preservation:

Glycerine (40%)
Propylene glycol (20–25%)
Butylene glycol (10–15%)
Ethanol (5–10%)
Caprylyl glycol (0.5–1.5%)

The first three substances listed work mostly by binding much of the available water, thereby reducing the water activity of the end product beyond the point where microorganisms can survive. Are they antimicrobial? There are many other substances that behave similarly over a range of different concentrations – at what point does the substance become antimicrobial?

It is possible to protect a product from microbial contamination without the use of 'legal' preservatives (in EU terms), but it is not possible to protect a product from microbial attack without the use of a preservation system (unless the product is totally anhydrous and, even in this instance, there is an argument for a preservation system). Below is a list of increasingly frequently used secondary preservatives with their 'primary' functions:

Caprylyl glycol (emollient)
Ethylhexylglycerine (emollient)
Pentylene glycol (emollient)
Levulinic acid (perfume)
p-Anisic acid (perfume)

It is perfectly legal to use these, and similar ingredients, provided there is a full justification for their inclusion. For example, it would be difficult to justify the use of an emollient in a hair colorant or a mouthwash, and the only possible explanation for the presence of caprylyl glycol would be for its antimicrobial activity. And this would not be legal within the EU.

The issue of preservative-free claims is a separate matter, in some respects. Whilst, from a legal point of view, a product preserved entirely with secondary preservatives may be 'preservative free', scientifically, it is preserved and contains a definable preservation system. 'Preservative free' is, therefore, a questionable position, but moreover, there are other implications. The use of this claim may be taken to imply that this has increased the safety of the product and, by further implication that product containing preservatives are, therefore, less safe. This is not the case. Continuing or increasing use of this claim may lead the EU Commission to look again at how preservatives are regulated within the Cosmetics Directive/Regulation.

23.11 Safety of Preservatives

Preservatives are biologically active substances and, therefore, have an inherent potential to have an adverse effect on any living cells, not only microbial cells. For this reason, it is obviously important to take all steps to ensure that preservatives are used safely. It is simply not possible to guarantee that no consumer will experience any adverse reaction (not only to preservatives – other ingredients may have the ability to elicit an adverse skin reaction – but their biological activity does increase the potential, as a general rule), but it is the case that all available information is evaluated prior to approval. Different markets have different ways of evaluating preservatives, but perhaps the most stringent is the European Union. The EU has appointed a specific body, the Scientific Committee for Consumer Safety (SCCS – also previously known as the SCCP and, before that, the SCCNFP), one of three safety groups set up to advise the EU Commission on safety matters [20]. The Committee provides opinions on health and safety risks (chemical, biological, mechanical and other physical risks) of non-food consumer products (e.g. cosmetic products and their ingredients, toys, textiles, clothing, personal care and household products) and services (e.g. tattooing, artificial sun tanning). A general video about the work of the three safety groups is available online [21].

The SCCS have evaluated all the preservatives listed on Annex VI since 1976, some of them on several occasions, and draw conclusions from all available data. The main role is to determine a maximum permitted concentration, but other restrictions may also be considered (e.g. specific product types, not for use on children under 3 years of age, etc.). This is usually based on allowing a margin of safety factor of at least 100 times the exposure of the lowest no observed adverse effect level (NOAEL) (if any) across all the available studies. The Final Opinion document produced by the SCCS contains a detailed discussion of the thorough process that led to the decision, where appropriate, and the details of the calculation employed, and examples may be found by following the link referenced below [22].

Successful preservation is a balance between controlling all potential contaminant microorganisms and ensuring that the risk of irritation or sensitisation is minimised. It is important to avoid over-preservation. The best method of achieving this is to test several different concentrations of one or more preservation systems. This will better optimise the preservation system. Most manufacturers tend to test only one preservation option, but this may be a false economy, especially when this increases the possibility of over-preservation.

23.12 Environmental Issues

If there is a failing in the EU Cosmetics Directive, it could be argued that it is the lack of consideration for possible environmental effects, both in general, and specifically for preservatives. Again, as with the aspect of human safety, preservatives are biologically active substances and, if they are entering the environment, there is a potential for adverse effects to aquatic species in particular. Preservatives are used at relatively low concentrations (rarely more than 1% in cosmetics), and when breakdown and dilution factors are taken into consideration, there is unlikely to be any measurable impact on the aquatic environment.

Taking the parabens as a useful example, given their status of being by far the most widely used preservatives [2], a study by Lee et al. measured the concentrations of the different parabens in the inflow of a sewage treatment facility and also at the outflow [23]. The highest concentration detected in the inflow to the sewage treatment plant was of propylparaben, rather than methylparaben, as might be anticipated from the known usage in cosmetics. The reason for the higher concentration of propylparaben may be due to its greater chemical stability, compared with methylparaben. The actual propylparaben concentration detected was 2.43 parts per trillion (0.000000000243%), and even more importantly, the concentration detected after treatment in the immediate outflow was reduced to 0.04 parts per trillion (ppt). The comparative figures for methylparaben were 1.47 ppt and 0.03 ppt, respectively. These concentrations are taken directly from the immediate vicinity of the outflow, and so much greater dilution follows on dispersion within the wider environment. These concentrations are many orders of magnitude below the levels where the substances have been shown to be toxic to aquatic organisms. For example, the acute fish toxicity for methylparaben is:

48 h LC_0 (Leuciscus idus – Golden Orfe)
50mg/l

50 mg/l is equivalent to 50 ppm – a figure approximately 1.67 trillion times higher than the concentration of methylparaben (0.03 ppt) detected in the sewage outflow. It may be concluded, therefore, that methylparaben is unlikely to have any measurable environmental impact.

Whilst it would be unwise to attempt to extrapolate these figures directly to all preservatives used in cosmetics, it does allow a sense of context, given the huge dilution factors involved.

General Note on Regulations

Science never stands still, and new data sometimes become available on substances that have been in use for many years, and the new data can potentially change the risk assessment of the substance in question. In such cases, the SCCS are asked to review the new information and consider whether the previous risk assessment is still valid. Where the SCCS determine that the risk has changed in the light of the new data, then the regulations may be changed to reflect this situation. For this reason, it is advisable to check the latest position with regard to SCCS opinions to confirm that the information provided on any specific preservative in this chapter remains up to date [22].

Take Home Messages

- Cosmetic products susceptible to microbial growth must be preserved for aesthetic reasons, but also, more importantly, for consumer safety.
- The combination of preservatives used must endow broad-spectrum protection against bacteria and fungi.
- Microbial challenge testing is vital to ensure that products are adequately protected against microbial growth.
- Preservative blends offer more robust protection than most single substances.
- Preservatives must be used carefully and at the lowest concentration required to achieve sufficient antimicrobial protection to ensure safety in use and to reduce the low risk of skin response even further, as much as possible.
- Preservatives are tightly regulated, and it is important to be aware of the restrictions in target markets and equally important to be aware of changes to regulations as they occur.
- 'Preservative free' claims are contentious and may be best avoided.
- There is no evidence of any adverse environmental impact resulting from the use of preservatives in cosmetics.

References

1. Engel LS, Hill JM, Moreau JM, Green LC, Hobden JA, O'Callaghan RJ (1998) Pseudomonas aeruginosa protease IV produces corneal damage and contributes to bacterial virulence. Invest Ophthalmol Vis Sci 39(3):662–665
2. Steinberg D (2010) Cosmetics & Toiletries magazine, 125:46–51
3. Azelis product literature http://azelis.com
4. Clariant product literature http://clariant.com
5. Tallon M, Merianos JJ, Subramanian S (2009) Non-destructive method for determining the actual concentration of free formaldehyde in personal care formulations containing formaldehyde donors. SOFW J 135(5):22–32
6. Winkelman JGM et al (2002) Kinetics and chemical equilibrium of the hydration of formaldehyde. Chem Eng Sci 57:4067–4076
7. http://personalcaretruth.com/2012/02/parabens-in-perspective-an-introduction/
8. http://personalcaretruth.com/2012/02/parabens-in-perspective-part-i/
9. http://personalcaretruth.com/2012/02/parabens-in-perspective-part-ii/
10. http://personalcaretruth.com/2012/02/parabens-in-perspective-part-iii/
11. http://personalcaretruth.com/2012/02/parabens-in-perspective-part-iv/
12. http://personalcaretruth.com/2012/02/parabens-in-perspective-part-v/
13. http://personalcaretruth.com/2012/02/parabens-in-perspective-part-vi/
14. http://personalcaretruth.com/2012/02/parabens-in-perspective-part-vii/
15. http://personalcaretruth.com/2012/02/parabens-in-perspective-part-viii/
16. http://personalcaretruth.com/2012/02/parabens-in-perspective-part-ix/
17. http://personalcaretruth.com/2012/02/parabens-in-perspective-part-x/
18. http://tiny.cc/o904y/2012/02
19. Gottschlack TE, Bailey JE (eds) (2012) International cosmetic ingredient dictionary and handbook. Personal Care Products Council, Inc, Washington
20. http://ec.europa.eu/health/scientific_committees/consumer_safety/index_en.htm/2012/02
21. http://ec.europa.eu/health/scientific_committees/videos/videos/video_committees_en.htm/2012/02
22. http://ec.europa.eu/health/scientific_committees/consumer_safety/opinions/index_en.htm/2012/02
23. Lee HB, Peart TE, Svoboda ML (2005) Determination of endocrine-disrupting phenols, acidic pharmaceuticals, and personal-care products in sewage by solid-phase extraction and gas chromatography-mass spectrometry. J Chromatogr A 1094:122–129

Potential Allergens in Moisturizing Creams

24

Ana Rita Travassos and An Goossens

24.1 Introduction

These days, everyone is using cosmetic products, and allergic reactions are increasingly observed [1]. Indeed, in our department during the last 11 years, 21% of the patients tested suffered from adverse reactions to cosmetics compared to 16% in the previous decade.

Contact allergic reactions to cosmetics may be delayed-type reactions resulting in allergic or photoallergic contact dermatitis. More exceptionally, immediate-type allergic reactions occur, such as the contact urticaria (syndrome).

The cosmetic allergens involved can reach the skin in several different ways: direct application; occasional contact with an allergen-contaminated surface; airborne contact; transfer by the hands to more sensitive areas (e.g., the eyelids), so-called ectopic dermatitis, by a product used by the partner, or any other person in close contact with (connubial or consort dermatitis); or photo-induced, resulting from contact with a photoallergen and exposure to sunlight (particularly UV-A light). An allergic contact dermatitis may sometimes spread to other areas of the body not in direct contact with the allergen, which is comparable to a reaction by systemic exposure (in which the allergen may reach the skin through the circulatory system and produce a systemic contact-type dermatitis), the latter being extremely rare with cosmetics [1].

In our Contact Allergy Unit in Leuven, we recorded using a standardized form [2] positive patch-test reactions or positive usage tests to cosmetic products (from different cosmetic categories) responsible for allergic contact dermatitis or contact urticaria, as well as positive reactions to specific ingredients in them. Moisturizers were the main causal cosmetic products involved, i.e., responsible for 33% of 992 allergic reactions, the results of which will be discussed here.

24.2 Allergic Contact Dermatitis (ACD) Due to Moisturizers

24.2.1 Diagnosis

Taking the history of the patient and inspecting the clinical symptoms and localization of the lesions frequently suggest the etiological

A.R. Travassos
Clínica Universitária de Dermatologia – Hospital de Santa Maria,
Avenida Professor Egas Moniz, 1649-035
Lisbon, Portugal
e-mail: ritatravassos@gmail.com

A. Goossens (✉)
Contact Allergy Unit – Department of Dermatology,
University Hospital St. Rafaël,
Katholieke Universiteit Leuven,
Kapucijnenvoer 33, B-3000, Leuven, Belgium
e-mail: an.goossens@uzleuven.be

M. Lodén, H.I. Maibach (eds.), *Treatment of Dry Skin Syndrome*,
DOI 10.1007/978-3-642-27606-4_24,

factor(s). Allergen identification for a patient with a possible allergic contact dermatitis from cosmetics is performed by means of patch testing with the baseline (standard) series, cosmetic series, and the product(s) used by the patient and, if possible, also with the ingredients present. If a photoallergic contact dermatitis is suspected, photopatch tests with the suspected agents are needed [3]. Moreover, semi-open tests (in case of possible irritants), usage tests, and repeated open application tests (ROAT) may also be performed [1]. Once an allergen has been identified, it is the dermatologist's task to provide specific advice about the products that can be used safely and the specific ingredients that must be avoided [1, 4].

24.2.2 Causal Allergens

According to our study, fragrances together with preservatives were the most frequent classes of allergens in moisturizers, followed by vehicle components, emulsifiers, and conditioning agents (Table 24.1). Figure 24.1 illustrates the relative frequency of reactions to the allergen's classes, while Tables 24.2 and 24.3 give the reactions to the individual "nonfragrance" and fragrance allergens, respectively, the first along with the corresponding literature references. The nature of the individual fragrances having caused reactions in moisturizers has been discussed in detail in a previous study [2].

24.3 Specific Allergens in Moisturizers

24.3.1 Fragrances

Currently, fragrance mix (FM) 1 and 2, *Myroxylon pereirae* and to a minor extent colophonium, are the diagnosis markers of perfume allergy in the baseline series [2].

FM 1 contains amyl cinnamal, cinnamal, cinnamyl alcohol, hydroxycitronellal, eugenol, isoeugenol, geraniol, and *Evernia prunastri* (oakmoss) and remains the best screening agent for contact allergy to perfumes because it is said to detect some 70–80% of all perfume allergies [51]. FM 2, which consists of hydroxyisohexyl 3-cyclohexene carboxaldehyde (HICC), farnesol, citral, citronellol, coumarin, and alfa-hexyl cinnamaldehyde [52], detects additional cases [2], underlining its importance as a screening agent [1].

Fragrance components may be allergenic by themselves, but may, as in the case of terpenes such as limonene [53] and linalool [54], form sensitizing oxidation products; they sometimes also contain contaminants. For example, resin acids and their oxidation products are the main allergens in colophonium and the widely used perfume ingredient *Evernia furfuracea* (or tree moss, also obtained from pine species); however, they were found as contaminants in *Evernia prunastri* (oakmoss), both in the qualities used by the fragrance industry and in patch-test materials. Besides, atranol and chloratranol have been identified as being the most potent allergens in oak moss ever described [1, 55].

Moreover, multiple positive patch-test reactions are frequently associated with fragrance allergy and often indicate the presence of common or cross-reacting ingredients in natural products [1, 56], cross-reactions between simple fragrance chemicals, or concomitant reactions.

Sensitization to fragrance components is most often induced by highly perfumed products, such as toilet waters, aftershave lotion, and deodorants [4], followed by moisturizers, in which they became relatively more important during the last decade (Table 24.1; Fig. 24.1). HICC and limonene were the most frequent individual fragrance allergens in them (Table 24.3; Fig. 24.2) [2].

24.3.2 Preservatives

Preservatives, used to prevent microbiological contamination that may spoil cosmetic or other products [57], are important sensitizers in water-based products, such as moisturizers. The proportion of positive reactions to them in moisturizers did not differ in the two periods studied (Table 24.1; Fig. 24.1). Historically, changing contact allergy epidemics have been observed [57], as well as variations between different countries in the spectrum of the allergenic preservatives [4]. During the last decades, a considerable number of newly developed preservatives, such as MCI/MI, formaldehyde releasers, and methyldibro glutaronitrile were found to be sensitizers and were added to the baseline series or to special patch-test series [13].

Table 24.1 Total number of positive reactions to allergens in moisturizers

Classes of allergens	2000–2005	2006–2010	Total (%)
Fragrances	9	108	117 (35.5)
Preservatives	23	90	113 (34.3)
Vehicle components and emulsifiers	22	40	62 (18.8)
Conditioning agents[a]	6	9	15 (4.5)
Plant extracts	9	4	13 (3.9)
Antioxidants	1	5	6 (1.8)
UV absorbers/filters	2	2	4 (1.2)
Totals	72	258	**330** (100)

[a]Conditioning agents are ingredients that may have several other functions, such as, for example, preservative (i.e., ethylhexylglycerin) or disinfectant properties (i.e., propolis extract)

24.3.2.1 Formaldehyde and Formaldehyde Releasers

The use of formaldehyde has decreased markedly in cosmetics, but at the same time, the use of formaldehyde releasers did increase [58]. In our department, 58% of allergic reactions to preservatives in moisturizers were due to formaldehyde and formaldehyde releasers (Fig. 24.3). They have been shown to be present, for example, in approximately 20% of cosmetics and personal care products in the USA [5] and 25% of cosmetics in Sweden [7].

Formaldehyde releasers are chemicals that in the presence of water release formaldehyde by hydrolysis [59]. The antimicrobial activity of these preservatives most likely results from formaldehyde release, but it has also been postulated that at least some of these substances both act as preservatives [60] and contact allergens independently [61].

Moreover, many patch-tested patients react both to the formaldehyde releasers diazolidinyl urea and imidazolidinyl urea [62], which may be explained by sharing a common metabolite: (4-hydroxymethyl-2,5-dioxo-imidazolidin-4-yl) urea (compound HU) [63].

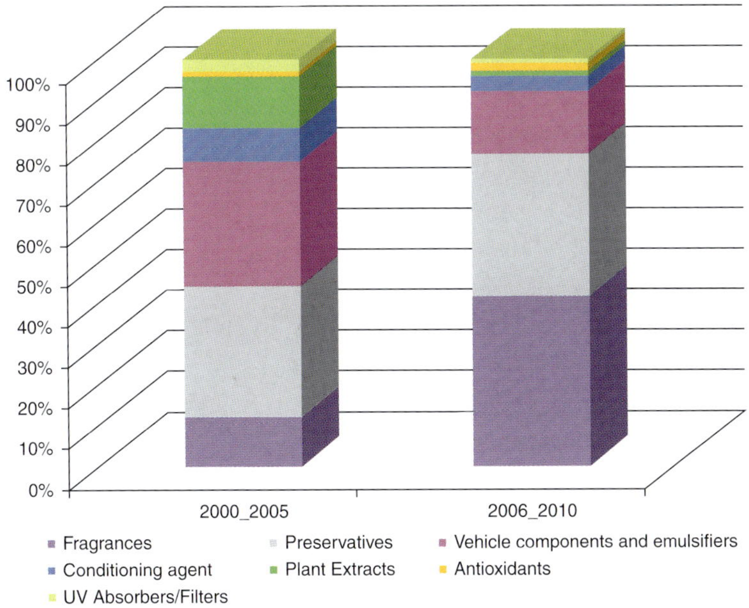

Fig. 24.1 Relative frequency (%) of allergens in moisturizers during the periods: 2000–2005 and 2006–2010

Table 24.2 Allergic reactions to nonfragrance allergens in moisturizers

Nonfragrance allergens	Literature references	2000–2005	2006–2010	Total
Preservatives				**(113)**
Benzoic acid	–	–	1	1
2-Bromo-2-nitropropane-1,3-diol	[5–7]	2	7	9
Chlorphenesin	[8, 9]	1	2	3
Diazolidinyl urea	[5–7]	2	12	14
Dichlorobenzyl alcohol	[10]	1	1	2
DMDM hydantoin	[5–7]	2	4	6
Farnesol[a]	[11, 12]	–	1	1
Formaldehyde	[5–7]	5	18	23
Imidazolidinyl urea	[5–7]	2	10	12
Methyldibromo glutaronitrile	[7, 13, 14]	3	2	5
Methylchloro- and methylisothiazolinone	[7, 13]	–	6	6
Methylisothiazolinone	[7, 13, 15, 16]	–	2	2
Parabens	[7, 17]	3	14	17
Phenoxyethanol	[7, 14, 18]	2	7	9
Potassium sorbate	[19, 20]	–	2	2
Quaternium-15	[5–7]	–	1	1
Vehicle components and emulsifiers				**(62)**
Arachidyl glucoside	–	–	1	1
Butyrospermum parkii butter	–	–	4	4
Cetearyl glucoside	[21]	–	1	1
Cetyl alcohol	[22]	–	4	4
Decyl glucoside	[23–25]	–	1	1
Hydroxyethyl acrylate	[26]	–	1	1
Isononyl isononanoate	[27]	–	2	2
Isopropyl myristate	[28]	–	1	1
Lanolin alcohols	[29, 30]	9	13	22
Lauroyl collagen amino acids	–	1	–	1
Lauryl alcohol	[31]	3	–	3
Methoxy peg-22/dodecyl glycol copolymer	[31, 32]	4	–	4
Propylene glycol	[33]	3	4	7
Tetrahydroxypropyl ethylenediamine	[34]	–	5	5
Sorbitan oleate	[35]	–	1	1
Sorbitan sesquioleate	[35]	2	2	4
Conditioning agents				**(15)**
Bisabolol	[36, 37]	1	2	3
Ethylhexylglycerin	[23, 38]	2	4	6
Panthenol	[39, 40]	2	2	4
Propolis extract	[41]	1	1	2
Plant extracts				**(13)**
Achillea millefolium extract	–	1	–	1
Arnica montana extract	[42]	1	–	1
Avena sativa extract[b]	[43]	–	1	1
Calendula officinalis extract	[42]	–	2	2
Compositae mixture	[42]	2	–	2
Euphorbia extract	–	1	–	1
Melaleuca alternifolia leaf oil	[44]	4	1	5

Antioxidants				**(6)**
Ascorbyl tetraisopalmitate	[45]	–	1	1
Propyl gallate	[46]	1	1	2
Sodium metabisulfite	[47]	–	1	1
Tocopherol	[48]	–	2	2
UV absorbers/filters				**(4)**
Benzophenone-3	[49]	–	1	1
Ethylhexyl methoxycinnamate	–	1	–	1
Methylene bis-benzotriazolyl tetramethylbutylphenol	[50]	–	1	1
Terephthalylidene dicamphor sulfonic acid	–	1	–	1
		63	**150**	**213**

[a]Farnesol, which is a fragrance allergen, has also antimicrobial properties
[b]Immediate type I reaction to *Avena sativa* extract

Table 24.3 Number of reactions to fragrance allergens in moisturizers

Fragrance allergens	Presence confirmed	Presence not confirmed	Total
FM 1	4	29	33
FM 2	10	11	21
Hydroxycitronellal	3	6	9
Geraniol	7	4	11
Eugenol	–	1	1
Isoeugenol	–	3	3
Oak Moss		3	3
Hydroxyisohexyl 3-cyclohexene carboxaldeyde (Lyral®)	11	10	21
Citral	2	–	2
Farnesol	1	1	2
Citronellol	3	1	4
Coumarin	1	–	1
Limonene	13	1	14
Linalool	4	–	4
Butylphenyl methylpropional	–	2	2
α-isomethyl ionone	1	–	1
Menthol	1	–	1
Perfume	7	–	7
Eucalyptus oil	1	4	5
Lavender oil	1	–	1
Neroli oil	2	2	4
Niaouli oil	1	–	1
Orange peel oil	1	–	1
Rose oil	2	–	2
Tea tree oil	1	–	1
	77	**78**	**155**

Adapted from [2]
The presence of a fragrance allergen was considered confirmed when, according to the label, it was present in the suspect product and not confirmed, when its presence was only suspected

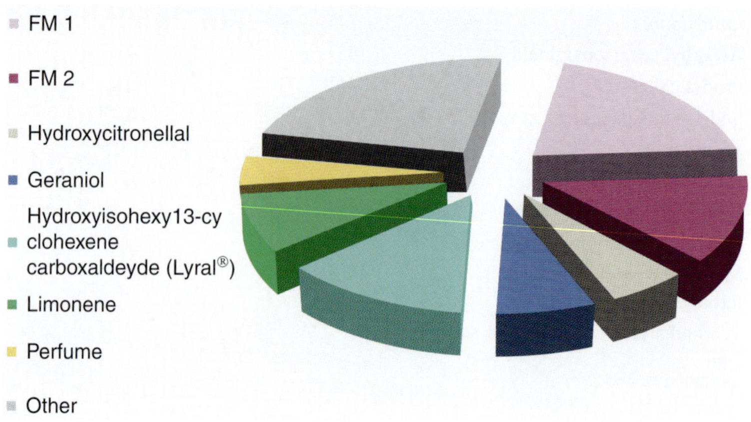

Fig. 24.2 Proportion of the reactions to fragrance allergens in moisturizers (Adapted from [2])

24.3.2.2 Methylchloro- and Methylisothiazolinone

Methylchloro- and methylisothiazolinone mixture (MCI/MI), commonly used since the 1980s, previously became an important cause of contact allergies, and its frequency is actually rising again. MCI/MI had been recommended (first up to 30, later 15 ppm) to be used only in rinse-off products; however, it is still found in several leave-on products, such as moisturizers [1].

Recently, it has been replaced by methylisothiazolinone (MI) alone, once thought to be a weaker allergen [1, 15]. However, MI is also a less efficient preservative, which requires larger use concentrations [1], i.e., in cosmetics it is allowed up to 100 ppm [16].

Sensitization seems to be particularly related to its presence in intimate hygiene products, i.e., wipes (or moist toilette paper) for babies and adults [1, 15], in which MCI/MI used to be the allergenic culprit previously. The use of such products (or any other leave-on product containing MCI/MI or MI) in nonkeratinized areas or under occlusion enhances their sensitizing potential [15].

24.3.2.3 Parabens

Parabens have a broad spectrum of activity, and enhancement of microbial coverage is achieved by combining them with other biocides (such as formaldehyde releasers, MCI/MI, or phenoxyetanol) [17]. In Sweden, methylparaben was the most frequently identified preservative in cosmetics and in 44% of the cosmetic products at least one paraben was present [7]; in the USA, this percentage was also more than 35% [64].

Parabens are rare causes of ACD, and when it occurs, the primary sensitization source is most often a topical pharmaceutical product [1, 4]. They are actually "banned" from use in cosmetics by several companies, which is a consumer and political issue since carcinogenic and estrogenic effects have not been demonstrated in humans and seem unlikely from its use in cosmetic [65]. However, in Denmark they are no longer allowed in products for children under the age of 3.

24.3.2.4 Other Preservatives

Methyldibromo glutaronitrile, used as a mixture with phenoxyethanol (Euxyl K400), became such an important allergen that it was banned from cosmetic products in the EU in 2007 [66], which was followed by a decrease of positive reactions observed [13].

Phenoxyetanol that is considered a rare allergen [18] was, in our department, responsible for 8% of the positive reactions to preservatives in moisturizers (Table 24.2; Fig. 24.3).

Chlorphenesin may cross-react with mephenesin, a rubefacient used in topical pharmaceutical products [9].

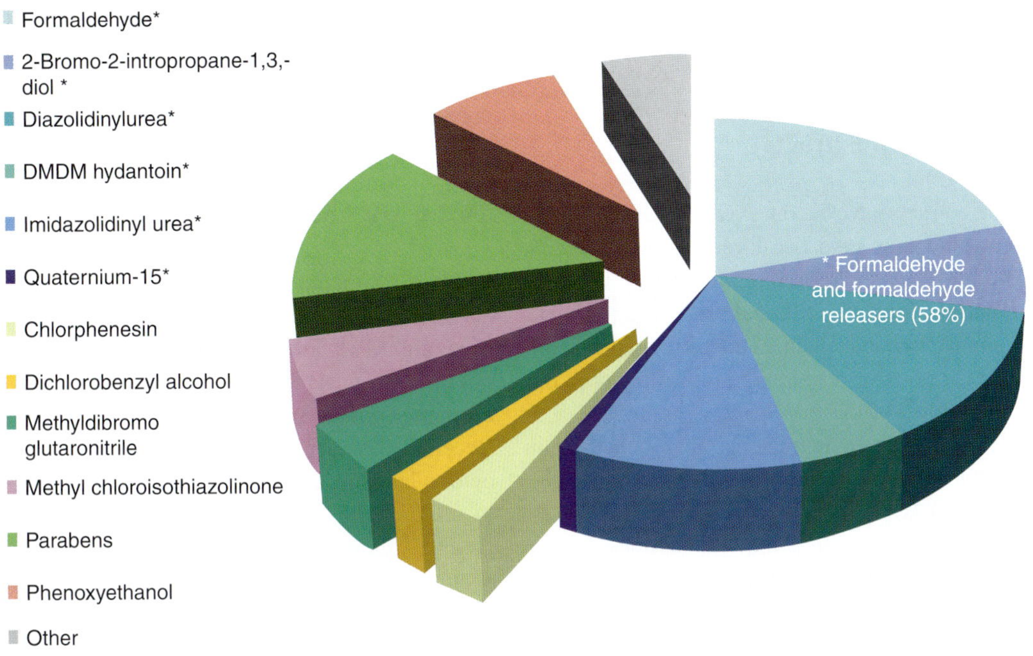

Fig. 24.3 Proportion of reactions to the preservative allergens in moisturizers

24.3.3 Vehicle Component, Emulsifiers, Humectants, and Conditioning Agents

The classical examples of potential allergenic vehicle components are lanolin alcohols (Table 24.2) [29, 30], fatty alcohols (e.g., cetyl alcohol) [22], and propylene glycol [33]. More recently, several esters such as dicaprylyl maleate [67], isononyl isononanoate and trioleyl phosphate [27], as well as humectants such as butylene glycol [68] and pentylene glycol [69] were identified as potential allergens.

Alkyl glucosides, i.e., condensation products of fatty alcohols with glucose such as coco- and lauryl glucosides [21] are often used as mild surfactants, but also as emulsifiers, particularly cetearyl- and decyl glucoside [24, 25]. They may cross-react with other alkyl glucosides and also with methyl glucoside dioleate (a chemically closely related surfactant) [23].

We also observed some cases of sensitization to bisabolol (Table 24.2), a monocyclic sesquiterpene alcohol derived from *Matricaria chamomilla* that has been included in several cosmetic products because of its anti-inflammatory and skin-soothing properties [36].

Other possible allergens include ethylhexylglycerin (syn.: octoxyglycerin), a skin conditioning agent [38], and copolymers, such as methoxy PEG-17 and PEG-22/dodecyl glycol copolymers (alkoxylated alcohols and synthetic polymers used as emulsion stabilizers, suspending and viscosity-increasing agents, and also as skin conditioners) [31, 32] and polyvinylpyrrolidone (PVP)/eicosene, which was reported as a cause of a generalized reaction [70]. We do not know whether allergic reactions are due to the copolymers themselves or to degradation products in them, larger molecules being less likely to induce sensitization.

Some other "rare" allergens in moisturizers reported are, for example, alkyl rhamnoside-C5 (a sugar derivate used as a cosurfactant for microemulsions) in a product particularly recommended for use in atopic skin [71] and phytantriol (3,7,11,15-tetramethylhexadecane-1,2,3-triol), a fatty alcohol used as a surfactant, penetration enhancer, and humectant in a facial cream [72].

24.3.4 Plant Extracts

Plant extracts have become very popular in recent years and may give rise to severe ACD [1, 73, 74]. *Melaleuca alternifolia*, frequently used for its antibacterial or antifungal properties [44], was the most frequent plant extract allergen responsible for positive reactions to moisturizers in our unit (Table 24.2).

Protein-derived ingredients are often used in moisturizers, for atopic skin (often in children). Oatmeal (Avena) [75], hydrolyzed wheat [76], or soybean extracts [77] may sometimes induce ACD, although immediate-type reactions are more frequently seen [1]. We observed an immediate-type reaction to *Avena sativa* (wild oat) extract from a moisturizer in an atopic patient. The diagnosis was confirmed by prick tests and detection of specific IgE antibodies (by ELISA) in the patient's serum [43]. In fact, the use of cosmetics with oat (or other flour extracts) in atopic patients is still controversial. Some authors suggest their avoidance, based on the possible risk of subsequent sensitization to food proteins [78], while others have considered the evidence for sensitization from these products to be insufficient [79, 80].

Tanacetum parthenium (feverfew) is a recognized Compositae plant sensitizer, especially due to its content of parthenolide. Recently, allergic reactions to a "parthenolide-free" feverfew extract, used because of its anti-inflammatory properties, have been reported, the presence of traces of parthenolide not being excluded [81]. Patients allergic to plants belonging to this family also often react to fragrance allergens, which is probably due to the common presence of (oxidized) terpenes [42].

24.3.5 Antioxidants

Certain antioxidants are used in moisturizing products to prevent aging, some of which responsible for ACD, i.e., tocoferol (vitamin E), retinol palmitate and acetate [48], ascorbic acid (vitamin C) [82], and its tetraisopalmitate ester [45]; also, ubiquinone and idebenone or hydroxydecyl ubiquinone (a synthetic analog of coenzyme Q10) are potential allergens [83–85].

24.3.6 UV Absorbers/Filters

Because of media attention being given to the carcinogenic and accelerated skin-aging effects of sunlight, UV absorbers are increasingly used, not only in sunscreen products, but also in other cosmetic products including moisturizers [1]. Recently, contact and photocontact allergy to octocrylene has been increasingly observed, also in children [86]. As with benzophenone compounds, photoallergic reactions to octocrylene occur particularly in patients previously photosensitized by ketoprofen, a nonsteroidal anti-inflammatory drug, which is attributed to cross-reactivity [1, 87].

Conclusion

In agreement with the literature, the main allergens in moisturizers were found to be fragrance components and preservative agents; hence, the most frequent allergens, such as HICC and limonene and MCI/MI and MI, respectively, should perhaps be avoided. Special care should be taken regarding products recommended for use in atopic skin, particularly those containing protein-derived materials. Indeed, their use is still controversial because of a possible risk of subsequent sensitization to food.

Take Home Messages

- Contact allergic reactions to cosmetics (such as moisturizers) are increasingly observed.
- The most frequent allergic reactions to moisturizers are allergic contact dermatitis (ACD), but also immediate-type reactions (such as contact urticaria syndrome) may occur.

- Patch tests are the gold standard for diagnosing contact dermatitis, while prick tests for contact urticaria.
- The most important sensitizing culprits in moisturizers are fragrances and preservatives.
- Currently, FM 1 and 2, *Myroxylon pereirae* and, to a lesser extent colophonium, are the diagnostic markers for perfume allergy in the baseline series. Although FM 1 can detect some 70–80% of all perfume allergies, testing with additional markers increases sensitivity.
- Variations in the spectrum of the allergenic preservatives are continuously observed. As new preservatives are introduced and found to be sensitizers, they are progressively added to the baseline or to special patch test series (i.e., MCI/MI and MI).
- Plant extracts and fragrances may contain common allergens; hence, patients may develop multiple allergies.
- Antioxidants and sunscreens have been progressively introduced into moisturizing products in order to prevent ageing; however, they add to the sensitization potential in them.

References

1. Goossens A (2011) Contact-allergic reactions to cosmetics. J Allergy 2011:467071. Epub 2011 Feb 21
2. Nardelli A, Drieghe J, Claes L, Boey L, Goossens A (2011) Fragrance allergens in 'specific' cosmetic products. Contact Dermatitis 64:212–219
3. Bruynzeel DP, Ferguson J, Andersen K, Gonçalo M, English J, Goossens A, Holzle E, Ibbotson SH, Lecha M, Lehmann P, Leonard F, Moseley H, Pigatto P, Tanew A, European Taskforce for Photopatch Testing (2004) Photopatch testing: a consensus methodology for Europe. J Eur Acad Dermatol Venereol 18: 679–682
4. Goossens AE (2006) Sensitizing substances. In: Loden M, Maibach HI (eds) Dry skin and moisturizers: chemistry and function. CRC Press, Boca Raton, pp 515–522
5. de Groot AC, White IR, Flyvholm MA, Lensen G, Coenraads PJ (2010) Formaldehyde-releasers in cosmetics: relationship to formaldehyde contact allergy. Part 1. Characterization, frequency and relevance of sensitization, and frequency of use in cosmetics. Contact Dermatitis 62:2–17
6. de Groot A, White IR, Flyvholm MA, Lensen G, Coenraads PJ (2010) Formaldehyde-releasers in cosmetics: relationship to formaldehyde contact allergy. Part 2. Patch test relationship to formaldehyde contact allergy, experimental provocation tests, amount of formaldehyde released, and assessment of risk to consumers allergic to formaldehyde. Contact Dermatitis 62:18–31
7. Yazar K, Johnsson S, Lind ML, Boman A, Lidén C (2011) Preservatives and fragrances in selected consumer-available cosmetics and detergents. Contact Dermatitis 64:265–272
8. Brown VL, Orton DI (2005) Two cases of facial dermatitis due to chlorphenesin in cosmetics. Contact Dermatitis 52:48–49
9. Wakelin SH, White IR (1997) Dermatitis from chlorphenesin in a facial cosmetic. Contact Dermatitis 37: 138–139
10. Thormann H, Kollander M, Andersen KE (2009) Allergic contact dermatitis from dichlorobenzyl alcohol in a patient with multiple contact allergies. Contact Dermatitis 60:295–296
11. Katsuyama M, Kobayashi Y, Ichikawa H, Mizuno A, Miyachi Y, Matsunaga K, Kawashima M (2005) A novel method to control the balance of skin microflora Part 2. A study to assess the effect of a cream containing farnesol and xylitol on atopic dry skin. J Dermatol Sci 38:207–213
12. Gilpin S, Maibach H (2010) Allergic contact dermatitis caused by farnesol: clinical relevance. Cutan Ocul Toxicol 29:278–287
13. Schnuch A, Lessmann H, Geier J, Uter W (2011) Contact allergy to preservatives. Analysis of IVDK data 1996 – 2009. Br J Dermatol 164:1316–1325. doi:10.1111/j.1365-2133.2011.10253.x, Epub ahead of print
14. Tosti A, Guerra L, Bardazzi F, Gasparri F (1991) Euxyl K 400: a new sensitizer in cosmetics. Contact Dermatitis 25:89–93
15. García-Gavín J, Vansina S, Kerre S, Naert A, Goossens A (2010) Methylisothiazolinone, an emerging allergen in cosmetics? Contact Dermatitis 63:96–101
16. Ackermann L, Aalto-Korte K, Alanko K, Hasan T, Jolanki R, Lammintausta K, Lauerma A, Laukkanen A, Liippo J, Riekki R, Vuorela AM, Rantanen T (2011) Contact sensitization to methylisothiazolinone in Finland – a multicentre study. Contact Dermatitis 64:49–53
17. Cashman AL, Warshaw EM (2005) Parabens: a review of epidemiology, structure, allergenicity, and hormonal properties. Dermatitis 16:57–66
18. Lovell CR, White IR, Boyle J (1984) Contact dermatitis from phenoxyethanol in aqueous cream BP. Contact Dermatitis 11:187
19. Raison-Peyron N, Meynadier JM, Meynadier J (2000) Sorbic acid: an unusual cause of systemic contact dermatitis in an infant. Contact Dermatitis 43: 247–248

20. Patrizi A, Orlandi C, Vincenzi C, Bardazzi F (1999) Allergic contact dermatitis caused by sorbic acid: rare occurrence. Am J Contact Dermat 10:52
21. Goossens A, Decraene T, Platteaux N, Nardelli A, Rasschaert V (2003) Glucosides as unexpected allergens in cosmetics. Contact Dermatitis 48:164–166
22. Kiec-Swierczynska M, Krecisz B, Swierczynska-Machura D (2005) Photoallergic and allergic reaction to 2-hydroxy-4-methoxybenzophenone (sunscreen) and allergy to cetyl alcohol in cosmetic cream. Contact Dermatitis 53:170–171
23. Pascoe D, Moreau L, Sasseville D (2010) Emergent and unusual allergens in cosmetics. Dermatitis 21: 127–137
24. Blondeel A (2003) Contact allergy to the mild surfactant decylglucoside. Contact Dermatitis 49:304–305
25. Andersen KE, Goossens A (2006) Decyl glucoside contact allergy from a sunscreen product. Contact Dermatitis 54:349–350
26. Lucidarme N, Aerts O, Roelandts R, Goossens A (2008) Hydroxyethyl acrylate: a potential allergen in cosmetic creams? Contact Dermatitis 59:321–322
27. Goossens A, Verbruggen K, Cattaert N, Boey L (2008) New cosmetic allergens: isononyl isononanoate and trioleyl phosphate. Contact Dermatitis 59:320–321
28. Bharati A, King CM (2004) Allergic contact dermatitis from isohexadecane and isopropyl myristate. Contact Dermatitis 50:256–257
29. Lee B, Warshaw E (2008) Lanolin allergy: history, epidemiology, responsible allergens, and management. Dermatitis 19:63–72
30. Warshaw EM, Nelsen DD, Maibach HI, Marks JG, Zug KA, Taylor JS, Rietschel RL, Fowler JF, Mathias CG, Pratt MD, Sasseville D, Storrs FJ, Belsito DV, DeLeo VA (2009) Positive patch test reactions to lanolin: cross-sectional data from the North American contact dermatitis group, 1994 to 2006. Dermatits 20:79–88
31. Goossens A, Armingaud P, Avenel-Audran M, Begon-Bagdassarian I, Constandt L, Giordano-Labadie F, Girardin P, Coz CJ, Milpied-Homsi B, Nootens C, Pecquet C, Tennstedt D, Vanhecke E (2002) An epidemic of allergic contact dermatitis due to epilating products. Contact Dermatitis 47:67–70
32. Le Coz CJ, Heid E (2001) Allergic contact dermatitis from methoxy PEG-17/dodecyl glycol copolymer (Elfacos OW 100). Contact Dermatitis 44:308–309
33. Warshaw EM, Botto NC, Maibach HI, Fowler JF Jr, Rietschel RL, Zug KA, Belsito DV, Taylor JS, DeLeo VA, Pratt MD, Sasseville D, Storrs FJ, Marks JG Jr, Mathias CG (2009) Positive patch-test reactions to propylene glycol: a retrospective cross-sectional analysis from the North American Contact Dermatitis Group, 1996 to 2006. Dermatitis 20:14–20
34. Goossens A, Baret I, Swevers A (2011) Allergic contact dermatitis caused by tetrahydroxypropyl ethylenediamine in cosmetic products. Contact Dermatitis 64:161–164
35. Pereira F, Cunha H, Dias M (1997) Contact dermatitis due to emulsifiers. Contact Dermatitis 36:114
36. Russell K, Jacob SE (2010) Bisabolol. Dermatitis 21:57–58
37. Wilkinson SM, Hausen BM, Beck MH (1995) Allergic contact dermatitis from plant extracts in a cosmetic. Contact Dermatitis 33:58–59
38. Linsen G, Goossens A (2002) Allergic contact dermatitis from ethylhexylglycerin. Contact Dermatitis 47:169
39. Roberts H, Williams J, Tate B (2006) Allergic contact dermatitis to panthenol and cocamidopropyl PG dimonium chloride phosphate in a facial hydrating lotion. Contact Dermatitis 55:369–370
40. Stables GI, Wilkinson SM (1998) Allergic contact dermatitis due to panthenol. Contact Dermatitis 38: 236–237
41. Ting PT, Silver S (2004) Allergic contact dermatitis to propolis. J Drugs Dermatol 3:685–686
42. Paulsen E, Chistensen LP, Andersen KE (2008) Cosmetics and herbal remedies with Compositae plant extracts – are they tolerated by Compositae-allergic patients? Contact Dermatitis 58:15–23
43. Vansina S, Debilde D, Morren MA, Goossens A (2010) Sensitizing oat extracts in cosmetic creams: is there an alternative? Contact Dermatitis 63:169–171
44. Fritz TM, Burg G, Krasovec M (2001) Allergic contact dermatitis to cosmetics containing *Melaleuca alternifolia* (tea tree oil). Ann Dermatol Venereol 128:123–126
45. Swinnen I, Goossens A (2011) Allergic contact dermatitis caused by ascorbyl tetraisopalmitate. Contact Dermatitis 64:241–242
46. Foti C, Bonamonte D, Cassano N, Conserva A, Vena GA (2010) Allergic contact dermatitis to propyl gallate and pentylene glycol in an emollient cream. Australas J Dermatol 51:147–148
47. Malik MM, Hegarty MA, Bourke JF (2007) Sodium metabisulfite – a marker for cosmetic allergy? Contact Dermatitis 56:241–242
48. Manzano D, Aguirre A, Gardeazabal J, Eizaguirre X, Díaz Pérez JL (1994) Allergic contact dermatitis from tocopheryl acetate (vitamin E) and retinol palmitate (vitamin A) in a moisturizing cream. Contact Dermatitis 31:324
49. Silva R, Almeida LM, Brandão FM (1995) Photoallergy to oxybenzone in cosmetic creams. Contact Dermatitis 32:176
50. González-Pérez R, Trébol I, García-Río I, Arregui MA, Soloeta R (2007) Allergic contact dermatitis from methylene-bis-benzotriazolyl tetramethylbutylphenol (Tinosorb M). Contact Dermatitis 56:121
51. Frosch PJ, Pilz B, Andersen KE et al (1995) Patch testing with fragrances: results of a multi-center study of the European Environmental and Contact Dermatitis Research Group with 48 frequently used constituents of perfumes. Contact Dermatitis 33:333–342
52. Frosch PJ, Johansen JD, Menné T et al (1999) Lyral is an important sensitizer in patients sensitive to fragrances. Br J Dermatol 141:1076–1083
53. Matura M, Goossens A, Bordalo O, Garcia-Bravo B, Magnusson K, Wrangsjo K, Karlberg AT (2003) Patch testing with oxidized R- (+)-limonene and its hydroperoxide fraction. Contact Dermatitis 49:15–21

54. Sköld M, Börje A, Matura M, Karlberg AT (2002) Studies on the autoxidation and sensitizing capacity of the fragrance chemical linalool, identifying a linalool hydroperoxide. Contact Dermatitis 46: 267–272
55. Johansen JD, Bernard G, Giménez-Arnau E et al (2006) Comparison of elicitation potential of chloroatranol and atranol – 2 allergens in oak moss absolute. Contact Dermatitis 54:192–195
56. Paulsen E, Andersen KE (2005) Colophonium and Compositae mix as markers of fragrance allergy: cross-reactivity between fragrance terpenes, colophonium and compositae plant extracts. Contact Dermatitis 53:285–291
57. Thyssen JP, Engkilde K, Lundov MD, Carlsen BC, Menné T, Johansen JD (2010) Temporal trends of preservative allergy in Denmark (1985–2008). Contact Dermatitis 62:102–108
58. Lundov MD, Johansen JD, Carlsen BC, Engkilde K, Menné T, Thyssen JP (2010) Formaldehyde exposure and patterns of concomitant contact allergy to formaldehyde and formaldehyde-releasers. Contact Dermatitis 63:31–36
59. Emeis D, de Groot AC, Brinkmann J (2010) Determination of formaldehyde in formaldehyde-releaser patch test preparations. Contact Dermatitis 63:57–62
60. Flyvholm M-A, Andersen P (1993) Identification of formaldehyde releasers and occurrence of formaldehyde and formaldehyde releasers in registered chemical products. Am J Ind Med 24:533–552
61. Kireche M, Gimenez-Arnau E, Lepoittevin JP (2010) Preservatives in cosmetics: reactivity of allergenic formaldehyde-releasers towards amino acids through breakdown products other than formaldehyde. Contact Dermatitis 63:192–202
62. García-Gavín J, González-Vilas D, Fernández-Redondo V, Toribo J (2010) Allergic contact dermatitis in a girl due to several cosmetics containing diazolidinyl-urea or imidazolidinyl-urea. Contact Dermatitis 63:49–50
63. Lehmann SV, Hoeck U, Breinholdt J, Olsen CE, Kreilgaard B (2006) Characterization and chemistry of imidazolidinyl urea and diazolidinyl urea. Contact Dermatitis 54:50–58
64. Lundov MD, Moesby L, Zachariae C, Johansen JD (2009) Contamination versus preservation of cosmetics: a review on legislation, usage, infections, and contact allergy. Contact Dermatitis 60:70–78
65. Revuz J (2009) Long live parabens. Ann Dermatol Venereol 136:403–404
66. European-Communities (2007) Directive EU 2007/17/EC 22 March 2007
67. Lotery H, Kirk S, Beck M, Burova E, Crone M, Curley R, Downs A, Hill G, Horne H, Iftikhar N, Lovell C, Malanin K, Orton D, Powell S, Sansom J, Sonnex T, Todd D, Tucker S, Wilkinson M, Haworth A (2007) Dicaprylyl maleate. Contact Dermatitis 57:169–172
68. Sugiura M, Hayakawa R, Kato Y, Sugiura K, Hashimoto R, Shamoto M (2001) Results of patch testing with 1,3-butylene glycol from 1994 to 1999. Environ Dermatol 8:1–5
69. Gallo R, Viglizzo G, Vecchio F, Parodi A (2003) Allergic contact dermatitis from pentylene glycol in an emollient cream, with possible co-sensitization to resveratrol. Contact Dermatitis 48:176–177
70. Gallo R, Sacco DD, Ghigliotti G (2004) Allergic contact dermatitis from VP/eicosene copolymer (Ganex V-220) in an emollient cream. Contact Dermatitis 50:261
71. Kügler K, Mydlach B, Frosch PJ (2009) Contact allergy from alkyl rhamnoside-C5. Contact Dermatitis 61:352–353
72. Brasch J, Lipowsky F, Kreiselmaier I (2008) Allergic contact dermatitis to phytantriol. Contact Dermatitis 59:251–252
73. Kiken DA, Cohen DE (2002) Contact dermatitis to botanical extracts. Am J Contact Dermat 13:148–152
74. Thomson KF, Wilkinson SM (2003) Allergic contact dermatitis to plant extracts in patients with cosmetic dermatitis. Br J Dermatol 142:84–88
75. Pazzaglia M, Jorizzo M, Parente G, Tosti A (2000) Allergic contact dermatitis due to avena extract. Contact Dermatitis 42:364
76. Sanchez-Pérez J, Sanz T, García-Díez A (2000) Allergic contact dermatitis from hydrolyzed wheat protein in a cosmetic cream. Contact Dermatitis 42:360
77. Shaffrali FC, Gawkrodger DJ (2001) Contact dermatitis from soybean extract in a cosmetic cream. Contact Dermatitis 44:51–52
78. Boussault P, Léauté-Labrèze C, Saubusse E, Maurice-Tison S, Perromat M, Roul S, Sarrat A, Taïeb A, Boralevi F (2007) Oat sensitization in children with atopic dermatitis: prevalence, risks and associated factors. Allergy 62:1251–1256
79. Goujon-Henry C, Hennino A, Nicolas J-F (2008) Do we have to recommend not using oat-containing emollients in children with atopic dermatitis? Allergy 63:781–782
80. Rancé F, Dargassies J, Dupuy P, Schmitt AM, Gúerin L, Dutau G (2001) Faut-il contre-indiquer l'utilisation des émollients à base d'avoine chez l'enfant atopique? Rev Fr Allergol Immunol Clin 41:477–483
81. Paulsen E, Christensen LP, Fretté XC, Andersen KE (2010) Patch test reactivity to feverfew-containing creams in feverfew-allergic patients. Contact Dermatitis 63:146–150
82. Belhadjali H, Giordano-Labadie F, Bazex J (2001) Contact dermatitis from vitamin C in a cosmetic anti-aging cream. Contact Dermatitis 45:317
83. Sasseville D, Moreau L, Al-Sowaidi M (2007) Allergic contact dermatitis to idebenone used as an antioxidant in an anti-wrinkle cream. Contact Dermatitis 56:117
84. Natkunarajah J, Ostlere L (2008) Allergic contact dermatitis to idebenone in an over-the-counter anti-ageing cream. Contact Dermatitis 58:239
85. Fleming JD, White JM, White IR (2008) Allergic contact dermatitis to hydroxydecyl ubiquinone: a

newly described contact allergen in cosmetics. Contact Dermatitis 58:245
86. Avenel-Audran M, Dutartre H, Goossens A, Jeanmougin M, Comte C, Bernier C, Benkalfate L, Michel M, Ferrier-Lebouëdec MC, Vigan M, Bourrain JL, Outtas O, Peyron JL, Martin L (2010) Octocrylene, an emerging photoallergen. Arch Dermatol 146:753–757
87. Karlsson I, Vanden Broecke K, Mårtensson J, Goossens A, Börje A (2011) Clinical and experimental studies of octocrylene's allergenic potency. Contact Dermatitis. doi:10.1111/j.1600–0536.2011.01899.x, Epub ahead of print

25 Formulating Moisturizers Using Natural Raw Materials

Swarnlata Saraf

25.1 Introduction

Traditionally, cosmetics were the substances applied to the human body for cleansing, beautifying, perfuming or changing the appearance except soap and must not cause damage to the human health. The use of herbal beauty products dates back to ancient times. In fact, virtually, every ancient culture recorded the use of native herbs for a beautiful healthy complexion. This evidence supports herbal skin care's efficacy, with recipes once highly reputed being lost for a time and rediscovered in recent history. Furthermore, modern science has evaluated and confirmed the cleansing, healing and protective qualities of many herbs. Herbs and spices have been used in maintaining and enhancing human beauty since naturals have a lot of properties like sunscreen effect, anti-ageing, moisturizing, antioxidant, anti-cellulite and antimicrobial effect. In early 1920s, a big population started using cosmetic preparations containing synthetic ingredients for their instant effects with some advantages like less time consuming, ease of application, high aesthetic appeal, ease to store, easy to carry, etc., with some limitations like sporadically deterioration, more unwanted after effects, skin allergies and cost effectiveness [2]. Natural raw materials used for formulating moisturizers could be of plant origin like dry exudates or herbal extracts, from animal origin like gelatine, cholesterol and lanolin; from marine sources like sphingolipids or from minerals like bentonite and Veegum.

As compared to synthetic cosmetic products, natural products are mild, biodegradable and have low toxicity profile. To enhance these properties, researches are being done in the development of newer approaches, which could improve both the aesthetic appeal and performance of a cosmetic product. But the latest trend is to combine clinically proven natural ingredients with patented delivery systems and the aesthetics of fine cosmetics [15].

The appearance and function of the skin are maintained by an important balance between the water content of the stratum corneum and skin surface lipids [36, 39]. When this balance is disrupted, skin mechanical properties and water content get disturbed; hence, skin becomes dry and loses its elasticity. In these cases, effective dermato-cosmetic products must be used to improve the skin hydration and viscoelasticity not only for aesthetic purposes but also to maintain the normal conditions of skin and to prevent dry skin alterations [30].

The stratum corneum is the main barrier of the skin and prevents dehydration. Water plays an important role in respect to the normal function of the epidermal barrier, which is also reflected in the differing water contents of the stratum corneum

S. Saraf
Department of Pharmacy,
Guru Ghasidas Central University,
Koni Bilaspur, Chhattisgarh 495009, India
e-mail: swarnlata_saraf@rediffmail.com

M. Lodén, H.I. Maibach (eds.), *Treatment of Dry Skin Syndrome*,
DOI 10.1007/978-3-642-27606-4_25, © Springer-Verlag Berlin Heidelberg 2012

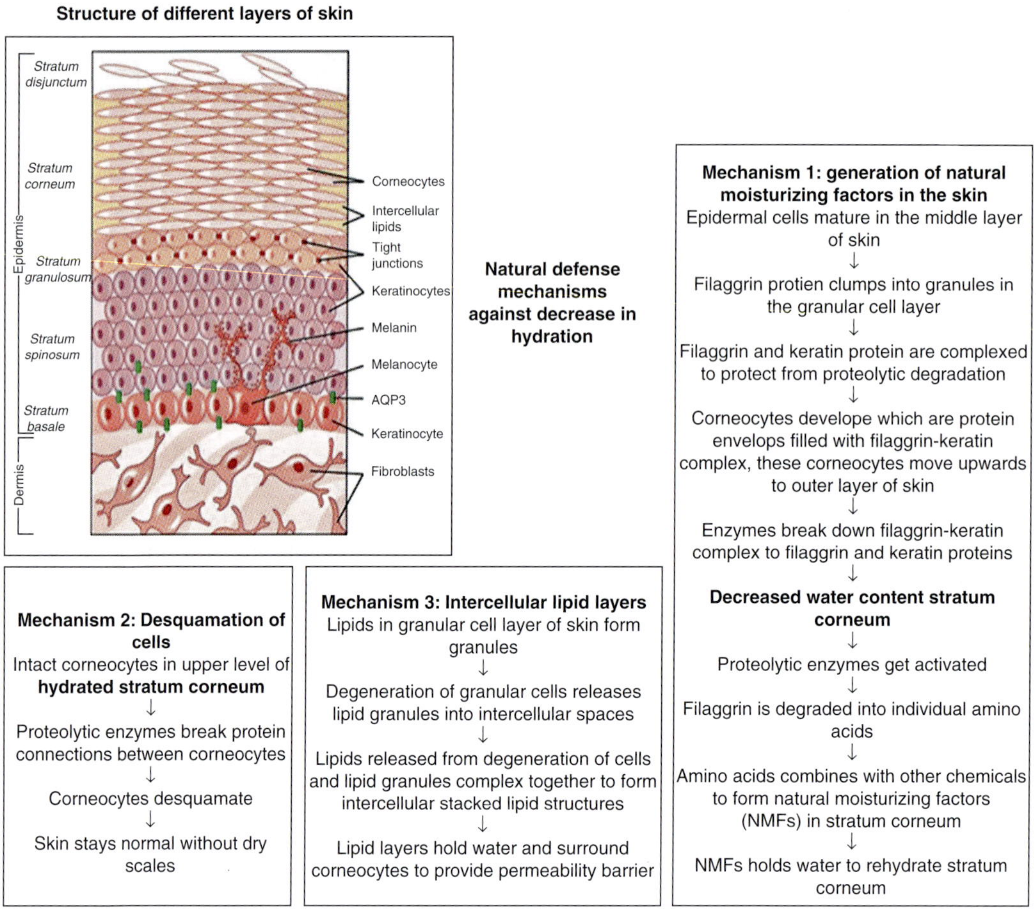

Fig. 25.1 Physiology of skin hydration and dehydration

(10–15%) and viable epidermis (about 60%). The water content in the stratum corneum is mostly bound to the head group of ceramides and to proteins and is an essential prerequisite for the barrier function. Thus, a decrease in water content below the minimum level is associated with skin malfunction [19]. The moisture content of the skin is of particular interest in cosmetic applications. Cosmetic care is therefore concerned to equilibrate the moisture balance of the skin (Fig. 25.1).

According to market survey, the global market for cosmetics and toiletries reached nearly $150 billion in 2004, increase by more than 4% from 2003, which highlights major growth in key developing markets. The herbal market has been boosted by increasing demand for natural alternative medicines. World demand for herbal products has been growing at a rate of 10–15% per annum. The medicinal plants-related trade in India alone is approximately Rs. 5.5 billion. World Health Organization (WHO) has forecasted that the global market for herbal products would be worth $5 trillion by the year 2050. Europe and the United States are the two major herbal products markets in the world, with a market share of 41% and 20%, respectively. According to the World Bank, the global market for medicinal plants and their products includes the potential sectors of pharmaceuticals, nutraceuticals and cosmeceutical to be estimated of worth US$ 62 billion and offers a plethora of opportunities for the Indian pharma and cosmetic companies [2].

By adopting proper methodologies and techniques, risk factors of ingredients incorporated in cosmetics can be determined and managed at safety level. The toxicological evaluation of a cosmetic product should be certainly carried out with full knowledge of the pharmacotechnical, toxicological, pharmacokinetic, regulatory, clinical phase's areas and Scientific Committee of Cosmetics and Non-Food Products Intended (SCCNFP), Organization for Economic Cooperation and Development (OECD), European Cosmetic, Toiletry and Perfumery Association (COLIPA), Cosmetics, Toiletries and Fragrances Association (CTFA), Bureau of Indian Standard (BIS) and World Health Organization (WHO) guidelines [17, 24, 25]. Cosmetic products are regulated in various countries according to their own legislations like EU Cosmetic Directives in European Union (EU), Food Drug and Cosmetics Act in USA, Pharmaceutical Affairs Law (PAL) in Japan and Legislations of Canada, India, Australia, China and other Asian countries [40].

25.2 Problems Related to Skin

Commonly, skin types are categorized as normal skin, dry skin, oily skin, combination skin and sensitive skin. The disturbance in balance between water content of the stratum corneum and skin surface lipids causes dry skin [5]. Dry skin could be caused by a dry climate, winter weather and deficiency of vitamin A, systemic illness, overexposure to sunlight, medication or by medical conditions like diabetes and psoriasis. The skin loses moisture resulting in crack and peel, or it may become irritated, inflamed, and itching, leading to serious skin problems. Dry skin is also observed in patients with atopic dermatitis [5]. When photo-stress is applied on the skin, the sebum quantity decreases, the hydration index reduces and the melanin index increases [47]. The hydration level of the stratum corneum affects its mechanical and electrical properties [52]. Age-related changes in the skin's appearance are dryness, wrinkling and laxity. Xerosis with pruritus and scleroderma like skin changes are observed in persons having diabetes mellitus [49]. Moisturizing formulations play significant aspect in rectifying dry skin by softening the skin as water is important for maintaining the flexibility and softness of skin. But specifically, the moisture-related skin types could be determined as very dry skin (corneometer unit below 30), dry skin (between 30 and 40) and normal skin (higher than 40 arbitrary units) [21]. The selection of moisturizing formulation is very important according to the skin type, condition and body part. Similarly, designing of safe and effective moisturizers with suitable raw materials is also a challenging aspect.

25.3 Natural Raw Materials Improving Skin Hydration

Various moisturizers are available under the label of natural, safe, organic and herbal, while the basic properties of humectancy, occlusivity and emolliency are consistent across all moisturizers. Most of the available moisturizers use synthetic adhesives, emulsifiers, perfuming agents, pigments, surfactants and thickeners to form the base. There is extensive need to replace toxic synthetic agent from base using natural agents [26]. Table 25.1 summarizes the category of natural substances associated with the enhancement of skin hydration through various mechanisms.

In the study of comparison of hydration effect of various moisturizers, it was observed that the formulation having wheat germ oil, *Aloe vera* and turmeric extract in combination showed significant moisturizing effects [44]. Wheat germ oil is rich in vitamins A, D and E, used for its antioxidant effects on free radicals in the skin as natural preservative. Herbs like *Aloe vera*, comfrey, calendula, dandelion, chamomile, fennel

Table 25.1 Natural moisturizing raw materials categorized on the basis of mechanism of action

Category	Mechanism of action	Examples
Moisturizers	They add moisture or water to the skin	D-Panthenol and sorbitol present in fruits and berries
Emollients	They soften and smoothen the skin and are used to correct dryness and scaling of the skin by preventing water loss	Jojoba oil, black cohosh, soy extract and vitamin A and E
Humectants	Are substances that have a molecular structure that enables them to retain water and bind it in the skin. Humectants are also capable penetrating the skin. They are introduced into the stratum corneum to increase its water-holding capacity	Glycerin, honey, silk protein and natural phospholipids, from lecithin
Occlusives	Provide a layer of oil on the surface of the skin to slow water loss and thus increase the moisture content of the stratum corneum	Paraffin oils/waxes
Substantives	Substantives are substances or ingredients that attach themselves very well to the surface of the skin, then spread across the skin to protect and to hydrate it	Algae products
Natural antioxidants	Natural antioxidants quench free radicals and are an essential component of anti-ageing formulations. They potentially offer protection against damage to the tissues by environmental and other agents	Flavonoids like apigenin, Catechin, Epicatechin, alpha glycosyl rutin and Silymarin are polyphenolic and antioxidant
		Vitamins: ascorbic acid, alpha-tocopherol, retinol
		Natural oils such as rapeseed oil, sunflower oil and soybean oil
Natural anti-inflammatory agents	They sooth, heal and protect skin tone and integrity	Liquorice (*G. glabra*), marigold (*C. officinale*), varuna (*C. nurvala*), etc. are the potent anti-inflammatory herbs
Anti-irritant	They improve hydration and elasticity and help to prevent skin breakdown	Essential fatty acids
Keratolytic agents	They prevent accumulation of excessive stratum corneum and remove the cohesive attachment of cornified cells	Glycolic acids, retinoic acids and lactic acid

and peppermint are very effective for preventing dry skin, soothing the discomfort of dry skin and healing the symptoms of dry skin, while essential oils help lubricate the skin to curb dryness, herbs work by softening and moisturizing the skin.

Vegetable oils like peanut oil, almond oil, sesame oil and olive oil are important oleaginous raw material used for the preparation of creams. Stearic acid is used as an emulsifier to develop consistency in the cream and to give a matt effect on the skin. Stearyl alcohol and cetyl alcohol are used as emollients and stabilizers. Waxes of animal and vegetable origin like lanolin, beeswax and carnauba wax also constitute important component in the formulation of moisturizing formulations. Natural gums are polysaccharides of natural origin, capable of causing a large viscosity increase in solution, even at small concentrations. They are used as thickening agents, gelling agents, emulsifying agents, binding agents and stabilizers. Natural gums could be obtained from sea weeds, bacterial fermentation and from non-marine botanical resources. Glycerin and sorbitol (70%) are used as humectants which enhance the spreadability, improve consistency and prevent the cream from drying out [31]. The raw materials could also be categorized on the basis of their source of origin as depicted in Table 25.2.

25.4 Herbal Extracts as Raw Materials for Moisturizing Formulations

Due to the harmful effects of chemicals, the researchers are shifting towards herbal cosmetics. The poly-herbal cosmetic formulations have been recommended for the management of skin properties for a long time, and their effects are also well accepted [3]. Formulating cosmetics using completely natural raw materials is a difficult task. The need is to substitute synthetic base from naturals while maintaining the same functional effects acquiring from synthetic one [26]. Extracts of many plants, citrus fruits and leafy vegetables as source of ascorbic acid, vitamin E and phenolic compounds and enzymes possess the ability to reduce the oxidative damage [29]. The formulations composed of such extracts could be utilized for the protection of photo-induced intrinsic oxidative stress as well as structural alteration in skin [4, 14]. It has been observed by our research group that the products which contains either herbal extract/seed/oil/juice/gel of aloe vera, grape, almond, olive, wheat germ, sandalwood and cucumber shown better viscoelastic and hydration effect as compared to other products [27]. The herbal cosmetic cream formulations were designed by Ashawat et al. [3] using ethanolic extracts of *Glycyrriza glabra*, *Curcuma longa* (roots), seeds of *Psorolea corylifolia*, *Cassia tora*, *Areca catechu*, *Punica granatum*, fruits of *Embelica officinale*, leaves of *Centella asiatica*, dried bark of *Cinnamon zeylanicum* and fresh gel of *Aloe vera* in varied concentrations (0.12–0.9%w/w) and observed the improvement in skin viscoelastic and hydration properties [3]. Table 25.3 shows some of the important herbs with their chemical constituents and functional properties that could be used to formulate herbal moisturizers.

In the study performed by Kapoor and Saraf, various marketed herbal moisturizers were compared and concluded that presence of *Aloe vera* (Ghrit kumari) extract, which is rich composition in hygroscope mono- and polysaccharides and in the amino acids, improves water retention in the stratum corneum [26]. The silica in cucumber (*Cucumis sativum*) is an essential component of healthy connective tissue, which includes muscles, tendons, ligaments, cartilage and bone, and is an excellent source of potassium, vitamin C and folic acid. The high water content makes cucumbers good for moisturizing effect. Methi (*Trigonella foenum-graecum*) seed extract contains 45–60% carbohydrates, 5–10% fixed oils (lipids), flavonoids and free amino acids that provide softening, cleansing and soothing properties to skin. Sandalwood (*Santalum alba*) the main constituent of sandalwood oil is santalol, credited for its moisturizing and viscoleastictity property. Almond oil (*Prunus amygdalus*) contains folic acid, alpha-tocopherol and zinc, which are useful in skin disorders. Wheat germ oil (*Triticum*

Table 25.2 Various types of raw materials based on origin constituting moisturizing formulations

Category/type	Name of materials	Source	Uses
Plant-originated raw materials	Acacia	Dry exudates from species of *Acacia*	Emulsifying agent
	Tragacanth	Dry gummy exudates from species of *Astragalus*	Stabilizer, thickener and emulsifier
	Agar, carrageenan and alginates	Extracted from sea weeds like red algae	Suspending and gelling agent
	Seed gum, guar gum, psyllium seed gum	Seed gums or extracts	Emulsifier
	Soy lecithin	Is manufactured from soybean oil seeds. The major phospholipids for soy lecithin are phosphatidylcholine, phosphatidylethanolamine and phosphatidylinositol	Emulsifiers, antioxidants, stabilizers and wetting agents
Animal-originated raw materials	Gelatin	Partial hydrolysis of collagen derived from skin, connective tissues and bones of animals	Stabilizer and thickener
	Cholesterol	Obtained by saponification and fractionation of wool fat	Stabilizers
	Lanolin and lanolin alcohols	Lanolin material derived from wool; it is a mixture of cholesterol esters and higher fatty acid esters.	Used as base of cosmetic formulations and emulsifiers
		Lanolin alcohols are obtained by hydrolysis of lanolin	
	Beeswax	Purified wax from the honeycomb of *Apis mellifera* bee	Emulsion stabilizer, skin-conditioning agent, thickening agent and has emollient, soothing and softening properties
	Egg lecithin	Produced from egg yolk and consists of phosphatidylethanolamine and phosphatidylcholine	Emulsifiers, soothing and softening properties
	Casein	Is a milk protein which can be prepared by isoelectric precipitation or enzyme precipitation	Emulsifiers, thickeners and gelling agents
	Chitosan	Natural polymer obtained by deacetylation of chitin. Present in shell fish	Gelling agent, increases viscosity

Mineral-originated raw materials	Bentonite	Is natural colloidal-hydrated aluminium silicate	Has swelling property and thickener, used in forming gels
	Veegum	Is colloidal magnesium aluminium silicate	Suspending agent and thickener
	Attapulgite	Obtained from Attapulgus and is hydrous magnesium aluminium silicate	Suspending agent and thickener
Fermentation product	Xanthan gum	Produced by culture fermentation of carbohydrate with *Xanthomonas campestris*	Stabilizer, thickener and emulsifier
Marine-originated raw materials	Marine phospholipids (eicosapentaenoic and docosahexaenoic acid)	Antartic krill (*Euphausia superba*) and fish Roe	Novel vesicular system development like Marinosomes
	Sphingolipid (sphingomyelin)	Mammals' milk, preferably bovine milk; brain; egg yolk and erythrocytes from animal blood, preferably sheep	Novel vesicular system development like Sphingosomes

Table 25.3 List of herbs with their chemical constituents and functional properties to formulate herbal moisturizers

Herbs	Chemical constituents	Functional properties
Aloe barbadensis (leaf extract)	Barbaloin, aloe emodin, aloesin, amino acid, enzymes, vitamin	Moisturizing agent and impart elasticity
Areca catechu (seeds)	High amounts of tannic acid and gallic acid. Polyphenols and tannins are the major constituent of the nut	Antimicrobial, anti-inflammatory, anti-melanogenesis, anti-elastase and antioxidant activity
Azadirachta indica (leaf extract)	Nimbin, nimbinin and nimbidin	Rejuvating and extrafoliating agent and as preservative
Centella asiatica (leaves)	Triterpene glycosides such as centella saponin, asiaticoside, madecassoside and sceffoleoside and also asiatic acid and madecassic acid	Antioxidant, wound healing, in skin improver tonics, anti-ageing and as cooling agents
Cinnamon zeylanicum (bark)	Phenolic compounds, such as catechin, epicatechin, and procyanidin B2, phenol polymers and polyphenols	Antioxidants, antiseptic, astringent, and antibacterial
Cocos nucifera (oil)	Lauric oils	Soothing agent
Cucumis sativus (main fruit juice)	Silica, vitamin C and folic acid	Moisturizing and firming agent
Curcuma caesia (rhizomes)	Oil of *Curcuma caesia* contain *ar*-turmerone, (*Z*)-β-ocimene, camphor, *ar*-curcumene, 1,8-cineole, β-elemene, borneol, bornyl acetate and γ-curcumene as the major constituents	Rhizomes are useful in treating leucoderma, tumours, inflammations and allergic eruptions
Emblica officinalis	Vitamin C	Antioxidant
Glycerrhiza glabra (bark extract)	Estragole, anethole, flavonoids	Astringent
Oleum olivae (oil)		Prevent drying and chafing
Prunus amygdalus (oil)	Amandin, folic acid, alpha-tocopherol and zinc	Hydrating and firming agent
Santalum alba (oil)	Santalol	Alleviate itching and cooling agent
Tamarindus indica (fruit)	Mineral elements, saponins alkaloids and glycosides and with a high antioxidant capacity associated with high phenolic including gallic acid	Anti-fungal, antibacterial, anti-inflammatory and antioxidant properties
Trigonella foenum-graecum (seed extract)	Carbohydrates, lipids, flavonoids and free amino acids	Softening and soothing agent
Triticum sativum (oil)	Vitamin E and carbohydrate	Nourishing and occlusive agent

sativum) is a rich source of tocopherols with high vitamin E potency that nourishes and prevents loss of moisture from the skin. Red apple (*Pyrus malus*) is a rich source of various vitamins, trace elements, amino acids and flavonoids due to which it acts as humectant and provides moisturizing and viscoelasticity property. Coconut (*Cocos nucifera*) oil helps keep skin soft and smooth. Lauric oils, the dominant fatty acid (45–48%) in coconut oil, are used in cosmetics. Yashtimadhu (*Glycyrrhiza glabra*) extract is helpful to formulate cosmetic products for the protection of skin and hair against oxidative processes. Grape seed (*Vitis vinifera*) contain pycnogeneol, which is responsible for its cosmetic properties [26].

25.5 Preparation of Moisturizing Formulations

Pharmaceutically, cosmetic moisturizers like creams, lotions and milks are emulsion systems varying in consistency and rheological character on the basis of their constituents and purpose. Creams are semisolid viscous with opaque appearance having apparent viscosity, while lotions are pourable with low viscosity. Gels are semisolid system in which a liquid phase is constrained within a 3-D polymeric matrix (consisting of natural or synthetic gum) having a high degree of physical or chemical cross-linking. Jellies are transparent or translucent non-greasy semisolids to thick viscous fluids that consist of submicroscopic particles in plastic or rigid baselike natural gums. The cosmetic emulsions could be oil-in-water type, water-in-oil type or oil-in-water-in-oil or water-in-oil-in-water type. All cosmetic formulations can be categorized into four major groups: cleansing, moisturizing, all-purpose and protective products based on their functional properties [32]. Majority of cosmetic creams and lotions contain lipid (oil) and water as their major components and other minor ingredients like surface active agents, moisturizers, emollients, waxes, thickeners, active ingredients, sunscreens, antioxidants, colours, preservative, etc. All of these substances collectively result in stable moisturizing formulations [1].

Development of moisturizing formulations taking natural raw materials is a challenging task. Since skin pH is towards acidic range [22], vegetable-oil-based formulations are developing as they are acidic in nature, easily biodegradable and skin lipid compatible, too [38]. Selection of emulsifying agent to prepare stable formulation is also important task. Hydrophilic lipophilic balance system of Griffin is very supportive in this contest and helps in deciding appropriate emulgents. Natural raw materials could be used as additives for the preparation of various moisturizing formulations, for example, spice extractives having aromatic principles could act as flavouring agents, gums as viscosity modifiers or thickeners, fruit acids for pH adjustment, vegetable oils as emollients and vehicles, waxes as thickeners and emollients, plant extracts as conditioners and vitamins and fatty acids as moisturizers and antioxidants. Caramel, carmine and beta-carotene are approved natural colourants. Natural preservatives include fruit extracts (grapefruit seed and rosemary), essential oils (tea tree, neem seed, thyme) and vitamins (vitamin E and vitamin C).

25.5.1 Techniques of Herbal Moisturizing Formulation

Moisturizing formulations could be prepared by using a phase inversion technique [18]. Initially, natural oil and other ingredients (like sesame oil, almond oil, cetyl alcohol, stearic acid, sorbitan stearate and sorbitan monooleate) are mixed using an overhead stirrer at 200 ± 25 rpm at 65–75°C on a hot plate. After the complete melting and homogenous mixing, a 50-ml portion of deionized water (70 ± 2°C) and glycerine are added at a rate of 30 ml/min^{-1} at increased speed (275 ± 25 rpm) along with the herbal extracts. When the temperature of the internal phase is reduced to 50°C, phase inversion occurs and the solution becomes viscous; the remaining aqueous phase containing propylene glycol is then added. When the temperature is reduced to 40°C, honey

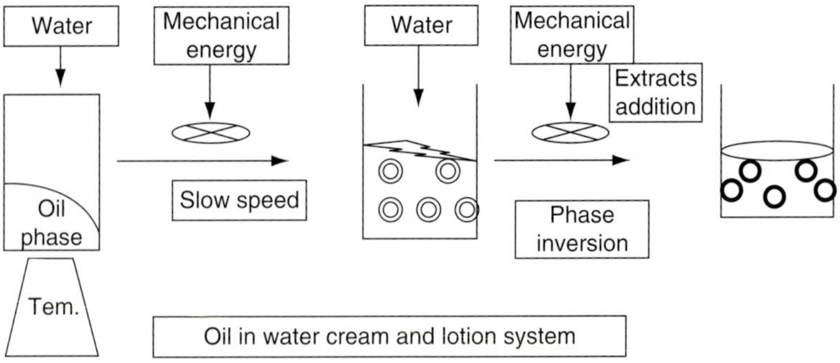

Fig. 25.2 Schematic representation of development of moisturizing formulation

is added to this mixture [3]. Schematic representation of development of cosmetic moisturizing formulation is shown in Fig. 25.2.

Another combination of natural raw materials for the preparation of water in oil emulsion cream is by initially melting bees wax at 60–70°C, then to this, added lanolin, almond oil, olive oil, neem oil and tocopherol. Then, aqueous phase along with neem extract is taken and heated at 50°C, to this, glycerine and rose water are added, and after cooling up to 40°C, sandalwood stick aq extract is added to it. Both the phases were mixed continuously for homogenous dispersion and cooled slowly for fragrance peppermint oil and sandalwood oil added [46].

25.5.2 Development of Herbal Moisturizing Formulations

Moisturizing formulations could be cream, lotion or milk preparation. For the development of herbal moisturizing formulation, first step is the extraction of herbal active constituents according to the well-established methods like hot extraction method for volatile constituents, cold maceration process for thermolabile phytoconstituents, etc. Then, the herbal extracts or juices obtained undergo qualitative and quantitative evaluation for the standardization and purity of the obtained phytoconstituents. Next step is preparation of cream base and inclusion of herbal extract/juices in that base. They could be either included during cream formation or could be incorporated in the prepared base cream. The prepared herbal cream formulation is then evaluated for stability, physicochemical evaluation and safety analysis. On the basis of these parameters, they are further taken for psychometric analysis, biological studies and bioengineering methods of evaluation. After the analysis of all the obtained evaluation parameters, the prepared moisturizing formulations are completely developed. The detailed steps are depicted in Fig. 25.3.

25.5.2.1 Example for the Development of Herbal Moisturizing Formulation

Preparation of Natural Base

Phase inversion technique was used to prepare natural base [M5]. The internal phase was prepared by using several ingredients, and emulsification was carried out in the mortar and pastel. Initially, grated and melted bees wax, natural oil of *T. sativum*, *C. nucifera*, *P. amygdalus*, *O. olivae* and *S. alba* and other ingredients acacia, soy lecithin and glycerin were mixed using an homogenizer at 200±25 rpm at 65–75°C. After the complete homogenous mixing, a 50-ml portion of triple distilled water [70±2°C] was added at a rate of 45 ml/min at increased speed [250±25 rpm]. When the temperature of the internal phase was reduced to 50°C, phase inversion took place and the solution became viscous. When the temperature was reduced to 40°C, honey [2% w/w] was added to this mixture [27].

Formulation of Herbal Moisturizer

Different concentrations, i.e., 0.135–0.9% w/w of *Cucumis sativus*, *Glycerrhiza glabra*, *Emblica officinalis*, *Azadirachta indica*, *Trigonella foenum-graecum*, *Aloe barbadensis* extracts, juice and gel prepared in ethanol were incorporated into the natural base and coded as M1. Natural

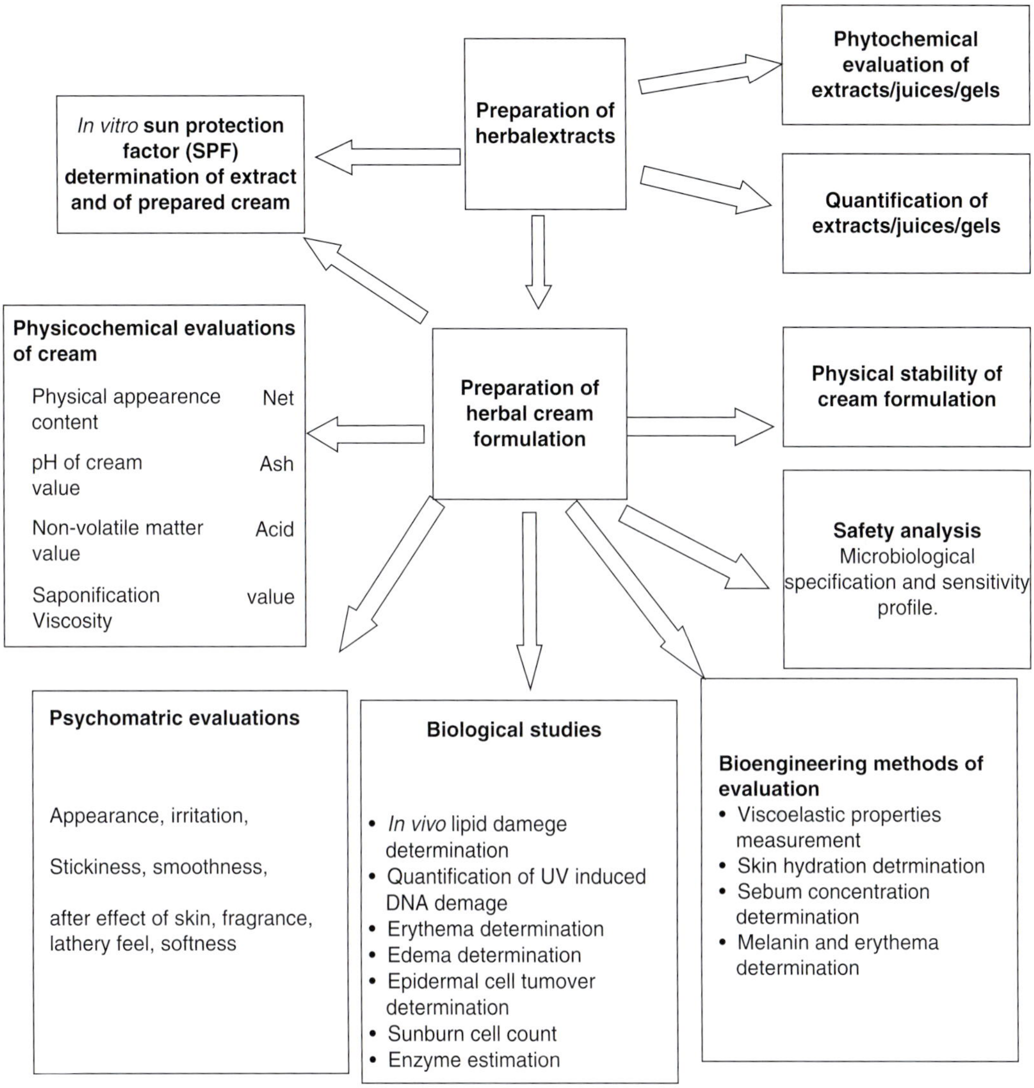

Fig. 25.3 Various steps for the development of herbal moisturizing formulation

base M5 was used as the control product, while commercial herbal moisturizer having similar ingredients with synthetic base was coded as M4.

Skin Viscoelasticity Evaluation of Herbal Moisturizer

Quantity of herbal constituents present in M1 are *Cucumis sativus* (0.70% w/w), *Glycerrhiza glabra* (0.75% w/w), *Emblica officinalis* (0.210% w/w), *Azadirachta indica* (0.75% w/w), *Trigonella foenum-graecum* (0.583% w/w) and *Aloe barbadensis* (0.78% w/w). Twenty subjects were enrolled in the study. The results showed that M1 and M4 had increased skin hydrations levels [30.97 ± 0.55% and 31.77 ± 0.59%], respectively, after 3 weeks which were more than the control formulation M5 [5.40 ± 2.51%]. The improvement in skin firmness was found to increase up to 30.46 ± 0.86% and 30.35 ± 0.91%, respectively, for M1 and M4. The improvement in the skin viscoelasticity was found to be increased for M1, 30.27 ± 0.55%, and M4, 29.69 ± 0.82% as compared to the control product M5, 5.76 ± 0.30%. These improvements may be

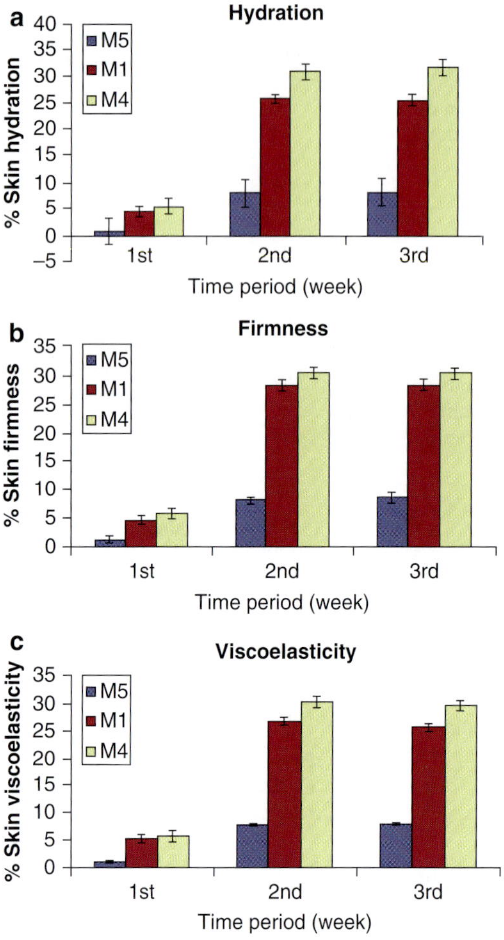

Fig. 25.4 (**a**) Increase in percentage of skin hydration. (**b**) Increase in percentage of skin firmness. (**c**) Increase in percentage of skin viscoelasticity after 3-week period [27]

due to the synergistic effects of active constituents present in the ethanolic extracts of selected herbs [27] (Fig. 25.4).

25.6 Novel Approaches for the Development of Moisturizing Formulations

Recent advances in nanotechnology show their promise as potential cosmetics for poorly soluble, poorly absorbed and labile herbal extracts and phytochemicals. The application of novel approaches retains moisture and restores the barrier functions of the skin. They deliver active ingredients to the skin with a continuous release over a prolonged time thus maintains skin appearance [41]. The formulation and selection of approach to be used for herbal cosmetics will depend upon purpose of preparation that is for topical or deep effect; inherent properties of drug or herb extract such as hydrophilic or hydrophobic; surface characteristics of a system-like permeability and charges; degree of biodegradability, biocompatibility and toxicity; release profile and size of the product required and anti-genicity of the final product [15]. Modified nanovesicles penetrate the stratum corneum and supply the nutrients to skin [8]. Important novel approaches that could be used for formulating moisturizers include microemulsions, multiple emulsions, liposomes transfersomes, lipid complex system, cubosomes and various other nanosystems [20, 37, 50]. By nanoparticles, controlled release of active ingredients, pigment effect and improved skin hydration and protection through film formation on the skin is obtained. The amalgamation of use of properties of phytoconstituents along with the characteristics of novel delivery systems are used as base for the formulation of moisturizing formulations with better an enhanced efficacy.

25.6.1 Various Novel Systems and Their Mechanism of Hydration

Vesicular systems are widely used in skin formulations due to the similarity of the bilayer structure of lipid vesicles to that of natural membranes. The ability of liposomal formulations, depending on lipid composition, to alter cell membrane fluidity and to fuse with cells help the delivering of active constituents to the target site and thereby improve skin properties. Specially designed lipid vesicles (transfersomes and ethosomes) penetrate into deeper layers of the skin. Ultradeformable vesicles are delivered to the deeper epidermal layers through dehydration of the lipid vesicles within the stratum corneum. Therefore, liposome uptake is driven by the hydration gradient that exists across the epidermis, stratum corneum and ambient atmosphere [53]. The presence of ethanol in ethosomes influences the stratum corneum penetration and permeation of drugs [54]. Liposomes as a drug delivery system can improve the therapeutic activity and safety of drugs, mainly by delivering them to their site of action and by maintaining therapeutic drug levels for prolonged periods of time. Complexation of herbal active constituents with certain other clinically useful nutrients like phospholipids improves their absorption and bioavailability.

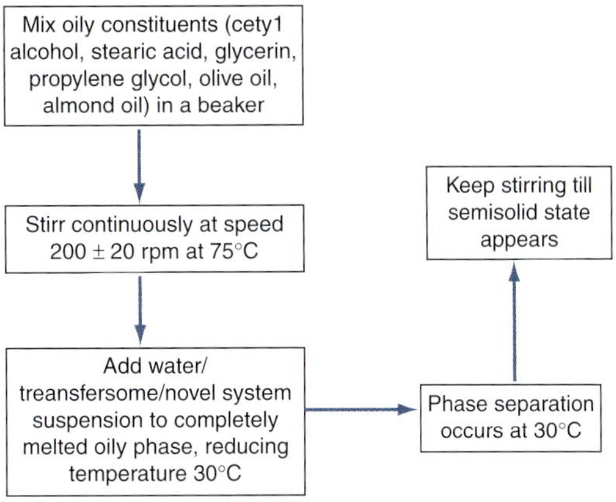

Fig. 25.5 Preparation of novel herbal moisturizing formulations

25.6.2 Role of Constituents of Novel Delivery Systems

The composition and properties of liposomes play an important role in their interaction with and possible penetration into the epidermis. In addition, liposomes provide valuable raw material for the regeneration of skin by replenishing lipid molecules and moisture. Lipids are well hydrated and, even in the absence of active ingredients, humidify the skin [9]. Liposome formulations have been implied for skin moisturization, due to the potential occlusive effect of the phospholipid film deposited on the skin surface. Egg and soya phospholipids are widely used natural lipids for formulating vesicular systems. An o/w microemulsion formulated using lecithin and an alkyl glucoside as mild, non-irritant surfactants was proposed as a cosmetic vehicle for arbutin and kojic acid, naturally occurring whitening agents. The stability of these compounds is higher in microemulsions than in aqueous solutions [11, 42]. By combining the emulsifying action of the phospholipids, with the standardized botanical extracts, the phytosome form provides dramatically enhanced bioavailability and delivers faster and improved absorption through the skin [34]. Transfersomes are applied in a non-occluded method to the skin, which permeate through the stratum corneum lipid lamellar regions as a result of the hydration or osmotic force in the skin. It can be applicable as drug carriers for a range of small molecules, peptides, proteins and nutraceuticals [12, 15]. Sphingosomes prepared from sphingolipids of natural origin are much more stable to acid hydrolysis, have better drug retention characteristics than liposomes and better skin compatibility with enhanced penetration [43].

25.6.3 Preparation of Herbal Novel Cosmetic Formulations

Initially, the herbal constituents are extracted, and novel systems are developed according to the solubility and nature of the extracts. Then, these novel systems are evaluated for their size, structure, surface properties, zeta potential, entrapment efficiency, drug release and stability. The stable herbal novel delivery systems are then incorporated into topical delivery systems like creams, gels or lotions. These developed herbal delivery system incorporated topical formulations are evaluated for physicochemical, psychometric and biological parameters, and the stable formulations are ready for use. Figure 25.5 depicts laboratory preparation of novel herbal cream formulations.

25.7 Quality Control Parameters of Formulations

Quality control evaluation is an important part of product/formulation development. The evaluation of a cosmetic product should be carried out with full knowledge of the pharmacotechnical, toxicological, pharmacokinetic, regulatory, clinical phase's areas and Scientific Committee of Cosmetics and Non-Food Products Intended [45], Organization for Economic Cooperation and Development (OECD), European Cosmetic, Toiletry and Perfumery Association [13], Cosmetics, Toiletries and Fragrances Association (CTFA), Bureau of Indian Standard [10] and World Health Organization [51] guidelines. To access the risk and the safety of cosmetic products, it is necessary to determine the characteristics and toxicological data of cosmetic ingredients. Risk factors for a cosmetic ingredient are calculated in terms of margin of safety, systemic exposure dosage and lifetime cancer risk [25].

Regulatory frameworks differ significantly between the different markets. Regulatory frameworks for cosmetics adopted by major markets (include EU, USA, Japan and Canada countries), emerging markets (include China, India, ASEAN, Mercosur and the Comunidad Andina countries) and third countries (include Russia, Ukraine, Korea and Taiwan) act as a model for other countries of the world [40].

25.7.1 Physicochemical Evaluations

The physical parameters of the formulations are evaluated to analyse the appearance and stability of the formulations. Colour and odour of the formulations is checked carefully, and net content is determined. Viscosity profile of cream formulation is to be measured using a Brookfield viscometer at 10–100 rpm. The pH, thermal stability, fatty content and non-volatile content of the prepared formulations could be determined according to Indian Standard Guideline (IS: 6608-1978B-1, IS: 6608-1978B-2, IS: 6608-19 78B-3). Human skin is covered with an acid mantle having acidic pH, but due to frequent washing and use of soap, the acidity is lost, and hence to normalize the skin, moisturizers used should have acidic range. Acceptable pH range of moisturizers should be 5–8. Other parameters include assessment of ash value, acid value, saponification value, spreadability and layer thickness [31]. The saponification value of the formulations reflects the presence of free esters, which may influence the formula stability, pH and cleansing properties. Spreadability and layer thickness are the measure of consistency of the product.

25.7.2 Physical Stability

Stability of prepared formulation is determined by centrifugation and freeze thaw method. During centrifugation study, cream is centrifuged at 3,500–13,500 rpm at the intervals of 500 rpm for 10 min and further observed for phase separation. In freeze thaw study, all the formulations are kept alternatively at 20°C and 40°C, then observed for colour change and phase separation. All evaluations were carried out in triplicate.

25.7.3 Safety Analysis

Safety analysis includes determination of microbiological specification and sensitivity profile. Microbial examination of 1-ml cream is tested according to COLIPA guidelines and Indian Standards methods IS 11648; 1999. Total numbers of viable mesophilic microorganism are recorded by using a colony counter. The sample is determined for the presence or absence of *Pseudomonas aeruginosa*, *Staphylococcus aureus* and *Candida albicans*. To ensure that formulation is free from any adverse effect, a sensitivity study using a patch-test design is conducted on all volunteers. After 24 h, volunteers are observed for any irritation, erythema score [redness] and oedema. Cream formulation is applied on the back of forearm with the help of surgical gauze (0.5 mg/cm^2), and the erythema score [redness] is determined using the scale defined in the Indian Standards. Average erythemal score = total score of each product/total number of volunteers. Erythema score 0 indicates that the formulation is free from irritation, and a score of 1 indicates slight redness of skin by visual observation according to COLIPA and BIS guidelines [3].

25.7.4 Psychometric Evaluations

The products are compared based on sensory evaluation, and ranking is done as per score obtained according to the hedonic scale. The cream formulations are applied twice a day once in morning and once in evening at the same time over volunteers up to 6 weeks, and observations are made by ranking method, various questions were asked to volunteers and according to their answers, ranking is done between 0 and 9 of hedonic scale; ranking is done as follows: 8–9 (extremely liking), 5–7 (medium), 1–3 (dislike), 6 (in between extreme liking and medium), 4 (in between medium and dislike), verbally for appearance, fragrance, lathery feel, softness, irritation, stickiness, smoothness and after-effect of skin [3, 23]. Overall ranking is done on the basis of average score of each product.

25.7.5 In Vitro Sun Protection Factor (SPF) Determination of Extracts and Formulation

For the development of moisturizers having sun protection properties, the extracts of photoprotective herbs like *Aloe vera*, *Curcuma longa*, *Punica granatum and Areca catechu* are included; further sun protection factor of these herbal extracts and the prepared herbal moisturizing formulations are evaluated in vitro and in vivo. Ratio of ultraviolet (UV) minimum erythemal doses protected to unprotected gives the SPF. The in vitro method measures the reduction of the irradiation by measuring the transmittance after passing through a film of product. The most common in vitro technique involves measuring the spectral transmittance at UV wavelengths from 280 to 400 nm [28, 35]. The observed absorbance values at 5-nm intervals are calculated using formula as follows:

$$\mathrm{SPF}_{\mathrm{spectrophotometric}} = \mathrm{CF} \times \sum_{290}^{320} \mathrm{EE}(\lambda) \times \mathrm{I}(\lambda) \times \mathrm{Abs}(\lambda),$$

where CF = correction factor (10), EE(l) = erythemogenic effect of radiation with wavelength l, $I(l)$ = intensity of solar light of wavelength l and Abs(l) = spectrophotometric absorbance values at wavelength l. The values of EE(l) × $I(l)$ are constant. They are determined by Sayre et al. [48]. The ultraviolet (UV) absorption ability of various volatile and non-volatile herbal oils used in sun-protective moisturizing formulations were evaluated and found that, among fixed oils taken, the SPF value of olive oil and coconut oil was high around 8 and, among essential oils taken, the SPF value of peppermint oil and tulsi oil was found around 7 [28]. These studies could be helpful while selection of oil phase in the designing of formulations.

25.7.6 In Vivo Method Sun Protection Factor (SPF) Determination

This method is based on subjective evaluation of human volunteers. The sun protection factor (SPF) value of a product is defined as the ratio of the minimal erythema dose on product protected skin (MEDp) to the minimal erythema dose on unprotected skin (MEDu) of the same subject [volunteer].

$$\mathrm{SPF} = \frac{\mathrm{MEDp\ [protected\ skin]}}{\mathrm{MEDu\ [unprotected\ skin].}}$$

The minimal erythema dose (MED) in human skin is defined as the lowest ultraviolet UV dose that produces the first perceptible unambiguous erythema with defined borders appearing over most of the field of UV exposure, 16–24 h after UV exposure [7, 23].

25.7.7 Bioengineering Methods of Evaluation

The evaluation of the effect of formulation on change in skin properties is determined by the application of formulation on the skin of human volunteers, and the change in skin viscoelasticity, skin hydration, sebum content, melanin and erythema are observed by the use of Cutometer and their probes.

The viscoelastic properties are measured using Cutometer® MPA 580 (Courage and Khazaka, Germany). The measuring principle is suction/elongation. An optical system detects the decrease of infrared light intensity depending on the distance the skin is being sucked into the probe. In this study, the strain time mode was applied. A probe with a 2-mm opening is used, and a pressure of 450–500 mbar is applied in order to suck the skin into the probe. Each measurement consisted of five suction cycles (2–3 s of suction followed by 2–3 s of relaxation) and is performed in triplicate on body skin (volar forearm). The following parameters (absolute and relative) are analyzed: Ue, elastic deformation; Uv, viscoelasticity; [R0] Uf, total deformation; Ur, retraction; [R2] Ua/Uf, overall elasticity of the skin; [R5] Ur/Ue, pure elasticity of the skin without viscous deformation; [R7] Ur/Uf, biological elasticity, i.e., the ratio of retraction to extension; [R6] Uv/Ue, the ratio of viscoelasticity to elastic deformation and R8 or (Ua), pliability, i.e. ability of the skin to return into its original state [16, 23].

Hydration of the epidermis (stratum corneum) is determined with a non-invasive, skin capacitance meter (Corneometer® CM 820, Courage Khazaka, Ko ln, Germany). Corneometry is an established method for the determination of skin hydration [6]. The acceptance is due to high reproducibility, easy handling, short measuring time and economy [21]. The device determines the water content of the superficial epidermal layers down to a depth of about 0.1 mm and expresses the values in arbitrary units. For single application studies after the baseline measurement, each formulation is applied to the volunteers, and measurements are carried out after 0.5, 1, 2 and 3 h of application. Similarly, for multiple application, formulations are applied twice daily, in the morning and in the evening; for 1, 2 and 6 weeks, the measurements are carried out.

Sebum consists of a mixture of lipids and cellular debris that form a lipidic film on the surface of the epidermis, which regulates the water content of the skin, its integrity, softness, plasticity, hydration and aspect [33]. The lipid concentration is measured using Sebumeter® SM 815 (Courage and Khazaka, Germany). The test product is applied twice daily to the body site (volar forearm or forehead) for a period of 6 weeks. A clinical assessment and instrumental measurements are done before and after the treatment period. Casual sebum level is determined. Mexameter® MX 18 is a narrow band reflectance spectrophotometer and measures the intensity of erythema and melanin pigmentation (Fig. 25.6).

25.7.8 Toxicological Profile Analysis

Cosmetic products should be free from side effects as their use is concern to human health. To access the risk and the safety of cosmetic products, it is necessary to determine the characteristics and toxicological data of cosmetic ingredients [25]. Important parameters for the determination of toxicological profile of the ingredients include acute toxicity, irritation and corrosivity, skin irritation and skin corrosivity, mucous membrane irritation, skin sensitization, dermal/percutaneous absorption, repeated dose toxicity, mutagenicity/genotoxicity, carcinogenicity, reproductive toxicity, toxicokinetic studies and photo-induced toxicity measured in terms of photoirritation and photomutagenicity of cosmetic ingredients [25].

25.7.9 Biological Studies

UV protecting effects of cream formulation is studied by estimation of biochemical parameters, i.e. catalase, superoxide dismutase, malondialdehyde, ascorbic acid and total protein in each set of experiment. Ultraviolet radiation induces changes in superoxide dismutases, catalase, malondialdehyde, ascorbic acid and total protein level in skin. Microscopically, as the skin ages normally, the des becomes hypocellular, the vasculature remains intact and collagen forms a stable with increased cross-linked matrix. By contrast, the epidermis of photoaged skin

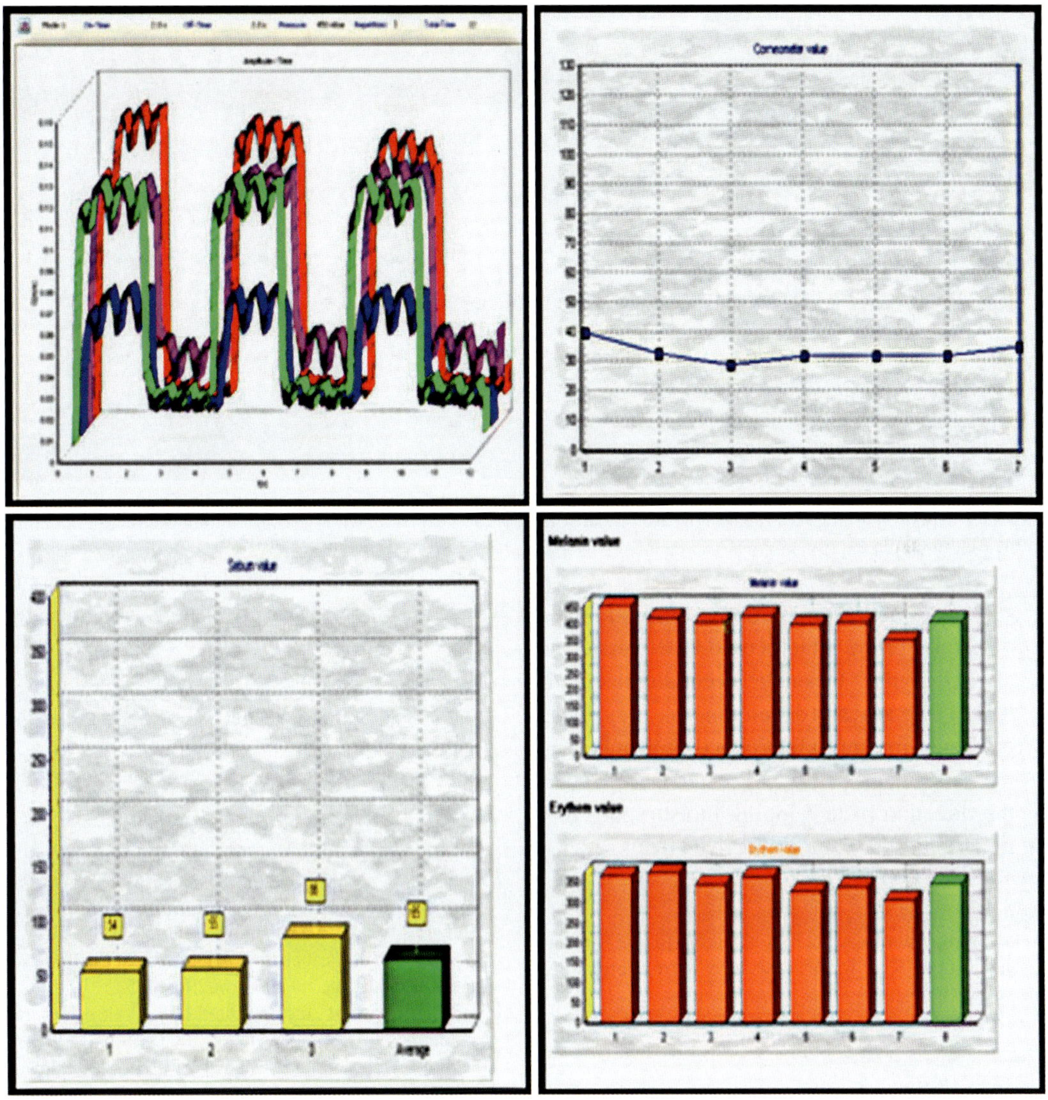

Fig. 25.6 Curves produced by Cutometer (skin viscoelasticity), Corneometer (skin hydration), Sebumeter (Sebum content) and Mexameter (melanin and erythema value)

becomes thickened and the vessels tortures. Antioxidants protect the human body against damage by reactive oxygen species [4].

Ashawat et al. prepared and characterized herbal cosmetic cream comprising extracts of *G. glabra*, *C. longa* (roots), seeds of *P. corlifolia*, *C. tom*, *A. catechu*, *P. granatum*, fruits of *E. officinale*, leaves of *C. asiatica*, dried bark of *C. zeylanicum* and fresh gel of *A. vera* for the protection of skin against UV-induced ageing and observed that treatment with such herbal extracts containing creams could be utilized for the protection of photo-induced intrinsic oxidative stress as well as structural alterations in skin (Fig. 25.7).

Conclusion

Formulation of moisturizing cosmetic formulations with the maximum use of natural raw materials is the present need for cosmeticians. Research is continuously been done to develop

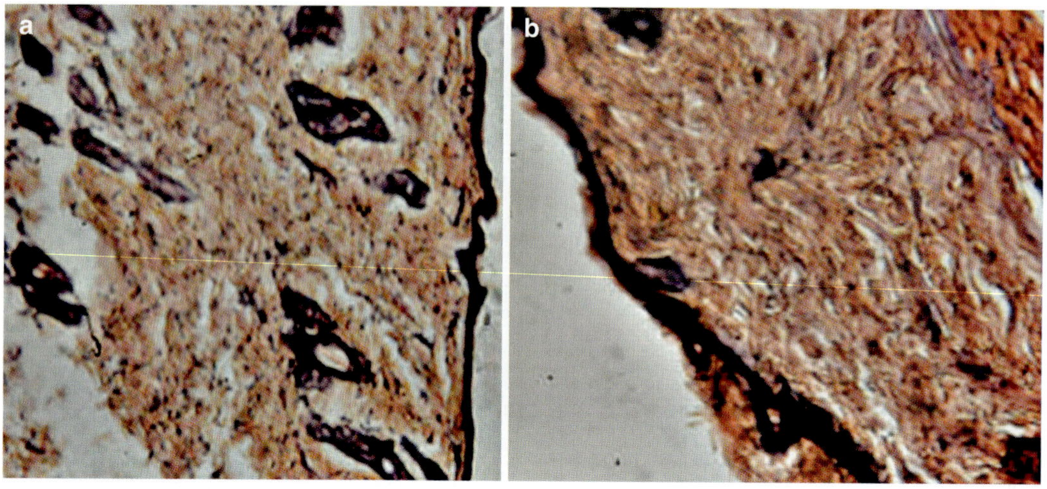

Fig. 25.7 Microphotograph of rat skin (**a**) after ultraviolet radiation exposure (**b**) after formulation pretreatment before ultraviolet radiation exposure

stable cosmetic formulations using additives of natural origin which could be effective for all skin types. Cosmetic formulations with herbal extracts are developing as they yield mild, non-irritant, safe products with enhancement of skin properties. Research is moving in the direction of developing moisturizing formulations with photoprotective effects.

Acknowledgements Author is thankful to the student Chanchal Deep Kaur for his assistance during formatting the work.

References

1. Andrade FF, Santos ODH, Oliveira WP, Rocha-Filho PA (2007) Influence of PEG-12 dimethicone addition on stability and formation of emulsions containing liquid crystal. Int J Cosmet Sci 29:211–218
2. Ashawat MS, Banchhor M, Saraf S et al (2009) Herbal cosmetics: trends in skin care formulation. Phcog Rev 3(5):72–79
3. Ashawat MS, Saraf S, Saraf S (2008) Preparation and characterisation of herbal creams for improvement of skin viscoelastic properties. Int J Cosmet Sci 30: 183–193
4. Ashawat MS, Saraf S, Saraf S (2007) Biochemical and histopathological studies of herbal cream against UV radiation induced damage. Trends Med Res 2(3):135–141
5. Belo SED, Gaspar LR, Campos RMBGM (2006) Moisturizing effect of cosmetic formulations containing *Aloe vera* extract in different concentrations assessed by skin bioengineering techniques. Skin Res Technol 12:241–246
6. Barel AO (1995) Clary's measurement of epidermal capacitance. In: Bioengineering of the skin: water and the stratum corneum. CRC Press, Boca Raton, pp 165–170
7. Bendova H, Akram J, Krejci A, Kubac L, Jirova D, Kejlova K, Kolarova H, Brabec M, Maly M (2007) In vitro approaches to evaluation of sun protection factor. Toxicol In Vitro 21:1268–1275
8. Benson HA (2006) Transferosomes for transdermal drug delivery. Expert Opin Drug Deliv 3(6):727–737
9. Betz G, Aeppli A, Menshutina N et al (2005) In vivo comparison of various liposome formulations for cosmetic application. Int J Pharm 296:44–54
10. BIS (Bureau of Indian standard) (2006) General guidelines for herbal cosmetics. PCD-19:6/T-1 C 1–6
11. Carlotti ME, Gallarate M, Rossatto V (2003) O/W microemulsion as a vehicle for sunscreens. J Cosmet Sci 54(5):451–462
12. Cevc G (2004) Lipid vesicles and other colloids as drug carriers on the skin. Adv Drug Deliv Rev 56(5):675–711
13. COLIPA (2001) Evaluation of the efficacy of cosmetic products. COLIPA Guidelines 1–16
14. Deep C, Saraf S (2009) Herbal photoprotective formulations and their evaluation. Open Nat Prod J 2:57–62
15. Deep C, Saraf S (2008) Novel approaches in herbal cosmetics. J Cosmet Dermatol 7:89–95
16. Escoffer C, Rigal JD, Rochefort R et al (1989) Age related mechanical properties of human skin: an in vivo study. J Invest Dermatol 93:353–357
17. European Chemicals Bureau, ECB (2003) Technical guidance document on risk assessment in support of Commission Directive 93/67/EEC on risk assessment for new notified substances, Commission Regulation (EC) No 1488/94 on risk assessment for existing

substances and Directive 98/8/EC of the European Parliament and of the Council concerning the placing of biocidal products on the market. Doc. EUR 20418 EN/1, European Communities
18. Forster T, Tesmann H (1991) Phase inversion emulsification. Cosmet Toil 11:106
19. Gregoriadis G (1994) Liposomes and anti-ageing creams: the facts beneath the face. Biochemist Feb/Mar
20. Gupta A, Ashawat MS, Saraf S, Swarnlata S (2007) Phytosome: a novel approach towards functional cosmetics. J Plant Sci 2(6):644–649
21. Heinrich U, Koop U, Leneveu Duchemin MC et al (2003) Multicentre comparison of skin hydration in terms of physical, physiological and product dependent parameters by the capacitive method (Corneometer CM 825). Int J Cosmet Sci 25:45–53
22. Jacobi O, Heinrich (1954) The acid mantle of the skin. Proceedings Science Sector of Toilet Goods Association, 21, 6
23. Kapoor S, Saraf S (2009) Age dependent studies as various skin parameters using cutometer. Indian J Pharm Educ Res 43(4):338–345
24. Kapoor S, Swarnlata S (2008) A note on dire need of harmonisation of cosmetic legislation. Int J Trade Glob Mark 1(4):419–431
25. Kapoor S, Saraf S (2008) Risk analysis tools for toxicological profile of cosmetics. Internet J Toxicol 5(2):1–13
26. Kapoor S, Saraf S (2010) Assessment of viscoelasticity and hydration effect of herbal moisturizers using bioengineering techniques. Phcog Mag 6(24):298–304
27. Kapoor S, Saraf S (2010) Formulation and evaluation of moisturizer containing herbal extracts for the management of dry skin. Phcog J 2(11):409–418
28. Kaur CD, Saraf S (2010) *In vitro* SPF determination of herbal oils used in cosmetics. Pharmacog Res 2(1):22–25
29. Kaur CD, Saraf S (2011) Photochemoprotective activity of alcoholic extract of *Camellia sinensis*. Int J Pharmacol 7(3):400–404
30. Lachapelle JM (1996) Efficacy of protective creams and/or gels. Prevention of contact dermatitis. Curr Probl Dermatol 25:182–192
31. Lachman L, Herbert AL, Joseph LK (1999) The theory and practice of industrial pharmacy, IIIth edn. Varghese Publ. House, Bombay, p 569
32. Latuen AR (1958) Fundamental and comparative actions of cleansing cream. Am Perfumes 72:29
33. Leydenn JJ (1995) New understanding of the pathogenesis of acne. J Am Acad Dermatol 32:S15–S25
34. Loggia RD, Sosa S, Tubaro A, Morazzoni P, Bombardelli E, Griffin A (1996) Anti-inflammatory activity of some Gingko biloba constituents and of their phospholipids- complexes. Fitoterapia 3: 257–273
35. Mansur JS, Breder MNR, Mansur MCA et al (1986) Determinação Do Fator De Proteção Solar Por Espectrofotometria. An Bras Dermatol 61:121–124
36. Marty JP (2002) NMF and cosmetology of cutaneous hydration. Ann Dermatol Venereol 129:131–136
37. Niemiec SM, Ramachandran C, Weiner N (1995) Influence of nonionic liposomal composition on topical delivery of peptide drugs into pilosebaceous units: an in vivo study using the hamster ear model. Pharm Res 12(8):1184–1188
38. Oyedeji FO, Okeke IE (2010) Comparative analysis of moisturising creams from vegetable oils and paraffin oil. Res J Appl Sci 5(3):157–160
39. Rawlings AV, Harding CR (2004) Moisturization and skin barrier function. Dermatol Ther 17:43–48
40. Saraf S, Kapoor S (2008) Cosmetic legislation, Istth edn. Nirali Prakashan, Pune. ISBN 978–81–96396–13–8
41. Saraf S, Kaur CD (2010) Phytoconstituents as photoprotective novel cosmetic formulations. Pharmacog Rev 4(7):1–11
42. Saraf S (2010) Application of nanosystem in cosmetics. In: Chaughule RS, Ramanujan RV (eds) Nanoparticles synthesis, characterization and applications. American Scientific Publication, Stevenson Ranch, pp 379–399. ISBN 1–58883–180–9
43. Saraf S, Paliwal S, Kaur CD, Saraf S (2011) Sphingosomes a novel approach to vesicular drug delivery. Res J Pharm Tech 4(5):661–666
44. Saraf S, Sahu S, Kaur CD, Saraf S (2010) Comparative measurement of hydration effects of herbal moisturizers. Pharmacog Res 2(3):146–151
45. Scientific Committee of Cosmetics and Non-Food Products (SCCNFP) (2003) Notes of guidance for testing of cosmetic ingredients and their safety evaluation by the SCCNFP. SCCNFP/0690/03 Final 1–102
46. Thomssen EG (2006) Modern cosmetics. Universal Publishing Corporation, Bombay, 101
47. Yamaguchi M, Tahara Y, Teruhiko M et al (2009) Comparison of cathepsin l activity in cheek and forearm stratum corneum in young female adults. Skin Res Technol 15:370–375
48. Sayre RM, Agin PP, Levee GJ et al (1979) Comparison of in vivo and in vitro testing of sunscreening formulas. Photochem Photobiol 29:559–566
49. Yoon HS, Baik SH, Oh CH (2002) Quantitative measurement of desquamation and skin elasticity in diabetic patients. Skin Res Technol 8:250–254
50. Khan Y, Talegaonkar A, Zeenat SI et al (2006) Multiple emulsions: an overview. Curr Drug Deliv 3(4):429–443
51. World Health Organization (WHO) (1998) Quality control methods for medicinal plant materials. WHO, Geneva, pp 1–122
52. Murray BC, Wickett RR (1996) Sensitivity of Cutometer data to stratum corneum hydration level. A preliminary study. Skin Res Technol 2:167–172
53. Cevc G, Blume G (1992) Lipid vesicles penetrate into intact skin owing to the transdermal osmotic gradients and hydration force. Biochim Biophys Acta 1104: 226–232
54. Touitou E, Dayan N, Bergelson L (2000) Ethosomes-novel vesicular carriers for enhanced delivery: characterization and skin penetration properties. J Control Rel (65)3: 403-418

Chemical and Physical Properties of Emollients

26

Jari T. Alander

26.1 Introduction

Emolliency can be translated as "softening ability," and emollients are substances that make something softer to the touch. In cosmetic and personal care applications, an emollient is usually an oily substance, which when applied to the skin, makes it softer and more lubricated, enhancing the sensory properties of the skin. Emolliency is also an important parameter in skin moisturization as many emollients also contribute to regulating the moisture balance in the skin. In clinical practice, the term emollient is also used for formulated products used for treating dry skin conditions.

Emollients are normally volume-wise the biggest ingredient group in a skin care formulation, after water. The emollient phase may comprise 5–30% of the formulation in oil-in-water emulsions. Anhydrous systems and water-in-oil emulsions can contain even higher emollient concentrations. Understanding the different emollient types and their chemical and physical behavior is consequently important for the formulator, especially when optimizing the emollient composition to meet requirements on functionality and cost.

This chapter reviews several emollient technologies used in skin care products and describes the similarities and differences between the different substances that are commonly used for emolliency. The focus is on chemical and physical parameters differentiating the different emollient types, with the purpose of giving the formulator better understanding of this ingredient group.

26.2 Emollient Functionality Is Complex

Emollients are, along with emulsifiers and actives, the most important functional ingredient groups in skin care formulations. The emollient will influence the performance of the formulation in several ways: consistency of the formulation, skin feel, moisturization and lubricity on skin, delivery of actives, and the marketability of the product. It is therefore important to be able to optimize the properties of the emollients phase and tailor-make it for the intended use.

26.2.1 Emollients Determine the Structure of the Formulation

In the formulation, the emollient phase composition will determine the consistency of the cream or lotion. The viscosity and polarity, together with the presence of solid emollients, can be used to make the formulation more fluid or more solid, depending on the intended use.

J.T. Alander
Lipids for Care, AarhusKarlshamn AB, Västra Kajen, Karlshamn, Sweden
e-mail: jari.alander@aak.com

M. Lodén, H.I. Maibach (eds.), *Treatment of Dry Skin Syndrome*,
DOI 10.1007/978-3-642-27606-4_26, © Springer-Verlag Berlin Heidelberg 2012

The emollient polarity will determine the solubility of active components, especially lipophilic ones. Correct choice of emollients can potentiate the activity of an active substance by controlling its bioavailability, by considering the properties of the active ingredient, stratum corneum and the formulation [1].

The interaction with emulsifiers and the choice of emulsifiers are also determined by the polarity and viscosity of the emollient. The solubility of the emulsifier and its ability to form liquid crystals and other surfactant aggregates are strongly dependent on the polarity of the oil phase in the system. This phenomenon is reflected in the use of the HLB system for characterizing emulsifiers as well as the phase inversion temperature (PIT) concept [2, 3].

26.2.2 Skin Feel Is Influenced by the Choice of Emollient

When applied to the skin, the polarity and viscosity of the emollient phase will determine "the skin feel." This elusive term is a concentrate of everything which can be classified as the sensory properties of the formulation: lubricity, spreadability, absorption into the skin, and duration on the skin surface. These factors are closely linked to the molecular structure of the emollients [4–6].

The functionality of the emollient when absorbed into the skin is also important to consider. In contrast to common belief, the emollient is seldom an inert substance that does not influence the physiology of the skin. The emollient may interact with the skin lipids and also be metabolized in the skin if the chemical structure is suitable [7, 8].

26.3 Principles for Emollient Classification

There are many reasons to classify emollients: for understanding the behavior of emollients in formulations, for simplifying formulations, for making alternative formulations, and for solving problems due to emollient behavior. The classification of emollients can be based on the chemistry of the substances used, but sometimes, especially when dealing with complex ingredients or mixtures of ingredients, a physicochemically based classification is more appropriate.

26.3.1 Emollient Classification Based on Molecular Structure

From a chemical point of view, most commercially available emollients come from three different types of chemistries: hydrocarbon based, ester based, or silicone based. Emollients utilizing moieties containing nitrogen and phosphorus are not common, and combinations with halogens are normally too toxic to be of interest. Table 26.1 illustrates some typical emollient structures and structural variations in each group.

Hydrocarbons, in this case without functional groups other than unsaturation and ring formation, are the common base for many classes of emollients. In this group, we find naturally occurring hydrocarbons such as squalene and squalane derived from biomaterials, simple hydrocarbons from mineral oil deposits (petroleum based), and synthetic hydrocarbons, normally derived from petroleum sources. Saturated hydrocarbons are usually chemically inert, being resistant to oxidation and hydrolysis.

Fatty alcohols such as oleyl alcohol or isostearyl alcohol are also frequently used as emollients or emollient modifiers in skin care formulations. These substances combine a long hydrocarbon chain with a primary hydroxyl group. In some cases, especially in short chain alcohols used in esters, the alcohol group can also be a secondary one.

Ester-based emollients combine a carboxylic acid with an alcohol. Depending on the chemical structure of the acid and the alcohol, we can talk about simple esters, polyhydric alcohol (polyol) esters, and complex esters. A specific group of polyhydric alcohol esters are the naturally occurring vegetable and animal oils and fats, which are based on fatty acid esters of glycerol. The common

Table 26.1 Grouping of commonly used skin care emollients and typical structural variations

Emollient type	Examples	Variations	Molecular structure
Mineral oil hydrocarbons	Paraffin oil	Chain length and branching	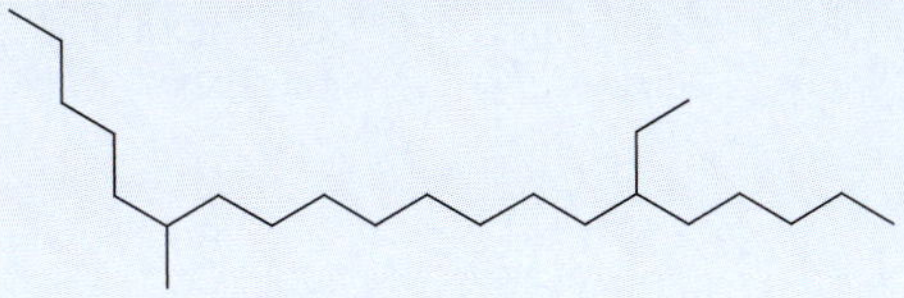
Naturally occurring hydrocarbons	Squalane	Unsaturation	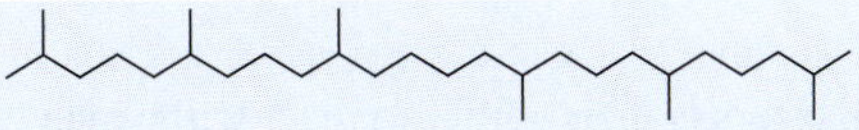
Synthetic hydrocarbons	Isohexadecane	Monomer type, chain length, and branching	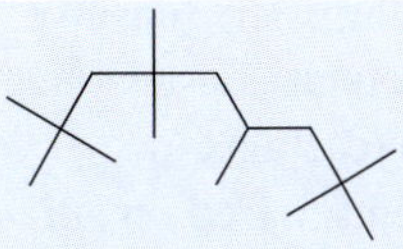
Fatty alcohols	Cetearyl alcohol	Chain length and unsaturation	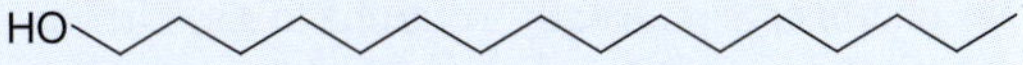
Guerbet and oxo alcohols	2-octyldodecanol	Chain length and branching	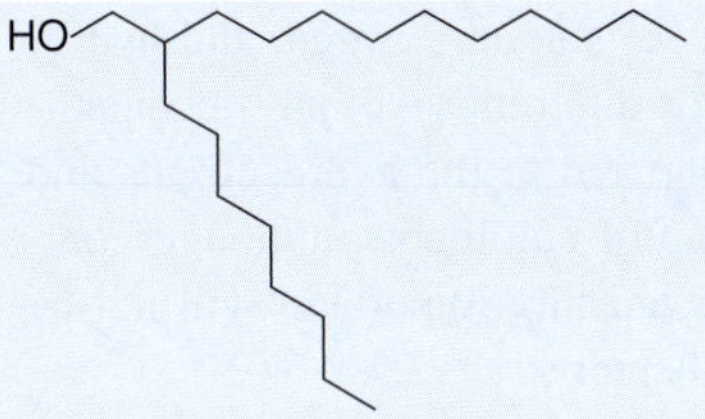
Natural fatty acids	Oleic acid	Chain length and unsaturation	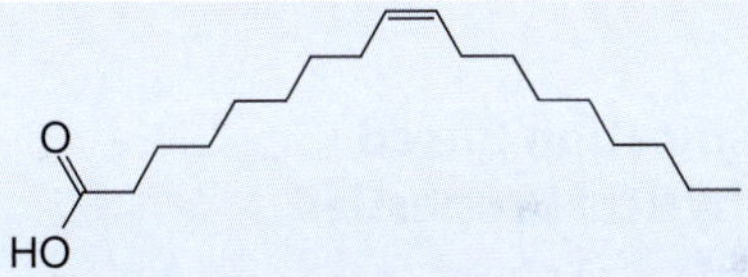
Synthetic fatty acids	Isostearic acid	Chain length and branching	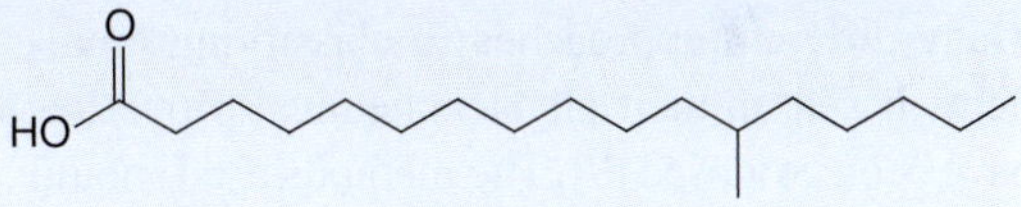
Simple esters	Isopropyl myristate	Acid and alcohol structure	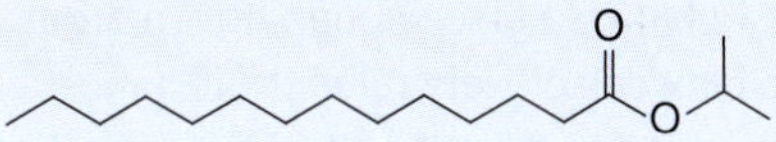
Natural triglycerides	Olive oil	Fatty acid and triglyceride composition	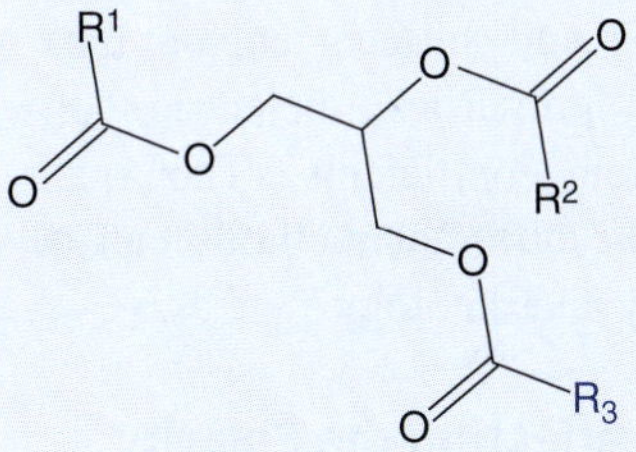
Synthetic triglycerides	Caprylic/capric triglyceride	Fatty acid type and ratio	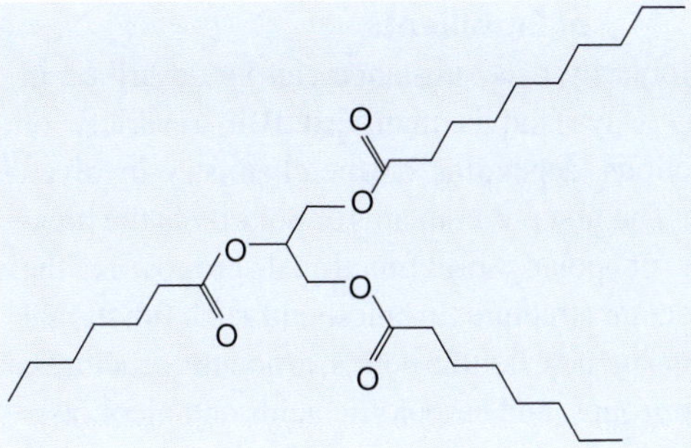

(continued)

Table 26.1 (continued)

Emollient type	Examples	Variations	Molecular structure
Complex esters	Diisopropyl adipate	Acid and alcohol structure	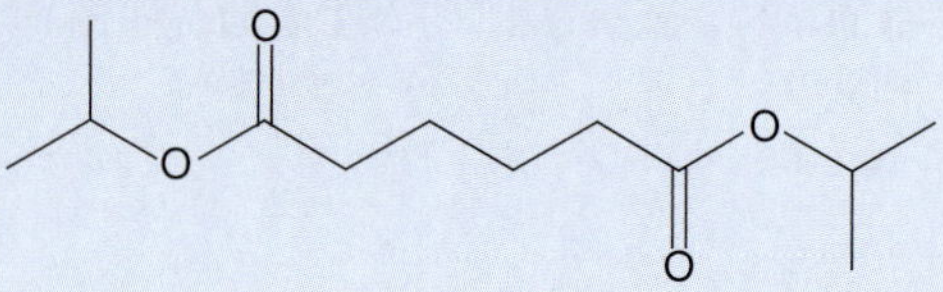

trait of all esters is their ability to react with water, releasing acid and alcohol, making esters sensitive to formulation conditions. Unsaturated esters are also sensitive towards oxidation reactions.

The fourth group of emollients, based on silicon chemistry, is usually referred to as silicone oils. More appropriately named siloxanes, they are combinations of silicon, oxygen, and hydrocarbons, offering a different set of physicochemical behavior compared to the hydrocarbons and esters. This group of emollients, although commercially and technically important, will not be covered in this chapter.

26.3.2 Classification Based on Physical Properties

Many different approaches to classifying emollients based on their physicochemical properties have been proposed [9]. The methods used should be easy to apply but also give enough information to distinguish between closely related substances. Methods proposed for the classification include rheology, interfacial and surface tension measurements, thermal properties, dielectric constants, and partition coefficients. The main directions for all the different methods can be divided into polarity and rheology.

26.3.2.1 Factors Affecting the Polarity of Emollients

The polarity of a substance can be described in many ways and is manifested in a variety of directions, depending on the chemistry involved [10]. The first prerequisite for polarity is the presence of polarizable functional groups in the molecular structure. In emollients such functional groups include double bonds, aromatic structures, ester groups, and carboxylic acids and alcohols.

The polarizability of double bonds increase in the following order: isolated double bonds < conjugated double bonds < aromatic double bonds as the presence of mobile electrons increases. Isolated ester bonds are less polarizable than conjugated ones of the same reason.

Polarizable groups can also present permanent dipoles if the functional groups are separated by an appropriate distance.

Permanent polarity is also caused by hydrogen bonding. Here, free carboxylic acid, alcohol, and amino groups are important functionalities to consider.

A classification of emollients based on polarity looks into the presence and concentration of these polarizable structural elements, permanent dipoles, and the presence or absence of hydrogen bonding.

26.3.2.2 Rheology as a Tool to Describe Emollients

The viscosity of a substance is to a large degree dependent on the size of the constituent molecules, larger molecules have larger surface areas, increasing the possibility of van der Waals interactions. Structural factors such as branching and cyclization will affect the molecular size and shape leading to effects on viscosity and self diffusion coefficients [11]. Increasing the molecular interactions by introducing polarizability and polarization will also strongly influence the rheological properties.

In complex emollient mixtures comprising solid crystals, such as in petrolatum, the rheology is more complex, and viscoelasticity is commonly encountered. For viscoelastic systems, viscosity as commonly measured is an insufficient tool to describe the rheological properties, and more sophisticated rheometers must be used to get a correct evaluation of such systems. The elastic modulus is often giving good correlation to formulation stability and to sensory properties [12].

Classification of emollients based on rheology is a simple tool and gives a rough guideline for the estimation of the applicability of each emollient.

26.4 Individual Emollient Groups

The commercially available emollients can be described in order of increased complexity, starting with simple hydrocarbons and adding functional groups to influence the physicochemical properties.

26.4.1 Hydrocarbon-Based Emollients

Although emollients based on vegetable and animal oils and fats were probably the first ones to be used in skin care, petroleum-based materials rapidly became the standard when the cosmetic industry developed in the early 1900s. Petroleum-based materials were abundant, had good technological properties, and gave an excellent moisturization and emolliency. Petrolatum and mineral oil are still the most commonly used emollients globally although alternative technologies are being developed, basically due to the nonrenewability of the petroleum resources.

26.4.1.1 Naturally Occurring Hydrocarbons

Squalane and Squalene

Squalene and squalane are naturally occurring hydrocarbons with a specific metabolic function, being precursors for the formation of steroidal components in animals and plants [13]. Pure squalene is extracted from shark liver oil and from olive oil processing residuals. The shark oil squalene is not a sustainable alternative due to overfishing of the shark, and most squalene on the market is now from vegetable sources. The main raw material is olive oil deodorizer distillate which can contain sufficiently high levels of squalene to be commercially viable [14].

Squalene is highly unsaturated and oxidizes rapidly. Oxidized squalene is associated with comedogenicity. Squalene with a high peroxide value was tested and shown to be comedogenic. After purification to remove the oxidized squalene, the comedogenicity disappeared, linking oxidized lipids to inflammatory reactions associated with comedogenesis [15–18].

The squalene is hydrogenated to produce squalane, a very stable, low-melting branched hydrocarbon with low viscosity. It is used to decrease the oiliness of the formulation, increasing the slip and for a generally pleasant and light skin feel.

Petrolatum and Mineral Oil

Petrolatum is a fraction of mineral oil with semisolid consistency. Physicochemically, it is an oleogel, an oil-based, lipophilic, gel stabilized by network forming crystals of high-melting hydrocarbons. The composition of petrolatum is usually complex, comprising hundreds of individual hydrocarbons [19, 20]. It is derived from paraffinic mineral oils which is purified and hydrogenated to remove unsaturation and improve stability and color. Liquid mineral oils or paraffin oils are chemically similar to petrolatum but do not contain the high-melting waxes that give petrolatum its consistency.

26.4.1.2 Synthetic Hydrocarbons

Synthetic hydrocarbons are obtained from simple building blocks such as ethene, propene, isobutene, and decene by oligomerization reactions. Ethene produces polyethylene which is a linear hydrocarbon resulting rapidly in high melting points with increased molecular weight while propene, isobutene, and decene can be used to make low-melting branched hydrocarbons. These saturated, branched, emollients are hydrophobic and stable against oxidation. Synthetic hydrocarbons can also be obtained by catalytic cracking of heavier mineral oils and fractional distillation to obtain fractions with desired melting points and viscosities.

26.4.2 Alcohol-Based Emollients

A few long chain alcohols are used as emollients on their own, but both long-chain and short-chain alcohols are important building blocks for ester-based emollients. They also introduce an important additional functionality to the hydrocarbons: the hydroxyl group. Free hydroxyl groups increase the polarity and have the capacity of forming hydrogen bonds with water, allowing alcohols to participate in liquid crystals and interact with skin lipids.

26.4.2.1 Long Chain Fatty Alcohols

Saturated fatty alcohols such as cetyl (palmitoyl), stearyl, or cetostearyl alcohols are not primarily used as emollients in skin care creams and lotions, their primary function being emulsion stabilizer and consistency factor. They do, however, contribute to the moisturization and emolliency by interacting with the emulsifier system when formulated at 1–2% in the formulation. These saturated alcohols are obtained from fully saturated palm oil, soybean oil, or animal fats after a catalytic reduction of the corresponding acids or methyl esters.

Oleyl alcohol is a constituent of some plant and animal waxes. A traditional source is whale oil which was obtained from the blubber of the sperm whale. Small amounts of oleyl alcohol are present in jojoba oil (*Simmondsia chinensis*) where the seed oil contains esters of unsaturated long chain alcohols with long chain fatty acids (wax esters) [21]. Most industrial oleyl alcohol is produced by catalytic reduction of oleic acid or its methyl esters. Oleyl alcohol is available in different grades characterized by the iodine value, reflecting the degree of unsaturation. Stearyl and palmitoyl alcohol are present as by-products, depending on the raw material origin (palm oil or animal fats).

Isostearyl alcohol is a branched fatty alcohol which is formed by a high-temperature isomerization reaction of unsaturated fatty acids, producing a mixture of randomly branched isomers. After hydrogenation to remove remaining double bonds and to convert the acid to alcohol, isostearyl alcohols with a low melting point and high stability are obtained.

Guerbet alcohols are a special class of branched alcohols formed from primary alcohols via an oxidation and aldol condensation mechanism [22]. The resulting alcohols are primary alcohols with a long hydrocarbon branching in the beta position. Typical Guerbet alcohols are 2-ethylhexanol (from *n*-butanol), 2-octyldodecanol (from *n*-decanol), and 2-hexyldecanol (from *n*-octanol). The branched Guerbet alcohols have lower melting points than their corresponding linear isomers with the same carbon number. Being saturated, Guerbet alcohols are normally resistant against oxidation.

Synthetic alcohols from petroleum sources include the oxo alcohols which are derived from unsaturated hydrocarbons by the addition of carbon monoxide and hydrogen in a hydroformulation process. The resulting aldehydes can further react by the aldol condensation forming branched alcohols after reduction of the aldehyde. Oxo alcohols are available in chain lengths from C8 (2-ethylhexanol) to C15.

26.4.3 Ester-Based Emollients

Esters are a popular and versatile group of emollients, due to the availability of a large number of ingredients with large differences in properties. This versatility can be used by the formulator to bring various functions to the skin care product, influencing stability, aesthetics, skin feel, and delivery of actives.

26.4.3.1 Simple Esters

Simple esters can be defined as esters of monohydric alcohols with acids with only one acid group. When used as emollients, the molecular weights, expressed as carbon numbers, range from C16 to C36, and the melting points from about −30°C up to 40°C. If the melting points exceed 40°C, the ingredients are often too waxy and hard to be used alone. However, high melting esters can be used at low concentration to modify the consistency and skin feel of the formulations.

Raw Materials for Simple Esters

Two types of raw materials are needed for ester production: an alcohol and a fatty acid. As there are numerous possibilities of combining an acid with an alcohol, a large variety in properties and behavior can be seen. Many groups of emollients are the result of the development of oleochemistry which combines a natural raw material with a synthetic one.

Carboxylic Acids for Ester Production

All types of carboxylic acids are useful reactants for the formation of esters. Emollient esters, however, are usually based on acids that are longer than 8 carbons due to the higher aggressiveness of shorter acids and due to the normally offensive smell associated with shorter fatty acids. These long chain carboxylic acids are normally called fatty acids, especially if they originate in natural raw materials.

Several types of structural variations are relevant when describing the fatty acids used in emollient esters: chain length, even/odd carbon chains, unsaturation, branching, position on the chain of various functional groups, and so on. All these parameters contribute to the performance of the resulting ester as a cosmetic emollient.

Natural Fatty Acids

Natural fatty acids are obtained from vegetable or animal oils and fats by splitting (hydrolysis) of the fat into glycerol and acids [23]. The most important sources for fatty acids are coconut/palm kernel oil for lauric and myristic acids, palm oil for palmitic and oleic acids, and soybean/rapeseed oil for oleic, linoleic, and linolenic acids. Palm oil, soybean oil, and rapeseed oil are also important sources of stearic acid after hydrogenation. Animal fats such as lard and tallow are sources of palmitic, oleic, and stearic acids but are also often used after hydrogenation producing palmitic and stearic acids.

Vegetable-derived fatty acids are usually even numbered with chain lengths ranging from C8 to C24, with predominance for C12–C18. Fatty acids derived from animal fats can also contain fatty acids with an uneven number of carbons, typically C15 and C17.

The longer chain length fatty acids, starting from C16, can contain one or more double bonds. The number of double bonds and their location are important characteristics for unsaturated fatty acids. In life sciences, the normally used nomenclature is the n-x or omega-x system which indicates the position of the first double bond, when calculated from the terminal end of the fatty acid chain. Oleic acid is thus an omega-9 fatty acid, linoleic acid an omega-6 fatty acid, and alpha-linolenic acid is an omega-3 fatty acid. Gamma-linolenic acid, in contrast, is an omega-6 fatty acid with three double bonds, changing its functionality and metabolism in the skin.

Unsaturated fatty acids from plants are normally in the all-cis configuration. Partially hydrogenated fatty acids and animal fatty acids can also contain trans-configured double bonds.

Natural-based fatty acids also comprise hydroxy acids which are found in, for example, castor oil and in lanolin (wool fat). Lanolin is also a source for branched fatty acids as well as dicarboxylic acids.

Synthetic Fatty Acids

Isostearic acid is produced as a by-product from oleic acid dimerization by a high-temperature reaction using montmorillonite clay or zeolites as catalyst [24]. Other long chain branched fatty acids are obtained by oxidation of the corresponding Guerbet alcohol or oxo alcohol.

Alcohol Sources for Esters

Alcohols and acids are related to each other in many ways. During chemical synthesis, an acid may be formed which is later reduced to an alcohol via an aldehyde. In a similar fashion, the first step in a chemical synthesis may result in an alcohol which later is oxidized to an acid. This means that for many alcohols and acids, there is a common hydrocarbon background, and the chemistry of these substances has many properties in common.

Low Molecular Weight Alcohols

Low molecular weight alcohols used in the manufacture of cosmetic emollients include isopropanol and ethanol as well as methanol and 2-ethylhexanol. Isopropanol and 2-ethylhexanol are obtained from petrochemistry while ethanol and methanol are also available through fermentation.

Low molecular weight polyhydric alcohols are also often used, for example, 1,2-propandiol (propylene glycol). Glycerol (1,2,3-propantriol) is available both from natural sources (vegetable and animal oils and fats) and from petroleum chemistry.

Long Chain Alcohols

All types of long chain fatty alcohols described above are also useful as reactants in ester formation. Branched alcohols are often used due to their stability and low melting points. The nomenclature does not always reveal if the alcohol is branched or not: octanol can be either n-octanol obtained from caprylic acid or 2-ethylhexanol obtained from petrochemical sources.

Production Methods

Classic Methods: Direct Esterification and Transesterification

Any carboxylic acid and alcohol may be used to produce an ester by direct esterification. Normally, catalysts such as strong acids or tin derivatives are used, together with a sufficiently high temperature to remove the water produced in the reaction. A more efficient route to esters is to do transesterification reactions starting from a vegetable or animal triglyceride-based oil [25]. In the first step, the oil can be reacted with methanol to produce methyl esters which can be further transesterified with other alcohols, releasing the methanol. The methanol is subsequently removed by distillation and recycled.

Esters of high molecular weight alcohols can also be produced by direct transesterification from the triglyceride oil, but reaction conditions and yields will be dependent on the structure of the alcohol used. Secondary alcohols will be less reactive in the transesterification process, and better yields are obtained via the methyl ester route.

New Developments in Esterification: Enzyme Catalysis

Biocatalysis, such as enzymatic catalysis using lipases supported by a carrier are increasingly used for the production of emollient esters. The reaction can be run at lower temperatures, saving energy but also leading to decreased formation of byproducts [26, 27].

26.4.3.2 Emollients Based on Triglycerides

Triglycerides are naturally occurring, renewable sources of emollients that can be used directly in skin care formulations. Plants and animals use triglycerides to store energy for future uses. The plants need energy in the seeds to produce a seedling that can start to photosynthesize. Animals store energy in fat depots to be used when the availability of food is scarce due to seasonal variations. Triglycerides are also a good source of raw materials for further processing to oleochemical derivatives.

Natural Oils and Fats

The fat depots in vegetable material and in animal material can be used to obtain triglyceride oils and fats that can be further developed into cosmetic ingredients. Many emollients and emulsifiers used in skin care formulations are derived from the easily accessible vegetable and animal oils and fats.

Due to purity and sustainability considerations, the vegetable fats have grown in importance over the last years and constitute an important raw material base for the cosmetic industry.

Raw Materials Based on Natural Oils and Fats

There are many possible raw materials available for making emollients based on natural oils and fats; however, most of them are produced in small quantities and are not always commercially feasible. Table 26.2 lists the vegetable oils and fats that are most common as raw materials for making cosmetic ingredients.

Animal fats are principally available from three sources: tallow from cattle, lard from pigs, and fish oil from marine fish species. Other sources do exist, but these are the main ones from an industrial point of view. Of these sources, the fish oil triglycerides are less common as very few fisheries remain to produce a cheap raw material. Lard and tallow are also less attractive today as raw materials due to issues related to sustainability, social, and cultural preferences.

The majority of industrially produced vegetable oils and fats come from four sources: *palm oil*, *soybean oil*, *rapeseed oil*, and *sunflower seed oil.*

Table 26.2 Approximative fatty acid composition ranges for commonly used vegetable oil raw materials

	C8	C10	C12	C14	C16	C18:0	C18:1	C18:2	C18:3	C22:1
Soybean oil					9–13	3–5	17–30	48–58	5–11	
Rapeseed oil (LEAR)					4–5	1–2	60–64	18–21	7–10	
Rapeseed oil (HEAR)					2–7	1–3	12–22	10–16	4–12	40–50
Rapeseed oil (HORO)					3–4	1–2	73–78	11–16	2–4	
Sunflower seed oil					4–9	1–7	14–40	48–74		
High-oleic SFO					2–4	3–4	80–84	7–10		
Shea butter					4–5	40–43	45–46	6–7		
Liquid shea butter					4–6	25–28	56–58	8–9		
Olive oil					7–20	0–4	56–85	4–20	0–1	
Sweet almond oil					4–9	0–3	62–86	17–30		
Palm oil				0–1	43–45	4–5	38–42	9–10		
Coconut oil	5–11	4–9	40–50	15–20	7–12	1–5	4–10	1–3		

Source: AarhusKarlshamn Sweden AB, Karlshamn, Sweden

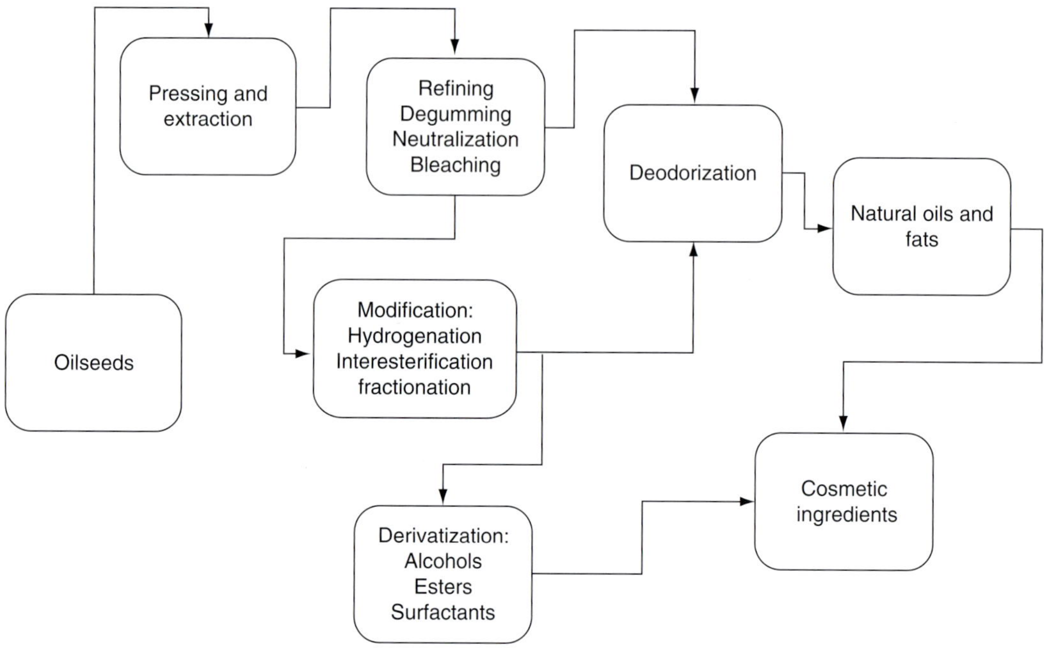

Fig. 26.1 Oilseeds of different kinds are converted to emollients, emulsifiers, and surfactants for skin care use via refining, modification, and derivatization steps

The three latter are liquid oils with high degree of unsaturation as they have high levels of linoleic (C18:2) and linolenic acids (C18:3). The unsaturation of soybean, rapeseed, and sunflower oil restricts their use in skin care as they are difficult to stabilize against oxidation. However, they are good starting points for modification as they are easily accessible and cost-effective.

Palm oil is a source for oleic (C18:1) and palmitic (C16:0) acids. It has a semisolid consistency at room temperature and is taken from the fruit pulp of the oil palm (*Elaeis guineensis*). The widespread cultivation of palm oil in Malaysia and Indonesia has lead to concerns about habitat destruction and deforestation, and mechanisms for sustainable production of palm oil have been implemented. The Round Table for Sustainable Palm Oil (RSPO) is a multistakeholder organization for promoting and certifying the production of palm oil which do not contribute to social and environmental degradation in the producing counties [28].

There are two major sources of short and medium chain fatty acids (C8, C10, C12, and C14): *palm kernel oil* and *coconut oil.* These two oils are the main raw material sources for producing surfactants and simple esters used in cosmetics and personal care applications.

Extraction, Purification, and Modification of Vegetable Oils and Fats

Naturals oils and fats which are used as cosmetic emollients need to be purified to remove undesired naturally occurring seed constituents and environmental pollutants [29]. Apart from undesired minor components, vegetable oils usually also contain functional lipids such as tocopherols (vitamin E) and phytosterols. A balanced production efficiently removes the contaminants but preserves the functional minor lipids in the oil. Figure 26.1 gives a simplified outline of the processing involved in converting oilseeds to cosmetic ingredients.

The first step in all oil processing is to remove the oil from the seeds, kernels, fruits, and nuts. This is usually done by decorticating and drying the seed raw material before crushing it by different types of mills. The resulting cake is pressed to extract the oil. For most seed materials, the resulting pressed seed cake is further extracted with a solvent, usually hexane. The crude oil is sometimes used as such, but normally the oil is further processed via refining, bleaching, and deodorization.

The refining of a vegetable oil can be regarded as a washing process using water with different pH values. The first washing, the degumming, is done using acidic water and removes phospholipids, gums, and sugars and decreases the level of metals and proteins present in the oil. The second washing is done with a weak alkali to remove free fatty acids. Again, water-soluble substances and metals are decreased. After drying, the oil is now ready for bleaching.

The bleaching step in vegetable oil refining comprises adding one or more absorbents to the oil and filtering off the absorbent after sufficient contact time. The absorbent is usually activated montmorillonite clay, also known as bleaching earth. The oil can also be treated with activated carbon to remove oil soluble contaminants. After the bleaching, the oil is free from phospholipids, free fatty acids, metal traces, protein residuals, and other degradation products and contaminants.

The final step in oil refining is the deodorization. This step, which is a steam distillation in vacuum, removes volatile components that cause odor and flavor. It also eliminates the last traces of free fatty acids. If done at too high temperature and extreme vacuum, this process also removes tocopherols and phytosterols, substances that are beneficial in skin care.

In case the properties of the oil are not suitable for the intended application, the vegetable oil can be modified using chemical and physical methods [30]. The most common method to modify the properties of unsaturated oils is to use hydrogenation. Hydrogen is added to the double bonds removing the unsaturation step by step. The melting point increases, but also the oxidative stability. Fully saturated vegetable oils are often used for further processing into esters and emulsifiers. Chain lengths from C14–C18 are preferred in this context.

Interesterification is another chemical modification method which is used to modify the melting and crystallization properties of oils and fats. This process rearranges the fatty acids on the glycerol backbone and with an altered triglyceride composition, the melting behavior and sensory properties are modified. Oxidative stability is not affected as the fatty acid composition is not changed.

The physicochemical properties as well as chemical behavior can also be modified using fractionation techniques [31]. Methods which can be used for low molecular weight substances, such as fatty acids, alcohols, and esters, are not suitable for triglyceride oils. The high boiling point of triglycerides is due to their large size and prevents separation based on distillation. Instead, high-melting solids can be frozen out of the oil phase by lowering the temperature. Dry fraction is the term used when the cooling of the oil is done without solvent and is frequently used for palm oil and its derivatives. Dry fractionation uses high-pressure filters to separate the solid and liquid fractions from each other. If a better separation of the solid and liquid fractions is needed, a solvent must be used for the fractionation process. Hexane or acetone is the industrially used solvent for this type of process.

After physical or chemical modification processes, the solvents, catalysts, and by-products are removed by bleaching and deodorization to produce an emollient with optimized properties and high purity.

Some Common Natural Oil-Based Emollients and Their Properties [23]

Soybean oil is the oil from the soya bean, Glycine soja, of the Leguminosae family. It is highly unsaturated and has a short shelf life in cosmetic applications. Soybean oil is a good source for linoleic and linolenic acids; tocopherols, especially gamma-tocopherol; and phytosterols. Soybean oil is frequently derived from GMO soybeans, and special care must be taken in sourcing if non-GMO soybean oil is required. Soybean oil can be used in skin care to provide essential fatty acids (linoleic and linolenic acids), but due to the low oxidative stability, the level in the formulation is usually lower than 1–2%.

Rapeseed oil is found at high concentration in the seeds of the oil rape, *Brassica campestris*. The dominant fatty acids are oleic acid and linoleic acid, but also, linolenic acid is abundant. Several varieties of oil rape have been developed over the years. Currently, at least three different types of rapeseed oil are available: low-erucic acid rapeseed (LEAR, canola oil), high-erucic acid rapeseed oil (HEAR), and high-oleic rapeseed oil (HORO). HEAR oil has a high level of the long-chain monounsaturated erucic acid (C22:1) while high-oleic rapeseed oil has a significantly lowered content of linolenic and linoleic acids for improved oxidation stability. Rapeseed oil is also rich in tocopherols and phytosterols. Hydrogenated and fractionated rapeseed oil having an elevated level of tocopherols and phytosterols can be used to increase recovery of surfactant damaged skin [32]. The high oleic and the hydrogenated rapeseed oil can be used at 1–5% in the formulation without adverse effects on smell and stability.

Sunflower seed oil is obtained from the seeds of the sunflower plant (*Helianthus annuus*). The traditional sunflower oil has a high content of linoleic acid and is prone to oxidation. Newer varieties with low-linoleic and high-oleic acid content are also available (high-oleic sunflower oil). Sunflower oil is rich in tocopherols but requires normally removal of the seed coat waxes by winterization to obtain clear oil. Sunflower seed oil of the traditional, high-linoleic acid type can be used to provide essential fatty acids to the formulation. Low oxidative stability limits the use to 1–2% in the formulation. High-oleic sunflower seed oil can be used as a basic emollient at higher concentrations.

Shea butter is a unique vegetable fat with a high functionality in skin care [33]. The main fatty acids are stearic (C18:0) and oleic (C18:1) acids. The triglyceride composition yields a solid fraction primarily comprising stearic-oleic-stearic triglycerides and a liquid fraction dominated by stearic-oleic-oleic triglycerides. This combination gives shea butter a semisolid consistency and high emolliency and moisturization when added to a skin care formulation. The uniqueness of shea butter also lies in the presence of high concentrations of triterpene cinnamates and acetates which are sometimes useful as bioactive additives in skin care [34]. A variety of shea butter, meeting the criteria on stability and low melting point, is liquid shea butter, obtained by fractionation of the semi-solid material. It has a high level of oleic acid but contributes also with a significant level of triterpene esters.

Two oils with a high content of monounsaturated fatty acids are *olive oil* and *sweet almond oil*. These oils are both popular in skin care formulations. Olive oil can be used as nonrefined but contributes with a typical greenish color and olive flavor to the formulation. These two oils are reasonably stable against oxidation due to the lack of sensitive linolenic acid and a moderate content of linoleic acid.

Numerous other vegetable oils are used in cosmetic formulations, mainly due to their usefulness as marketing ingredients. The composition normally falls into one of the four groups described above. In this group, we find vegetable oils and fats such as cocoa butter, murumuru butter, avocado oil, and babassu oil.

Synthetic Triglycerides and Analogues

The most common synthetic triglyceride used as emollient in skin care formulations is "caprylic/capric triglyceride," also known as medium chain triglyceride (MCT). This synthetic triglyceride has intermediate viscosity and polarity and a high resistance against oxidation as it is fully saturated.

Caprylic/capric triglycerides are produced by esterification of glycerol by a mixture of caprylic and capric acids. Coconut oil or palm kernel oil is hydrolyzed to fatty acids and glycerol; the fatty acids are separated by distillation into fractions (C8–C10, C12–C14, and C16–C18). The C8–C10 fraction is added to glycerol, and the esterification reaction is carried out by removing reaction water. The process can be run without added catalyst or using tin-based acidic catalysts. After reaction, the oil can be deodorized to improve flavor and odor.

Emollients which are analogues to the caprylic/capric triglycerides are, for example, diesters of propylene glycol and triesters of glycerol and synthetic ethylhexanoic acid ("octanoic acid").

26.4.3.3 Complex Esters

Esters with poorly defined compositions and which are often made from constituents with several reaction centers can be summarized by the name complex esters. This group also comprises lanolin, which is a natural product with complex composition.

Polyacid and Polyhydric Esters

In the last years, a new group of emollient esters have been introduced. These complex esters are based on different combinations of polybasic acids and polyhydric alcohols and are usually more viscous than traditional esters. They have also higher molecular weights, and by the selection of constituents, the polarity can be modified.

Esters based on polyhydric alcohols such as trimethylolpropane (three hydroxyl groups) and pentaerythritol (four hydroxyl groups) are also available. These complex esters are normally produced using branched fatty acids or unsaturated acids as the long chain linear esters tend to become too high melting.

Esters based on polycarboxylic acids with simple alcohols are also available. In this case, the viscosities are low, and the polarity is high due to the presence of several ester groups. Examples of this category include esters of adipic acid and citric acid with low molecularweight alcohols.

Lanolin and Lanolin Derivatives

Lanolin is another naturally occurring oleogel, characterized by having a high content of cholesterol and lanosterol esters. It is also rich in esters between dicarboxylic acids, long-chain diols, and hydroxy acids. Lanolin can be fractionated to yield different qualities of emollients, and it can be derivatized to increase and tailor-make the functionality for different applications [35–38].

26.5 Important Properties to Consider When Selecting Emollients

When formulating skin care products, the emollient is often combined with water, actives, and emulsifiers. In the formulation, several aspects must be optimized: stability, aesthetics, and delivery of actives. By a careful selection of emollients and by systematic variation of the emollient composition, formulations meeting the desired characteristics may be developed.

26.5.1 Compositional Aspects of Emollient Selection

The composition of commercially available emollients is usually difficult to investigate and analyze. Two emollients with the same INCI name, for example, "isopropyl palmitate" may differ in properties because the "palmitate" part may be derived from different starting materials. The palmitic acid used for this ester is seldom pure, and various amounts of stearic acid may be present as well as shorter fatty acids such as myristic and lauric. If the palmitic acid is derived from animal fats, it may also contain fatty acids with 15 and 17 carbons as well as branched fatty acids.

Many other types of emollients are equally difficult to characterize due to the complex composition of structurally similar and isomeric forms. This can be the case with petrolatum and mineral oils which can have different compositions depending on their origin. For this reason, it is important to remember that there cannot be a direct comparison from a technological point of view of two emollients, even if they are nominally the same and fulfill the same specification.

26.5.1.1 Contaminants: Environmental and Processing Dependent

All raw materials can be more or less contaminated with environmental pollutants. Such pollutants come from the soil, from air, from the processing, and from transports of raw materials and intermediates. Contaminants can also leach into the emollient from packaging materials and from process equipment. Since contaminants of different types are ubiquitous and often represent higher toxicity than the emollients themselves, monitoring the presence of contaminants is important and constitute a part of the new Cosmetic Regulation of the European Union [39].

Contaminants which are of specific concern for emollients are heavy metals, pesticide residuals for plant derived materials, and polyaromatic hydrocarbons. Allergens, both those associated with skin sensitization as well as food allergens, should be absent. Even if emollients normally do not sustain microbial growth due to low water activity in the ingredient itself, packaging materials, and insufficiently heated materials can cause transfer of microbial contamination.

26.5.1.2 By-Products, Processing Aids, and Other Residues from Manufacturing

Normally, emollients do not contain high levels of toxic or irritating by-products from the reactions used to manufacture the ingredient, unless the material is highly unsaturated or has been subjected to very high temperatures for a prolonged time. It is important to check the level of residual processing aids and catalysts. Processing aids include solvents, filter aids, and acids/alkalis used to neutralize the material after esterification or other reactions. Catalyst residuals may be strongly acidic or alkaline or contain heavy metals such as nickel or tin.

26.5.2 Chemical Properties to Consider when Selecting Emollients

Chemical reactions usually need a reaction center and one or more reactants and frequently the presence of a catalyst. In emollients, the reaction centers can either be located in the hydrocarbon chain or it can be one or more of the functional groups present in the structure. Only two reactants will be considered in this review: oxygen and water. The two reaction types are consequently oxidation and hydrolysis, two reactions that degrade the emollients and can have large impact on the quality and shelf life of the formulation.

26.5.2.1 Oxidation: Rancidity and Skin Damage

In emollient technology, oxidation can be regarded as a simple reaction between oxygen and the emollient. The oxidation results in breakdown products which can be smelly or irritating, depending on their size and volatility. Oxidation can also cause changes in the color and appearance of the formulation. In the worst case, oxidation can cause changes in metabolic pathways in the skin, resulting, for example, in inflammatory reactions, mutations, and apoptosis [40, 41]. Understanding emollient oxidation is therefore important for the formulator and product designer.

Oxidation requires an activated reaction center to proceed rapidly. Saturated hydrocarbons contain few activated carbons that can serve as reaction centers and are usually resistant against oxidation. The introduction of one double bond creates two active reaction centers adjacent to the double bond, and oxidation rates are more than doubled. When more double bonds are added, more active reaction centers are introduced and the oxidative stability decreases rapidly. Carboxylic acids and hydroxyl groups also contribute to active reaction centers. In case an oxygen molecule reacts with an activated carbon moiety, a hydroperoxide is formed. This hydroperoxide is a primary oxidation product and is measured by the "peroxide value" which is normally stated as a quality parameter for emollients.

If more oxygen is available, the oxidation process can proceed in two directions: formation of additional hydroperoxides or further oxidation of the hydroperoxide to form aldehydes, ketones, and hydrocarbons. This secondary oxidation breaks the hydrocarbon chains and produces fragments of different sizes and polarities. Fragments with low molecular weights are volatile and enter the headspace above the emollient. These volatile aldehydes and hydrocarbons have low odor thresholds and can be detected by the human nose in concentrations that are in the ppb-ppm range. If the oxidized fragment is larger, it does not volatilize and stays in the emollient. These components are usually not smelly, but they can contribute to skin irritation.

Oxidation is catalyzed by metal ions, by certain enzymes and by the presence of oxidation products (autocatalysis) [42]. Iron and copper are the most active oxidation catalysts seen in emollient systems, and already, ppm levels of these metals can cause problems. Oxidation is also catalyzed by UV radiation and by visible light (photooxidation). Unstable emollients, such as highly unsaturated oils, as well as sensitive actives need to be formulated with care and the product packaged in opaque packaging to prevent photooxidation.

Oxidation can be prevented by the use of antioxidants. Most antioxidants are free radical scavengers and will eliminate the oxygen before it reacts with the activated reaction centers, alternatively deactivating the hydroperoxide and preventing the secondary oxidation. A good principle to prevent oxidation in formulations is to combine a water-soluble antioxidant with an oil-soluble one. Further protection is obtained if a surface active antioxidant is added to act at the interface between oil and water. The choice of antioxidant is often regulated by the legal restrictions, and care must be taken to use only permitted antioxidants.

Avoiding oxidation is also important from a product safety aspect. Free radicals and reactive oxygen species can start and maintain inflammatory reactions in the skin. They can also contribute to the oxidation of proteins and structural lipids in the skin, reducing the ability of the skin to maintain its elasticity and moisture barrier properties.

26.5.2.2 Hydrolysis of Esters Gives Texture Changes in the Formulation

A second chemical reaction of importance for ester-based emollients is hydrolysis. Obviously, hydrocarbons and alcohols do not react with water, but all esters are more or less sensitive towards hydrolysis. The hydrolysis is the reversed version of the esterification reaction: water reacts with the ester bond and liberates the acid and the alcohol. As this is an equilibrium reaction, esterification occurs if the water is continuously removed while the hydrolysis takes place when there is an excess of water. Hydrolysis of esters is catalyzed by strong alkalis, strong acids, and by enzymes such as lipases and esterases. Most esters are stable in the pH range 5–8, especially if they are encapsulated inside emulsion droplets. Hydrolysis of esters in skin care formulation can cause the emulsion structure to change, leading to texture changes and instability. The pH value of the formulation drops, and the liberated acid or alcohol can increase the irritancy of the formulation. High molecular weight esters with low polarity have better hydrolysis resistance as the ester bond concentration is lower and because water solubility in the ester is restricted. Formulating with barrier forming emulsifiers and polymers can also protect the oil phase against hydrolysis.

26.5.3 Selecting Emollients Based on Physicochemical Behavior

Controlling the polarity and rheology of the emollient blend in a formulation is necessary in order to obtain the desired skin feel and stability of the product. Many practical emollient mixtures contain high- and intermediate-melting components which give a semisolid consistency to the ingredient. Understanding crystallization and melting behavior for texture and rheology control is important, especially when formulating anhydrous ointments and high emollient content W/O emulsions.

26.5.3.1 Melting Points Versus Melting Ranges

For many semisolid emollients and for mixtures of emollients, the melting behavior is an important selection criterion. As most emollients and emollient mixtures have complex compositions, the melting point is no longer a good characteristic for comparison. In this case, the melting range or the melting profile is a more appropriate parameter. The melting profiles can easily be measured using differential scanning calorimetry

(DSC), also in formulations. The DSC results, when standardized, give a direct comparison of the melting behavior of an emollient mixture and can also give insight into interactions between the emollients and emulsifiers. Pure emollients and emollient blends can be characterized using low-resolution NMR techniques. These measurements are strongly influenced by water so the measurements are restricted to dry emollients and to anhydrous systems.

Analysis of the emollient melting behavior can be used to optimize the formulation properties. Important temperature ranges to consider are storage temperatures (normal, too low, too high), body temperature, and temperatures during product stability testing. The formulation should be possible to dispense from its container (at storage temperature), meaning that the solids content must not be too high. On the other hand, in order to achieve high temperature stability and stability at varying storage conditions, increasing the solids content can be the solution as the solids will help the emulsifier and stabilizer system to maintain consistency. Finally, the solids can also be used to modify skin feel and moisturization. The higher the solids content, the heavier the skin feel is, but the perceived moisturization is improved.

26.5.3.2 Optimizing the Polarity by Mixing Emollients

As the polarity of an emollient or an emollient mixture is difficult to measure directly, the selection of emollients to optimize properties is at best a semiempirical procedure. In general, the polarity is additive, meaning that mixtures of emollients have properties proportional to the mixing proportions. However, some properties associated with polarity are strongly influenced by the purity of the system. For example, interfacial and surface tension of an emollient is sometimes used to evaluate polarity. These two parameters are strongly influenced by the presence of small amounts of surface active contaminants, and the measured values can be strongly misleading if the emollients are not properly purified before the measurements are taken.

In order to manipulate the skin feel and the solubility of actives, changing the polarity of the emollient system is a useful tool. A hydrocarbon-based emollient is normally nonpolar, and adding a more polar emollient such as an ester or a fatty alcohol can strongly influence the behavior.

26.5.3.3 Controlling Viscosity and Lubricity for Improved Skin Feel

Viscosities of emollient blends in the liquid state are normally additive, and the viscosity of the blend usually reflects the composition of the mixture and its individual constituents. Viscosity and perceived lubricity are often connected, but quite often there is an optimal viscosity associated with best skin feel and other sensory properties. If the emollient viscosity is too low, the skin feel is thin and watery while too high viscosities are perceived greasy and unpleasant. For sensitive skin, a high viscosity can also be disadvantageous as the drag will be perceived as irritating. High emollient viscosity is often preferred to reduce emulsifier and stabilizer content. High-viscosity oils can reduce emulsion instability, especially as higher viscosity is also often associated with higher density.

26.5.3.4 Spreading and Spreadability

Spreading and spreadability of the formulation on skin are important parameters for consumer appeal and acceptance. A formulation should be easy to apply, spread rapidly on the skin, and give a rapid disappearance from the skin surface. The spreading ability of emollients and emollient mixtures directly on skin is difficult to measure accurately, and various techniques have been applied to estimate the spreading properties [10, 43]. Spreadability and viscosity are dependent on each other as a rapid spreading is often observed for low-viscosity emollients. The rapid spreading is also associated with lubricity or slip, again favoring emollients of low viscosity. Equilibrium spreadability, on the other hand, is a different parameter and also important for the perceived emolliency of the formulation. High equilibrium spreading will yield a thin film on the skin surface and may lead to a disappearance of the perceived emolliency and moisturization over time.

26.5.4 Environmental Properties

Although the environmental properties of emollients are usually not considered to be a primary concern for skin care products, recent changes in legislation, especially in Europe, has brought the focus to this issue. When considering the use of skin care product, it is obvious that part of the emollients and other ingredients are absorbed into the skin, while other parts are rubbed off into clothes or washed off during showering and cleansing procedures. Other aspects concern the manufacturing, storage, and transport of emollients in large scale and the results locally and regionally of accidental discharge of chemicals into the environment. All this points to the importance of environmentally safe ingredients, and emollients, being used in relatively high concentrations in the formulations, are of special concern.

Biodegradability has become an important property for emollients and other cosmetic ingredients in the past few years. In a sustainability perspective, with life cycle analysis as a defining principle, not only the production and use of chemical substances but also the disposal after use and accidental discharge into the environment have become important to consider. Most straight-chain hydrocarbon-based emollients are readily degraded by sewage bacteria and can be considered readily biodegradable. This is also the case for straight chain fatty acids and alcohols. Esters are usually first hydrolyzed to the constituents which are then degraded. High-melting and high molecular weight substances are generally degraded more slowly due to low solubility and bioavailability. Although ultimately biodegradable, they can sometimes cause visible problems and disturb flora and fauna locally.

Another aspect of biological degradation is the possibility for substances to accumulate in the environment. Lipophilic substances, such as emollients, have a higher potential for bioaccumulation. However, since chemical structures that are known to cause toxic metabolites and show a high tendency to accumulate in the environment are today not used as emollients, most cosmetics are also safe in this aspect. Again, high molecular weight lipophilic substances with high melting points are more of a problem, especially since the data available is scarce.

Conclusions

Emollients are necessary ingredients for skin care preparations, and the selection of ingredients is a difficult task when optimizing properties and performance. This chapter has reviewed hydrocarbons, alcohols, and esters used for emolliency and pointed to important chemical and physical properties that must be considered when selecting emollients.

Each group of emollient technologies has its benefits and disadvantages, and it is obvious that the perfect emollient does still not exist. A skilled formulator can utilize the benefits of each emollient while minimizing the adverse effects. It is also evident that many of the properties of a finished formulation are the result of ingredient interactions, and the winning formulation is often achieved by skillful manipulation of the interactions.

Take Home Messages

When reading this chapter you should learn about the following points:

- Emollient classification based on chemistry of physical properties
- The importance of optimizing physical properties for the application
- The chemical reactions that must be considered for emollients
- How emollients are produced
- Different raw materials for emollients
- Considerations when selecting emollients

References

1. Wiechers JW, Kelly CL, Blease TG, Dederen JC (2004) Formulating for efficacy. Int J Cosmet Sci 26:173–182
2. Shinoda K, Friberg S (1986) Concepts of HLB, HLB temperature and HLB number. In: Emulsions and solubilization. Wiley, New York, pp 55–93

3. Shinoda K, Kunieda H (1983) Phase poperties of emulsions: PIT and HLB. In: Becher P (ed) Encyclopedia of emulsion technology, vol 1. Marcel Dekker, Inc, New York, pp 337–368
4. Parente ME, Gambaro A, Solana G (2005) Study of sensory properties of emollients used in cosmetics and their correlation with physicochemical properties. Int J Cosmet Sci 27:354
5. Goldemberg RL, de la Rosa CP (1971) Correlation of skin feel of emollients to their chemical structure. J Soc Cosmet Chem 22:635–654
6. Wortel VAL, Verboom C, Wiechers JW (2005) Linking sensory and rheology characteristics. Cosmet Toiletries 120:57–66
7. Otto A, Du Plessis J, Wiechers JW (2009) Formulation effects of topical emulsions on transdermal and dermal delivery. Int J Cosmet Sci 31:1–19
8. Friberg SE (1990) Micelles, microemulsions, liquid crystals, and the structure of stratum corneum lipids. J Soc Cosmet Chem 41:155–171
9. Hughes KJ, Lvovich VF, Woo J, Moran B, Suares A, Truong MHT (2006) Novel methods for emollient characterisation. Cosmet Toiletries Manuf Worldwide 93:19–24
10. Gorcea M, Laura D (2010) Evaluating the physiochemical properties of emollient esters for cosmetic use. Cosmet Toiletries 125:26–33
11. Iwahashi M, Kasahara Y (2007) Effects of molecular size and structure on self-diffusion coefficient and viscosity for saturated hydrocarbons having six carbon atoms. J Oleo Sci 56:443–448
12. Barry BW (1975) Viscoelastic properties of concentrated emulsions. Adv Colloid Interface Sci 5: 37–75
13. Huang Z-R, Lin Y-K, Fang JY (2009) Biological and pharmacological activities of squalene and related compounds: potential uses in cosmetic dermatology. Molecules 14:540–554
14. Bondioli P, Mariani C, Lanzani A, Fedeli E, Muller A (1993) Squalene recovery from olive oil deodorizer distillates. J Am Oil Chem Soc 70:763–766
15. Chiba K, Yoshizawa K, Makino I, Kawakami K, Onoue M (2000) Comedogenicity of squalene monohydroperoxide in the skin after topical application. J Toxicol Sci 25:77–83
16. Motoyoshi K (1983) Enhanced comedo formation in rabbit ear skin by squalene and oleic acid peroxides. Br J Dermatol 109:191–198
17. Saint-Leger D, Bague A, Lefebvre E, Cohen E, Chivot M (1986) A possible role for squalene in the pathogenesis of acne. II. In vivo study of squalene oxides in skin surface and intra-comedonal lipids of acne patients. Br J Dermatol 114:543–552
18. Saint-Leger D, Bague A, Cohen E, Chivot M (1986) A possible role for squalene in the pathogenesis of acne. I. In vitro study of squalene oxidation. Br J Dermatol 114:535–542
19. Barry BW, Grace AJ (1971) Structural rheological and textural properties of soft paraffins. J Texture Stud 2:259–279
20. Morrison DS (1996) Petrolatum: a useful classic. Cosmet Toiletries 111:59–69
21. Busson-Breysse J, Farines M, Soulier J (1994) Jojoba wax: its esters and some of its minor components. J Am Oil Chem Soc 71:999–1002
22. O'Lenick A (2001) Guerbet chemistry. J Surfactants Deterg 4:311–315
23. Gunstone FD, Harwood JL (2007) Occurrence and characterisation of oils and fats. In: Gunstone FD, Harwood JL, Dijkstra AJ (eds) The lipid handbook with CD-ROM. CRC Press, Boca Raton, pp 37–142
24. Biermann U, Metzger JO (2008) Synthesis of alkyl-branched fatty acids. Eur J Lipid Sci Technol 110:805–811
25. Schuchardt U, Sercheli R, Matheus Vargas R (1998) Transesterification of vegetable oils: a review. J Braz Chem Soc 9:199–210
26. Thum O, Oxenboll KM (2008) Biocatalysis: a sustainable process for production of cosmetic emollient esters. SÖFW-J 134:44–47
27. Hills G (2003) Industrial use of lipases to produce fatty acid esters. Eur J Lipid Sci Technol 105:601–607
28. RSPO – promoting the growth and use of sustainable palm oil (2011) http://www.rspo.org/[On-line]
29. Dijkstra AJ, Segers JC (2007) Production and refining of vegetable oils. In: Gunstone FD, Harwood JL, Dijkstra AJ (eds) The lipid handbook with CD-ROM. CRC Press, Boca Raton, pp 143–262
30. Dijkstra AJ (2007) Modification processes and food uses. In: Gunstone FD, Harwood JL, Dijkstra AJ (eds) The lipid handbook with CD-ROM. CRC Press, Boca Raton, pp 263–354
31. Padley FB (1994) Fractionated products: a brief survey of the application of fractions of edible oils and fats. Society of Chemical Industry, London, 22pp
32. Loden M, Andersson AC (1996) Effect of topically applied lipids on surfactant-irritated skin. Br J Dermatol 134:215–220
33. Alander J (2004) Shea butter - a multifunctional ingredient for food and cosmetics. Lipid Technol 16:202–205
34. Akihisa T, Kojima N, Kikuchi T, Yasukawa K, Tokuda H, Masters T, Manosroi A, Manosroi J (2010) Anti-inflammatory and chemopreventive effects of triterpene cinnamates and acetates from shea fat. J Oleo Sci 59:273–280
35. Motiuk K (1979) Wool wax alcohols: a review. JAOCS 56:651–658
36. Motiuk K (1979) Wool wax acids: a review. JAOCS 56:91–97
37. Schlossman M, McCarthy J (1978) Lanolin and its derivatives. J Am Oil Chem Soc 55:447–450
38. Motiuk K (1980) Wool wax hydrocarbons: a review. J Am Oil Chem Soc 57:145–146

39. Regulation (EC) No 1223/2009 of the European Parliament and of the Council of 30 November 2009 on cosmetic products (2009) Official Journal of the European Union [On-line], L 342/59, 59–209
40. Kohen R (1999) Skin antioxidants: their role in aging and in oxidative stress–new approaches for their evaluation. Biomed Pharmacother 53:181–192
41. Thiele JJ, Schroeter C, Hsieh SN, Podda M, Packer L (2001) The antioxidant network of the stratum corneum. Curr Probl Dermatol 29:26–42
42. Shahidi F, Zhong Y (2010) Lipid oxidation and improving the oxidative stability. Chem Soc Rev 39:4067–4079
43. Bruns C, Müller RH, Prinz D, Kutz G (2006) Identification of topical excipients with high performance spreadability. Poster, 5th world meeting on pharmaceutics, Biopharmaceutics and Pharmaceutical Technology, Geneva

27 Polyfunctional Vehicles by the Use of Vegetable Oils

Luigi Rigano and Chiara Andolfatto

27.1 Introduction

Skin is regularly softened and lubricated by the water arriving from deep dermis or produced from sweat glands. Some water content is released to the external environment, determining a dynamic equilibrium. Water loss by evaporation is regulated by the physiological cutaneous barrier that lays at the horny layer level. The horny layer is made of corneocytes, keratinocytes that have reached the final differentiation steps. They are rich in keratin, responsible of the mechanical resistance of the skin and immersed in a permeable matrix. This last one is formed by water emulsified by substances of fatty nature, produced by the sebaceous glands, deriving from the degradation of mature skin cells reaching the stratum corneum level or directly synthesized by keratinocytes [6]. It consists of lipids and amphiphile molecules, like cholesterol (25%), ceramides (50%) and free fatty acids (15%) especially those bearing unsaturated chains [10] [5]. Moreover, squalene and small amounts of phospholipids are also present. They create an ordered structure with the aqueous phase, forming a series of bilayers (aqueous and lipid) that protect the skin and guarantee its metabolic functions [22]. Therefore, the epidermal horny layer consists of keratinized cells surrounded by a lipid matrix that hinders water evaporation and the diffusion of water and electrolytes. Such structure builds the permeable moisturizing barrier of the skin [4].

27.2 Cutaneous Lipids and Moisturization

The main responsible of the cutaneous modification which leads to dryness is the hydro-lipidic unbalance, both qualitative and quantitative, of the more external cutaneous layers. Moisturization and barrier effects being strictly related to the lipids of the horny layer are supported by the fact that increased permeability of the cutaneous barrier is induced by its disruption after lipids removal by means of organic solvents (i.e. acetone), following mechanical stress (i.e. sequential tape stripping) or the action of cleansing surfactants (i.e. SLS). This is evidenced by an increase of trans-epidermal water loss and of newly produced epidermal lipids [5]. The level of stimulation of the lipid synthesis is related to the extent of damage of the skin barrier. Moreover, when the cutaneous barrier functionality is recovered, also the synthesis of epidermal lipids turns to its average normal values. The re-establishment of the equilibrium water content in the horny layer, on the other side, takes place proportionally and as the last step [6].

L. Rigano (✉) • C. Andolfatto
Rigano Industrial Consulting and Research, via Bruschetti 1, 20125 Milano, Italy
e-mail: rigano@thecosmetologist.com

M. Lodén, H.I. Maibach (eds.), *Treatment of Dry Skin Syndrome*,
DOI 10.1007/978-3-642-27606-4_27, © Springer-Verlag Berlin Heidelberg 2012

The external supplement of topically applied oils may solve the problems of disequilibrium of the cutaneous hydro-lipidic film. The main evidences derive from studies carried out with newborns and premature babies. Indeed, their skin structure is not yet completely developed, and they have reduced barrier function. It has been shown that the cutaneous application of vegetal oils, followed by massage, can significantly increase moisturization and improve their barrier function. As a positive set of accompanying effects, this compensates the deficiency of essential fatty acids, reduces the nosocomial infections (verified with sunflower oil), improves the somatic cells growth (verified with soy oil) and quickly re-equilibrates the cutaneous comfort in cases of dermatological affections [20].

As oils have hydrophobic nature, moisturization does not derive from an external water supply but is given by the integration with lipids already existing in the epidermis. The use of non-physiological lipids as petrolatum, lanolin or beeswax may quickly restore the normal permeability of the cutaneous barrier but only at a partial level [5]. Clinical studies confirm that, following the application of a vegetal oil (sweet almond oil) and of a liquid vegetal wax (jojoba oil), a mild but significant increase of total lipids in the first 6–8 μm of the horny layer can be measured [18].

A support to the barrier effect is so obtained: the water content in the horny layer changes following the application of oils onto the skin surface. Oils determine an emollient effect on the skin, they modify its physical properties and make the skin softer and more even. An interesting antimicrobial activity has been associated to some specific fatty acids [4].

27.3 Vegetal Oils

Fats, oils and waxes represent for plants a way to store energy, in a concentrated and little voluminous way, that is necessary for seeds germination. Moreover, they can play the role of a protective coating layer, especially for their hydro-repellency and thermal insulation property. In general, all small seeds contain fatty materials. In general, cells generally contain more oils when they belong to the aleuronic layer that coats the cereal grains of the germ and the seed. Oils are reserve substances accumulated by the plants in variable extent in dependence of the involved vegetal species, during growth. Moreover, they are found in the pericarp of some fruits and, to a lower degree, in pollens, spores and vegetative organs.

All lipid molecules in the vegetal world are fundamentally characterized by the content of one or more fatty acids with aliphatic chains, i.e. aliphatic carboxylic acid with an even number of carbon atoms.

When taking into account the lipid storage reserves localized in plants, except palm and coconut oil, the other vegetal oils are dominated by the group of unsaturated fatty acids with 18 carbon atoms. Indeed, for each oleaginous plant species actually used, more than 80% of the fatty acids content is generally represented by oleic (C18:1), linoleic (C18:2) and linolenic (C18:3). The same prevalence of fatty acids C18 mono-, di-, and tri-unsaturated, about 60% of the total fatty acids, is observed in the seed of cereals [14].

27.3.1 Triglycerides

Vegetal oils are formed by about 95% of a blend of triglycerides that altogether represent a fairly homogenous complex, from the chemical point of view, called ‘saponifiable fraction’ [8]. Indeed, triglycerides treated with concentrated aqueous alkali give rise to soaps, i.e. the alkaline salts of fatty acids, and to glycerine. The remaining part is called ‘unsaponifiable’, as it cannot react with alkali and therefore does not give rise to soaps. Vegetal triglycerides structurally are triesters of the polyol (polyalcohol) glycerine, with long-chain mono-carboxylic fatty acids. Other glycerides, that are present in minor amounts in the saponifiable fraction of oils, are mono- and diglycerides, compounds where glycerine is esterified only with one, or respectively two, fatty acid molecules. Consequently, the glycerides category is subdivided, in increasing polarity order, in:

- Triglycerides: three fatty acid chains are bound to glycerine, three ester bonds, no free alcohol group
- Diglycerides: two fatty acid chains are bound to glycerine, two ester bonds and one free alcohol group
- Mono-glycerides: only one fatty acid bound to glycerine, one ester bond and two free alcohol groups in the structure

In spite of the increasing polarity of the molecules in this series and the consequent possibility of establishing some attraction forces for water molecules, all these substances are insoluble in water but soluble in several organic solvents, at room temperature. Nevertheless, at high temperature, melted mono- and diglycerides can be easily dispersed in water.

The different chemical and physical characteristics of the different glycerides need to be ascribed to the different nature of the esterifying acids, to the substitution degree of the alcohol groups in glycerine and to the mutual position of the acyl chains within the molecule. Differences are even more detectable in the solid state, as all glycerides exhibit polymorph, temperature and cooling-rate dependant crystallization states. Acids participating to the formation of glycerides possess more frequently a linear alkyl chain, with an even number of carbon atoms. In nature, we find fatty acids with a number of carbon atoms varying from 2 to 30, but the most represented are the 18 or 16 carbon atom chains. Differences of relevant properties, in all those cases, are only related to the chain lengths, to the presence or absence of double bonds and their position in the acyl chains.

Fatty acids can be saturated or unsaturated. In the saturated acids family, the acyl chain does not have any double bond between carbon atoms, while unsaturated acid possess one or more double bonds. When containing one double bond only, they are called monounsaturated fatty acids, while the definition of polyunsaturated characterizes those having two or more double bonds in one acyl chain. In nature, the unsaturated fatty acids with *cis* configuration (when both chains separated by the double bond lie on the same side of a plane) are very abundant, while the *trans* configuration may be produced following modification induced by physico-chemical treatments, as those taking place during some oils refining process.

An additional subdivision applies to unsaturated fatty acids, according to the position of the double bond in the alkyl chain. The most widespread in the vegetal world are three, all related in the plants biosynthesis, i.e. the family of ω_9, ω_6 and ω_3 fatty acids. The official nomenclature applies the Greek letter 'omega' ω to the distance of the first double bond from the first terminal methyl group in the chain, and the accompanying number gives the position of the double bond. For instance, the symbol ω_3 indicates that the first position where the double bond is found is situated on the third carbon atom, starting the count of carbon atoms from the first methyl group. The position of the double bond, together with the special configuration (*cis* or *trans*) determine the biological properties of unsaturated fatty acids.

The family of ω_9 fatty acids includes monounsaturated structures, where the *cis* configuration of the molecule, from the point of view of the alkyl chains attached to the double bond, is necessary in order to guarantee the correct smoothness to the membranes of vegetal cells. Indeed, they are essential components of such membranes, and oleic acid is the most abundant representative of this category.

Vegetal polyunsaturated fatty acids belong to the groups ω_6 and ω_3. Linoleic acid, that is contained in oil seeds at high percentage and at a fairly good amount also in olive oil, and γ-linolenic acid belong to the ω_6 family, while α-linolenic acid, that is very abundant in linseeds, eicosapentaenoic acid (EPA) and docosaesaenoic acid (DHA) are in the ω_3 group.

The presence of one or more double bonds makes the unsaturated fatty acid very sensitive to auto-oxidation reactions that are the ground of the oxygen-induced degradation of oils. The triglycerides of unsaturated fatty acids go rancid very easily, especially when exposed to sunlight and atmospheric oxygen. The reaction is catalyzed by the presence of traces of metallic ions. As smaller dimensions, volatile molecules are formed in the process, the peroxidation of double bonds is accompanied by the development

Table 27.1 The most represented fatty acids in plants

Designation (C atoms n°: double bonds n°)	Traditional name	Chemical name	Formula
6:0	Caproic acid	Hexanoic acid	$C_6H_{12}O_2$
8:0	Caprylic acid	Octanoic acid	$C_8H_{16}O_2$
10:0	Capric acid	Decanoic acid	$C_{10}H_{20}O_2$
12:0	Lauric acid	Dodecanoic acid	$C_{12}H_{24}O_2$
14:0	Myristic acid	Tetradecanoic acid	$C_{14}H_{28}O_2$
14:1	Myristoleic acid	Tetradec-9-enoic acid	$C_{14}H_{26}O_2$
16:0	Palmitic acid	Hexadecanoic acid	$C_{16}H_{32}O_2$
16:1	Palmitoleic acid	Hexadec-9-enoic acid	$C_{16}H_{30}O_2$
18:0	Stearic acid	Octadecanoic acid	$C_{18}H_{36}O_2$
18:1	Oleic acid	Cis-9-octadecenoic acid	$C_{18}H_{34}O_2$
18:2	Linoleic acid	All-cis-9,12-octadecadienoic acid	$C_{18}H_{32}O_2$
18:3	Linolenic acid	All-cis-9,12,15-octadecatrienoic acid	$C_{18}H_{30}O_2$
20:0	Arachidic acid	Eicosanoic acid	$C_{20}H_{40}O_2$
20:1	Gadoleic acid	Cis-11-eicosenoic acid	$C_{20}H_{38}O_2$
22:0	Behenic acid	Docosanoic acid	$C_{22}H_{44}O_2$
22:1	Erucic acid	Cis-13-docosenoic acid	$C_{22}H_{42}O_2$
24:0	Lignoceric acid	Tetracosanoic acid	$C_{24}H_{48}O_2$

of bad smell. Consequently, the oxidative stability of vegetal oils is determined by their fatty acids composition, in particular by the unsaturation degree and, to a lesser extent, by the position of double bonds inside the triglyceride molecule. A fundamental role in this process is played by the system of antioxidant molecules present in vegetal oils, such as those of the vitamin E group, which belongs to the unsaponifiable fraction [8].

The most common fatty acids in the vegetal domain are reported in Table 27.1.

In general, a vegetal oil is a complex blend of triglycerides, where fatty acids that esterify the alcohol functions of glycerine vary in their acyl chain length and for their unsaturation degree and position of double bonds. In other words, triglycerides in vegetal oils are heterogeneous. The composition of fatty acids in any specific oil type is variable in a determined interval. This mainly depends on the *cultivated variety* and from the temperature in the area of farming of the plant. Moreover, the ripening degree is a contributing factor in determining the composition of the fatty acids blend. The higher the unsaturation, the lower the melting point: Oils are by definition liquid at room temperature, while triglycerides rich in saturated fatty acids are consistent or solid and are called 'butters'. Oils can be transformed in solid fats via saturation of the double bonds of the fatty acids in a more or less complete process of hydrogenation.

Indeed, the so-called saponifiable fractions do not include only the esters of fatty acids with glycerine, even if they represent the absolute majority, but also the esters of different alcohols or sterols, phospholipids and glycolipids (accompanying ingredients) [15].

27.3.2 Secondary Ingredients

Secondary ingredients in vegetal oils are generally present in moderate amounts and represent the non-glyceride fraction. We could subdivide these secondary ingredients in saponifiable components (phospholipids, waxes and sphingolipids, for instance) and in unsaponifiable ingredients (hydrocarbons, tocopherols and tocotrienols, superior fatty alcohols, sterols, methyl sterols, diterpene and triterpenes alcohols, vitamins, pigments and ubiquinones).

Similarly to triglycerides, phospholipids are made essentially of glycerine, fatty acids, a phosphoric group and a hydroxylated compound, frequently choline, cholamine or serine, all bound together by ester bonds. Consequently, phospholipids can be considered as derivatives of the glycerophosphoric acid, such as phosphatidylcholine and phosphatidylethanolamine: They are present variable amounts, but never abundant, in vegetal oils.

Glycolipids and sulpholipids are compounds where two hydroxyl groups of glycerine are esterified by fatty acids, while the third engaged in a glycoside bond with galactose or one of its derivatives. Finally, sphingolipids are combinations were one molecule of fatty acid is bound to a long-chain amino alcohol (sphingosine and derivatives) to form a ceramide.

Waxes are complex blends of esters of long-chain fatty acids with higher alcohols, such as docosanol, tetracosanol and esacosanol.

The unsaponifiable fraction is represented by substances which do not undergo any modification, when submitted to the action of concentrated alkali. The ingredients in the unsaponifiable fraction are low molecular-weight compounds, lipophilic or amphiphilic, that may noticeably influence the oxidation speed of vegetal oils [15].

27.3.2.1 Hydrocarbons

Hydrocarbons are minor components of the unsaponifiable fraction, a heterogeneous group of saturated and unsaturated molecules that are present in vegetal fatty materials. Among the unsaturated hydrocarbons, the most frequently found molecule is squalene, a terpene with 30 carbon atoms with six double bonds. This substance is outstandingly important from the human biology point of view, as it is the biosynthetic precursor of all sterols.

27.3.2.2 Pigments

Also, pigments belong to the group of the minor ingredients in vegetal oils. Pigments can be subdivided into two main categories: carotenoids and chlorophyll (a and b types chlorophylls and a and b type pheophytins) that are responsible of yellow tones (the first ones) and of the green hues (the second category). The carotenoids fraction includes β-carotene, lutein, neoxanthine and violet xanthine. While carotenoids develop an antioxidant action by neutralizing the singlet oxygen, chlorophylls perform pro-oxidant properties, as they catalyze the formation of singlet oxygen species under the action of sunlight. Therefore, a right ratio between chlorophyll and carotenoids pigments is essential for an adequate oil fastness toward oxidation. ß-carotene, or pro-vitamin A, is responsible for the yellow colour that is characteristic of olive oils and many other vegetal oils. Corn oil is one of the richest oils in beta-carotene; nevertheless, the industrial refining process can deplete the oil of this substance, resulting in a colourless appearance.

27.3.2.3 Vitamin E

Natural vitamin E, as synthesized by plants, is a mix of tocopherols and tocotrienols, that can be distinguished according to the number and positions of the methyl groups attached to the chroman ring. The different isomers take the names of α-, β-, γ- and δ-tocopherol and of α-, β-, γ- and δ-tocotrienol, respectively. They are very powerful vegetal antioxidants that hinder the developments of oil rancidity. Among tocopherols, α-tocopherol is considered to have superior biological activity and is also by far the most abundant isomer in human plasma and tissues. Many recent studies evidence that the biological activity of tocotrienols is higher in comparison to that of tocopherols (40–60 times higher than that of α-tocopherol).

All molecules belonging to the family of vitamin E are very powerful antioxidant. They participate in many metabolic processes of human tissues and prevent the oxidative damages of induced by UV rays exposure. In particular, vitamin E is involved in the biochemical protection strategy of lipoproteins from oxidation. Its 'radicals trap' action (radical scavenging + quenching) is synergic with that of beta-carotene, of vitamin C and of glutathione that are normally present in biological tissues. Vitamin C functions with a different mechanism: It operates as a regenerative player for vitamin E from its tocopheryl radical that is formed following the elimination of peroxide radicals.

27.3.2.4 Phytosterols

Phytosterols are lipophilic compounds of the triterpenes family. They possess a structure similar to that of cholesterol. It is made of tetracyclic ring and a long flexible side chain at the C-17 carbon atom site. They are different from cholesterol for the presence of methyl or ethyl groups in the side chain attached to the C-24 carbon atom. Saturated sterols, called stanols, are also present in vegetal oils. They are characterized by the absence of the double bond at the position Δ-5 of the sterol ring and are less abundant in nature of the corresponding unsaturated parents [9] [13]. In common sense, the term phytosterols is generally used to denote altogether sterol and stanols. Although more than 250 different phytosterols have been identified, the most common are sitosterol, campesterol and stigmasterol [12]. The composition of the sterols fraction may change consistently from plant to plant: For this reason, phytosterols constitute a kind of vegetal fingerprint of each vegetal oil. Indeed, some sterols are specific of unique vegetal oils.

27.3.2.5 Polyphenols

The term polyphenols includes several classes of compounds sharing a common chemical structure: They are benzene derivatives with one or more hydroxyl groups associated to the aromatic ring. Such structures allow these compounds to work actively as *radical scavenger* and to stabilize free radicals, as reducing agents, as chelating compounds of the pro-oxidant metals and as *quenchers* of the process of formation of singlet oxygen. They are necessary to the plant metabolism in order to avoid the auto-oxidation of the oil. In general, the richer in unsaturated triglycerides a vegetal oil is, the higher its content of polyphenols. The main classes of polyphenols are separated into flavonoids, phenolic acids, stilbenes and lignans, as a function of the number of phenolic rings and of the structural elements binding such rings. The most common vegetal polyphenols are derivatives of benzoic and cinnamic acids, or of tirosol and hydroxytirosol [3].

27.3.2.6 Triterpene Alcohols

Simple alcohols and diols belong to the group of terpene alcohols, having complex chemical structures. The composition of their typical blend among the unsaponifiable matters characterizes the different vegetal oil. Some of them are intermediates in the biosynthesis of sterols [15]; some others posses anti-inflammatory and germicide properties. γ-oryzanol is a group of ferulic esters of triterpene alcohols, present in rice oil. The anti-inflammatory properties of this cosmetic ingredient are attributed to the cinnamates of triterpene alcohols present in shea butter [17].

27.4 Vegetal Oils of Common Cosmetic Use

27.4.1 Corn Oil

Corn oil is obtained from the annual plant *Zea mays* that is mainly harvested for fodder but also for human consumption and industrial uses. Corn is a cereal of cosmetic interest for getting starch and its derivatives. During the process of starch preparation, corn germs are recovered, that are rich of oil. The crude oil has a dark amber-red colour and contains high amounts of phospholipids, together with traces of waxes. The refined oil, devoid of waxes and phospholipids, is one of the seed oils most frequently used in the food industry. The glyceride fraction is rich in linoleic (45–62%), oleic (24–33%), palmitic (8–13%) and linolenic acid (~1%). The unsaponifiable fraction can represent up to 2% of the oil and is characterized by the presence of fairly high amounts of beta-sitosterol, campesterol and γ- and α-tocopherol [2].

27.4.1.1 Cosmetic Use

Corn oil is used as emollient and moisturizer in emulsions and cosmetic oils. It is frequently employed as vehicle to dissolve lipo-soluble active ingredients (e.g. retinol).

27.4.2 Coconut Oil

Cocoa butter, better known as coconut oil, is obtained from the endosperm of the fruit, i.e. the white flesh of the nut of the plant *Cocos nucifera*

L. Below 25–27°C, it is an ivory coloured solid, with a characteristic pleasant odour. Its unsaponifiable fraction is very low (0.1–0.3%), while the trigliceride fraction is rich of saturated fatty acids (about 95%) as lauric (45–51%), myristic (17–20%), caprylic (7–10%), capric (4–11%) and palmitic acid (4–9%). It contains only a modest amount of unsaturated fatty acids, like oleic (2–11%).

27.4.2.1 Cosmetic Use

Triglycerides obtained from coconut oil are used mainly as they show marked sebum-restitution properties. For its high amount of lauric acid and also of short chain fatty acids, coconut oil is largely used on a world scale as intermediate for the preparation of surfactants [16].

27.4.3 Palm Oil

Palm oil is obtained from the plant *Elaeis guineensis*, native of the African continent, but successively widespread also in Asia and south and central America. The fruit is a bunch made of 20–200 individual fruits: From their mesocarp, the palm oil is obtained, while palm kernel oil comes from the fruit stones. Raw palm oil, obtained both via centrifugation or by hydraulic compression of the pulp, is orange red for its high amount of carotenoids. Its viscosity is variable according to the extraction process used. The raw oil is normally neutralized, bleached and deodorized in one step. It is mainly made of oleic (40–50%) and palmitic acids (32–47%), but it also contains linoleic (5–12%), stearic (1–9%) and myristic acid, (~1%) together with 1% unsaponifiable matters. Palm kernel oil, obtained from the nut of the seeds, is very similar to coconut oil, for its physico-chemical characteristics and as it contains lauric (46–52%), myristic (14–17%), oleic (13–19%) and palmitic acids (6–9%) [11].

27.4.3.1 Cosmetic Use

It is mainly used as a starting material for the industrial production of chemical derivatives (fatty acids, alcohols, esters and glycerine) which show a wide range of application. Among them, the production of surfactants, emulsifiers, cleansing products and skin care emulsions [7].

27.4.4 Soybean Oil

Soybean oil is derived from one of the most ancient plants cultivated by man, diffused in Asia, Europe and America. The crude oil is mainly obtained by solvent extraction (especially *n*-hexane) of seeds, with a yield of 18–22%. The residue from extraction is a flour, constituting the main protein source for animal farming. The raw oil deriving from gone bad seeds has a dark colour, high content of free fatty acids and modified lipids. When the quality of the seeds is good, it has an amber colour. The strong tendency of soybean oil to oxidize is due mainly to its high linolenic acid content (~6%); this is decreased when the oil is submitted to partial hydrogenation. It is also rich in oleic (~29%), linoleic (~54%), palmitic (~7%) and stearic acids (~4%) [2] [11].

27.4.4.1 Cosmetic Use

For its sensitivity to oxidation, soybean oil is quite unstable to light and heat; therefore it is not frequently used as such in cosmetic formulations, as it increases their potential development of rancidity.

27.4.5 Olive Oil

Virgin olive oil is obtained from olives, drupe of the plant *Olea europea* L, belonging to the family of Oleacee. The cultivation of olive trees dates back to ancient era but remains till now in the Mediterranean 'continent' a very common agricultural practice, together with the related production of the oil. Fatty acids contained in olive oil have a medium unsaturation degree, with a low content of saturated fatty acids. Oleic acid (C18:1) is the most abundant among the constituent fatty acids (70–80%). The high level of this monounsaturated fatty acid makes the olive oil particularly stable toward oxidative degradation. In the composition, also linoleic (4–7%), palmitoleic (0.5–1%), palmitic (7–11%) and stearic acids are well represented (1–4%). The unsaponifiable fraction of olive oil (0.5–1.5%) is made by more than 80% by squalene.

27.4.5.1 Cosmetic Use

Squalene being one of the main constituents of human sebum, the unsaponifiable fraction of olive oil is especially interesting for the sebum-restitutive and emollient action. Its stimulating power for the cutaneous reparation process has been demonstrated, together with a protective action from sunburn. Olive oil fats are also used for preparing 'green' surfactants and emulsifiers characterized by low irritation power and good cutaneous compatibility [16].

27.4.6 Avocado Oil

Avocado oil is obtained from the dried pulp of the fruit of *Persea americana Mill.* The plant, an evergreen tree native of central America, is now widely cultivated in all tropical areas. Avocado oil is made of oleic (55–74%), linoleic (10–14%), palmitic (9–22%) and palmitoleic acid (3–7%) glycerides. Nevertheless, the most interesting component of avocado oil is its abundant unsaponifiable fraction (2–12%) rich in branched chain hydrocarbons, phytosterols, terpene alcohols, avocatine, volatile acids and vitamins.

27.4.6.1 Cosmetic Use

While the triglycerides are responsible for the sebo-restitutive properties of avocado oil, its unsaponifiable fraction is frequently used, after separation from the oil, in moisturizing cosmetics and for the protection from environmental damages (e.g. UV rays) for the normalizing properties of the hydro-lipidic barrier. Avocado oil unsaponifiable is mainly made of saturated and unsaturated hydrocarbons, terpenes like carotenoids, sterols, triterpenes and fatty alcohols, tocopherols and tocotrienols. The functional substances of the unsaponifiable fraction can stimulate the dermal fibroblasts activity, therefore promoting the collagen neo-synthesis and inhibiting the activity of collagenase enzymes that degrade the collagen fibres (activity specific of avocatine). The result is the effective stimulation to the cutaneous turn over, improving skin moisturization and elasticity. Tocopherols in the unsaponifiable fraction, performing antioxidant and anti-free radicals activity, defend the skin in inflammatory process, thus reducing the cell and tissues damages induced by radical species, and improve skin properties as they promote the firmness of epidermis. Avocado unsaponifiable can therefore be seen as a special blend with antioxidant, protective and lenitive system. For these characteristics, cosmetics containing avocado oil and its unsaponifiable fraction are especially used in anti-age and anti-striae treatments, firming and sun protection products [16].

27.4.7 Borage and Evening Primrose Oils

Borage (*Borrago officinalis L.*) is a Mediterranean plant cultivated for its seed oil and for decorative reasons. Borage oil, obtained by cold pressing from the seeds, is very rich in polyunsaturated fatty acids. Moreover, some of them are essential for the human organism, in particular those belonging to the series ω_6. Essential fatty acids are so-called as the body cannot synthesize them but is obliged to have them with the diet. Linoleic and α-linolenic acid are the true essential fatty acids. They are key components of cell membranes and the hydro-lipidic film on the skin surface. They play an essential role in the cutaneous barrier and are precursors for the synthesis of other key molecules for the cutaneous tissues. Borage oil is therefore a natural precious source of linoleic (32–38%), oleic (14–23%), γ-linolenic (22–25%), palmitic (11–14%), and stearic acids (~5%).

Evening primrose oil is extracted from the seeds of the plant *Oenothera biennis L.* Its glycerides profile resembles borage oil: Rich in essential fatty acids, especially the ω_6 family, it is an excellent source of γ-linolenic (7–10%) and linoleic acid (up to 70%) [19]. For their high content of polyunsaturated fatty acids, oils of borage and evening primrose exhibit oxidative stability which is highly dependent on their content of antioxidant polyphenols [21].

27.4.7.1 Cosmetic Use

ω_6 fatty acids of which borage oil is rich contribute to the maintenance of normal barrier function and perform moisturizing and restitutive action, thereby facilitating the physiological restoration of chapped and dry skin. It has been shown that ω_6 fatty acids, after topical application, are integrated directly into the hydro-lipid film of the skin, where they improve the state of dryness, reduce irritation and strengthen the barrier function, which is regulated by lipid structure. It has also been shown that oils rich in ω_6 fatty acids oppose the excessive trans-epidermal water loss and improve skin moisturization and elasticity. The use of borage and enothera oil is therefore particularly advisable in many states of imbalance in the skin, caused for example by excessive exposure to sunlight, environmental stress and aging. These oils are used in cosmetic products for problem skin, seborrhoeic dermatitis, atopic skin, psoriasis, chronic irritation and flaking of the skin for their soothing and decongestant effect [16].

27.4.8 *Limnanthes alba* Oil

The oil of *Limnanthes alba* is also called Meadowfoam (seed) oil because after the winter growth in mild climates of the northwest USA, the plant blooms in May, densely covering the fields with small white flowers that seem to foam. A bright yellow oil is extracted from the seeds, accounting for more than 90% of long-chain monounsaturated fatty acids (C20–C22). The oil is also rich in antioxidants such as gamma-tocopherol (0.02–0.05%). For this particular composition, the oil is very stable to oxidation and rancidity.

27.4.8.1 Cosmetic Use

The long-chain fatty acids of *Limnanthes alba* oil are similar to sebum like and easily penetrate into the skin through pores and interstices of the stratum corneum cell. Its rapid absorption makes it a non-occlusive emollient oil, restorative and moisturizing [16].

27.4.9 Shea Butter

The shea tree (*Vitellaria paradoxa*) produces a nut that is very rich in fatty materials. Shea (also called karité) butter is a slightly yellowish or ivory pasty material, obtained from the nuts by crushing, roasting, boiling in water and stirring. Water is then separated and evaporated. Shea fats melt at about 30–35°C [1]; therefore their blend is indeed a butter that may also be used in food preparation. It contains oleic (40–60%), stearic (20–50%), linoleic (3–11%), pamitic (2–9%) linolenic and arachidic acids (<1%), but of outmost importance is its high unsaponifiable fraction (8%) with triterpene alcohols cinnamate, tocopherols (100–150 ppm). Triterpene alcohols such as lupeol and alpha-/beta-amyrin have been shown to possess anti-inflammatory effects, especially in their esterified forms, which can be only ten times lower than those of hydrocortisone.

27.4.9.1 Cosmetic Use

It is widely used in cosmetics as a moisturizer, emollient and healing agent, also in sunburn cases. It has been claimed that its use is helpful in diseased skin conditions, like eczema, burn and rashes and for the reduction of psoriasis discomfort. It is absorbed easily into the skin, without leaving any greasy feel and reduces severe skin dryness. It can also be introduced in soaps a super-fatting agent.

27.4.10 Other Oils

All seeds used in the food industry are used in cosmetics also for their moisturizing properties. They share the favourable toxicology profile, their comparably high polarity in comparison to other fatty esters, the frequently interesting content in unsaponifiable fractions which interact positively with the skin properties. Here, it can be mentioned that *Argania spinosa* oil, Macadamia oil and Jojoba oil are exotic sources while sweet almond oil and wheat germ oil are more common in the western countries. Rice oil is also an interesting moisturizing emollient from Asia and also some European countries. The long history of familiarity of mankind with edible oils accounts for their safe use and high tolerability. Indeed, they are very powerful tool for skin maintenance and protection.

Take Home Messages

- State of the art: Keratinocytes that have reached the final differentiation stage, surrounded by a lipid matrix that hinders water evaporation and the diffusion of water and electrolytes, form the epidermal horny layer. Epidermal moisturization level and barrier effects are strictly related to the amount and structure of lipids in such layer. The supplement of topically applied oils may solve the disequilibrium problems of the hydro-lipidic film in the horny layer.
- Function and composition of vegetal oils: Vegetal oils are complex blend of triglycerides, where fatty acids that esterify glycerine vary for (1) their acyl chain length, (2) their insaturation degree and (3) position of double bonds. Vegetal oils triglyceride composition is dominated by the group of unsaturated fatty acids derivatives.
- Vegetal triglycerides: Vegetal triglycerides are triesters of the polyalcohol glycerine, with several types of long-chain mono-carboxylic fatty acids.
- Accompanying ingredients: Secondary ingredients in vegetal oils represent the non-glyceride (unsaponifiable) fraction, generally present in moderate amounts. Such ingredients may noticeably influence the oxidation speed of vegetal oils.
- In vegetal oils, an equilibrated ratio between chlorophyll and carotenoid pigments is essential for an adequate oil fastness toward oxidation. All molecules in the unsaponifiable fraction belonging to the family of vitamin E are very powerful antioxidant. Phytosterols constitute a kind of vegetal fingerprint of each vegetal oil. Polyphenols work actively as *radical scavengers*.
- Vegetal oils of common cosmetic use: Corn oil, coconut oil, palm oil, soybean oil, olive oil, avocado oil, borage oil, evening primrose oil, *Limnanthes alba* oil and shea butter are among the most frequently used vegetal oils in cosmetics.

References

1. Alander J, Andersson AC, Lindstrom C (2006) Cosmetic emollients with high stability against photo-oxidation. Lipid Technol 18:226–230
2. Bruneton J (1999) Pharmacognosie: Phytochimie, Plantes médicinales, 3rd edn. Editions Tec & Doc Lavoisier, Paris
3. Carratù B, Sanzini E (2005) Biologically active substances present in vegetal derived food. Ann Ist Super Sanita 1:7–16 (in Italian)
4. Drake DR, Brogden KA, Dawson DV, Wertz PW (2008) Antimicrobial lipids at the skin surface. J Lipid Res 49:4–11
5. Feingold KR (2007) The role of epidermal lipids in cutaneous permeability barrier homeostasis. J Lipid Res 48:2531–2546
6. Grubauer G, Elias PM, Feingold KR (1989) Transepidermal water loss: the signal for recovery of barrier structure and function. J Lipid Res 30: 323–333
7. Gunstone FD (2001) Palm oil supplying much of world demand for fats and oil. Inform 12:141–146
8. Kamal-Eldin A (2006) Effect of fatty acids and tocopherols on the oxidative stability of vegetable oils. Eur J Lipid Sci Technol 58:1051–1061. doi:10.1002/ejlt.200600090
9. Moreau RA, Whitaker BD, Hicks KB (2002) Phytosterols, phytostanols, and their conjugates in foods: structural diversity, quantitative analysis, and health-promoting uses. Prog Lipid Res 41(6):457–500
10. Nikkari T, Schreibman PH, Ahrens EH Jr (1974) In vivo studies of sterol and squalene secretion by human skin. J Lipid Res 15:563–573
11. O'Lenick AJ, Steinberg DC, Klein K, LaVay C (2008) Oils of nature. Allured, Carol Stream
12. Patel MD, Thompson PD (2006) Phytosterols and vascular disease. Atherosclerosis 186:12–19
13. Piironen V et al (2000) Plant sterols: biosynthesis, biological function and their importance to human nutrition. J Sci Food Agric 80:939–966
14. Quarantelli A et al (2003) Oxidation process in vegetal derived food. Ann Fac Medic Vet Parma XXIII: 181–202 (in Italian)

15. Radaelli R (1986) Fundamentals of vegetal chemistry (in Italian). Edagricole, Bologna
16. Rigano L, Boncompagni E, Giogli A, Occhionero G (2003) Vegetal substances in cosmetics (in Italian). Aboca S.p.A, Sansepolcro
17. Safayhi H, Sailer ER (1997) Anti-inflammatory actions of pentacyclic triterpenes. Planta Med 63: 487–493
18. Stamatas GN, Sterke JD, Hauser M, Stetten OV, Pol AVD (2008) Lipid uptake and skin occlusion following topical application of oils on adult and infant skin. J Dermatol Sci 50:135–142
19. Szterk A, Roszko M, Sosin'ska E, Derewiaka D, Lewicki PP (2010) Chemical composition and oxidative stability of selected plant oils. J Am Oil Chem Soc 87:637–645
20. Vaivre-Douret L, Oriot D, Blossier P, Py A, Kasolter-Péré M, Zwang J (2008) The effect of multimodal stimulation and cutaneous application of vegetable oils on neonatal development in preterm infants: a randomized controlled trial. Child Care Health Dev 35(1):96–105
21. Wang M, Li J, Shao Y, Huang TC, Huang MT, Chin CK, Rosen RT, Ho CT (1999) Antioxidants of evening primrose. In: Shahidi F, Ho CT (eds) Phytochemicals and phytopharmaceuticals. AOCS Press, Champaign
22. Ziboh VA, Miller CC, Cho Y (2000) Metabolism of polyunsaturated fatty acids by skin epidermal enzymes: generation of anti-inflammatory and antiproliferative metabolites. Am J Clin Nutr 71(Suppl 1):361S–366S

The Effect of Natural Moisturizing Factors on the Interaction Between Water Molecules and Keratin

28

Noriaki Nakagawa

28.1 Introduction

The stratum corneum (SC) is the outermost layer of the skin and plays the role of a barrier between the interior of the body and the external environments. SC plasticity is maintained by its water content, which makes the SC flexible in the face of external physical stress. Natural moisturizing factors (NMFs) play a major role in maintaining the water content and the physical properties of the SC [1–3]. For example, the water content and elastic properties of the NMF-extracted SC were significantly decreased (Figs. 28.1 and 28.2) and the stiffness of the NMF-extracted SC was significantly increased, compared with no-treatment SC (Fig. 28.1) [1]. NMFs are composed of water-soluble compounds, such as amino acids, pyrrolidone carboxylic acid (PCA), urea, lactate, inorganic ions, etc. [4, 5].

Of the various NMFs, many researchers have focused mainly on amino acids. Amino acids are degraded from filaggrin in the SC during cornification [5, 6] and play the role of an NMF. For example, the amino acid content of the SC was lower in diseases displaying symptoms of dry skin, such as atopic dermatitis and atopic respiratory disease [7, 8]. Recently, it was reported that filaggrin mutation was a predisposing factor for atopic dermatitis and ichthyosis [9] and that the amino acid content of the SC was lower in carriers of filaggrin mutation than in healthy subjects [10]. The sodium salt of PCA, a derivative of amino acid, also increased the water content of the dry skin [11]. Urea is also known as an NMF. The urea content in the SC was significantly decreased in patients with atopic dermatitis [12], and an increase in SC water content as a result of the topical application of urea [13] has been reported by earlier studies.

Another NMF, lactate, also has a moisturizing effect on the SC. Lactate treatment alleviated symptoms of dry skin [14, 15]. Treatment using lactate salts softened the SC [16] and increased its water retention [17]. Among healthy subjects, the lactate content was higher in young subjects than in old subjects [18]. Previously, we demonstrated that potassium lactate plays an important role in maintaining the SC physical properties as an NMF and that potassium lactate increased the water content of the SC more than sodium lactate did [1]. Moreover, to evaluate the change of elastic properties of the SC due to potassium lactate, we examined whether potassium lactate changed the tan δ of the plantar SC. The tan δ represents the ratio between the dynamic elastic modulus and the dynamic loss modulus. The higher the tan δ is, the higher the elastic properties are. As a result, the tan δ of the SC treated with potassium lactate increased more than that of NMF extraction and was the same as that of nontreated SC

N. Nakagawa
Innovative Beauty Science Laboratory, Kanebo Cosmetics Inc.,
3-28, 5-Chome, Kotobuki-Cho, Odawara-Shi, Kanagawa-Ken 250-0002, Japan
e-mail: nakagawa.noriaki@kanebocos.co.jp

M. Lodén, H.I. Maibach (eds.), *Treatment of Dry Skin Syndrome*,
DOI 10.1007/978-3-642-27606-4_28, © Springer-Verlag Berlin Heidelberg 2012

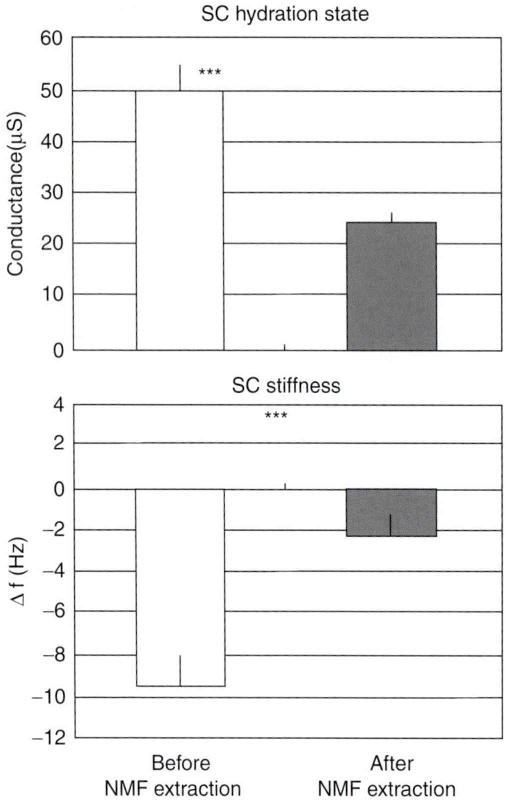

Fig. 28.1 The effect of NMF extraction on the SC physical properties

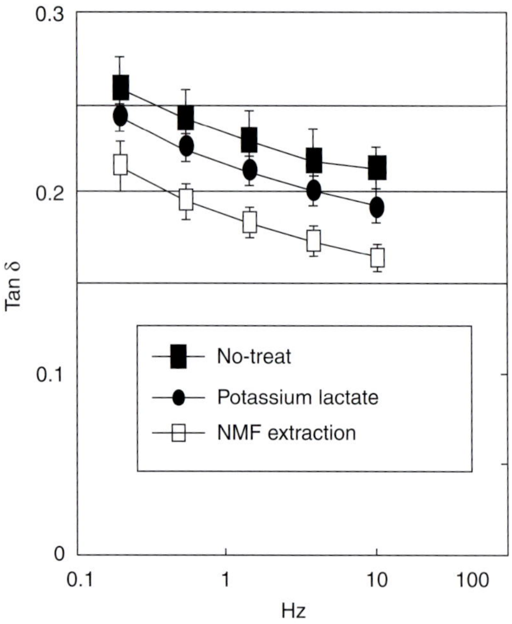

Fig. 28.2 The effect of potassium lactate on the SC elastic properties

(Fig. 28.2), suggesting that the treatment of potassium lactate on the SC increased the elastic properties of the SC more than that of NMF extraction, and that the elastic properties of the SC treated with potassium lactate were the same as that of nontreated SC.

On the other hand, there are some reports regarding the bound water content of the SC. For example, the bound water content of the SC was lower in subjects with diseases displaying dry skin symptoms than in healthy subjects [19], and the carbonylation of the SC caused a reduction in its bound water content [20] and changed the keratin structure [21]. These results suggest that the interaction of bound water with the SC keratin may contribute to the moisturization of the SC.

In the SC, 10-nm keratin filaments are composed of two types of keratins, K1 and K10. The secondary structure of keratin consists of three domains: the α-helical central rod domain, the nonhelical amino terminal domain, and the carboxyl terminal domain. It is known that keratin gene mutations cause dry skin symptoms such as epidermolytic hyperkeratosis [22–24], nonepidermolytic palmar-plantar keratoderma [25], and epidermolytic hyperkeratosis [26], suggesting that keratin structure also affects the moisturization of the SC.

Research into the mechanism of the moisturization of the SC is, however, sparse. Jokura et al. [4] reported that keratin became flexible with an increase in water content and that the nonhelical domain of keratin became more flexible than the α-helical domain with the increase in the water content. Yadav et al. [27] reported that water sorption converted a fraction of keratin α-helix to β-sheets, turns, and random coils. These results suggest that the moisturization of the SC may be caused due to an increase in the water molecules interacting with SC keratin associated with its structural change. Recently, we [28] have reported the mechanism of the moisturizing effect of potassium lactate on the SC in more detail. In this chapter, comments on the mechanism of the moisturizing effect of potassium lactate as an NMF are provided.

28.2 The Effect of Natural Moisturizing Factors on the Interaction Between Water Molecules and Keratin

We have demonstrated that potassium lactate plays an important role in maintaining the SC physical properties as an NMF [1] and that potassium lactate increased the water-holding capacity (WHC) of the SC more than sodium lactate did [28]. Therefore, we have examined the effect of potassium lactate on the interaction between water molecules and the SC keratin by comparing it with that of sodium lactate. We used two methods. The bound water content of the SC was lower in subjects with diseases displaying dry skin symptoms than in healthy subjects [19], suggesting that the interaction of bound water with the SC may contribute to the moisturization of the SC. We used differential scanning calorimetry (DSC) to examine whether potassium lactate increased the bound water content of the SC more than sodium lactate did. Keratin became flexible with the increase in its water content [4], suggesting that the component interacting with water molecules may be the SC protein. To examine whether the SC protein interacts with water molecules, we used the attenuated total reflectance infrared (ATR-IR) spectroscopy with hydrogen/deuterium exchange.

28.2.1 The Bound Water Content of the SC Treated with Potassium Salts

We [1, 28] demonstrated that potassium lactate increased the WHC of the SC more than sodium lactate did. This result does not, however, explain whether the increased WHC of the SC was due to the WHC of potassium lactate itself or the WHC of SC components. The DSC experiment was performed in an effort to gain a clear understanding of the cause of the increased WHC of the SC. We found that both potassium lactate and sodium lactate treatment caused a significant increase in the bound water content compared with NMF extraction (Table 28.1). Moreover, potassium lactate increased the bound water content significantly more than sodium lactate did (Table 28.1). However, the bound water content of potassium lactate in aqueous solution was less than that of sodium lactate (Table 28.2). These results suggest that the WHC of potassium lactate itself is not related to the WHC of the SC and that potassium lactate interacts with SC components and increases their bound water content. Takenouchi et al. [19] reported that the SC-bound water content was lower in subjects with dry skin disease conditions than in healthy subjects. They pointed out that the low WHC of the pathologic SC was due to its smaller capacity for bound water. Therefore, the interaction of bound water with the SC components may contribute to the moisturization of the SC.

Table 28.1 The bound water content of the SC treated with lactate salts

Treatment of SC	The bound water content (%; mg/mg dry SC)
Potassium lactate	37.7
Sodium lactate	33.3
NMF extraction	29.2

Table 28.2 The bound water content of lactate salts in aqueous solution

Aqueous solutions	The bound water content (%)
Potassium lactate	39.1
Sodium lactate	51.1

28.2.2 The Domain of Keratin Interacted with Water Molecules

Keratin became more flexible with an increase in water content [4], suggesting that hydrophilic amino acids in keratin may be interacting with the water molecules. In the nonhelical domain of keratins K1 and K10, the amino acid composition ratio of serine is 23%, the highest ratio among hydrophilic amino acids [29, 30]. From these facts, we hypothesized that the OH group of serine in keratin interacted with the water molecules. Because the absorption region of the OH group of alcohol is from 1,390 to 1,280 cm^{-1} [31], there was a possibility that the 1,340-cm^{-1} band

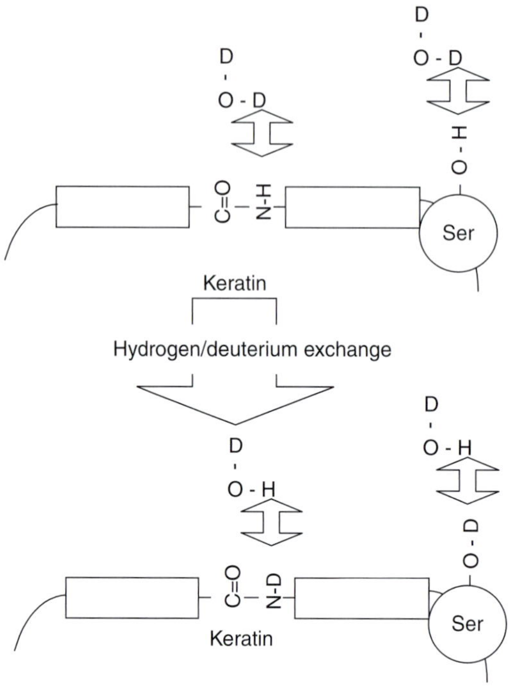

Fig. 28.3 The scheme of hydrogen/deuterium exchange

(Fig. 28.4) was derived from the OH group of amino acids in the SC protein. To prove the above hypothesis, we used ATR-IR spectroscopy with hydrogen/deuterium exchange.

The principle of ATR-IR spectroscopy with hydrogen/deuterium exchange can be explained as follows: The hydrogen/deuterium exchange represents a change of the hydrogen of NH, COOH, and OH groups, etc., to deuterium by exposing a protein to deuterium oxide (Fig. 28.3). This hydrogen/deuterium exchange had a significant effect on the IR spectrum (Fig. 28.4b) because the absorbance of these groups decreases and the absorbance of ND, COOD, and OD groups increases. Therefore, the ratio of absorbance before and after hydrogen/deuterium exchange represents the degree of the interaction between water molecules and the functional group in a protein. In this study, the ratio of hydrogen/deuterium exchange was calculated as follows:

The ratio = absorbance after deuterium oxide treatment/absorbance before deuterium oxide treatment

A decrease in this ratio means an increase in the ratio of hydrogen/deuterium exchange.

NMF extraction caused a change in the SC spectrum and a reduction in the absorbance of the 1,340-cm^{-1} band (Fig. 28.4a). However, even after the extraction of lipids and NMFs, a portion of the 1,340-cm^{-1} band still remained (Fig. 28.4a). These results suggest that the compound in the 1,340-cm^{-1} band is derived from SC protein and NMFs in a nontreated SC. In the case of NMF-extracted SC, however, the compound in the 1,340-cm^{-1} band is derived from SC protein. Moreover, the absorbance of the 1,340-cm^{-1} band in the NMF-extracted SC decreased as a result of hydrogen/deuterium exchange (Fig. 28.4b), suggesting that SC protein in the 1,340-cm^{-1} band interacts with water molecules.

To confirm that the 1,340-cm^{-1} band was derived from the OH group of serine, we made a comparison of the spectral changes in amino acids with an OH group before and after hydrogen/deuterium exchange. Our results showed that near the 1,340-cm^{-1} band, a band in the spectrum of serine and threonine was found before hydrogen/deuterium exchange (Fig. 28.5). The band of serine was nearest to 1,340 cm^{-1} among these bands. Moreover, as a result of hydrogen/deuterium exchange, the absorbance of the serine band decreased, but that of the threonine band did not (Fig. 28.5), suggesting that the 1,340-cm^{-1} band is derived from the OH group of serine. The composition ratio of serine among free amino acids in the NMF is 30% [32] and the decreased absorbance of the 1,340-cm^{-1} band after NMF extraction also supported the theory that this band consists of the OH group of serine. Our results suggest that the OH group of serine in the SC protein interacts with water molecules. The composition ratio of keratin and filaggrin were about 60% and less than 40% (by weight) respectively in the entire SC layer of mice [33], and filaggrin is degraded during cornification [5, 6]. These findings suggest that the protein component of the superficial SC is mainly keratin. Because the measurement range of depth by ATR-IR spectroscopy was less than 1.5 μm [34], the 1,340-cm^{-1} band of the NMF-extracted SC is mostly derived from keratin. Seventy-six percent of the

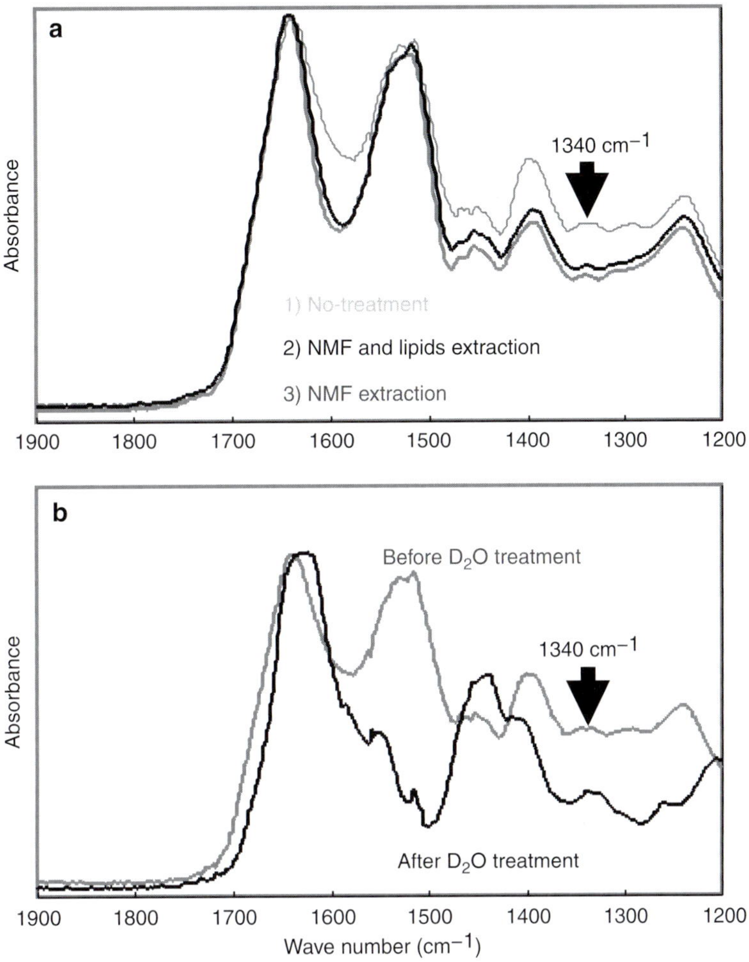

Fig. 28.4 (**a**) Spectra of plantar SC. *Thin Gray line*: no-treatment, *Thick gray line*: NMF extraction, *Black line*: NMF and lipids extraction. (**b**) Spectra of NMF extracted SC before or after deuterium oxide treatment. *Gray line*: before treatment, *Black line*: after treatment.

serine residue in keratins K1 and K10 exists in the nonhelical domain [29, 30]. The nonhelical domain of keratin became more flexible than the α-helical domain with the increase in the water content [4], suggesting that water molecules may interact with the OH group of serine in the nonhelical domain of keratin.

28.2.3 The Effect of NMF on the Interaction Between Water Molecules and Keratin

With the 1,340-cm^{-1} band, we elucidated the efficacy of potassium lactate in the interaction between water molecules and the OH group of serine in the SC keratin. We found that potassium lactate increased the exchange ratio at 1,340 cm^{-1} significantly more than sodium lactate and NMF extraction did (Fig. 28.6). Sodium lactate also increased the exchange ratio at 1,340 cm^{-1} significantly more than NMF extraction did (Fig. 28.6). These results suggest that potassium lactate increases the interaction between water molecules and serine in the SC keratin to a greater extent than sodium lactate or NMF extraction. This result corresponds with the result of the bound water content by DSC experiment (Table 28.1). These findings suggest that potassium lactate as an NMF increases the WHC of the SC by increasing the interaction between water molecules and the OH group of serine in the SC keratin. We also found that the exchange ratios at amide II of the SC treated with lactate salts and NMF-extracted SC were not different from each other [28], suggesting that the change in exchange ratio was not due

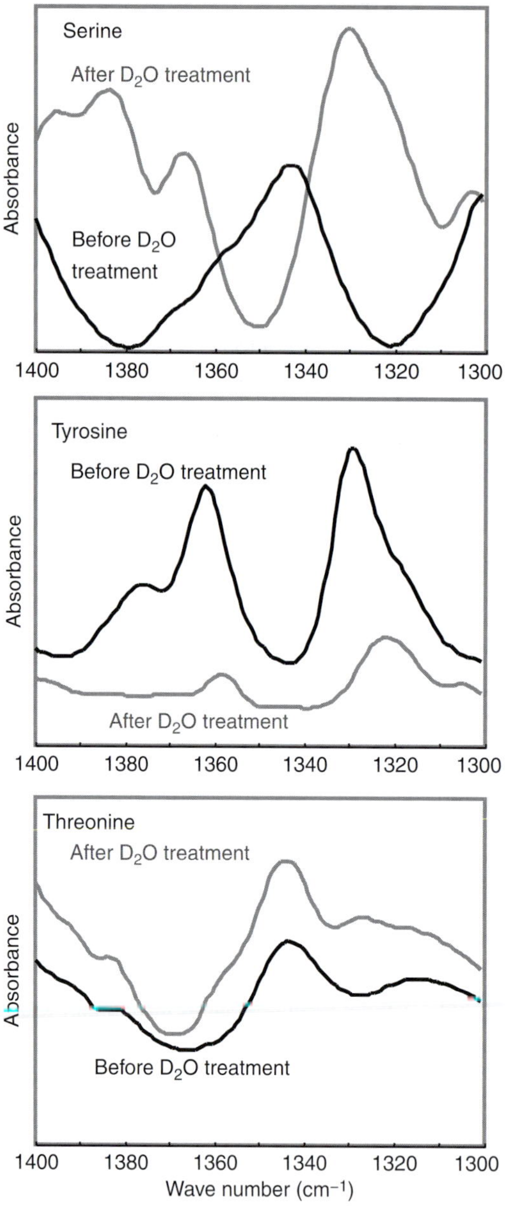

Fig. 28.5 The spectra of the amino acids with OH group before and after deuterium oxide treatment

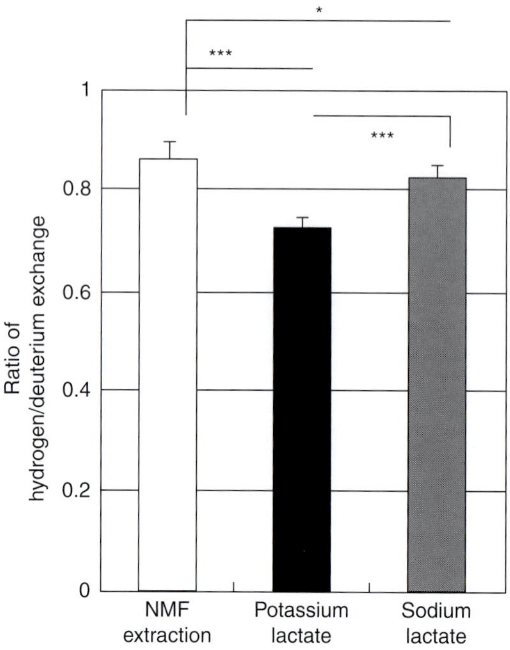

Fig. 28.6 The effect of potassium lactate on the ratio of hydrogen/deuterium exchange

to a change in the overall structure of an SC protein but due to the structural change in a specific domain of an SC protein.

Monovalent cations change the structure and activity of various enzymes according to the Hofmeister series. For example, lysozyme was more soluble in the presence of potassium than in the presence of sodium [35]. Glucose oxidase was more stable against thermal denaturation in the presence of potassium than in the presence of sodium [36]. Recently, ion-protein interaction according to the Hofmeister series was explained using computational chemistry techniques, such as classical molecular dynamics simulation. The binding activity between potassium and the carboxyl group was weaker than that of sodium with the same [37, 38]. The affinity of sodium to glutamate and aspartate was higher than that of potassium [39]. Glutamate and aspartate are the components of the nonhelical domain of keratins K1 and K10 [29, 30]. These findings suggest that, in the presence of sodium, the structure of the nonhelical domain of keratin may be more cohesive due to the strong interaction of sodium to glutamate and/or aspartate than in the presence of potassium and that the OH group of serine in the presence of sodium may interact with water molecules less than in the presence of potassium. However, further study will be needed to elucidate the difference in the mechanism by which potassium lactate and sodium lactate enhance the WHC of the SC.

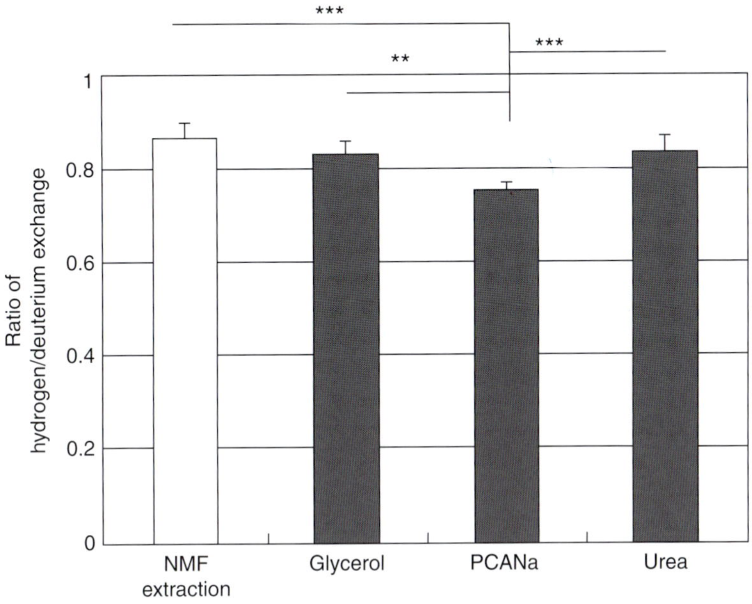

Fig. 28.7 The effect of other NMFs on the ratio of hydrogen/deuterium exchange

We made a preliminary examination to elucidate the efficacy of other NMFs, such as glycerol, sodium salt of PCA, and urea. We found that three NMFs increased the exchange ratio at 1,340 cm^{-1} more than NMF extraction did, but the difference was not significant (Fig. 28.7). Only sodium salt of PCA increased the exchange ratio at 1,340 cm^{-1} significantly more than the other treatment did (Fig. 28.7), suggesting that the mechanism of moisturizing effect may be different from each NMF. It is known that glycerol itself has a high WHC. Glycerol may have a moisturizing effect on the SC due to its own WHC. Urea is known as a denaturing agent of protein. The moisturizing effect of urea on the SC may be due to the overall structural change of an SC keratin, which may cause the increase in the interaction between water molecules and the other domain of SC keratin. However, this experiment was done at a concentration of 100 mM. Further study, such as experiments at higher doses, is needed in order to make conclusions about the mechanism of the moisturizing effect of these NMFs.

Conclusion

We demonstrated that potassium lactate as an NMF interacts with the SC protein and increases its WHC by increasing the interaction between water molecules and the OH group of serine in the SC keratin. Other NMFs, such as sodium salt of PCA, also increase the interaction, but the mechanism of moisturizing effects may differ from one NMF to another. In the future, the experiments on the structural change of keratin by NMFs will be needed in order to reveal the precise mechanism of the moisturizing effect of NMFs.

Take Home Messages

- Natural moisturizing factors (NMFs) play a major role in maintaining the water content and the physical properties of the SC. Among NMFs, potassium lactate plays an important role in maintaining the SC physical properties as an NMF.
- The interaction of bound water with the SC keratin may contribute to the moisturization of the SC. Keratin structure also affects the moisturization of the SC.
- Potassium lactate interacts with SC components and increases their bound water content.
- Potassium lactate increases the bound water of the SC by increasing the inter-

action between water molecules and the OH group of serine in the SC keratin associated with its structural change.

- The mechanism of moisturizing effect may differ from one NMF to another.
- In the future, the experiments on the structural change of keratin by NMFs will be needed in order to reveal the precise mechanism of the moisturizing effect of NMFs.

References

1. Nakagawa N, Sakai S, Matsumoto M, Yamada K, Nagano M, Yuki T et al (2004) Relationship between NMF (lactate and potassium) content and the physical properties of the stratum corneum in healthy subjects. J Invest Dermatol 122:755–763
2. Visscher MO, Tolia GT, Wickett RR, Hoath SB (2003) Effect of soaking and natural moisturizing factor on stratum corneum water-handling properties. J Cosmet Sci 54:289–300
3. Robinson M, Visscher M, Laruffa A, Wickett R (2010) Natural moisturizing factors (NMF) in the stratum corneum (SC). II. Regeneration of NMF over time after soaking. J Cosmet Sci 61:23–29
4. Jokura Y, Ishikawa S, Tokuda H, Imokawa G (1995) Molecular analysis of elastic properties of the stratum corneum by solid-state 13C-nuclear magnetic resonance spectroscopy. J Invest Dermatol 104:806–812
5. Rawlings AV, Harding CR (2004) Moisturization and skin barrier function. Dermatol Ther 17:43–48
6. Kamata Y, Taniguchi A, Yamamoto M, Nomura J, Ishihara K, Takahara H et al (2009) Neutral cysteine protease bleomycin hydrolase is essential for the breakdown of deiminated filaggrin into amino acids. J Biol Chem 284:12829–12836
7. Tanaka M, Okada M, Zhen YX, Inamura N, Kitano T, Shirai S, Sakamoto K, Inamura T, Tagami H (1998) Decreased hydration state of the stratum corneum and reduced amino acid content of the skin surface in patients with seasonal allergic rhinitis. Br J Dermatol 139:618–621
8. Tagami H, Kobayashi H, O'goshi K, Kikuchi K (2006) Atopic xerosis: employment of noninvasive biophysical instrumentation for the functional analyses of the mildly abnormal stratum corneum and for the efficacy assessment of skin care products. J Cosmet Dermatol 5:140–149
9. Sandilands A, Sutherland C, Irvine AD, McLean WH (2009) Filaggrin in the frontline: role in skin barrier function and disease. J Cell Sci 122:1285–1294
10. Kezic S, Kemperman PM, Koster ES, de Jongh CM, Thio HB, Campbell LE et al (2008) Loss-of-function mutations in the filaggrin gene lead to reduced level of natural moisturizing factor in the stratum corneum. J Invest Dermatol 128:2117–2119
11. Middleton JD, Roberts ME (1978) Effect of a skin cream containing the sodium salt of pyrrollidone carboxylic acid on dry and flaky skin. J Soc Cosmet Chem 29:201
12. Wellner K, Wohlrab W (1993) Quantitative evaluation of urea in stratum corneum of human skin. Arch Dermatol Res 285:239–240
13. Grice K, Sattar H, Baker H (1973) Urea and retinoic acid in ichthyosis and their effect on transepidermal water loss and water holding capacity of stratum corneum. Acta Derm Venereol 53:114–118
14. Dahl MV, Dahl AC (1983) 12% lactate lotion for the treatment of xerosis. Arch Dermatol 119:27–30
15. Van Scott EJ, Yu RJ (1984) Hyperkeratinization, corneocyte cohesion, and alpha hydroxy acids. J Am Acad Dermatol 11:867–879
16. Takahashi M, Machida Y (1985) The influence of hydroxy acids on the rheological properties of stratum corneum. J Soc Cosmet Chem 36:177–187
17. Gournay A, Navarro R, Mathieu J, Riviere M (1995) Water retention of treated stratum corneum measured by a coupling method: thermal desorption-mass spectrometry. Int J Cosmet Sci 17:165–172
18. Egawa M, Tagami H (2008) Comparison of the depth profiles of water and water-binding substances in the stratum corneum determined in vivo by Raman spectroscopy between the cheek and volar forearm skin: effects of age, seasonal changes and artificial forced hydration. Br J Dermatol 158:251–260
19. Takenouchi M, Suzuki H, Tagami H (1986) Hydration characteristics of pathologic stratum corneum – evaluation of bound water. J Invest Dermatol 87:574–576
20. Iwai I, Hirao T (2008) Protein carbonyls damage the water-holding capacity of the stratum corneum. Skin Pharmacol Physiol 21:269–273
21. Iwai I, Ikuta K, Murayama K, Hirao T (2008) Change in optical properties of stratum corneum induced by protein carbonylation in vitro. Int J Cosmet Sci 30:41–46
22. Yang JM, Chipev CC, DiGiovanna JJ, Bale SJ, Marekov LN, Steinert PM et al (1994) Mutations in the H1 and 1A domains in the keratin 1 gene in epidermolytic hyperkeratosis. J Invest Dermatol 102: 17–23
23. Yang JM, Nam K, Park KB, Kim WS, Moon KC, Koh JK et al (1996) A novel H1 mutation in the keratin 1 chain in epidermolytic hyperkeratosis. J Invest Dermatol 107:439–441
24. Chipev CC, Korge BP, Markova N, Bale SJ, DiGiovanna JJ, Compton JG et al (1992) A leucine proline mutation in the H1 subdomain of keratin 1 causes epidermolytic hyperkeratosis. Cell 70:821–828
25. Kimonis V, DiGiovanna JJ, Yang JM, Doyle SZ, Bale SJ, Compton JG (1994) A mutation in the V1 end

domain of keratin 1 in non-epidermolytic palmar-plantar keratoderma. J Invest Dermatol 103:764–769
26. Sprecher E, Yosipovitch G, Bergman R, Ciubutaro D, Indelman M, Pfendner E et al (2003) Epidermolytic hyperkeratosis and epidermolysis bullosa simplex caused by frameshift mutations altering the v2 tail domains of keratin 1 and keratin 5. J Invest Dermatol 120:623–626
27. Yadav S, Wickett RR, Pinto NG, Kasting GB, Thiel SW (2009) Comparative thermodynamic and spectroscopic properties of water interaction with human stratum corneum. Skin Res Technol 15:172–179
28. Nakagawa N, Naito S, Yakumaru M, Sakai S, IO (2011) Hydrating effect of potassium lactate is caused by increasing the interaction between water molecules and the serine residue of the stratum corneum protein. Exp Dermatol 20:826–831. doi:doi: 10.1111/j.1600–0625.2011.01336.x
29. Zhou XM, Idler WW, Steven AC, Roop DR, Steinert PM (1988) The complete sequence of the human intermediate filament chain keratin 10. Subdomainal divisions and model for folding of end domain sequences. J Biol Chem 263:15584–15589
30. Steinert PM, Parry DA, Idler WW, Johnson LD, Steven AC, Roop DR (1985) Amino acid sequences of mouse and human epidermal type II keratins of Mr 67,000 provide a systematic basis for the structural and functional diversity of the end domains of keratin intermediate filament subunits. J Biol Chem 260:7142–7149
31. Socrates G (2001) Hydroxyl group compounds: O-H group. In: Socrates G (ed) Infrared and Raman characteristics group frequencies: tables and charts. Wiley, West Sussex, pp 94–100
32. Jacobson TM, Yüksel KU, Geesin JC, Gordon JS, Lane AT, Gracy RW (1990) Effects of aging and xerosis on the amino acid composition of human skin. J Invest Dermatol 95:296–300
33. Steinert PM, Cantieri JS, Teller DC, Lonsdale-Eccles JD, Dale BA (1981) Characterization of a class of cationic proteins that specifically interact with intermediate filaments. Proc Natl Acad Sci USA 78: 4097–4101
34. Brancaleon L, Bamberg MP, Sakamaki T, Kollias N (2001) Attenuated total reflection-Fourier transform infrared spectroscopy as a possible method to investigate biophysical parameters of stratum corneum in vivo. J Invest Dermatol 116:380–386
35. Annunziata O, Paduano L, Pearlstein AJ, Miller DG, Albright JG (2006) The effect of salt on protein chemical potential determined by ternary diffusion in aqueous solutions. J Phys Chem B 110:1405–1415
36. Ahmad A, Akhtar MS, Bhakuni V (2001) Monovalent cation-induced conformational change in glucose oxidase leading to stabilization of the enzyme. Biochemistry 40:1945–1955
37. Jagoda-Cwiklik B, Vacha R, Lund M, Srebro M, Jungwirth P (2007) Ion pairing as a possible clue for discriminating between sodium and potassium in biological and other complex environments. J Phys Chem B 111:14077–14079
38. Hess B, van der Vegt NF (2009) Cation specific binding with protein surface charges. Proc Natl Acad Sci USA 106:13296–13300
39. Vrbka L, Vondrášek J, Jagoda-Cwiklik B, Vácha R, Jungwirth P (2006) Quantification and rationalization of the higher affinity of sodium over potassium to protein surfaces. Proc Natl Acad Sci USA 103: 15440–15444

Impact of Stratum Corneum Damage on Natural Moisturizing Factor (NMF) in the Skin

29

Lisa M. Kroll, Douglas R. Hoffman, Corey Cunningham, and David W. Koenig

29.1 Introduction

The stratum corneum (SC) is a complex structure that protects our bodies and makes it possible for mammalian life on this planet. The SC employs a combination of both physical and biochemical processes to limit the movement of water in and out of the body although clearly it is the latter that is of most importance. The SC can be disturbed by comparatively minor injury caused by mechanical, occlusive, enzymatic, and chemical damages. Lipids and a family of hygroscopic molecules known as natural moisturizing factor (NMF) are vital to the SC's ability to regulate epidermal permeability. This chapter reviews what is known about the impact of barrier disruption on key skin components and provides new insights into NMF responses following damage induced by sodium lauryl sulfate (SLS).

L.M. Kroll • D.R. Hoffman • C.T. Cunningham • D.W. Koenig (✉)
Corporate Research & Engineering, Kimberly-Clark Corporation, 2100 Winchester Road, Neenah 54956, WI, USA
e-mail: lmkroll@kcc.com; douglas.r.hoffman@kcc.com; ccunning@kcc.com; dwkoenig@kcc.com

29.2 Mechanisms and Impact of Stratum Corneum Damage

Damage to the SC can lead to multiple skin health impairments including increased transepidermal water loss, redness, and susceptibility to infection or irritation by external factors. The magnitude of these injuries is often influenced by the mechanism of SC damage, chronic or acute exposure, and the anatomical location of the damage. Underlying deficiencies in the processes responsible for development of a normal, healthy SC barrier have been linked to the etiology of skin disorders including psoriasis, eczema, and atopic dermatitis [1–4].

Mechanical damage is one mechanism that can impact skin barrier function by damaging the skin through actions such as scraping, abrasion, or removal of SC by adhesives. The end result of these actions is the physical removal of corneocytes from the skin surface and increased barrier permeability. Maintaining adequate skin flexibility and elasticity is a primary defense against mechanical damage. Aging decreases the skin's flexibility and elasticity, increasing susceptibility to mechanical damage [5].

Overhydration and ultraviolet (UV) damage the skin in a more complex way involving both biochemical and chemical changes. Occlusion or excessive water exposure disrupts the SC water balance increasing its permeability and susceptibility to irritation [6]. Exposure to UV radiation represents a common type of SC damage. UV exposure induces oxidation and subsequent loss

M. Lodén, H.I. Maibach (eds.), *Treatment of Dry Skin Syndrome*,
DOI 10.1007/978-3-642-27606-4_29, © Springer-Verlag Berlin Heidelberg 2012

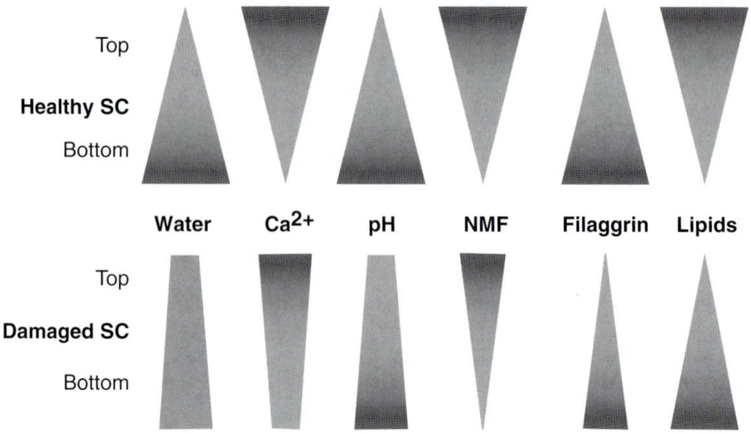

Fig. 29.1 Stylized diagram of biochemical changes associated with barrier damage. Shape is an approximate representation of the amount of each component relative to position in the stratum corneum (*SC*). *Top* = SC surface. *Bottom* = SC viable epidermal interface

of functionality of SC lipids, proteins, and antioxidants. Reductions in SC antioxidant levels, including α-tocopherol, the most predominant antioxidant in the SC, have been reported with UV exposure [7–9].

Biochemically induced SC damage such as enzymatic degradation of lipids and proteins can eventuate in damage to skin barrier function. For example, enzyme-induced damage is commonly associated with the use of absorbent articles for fecal incontinence [10]. Feces contain a number of proteases and lipases that can degrade key SC components, resulting in loss of barrier function. Serine proteases such as trypsin and chymotrypsin are the most prevalent enzymes present in fecal insults [10].

Surfactants and solvents are a common chemical means of SC damage. In consumer markets, exposure to surfactants and solvents are commonly the result of using personal hygiene products such as soaps, cleansers, and acne treatments. Likewise, workplace exposures are not uncommon. Frequent hand washing in health care, the daily work of hair dressers, and food and metal workers are examples of occupations that frequently experience skin damage due to routine chemical exposures. Surfactants impact barrier function by several means including damage to SC proteinaceous material and lipids [11]. The net charge and micelle size affect the likelihood of surfactants to cause damage, with anionic surfactants (e.g., sodium lauryl sulfate, sodium dodecyl sulfate) that form small micelles (<2.9 nm) being the most damaging [12]. Alcohol and acetone are common solvents encountered. The primary mechanism for solvent-induced damage is disruption of SC lamellae resulting in increased solute permeability into the epidermis [13].

Barrier disruption, whether caused by chemical, physical, or biochemical means, alters the SC composition and structure required to maintain barrier homeostasis. The water gradient, pH gradients, ion gradients, NMF, and lipid configurations, are all impacted by barrier disruption (Fig. 29.1). The impact of disruption on SC lipids is well documented [14–22]. A significant reduction in ceramide, cholesterol, and free fatty acid concentrations occurs after disruption followed by a rapid secretion of lipids to the upper SC as an initial step towards reestablishing healthy barrier homeostasis.

Disruption has also been shown to alter pH and ion gradients, both of which can impact the functionality of key enzymes involved in epidermal differentiation and lipid processing [23–26]. Under normal conditions, the surface of the SC maintains a slightly acidic (~4–6) pH. Following barrier disruption, the SC surface pH increases, dissolving the pH gradient throughout the SC. Lipid processing is dependent on two pH-dependent lipid hydrolases (β-glucocerebrosidase and acid sphingomyelinase). These enzymes are activated by the acidity in the extracellular spaces and lose activity as pH increases. Not only does an increased pH render these enzymes inactive but it also activates other enzymes (serine proteases) which degrade corneodesmosomes, resulting in loss of SC integrity [23–25].

Skin barrier disruption can also disturb ion gradients present in the SC. Changes in the Ca^{2+}, K^+, and Cl^- ionic gradients following barrier disruption have been shown to impact the secretion of lamellar bodies (LB) into extracellular spaces [23, 25]. Influx of cytosolic Ca^{2+} into epidermal keratinocytes inhibits LB secretion and delays epidermal recovery. Exposure to a high level of Ca^{2+} following barrier disruption has a similar effect [25], indicating normal barrier function is dependent on a specific Ca^{2+} range. Epidermal Ca^{2+} levels are also associated with a decrease in mRNA levels for specific differentiation-linked proteins such as loricrin [25]. Increased extracellular K^+ shows similar effects. Conversely, the influx of Cl^- into keratinocytes accelerates LB secretion and consequently barrier recovery rate after disruption [23].

29.3 Impact of Stratum Corneum Damage on Natural Moisturizing Factor

Less understood is the effect of acute disruption on NMF and its precursors, profilaggrin and filaggrin. NMF serves as the primary humectant in skin. It is principally comprised of hygroscopic amino acids and derivatives that absorb moisture from the surrounding environment and retain the water inside the lipid-protected corneocytes [27]. NMF is derived from a large histidine-rich protein called filaggrin, which functions to aggregate keratin in the final stages of epidermal differentiation [28]. After undergoing internal charge reorganization during differentiation, filaggrin is no longer bound to the keratin of the keratinocytes. The result is filaggrin is susceptible to protease activity and subsequently is hydrolyzed into individual amino acids and derivatives.

The importance of the NMF contribution to barrier homeostasis is evidenced by reported links between abnormalities in profilaggrin/filaggrin production and/or processing with skin conditions such as ichthyosis, atopic dermatitis, and scaling disorder [28–30]. In addition to amino acids, other key components of NMF include lactate, urea, and sugars. The amino acid fraction of NMF primarily exists within corneocytes following filaggrin degradation whereas lactate, urea, and sugars are derived from and exist in extracellular spaces [31]. In concert with lipids, which slow water diffusion by providing the SC with a torturous hydrophobic path, NMF help corneocytes hold a normal flattened, elongated shape by selectively binding and retaining water. The planar geometry of corneocytes is a key factor in maintaining the tortuous path; the flattened, elongated shape allows corneocytes to maintain a strong attachment to each other via corneodesmosomes [32]. The ability to maintain cell shape also makes NMF a key contributor to maintaining skin flexibility [33].

Changes in filaggrin processing and NMF concentrations have been reported following acute barrier disruption induced by physical or chemical means [34–40]. Different types of damage induce different effects on specific NMF components (Table 29.1).

Literature suggests that many key SC NMF components are reduced following barrier disruption [34–37, 40]. A study was recently completed to investigate the impact of SLS barrier disruption on NMF using noninvasive measurements (Fig. 29.2) [35]. In agreement with previous reports [34, 36], results suggest that SLS-induced damage decrease SC levels of alanine, glycine, pyrrolidone carboxylic acid (PCA), and serine. *trans*-Urocanic acid is also reduced along with its precursor histidine [34–36].

Other studies have also developed evidence to suggest that other types of barrier damage can impact NMF levels [37, 40]. For instance, tape stripping followed by occlusion was found to reduce levels of SC free amino acids including citrulline [40]. Repeated UV irradiation lowered SC concentrations of glutamic acid, arginine, citrulline, and histidine by ~20% but had no effect on urea, serine, glutamine, and tyrosine levels [37].

However, some NMF components do increase after barrier damage. Most notably, specific types of damage appear to increase the concentration of products and intermediates of urea cycling.

Table 29.1 Barrier disruption and impact on natural moisturizing factor (NMF)

		NMF Response		
Reference	Damage Mechanism	Increase	Decrease	No Change
Koyama [34][a] Kroll [35][b] Porcheron [36][c]	Surfactant (SLS)	Lactate[b] Ornithine[a,b,c] Proline[a,b] Urea[a,b]	Alanine[b,c] Arginine[a] Citrulline[a] Glycine[b,c] Histidine[a,b,c] PCA[b] Serine[b,c] Urocanic acid[a,b]	Lactate[c]
Pratzel [37]	Ultraviolet irradiation	Glycine Isoleucine Proline Urocanic acid Valine	Arginine Citrulline Glutamic acid Histidine	Glutamine Serine Tyrosine Urea
Visscher [40]	Tape stripping	Glutamic acid	Citrulline Histidine Serine	–
Visscher [40]	Tape stripping followed by occlusion	–	Citrulline Glutamic acid Histidine Serine	–

SLS sodium lauryl sulfate, *PCA* pyrrolidone carboxylic acid

Both urea and ornithine have been reported to increase following SLS-induced barrier perturbation [34–36]. An increase in lactate was reported by Kroll [35]; however, Porcheron [36] found no impact on SC lactate. Increases in proline have also been observed [34, 35]. Tape stripping followed by occlusion increased glutamic acid levels [40] while UV irradiation increased SC levels of urocanic acid, proline, glycine, valine, and isoleucine by ~20% [37].

29.4 Sodium Lauryl Sulfate Impact on Natural Moisturizing Factor Processing

Continued research to understand the biochemistry of NMF production is essential to fully appreciate its role in barrier disruption and repair. While the entire process has not been fully elucidated, Fig. 29.3 provides a plausible pathway for NMF generation. Profilaggrin/filaggrin processing is a complex process involving multiple enzymes [41], and barrier disruption likely impacts the stability and/or activity of each. During normal epidermal differentiation, profilaggrin is dephosphorylated and cleaved to filaggrin monomers [42–47]. Filaggrin monomers are deiminated by the peptidylarginine deiminases (PAD1 and PAD3), converting filaggrin-associated arginine residues to citrulline [48–50]. The deiminated filaggrin is then hydrolyzed into peptide fragments and eventually to individual amino acids and derivatives likely involving multiple enzymatic steps [51–56]. A recent study has shown bleomycin hydrolase (BH), a neutral cysteine protease identified in the rat epidermis, likely plays a substantial role in the final stages of NMF generation. BH was found to readily hydrolyze deiminated filaggrin that was partially degraded by a calcium-dependent cysteine protease called calpain 1 [56].

SLS-induced barrier disruption has been reported to reduce the expression of profilaggrin genes within 6 h of exposure [39]. However, this

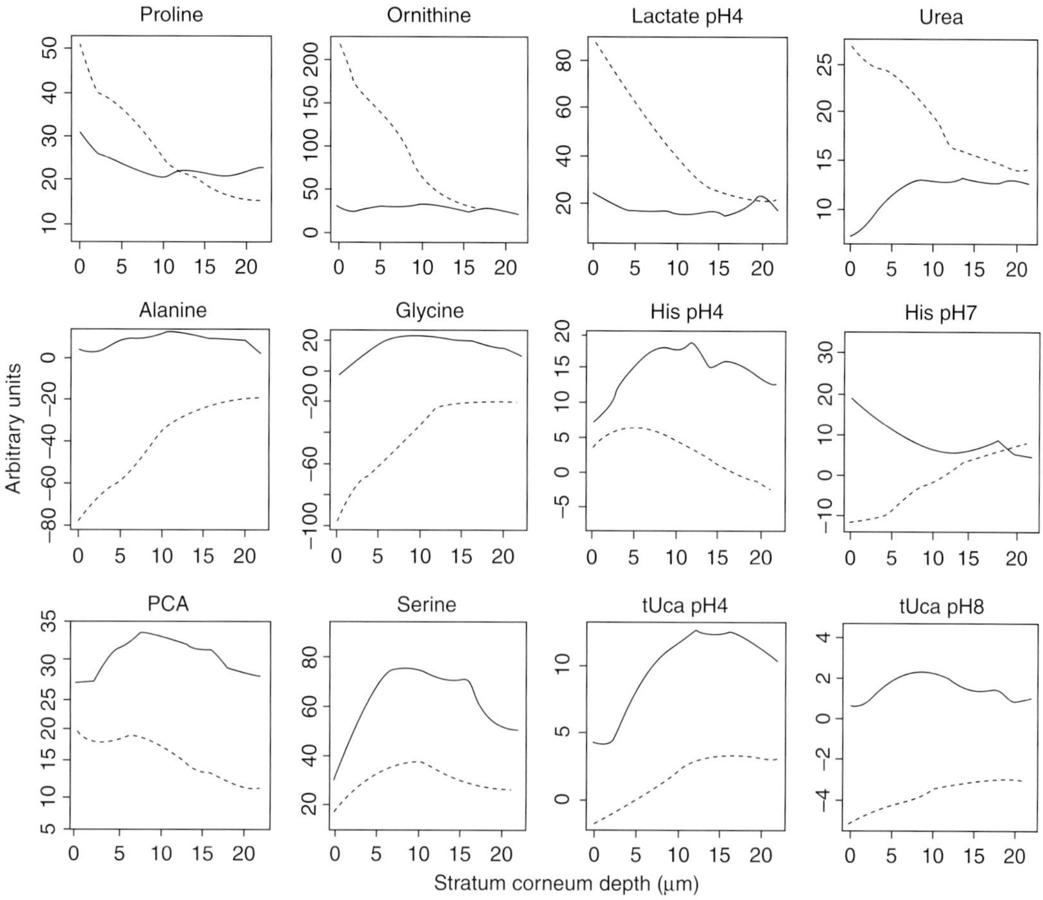

Fig. 29.2 Raman profiles of natural moisturizing factor (*NMF*) components after sodium lauryl sulfate (*SLS*) exposure. *Dashed line* = SLS-exposed stratum corneum (*SC*). *Solid line* = water-exposed stratum corneum. Forearm sites were patched with 1% SLS or water for 24 h. Patches were removed, sites were allowed to acclimate for 30 min, and the distribution of key SC NMF constituents determined using in vivo confocal Raman spectroscopy [35]. *His* Histidine, *PCA* pyrrolidone carboxylic acid, *tUCA trans*-Urocanic acid

observation did not translate to the protein level as no change in filaggrin levels was detected. This implies the most prominent effect of SLS disruption on NMF generation is in the deimination and/or hydrolysis of filaggrin. The NMF responses to barrier damage (Table 29.1) infer that the activity of key enzymes may be universally reduced by barrier disruption. Reductions in histidine, citrulline, serine, and arginine appear to be most common irrespective of the mechanism of barrier disruption, suggesting the enzymes involved in their release may be more susceptible to loss of activity. Another possibility is that the substrates are altered or that the downstream enzymes capable of utilizing these amino acids as substrates have increased kinetics following disruption. These types of responses may help explain the NMF concentrations observed following SLS-induced disruption, specifically those NMF components derived from urea cycling (Fig. 29.4).

A reduction in arginine following SLS exposure appears to coincide with an increase in ornithine and urea [34–36], the products of arginase-mediated breakdown of arginine [55]. This suggests an increase in arginase activity. Alterations in arginase activity as a function of barrier damage have not been investigated to date and warrant

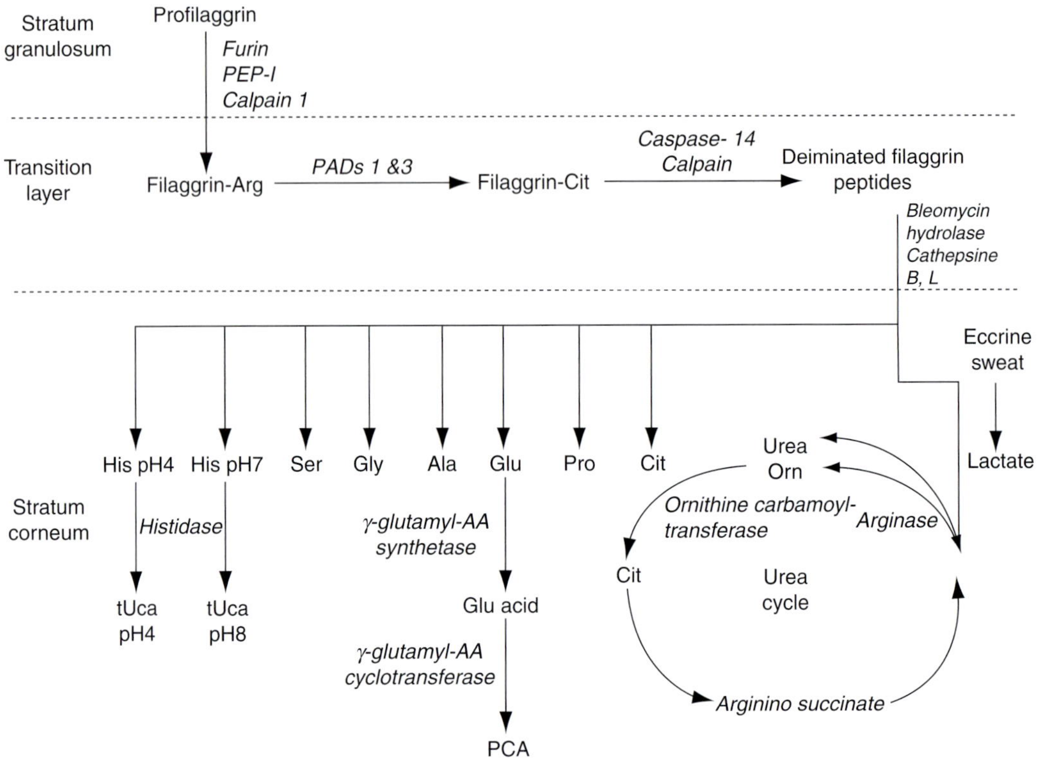

Fig. 29.3 Putative pathway for natural moisturizing factor production. *PEP1* profilaggrin endoproteinase 1, *PAD* peptidylarginine deiminase, *Arg* arginine, *Cit* citrulline, *Orn* ornithine, *Pro* proline, *Glu* glutamine, *Glu acid* glutamic acid, *PCA* pyrrolidone carboxylic acid, *Ala* alanine, *Gly* glycine, *Ser* serine, *His* histidine, *tUca trans*-Urocanic acid

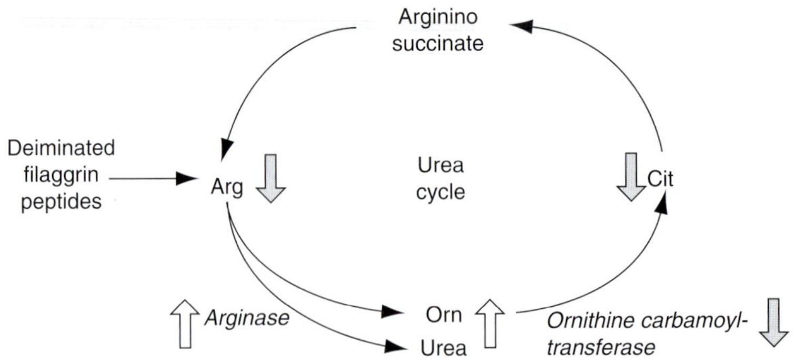

Fig. 29.4 Hypothetical model of sodium lauryl sulfate (*SLS*) mediated impact on stratum corneum (*SC*) natural moisturizing factor derived from urea cycling. Forearm sites were patched with 1–10% SLS for up to 24 h and compared to a site patched with water alone. *Open, upward facing arrows* represent amino acids that increased with SLS exposure or enzymes hypothesized to have higher kinetics with SLS. Similarly, *filled, downward facing arrows* represent amino acids that decreased or enzymes hypothesized to have lower kinetics. Decreased arginine and increased ornithine/urea levels may be due to increased arginase activity following disruption. Conversely, reduced citrulline levels may result from reduced activity of ornithine carbamoyltransferase. *Arg* arginine, *Cit* citrulline, *Orn* ornithine (Model derived from observations reported in Koyama [34], Kroll [35], and Porcheron [36])

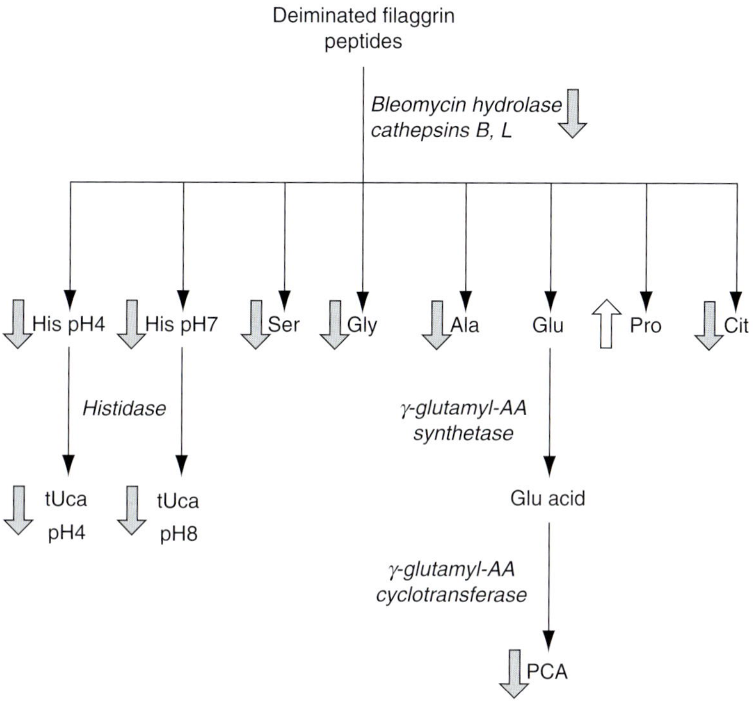

Fig. 29.5 Hypothetical model of sodium lauryl sulfate (*SLS*) mediated impact on stratum corneum (*SC*) natural moisturizing factors derived from bleomycin hydrolase (*BH*), cathepsin B, and cathepsin L-mediated hydrolysis of filaggrin Forearm sites were patched with 1–10% SLS for up to 24 h and compared to a site patched with water alone. Open, upward facing arrows represent amino acids that increased following SLS exposure or enzymes hypothesized to have higher kinetics with SLS. Similarly, filled, downward facing arrows represent amino acids that decreased or enzymes hypothesized to have lower kinetics. Other than proline, all amino acids are decreased following SLS exposure. This would imply proline is released in the SC independent of or downstream of the other amino acids and the mechanism of its release is enhanced by SLS exposure. Alternatively, increased proline may be attributed to SLS-induced denaturation of small proline-rich proteins (*SPRPs*) that provide structural support to the cornified envelope. *Cit* Citrulline, *Pro* Proline, *Glu* Glutamine, *Glu acid* Glutamic acid, *PCA* Pyrrolidone carboxylic acid, *Ala* Alanine, *Gly* Glycine, *Ser* Serine, *His*=Histidine, *tUca*=*trans*-Urocanic acid (Model derived from observations reported in Koyama [34], Kroll [35] and Porcheron [36])

further research. Altered conditions of pH, ion concentrations, or substrate may explain the increase in arginase activity under damaged conditions. Also coinciding with decreased arginine and increased ornithine levels is a decrease in citrulline, implying a reduction in the activity of ornithine carbamoyltransferase, the enzyme responsible for converting ornithine to citrulline during urea cycling [55]. A similar response is observed following UV damage, with increased *trans*-Urocanic levels coinciding with decreased histidine [37], implying an increase in histidine breakdown with UV-mediated disruption (Fig. 29.5).

Following SLS exposure, the majority of NMF derived components outside of urea cycling are at reduced levels in the SC (histidine, serine, glycine, alanine, PCA, and citrulline) (Table 29.1 and Fig. 29.2). This observation could be attributed to direct enzyme inactivation by SLS or SLS-mediated denaturation of filaggrin at enzyme recognition sites, or other pleiotropic events that have yet to be elucidated. Levels of the downstream breakdown products of these amino acids are also decreased (*trans*-Urocanic acid and PCA), likely due to lack of substrate amino acids or enzyme inactivation by SLS.

Proline levels in the SC appear to increase following SLS exposure (Table 29.1 and Fig. 29.2). It is not known which specific enzyme is responsible for generating free proline during normal epidermal differentiation. Recent analyses of BH activity against aminoacyl-β-naphthylamide substrates indicate that it is capable of releasing all amino acids except proline [56]. Additionally, experiments investigating BH hydrolysis of recombinant filaggrin failed to detect released proline. This implies free SC proline may be generated independent of or downstream of BH-mediated filaggrin hydrolysis. Alternatively, increased proline may be arising from the breakdown or denaturation of proteins other than filaggrin. The cornified envelope is partially comprised of the structural pancorulin and cornifin proteins which are predominantly comprised of proline, commonly referred to as small proline-rich proteins (SPRPs). SLS-mediated denaturation of these SPRPs may contribute to the observed SC proline increase.

29.5 Implications for Future Research

Mammalian skin is a complex organ with an innate ability to respond to its environment. SC damage by chronic or acute exposure to chemical, physical, or biochemical agents initiates an important repair process. For mammals, this repair function is an absolute requirement for survival. Accordingly, these processes are presumed to be highly conserved and tightly controlled.

With regard to surfactant damage to the SC, at least two intersecting research avenues are envisioned to investigate both the impact of damage on SC biochemistry and subsequent SC repair. The first avenue includes work to elucidate the regulation and control of SC enzymology as a function of factors including pH, ion concentration, substrate availability, and the absence/presence of inhibitors. The second avenue is to better appreciate the alteration of the viable epidermis with regard to cell metabolism and gene expression. Both avenues are important in understanding the control of NMF processing during SC development and repair.

With damage the skin loses direct control of factors such as pH and ion gradients; however, the skin can rebalance these factors during repair. This rebalancing requires an orchestrated execution of enzyme activity as well as the availability of respective substrates. Surfactants can alter the tertiary structure of both the enzymes and substrates involved in this rebalancing process, thus changing enzyme kinetics and, in some cases, substrate recognition.

The second research avenue of SC damage and repair is associated with alterations in gene expression and cellular functions important to repair processes. Barrier disruption can have an effect beyond the SC, directly impacting cellular function in the viable epidermis [39, 57, 58]. It is expected that both chemical and biochemical insults will have a greater influence on cellular functions than would mechanical insults such as abrasion. Unlike mechanical insults whose disruption is by and large focused on the upper SC, chemical and biochemical insults permeate the SC providing a greater ability to impact cellular processes. The effective concentration of the insult reaching the cells will be paramount in the type and magnitude of damage and cellular response.

Specifically looking at the impact of surfactants on the damage and repair of the SC, it would appear that both cellular and biochemical regulatory pathways are impacted. The loss of enzyme functionality can address some of the observed changes in the NMF products. However, alterations in NMF processing enzymology alone seem unlikely to completely account for the observed outcomes of SC damage by SLS. It is anticipated that cellular responses to SLS occurs and further studies are required to elucidate these mechanisms.

To dissect the impact of SLS on SC enzymology, it may be necessary to provide chronic exposure to lower levels of SLS and measure NMF responses. The studies presented in Table 29.1 employed an acute exposure to a relatively large amount of SLS. This method of exposure likely impacted cellular functions beyond the SC, making it difficult to isolate a direct impact to enzyme processes specific to the SC. Nondestructive in vivo measurements such as Raman spectroscopy can be used to measure these responses. In parallel, changes in gene expression using gene arrays can provide a means to measure cellular responses to these insults.

The advancement of knowledge on the biochemical processes and repair functions of the SC are an important study area impacting the study of both cosmetic and dermatological skin conditions. Elucidating the enzymology and cellular aspects of NMF processing is a key step in reaching that goal. More studies are needed that utilize a systems biology approach to provide a holistic view of SC damage and repair processes. Understanding these processes at a cellular and biochemical level will provide new opportunities to give comfort to those with cosmetic skin issues as well as those suffering from dermatological diseases.

Take Home Messages

- Skin barrier disruption, whether caused by chemical, physical, or biochemical means, alters the SC composition and structure required to maintain barrier homeostasis. The water gradient, pH gradient, ion gradients, NMF, and lipid configurations are all impacted by barrier disruption.
- NMF serves as the primary humectant in skin. It is principally comprised of hygroscopic amino acids and derivatives that absorb moisture from the surrounding environment and retain water inside the lipid-protected corneocytes.
- During normal epidermal differentiation, profilaggrin is processed to NMF via a cascade of multiple enzymatic activities.
- Different types of barrier disruption induce different effects on specific NMF components. Many key NMF components are reduced following barrier disruption while some increase.
- Changes in the activity of key enzymes and/or the availability of substrates likely impact observed changes in NMF concentrations.
- Further research is needed to elucidate the regulation and control of SC enzymology as a function of factors including pH, ion concentration, substrate availability, and the absence/presence of inhibitors.
- Continued work is also needed to better understand the alteration of the viable epidermis following barrier damage and during repair with regard to cell metabolism and gene expression.
- More studies are needed that utilize a systems biology approach to provide a holistic view of SC damage and repair processes.

Abbreviations

Ala	Alanine
BH	Bleomycin hydrolase
Cit	Citrulline
FFA	Free fatty acids
Gly	Glycine
His pH4	Histidine pH4
His pH7	Histidine pH7
LB	Lamellar bodies
NMF	Natural moisturizing factor
PAD1 and PAD3	Peptidylarginine deiminases
PCA	Pyrrolidone carboxylic acid
Ser	Serine
SPRPs	Small proline-rich proteins
SLS	Sodium lauryl sulfate
SC	Stratum corneum
tUca	*trans*-Urocanic acid
UV	Ultraviolet

References

1. Motta S, Monti M, Sesana S, Caputo R, Carelli S, Ghidoni R (1993) Ceramide composition of the psoriatic scale. Biochim Biophys Acta 1182(2):147–151
2. Cookson WO, Ubhi B, Lawrence R, Abecasis GR, Walley AJ, Cox HE, Coleman R, Leaves NI, Trembath RC, Moffatt MF, Harper JI (2001) Genetic linkage of childhood atopic dermatitis to psoriasis susceptibility loci. Nat Genet 27(4):372–373

3. Sator PG, Schmidt JB, Hönigsmann H (2003) Comparison of epidermal hydration and skin surface lipids in health individuals and in patients with atopic dermatitis. J Am Acad Dermatol 48(3):352–358
4. Proksch E, Elias PM (2002) Epidermal barrier in atopic dermatitis. In: Beiber T, Leung DY (eds) Atopic dermatitis. Marcel Dekker, New York
5. Schulze C, Wetzel F, Kueper T, Malsen A, Muhr G, Jaspers S, Blatt T, Wittern KP, Wenck H, Käs JA (2010) Stiffening of human skin fibroblasts with age. Biophys J 99(8):2434–2442
6. Fluhr JW, Akengin A, Bornkessel A, Fuchs S, Praessler J, Norgauer J, Grieshaber R, Kleesz P, Elsner P (2005) Additive impairment of the barrier function by mechanical irritation, occlusion, and sodium lauryl sulphate in vivo. Br J Dermatol 153(1):125–131
7. Shindo Y, Witt E, Han D, Packer L (1994) Dose–response effects of acute ultraviolet irradiation on antioxidants and molecular markers of oxidation in murine epidermis and dermis. J Invest Dermatol 102(4):470–475
8. Shindo Y, Witt E, Packer L (1993) Antioxidant defense mechanisms in murine epidermis and dermis and their responses to ultraviolet light. J Invest Dermatol 100(3):260–265
9. Thiele JJ, Traber MG, Packer L (1998) Depletion of human stratum corneum vitamin E: an early and sensitive in vivo marker of UV-induced photooxidation. J Invest Dermatol 110(5):756–761
10. Andersen PH, Bucher AP, Saeed I, Lee PC, Davis JA, Maibach HI (1994) Faecal enzymes: in vivo skin irritation. Contact Dermatitis 30(3):152–158
11. Törmä H, Berne B (2009) Sodium lauryl sulphate alters mRNA expression of lipid-metabolizing enzymes and PPAR signaling in normal human skin in vivo. Exp Dermatol 18(12):1010–1015
12. Moore PN, Shiloach A, Puvvada S, Blankschtein D (2003) Penetration of mixed micelles into the epidermis: effect of mixing sodium dodecyl sulfate with dodecyl hexa (ethylene oxide). J Cosmet Sci 54(2):143–159
13. Fartasch M (1997) Ultrastructure of the epidermal barrier after irritation. Microsc Res Tech 37(3):193–199
14. Feingold KR (1991) The regulation of epidermal lipid synthesis by permeability barrier requirements. Crit Rev Ther Drug Carrier Syst 8(3):193–210
15. Grubauer G, Feingold KR, Harris RM, Elias PM (1989) Lipid content and lipid type as determinants of the epidermal permeability barrier. J Lipid Res 30(1):89–96
16. Harris IR, Farrell AM, Grunfeld C, Holleran WM, Elias PM, Feingold KR (1997) Permeability barrier disruption coordinately regulates mRNA levels for key enzymes of cholesterol, fatty acid, and ceramide synthesis in the epidermis. J Invest Dermatol 109(6):783–787
17. Holleran WM, Takagi Y, Menon GK, Jackson SM, Lee JM, Feingold KR, Elias PM (1994) Permeability barrier requirements regulate epidermal β-glucocerebrosidase. J Lipid Res 35(5):905–912
18. Lasch J, Schönfelder U, Walke M, Zellmer S, Beckert D (1997) Oxidative damage of human skin lipids. Dependence of lipid peroxidation on sterol concentration. Biochim Biophys Acta 1349(2):171–181
19. Mao-Qiang M, Elias PM, Feingold KR (1993) Fatty acids are required for epidermal permeability barrier function. J Clin Invest 92(2):791–798
20. Mao-Qiang M, Feingold KR, Jain M, Elias PM (1995) Extracellular processing of phospholipids is required for permeability barrier homeostasis. J Lipid Res 36(9):1925–1935
21. Proksch E, Holleran WM, Menon GK, Elias PM, Feingold KR (1993) Barrier function regulates epidermal lipid and DNA synthesis. Br J Dermatol 128(5):473–482
22. Takagi Y, Kriehuber E, Imokawa G, Elias PM, Holleran WM (1999) β-Glucocerebrosidase activity in mammalian stratum corneum. J Lipid Res 40(5):861–869
23. Choi EH, Man MQ, Xu P, Xin S, Liu Z, Crumrine DA, Jiang YJ, Fluhr JW, Feingold KR, Elias PM, Mauro TM (1991) Stratum corneum acidification is impaired in moderately aged human and murine skin. J Invest Dermatol 127(12):2847–2856
24. Denda M, Tsutsumi M, Inoue K, Crumrine D, Feingold KR, Elias PM (2007) Potassium channel openers accelerate epidermal barrier recovery. Br J Dermatol 157(5):888–893
25. Elias PM, Ahn SK, Denda M, Brown BE, Crumrine D, Kimutai LK, Kömüves L, Lee SH, Feingold KR (2002) Modulations in epidermal calcium regulate the expression of differentiation-specific markers. J Invest Dermatol 119(5):1128–1136
26. Mauro T, Holleran WM, Grayson S, Gao WN, Man MQ, Kriehuber E, Behne M, Feingold KR, Elias PM (1998) Barrier recovery is impeded at neutral pH, independent of ionic effects: implications for extracellular lipid processing. Arch Dermatol Res 290(4):215–222
27. Rawlings AV, Scott IR, Harding CR, Bowser PA (1994) Stratum corneum moisturization at the molecular level. J Invest Dermatol 103(5):731–741
28. Sandilands A, Sutherland C, Irvine AD, McLean WH (2009) Filaggrin in the frontline: role in skin barrier function and disease. J Cell Sci 122(Pt 9):12851294
29. McGrath JA, Uitto J (2008) The filaggrin story: novel insights into skin-barrier function and disease. Trends Mol Med 14(1):20–27
30. Palmer CN, Irvine AD, Terron-Kwiatkowski A, Zhao Y, Liao H, Lee SP, Goudie DR, Sandilands A, Campbell LE, Smith FJ, O'Regan GM, Watson RM, Cecil JE, Bale SJ, Compton JG, DiGiovanna JJ, Fleckman P, Lewis-Jones S, Arseculeratne G, Sergeant A, Munro CS, El Houate B, McElreavey K, Halkjaer LB, Bisgaard H, Mukhopadhyay S, McLean WH (2006) Common loss-of-function variants of the epidermal barrier protein filaggrin are a major predisposing factor for atopic dermatitis. Nat Genet 38(4):441–446
31. Rawlings AV (2006) Sources and role of stratum corneum hydration. In: Elias PM, Feingold KR (eds) Skin barrier. Taylor & Francis, New York
32. Harding CR, Watkinson A, Rawlings AV, Scott IR (2000) Dry skin, moisturization and corneodesmolysis. Int J Cosmet Sci 22(1):21–52

33. Nakagawa N, Sakai S, Matsumoto M, Yamada K, Nagano M, Yuki T, Sumida Y, Uchiwa H (2004) Relationship between NMF (lactate and potassium) content and the physical properties of the stratum corneum in healthy subjects. J Invest Dermatol 122(3):755–763
34. Koyama J, Horii I, Kawasaki K (1984) Free amino acids of stratum corneum as a biochemical marker to evaluate dry skin. J Cosmet Chem Japan 35(4):183–195
35. Kroll LM, Hoffman DR, Basehoar A, Cunningham C, Reece B, Koenig DW (2011) Confocal Raman study of stratum corneum changes after damage with sodium lauryl sulfate. In: International Society for Biophysics and Imaging of the Skin (ISBS). US technical symposium of ISBS, Tampa Bay, 6–9 Apr 2011
36. Porcheron A, Mauger E, Guinot C, Tschachler E, Morizot F (2007) Abstracts from the stratum corneum V conference 2007. Int J Cosmet Sci 29(3):219–228
37. Pratzel H, Fries P (1977) Modification of relative amount of free amino acids in the stratum corneum of human epidermis by special factors of the environment. I. The influence of UV irradiation. Arch Dermatol Res 259(2):157–160
38. Scott IR (1986) Alterations in the metabolism of filaggrin in the skin after chemical- and ultraviolet-induced erythema. J Invest Dermatol 87(4):460–465
39. Törmä H, Lindberg M, Berne B (2008) Skin barrier disruption by sodium lauryl sulfate-exposure alters the expressions of involucrin, transglutaminase 1, profilaggrin, and kallikreins during the repair phase in human skin *in vivo*. J Invest Dermatol 128:1212–1219
40. Visscher M, Robinson M, Wickett R (2011) Stratum corneum free amino acids following barrier perturbation and repair. Int J Cosmet Sci 33(1):80–89
41. Presland RB, Rothnagel JA, Lawrence OT (2006) Profilaggrin and the fused S100 family of calcium-binding proteins. In: Elias PM, Feingold KR (eds) Skin barrier. Taylor & Francis, New York
42. Presland RB, Kimball JR, Kautsky MB, Lewis SP, Lo CY, Dale BA (1997) Evidence for specific proteolytic cleavage of the *N*-terminal domain of the human profilaggrin during epidermal differentiation. J Invest Dermatol 108(2):170–178
43. Pearton DJ, Nirunsuksiri W, Rehemtulla A, Lewis SP, Presland RB, Dale BA (2001) Proprotein convertase expression and localization in epidermis: evidence for multiple roles and substrates. Exp Dermatol 10(3):193–203
44. Resing KA, Walsh KA, Haugen-Scofield J, Dale BA (1989) Identification of proteolytic cleavage sites in the conversion of profilaggrin to filaggrin in mammalian epidermis. J Biol Chem 264(3):1837–1845
45. Resing KA, al-Alawi N, Blomquist C, Fleckman P, Dale BA (1993) Independent regulation of two cytoplasmic processing stages of the intermediate filament-associated protein filaggrin and role of Ca2+ in the second stage. J Biol Chem 268(33):25139–25145
46. Resing KA, Thulin C, Whiting K, al-Alawi N, Mostad S (1995) Characterization of profilaggrin endoproteinase 1. A regulated cytoplasmic endoproteinase of epidermis. J Biol Chem 270(47):28193–28198
47. Yamazaki M, Ishidoh K, Suga Y, Saido TC, Kawashima S, Suzuki K, Kominami E, Ogawa H (1997) Cytoplasmic processing of human profilaggrin by active mu-calpain. Biochem Biophys Res Commun 235(3):652–656
48. Tarcsa E, Marekov LN, Mei G, Melino G, Lee SC, Steinert PM (1996) Protein unfolding by peptidylarginine deiminase. Substrate specificity and structural relationships of the natural substrates trichohyalin and filaggrin. J Biol Chem 271(48): 30709–30716
49. Vossenaar ER, Zendman AJ, van Venrooij WJ, Pruijn GJ (2003) PAD, a growing family of citrullinating enzymes: genes, features and involvement in disease. Bioessays 25(11):1106–1118
50. Chavanas S, Méchin MC, Nachat R, Adoue V, Coudane F, Serre G, Simon M (2006) Peptidylarginine deiminases and deimination in biology and pathology: relevance to skin homeostasis. J Dermatol Sci 44(2):63–72
51. Elias PM (2004) The epidermal permeability barrier: from the early days at Harvard to emerging concepts. J Invest Dermatol 122(2):xxxvi–xxxix
52. Kawada A, Hara K, Hiruma M, Noguchi H, Ishibashi A (1995) Rat epidermal cathepsin L-like proteinase: purification and some hydrolytic properties toward filaggrin and synthetic substrates. J Biochem 118(2): 332–337
53. Kawada A, Hara K, Morimoto K, Hiruma M, Ishibashi A (1995) Rat epidermal cathepsin B: purification and characterization of proteolytic properties toward filaggrin and synthetic substrates. Int J Biochem Cell Biol 27(2):175–183
54. Benavides F, Starost MF, Flores M, Gimenez-Conti IB, Guénet JL, Conti CJ (2002) Impaired hair follicle morphogenesis and cycling with abnormal epidermal differentiation in nackt mice, a cathepsin L-deficient mutation. Am J Pathol 161(2):693–703
55. Tabachnick J, LaBadie JH (1970) Studies on the biochemistry of epidermis. IV. The free amino acids, ammonia, urea, and pyrrolidone carboxylic acid content of conventional and germ-free albino guinea pig epidermis. J Invest Dermatol 54(1):24–31
56. Kamata Y, Taniguchi A, Yamamoto M, Nomura J, Ishihara K, Takahara H, Hibino T, Takeda A (2009) Neutral cysteine protease bleomycin hydrolase is essential for the breakdown of deiminated filaggrin into amino acids. J Biol Chem 284(19): 12829–12836
57. Gibson WT, Teall MR (1983) Interactions of C12 surfactants with the skin: changes in enzymes and visible and histological features of rat skin treated with sodium lauryl sulphate. Food Chem Toxicol 21(5):587–594
58. Le M, Schalkwijk J, Siegenthaler G, Van De Kerkhof PCM, Veerkamp JH, Van Der Valk PGM (1996) Changes in keratinocyte differentiation following mild irritation by sodium dodecyl sulfate. Arch Dermatol Res 288(11):684–690

Water and Minerals in the Treatment of Dryness

30

Ronni Wolf, Danny Wolf, Donald Rudikoff, and Lawrence Charles Parish

Part of this article was adapted with permission from: Wolf R, Parish LC, Davidovici B, et al (2007) Drinking 6 to 8 glasses of water a day is essential for skin hydration: myth or reality? Skinmed 6:90–91.

30.1 The Apparent Paradox

There is no generally accepted definition of what constitutes dry skin, but low water content of the stratum corneum (SC) and lower layers of the skin definitely play a role in the pathomechanism. Therefore, it would seem obvious that the right way to combat and reverse dry skin is by giving it what it lacks—water. Put another way, if dry skin is deficient of water, it makes sense that hydrating/wetting it is the most direct way of reversing the condition. But, is it? The present chapter will deal with the issues of internal water consumption and external application of water and their effects (or lack of) on dry skin.

R. Wolf, M.D. (✉)
The Dermatology Unit, Kaplan Medical Center, 76100, Rechovot, Israel

Hebrew University – Hadassah Medical School, Jerusalem, Israel
e-mail: wolf_r@netvision.net.il

D. Wolf, M.D.
Pediatric Outpatient Clinic, Sherutei Briut Clalit, Hasharon Region, Natanya, Israel

D. Rudikoff, M.D.
The Division of Dermatology, Bronx Lebanon Hospital Center, Albert Einstein College of Medicine, Bronx, NY, USA

L.C. Parish, M.D., M.D. (Hon)
The Department of Dermatology and Cutaneous Biology and the Jefferson Center for International Dermatology, Jefferson Medical College of Thomas Jefferson University, Philadelphia, PA, USA

30.2 Drinking Water and Skin Hydration

30.2.1 The Media

The sanctity of the sacred cow has been challenged! We will start with a few among dozens of links extolling the beneficial effect of drinking eight glasses of water on skin before we put in our 2 cents' worth.

http://whatscookingamerica.net/HealthBeauty/Water-TheFountainOfYouth.htm

> Now that I have hopefully convinced you of the benefits of drinking water for your skin and health, how much should your drink a day? The Mayo Clinic suggests using "8×8" as a guideline: 8 glasses (8 ounces each) = a minimum of 64 ounces of fluid (water) daily. You may need even more as exercising, hot weather, offices with exposure to central heating, air conditioning, and electrical equipment all cause your body to lose water.

http://www.happyhealthylonglife.com/happy_healthy_long_life/2008/06/how-much-water-do-i-need-to-drink-what-the-experts-say.html

> Now all of a sudden the press is saying "Forget about forcing down those 8 glasses of 8!" I decided to read the studies myself and separate the truth from the fiction. I also know how I feel when I drink my usual 64 ounces (8 glasses) of water (& other fluids) a day, and when I don't. For me, it's all about "evidence-based living"! Last weekend in Chicago, I didn't lug around my "stainless steel" water bottle, or down nearly enough liquid to fill my usual quota. And yes, my body noticed it. Won't do that again! Needless to say, my trips to the bathroom were not what they should have been. And as Dr. Goldfarb would say, "There was

M. Lodén, H.I. Maibach (eds.), *Treatment of Dry Skin Syndrome*,
DOI 10.1007/978-3-642-27606-4_30, © Springer-Verlag Berlin Heidelberg 2012

> definitely less turgor in my skin." (I looked wrinkled.) As far as I'm concerned, water works! I look better, my digestion is better, I feel better & even think better. You can decide for yourself, but here's what I learned about water.

http://www.smartskincare.com/nutrition/diet.html

> A well-moisturized skin is somewhat less prone to developing of wrinkles. Drinking plenty of fluids throughout the day ensures proper hydration of the body and helps reduce skin dryness. Experts usually recommend drinking 6–8 glasses of water a day.

http://www.iloveindia.com/nutrition/water/index.html

> Water forms a major part (2/3) of our body weight. Blood is 83% water, muscles are 75% water, brain is 74% water and bone is 22% water. Water is necessary for the very survival of human beings, as it ensures the smooth functioning of body systems. Skin cells, like any other cell in the body, are almost entirely made up of water. Without water the organs in the body - and the skin is the biggest – will not function properly. Loss of hydration in the skin is expressed in a variety of ways, such as dryness, tightness, flakiness. Dry skin has less resilience and is more prone to wrinkling. Water is essential to maintain skin moisture and is the vehicle for delivering essential nutrients to the skin cells. Given that water is lost in large quantities every day, it stands to reason that it needs to be replaced somehow.

In summary, the argument for high water intake, as presented in the media, is: because our body is almost entirely made up of water and because water is essential for living tissues and humans cannot survive for more than a few days without ingesting water, we, therefore, need to drink large quantities of water, and the more the better. Applying this kind of logic to gasoline and motor vehicles, the reasoning would be: because gasoline is essential for the car to function, we need to maintain large amounts of gasoline in the vehicle's tank, and the more the better.

30.2.2 The Alleged Beneficial Effect of Extra Fluid Intake on General Health

An excellent editorial recently published in the *Journal of the American Society of Nephrology* critically reviewed this issue [1]. The question asked was: "There are certainly well-recognized disease states, such as nephrolithiasis, for which increased fluid intake is therapeutic, but do average, healthy individuals living in temperate climate need to drink extra fluid – even when not thirsty – to maintain health?" The authors examined several claims of a benefit for extra water drinking, e.g., it leads to more toxin excretion through the kidneys; it improves skin tone, and it reduces hunger and headache frequency. They came to the conclusion that "There is no clear evidence of benefit from drinking increased amounts of water. Although we wish we could demolish all of the urban myths found on the Internet regarding the benefits of supplemental water ingestion, we concede there is also no clear evidence of lack of benefit. In fact, there is simply a lack of evidence in general." We could not agree more with those authors.

The conclusions of another review article [2] were similar: "Thus I have found no scientific proof that we must 'drink at least eight glasses of water a day', nor proof, it must be admitted, that drinking less does absolutely no harm. However, the published data available to date strongly suggest that, with the exception of some diseases and special circumstances, such as strenuous physical activity, long airplane flights, and climate, we probably are currently drinking enough and possibly even more than enough." The authors continues with "... osmotic regulation of vasopressin secretion and thirst is so sensitive, quick, and accurate that it is hard to imagine that evolutionary development left us with a chronic water deficit that has to be compensated by forcing fluid intake."

30.2.3 The Alleged Beneficial Effect of Drinking 8 × 8 Glasses of Water on the Skin

We are aware of only one study [3] relating to the effect of long-term water intake (2.25 L/day of either mineral water or tap water) on skin physiology. After 4 weeks of drinking water in excess, the mineral water group measurements revealed a significant decrease in skin density and an increased skin thickness (significantly only in the subjects who routinely drank comparably little before the start of the study). Skin density increased significantly, and skin thickness decreased significantly in the tap water group. Finger circumference decreased noticeably in the mineral water group and increased in tap water group. Objective skin surface morphology did not change in any group. As the authors admitted, "...not all of the objectively measured changes can be explained straightforwardly, as the exact mechanisms necessitate further research in this area." This report leaves more questions than answers, particularly concerning the differences and contradictory results between measurements of the group that drank mineral water compared to the group that drank tap water. The clinical relevance of the results is unclear; however, the study is important by being the first to demonstrate that the consumption of more than 2 L of water per day can have a measurable influence on skin physiology in healthy volunteers. Noteworthy, objective assessment of the skin surface profile did not reveal any significant changes in either group. "This is interesting," the authors noted, "as it is generally claimed that drinking lots of water might reduce visible signs of cutaneous ageing such as wrinkles and lines. We could not confirm any objective improvement of wrinkles or skin surface roughness after increasing the daily water uptake to more than 2 liters over weeks" (our underline).

In our opinion, the lack of association between excessive fluid intake and skin surface profile (e.g., wrinkles, skin surface roughness) as demonstrated in Williams et al.'s study [3] provides the main take-home message of the current presentation as well. The lack of any convincing evidence for a benefit of the 8×8 rule in other fields also applies to dermatology, including skin wrinkling and surface roughness in otherwise healthy people.

We are taught in medical school how to evaluate dehydration by assessing skin turgor. The skin should be pinched and lifted to create a fold over the sternum, the abdomen, or the arm. In cases of decreased skin turgor, the skin fold will "hold" or "tent" for up to 30 s, whereas in normal conditions, it returns immediately to its original state [4–6]. Does the fact that severe dehydration can decrease skin turgor indicate that excessive fluid intake in otherwise healthy individuals over a long period of time will do the opposite, namely, increase turgor? The answer is a resounding "No!"

30.2.4 Starling's Equation

Although the main water reservoir of the skin is the dermis, it is the SC water content which plays a crucial role in maintaining many of the skin's biophysical properties, such as elasticity and surface roughness. The connective tissue of the skin is crucial for water storage in the body. The skin tissue volume of a man with a body weight of 70 kg is about 7 L. The extracellular matrix comprises two-thirds of this volume and consists of about 50% fluid. Thus, one-third of the tissue layer consists of interchangeable water. Proteoglycans, a major component of the extracellular matrix, can bind one-third of the total interstitial amount of fluid [7]. It is noteworthy that this interstitial fluid confers a degree of turgor to the skin. Although modest expansion of interstitial fluid volume may not be detected, an excess of several liters causes visible and palpable swelling termed "edema." The interstitial fluid volume and the net flux through the capillary wall are regulated by the forces of the Starling equation, according to which the movement of fluid depends on six variables: (1) capillary hydrostatic pressure, (2) interstitial hydrostatic pressure, (3) capillary oncotic pressure, (4) interstitial oncotic pressure, (5) filtration coefficient (of the capillary wall), and (6) reflection coefficient (a "correction factor" that also describes the permeability of the capillary wall). The main value of this equation lies in its didactic logical explanation of the forces involved in fluid movement from one compartment to another—in our case, from blood vessels to the interstitial spaces of the skin—especially when pathologic processes grossly alter one or more of the variables. The equation is not meant to be used for clinical purposes because it is almost impossible to measure all six variables together in actual patients.

According to Starling's equation, increasing capillary hydrostatic pressure and decreasing colloid osmotic pressure or increased permeability of the capillary wall leads to increasing fluid shift from the intravascular space to the interstitial tissue. There is enough evidence to show that excessive and rapid fluid intake/infusion may lead to increasing interstitial volume and edema. In a recent study using a canine model [8], dermal echogenicity decreased significantly (Note: dermal water content is negatively correlated with dermal echogenicity due to interstitial edema, which leads to a decrease in the strong echogenicity of collagen bundles) and skin thickness increased significantly after hydration via intravenous administration of an isotonic crystalloid solution (30 mL/kg/h for 30 min). In another study on 20 healthy men, dermal thickness increased significantly 30 min after infusion of 10 mL/kg body weight of Ringer's solution given over 15 min [7], whereas rapid removal of fluids and water from the body during dialysis had an opposite effect. Removal of fluid after hemodialysis was associated with a significant decrease in skin thickness, skin elasticity, stratum corneum water content, and skin distensibility [9].

Does the fact that changes in plasma colloid osmotic pressure after excessive and abrupt fluid intake (a change that may also be detected by hematocrit and electrolyte changes, as well as changes in the variables of Starling's equation) may influence water content of the skin indicate that excessive fluid intake throughout the day and over long periods of time do the same? No! There is no scientific proof that drinking habits may intervene or cause a change in Starling's equation and thus that they have any influence on the water content of the skin.

30.3 Applying Water Externally, Hydrotherapy, and Skin Hydration

The issues concerning the effect of water applied to the skin externally on skin hydration are entirely different than those associated with water consumption. Water applied externally through bathing/immersion has historically been considered an important therapeutic tool, especially in the management of patients suffering from chronic inflammatory diseases (e.g., rheumatoid conditions) or skin diseases (e.g., atopic dermatitis or psoriasis). Notably, this was before active and specific drugs became available. Depending on the culture of individual countries, hydrotherapeutic approaches were endorsed by physicians, health care personnel, patients, and the media. There has recently been a resurgence of interest in the role of water in the treatment of several skin diseases, as witnessed by the tremendous increase in the popularity and demand for hydrotherapy, perhaps as part of the general tendency to switch to complementary, alternative, and unconventional medicine.

Various researchers [10–13] were able to show the manifold effect of spa waters on various components of the skin, particularly on the immune system (on TNF-alpha, interleukin [IL]-8, IL-6) on endorphin levels, on keratinocyte differentiation via receptor potential vanilloid (TRPV6), on free radical levels, and many others.

With all these therapeutic effects on various chronic inflammatory skin diseases, the immune-modulating effects, and other beneficial and valuable biological properties of mineral waters notwithstanding, we found no specific claim on their effect on skin moisture or hydrating properties. This is particularly germane to the treatment of atopic dermatitis. Although dry skin is a hallmark of atopic dermatitis and plays a major role in its pathogenesis, the therapeutic effects of thermal waters on the disease is attributed mainly to their immune-modulatory, anti-inflammatory, antibacterial, and vasoactive properties and not to their effect on skin moisture/hydration. Historically, there have been multitudinous variations in "expert recommendations" for optimal bathing practices in the management of atopic dermatitis. The most widely accepted recommendation in recent times was that of daily bathing followed by immediate application of topical emollient or topical medication. This is what we, the authors, also recommend to our patients. It is our empirical (not evidence-based) experience that application of a moisturizer directly onto the moist skin within 3 min after bathing will soothe the skin and keep it hydrated. However, Chiang and Eichenfield's recent study [14] analyzed this precise issue, and their findings did not support the postbathing moisturizer approach. According to those authors, bathing without moisturizer may compromise skin hydration, and bathing followed by moisturizer application provides modest hydration benefits, though less than that of simply applying moisturizer alone. Whatever the conclusions on the values of moisturizers, the study results showed that bathing per se does not add hydration to the skin.

Finally, we are all aware of the ancient treatment principle of "wet-to-moist" dressings aimed at irrigating, cleaning, absorbing exudate, and drying the surface of the skin. We would be hard pressed to find a better way to emphasize that putting water/saline on the skin and allowing it to evaporate will have the effect of drying the skin by transferring the water/fluid from the skin to the air and not hydrating it.

Take Home Messages

- Although there is no generally accepted definition of what constitute dry skin, low water content probably plays a role.
- The media is saturated with assays/articles about the beneficial effect of drinking eight glasses of water on our skin and skin hydration.
- The Mayo Clinic favors the "8×8 rule" for drinking, translated into the consumption of 8 glasses×8 ounces each daily, but rules out any effect on the skin.
- There is no convincing evidence that water drinking habits have any effect on our skin, including skin wrinkling and surface roughness, in otherwise healthy people.
- Bathing, particularly in mineral and thermal waters, has historically been considered an important therapeutic tool in the management of musculoskeletal/rheumatoid conditions and various skin diseases.
- Modern research has provided evidence to scientifically confirm the numerous beneficial effects of spa waters on various components of the skin, the immune system and the vasculature, as well as a significant therapeutic effect on various inflammatory skin diseases.
- There is no convincing evidence that water applied externally has any effect on skin moisture or skin hydration.

References

1. Negoianu D, Goldfarb S (2008) Just add water. J Am Soc Nephrol 19:1041–1043
2. Valtin H (2002) "Drink at least eight glasses of water a day." Really? Is there scientific evidence for "8 × 8"? Am J Physiol Regul Integr Comp Physiol 283:R993–R1004
3. Williams S, Krueger N, Davids M et al (2007) Effect of fluid intake on skin physiology: distinct differences between drinking mineral water and tap water. Int J Cosmet Sci 29:131–138
4. Otieno H, Were E, Ahmed I et al (2004) Are bedside features of shock reproducible between different observers? Arch Dis Child 89:977–979
5. McGarvey J, Thompson J, Hanna C et al (2010) Sensitivity and specificity of clinical signs for assessment of dehydration in endurance athletes. Br J Sports Med 44:716–719
6. Aguilar OM, Albertal M (1998) Images in clinical medicine. Poor skin turgor. N Engl J Med 338:25
7. Eisenbeiss C, Welzel J, Eichler W et al (2001) Influence of body water distribution on skin thickness: measurements using high-frequency ultrasound. Br J Dermatol 144(5):947–951
8. Diana A, Guglielmini C, Fracassi F et al (2008) Use of high-frequency ultrasonography for evaluation of skin thickness in relation to hydration status and fluid distribution at various cutaneous sites in dogs. Am J Vet Res 69(9):1148–1152
9. Brazzelli V, Borroni G, Vignoli GP et al (1994) Effects of fluid volume changes during hemodialysis on the biophysical parameters of the skin. Dermatology 188:113–116
10. Bieber T (2011) Evidence-based efficacy of Avene thermal spring water. J Eur Acad Dermatol Venereol 25:1–34
11. Ghersetich I, Freedman D, Lotti T (2000) Balneology today. J Eur Acad Dermatol Venereol 14:346–348
12. Chiarini A, Dal PI, Pacchiana R et al (2006) Comano's (Trentino) thermal water interferes with interleukin-6 production and secretion and with cytokeratin-16 expression by cultured human psoriatic keratinocytes: further potential mechanisms of its anti-psoriatic action. Int J Mol Med 18:1073–1079
13. Dal PI, Chiarini A, Pacchiana R et al (2007) Comano's (Trentino) thermal water interferes with tumour

necrosis factor-alpha expression and interleukin-8 production and secretion by cultured human psoriatic keratinocytes: yet other mechanisms of its anti-psoriatic action. Int J Mol Med 19:373–379

14. Chiang C, Eichenfield LF (2009) Quantitative assessment of combination bathing and moisturizing regimens on skin hydration in atopic dermatitis. Pediatr Dermatol 26:273–278

Hyaluronan Inside and Outside of Skin

31

Aziza Wahby, Kathleen Daddario DiCaprio, and Robert Stern

31.1 Introduction

The glycosaminoglycan hyaluronic acid (also called hyaluronan or hyaluronate and abbreviated as HA) is a major component of the extracellular matrix (ECM) of skin and plays an important role in the metabolism of both the epidermis and dermis. Hyaluronan is responsible for hydration, nutrient exchange, and protects against free radical damage via a multitude of signaling pathways. It is also involved in basic biologic processes such as cell differentiation and motility. An overview is provided here that provides recent information, bringing up-to-date advances in matrix biology relevant for dermatology and skin care, with a particular emphasis on skin moisture.

31.2 Hyaluronan

Hyaluronan is a highly anionic molecule. At the body's pH, it is one of the most highly charged molecules in biology, which provides HA with some of its unique qualities. A massive cloud of water surrounds the molecule in an attempt to neutralize the charge. It is this particular quality which provides the hydrating functions of HA, with the simultaneous ability to expand tissues and to open spaces for cell movement.

Extrinsic aging in the human skin, compared with photo-protected skin is associated with alterations in the expression of HA and its metabolizing enzymes, both the hyaluronidases and the HA synthase complex of enzymes [58], as described below. It is clear that the "dried" appearance of aging skin is intimately associated with changes in apparent levels and types of HA deposition, dependent on changes in controls of its underlying metabolism.

Hyaluronan is involved in multiple aspects of skin biology, responsible not only for skin hydration but also for nutrient exchange, tissue homeostasis, repair processes, protection against free radical damage, cell differentiation, and cell motility. Native and formulated preparations of HA, applied exogenously, help skin regain elasticity, turgor, as well as moisture. Understanding HA metabolism may provide clues for reversing some of the processes that lead to skin aging, loss of moisture, and wrinkling.

31.3 Hyaluronan in Skin

There are numerous reports of decreased amounts of HA in aging skin. These observations are based on histochemical stains, such as Alcian blue, and affinity histochemistry with the

A. Wahby • K.D. DiCaprio • R. Stern (✉)
Department of Basic Medical Sciences,
Touro College of Osteopathic Medicine,
New York, NY 10027, USA
e-mail: robert.stern@touro.edu

M. Lodén, H.I. Maibach (eds.), *Treatment of Dry Skin Syndrome*,
DOI 10.1007/978-3-642-27606-4_31, © Springer-Verlag Berlin Heidelberg 2012

HA-binding peptide. However, actual biochemical extraction techniques, using progressively potent extraction solutions, indicate that the HA content remains constant with age. The difference is that the HA becomes increasingly tissue associated, becoming more and more resistant to extraction [32]. The apparent results from histochemical investigations are perhaps best explained by increasing competition between tissue proteins for HA binding sites and the HA-binding peptide as a function of age. The HA, encased within tissue proteins, may be restricted from functioning as a hydrating molecule. This proviso also indicates that the HA-staining procedure, as normally performed with an HA-binding peptide, is not a quantitative procedure.

31.3.1 Distribution of Hyaluronan in Skin

Hyaluronan in skin occurs in both dermis and epidermis, with dermis containing the greater proportion. Epidermal HA is more loosely associated and is more easily extracted from tissue. Formalin, an aqueous fixative, easily removes most of the HA from epidermis. It is less able to extract HA from dermis. Alcoholic formalin enhances histolocalization of epidermal HA and indicates considerable levels are contained therein [30].

Skin HA has a very rapid turnover, with a half-life of 1–2 days in the epidermis [47]. The turnover rate in the dermis is similar, with catabolism occurring in liver and lymph nodes, following lymphatic drainage [46].

The turnover mechanism in the epidermis is not clear and may be a combination of free radical fragmentation, stimulated by UV light, and enzymatic degradation (*vide infra*).

31.3.1.1 Hyaluronan in the Epidermis

Until recently, it was assumed that only mesenchymal cells were capable of synthesizing HA. With newer techniques, evidence for HA being made in the epidermis became apparent. Techniques for separating dermis and epidermis facilitated detection of HA in each compartment. Hyaluronan is most prominent in the upper spinous and granular, where much of it is extracellular. In the basal layer, HA is predominantly intracellular and is not easily eluted out during aqueous fixation. Basal keratinocyte HA is involved in mitotic events, presumably, while extracellular HA in the upper layers of the epidermis is involved in barrier disassociation and sloughing of cells.

Tissue cultures of keratinocytes have facilitated studies of epithelial HA metabolism. These cultured cells synthesize large quantities of HA. When Ca^{++} concentrations of the culture medium are increased from 0.05 to 1.20 mM, basal-like cells begin to differentiate, HA synthesis levels drop, and hyaluronidase activity is induced [28, 57]. This increase in calcium that appears to simulate in culture the natural in situ differentiation of basal keratinocytes parallels the increasing calcium gradient observed in the epidermis. There may be intracellular stores of calcium that are released as keratinocytes mature. Alternatively, the calcium stores may be concentrated by lamellar bodies from the intercellular fluids released during terminal differentiation. The lamellar bodies are thought to be modified lysosomes containing hydrolytic enzymes and a potential source of the hyaluronidase activity.

The lamellar bodies fuse with the plasma membranes of the terminally differentiating keratinocytes, increasing the plasma membrane surface area. Lamellar bodies are also associated with proton pumps that enhance acidity. A proton pump, specifically Na^+-H^+ exchanger1 (NHE1), is part of a complex involved in the internalization and degradation of HA of the ECM [10]. This same pump also creates localized areas of acidity on the cell surface, presumably within lipid rafts where CD44, the predominant HA receptor, is localized [39].

The lamellar bodies also acidify, and their polar lipids become partially converted to neutral lipids, thereby participating in skin barrier function. Diffusion of aqueous material through the epidermis is blocked by these lipids synthesized by keratinocytes in the stratum granulosum, the boundary corresponding to the level at which HA-staining ends. This constitutes part of the barrier function of skin. The HA-rich area inferior to this layer may obtain water from the moisture-rich dermis. And the water contained therein cannot penetrate beyond the lipid-rich stratum granulosum. The HA-bound water in both the dermis and in the vital area of the epidermis is critical for skin hydration. And the stratum granulosum is essential for maintenance of that hydration, not only for the skin, but also for the body in general. Profound dehydration is a serious clinical problem in burn patients with extensive losses of the stratum granulosum.

Hyaluronan of the epidermal ECM forms two different structures: a pericellular coat close to the plasma membrane, forming an intimate pericellular matrix, and HA chains that coalesce into large cables. Such cables, induced by inflammatory agents, bind leukocytes, whereas the pericellular HA does not. Thus, under inflammatory conditions, epidermal keratinocytes are able to form HA cables that can bind leukocytes [26].

31.3.1.2 Hyaluronan in the Dermis

The HA content of the dermis is far greater than that of the epidermis and accounts for most of the 50% of total body HA present in skin. The papillary dermis has a more prominent level of HA than does the reticular dermis. The HA of the dermis is in direct continuity with both the lymphatic and vascular systems, which epidermal HA apparently does not.

Exogenous HA is cleared from the dermis and rapidly degraded [46]. The dermal fibroblast provides the synthetic machinery for endogenous dermal HA, and should be the target for any pharmacological attempts to enhance skin hydration. The fibroblasts of the body, the most banal of cells from a histologic perspective, are probably the most diverse of all vertebrate cells with the broadest repertoire of biochemical reactions and potential pathways for differentiation. Much of this diversity is site-specific. What makes the papillary dermal fibroblast different from other fibroblasts is not known. However, these cells have an HA synthetic capacity similar to that of the fibroblasts that line joint synovium or the hyalocytes of the eye, responsible for the HA-rich synovial fluid and the vitreous of the ocular chambers, respectively.

A clue to the vigorous HA synthetic capacity of dermal fibroblasts comes from an unexpected direction. Adiponectin, a cytokine produced by adipose tissue, stimulates HA synthesis in dermal fibroblasts [3]. Sebaceous glands of the skin produce adiponectin as well, and dermal fibroblasts are demonstrated to have specific adiponectin receptors, producing HA by upregulation of their HA synthase 2 (HAS2). The female breast is a modified sebaceous gland, with associated lipid tissue. The body's fat tissue is an endocrine gland that is largely overlooked. The sebaceous glands of the skin may hold a key to the problem of loss of skin moisture, in light of the observation that adiponectin levels decrease markedly with age.

31.3.2 Hyaluronan in the Basal Lamina

Hyaluronan deposition occurs most prominently in the papillary dermis and in the basement membrane zone of skin. Hyaluronan is a component of all basement membranes, but its role in that barrier between dermis and epidermis is entirely unknown. Ultrastructural and immunohistochemical studies have not contributed to our understanding of HA in basement membrane, nor is the relationship between HA and other components of that structure known, such as type IV collagen, laminins, and fibronectin. Stoichiometric measurements make no sense, given that HA is a polymer that varies so widely in size. Decreased levels of HA and decreased thickness of the basal lamina occur in diabetic skin, contributing to "thick skin" syndrome [8]. Hyaluronan has a key role in cell motility. Penetration and movement of tumor cells from epidermis to dermis through the basal lamina defines a key event in the metastatic spread of a malignancy. Understanding the nature of HA in basement membranes and identifying its interactions with proteins and other matrix polymers would seem to be an important matter.

Addition of exogenous HA to an organotypic keratinocyte-fibroblast coculture model enhances epidermal proliferation, resulting in a thicker epidermis. Hyaluronan also improves basement membrane assembly as evidenced by an increased expression of laminin-332 and collagen type IV at the epidermal-dermal junction. Furthermore, development of the epidermal lipid barrier structure is enhanced [19].

31.4 Hyaluronan and Edema

Hyaluronan in skin becomes much more prominent with edema. Tissue swelling is one of the five cardinal signs of inflammation, and that swelling is comprised predominantly of HA [37, 52, 61]. This is a concept not sufficiently appreciated. Indeed, many of the inflammatory cytokines induce HA production, and conversely, HA fragments induce such cytokine synthesis in a self-stimulatory cycle [22, 25]. The HA content of the various bullous lesions of skin is another area of potential importance. High levels of HA have been documented in the blister fluid from patients with active psoriatic lesions [31].

31.5 Hyaluronan and Fragment Size

Despite its simple repeating structure, HA has a wide range and occasionally contradictory functions, even though it is without branch points and without sulfation or other secondary modifications. The multiple functions are in part attributed to variations in chain length. The variation in size is an extraordinarily rich informational system [53, 56]. In general, high molecular weight HA occurs in normal healthy tissues, while fragmented HA is highly inflammatory, angiogenic, and immune-stimulatory, a reflection of tissues under stress. The large HA polymers are, in marked contrast, anti-inflammatory, antiangiogenic, and immunosuppressive.

Many injectable cosmetic and dermal preparations contain HA in various concentrations and cross-linked using a number of reactions. There is an intrinsic need to ensure that such materials do not contain short HA chains that could stimulate an inflammatory response. An additional caution is the generation of short HA fragments that could be cleaved from those cross-linked polymers and that could also be highly inflammatory.

A major conundrum remains regarding the hydration properties of HA. The number of water molecules in the hydration shell of HA of different molecular sizes and in the presence of various counterions has not been determined. It is certain to be a nonlinear relationship. Intuitively, it is predicted that large HMW chains of HA are more effective hydrating molecules, that they carry larger numbers of water molecules per disaccharide unit. But this must be demonstrated experimentally. An approach to this question has been described, though no clear relationship was demonstrated [45]. A caveat in such studies, and a major experimental problem, is that the results are highly dependent upon the methods used to isolate and prepare the HA [20].

31.6 CD44

The most prominent receptor for HA is CD44, a transmembrane glycoprotein that occurs in a wide variety of isoforms, products of a single gene with variant exon expression, all inserted into a single extracellular position near the membrane insertion site. CD44 is coded for by 10 constant exons, plus from 0 to 10 variant exons. The standard form, CD44s, contains no variant exons and is distributed exclusively on the cell surface, while variant exon-bearing isoforms can have additional intracellular localization (unpublished observations). CD44 is able to bind a variety of other ligands including fibronectin, collagen, and heparin-binding growth factors. CD44 is distributed widely, being found on virtually all cells. It participates in cell adhesion, migration, lymphocyte activation and homing, and in cancer metastasis. The appearance of HA in dermis and epidermis parallels the histolocalization of CD44.

The nature of the CD44 variant exons in skin at each location has not been determined. It would be important to establish whether modulation occurs in CD44 variant exon expression with changes in the state of skin hydration and as a function of age, particularly in wrinkled and UV-exposed skin.

31.7 RHAMM

Another receptor for HA is the receptor for HA-mediated motility (RHAMM). This receptor is involved in cell locomotion, focal adhesion turnover, and contact inhibition. Like CD44, it also is expressed in a number of variant isoforms and occurs as a cell surface receptor as well as having multiple intracellular isoforms. The interactions between HA and RHAMM regulate locomotion of cells by a complex network of signal transduction events and interaction with the cytoskeleton of cells. It is also an important regulator of cell growth.

In a murine system, blocking expression of the RHAMM protein, either by gene deletion or by a blocking reagent, selectively induces the generation of fat cells to replace those lost in the aging process. This has promise as a technique to improve the appearance of aging skin and a potential source of the adiponectin, as discussed below.

31.8 The Hyaluronan Synthases

Three isoforms of a single enzyme synthesize HA. These are dual-headed transferases that utilize as substrates alternately UDP-glucuronic acid, and UDP-*N*-acetylglucosamine. These are membrane proteins, located on the inner surface of the plasma membrane. They extrude their product through the plasma membrane into the extracellular space as the HA is being synthesized. This permits unconstrained polymer growth, without destruction of the cell. There are three synthase genes in the mammalian genome, coding for HAS1, HAS2, and HAS3. They are located on three separate chromosomes and are differentially regulated, with each producing a different size polymer (for review, see [24, 62]). These homologous isoenzymes contain seven membrane-associated regions and a central cytoplasmic domain possessing several consensus sequences that are substrates for phosphorylation by protein kinase C. The HAS1 and HAS2 genes are upregulated in skin by TGF-β in both dermis and epidermis, but there are major differences in the kinetics of the TGF-β response between HAS1 and HAS2 and between the two compartments, suggesting that the two genes are regulated independently.

31.9 The Hyaluronidases

Hyaluronan is very metabolically active, with a half-life of 3–5 min in the circulation, less than 1 day in skin, and in, apparently, an inert a tissue such as cartilage, the HA turns over with a half-life of 1–3 weeks. This catabolic activity is primarily the result of hyaluronidases, endoglycolytic enzymes with a specificity, except for the leech enzyme, for the β1–4 glycosidic bonds. The human genome project has also promoted explication at the genetic level, and a virtual explosion of information has ensued [55].

The mammalian hyaluronidases are endo-β-hexosaminidases and function as hydrolases, in contrast to prokaryotic hyaluronidases that cleave the glycosidic bond using an eliminase mechanism of action. They lack substrate specificity, able to digest chondroitin sulfates (CS), albeit at a slower rate.

Six hyaluronidase-like sequences are present in the human genome, while most other mammals have seven such sequences. All are transcriptionally active with unique tissue distributions. In the human, three genes (*HYAL1*, *HYAL2*, and *HYAL3*) are found tightly clustered on chromosome 3p21.3. Another three genes *HYAL4, PHYAL1* (a pseudogene), and PH20 and sperm adhesion molecule1 (*SPAM1*) are clustered similarly on chromosome 7q31.3.

The enzymes HYAL1 and HYAL2 constitute the major hyaluronidases in somatic tissues; HYAL1, an acid-active lysosomal enzyme, was the first somatic hyaluronidase to be isolated and characterized. Why an acid-active hyaluronidase should occur in plasma is not clear. HYAL1 is able to utilize HA of any size as a substrate and generates predominantly tetrasaccharides. HYAL2 is also acid-active, anchored to plasma membranes by a GPI (glycosylphosphatidylinositol)-link. HYAL2 cleaves high molecular weight HA to a limit product of approximately 20 kDa, or about 50 disaccharide units.

Not all tissues that contain HYAL1 activity synthesize that enzyme. Active endocytosis of the protein from the circulation occurs [17]. Monocytes contain no mRNA for HYAL1, yet have very high levels of enzyme activity (unpublished observations). Megakaryocytes and platelets contain no HYAL1, [12] perhaps because they lack the receptors for endocytosis of circulating HYAL1.

31.10 The Hyaluronasome

It is possible to invoke the existence of a new and novel organelle, the hyaluronasome. Parallels between glycogen and HA metabolism are the basis of such a formulation. Both are monotonous, unadorned carbohydrate polymers of repeating sugars. A glycogen organelle can be visualized in liver, where it is prominent following a period of starvation or prolonged intravenous feeding, when the organelles have been emptied of their glycogen substrate.

> Readily visualized by the electron microscope, glycogen granules appear as bead-like structures localized to specific subcellular locales. Each glycogen granule is a functional unit, not only containing carbohydrate, but also enzymes and other proteins needed for its metabolism. These proteins are not static, but rather associate and dissociate, depending on the carbohydrate balance of the tissue. Regulation takes place not only by allosteric regulation of enzymes, but also due to other factors, such as sub-cellular location, granule size, and association with various related proteins. (Shearer and Graham [51])

Such observations may be applicable to HA and the proteins related to its metabolism and regulation in an organelle termed "the hyaluronasome". Indeed, such a complex was described in fibroblasts several decades ago for the synthetic apparatus [33, 34]. This may be a component of an even larger complex that contains not only the synthetic but also the degradative enzymes, associated regulatory proteins and peptides, as well as receptors and other binding proteins. A quasi-complex has been described for the apparatus that brings HA chains into the cells for degradation, containing HA, the CD44 receptor, HYAL2, and a Na^{+}-H^{+} exchanger (NHE1) for creating acidic foci on plasma membrane indentations termed lipid rafts [10]. This putative cell organelle could be a functional unit that provides response mechanisms dependent on the metabolic state of the cell. A search should be taken for such an organelle in the robust HA synthesizing fibroblasts of the papillary dermis.

Suggestive evidence for the existence of the hyaluronasome comes from several sources. Treating cultured cells with very low concentrations of hyaluronidase has the anomalous effect of increasing levels of HA synthesis [29, 43, 44]. Even treatment of isolated membrane preparations with low levels of hyaluronidase has a similar effect [43], suggestive of a feedback mechanism that instructs the cell on how much HA has been made. Constant clipping of the polymer as it is being extruded from the cell provides the misinformation that little HA has been deposited into the extracellular space. The plasma membrane-bound receptor CD44 is an ideal candidate for providing such a feedback mechanism.

Treating cells with higher levels of hyaluronidase modulates the expression profile of the variant exons of CD44, thus providing exquisite control mechanisms for the metabolic control of HA deposition [54]. An organelle in which all components are tethered together would provide the structural organization for such reactions to occur with maximum efficiency.

31.11 Hyaluronan Protects Against UV Damage

UVB represents only 0.5% of the sunlight that reaches the Earth's surface, but accounts for much of the acute and chronic sun-related damage to skin. UVB-irradiation accelerates skin aging, in part by disruption of the turnover of its ECM. Among the changes that have been documented are enhanced expression of the MMPs (matrix metalloproteinases), the attendant cleavage of collagen, and reduced levels of HA. The collagen fragments themselves are a component of the mechanism for the suppression of HA deposition; a direct effect on HAS2 expression has been documented [11, 49]. Chronic UVB irradiation causes loss of HA from mouse dermis because of downregulation of HA synthase expression. Exogenous HA minimizes the effects of UV irradiation when added to cultures of human keratinocytes, protecting against the suppression of CD44 and TLR-2 expression [21].

31.12 Hyaluronan Protects Against Free Radical and Reactive Oxygen Species Damage

Reactive oxygen species (ROS) are generated during the metabolic reactions in which oxygen participates. These ROS moieties facilitate the catabolism of HMW HA within dermis and epidermis by mechanisms that are not well understood [2]. The proportion of HA degradation between enzymatic catalysis and ROS scission is also unknown. There are low levels of HYAL1 and HYAL2 in skin, as established in an expression library. Effectiveness of ROS is enhanced by iron and copper ions, as well as by ions of other transition metals, especially in the presence of ascorbic acid. Part of this is offset by the ability of Vitamin C to enhance the activity of hyaluronidase inhibitors [9, 35, 55]. There is apparently an entire system of checks and balances for maintaining levels of HA deposition in skin that is unknown. Many commercial skin serums contain high levels of Vitamin C. Their effectiveness may be due to the ability to tilt the balance toward enhanced HA deposition, an effect achieved entirely by accident.

The ROS free radicals are highly unstable, reactive, and toxic. It is hardly conceivable that they participate as intermediates or as regulatory agents in biologic reactions. Yet, their high levels in skin and their generation with the constant skin bombardment by UV irradiation suggests their involvement in such reactions occurs through evolutionary forces. Controlled oxidative-reductive degradation of HA chains by the combined effect of oxygen, transition metal cations, and ascorbate is entirely plausible. Reduction of oxidized transitional metal ions occurs in the presence of ascorbate, a reaction that may occur at a greater level in skin than in any other tissue.

It would be of intrinsic interest to examine levels of HA in the skin of severely ascorbate deficient or anemic patients. Human beings are among the few vertebrates in whom the enzymatic pathway for ascorbate synthesis has been inactivated. Our hairlessness may be the basis of this mutation, as a selective force, as a survival mechanism. In humans, the entire pathway is extant, except for the final enzymatic step. Could this inactivation have correlated with loss of body hair in the course of human evolution?

Another concept to be kept in mind is that products of enzymatic cleavage of HMW HA generate products that have structures that are, excepting for chain length, identical to the original substrate. On the other hand, the products of free radical cleavage contain oxidized carboxyl and hydroperoxide functional groups. These are reactive moieties that can interact with other tissue molecules. This may be the basis of the sequentially more insoluble HA content of skin, the HA that becomes increasingly resistant to extraction as a function of age [32]. This also suggests that the proportion of HA degraded by oxidative reactions generates a greater portion of permanent structural tissue HA than that degraded enzymatically. Further documentation of this sequestering of HA phenomenon as a function of age has been documented. The apparent decrease in HA staining of skin with age [38] can be explained. Binding sites on the HA substrate for the biotinylated HA-binding peptide, the basis of the staining reaction, become progressively less available with age.

Extrinsic aging in human skin is associated with alterations in the metabolizing enzymes of HA. There is considerable increase in HA of lower molecular mass with aging, and with UV exposed skin, compared to photo-protected skin of the buttocks. This increase is associated with decreased HAS1 expression and increased expression of HYAL1-3. The receptors CD44 and RHAMM are also significantly downregulated [58].

Inspection of the images of HA staining in formalin-fixed skin, compared to alcoholic-acid formalin fixed skin, demonstrates that epidermis contains HA that is easily eluted, barely surviving the aqueous formalin fixation. The dermal HA remains more tissue associated, the greater portion remaining present following aqueous fixation. From this, it follows that dermal HA, the more tissue associated, may be the result of a greater proportion being modified by free radicals.

Another proviso is that free radicals, and particularly ROS cleave HA, and the fragments generated are more susceptible to subsequent hyaluronidase cleavage than are the parent polymers [13].

31.13 Stem Cells of Skin and the Hyaluronan Connection

Hyaluronan has a general effect of suppressing differentiation. Hyaluronan suppresses epidermal differentiation in organotypic cultures of rat keratinocytes [40]. The concentration of HA is most prominent in tissues undergoing rapid growth and has been identified in the stem cell niche. Hyaluronan provides an environment for maintaining the undifferentiated stem cell state, as well as expansion of the stem cell population. Cells must exit from this HA-rich environment in order to undergo differentiation. The reservoir of stem cells for skin occurs in the bulge regions of hair follicles. They exit the bulge and migrate to areas where skin cell expansion and growth must occur [59]. One of the unsolved mysteries in dermatology is the source of skin stem cells in patients with alopecia areata. They appear to be spared in this disorder.

31.14 Retinoids

The synthesis of HA in vitro can be stimulated by several growth factors, including retinoids, dibutyryl cyclic adenosine monophosphate, and peroxisome proliferator-activated receptor-α agonists. The effect of retinyl retinoate, a novel retinol derivative, on HA expression, was examined in primary human keratinocytes cultures and in hairless mouse epidermal skin. Histochemistry indicated that topical retinyl retinoate increased HA staining in the murine skin. Moreover, topical retinyl retinoate increased CD44 expression. Using reverse transcription polymerase chain reaction, the expression level of the *HAS2* gene in primary human keratinocytes and in hairless mouse epidermal skin was assessed. It was found that retinyl retinoate upregulates mouse and human *HAS2* mRNAs. Application of retinyl retinoate induced increasing transepidermal water loss less than retinol, retinoic acid, and retinaldehyde. Taken together, retinyl retinoate is more effective on HA production and less of an irritant than other retinoids. But the proper form of Vitamin A for human oral consumption and for maximal effect has still not been established.

Synergistic effects of hyaluronate fragments occur in retinaldehyde-induced skin hyperplasia, which appears to be a CD44-dependent phenomenon [6].

31.15 Corticosteroids and Skin Atrophy

Systemic corticosteroids induce skin dehydration and atrophy, as does topical applications. The parallel decrease with HA concentrations indicates a cause and effect relationship, as confirmed in a skin organ culture system [1]. Topical application of glucocorticoids causes a rapid reduction of dermal HA, a phenomenon caused by suppressed HA synthase activity, without an effect on hyaluronidase [18]. Glucocorticoids induce a nearly total inhibition of HAS2 mRNA in dermal fibroblasts, the predominant HA synthase therein [4].

31.16 Estrogen Effects

The influence of estrogen on aging has been examined in many organ systems, but there is surprisingly little information on the effect of estrogen on skin HA [50]. As the population ages, interest in skin moisture in postmenopausal women grows proportionately, as does the effect of estrogen on preventing skin aging.

This estrogen effect is best exemplified by the aging and drying of skin after menopause, when ovarian estrogen synthesis ceases. Women with full figures have increased levels of estrogens in their fat stores. These act as estrogen slow-release capsules long after ovaries stop estrogen production. This accounts in part for the moisture and more youthful appearing skin of such women.

Another example of the natural estrogen effect on skin is the sex skin of baboons. The increased redness and fullness of the female sex skin is largely HA and its associated solvent water [7]. From this, it is possible to extrapolate that the fullness of the perineal skin of the sexually aroused female primate is also based on HA. The fullness of the perilabial and perineal skin may also serve the secondary purpose of holding on to the male member more firmly. Direct experimental evidence also comes from observations that HA synthase levels are induced by estrogens in mouse skin [60].

31.17 Vitamin C (Ascorbic Acid)

Vitamin C is added to many skin preparations that promise moisturizing effects, occurring occasionally at very high concentrations. The mechanisms of action behind such assurances are varied. Vitamin C has pronounced HA-stimulating effects in fibroblasts. The deposition of HA is stimulated when Vitamin C is added to cultured fibroblasts. The most profound changes occur in the compartmentalization of HA. The preponderance of the enhanced HA becomes cell layer instead of being secreted into the medium [23, 27]. The chemical reactions catalyzed by ascorbic acid that bind HA to cell or matrix components are undefined. Derivatives of Vitamin C and their analogs can function as hyaluronidase inhibitors, in particular l-ascorbic acid-6-hexadecanoate [9]. Some of the ability of Vitamin C to enhance HA deposition may be attributed to its inhibition of hyaluronidase activity. But its oxidizing activity, in the presence of divalent cations, particularly iron and copper, complicates the role of Vitamin C in HA metabolism.

31.18 Applications of Hyaluronan from Outside Skin

In cultured fibroblasts, exogenously added HA is incorporated into fine HA filaments of the pericellular fibroblast matrix. This indicates that soluble HA facilitates assemble of a supramolecular pericellular structure [48]. Whether cross-linked HA has this property has not been established, nor whether injected stabilized HA can perform such functions. It would also be important to determine whether any topically applied HA to skin in vivo has this effect, whether it is size dependent, and whether any such materials can permeate human skin.

31.18.1 Cross-Linked Hyaluronan and Injectable Fillers

In its natural state, HA exhibits poor biomechanical properties as a dermal filler. As a soluble polymer, it is cleared rapidly when injected into normal skin. To provide the ability fill wrinkles in skin, several chemical modifications have been employed. The two most common functional groups that can be modified are the carboxylic acid and the hydroxyl alcohol moieties. Many methods for cross-linking HA are available using these two reactive groups. Biomaterials have been produced through modification of the carboxyl acid group by esterification and through the use of cross-linkers such as dialdehydes and disulfides. The most commonly employed cross-linkers for dermal fillers are divinyl sulfone and diglycidyl ethers (Restylane®) and bis-epoxides. The Restylane® family of products is the first HA-derived materials to be approved by the FDA for skin injection.

Additional injectable, long-lasting, resorbable HA-modified fillers have recently become available, such as Juvéderm™ Voluma™, though the nature or number of the cross-links have not become available [15]. The manufacturers claim it is a novel version of the usual HA filers comprised of a homogenized gel that is not a gel-particle suspension. It uses a high concentration of cross-links and manages to retain a gelatinous texture. Interestingly, it has been effective in the treatment of focal steroid atrophy [14].

31.18.2 Topical Applications of Hyaluronan

A new HylaSponge® system promises to be an effective treatment modality for moisturizing skin [5, 41, 42]. Topical application of the HylaSponge® system enhances the moisture of underlying epidermis and extends down into the upper layers of the dermis. A free radical polymerization process is used to cross-link high molecular weight HA polymers into a coil-coil system generating spheres of infinite size. These dry sponge-like spheres, applied to the skin, take on large volumes of water that remain associated with the skin. The nonhydrates spheres are 20–50 μm in diameter and grow typically to 400 × 800 μm spheres when hydrated, the hydrated sphere being less than 1% HA, and the rest, water, i.e., the sponges, take on 100 times their weight in water. The fully hydrated sponges constitute an HA gel system that retains moisture in intimate contact with the skin surface.

A new potential for the application of HA to skin has been initiated with studies on transdermal delivery of nanoparticles. Successful treatment of photo-damaged skin was accomplished using nanoscale retinoic acid particles in a novel transdermal delivery system [63]. Whether HA-coated nanoparticles can be used in a similar system to enhance skin moisture and overall appearance of aging and photo-damaged skin awaits further studies.

31.19 Systemic Administration of Hyaluronan

An interesting era of HA biology has begun, with the documentation that systemic administration of HA can have system-wide effects. Intraperitoneal injection of HMW HA stimulates wound healing in diabetic mice [16]. Administration of HA also suppresses tumor growth [36]. It would be essential that the turnover of such HA be measured in an experimental animal system, accompanied by observations on chain length. Whether the systemic administration of HA can enhance skin hydration to any degree would be the next step.

31.20 Oral Administration of Hyaluronan

The literature on the effects of orally administered HA is vast, contradictory, and very confusing. Chain lengths of the polymer used in such studies are often not provided. As documented, this may be the source of much confusion. Controlled, prospective clinical trials are necessary with a need to demonstrate strict dose-dependent effects. It has not been established whether HA survives oral administration and whether absorption through the small intestine takes place. And, whether skin moisture can be modified by oral HA is the critical question.

Conclusion

Skin contains 50% of body HA. It is a major component of the ECM of skin, appearing in epidermis, dermis, as well as in the basal lamina that lies between. Hyaluronan is also observed intracellularly. This GAG plays an important role in metabolism, cell turnover, differentiation, cell movement, tissue repair, hydration, nutrient exchange, and protection against free radical damage. Its rapid turnover suggests that it may also be important as a conduit for the removal of toxic materials. It plays key roles in signal transduction pathways, an area of the literature that is so voluminous that it could not be summarized in the present communication. Native HA as well as modified cross-linked HA has been employed to help skin maintain and even regain elasticity, turgor, as well as moisture. The literature on HA is growing rapidly. Dermatology benefits disproportionately as new breakthroughs occur.

References

1. Agren UM, Tammi M, Tammi R (1997) Hydrocortisone regulation of hyaluronan metabolism in human skin organ culture. J Cell Physiol 164(2):240–248
2. Agren UM, Tammi RH, Tammi MI (1997) Reactive oxygen species contribute to epidermal hyaluronan catabolism in human skin organ culture. Free Radic Biol Med 23(7):996–1001
3. Akazawa Y, Sayo T, Sugiyama Y, Sato T, Akimoto N, Ito A, Inoue S (2011) Adiponectin resides in mouse skin and upregulates hyaluronan synthesis in dermal fibroblasts. Connect Tissue Res 52(4):322–328
4. Averbeck M, Gebhardt C, Anderegg U, Simon JC (2010) Suppression of hyaluronan synthase 2 expression reflects the atrophogenic potential of glucocorticoids. Exp Dermatol 19(8):757–759
5. Balazs EA (1981) Hyaluronan-based composition and cosmetic formulations containing same. US Patent #4,303,676
6. Barnes L, Tran C, Sorg O, Hotz R, Grand D, Carraux P, Didierjean L, Stamenkovic I, Saurat JH, Kaya G (2010) Synergistic effect of hyaluronate fragments in retinaldehyde-induced skin hyperplasia which is a CD44-dependent phenomenon. PLoS One 5(12):e14372
7. Bentley JP, Brenner RM, Linstedt AD, West NB, Carlisle KS, Rokosova BC, MacDonald N (1986) Increased hyaluronate and collagen biosynthesis and fibroblast estrogen receptors in macaque sex skin. J Invest Dermatol 87(5):668–673
8. Bertheim U, Engström-Laurent A, Hofer PA, Hallgren P, Asplund J, Hellström S (2002) Loss of hyaluronan in the basement membrane zone of the skin correlates to the degree of stiff hands in diabetic patients. Acta Derm Venereol 82(5):329–334
9. Botzki A, Rigden DJ, Braun S, Nukui M, Salmen S, Hoechstetter J, Bernhardt G, Dove S, Jedrzejas MJ, Buschauer A (2004) L-ascorbic acid 6-hexadecanoate, a potent hyaluronidase inhibitor. X-ray structure and molecular modeling of enzyme-inhibitor complexes. J Biol Chem 279(44):45990–45997
10. Bourguignon LY, Singleton PA, Diedrich F, Stern R, Gilad E (2004) CD44 Interaction with Na+-H+exchanger (NHE1) creates acidic microenvironments leading to hyaluronidase-2 and cathepsin B activation and breast tumor cell invasion. J Biol Chem 279(26):26991–27007
11. Dai G, Freudenberger T, Zipper P, Melchior A, Grether-Beck S, Rabausch B, de Groot J, Twarock S, Hanenberg H, Homey B, Krutmann J, Reifenberger J, Fischer JW (2007) Chronic ultraviolet B irradiation causes loss of hyaluronic acid from mouse dermis because of down-regulation of hyaluronic acid synthases. Am J Pathol 171(5):1451–1461
12. de la Motte C, Nigro J, Vasanji A, Rho H, Kessler S, Bandyopadhyay S, Danese S, Fiocchi C, Stern R (2009) Platelet-derived hyaluronidase 2 cleaves hyaluronan into fragments that trigger monocyte-mediated production of proinflammatory cytokines. Am J Pathol 174(6):2254–2264
13. Duan J, Kasper DL (2011) Oxidative depolymerization of polysaccharides by reactive oxygen/nitrogen species. Glycobiology 21(4):401–409
14. Elliott L, Rashid RM, Colome M (2010) Hyaluronic acid filler for steroid atrophy. J Cosmet Dermatol 9: 253–255
15. Fischer TC (2010) A European evaluation of cosmetic treatment of facial volume loss with Juvéderm™ Voluma™ in patients previously treated with Restylane SUB-Q™. J Cosmet Dermatol 9(4):291–296
16. Galeano M, Polito F, Bitto A, Irrera N, Campo GM, Avenoso A, Calò M, Cascio PL, Minutoli L, Barone M, Squadrito F, Altavilla D (2011) Systemic administration of high-molecular weight hyaluronan stimulates wound healing in genetically diabetic mice. Biochim Biophys Acta 1812(7):752–759
17. Gasingirwa MC, Thirion J, Mertens-Strijthagen J, Wattiaux-De Coninck S, Flamion B, Wattiaux R, Jadot M (2010) Endocytosis of hyaluronidase-1 by the liver. Biochem J 430(2):305–313
18. Gebhardt C, Averbeck M, Diedenhofen N, Willenberg A, Anderegg U, Sleeman JP, Simon JC (2010) Dermal hyaluronan is rapidly reduced by topical treatment with glucocorticoids. J Invest Dermatol 130(1): 141–149
19. Gu H, Huang L, Wong YP, Burd A (2010) HA modulation of epidermal morphogenesis in an organotypic keratinocyte-fibroblast co-culture model. Exp Dermatol 19(8):336–339
20. Hargitai I, Hargittai M (2008) Molecular structure of hyaluronan: an introduction. Struct Chem 19: 697–717
21. Hašová M, Crhák T, Safránková B, Dvo áková J, Muthný T, Velebný V, Kubala L (2011) Hyaluronan minimizes effects of UV irradiation on human keratinocytes. Arch Dermatol Res 303(4):277–284
22. Heldin P, Karousou E, Bernert B, Porsch H, Nishitsuka K, Skandalis SS (2008) Importance of hyaluronan-CD44 interactions in inflammation and tumorigenesis. Connect Tissue Res 49(3):215–218
23. Huey G, Moiin A, Stern R (1990) Levels of [3H]glucosamine incorporation into hyaluronic acid by fibroblasts is modulated by culture conditions. Matrix 10(2):75–83
24. Itano N, Sawai T, Yoshida M, Lenas P, Yamada Y, Imagawa M, Shinomura T, Hamaguchi M, Yoshida Y, Ohnuki Y, Miyauchi S, Spicer AP, McDonald JA, Kimata K (1999) Three isoforms of mammalian hyaluronan synthases have distinct enzymatic properties. J Biol Chem 274(35):25085–25092
25. Jiang D, Liang J, Noble PW (2011) Hyaluronan as an immune regulator in human diseases. Physiol Rev 91(1):221–264
26. Jokela TA, Lindgren A, Rilla K, Maytin E, Hascall VC, Tammi RH, Tammi MI (2008) Induction of hyaluronan cables and monocyte adherence in epidermal keratinocytes. Connect Tissue Res 49(3):115–119
27. Kao J, Huey G, Kao R, Stern R (1990) Ascorbic acid stimulates production of glycosaminoglycans in cultured fibroblasts. Exp Mol Pathol 53(1):1–10

28. Lamberg SI, Yuspa SH, Hascall VC (1986) Synthesis of hyaluronic acid is decreased and synthesis of proteoglycans is increased when cultured mouse epidermal cells differentiate. J Invest Dermatol 86(6):659–667
29. Larnier C, Kerneur C, Robert L, Moczar M (1989) Effect of testicular hyaluronidase on hyaluronate synthesis by human skin fibroblasts in culture. Biochim Biophys Acta 1014(2):145–152
30. Lin W, Shuster S, Maibach HI, Stern R (1997) Patterns of hyaluronan staining are modified by fixation techniques. J Histochem Cytochem 45(8):1157–1163
31. Lundin A, Engström-Laurent A, Michaëlsson G, Tengblad A (1987) High levels of hyaluronate in suction blister fluid from active psoriatic lesions. Br J Dermatol 116(3):335–340
32. Meyer LJ, Stern R (1994) Age-dependent changes of hyaluronan in human skin. J Invest Dermatol 102(3): 385–389
33. Mian N (1986) Analysis of cell-growth-phase-related variations in hyaluronate synthase activity of isolated plasma-membrane fractions of cultured human skin fibroblasts. Biochem J 237(2):333–342
34. Mian N (1986) Characterization of a high-Mr plasma-membrane-bound protein and assessment of its role as a constituent of hyaluronate synthase complex. Biochem J 237(2):343–357
35. Mio K, Stern R (2002) Inhibitors of the hyaluronidases. Matrix Biol 21(1):31–37
36. Mueller BM, Schraufstatter IU, Goncharova V, Povaliy T, DiScipio R, Khaldoyanidi SK (2010) Hyaluronan inhibits postchemotherapy tumor regrowth in a colon carcinoma xenograft model. Mol Cancer Ther 9(11):3024–3032
37. Nettelbladt O, Tengblad A, Hällgren R (1989) Lung accumulation of hyaluronan parallels pulmonary edema in experimental alveolitis. Am J Physiol 257(6 Pt 1):L379–L384
38. Oh JH, Kim YK, Jung JY, Shin JE, Chung JH (2011) Changes in glycosamino-glycans and related proteoglycans in intrinsically aged human skin in vivo. Exp Dermatol 20(5):454–456
39. Oliferenko S, Paiha K, Harder T, Gerke V, Schwärzler C, Schwarz H, Beug H, Günthert U, Huber LA (1999) Analysis of CD44-containing lipid rafts: recruitment of annexin II and stabilization by the actin cytoskeleton. J Cell Biol 146(4):843–854
40. Passi A, Sadeghi P, Kawamura H, Anand S, Sato N, White LE, Hascall VC, Maytin EV (2004) Hyaluronan suppresses epidermal differentiation in organotypic cultures of rat keratinocytes. Exp Cell Res 296(2): 123–134
41. Phillips GO, du Plessis TA, Al-Assaf S, Williams PA (2003) US Patent #6,610,810
42. Phillips GO, du Plessis TA, Al-Assaf S, Williams PA (2005) US Patent #6,841,644
43. Philipson LH, Schwartz NB (1984) Subcellular localization of hyaluronate synthetase in oligodendroglioma cells. J Biol Chem 259(8):5017–5023
44. Philipson LH, Westley J, Schwartz NB (1985) Effect of hyaluronidase treatment of intact cells on hyaluronate synthetase activity. Biochemistry 24(27): 7899–7906
45. Prusova A, Smejkolova D, Chytil M, Velebny V, Kucerik J (2010) An alternative DSC (differential scanning colorimetry) approach to study the hydration of hyaluronan. Carbohydr Polym 52(2):498–503
46. Reed RK, Laurent UB, Fraser JR, Laurent TC (1990) Removal rate of [3H] hyaluronan injected subcutaneously in rabbits. Am J Physiol 259(2 Pt 2): H532–H535
47. Reed RK, Lilja K, Laurent TC (1988) Hyaluronan in the rat with special reference to the skin. Acta Physiol Scand 134(3):405–411
48. Röck K, Fischer K, Fischer JW (2010) Hyaluronan used for intradermal injections is incorporated into the pericellular matrix and promotes proliferation in human skin fibroblasts in vitro. Dermatology 221:219–228
49. Röck K, Grandoch M, Majora M, Krutmann J, Fischer JW (2011) Collagen fragments inhibit hyaluronan synthesis in skin fibroblasts in response to UVB: new insights into mechanisms of matrix remodelling. J Biol Chem 286(20):18268–18276
50. Shah MG, Maibach HI (2001) Estrogen and skin. An overview. Am J Clin Dermatol 2(3):143–150
51. Shearer J, Graham TE (2002) New perspectives on the storage and organization of muscle glycogen. Can J Appl Physiol 27(2):179–203
52. Stair S, Carlson KW, Shuster S, Wei ET, Stern R (2002) Mystixin peptides reduce hyaluronan deposition and edema formation. Eur J Pharmacol 450(3):291–296
53. Stern R, Asari AA, Sugahara KN (2006) Hyaluronan fragments: an information-rich system. Eur J Cell Biol 85(8):699–715
54. Stern R, Shuster S, Wiley TS, Formby B (2001) Hyaluronidase can modulate expression of CD44. Exp Cell Res 266(1):167–176
55. Stern R, Jedrzejas MJ (2006) Hyaluronidases: their genomics, structures, and mechanisms of action. Chem Rev 106(3):818–839
56. Sugahara KN (2009) Hyaluronan fragments: informational polymers commandeered by cancers. In: Stern R (ed) Hyaluronan in cancer biology. Academic, San Diego, pp 221–254. ISBN 978–0–12–374178–3
57. Tammi R, Säämänen AM, Maibach HI, Tammi M (1991) Degradation of newly synthesized high molecular mass hyaluronan in the epidermal and dermal compartments of human skin in organ culture. J Invest Dermatol 97(1):126–130
58. Tzellos TG, Klagas I, Vahtsevanos K, Triaridis S, Printza A, Kyrgidis A, Karakiulakis G, Zouboulis CC, Papakonstantinou E (2009) Extrinsic ageing in the human skin is associated with alterations in the expression of hyaluronic acid and its metabolizing enzymes. Exp Dermatol 18(12):1028–1035

59. Underhill CB (1993) Hyaluronan is inversely correlated with the expression of CD44 in the dermal condensation of the embryonic hair follicle. J Invest Dermatol 101(6):820–826
60. Uzuka M, Nakajima K, Ohta S, Mori Y (1981) Induction of hyaluronic acid synthetase by estrogen in the mouse skin. Biochim Biophys Acta 673(4):387–393
61. Waldenström A, Martinussen HJ, Gerdin B, Hällgren R (1991) Accumulation of hyaluronan and tissue edema in experimental myocardial infarction. J Clin Invest 88(5):1622–1628
62. Weigel PH, Hascall VC, Tammi M (1997) Hyaluronan synthases. J Biol Chem 272(22):13997–14000
63. Yamaguchi Y, Nagasawa T, Nakamura N, Takenaga M, Mizoguchi M, Kawai S, Mizushima Y, Igarashi R (2005) Successful treatment of photo-damaged skin of nano-scale atRA particles using a novel transdermal delivery. J Control Release 104(1):29–40

Glycerol as a Skin Barrier Influencing Humectant

32

Laurène Roussel, Nicolas Atrux-Tallau, and Fabrice Pirot

Glycerol, also named glycerin, is found in many industries as nitroglycerin production in explosives manufacture, as food preservative, sweetening agent, and solvent in food industries. Due to its high hygroscopic and hyperosmotic properties, glycerol is widely used in cosmetic and pharmaceutical formulations (*e.g.*, as laxative in suppositories, as brain edema treatment in infusion, and mainly as humectant in topical preparations).

The glycerol physicochemical properties will be defined as its synthesis, metabolism, and medicinal uses.

In the skin, endogenous glycerol has been identified. The understanding of its effects, into the skin, is important to promote the glycerol cutaneous application. The properties of glycerol will be defined to explain the role of glycerol in the skin.

L. Roussel • N. Atrux-Tallau • F. Pirot (✉)
Laboratoire de Recherche de Développement de Pharmacie Galénique Industrielle, EA 4169 Lyon, France

Université Lyon 1, 8 Avenue Rockefeller, 69373 Lyon Cedex 08, France

Université Claude Bernard Lyon, Lyon, France
e-mail: laurene.roussel@univ-lyon1.fr; nicolas.atrux@gmail.com; fabrice.pirot@univ-lyon1.fr

32.1 Fundamentals About Glycerol

Glycerol, etymologically from Greek word "sweet," also called glycerin (propane-1,2,3-triol), is a natural compound found in living organisms and extensively used in pharmaceutical and cosmetic formulations. Main physicochemical properties of glycerol are reported in Table 32.1. Glycerol has three hydrophilic hydroxyl groups that are responsible for its hygroscopicity and excellent water solubility. Glycerol can be dissolved easily into alcohols (*e.g.*, ethanol and methanol) and water but not into oils. Glycerol is widely used as antimicrobial preservative, emollient (*i.e.*, having the power of softening or relaxing the skin), and humectant (*i.e.*, water absorption tendency of a substance from the surroundings) (Table 32.2). Furthermore, glycerol might be handled with many other substances. It is a product which is viscous, odorless, and sweet-tasting fluid.

Glycerin is nontoxic to the environment and to human health; it presents few side effects. It has nonirritating effect when applied externally. It is biocompatible and considered as a safe chemical agent by the Food and Drug Administration.

32.2 Glycerol Production and Metabolism

Glycerin is produced either by hydrolysis or saponification of oils or fats (Fig. 32.1). Alternatively, alcoholic fermentation of sugar

M. Lodén, H.I. Maibach (eds.), *Treatment of Dry Skin Syndrome*,
DOI 10.1007/978-3-642-27606-4_32, © Springer-Verlag Berlin Heidelberg 2012

Table 32.1 Physicochemical properties of glycerol

Physicochemical propertie	Value
Chemical formula	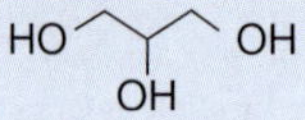
Molecular weight	92.09 $g \cdot mol^{-1}$
Density	1.26 $g \cdot cm^{-3}$ at 25°C
Boiling point	290°C
Melting point	17.8°C
Surface tension	63.4 $mN \cdot m^{-1}$ at 20°C
Dynamic viscosity at 20°C	5% aqueous solution (w/w): 1.14 mPa·s
	83% aqueous solution (w/w): 111 mPa·s
Water solubility	1,000 $g \cdot L^{-1}$ at 20°C
Acetone solubility	Slightly soluble at 20°C
Oil solubility	Practically insoluble at 20°C
Ethanol (95°) and methanol solubility	Soluble at 20°C
Osmolarity	2.6% (v/v) aqueous solution is isosmotic with serum
pK_a	14.4
Log K (octanol/water)	−1.98
Log K_p	−8.27

Adapted from [40]

Log K (octanol/water) is octanol/water partition, determined by using ProLog® software (ChemCAD, Obernai, France)

Permeability coefficient of glycerol within the SC calculated as [39]: $\log K_p\ (cm \cdot s^{-1}) = -6.3 + 0.71 \log K - 0.0061\ MW$

Table 32.2 Uses of glycerol

Use	Concentration (%)
Humectant	≤30
Emollient	≤30
Antimicrobial preservative	<20

Adapted from [40]

gives glycerol, especially when the reaction is done in presence of sodium sulphite (Na_2SO_3). Industrial production is based essentially on different reactions from propylene (chlorination and saponification) [16].

In living organisms, glycerol results from fat hydrolysis [27]. Lipolysis in adipocytes is activated during fasting or exercise for giving energy. A phosphorylated hormone-sensitive lipase hydrolyzes triglycerides to free fatty acid and glycerol, and both are released into the bloodstream. Serum glycerol concentrations approximate 0.05 $mmol \cdot L^{-1}$ at rest and can increase up to 0.30 $mmol \cdot L^{-1}$ during increased lipolysis [44]. Then, glycerol could be used for gluconeogenesis in the liver.

32.3 Glycerol Therapeutic Uses

Glycerol can be useful for the treatment of some diseases. In fact, glycerol, as hyperosmolar agent, has been used in research settings in the short-term treatment of cerebral edema resulting from ischemic stroke [42, 43]. Glycerol's infusion has become a standard practice for the management of head-injured patients with suspected or actual intracranial hypertension [10].

Glycerol ingestion with added fluid has been used to create an osmotic gradient in the circulation favoring fluid retention, thereby facilitating hyperhydration. Thus, glycerol provides benefits during endurance exercise or exposure to warm environments by inducing hyperhydration and rehydration [22].

Glycerol-preserved skin allografts (GPA) are mainly used in the management of severe burn injuries, chronic ulcers, and complex, traumatic wounds. The selective and strategic use of the GPA in major burn patients ensures optimal benefits in the management of burns [28].

50% Glycerol has been used for a long time as a viral preservation medium in tissue samples [53]. Preservation in 85% glycerol allowed to GPA to maintain its suppleness mandatory during surgery.

32.4 Endogenous Glycerol Content into the Skin

Endogenous glycerol is actually known to be an essential component to maintain stratum corneum (SC) hydration. In humans, glycerol skin content differs as a function of the body site. Onto the cheek, concentration is around 0.7 $\mu g \cdot cm^{-2}$ while in the forearm, glycerol content reaches 0.2 $\mu g \cdot cm^{-2}$. Glycerol content seems dependent on the sebaceous gland density [54].

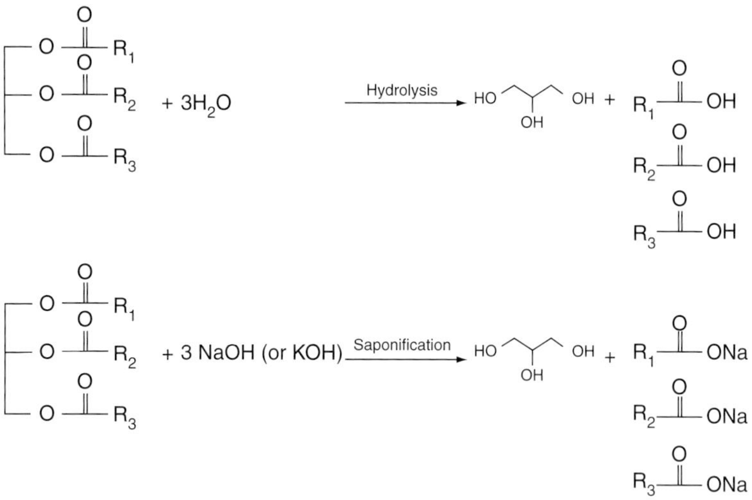

Fig. 32.1 Synthesis of glycerol

Glycerol is a byproduct of the triglycerides lipolysis within pilosebaceous gland [33]. The lipolysis of triglycerides is more efficient within the pilosebaceous apparatus than within the SC [52]. In the SC, the level of triglycerides available for lipolysis is low [47].

It is also possible that there are sources of glycerol in SC other than those derived from sebaceous glands. Indeed, SC phospholipid catabolism generates a family of nonessential free fatty acids required for the barrier function which might simultaneously generate glycerol in the SC interstices. The glycerol is formed by the breakdown of phospholipids by phospholipases [15].

Glycerol diffuses from the dermis and is transported into basal cells of the epidermis through aquaporin 3 (AQP3), a transmembrane water/glycerol transporting protein. Indeed, in AQP3 knockout mice [25], deletion produced a significant reduction in glycerol content in SC and epidermis but not in dermis or blood. Therefore, glycerol transport via AQP3 occurs solely across the relatively glycerol-impermeable basal layer of epidermis in response to a steady-state dermal-to-epidermal glycerol gradient.

AQP3 is expressed in the innermost layer of keratinocytes in mammalian epidermis. By indirect immunofluorescence and electron microscopy gold labeling on human epidermis sections, AQP3 was primarily and abundantly localized in plasma membrane of the keratinocytes in epidermal human skin [49, 50].

AQP3 synthesis appears to occur early in basal cells with a predominant cytoplasmic distribution, and the differentiation process could induce AQP3 translocation to the plasma membrane [49].

The importance of endogenous glycerol is now established in the SC hydration. Glycerol belongs to the natural moisturizing factor (NMF).

The decrease of the endogenous glycerol in SC is correlated to a decrease in SC hydration [16, 18, 26]. Choi [13] confirmed that variation in SC hydration is correlated with variations in both blood and sebaceous gland glycerol content.

In asebia mice [18], with a large depletion of sebaceous gland, the SC hydration was also decreased. As well, the glycerol content in SC decreased by 83%. The addition of sebum-like lipids (triglycerides) did not restore the normal SC hydration while topical addition of glycerol did.

In AQP3 deficient mice, the glycerol content decreased by 50% in the SC as compared to wild-type mice and by 37% in the epidermis. Additional skin phenotype analysis highlighted a delayed barrier recovery after SC removal by tape stripping in AQP3 null mice, as well as delayed wound healing [25].

Reduction in skin conductance in AQP3 null mice was not corrected by occlusion or exposure to a humidified atmosphere, suggesting an intrinsic defect in SC water-holding capacity (WHC). Thus, the water transporting function of AQP3 did not appear to be responsible for the reduced superficial skin conductance. However, when glycerol is topically added, the hydration defect is corrected in AQP3 knockout mice [26]. Glycerol improvement by topical routes increased SC water content, with excellent correlation between SC water and glycerol content in AQP3 null mice.

The relationship between AQP3 and skin disorders associated with abnormal water homoeostasis (atopic dermatitis, psoriasis, xeroderma, and ichthyosis) needs to be investigated.

Modulation of AQP3 functions by different compounds could be interesting in activating the water/glycerol transport from the dermis to the basal layers of epidermis. An AQP3 upregulation may increase SC water content and improve the barrier function.

Hara-Chikuma and Verkman [24] provided evidence for involvement of AQP3-facilitated water transport in epidermal cell migration and for AQP3-facilitated glycerol transport in epidermal cell proliferation during repair of skin wounds. Pharmacological modulation of AQP3 could be also therapy to accelerate wound healing in traumas, burns, and other forms of injury.

32.5 Effects of Cutaneous Exposure to Glycerol

Glycerol is widely used in different dermatological and cosmetic preparations. It acts as natural moisturizer and preserves the SC barrier function. It also influences the skin surface mechanical properties by plasticizing SC and inducing smoothing effect [9, 36] (by cell shrinking of the superficial corneocytes). It can also increase skin elasticity [36].

It is actually known that the skin care benefits of glycerol are due to different properties of the compounds: attraction of moisture, maintenance of crystallinity/fluidity of cell membranes and intracellular lipids [31], keratolytic effect, and its ability to diffuse and penetrate into the SC [6].

Glycerol is a hygroscopic compound, limiting thus water evaporation and improving SC hydration. Glycerol efficiency is also due to its capacity to diffuse and accumulate in the entire thickness of the SC in a high proportion [35]. Indeed, *in vivo* determination of skin water content with a confocal Raman optical microprobe, revealed an increase of the water content after glycerol application with no dependence on the SC depth [14].

Nevertheless, in guinea pig model, diglycerol and triglycerol, with a higher humectant activity *in vitro* than glycerol, showed less effective action on skin dryness improvement as compared to glycerol [46]. The chemical properties determined *in vitro* could not be sufficient to predict the molecule effect on SC hydration.

The SC water content in a healthy skin is around 20–30% by weight [48]. The SC needs to be hydrated to maintain its integrity. SC hydration variations can influence the SC barrier function [16].

Glycerol prevents damaging effect on the SC. Glycerol pretreatment decreases irritancy caused by alkali solution (*e.g.*, sodium hydroxide), dimethyl sulfoxide, and sodium lauryl sulphate (SLS) [16].

Glycerol leads to a more rapid reconstitution of the protective skin barrier following mechanical (tape stripping) or chemical (repeated SLS application, acetone) damage. It can absorb water and thus creating water flux in the SC which may lead to a stimulus for barrier repair [17]. In Andersen *et al.* studies [1–3], only glycerol treatment improved skin barrier recovery after acute and cumulative irritations induced by SLS or nonanoic acid applications in hairless guinea pig model and in human volunteers. The high hygroscopicity of glycerol can be involved in this action, supporting transepidermal water loss (TEWL) and ion movement (especially calcium) [8].

In the case of aqueous solution, after SLS-induced irritation on skin, it appears that glycerol efficacy on hydration (evaluated by capacitance measurement) and TEWL reached a plateau phase when enhancing glycerol concentration, resulting in a maximal WHC value [5]. The recovery of the water barrier function with glycerol by skin rehydration is thus saturable. The WHC of stratum corneum is related to hygroscopic compounds and to SC osmotic pressure. The WHC and skin hydration were found to be correlated with SC osmolality, varied as a function of the osmolality of solutions (Fig. 32.2), and the SC permeability of osmolytes [37, 38].

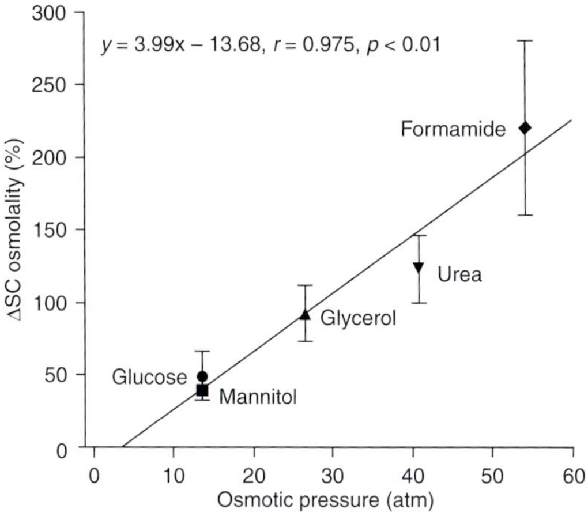

Fig. 32.2 Linear relationship between ΔSC osmolality (%) and the osmotic pressure (atm) of donor solutions. Each data point is the mean ± standard deviation of 3 or 5 experimental determinations [38]. ■ = Mannitol, ● = Glucose, ▲ = Glycerol, ▼ = Urea, ♦ = Formamide

A low-dose topical application of glycerol was shown to restore the water barrier function of SLS-damaged skin. The beneficial effect of glycerol on skin barrier function, disrupted by acute chemical, acts throughout the increase of WHC [5]. WHC reflects an equilibrium between bound and free water determined, respectively, by hydration measurement and TEWL.

In normal SC, it is thought that the ratio of lipids in ordered and disordered (liquid crystalline) phases modulates the SC barrier function properties [11].

The entity of the skin barrier is ensured by the optimal organization and the interactions of the SC components, *i.e.*, corneocytes and the intercellular lipids bilayers. The lipid bilayers disorganization, rather than lipid extraction, is responsible for barrier impairment.

A pure liquid crystal system, produced by an all-unsaturated fatty acid mixture, allows a rapid water loss through the bilayers with a moderate barrier action. The solid system produced with an all-saturated fatty acid mixture causes an extreme water loss due to breaks in the solid crystal phase [16]. Maintaining the balance between the two phases is required for optimal barrier function in preventing water loss [51].

Thus, the proportion of lipophilic components in solid state was noted in skin exhibiting SC barrier damage [19].

Froebe *et al.* [19] showed, from an *in vitro* experiment, that by glycerol adding to the SC lipids, the transition of the lipophilic components from the liquid crystalline phase to the solid crystalline phase can be prevented at low relative humidity. It has been hypothesized that glycerol can interact with polar head groups of the lipid bilayers rather than by penetrating the alkyl chains. Consequently, maintaining the fluidity of the lipid membrane improves skin conditions in dry climates. Thus, glycerol decreases SC permeability to water but enhances SC barrier function.

Batt and Fairhurst [7] postulated that a depot formation of glycerol in the depth of the horny layer lipids occurs because of glycerol persistent effects after discontinuation of the therapy over 24 h. This would suggest that the effect on the SC lipids is present not only to the upper layers, but also to the SC lipids deeper layers.

Glycerol-containing moisturizers continue to improve barrier function for at least a week after cessation of treatment [4].

Furthermore, 10% glycerol addition in an aqueous solution of SLS prevents the skin barrier perturbation induced by the surfactant *in vitro* by reducing the skin aqueous pore radius and the aqueous pore number density [20]. Glycerol present in the SC is able to bind water in the SC and thus reduce the mobility of water. In hydrated skin, aqueous pores are constituted by lacunar domains within water is mobile. The limited mobility of water may result in lacunar domains structural continuity loss within the SC extracellular lipid bilayers [34]. Ghosh *et al.* [20] suggested that it may involve the reduction of the radius of the aqueous pore if the loss of continuity is partial and the reduction of the aqueous pore number density if the loss is complete. Moreover, the glycerol property to maintain the intercellular lipid mortar in liquid phase can also lead to minimize the lacunar domains and thus reduce the continuity of it.

The glycerol-hydrating property occurs not only on healthy skin but also on skin affected by xerosis.

The understanding of skin moisturization disturbances is of major importance for new treatment of pathologies such as atopic dermatitis, eczema.

Glycerol seems to be a relevant treatment in atopic dermatitis (AD). However, Lodén *et al.* [30] were not able to detect differences in the biophysical assessment of epidermal functions in a placebo-controlled AD study. Thirty days glycerin treatment versus placebo in atopic dermatitis patient showed no differences in TEWL.

Breternitz *et al.* [12] investigated lesional skin of atopic patients and detected a positive (but not significant) effect of glycerol for recovery of altered epidermal barrier function. Concerning hydration, glycerol cream has significant advantages as compared to the glycerol-free formulation. The erythema values as a marker of skin irritation or inflammation were slightly lower in the group of patients treated with glycerol. However, any significant differences were distinguished between the glycerol-based formulation and glycerol-free formulation regarding improvement of epidermal barrier function, irritation parameters, surface pH, and clinical scores.

The recent observation that xerotic skin is associated with incomplete desmosome digestion suggests that moisturizers improve the desquamation process in such conditions.

Glycerol seems to have keratolytic properties. After first week of glycerol treatment, an activation of SC protease activity occurs (simply by elevated water activity). This protease is responsible of the regulation of corneocytes desquamation, resulting in more efficient reduction in SC thickness. The desmosome degradation is essential to maintain a healthy skin which requires an equilibrium between degradation and synthesis of desmosome. Furthermore, glycerol desmolytic effect, demonstrated by Rawlings *et al.* [41], causes a decrease in intraepidermal pressure on the bilamellar intercellular lipids and, therefore, indirectly causes an increase in the liquid crystalline state lipids. The dry skin scaliness is thus reduced, and the SC barrier is maintained in xerotic skin.

Investigations on the influence of the vehicle used showed that the beneficial effect of glycerol on skin was more pronounced in using oil in water emulsion compared with water in oil emulsion [21, 23]. The quantity of absorbed humectant in the SC influences the glycerol moisturization effect [35]. Furthermore, glycerol moisturizing efficiency depends on solvents in which it is dissolved. Therefore, glycerol acts as an effective humectant only when it is dissolved in water [45].

Gloor [21] showed that the pretreatment with oil in water emulsions containing glycerol prevents dehydration, barrier perturbation, and irritation caused by washing with SLS. In the case of oil in water emulsions, the proportion of glycerol should not be less than 8.5%. However, glycerol high concentration application results in dehydration of the skin because of the osmotic water extraction from the SC caused by glycerol.

However, in aqueous solution, glycerol concentration must not exceed 5% to restore barrier function [5].

In addition, it has been reported that glycerol facilitated skin penetration of topically applied drugs [17, 29]. After tape stripping, glycerol could have penetration-enhancing effect mainly by the glycerol action on SC lipid organization [8], whereas protective and curative effect against irritants was reported [16].

Recently, glycerol-derived compounds have been identified and could be efficient as moisturizer treatment: Glycerol quat® (dihydroxypropyltrimonium chloride) is a combination of glycerin and a quat (*i.e.*, a positively charged group of molecules attached to negatively charged skin proteins). Such compound is less lipophilic (allowing it to remain at the outermost layers) and binds four times more water molecules than glycerol. The objective is to compensate glycerol poor moisturizing efficiency at skin surface outermost layers [32].

Take Home Messages

- Endogenous glycerol represents an interesting compound in the epidermis. It maintains the hydration properties of the SC and thus the barrier function.
- The AQP3 functions modulation by different compounds could be interesting in order to activate the water/glycerol

transport from the dermis to the epidermis basal layers.

- AQP3 expression pharmacological modulation could be benefit in a number of skin disorders, burn repair, and other wounds.
- Glycerol, by its high hygroscopic properties, acts as a humectant.
- Glycerol leads to maintain crystallinity/fluidity of cell membranes and intracellular lipids.
- Glycerol prevents damaging effect induced by alkali, surfactant, and organic solvent on the SC.
- The recovery of the water barrier function induced by glycerol after chemical damage can be explained by the improvement of WHC and skin hydration which are correlated with SC osmolality and the SC permeability of osmolytes.
- In xerotic skin, its keratolytic property confers to glycerol the capacity to improve skin barrier function and decrease its scaliness.

References

1. Andersen F, Hedegaard K, Fullerton A et al (2006) The hairless guinea-pig as a model for treatment of acute irritation in humans. Skin Res Technol 12:183–189
2. Andersen F, Hedegaard K, Petersen TK et al (2006) Anti-irritants I: dose–response in acute irritation. Contact Dermatitis 55:148–154
3. Andersen F, Hedegaard K, Petersen TK et al (2006) Anti-irritants II: efficacy against cumulative irritation. Contact Dermatitis 55:155–159
4. Appa Y, Hemingway L, Orth D et al (1997) High glycerine therapeutic moisturizers. In: Poster presented at the 55th annual meeting of the American Academy of Dermatology, San Francisco, CA
5. Atrux-Tallau N, Romagny C, Padois K et al (2010) Effects of glycerol on human skin damaged by acute sodium lauryl sulphate treatment. Arch Dermatol Res 302:435–441
6. Batt MD, Davis WB, Fairhurst E et al (1988) Changes in the physical-properties of the stratum-corneum following treatment with glycerol. J Soc Cosmet Chem 39:367–381
7. Batt MD, Fairhust E (1986) Hydration of the stratum corneum. Int J Cosmet Sci 8:253–264
8. Bettinger J, Gloor M, Peter C et al (1998) Opposing effects of glycerol on the protective function of the horny layer against irritants and on the penetration of hexyl nicotinate. Dermatology 197:18–24
9. Bettinger J, Gloor M, Vollert A et al (1999) Comparison of different non-invasive test methods with respect to the different moisturizers on skin. Skin Res Technol 5:21–27
10. Biestro A, Alberti R, Galli R et al (1997) Osmotherapy for increased intracranial pressure: comparison between mannitol and glycerol. Acta Neurochir (Wien) 139:725–732; discussion 732–723
11. Boncheva M, Damien F, Normand V (2008) Molecular organization of the lipid matrix in intact Stratum corneum using ATR-FTIR spectroscopy. Biochim Biophys Acta 1778:1344–1355
12. Breternitz M, Kowatski D, Langenauer M et al (2008) Placebo controlled, double blind, randomized prospective study of a glycerol-based emollient on eczematous skin in atopic dermatitis: biophysical and clinical evaluation. Skin Pharmacol Physiol 21:39–45
13. Choi EH, Man MQ, Wang FS et al (2005) Is endogenous glycerol a determinant of stratum corneum hydration in humans? J Invest Dermatol 125: 288–293
14. Chrit L, Bastien P, Sockalingum GD et al (2006) An in vivo randomized study of human skin moisturization by a new confocal Raman fiber-optic microprobe: assessment of a glycerol-based hydration cream. Skin Pharmacol Physiol 19:207–215
15. Feingold KR (2007) Thematic review series: skin lipids. The role of epidermal lipids in cutaneous permeability barrier homeostasis. J Lipid Res 48:2531–2546
16. Fluhr JW, Darlenski R, Surber C (2008) Glycerol and the skin: holistic approach to its origin and functions. Br J Dermatol 159:23–34
17. Fluhr JW, Gloor M, Lehmann L et al (1999) Glycerol accelerates recovery of barrier function in vivo. Acta Derm Venereol 79:418–421
18. Fluhr JW, Mao-Qiang M, Brown BE et al (2003) Glycerol regulates stratum corneum hydration in sebaceous gland deficient (asebia) mice. J Invest Dermatol 120:728–737
19. Froebe CL, Simion AF, Ohlmeyer H et al (1990) Prevention of stratum corneum lipid phase transitions in vitro by glycerol ± an alternative mechanism for skin moisturization. J Soc Cosmet Chem 41:51–65
20. Ghosh S, Blankschtein D (2007) The role of sodium dodecyl sulfate (SDS) micelles in inducing skin barrier perturbation in the presence of glycerol. J Cosmet Sci 58:109–133
21. Gloor M (2004) How do dermatological vehicles influence the horny layer? Skin Pharmacol Physiol 17:267–273
22. Goulet ED, Robergs RA, Labrecque S et al (2006) Effect of glycerol-induced hyperhydration on thermoregulatory and cardiovascular functions and endurance performance during prolonged cycling in a 25

degrees C environment. Appl Physiol Nutr Metab 31:101–109
23. Grunewald AM, Lorenz J, Gloor M et al (1996) Lipophilic irritants. Protective values of urea and glycerol containing oil in water emulsions. Dermatosen 44:81–86
24. Hara-Chikuma M, Verkman AS (2008) Aquaporin-3 facilitates epidermal cell migration and proliferation during wound healing. J Mol Med 86:221–231
25. Hara M, Ma T, Verkman AS (2002) Selectively reduced glycerol in skin of aquaporin-3-deficient mice may account for impaired skin hydration, elasticity, and barrier recovery. J Biol Chem 277:46616–46621
26. Hara M, Verkman AS (2003) Glycerol replacement corrects defective skin hydration, elasticity, and barrier function in aquaporin-3 deficient mice. Proc Natl Acad Sci USA 100:7360–7365
27. Hibuse T, Maeda N, Nagasawa A et al (2006) Aquaporins and glycerol metabolism. Biochim Biophys Acta 1758:1004–1011
28. Khoo TL, Halim AS, Saad AZM et al (2010) The application of glycerol-preserved skin allograft in the treatment of burn injuries: an analysis based on indications. Burns 36:897–904
29. Kiwada H, Barichello JM, Yamakawa N et al (2008) Combined effect of liposomalization and addition of glycerol on the transdermal delivery of isosorbide 5-nitrate in rat skin. Int J Pharm 357:199–205
30. Lodén M, Andersson AC, Andersson C et al (2001) Instrumental and dermatologist evaluation of the effect of glycerine and urea on dry skin in atopic dermatitis. Skin Res Technol 7:209–213
31. Lodén M, Maibach HI (2000) Dry skin and moisturizers: chemistry and function. CRC Press, Boca Raton
32. Lu N, Chandar P, Nole G et al (2010) Development and clinical analysis of a novel humectant system of glycerol, hydroxyethylurea, and glycerol quat. Cosmet Dermatol 23:86–94
33. Marples RR, Kligman AM, Downing DT (1971) Control of free fatty acids in human surface lipids by corynebacterium-acnes. J Invest Dermatol 56:127–131
34. Menon GK, Elias PM (1997) Morphologic basis for a pore-pathway in mammalian stratum corneum. Skin Pharmacol 10:235–246
35. Okamoto T, Inoue H, Anzai S et al (1998) Skin-moisturizing effect of polyols and their absorption into human stratum corneum. J Cosmet Chem 49:57–58
36. Olsen OL, Jemec GBE (1993) The influence of water, glycerin, paraffin oil and ethanol on skin mechanics. Acta Derm Venereol 73:404–406
37. Pirot F, Falson F, Pailler-Mattéi C et al (2004) Stratum corneum: an ideal osmometer? Exog Dermatol 3:339–349
38. Pirot F, Morel B, Peyrot G et al (2003) Effects of osmosis on water-holding capacity of stratum corneum and skin hydration. Exog Dermatol 2:252–257
39. Potts RO, Guy RH (1992) Predicting skin permeability. Pharm Res 9:663–669
40. Price J (2005) Glycerin. In: Rowe RC, Sheskey P, Owen SC (eds) Handbook of Pharmaceutical Excipients. Fifth edition, p 301–303
41. Rawlings A, Harding C, Watkinson A et al (1995) The effect of glycerol and humidity on desmosome degradation in stratum corneum. Arch Dermatol Res 287:457–464
42. Righetti E, Celani MG, Cantisani T et al (2004) Glycerol for acute stroke. Cochrane Database Syst Rev (2):CD000096
43. Righetti E, Celani MG, Cantisani TA et al (2002) Glycerol for acute stroke: a cochrane systematic review. J Neurol 249:445–451
44. Robergs RA, Griffin SE (1998) Glycerol. Biochemistry, pharmacokinetics and clinical and practical applications. Sports Med 26:145–167
45. Sagiv AE, Dikstein S, Ingber A (2001) The efficiency of humectants as skin moisturizers in the presence of oil. Skin Res Technol 7:32–35
46. Sagiv AE, Marcus Y (2003) The connection between in vitro water uptake and in vivo skin moisturization. Skin Res Techol 9:306–311
47. Schurer NY, Plewig G, Elias PM (1991) Stratum-corneum lipid function. Dermatologica 183:77–94
48. Silva CL, Topgaard D, Kocherbitov V et al (2007) Stratum corneum hydration: phase transformations and mobility in stratum corneum, extracted lipids and isolated corneocytes. Biochim Biophys Acta 1768:2647–2659
49. Sougrat R, Morand M, Gondran C et al (2002) Functional expression of AQP3 in human skin epidermis and reconstructed epidermis. J Invest Dermatol 118:678–685
50. Sugiyama Y, Ota Y, Hara M et al (2001) Gene expression of the water channels, aquaporins, in human keratinocyte and skin-equivalent cultures, and osmotic stress induction of aquaporin-3 mRNA in cultured keratinocytes. J Invest Dermatol 117:410
51. Thau P (2002) Glycerin (glycerol): current insights into the functional properties of a classic cosmetic raw material. J Cosmet Sci 53:229–236
52. Thody AJ, Shuster S (1989) Control and function of sebaceous glands. Physiol Rev 69:383–416
53. Vanbaare J, Buitenwerf J, Hoekstra MJ et al (1994) Virucidal effect of glycerol as used in donor skin preservation. Burns 20:S77–S80
54. Yoneya T, Nishijima Y (1979) Determination of free glycerol on human skin surface. Biol Mass Spectrom 6:191–193

The Use of Urea in the Treatment of Dry Skin

33

Marie Lodén

33.1 Introduction

Moisturizing creams contain a great variety of ingredients. They also have different effects on the skin structure and function. Their influence on skin barrier function has become more important after the findings that mutations in the filaggrin gene may weaken skin barrier function and cause eczema [1]. Mutations in the filaggrin gene have been identified as the major predisposing factor for atopic eczema [1, 2]. Filaggrin forms the natural moisturizing factor (NMF) in the stratum corneum and is essential during formation of the cornified envelope of corneocytes [3, 4]. Individuals with mutations in the filaggrin gene are more likely to report skin dryness [5]. Therefore, moisturizers that not only diminish the signs of dryness but also strengthen skin barrier function are likely to reduce the prevalence of inflammatory dermatosis [6, 7]. Thus, measurement of skin barrier function may be a relevant surrogate parameter for the changed risks for eczema.

This chapter will review the data on the influence of urea on the skin. Folklore is rich in references to the healing properties of urea. The Babylonians of about 800 bc are known to have used it. In the beginning of this century, urea was employed in the treatment of infections, particularly those involving wounds and ulcers, the ears, tooth sockets, malignant growths and of burns [8, 9]. This chapter will focus on more recent clinical findings, such as the effects on dry skin disorders and the effects on barrier function.

33.2 Chemistry

Urea (carbamide, carbonyl diamide, CAS no. 57-13-6, molecular weight 60.1) is a colourless or white, crystalline powder. Soluble 1 in 1.5 of water, 1 in 10 of alcohol and 1 in 1 of boiling alcohol, practically insoluble in chloroform and in ether. Solutions are neutral to litmus. Urea is readily incorporated in topical formulations by virtue of its solubility. However, urea gradually develops carbon dioxide and ammonia [10]. Unstable preparations may need to be stored in a refrigerator.

33.3 Biochemistry

Urea is a physiological substance occurring in human tissues, blood and urine [10]. The amount in urine is of the order of 2%. The extraction of

M. Lodén
Evidetm Institute AB, Research and Development,
Bergshamra Allé 9,
SE-17077 Solna, Sweden
e-mail: marie.loden@eviderm.se

M. Lodén, H.I. Maibach (eds.), *Treatment of Dry Skin Syndrome*,
DOI 10.1007/978-3-642-27606-4_33, © Springer-Verlag Berlin Heidelberg 2012

pure urea from urine was first accomplished by Proust in 1821, and urea was first synthesized by Wöhler in 1828 [11].

Urea is a major constituent of the water-soluble fraction of the stratum corneum. It is present there as a major component of NMF [12]. Filaggrin is the main source of NMF, and the levels of filaggrin degradation products are influenced by both filaggrin genotype and atopic dermatitis severity [13]. In patients with atopic dermatitis, the content of urea in the stratum corneum is significantly reduced [14].

Urea attracts water, and immersion of psoriatic and ichthyotic scales in 5 M urea shows that they will absorb 38% of water at 85% relative humidity [15]. Furthermore, the water-holding capacity of ichthyotic scales has been shown to increase from 9% to 18% by the treatment with a urea cream (10%) for 3 weeks [16].

Urea can cause uncoiling of DNA, a property used in many DNA studies, but this in vitro activity is not linked to any in vivo genotoxic activity [17]. Urea also unfolds proteins, thus solubilizing and/or denaturing them [9, 18, 19]. Pieces of upper epidermis kept in saturated urea solutions lose their original quaternary structure and change mechanically [18]. High concentrations of urea (20–40%) are used to detach dystrophic nails [20]. However, no changes in the binding forces within the stratum corneum have been found after exposure of normal skin to 10% for 6 h [21]. The lipid matrix of the skin seems not to be affected by urea since the transition temperatures of mouse skin lipids was not changed by exposure to 12% urea [22]. Urea could also protect against osmotic stress by replacing water and retaining the liquid crystalline phase at lower humidity [23].

Treatment of hyperkeratotic skin with 10% urea reduces the number of stratum corneum cell layers [24, 25]. Urea influences epidermal proliferation in healthy human skin and in guinea pigs [26, 27]. After short-term contact with a saturated urea solution, incorporation of thymidine in DNA was reduced, and a thinning of the epidermis was found. After exposure to urea for more than 2–6 weeks, no further thinning occurred, and

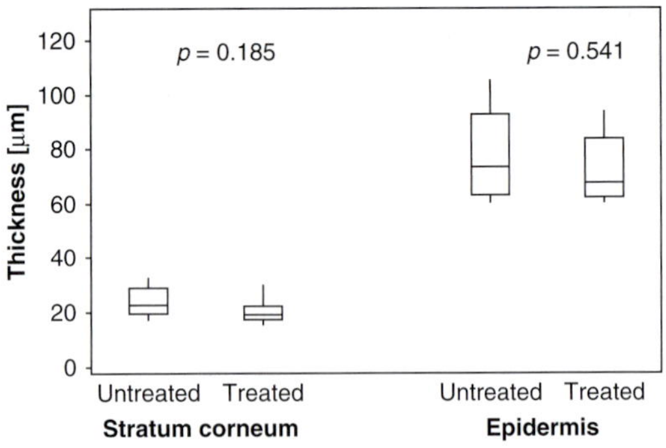

Fig. 33.1 Thickness of stratum corneum and epidermis in untreated and in barrier-improved normal skin after treatment with 5% urea in a medicinal cream (Modified from Buraczewska et al. [31])

there was no tendency for atrophy during this period [26, 27].

Reduction in epidermal DNA synthesis and epidermal proliferation in psoriasis has also been reported, measured as an altered expression of involucrin and cytokeratins [28]. Involucrin is involved in the assembly of the densely packed cornified cell envelope and functions as a scaffold for lipid and protein attachment. Decreased involucrin [29] expression and incomplete maturation of the cornified envelope [30] are observed in atopics.

Treatment of normal skin with 5% urea in a medicinal cream has repeatedly been shown to improve skin barrier function (see later part of this chapter). This improvement appears not to be accompanied by significant changes in the thickness of the stratum corneum or of the epidermis, Fig. 33.1 [31]. Moreover, immunofluorescence staining of skin biopsies did not show any changes in the protein expression of involucrin and transglutaminase, although a slight tendency of increased filaggrin level was noted ($p=0.07$) [31]. Furthermore, no changes in the mRNA expression of genes involved in synthesis of involucrin, transglutaminase and filaggrin and in the genes involved in the process of desquamation (SCCE and SCTE) were found [31]. Only cyclin-dependent kinase inhibitor 1A (also known as p21, WAF1/CIP1) was slightly decreased [31]. The cyclin-dependent kinase inhibitor 1A modulates cell cycle, apoptosis, senescence and differentiation.

33.4 Side Effects

Urea is a normal physiological metabolite and is generally regarded as safe as used in topical products [17]. No report on sensitization has been found despite its wide use in dermatological preparations. In 1943, Rattner patch tested 500 hospital patients, 66 of whom had skin disease, with a 3% urea cream and found no adverse reaction [8]. Clinical and patient assessments of the use of creams with 10% urea or lower showed no evidence of inflammation and barrier damage [32], although occlusive exposure to 20% urea in petrolatum for 24 h causes significant inflammation (i.e. increase in blood flow and skin thickness) and increases TEWL [33]. Despite these studies, some patients reported disagreeable skin sensations from urea treatments, such as redness, stinging and smarting [15, 32, 34–38]. Application of urea to freshly excoriated areas and to skin lesions can give burning sensations [39]. This is not irritation in the ordinary sense and usually does not cause clinically noticeable damages to the skin, but the disagreeable sensations will reduce compliance, especially in children [11]. Furthermore, it may be difficult to treat sensitive body areas, for example, the face, since stinging and other side effects from topical treatment are mainly perceived there [40, 41]. A recent study suggests that urea affects cutaneous arterial sympathetic nerve activity and elevates blood flow via histaminergic H3 receptor [42].

33.5 Clinical Effects in Dry Skin Disorders by Urea

The clinical efficacy of 4–10% urea in the treatment of dry skin in patients with atopic dermatitis is demonstrated in several studies, Table 33.1 [37, 43–46, 48, 49]. In a study on atopic dry skin, a 4% urea formulation was superior to a glycerin-containing cream to reduce clinical symptoms of dryness [49]. A 10% urea cream produced improvement of the xerosis and the pruritus, but somewhat less of erythema compared to those of a base cream [37]. A 5% urea cream increased skin hydration (measured as capacitance) [48] and showed similar efficacy to a 4% urea cream in a double-blind study on 48 atopic patients [46]. The clinical and instrumental assessment showed improvements in both groups during the treatment period [46]. A water-in-oil emulsion with 10% urea induced significantly higher skin capacitance than the corresponding placebo lotion [45]. Improvement in clinical skin condition could be observed in parallel to the increase in skin hydration [45].

Several studies also support clinical efficacy of 10% urea in the treatment of psoriasis vulgaris [15, 28, 44, 50] and ichthyosis [11, 15, 16, 34, 44, 51, 52], Table 33.2. In the treatment of psoriasis, five psoriatic patients with chronic therapy-resistant lesions obtained soft and pliable skin after treatment with 10% urea, but no effect on erythema was observed [15]. Psoriatic lesions on

Table 33.1 Treatment of atopic dermatitis with urea formulations

Design (number of patients)	Conc. %	Outcomes
Open, uncontrolled	5, 10	Urea formulations increase skin hydration [43]
Randomized, double-blind, bilateral (18)	10	No difference to aqueous cream [44]
Single-blind, 'placebo'-controlled (20)	10	Clinical improvement, decreased TEWL [37]
Randomized, bilateral, double-blind, placebo (38)	10	Clinical improvement, increased hydration (capacitance) [45]
Randomized, double-blind, parallel, 4% vs. 5% (48)	4, 5	Clinical improvements, no difference between products[46]
Randomized, double-blind, parallel, 5% vs. 10% (100)	5, 10	Clinical improvement, no difference between products [47]
Bilateral, blind evaluation, untreated control (15)	5	Increased hydration (capacitance) reduced susceptibility to sodium lauryl sulphate (SLS) [48]
Randomized, double-blind, parallel, vs. two reference creams (109)	4	Clinical improvement, urea superior[49]

Table 33.2 Treatment of psoriasis vulgaris and ichthyosis with urea formulations

Diagnosis	Design (number of patients)	Conc. %	Outcomes
Psoriasis	Open (5)	10	Softening effects [15]
Psoriasis	Randomized, double-blind, bilateral, vs. reference (4)	10	No difference to aqueous cream [44]
Psoriasis	Randomized, bilateral (10)	10	Increased hydration compared to petrolatum [50]
Psoriasis	Randomized, bilateral, double-blind, placebo (10)	10	Clinical evaluation and capacitance measurement show superiority to placebo [28]
Ichthyosis	Open, bilateral (7)	10	Improvement, better than control cream [15]
Ichthyosis	Open, no control (17)	10	Improvement [11]
Ichthyosis	Randomized, double-blind, parallel, vs. references (84)	10	Better than other preparations [51]
Ichthyosis	Randomized, double-blind, bilateral, vs. reference (7)	10	No difference to aqueous cream [44]
Ichthyosis	Randomized, double-blind, bilateral (14)	10	Better than placebo [16]
Ichthyosis	Randomized, double-blind, bilateral, reference cream with 10% urea (30)	10	Both creams effective, the one with pH 6 preferred to the one with pH 3 [34]
Ichthyosis	Randomized, double-blind, bilateral (60)	10	Better than placebo [52]

the extremities also showed clinical improvement after treatment with an ointment containing 10% urea in a placebo-controlled study on ten patients [28]. Higher values of skin capacitance were noted on urea-treated areas. Increased hygroscopicity and water content were also obtained after treatment with 10% urea ointment in patients with psoriasis vulgaris [50]. However, early data from a clinical study on various types of hyperkeratosis showed no superior effects from a 10% urea cream compared to aqueous cream [44].

The efficacy of urea in the treatment of ichthyosis has been investigated in several clinical studies. In seven patients with severe ichthyosis, a pronounced keratolytic effect was noticed after treatment with high concentrations (about 10%) [15]. The number of stratum corneum cell layers was reduced in 6 of 11 patients with ichthyosis after treatment with 10% urea [24]. In a double-blind trial on 84 outpatients with ichthyosis vulgaris or X-linked ichthyosis, a 10% urea cream was better in controlling the clinical signs of ichthyosis than three other preparations (salicylic acid ointment, an oily cream and another cream) [51]. The clinical results showed a statistically significant improvement, although the patient's assessment did not reveal any statistically significant difference between the groups. Significant clinical improvement was also noted in 14 patients with ichthyosis after treatment for 3 weeks with 10% urea compared with treatment with the base [16]. In another study, 60 children with ichthyosis showed pronounced improvement in the area treated with a 10% urea lotion compared to the corresponding placebo-treated area [52].Two preparations containing 10% urea tested on 30 patients with ichthyosis associated with atopic dermatitis showed improved skin conditions equally well [34].

Studies also show evidence for clinical efficacy of 4–10% urea in hands, feet and legs of elderly patients, Table 33.3. Creams containing 4% urea [38] or 10% [53, 54] were significantly better than corresponding placebo in improving dry legs. Moreover, studies on hyperkeratosis in feet support the use of urea (10–40%). In volar forearms, creams with 3% and 10% urea improved the skin with respect to dryness characteristics [32]. In one of the first clinical studies on urea, published 1943, its effect on hand eczema was

Table 33.3 Treatment of other types of dryness with urea formulations

Diagnosis	Conc. %	Design (number of individuals)	Outcomes
Dry skin	3, 10	Randomized, blind evaluation, untreated control (47)	Less scaling, improved hydration [32]
Dry senescent skin	4	Randomized, double-blind, bilateral, placebo-controlled (26)	Clinical improvement, urea cream better than placebo [38]
Dry senescent skin	10	Randomized, double-blind, bilateral, placebo-controlled (36+36)	Clinical improvement in both groups, higher moisture values in active [53]
Dry senescent skin	10	Randomized, double-blind, bilateral, placebo-controlled (60)	Differences in skin capacitance, not clinically [54]
Dry senescent skin	4	Randomized, bilateral, double-blind (23)	Improved, no difference to reference cream without sodium chloride [55]
Hyperkeratosis feet	40	Randomized, bilateral, double-blind vs. reference with 12% ammonium lactate (18)	More rapid effect from urea [56]
Hyperkeratosis feet	10	Randomized, double-blind, bilateral (8)	No difference to aqueous cream [44]
Hyperkeratosis feet	10	Randomized, bilateral, double-blind (40)	Urea superior [57]
Hyperkeratosis feet	30	Randomized, bilateral, double-blind	Urea superior to comparator [58]
Hyperkeratosis feet	10	Open (24)	Decreased thickness [25]
Hyperkeratosis	30	Observational, prospective, open-label case study (10)	Significant improvement [59]
Dry hands	3	Bilateral, placebo (250)	Urea cream better [8]
Dry hands	10	Randomized, double-blind, bilateral (18)	No difference to aqueous cream [44]
Dry hands	10	Randomized, double-blind, bilateral, reference cream with 10% urea (30)	Both creams effective, the one with pH 6 preferred to the one with pH 3 [34]

investigated [8]. Two hundred and twenty-five hospital personnel were given two jars of cream, one with 3% urea and one without urea, and were requested to use one on each hand. Both the investigators and the patients experienced better results with the urea cream, in that the skin seemed softer, smoother and even whiter [8]. Patches of slight dermatitis were reported to improve by the application of urea cream [8]. However, in a more recent clinical study from 1973, on cracked, chapped hands, the effect from a 10% urea cream was not superior to that of aqueous cream [44].

In other types of dryness diseases, 3% urea has been shown to reduce the incidence and severity of radio-induced dermatitis, which is a frequent side effect of radiotherapy. Intensive use of the lotion doubled the likelihood that breast cancer patients will not developed radio-dermatitis during radiotherapy [60]. A urea/lactic acid-based topical keratolytic moisturizer did not prevent capecitabine-induced hand-foot syndrome in a double-blind, placebo-controlled trial [61].

33.6 Combinations with Corticosteroids

The beneficial effects of corticosteroids in inflammatory skin conditions are well known, but corticosteroids reduce barrier lipid synthesis and the density of corneodesmosomes, which leads to an increased skin sensitivity and a weakened cutaneous permeability barrier homeostasis [62–65]. Therefore, the combination of moisturizers with corticosteroids could be of clinical significance.

Urea has been studied in combination with steroids. In a recent study on hand eczema, a larger clinical benefit was obtained when the morning application of betamethasone was replaced by a 5% urea cream, i.e. once daily treatment with betamethasone combined with 5% urea cream was superior to twice daily application of betamethasone [66]. This finding was especially pronounced in the group of patients with moderate eczema at inclusion [66].

The addition of 10% urea to a betamethasone cream also gave superior results compared to the steroid cream alone in subacute atopic eczema [67]. Moreover, treatment with a 10% urea cream-containing hydrocortisone has been shown to be clinically better than treatment with other hydrocortisone preparations in a single-blind and bilateral study on 12 patients with atopic eczema [15]. All patients became more soft and smooth in the skin. A 4% urea cream in combination with hydrocortisone was also superior to an ordinary hydrocortisone cream in the treatment of dry eczema [38]. A combination of a 10% urea moisturizer and one hydrocortisone preparation with 10% urea was evaluated in an open, uncontrolled, multicenter study on 1,905 patients with atopic dermatitis [35]. Over the 12-month observational period, a total of 84% of the patients were exclusively treated with the two trial preparations, and only 16% required additional treatment with other corticosteroids.

33.7 Influences on Normal Skin Barrier Function by Urea

Urea is easily absorbed into normal skin [14, 21] and has been reported to promote the absorption of different drugs, for example, hydrocortisone, triamcinolone acetonide, dithranol and retinoic acid [68–73]. The penetration of ketoprofen through isolated rat skin was also enhanced by the addition of urea [72]. Furthermore, it has been shown that the time of onset of erythema, induced by hexyl nicotinate, is reduced by simultaneous exposure to an oily cream-containing urea [71].

However, not all studies support the belief that urea is an effective penetration promoter [22, 74–77]. For instance, the latency time to induce erythema was not changed by 3-weeks treatment with a moisturizer containing 5% urea [78] or by pretreatment of forearm skin with an aqueous solution of 10% urea [75]. Moreover, urea (10%) had a minimal effect on the penetration of hydrocortisone through excised human and guinea pig skin [74]. Hydrocortisone acetate was even retarded through hairless mouse skin with increasing concentrations of urea (up to 12%) [22].

Measurement of TEWL is another way to study the effect on skin barrier function by various treatments. In vitro measurements on piglet stratum corneum suggest that urea markedly decreases TEWL [77]. Studies on humans indicate that treatment for a limited number of days (1 to 2 days) with 5–10% urea may increase TEWL, whereas longer treatment periods (10–20 days) decrease TEWL, Table 33.4 [37, 79–81].

Measurements of TEWL have also been combined with skin challenge by an irritant (sodium lauryl sulphate, SLS) to elucidate possible changes in susceptibility to irritation [80, 81]. These studies show that the irritant reaction after exposure to SLS was significantly lower after urea treatment compared to the untreated skin [80, 81]. A decreased susceptibility to SLS was also noticed after three applications of both 5% and 10% urea moisturizers, although this decrease in susceptibility was not accompanied by a prior reduction in TEWL [80]. The improvement in skin barrier function has been confirmed in a placebo-controlled study, where a significantly lower TEWL and reduced susceptibility to SLS were found in the urea-treated skin compared to the placebo-treated skin [83]. However, no change in skin reactivity to nickel in sensitized individuals was found after 3-week treatment with 5% urea [79].

Hence, evidence exists for lowering of TEWL and decreased susceptibility to SLS of 4–10% urea in normal skin, Table 33.4. Evidence for changed susceptibility to other noxious substances is scarcer.

33.8 Changes in Skin Barrier Function in Diseased and Experimentally Damaged Skin

In several, but not in all studies on barrier damaged skin, urea has been shown to improve barrier function, Table 33.5. In ichthyotic skin, TEWL has been found to be slightly reduced by the application of 10% urea for 3 weeks [16]. Moreover, in patients with dry atopic skin, a 5% urea cream has been found to reduce TEWL on the back of the hands [46] and also to make skin less susceptible to irritation by SLS [48]. In

Table 33.4 Influence of urea treatment on skin barrier function in normal skin

Design (number of individuals)	Conc. %	No. of days of treatment	Marker of barrier function	Outcomes
Randomized, untreated control, blind evaluation (28)	5, cream	20	Time to erythema from hexyl nicotinate	No difference [78]
Bilateral, water control (10)	10, solution	One exposure	Time to erythema from benzyl nicotinate	No difference [75]
Not reported (20)	5, 10, cream	Simultaneous exposure	Time to erythema from hexyl nicotinate	Shorter from 10% [71]
Randomized, untreated control, blind evaluation (25)	5, cream	20	TEWL, nickel reactivity	Reduced TEWL, no change in reactivity [79]
Randomized, controlled, bilateral, double-blind vs. placebo (28)	5, lotion	14	TEWL, SLS reactivity	Reduced TEWL and reduced reactivity [83]
Randomized, untreated control, blind evaluation (12)	10, cream	20	TEWL, SLS reactivity	Reduced TEWL days 10 and 20. Reduced reactivity day 20 [80]
Randomized, untreated control, blind evaluation (14)	10, gel	20	TEWL, SLS reactivity	Reduced TEWL days 10 and 20. Reduced reactivity day 20 [80]
Randomized, untreated control, blind evaluation (13)	5, cream	14	TEWL, SLS reactivity	Reduced TEWL, reduced reactivity [81]
Randomized, double-blind (12)	5, gel	1,5	TEWL, SLS reactivity	Reduced TEWL, reduced reactivity [80]
Randomized, double-blind (12)	10, gel	1,5	TEWL, SLS reactivity	No change in TEWL, reduced reactivity [80]
Randomized, untreated control	5	49	TEWL, SLS reactivity	Increased TEWL and reactivity [82]
Randomized	5	49	TEWL, SLS reactivity	Decreased TEWL and reactivity [82]

Table 33.5 Influence of urea treatment on skin barrier function in dry skin disorders

Disorder	Design (number of patients)	Conc. %	No. of days of treatment	Outcomes
Psoriasis	Randomized, double-blind, bilateral (10)	10	14	Decrease, not significant [28]
Ichthyosis	RCT, double-blind, bilateral (14)	10	21	Reduced TEWL [16]
Atopics	Single-blind, 'placebo'-controlled (14)	10	7	Reduced TEWL [37]
Atopic	Randomized, parallel, double-blind, 4% urea reference (48)	5	30	Reduced TEWL [46]
Atopic	Randomized, parallel, three groups, glycerin-controlled (109)	4	30	Reduced TEWL [49]
Atopic	Randomized (22)	4	14	No change [84]
Dry skin	Randomized, untreated control, bilateral (23+24)	3, 10	21	No change from 3%, but 10% decreased [32]
Hyperkeratosis feet	Randomized, double-blind, bilateral, vs. 12% ammonium lactate (25)	40	14	No change in TEWL [56]

another double-blind study on atopic patients, a 4% urea formulation was superior to a 20% glycerin moisturizer in lowering TEWL [49]. Two days treatment of atopic patients with 10% urea cream tended to increase TEWL, which then significantly decreased after 7 days of treatment [37]. In dry skin of environmental origin, no influence on TEWL was noted after treatment with a 3% urea cream, whereas TEWL decreased in skin treated with 10% urea cream [32].

In SLS-damaged skin, a 5% urea cream has been shown to promote barrier recovery, measured as TEWL [81, 83]. Furthermore, in a placebo-controlled study, it has been shown that urea was responsible for the accelerated barrier recovery and decreased susceptibility to SLS [83]. Twice daily exposures to SLS and treatment with a 5% urea cream for 15 days induced a slight but significant barrier damage, measured as TEWL, but the urea-treated sites appeared less damaged than the vehicle-treated areas [83].

33.9 Prevention of Eczema

Atopic dermatitis affects health and quality of life and has great impact on both health-care costs and costs to the society. Health-care professionals emphasize the use of moisturizers in treating eczema, even when the eczema is cleared. However, to our knowledge, there is only one clinical study available where the preventative effect on the recurrence of eczema in atopic patients has been investigated [85]. In that study, the patients were instructed to use the 5% urea cream at least twice daily or abstain from using any moisturizer after clearance of the eczema with strong corticosteroid cream (betamethasone valerate). The time until recurrence of eczema was then measured during a maximum period of 6 months. Within a 6-month period, approximately 35% of the cream-treated patients reported eczema, whereas twice as many obtained eczema in the untreated group during the same time period. The medium number of eczema-free days was more than 180 in the cream group and 18 in the control group. The probability of not having a relapse during the 26-week period was 68% in the moisturizer group and 32% for those not using the moisturizer, which resulted in a 53% relative risk reduction and 36% absolute risk reduction. Whether a similar delay in the flare-up of eczema in atopics should have been noted with a moisturizer without barrier-improving properties has yet to be studied.

The costs for the maintenance treatment with the 5% urea cream have also been evaluated using a Markov simulation model. The results showed the maintenance treatment to be a cost-effective option compared with no treatment in eczema-free periods in adult patients with atopic dermatitis in the four Nordic countries [86].

In another clinical study, patients with hand eczema prolonged the time to eczema relapse by the use of a urea-containing cream [87]. The median time to relapse showed a tenfold difference between the urea moisturizer and no treatment (20 days vs. 2 days, respectively). The shorter time to relapse in the hand eczema patients compared to the atopic patients was likely due to the higher vulnerability of hands, which are frequently exposed to external stressors.

33.10 Discussion and Conclusion

Clinical studies demonstrate beneficial effects of urea-containing moisturizers in the treatment of dry skin conditions. Urea formulations are effective for the symptomatic relief of psoriasis, ichthyosis, dry atopic skin and senescent skin. Furthermore, evidence shows barrier-improving effects of urea in both normal and in dry skin disorders (atopic skin, ichthyosis). Since the barrier abnormality is considered a critical exacerbant of the dermatitis, urea-containing moisturizers may also reduce the prevalence of certain dermatitis by strengthening of the skin barrier function. This has also been proven in two clinical studies on a urea moisturizer, where the recurrence of eczema was delayed by the treatment.

However, conflicting results have been reported from clinical studies. These may be due to differences in the compositions of the urea formulations. Moisturizers show large variability in compositions, and not only the concentration of urea but also the types of emulsions and stabilizers differ between moisturizers. For example, pH and the formation of ammonia have to be taken into account in urea-containing products. Moreover, the content of emulsifiers, lipids, chelators and preservatives may influence the effect [88]. Failure to strengthen the barrier is most likely due to the impact on the skin from the other ingredients in the formulation.

Urea is a promising tool in the treatment of dry skin disorders; however, more work is needed to fully understand the mechanisms for its effects and to optimize its efficiency on the skin barrier function.

Take Home Messages

- A defect skin barrier function is considered to be a critical exacerbant of dermatitis.
- Moisturizing creams contain a great variety of ingredients and induce different types of effects on the skin structure and function.
- The content of the humectant urea in the stratum corneum is decreased in certain dry skin conditions.
- Topically applied urea influences the expression of enzymes in the skin and the epidermal proliferation.
- Urea has been reported to be a penetration enhancer but also to retard penetration.
- A urea-containing moisturizer has been shown to prevent relapse of eczema in atopic patients and in those with hand eczema.
- The maintenance treatment with the moisturizing cream during eczema-free periods in patients with atopic dermatitis has been found cost-effective compared with no treatment in the four Nordic countries.

References

1. Palmer CN et al (2006) Common loss-of-function variants of the epidermal barrier protein filaggrin are a major predisposing factor for atopic dermatitis. Nat Genet 38(4):441–446
2. Weidinger S et al (2006) Loss-of-function variations within the filaggrin gene predispose for atopic dermatitis with allergic sensitizations. J Allergy Clin Immunol 118(1):214–219
3. Rawlings AV, Harding CR (2004) Moisturization and skin barrier function. Dermatol Ther 17(Suppl 1):43–48
4. Candi E, Schmidt R, Melino G (2005) The cornified envelope: a model of cell death in the skin. Nat Rev Mol Cell Biol 6(4):328–340
5. Ginger RS et al (2005) Filaggrin repeat number polymorphism is associated with a dry skin phenotype. Arch Dermatol Res 297(6):235–241
6. Taieb A (1999) Hypothesis: from epidermal barrier dysfunction to atopic disorders. Contact Dermatitis 41(4):177–180

7. Elias PM, Wood LC, Feingold KR (1999) Epidermal pathogenesis of inflammatory dermatoses. Am J Contact Dermat 10(3):119–126
8. Rattner H (1943) Use of urea in hand creams. Arch Dermatol Syph 48:47–49
9. Ashton H, Frenk E, Stevenson CJ (1971) Therapeutics XIII. Urea as a topical agent. Br J Dermatol 84: 194–196
10. Sweetman SC (ed) (2005) Martindale: the complete drug reference. Pharmaceutical Press, London
11. Rosten M (1970) The treatment of ichthyosis and hyperkeratotic conditions with urea. Australas J Dermatol 11:142–144
12. Jacobi OK (1959) Moisture regulation in the skin. Drug Cosmet Ind 84:732–812
13. Kezic S et al (2011) Levels of filaggrin degradation products are influenced by both filaggrin genotype and atopic dermatitis severity. Allergy 66(7): 934–940
14. Wellner K, Wohlrab W (1993) Quantitative evaluation of urea in stratum corneum of human skin. Arch Dermatol Res 285:239–240
15. Swanbeck G (1968) A new treatment of ichthyosis and other hyperkeratotic conditions. Acta Derm Venereol Suppl (Stockh) 48:123–127
16. Grice K, Sattar H, Baker H (1973) Urea and retinoic acid in ichthyosis and their effect on transepidermal water loss and water holding capacity of stratum corneum. Acta Derm Venereol Suppl (Stockh) 54: 114–118
17. CIR Expert Panel. (2005) Final report of the safety assessment of urea. Int J Toxicol 24(Suppl 3): 1–56
18. Hellgren L, Larsson K (1974) On the effect of urea on human epidermis. Dermatologica 149:89–93
19. Kunz D, Brassfield TS (1971) Hydration of macromolecules. II. Effects of urea on protein hydration. Arch Biochem Biophys 142:660–664
20. Farber EM, South DA (1978) Urea ointment in the nonsurgical avulsion of nail dystrophies. Cutis 22: 689–692
21. Lodén M, Bostrom P, Kneczke M (1995) Distribution and keratolytic effect of salicylic acid and urea in human skin. Skin Pharmacol 8(4):173–178
22. Bentley MVLB et al (1997) The influence of lecithin and urea on the in vitro permeation of hydrocortisone acetate through skin from hairless mouse. Int J Pharm 146:255–262
23. Costa-Balogh FO et al (2006) How small polar molecules protect membrane systems against osmotic stress: the urea-water-phospholipid system. J Phys Chem B 110(47):23845–23852
24. Blair C (1976) The action of a urea-lactic acid ointment in ichthyosis. With particular reference to the thickness of the horny layer. Br J Dermatol 94: 145–153
25. Borelli C et al (2011) Cream or foam in pedal skin care: towards the ideal vehicle for urea used against dry skin. Int J Cosmet Sci 33(1):37–43
26. Wohlrab W, Schiemann S (1976) Investigations on the mechanism of the activity of urea upon the epidermis [author's transl]. Arch Dermatol Res 255(1):23–30
27. Wohlrab W, Bohm W (1975) Reaction of epidermis after long-term action of urea. Dermatologica 151(3):149–157
28. Hagemann I, Proksch E (1996) Topical treatment by urea reduces epidermal hyperproliferation and induces differentiation in psoriasis. Acta Derm Venereol Suppl (Stockh) 76:353–356
29. Sugiura H et al (2005) Large-scale DNA microarray analysis of atopic skin lesions shows overexpression of an epidermal differentiation gene cluster in the alternative pathway and lack of protective gene expression in the cornified envelope. Br J Dermatol 152(1):146–149
30. Hirao T et al (2003) Ratio of immature cornified envelopes does not correlate with parakeratosis in inflammatory skin disorders. Exp Dermatol 12(5): 591–601
31. Buraczewska I, 2 et al (2009) Long-term treatment with moisturizers affects keratinocyte differentiation and desquamation on the mRNA level. Arch Dermatol Res 301:175–181 [Epub 2008 Oct 11]
32. Serup J (1992) A double-blind comparison of two creams containing urea as the active ingredient. Assessment of efficacy and side-effects by non-invasive techniques and a clinical scoring scheme. Acta Derm Venereol 177:34–43
33. Agner T (1992) An experimental study of irritant effects of urea in different vehicles. Acta Derm Venereol Suppl (Stockh) 177:44–46
34. Fredriksson T, Gip L (1975) Urea creams in the treatment of dry skin and hand dermatitis. Int J Dermatol 32:442–444
35. Burkard G, Schmitt S (1992) Langzeitstudie Neurodermitis-Therapie mit harnstoffhaltigen externa. Hautarzt 43:13–17
36. Lodén M, Andersson A-C, Lindberg M (1999) The effect of two urea-containing creams on dry, eczematous skin in atopic patients. II. Adverse effects. J Dermatolog Treat 10:171–175
37. Pigatto PD et al (1996) 10% urea cream (Laceran) for atopic dermatitis: a clinical and laboratory evaluation. J Dermatolog Treat 7:171–175
38. Frithz A (1983) Investigation of Cortesal®, a hydrocortisone cream and its water-retaining cream base in the treatment of xerotic skin and dry eczemas. Curr Ther Res 33:930–935
39. Gabard B, Nook T, Muller KH (1991) Tolerance of the lesioned skin to dermatological formulations. J Appl Cosmetol 9:25–30
40. Frosch PJ, Kligman AM (1977) A method for appraising the stinging capacity of topically applied substances. J Soc Cosmet Chem 28(28):197–209
41. De Groot AC et al (1988) Adverse effects of cosmetics and toiletries: a retrospective study in the general population. Int J Dermatol Sci 9:255–259

42. Horii Y et al (2011) Skin application of urea-containing cream affected cutaneous arterial sympathetic nerve activity, blood flow, and water evaporation. Skin Res Technol 17(1):75–81
43. Taube KM (1992) Moisture retaining effect and tolerance of urea-containing Externa in neurodermatitis patients. Hautarzt 43(Suppl 11):30–32 [Article in German]
44. Baillie ATK et al (1973) General practitioner research group. Carbamide in hyperkeratosis. Report no 179. Practitioner 210:294–296
45. Bohnsack K et al (1997) Wirksamkeit auf das symptom 'trockene haut' und langzeitverträglichkeit von Laceran lotion 10% urea bei patienten mit atopischem ekzem. Z Hautkr 72:34–39
46. Andersson A-C, Lindberg M, Lodén M (1999) The effect of two urea-containing creams on dry, eczematous skin in atopic patients. I. Expert, patient and instrumental evaluation. J Dermatolog Treat 10: 165–169
47. Bissonnette R et al (2010) A double-blind study of tolerance and efficacy of a new urea-containing moisturizer in patients with atopic dermatitis. J Cosmet Dermatol 9(1):16–21
48. Lodén M, Andersson A-C, Lindberg M (1999) Improvement in skin barrier function in patients with atopic dermatitis after treatment with a moisturizing cream (Canoderm®). Br J Dermatol 140:264–267
49. Lodén M et al (2001) Instrumental and dermatologist evaluation of the effect of glycerine and urea on dry skin in atopic dermatitis. Skin Res Technol 7(4): 209–213
50. Sasaki Y, Tadaki T, Tagami H (1989) The effects of a topical application of urea cream on the function of pathological stratum corneum. Acta Dermatol Kyoto 84(1989):581
51. Pope FM et al (1972) Out-patient treatment of ichthyosis: a double-blind trial of ointments. Br J Dermatol 86:291–296
52. Kuster W et al (1998) Efficacy of urea therapy in children with ichthyosis. A multicenter randomized, placebo-controlled, double-blind, semilateral study. Dermatology 196:217–222
53. Schölermann A et al (1999) Wirksamkeit und verträglichkeit von Eucerin salbe 10% urea bei xerotischer altershau.: Ergebnisse einer vehikel-kontrollierten klinischen doppelblindstudie. Z Hautkr 74:557–562
54. Schölermann A et al (1998) Efficacy and safety of Eucerin 10% urea lotion in the treatment of symptoms of aged skin. J Dermatolog Treat 9:175–179
55. Kuzmina N, Hagstromer L, Emtestam L (2002) Urea and sodium chloride in moisturisers for skin of the elderly – a comparative, double-blind, randomised study. Skin Pharmacol Appl Skin Physiol 15(3):166–174
56. Ademola J et al (2002) Clinical evaluation of 40% urea and 12% ammonium lactate in the treatment of xerosis. Am J Clin Dermatol 3:217–222
57. Pham HT et al (2002) A prospective, randomized, controlled double-blind study of a moisturizer for xerosis of the feet in patients with diabetes. Ostomy Wound Manage 48(5):30–36
58. Sadick NS et al (2010) Efficacy and safety of a new topical keratolytic treatment for localized hyperkeratosis in adults. J Drugs Dermatol 9(12):1512–1517
59. Goldstein JA, Gurge RM (2008) Treatment of hyperkeratosis with Kerafoam emollient foam (30% urea) to assess effectiveness and safety within a clinical setting: a case study report. J Drugs Dermatol 7(2): 159–162
60. Pardo Masferrer J et al (2010) Prophylaxis with a cream containing urea reduces the incidence and severity of radio-induced dermatitis. Clin Transl Oncol 12(1):43–48
61. Wolf SL et al (2010) Placebo-controlled trial to determine the effectiveness of a urea/lactic acid-based topical keratolytic agent for prevention of capecitabine-induced hand-foot syndrome: North Central Cancer Treatment Group Study N05C5. J Clin Oncol 28(35):5182–5187
62. Demerjian M et al (2009) Activators of PPARs and LXR decrease the adverse effects of exogenous glucocorticoids on the epidermis. Exp Dermatol 18(7): 643–649
63. Jensen JM et al (2009) Different effects of pimecrolimus and betamethasone on the skin barrier in patients with atopic dermatitis. J Allergy Clin Immunol 124(3 Suppl 2):R19–R28
64. Kao JS et al (2003) Short-term glucocorticoid treatment compromises both permeability barrier homeostasis and stratum corneum integrity: inhibition of epidermal lipid synthesis accounts for functional abnormalities. J Invest Dermatol 120(3): 456–464
65. Kolbe L et al (2001) Corticosteroid-induced atrophy and barrier impairment measured by non-invasive methods in human skin. Skin Res Technol 7(2): 73–77
66. Loden M et al (2011) The effect of a corticosteroid cream and a barrier-strengthening moisturizer in hand eczema. A double-blind, randomized, prospective, parallel group clinical trial. J Eur Acad Dermatol Venereol. doi:10.1111/j.1468-3083.2011.04128.x [Epub ahead of print]
67. Hindson MTC (1971) Urea in the topical treatment of atopic eczema. Arch Dermatol 104:284–285
68. Wohlrab W (1990) The influence of urea on the penetration kinetics of vitamin-A-acid into human skin. Z Hautkr 65:803–805
69. Wohlrab W (1984) The influence of urea on the penetration kinetics of topically applied corticosteroids. Acta Derm Venereol 64(3):233–238
70. Wohlrab W (1989) Significance of urea in external therapy. Hautarzt 40(Suppl 9):35–41
71. Beastall J et al (1986) The influence of urea on percutaneous absorption. Pharm Res 3:294–297

72. Kim CK et al (1993) Effect of fatty acids and urea on the penetration of ketoprofen through rat skin. Int J Pharm 99:109–118
73. Allenby AC et al (1969) Mechanism of action of accelerants on skin penetration. Br J Dermatol 81(suppl 4):47–55
74. Wahlberg JE, Swanbeck G (1973) The effect of urea and lactic acid on the percutaneous absorption of hydrocortisone. Acta Derm Venereol 53(3): 207–210
75. Lippold BC, Hackemuller D (1990) The influence of skin moisturizers on drug penetration in vivo. Int J Pharm 61:205–211
76. Stuttgen G (1989) Penetrationsförderung lokal applizierter Wirkstoffe durch Harnstoff. Hautarzt 40(Suppl 9):27–31
77. McCallion R, Po ALW (1994) Modelling transepidermal water loss under steady-state and non-steady-state relative humidities. Int J Pharm 105:103–112
78. Duval D et al (2002) Differences among moisturizers in affecting skin susceptibility to hexyl nicotinate, measured as time to increase skin blood flow. Skin Res Technol 8:1–5
79. Kuzmina N et al (2004) Effects of pre-treatment an emollient containing urea on nickel allergic skin reactions. Acta Derm Venereol 84:1–4
80. Lodén M (1996) Urea-containing moisturizers influence barrier properties of normal skin. Arch Dermatol Res 288(2):103–107
81. Lodén M (1997) Barrier recovery and influence of irritant stimuli in skin treated with a moisturizing cream. Contact Dermatitis 36(5):256–260
82. Buraczewska I et al (2007) Changes in skin barrier function following long-term treatment with moisturizers, a randomized controlled trial. Br J Dermatol 156(3):492–498
83. Lodén M et al (2004) The influence of urea treatment on skin susceptibility to surfactant-induced irritation: a placebo-controlled and randomized study. Exogen Dermatol 3:1–6
84. Hagströmer L, Nyrén M, Emtestam L (2001) Do urea and sodium chloride together increase the efficacy of moisturizers for atopic dermatitis skin. A comparative, double-blind and randomised study. Skin Pharmacol Appl Skin Physiol 14:27–33
85. Wirén K et al. (2009) Treatment with a barrier-strengthening moisturizing cream delays relapse of atopic dermatitis. A prospective and randomized controlled clinical trial. JEADV, 23:1267–1272.
86. Hjalte F, Asseburg C, Tennvall GR (2010) Cost-effectiveness of a barrier-strengthening moisturizing cream as maintenance therapy vs. no treatment after an initial steroid course in patients with atopic dermatitis in Sweden – with model applications for Denmark, Norway and Finland. J Eur Acad Dermatol Venereol 24(4):474–480
87. Loden M et al (2010) Treatment with a barrier-strengthening moisturizer prevents relapse of hand-eczema. An open, randomized, prospective, parallel group study. Acta Derm Venereol 90(6):602–606
88. Lodén M (2003) Role of topical emollients and moisturizers in the treatment of dry skin barrier disorders. Am J Clin Dermatol 4(11):771–788

34 Urea and Skin: A Well-Known Molecule Revisited

Alessandra Marini, Jean Krutmann, and Susanne Grether-Beck

34.1 The Importance of Urea in Topical Treatment

Since topical treatment is fundamental to maintain skin functions and to treat skin diseases, many strategies have been developed to repair the barrier or prevent barrier dysfunction. However, many patients overlook the importance of moisturizers considering them not real treatments. Patient adherence and compliance is a great challenge faced in the management of skin diseases. Strong odor, low pH, and sensory reactions may reduce patient acceptance [1]. Urea has been used for over a century in topical preparation to improve the surface properties of human skin in strengths ranging from 3% to 50% including cream, lotion, shampoo, gel, gel stick, wipe, emulsion, solution, suspension, spray, ointment, paste, foam, and shower/bath wash [2]. Side effects of urea are mild and may include cutaneous eruptions, stinging, irritation, and allergic contact dermatitis [3]. In addition to urea, other humectants include amino acids, propylene glycol, and glycerin. The chemical and physical characteristics of the individual ingredients determine the performance of the formulation and their influence on the superficial and deep layers of the skin [1]. Large differences exist between the different moisturizers. Leite and coworkers [4] evaluate *in vivo stratum corneum* hydration after treatment with different moisturizers presented in gel base. In this study, urea, a herbal extract from *Imperata cylindrical*, the components of the natural moisturizing factors, and carbohydrate derivate compound such as xylitylglucoside, anhydroxylitol, and xylitol were used as active substances. The gel-containing urea and the carbohydrate derivate compound gel promoted the most intense moisture effect compared with the other formulations [4].

Penetration of the moisturizers in the layers of the *stratum corneum* is also dependent on the vehicle. The galenics play an important role, and an unbalanced composition can lead to poor results [5]. Savica and coworkers [6] showed that barrier-improving and hydrating abilities of urea are bidirectional and dependent on the appropriate vehicle and the state of skin. Moreover, if the moisturizers are used in not appropriate quantities, they will have limited value. During the years, a variety of studies have assessed the utility of urea in a variety of different formulations. In addition, new vehicles have been developed to make urea more cosmetically acceptable. Moreover, studies supporting the beneficial effects of urea have been performed. In a 3-h short-term test and in a 7-day long-term test, Taube [5]

A. Marini, M.D. • J. Krutmann, M.D. (✉) •
S. Grether-Beck, Ph.D.
IUF – Leibniz Research Institute for Environmental Medicine at the Heinrich-Heine-University Düsseldorf, Auf'm Hennekamp 50, D-40225 Düsseldorf, Germany
e-mail: alessandra.marini@uni-duesseldorf.de; krutmann@uni-duesseldorf.de; grether-beck@uni-duesseldorf.de

M. Lodén, H.I. Maibach (eds.), *Treatment of Dry Skin Syndrome*,
DOI 10.1007/978-3-642-27606-4_34, © Springer-Verlag Berlin Heidelberg 2012

assessed the moisture level of the corneal layer and showed that urea in hydrous topical agents ensures acceleration of corneal hydration and helps retain water in the corneal layer. A significant increase in skin moisture and an improvement in skin's smoothness after application of a urea-containing cream were noticed in a large number of volunteers with healthy skin and in atopic dermatitis patients compared with untreated skin and with the placebo [7].Treatment of 25 patients with moderate to severe xerosis shows that an improvement of the skin is achieved quicker with 40% urea cream than with 12% ammonium lactate lotion [8]. A 40% urea emulsion in a vehicle system containing *Butyrospermum parkii* fruit oil, *Helianthus annuus* oil, glycine soja sterol, and stearic acid significantly improves barrier function in the *stratum corneum* after tape stripping [9]. Used in women presenting with a chronically dry, rough, thick, scaly skin, this preparation decreased roughness, pigmentation, and microtopography of the legs with no reports of side effects [10]. A 40% urea foam formulation reduced the signs and symptoms associated with dry skin [11]. Based on the patient assessment, urea foam formulation increased acceptance and patients compliance because of the attributes: creaminess, lack of oiliness, lack of stickiness, ease of rub in, and overall feel [12].

34.2 Urea and Skin Diseases: Overview of Clinical Studies

Urea has been shown useful in treating many skin diseases (Fig. 34.1). Urea is a natural compound synthesized mainly in the liver serving to excrete nitrogen via the kidneys. In addition, urea is also found in the outermost layer of skin as part of the natural moisturizing factor consisting besides urea of amino acids, their derivatives, lactic acid, sugars, and pyrrolidone carboxylic acid [13–15].

Healthy epidermis presents a concentration of urea of about 28 μg per square inch, while in xerotic skin the urea concentration is cut in half, in psoriatic and in actively atopic skin is decreased by 40% and by 85%, respectively [2]. During the years, a variety of studies have assessed the utility of urea as a moisturizer, keratinolytic product and as an extraordinary therapeutic agent for different skin disorders such as atopic dermatitis, psoriasis, and ichthyosis in a variety of formulations [16]. Corticosteroids represent the standard treatment for a wide range of inflammatory and proliferative dermatoses; urea is often added as important treatment adjunct. Stüttgen used for the treatment of 1,905 patients ranging from small children to adults suffering from atopic dermatitis a combination of urea and hydrocortisone to treat acute attacks and urea ointment for the chronic therapy [17]. Eighty-four percent of the patients showed good to very good results. Urea is often added to a variety of formulations to enhance their effects. Emollients can damage the *stratum corneum* and lead to desiccation and a disturbance of the barrier [18]. The damaging effect of O/W emulsions, which dry the skin, can be reduced by the addition of urea and glycerol [18].

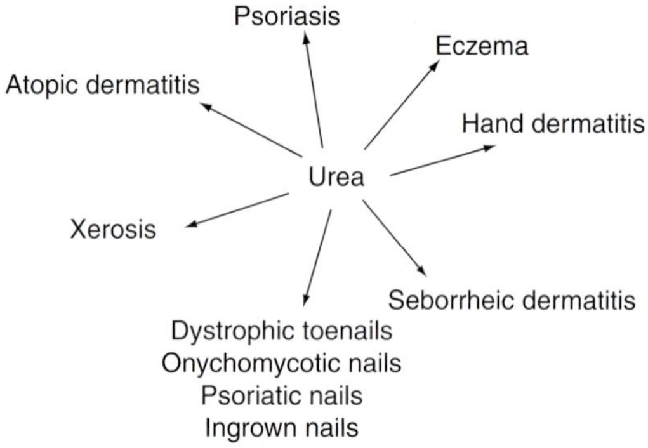

Fig. 34.1 Urea: a therapeutic agent for many skin disorders. Urea has been shown useful in treating many skin diseases. Some of those are schematic summarized

Urea has been used to treat hand dermatitis [19], scalp seborrheic dermatitis [20], and psoriasis [21]. Topical treatment by 10% urea significantly reduces epidermal hyperproliferation and induces differentiation in plaque type psoriasis versus the vehicle treatment in ten patients [21]. Küster [22] shows that 10% urea lotion has a strong positive effect on generalized ichthyotic keratinization disorders in childhood in a multicenter randomized, placebo-controlled, double-blind, semilateral study. Accordingly, 60 children between 1 and 16 years were treated with 10% urea lotion over 8 weeks. The response rates were 65% after 4 weeks and 78% after 8 weeks for 10% urea lotion, 50% after 4 weeks and 72% after 8 weeks for the urea-free lotion base [22]. Topical urea is useful for the debridement and promotion of normal healing of hyperkeratotic surface lesions [2]. In a prospective, randomized, controlled double-blind study, enrolling 40 patients a moisturizer for xerosis of the feet in patients with diabetes was studied [23]. The verum consisting of 10% urea and 4% lactic acid in patients with diabetes provided faster and better improvement after 4 weeks of treatment. In addition, significantly less xerosis regression than its emulsion base was determined after 2 weeks following discontinuation of the treatments [23]. Borelli [24] evaluated different urea-containing cosmetic preparations designed for foot care in diabetic patients reporting that the cream vehicles would be the better choice compared to the foam formulation. The first study in which the potential of a moisturizer to prevent relapse of hand eczema in patients with a controlled state of their eczema was addressed has been examined in 1943. Urea-containing moisturizer was found to be superior to a urea-free cream in inducing softer, smoother, and even whiter hands in 225 hospital personnel [25]. Since then, a large number of studies on the efficacy of moisturizers in the treatment of dry skin have been published. Wirén [26] demonstrated that maintenance treatment with a barrier-improving urea moisturizer on previous eczematous areas reduced the risk of relapse to approximately one third of that of no treatment. Recently, Lodén [27] investigated the time to relapse of eczema during treatment with a barrier-strengthening moisturizer (5% urea) in 53 randomized patients with successfully treated hand eczema. In this study, application of urea-containing moisturizer seems to prolong the disease-free interval in patients with controlled hand eczema [27].

Urea has been used in topical preparation in strengths ranging from 1% to 50%. In lower concentrations of 1–20%, urea acts as a humectant and has the most cosmetic benefits. In higher concentrations, urea also has concentration-dependent keratolytic effects. Products with urea concentrations of 40–50% often cannot be tolerated by the bodies and serve as a debriding agent in diseases such as dystrophic toenails, onychomycotic nails, psoriatic nails, and ingrown nails [2, 28, 29]. In this chapter, only a few studies are mentioned despite the great variety of research assessing the utility of urea. In summary, urea represents in the right concentration, quantity and vehicle an extraordinary therapeutic agent for skin disorders.

34.3 Molecular Approaches to Understand the Effects of Urea on Skin

It is widely assumed that urea acts by virtue of its capacity as a natural moisturizing factor [14, 30, 31]. Recent findings, however, indicate that urea may have more pronounced effects in the skin than previously considered. Accordingly, we have shown that this well-known molecule possesses gene regulatory activities and affects mRNA expression of certain genes involved in keratinocyte differentiation which can be used to enhance barrier function and innate immunity of human skin especially in patients suffering from atopic dermatitis [32].

According to the so-called brick and mortar model of permeability barrier in the *stratum corneum*, protein-enriched corneocytes are embedded in a continuous lipid-enriched, intercellular matrix [33]. The constantly renewing epidermis is formed via a differentiation process where constantly dividing basal keratinocytes form asymmetric daughter cells: one daughter cell retains stem cell characteristics and one daughter cell joins the pathway towards differentiation moving from the basal layer at the innermost location to the *stratum corneum* at the outermost layer of the epidermis. During this process of differentiation, the nucleus of keratinocytes degenerates and large keratin macromolecules align in parallel to the keratinocyte membrane and cross-linking enzymes interconnect the various proteins to the cell membranes creating the so-called cornified envelope. While differentiating, the cells change morphology from a small and round shape to a larger size and even more dramatic change their metabolic activity. Genes encoding proteins being used for creation of the fully keratinized epidermis—such as involucrin, loricrin, filaggrin, and transglutaminase 1—start to be expressed in the spinous layer during this differentiation process [34]. Involucrin, one of the earliest markers of terminal differentiation, serves as a scaffolding component of the cornified envelope structure, which replaces as a complex protein-lipid composite the plasma membrane of terminally differentiated keratinocytes and originates from the cross-linkage of precursor proteins including involucrin, small proline rich proteins, and loricrin. Transglutaminase 1 serves as a membrane-bound keratinocyte specific transglutaminase which is largely responsible for the cross-linking of involucrin and loricrin to form the cornified envelope.

Antimicrobial peptides such as LL-37 processed from cathelicidin and β-defensin-2, which are expressed in the outer layers of human epidermis and secreted into the *stratum corneum* interstices, are an evolutionarily conserved component of the innate immune response. β-defensins are small cysteine-rich cationic proteins expressed by leucocytes and keratinocytes and can form pore-like membrane defects in bacteria, fungi, and many viruses. From this location in the *stratum corneum* interstices, they are positioned to interdict invading pathogens. Importantly, at least LL-37 is also necessary for normal permeability barrier function, demonstrating the convergence of these two critical defense functions [33, 35].

Urea appears to be a highly active substance; it stimulates epidermal differentiation and lipid synthesis and increases the synthesis of antimicrobial peptides in the epidermis which in turn helps to reinforce skin's immune system [32]. Accordingly, in vitro stimulation of primary human epidermal keratinocytes with physiological doses of urea in the low millimolar range induced an increased transcriptional expression of transglutaminase 1, involucrin, filaggrin, and loricrin, i.e., genes, which play an important role in keratinocyte differentiation, and the antimicrobial peptides β-defensin-2 and the LL-37 precursor cathelicidin, which are expressed in the outer layers of the epidermis [36]. In addition, expression of enzymes involved in sphingolipid metabolism such as serine palmitoyltransferase ½ and acidic sphingomyelinase, and also the rate-controlling enzyme of the cholesterol synthesis 3-hydroxy-3-methylglutaryl-CoA reductase were found to be upregulated. Essentially identical data were obtained if normal human skin was topically treated with urea in a vehicle-controlled, double-blinded study enrolling 21 volunteers with healthy skin once daily during 4 weeks. Accordingly, 10% urea treatment caused a significant upregulation of skin differentiation markers such as transglutaminase 1, involucrin, filaggrin, and loricrin on the mRNA level versus untreated and, more importantly, versus vehicle-treated skin. In addition, a significant increase of cathelicidin and β-defensin-2 mRNA was observed in the same samples versus untreated and vehicle-treated skin. Moreover, histochemical analysis of the named markers on the protein level and of total lipid content also indicated an increase upon treatment with 10% urea as compared to the vehicle treatment. These changes on the molecular level were determined on the buttock of the volunteers. Skin physiological parameters such as the gold standard for barrier function that is transepidermal water loss were measured on the volar forearm. While a 10% urea treatment only resulted in a slight decrease of transepidermal water loss, a 20% urea treatment significantly diminished this parameter for skin barrier function.

The mechanism underlying these gene regulatory activities was found to be specific. Urea-induced gene regulation was not due to a urea-induced osmotic stress response [37, 38], but mediated by specific urea transporters [32]. In many cells, exogenous urea is taken up by specific urea transporters (UT). Two genes specific for these transporters have been identified in mammals, the renal UT-A (*slc14a2*) subfamily, and the erythrocyte UT-B (*slc14a1*) family [39], both expressing several isoforms. Grether-Beck et al. showed that normal human keratinocytes take up urea via a specific mechanism involving UTA1 and UTA2 and that urea uptake increased the expression of those urea transporters [32]. Hints that besides these urea transporters *senso stricto*, also other transporters might be involved in urea uptake in keratinocytes came from experiments where uptake of radio-labelled urea could only be partially inhibited by classic inhibitors of urea uptake such as thiourea and phloretin. In this context, we have to remind that urea can also be transported by a subgroup of the water-transporting aquaporin family, the so-called aquaglyceroporins which can be inhibited by mercury or copper [40]. Accordingly, basal human keratinocytes express mainly UTA1,

UTA2, and aquaglyceroporin 3, while expression of aquaglyceroporins 7 and 9 plays only a minor role [32]. Evidence for the functional relevance of these transporters for urea-induced skin differentiation and expression of antimicrobial peptides comes from inhibitor experiments where urea-induced upregulation of skin differentiation markers and antimicrobial peptides was assessed in the presence of thiourea, phloretin, mercury, or copper. Interestingly, urea-induced upregulation of the skin differentiation markers transglutaminase 1, involucrin, filaggrin, and loricrin could completely be inhibited by thiourea or phloretin but only partially by mercury and copper. In contrast, urea-induced mRNA expression of cathelicidin or β-defensin-2 was decreased by about 50% no matter which of the named inhibitors has been employed [36].

Involucrin and loricrin mRNA and protein expression are diminished in affected, but also in unaffected skin of atopic dermatitis patients [41]. The observations from Grether-Beck provide a rational for the beneficial effects of urea treatment in atopic dermatitis and other skin diseases. Interestingly, filaggrin expression showed the strongest upregulation upon urea treatment as compared to transglutaminase 1, filaggrin, and loricrin [32]. Loss-of-function mutations in the profilaggrin gene are associated with ichthyosis vulgaris and atopic dermatitis [42]. Mildner demonstrated that knockdown of filaggrin expression in an organotypic skin model reproduced epidermal alterations caused by filaggrin mutations in vivo. Filaggrin-deficient skin models presented a loss of keratohyalin granules, impaired lamellar body formation, and a disturbed barrier function [42]. In order to address whether urea might be helpful in atopic conditions, this molecule has been topically applied on a murine hairless mouse atopic dermatitis model. In this model, atopic dermatitis-like dermatoses can be generated by nine to ten repeated oxazolone challenges resulting among others in permeability barrier abnormality and a decrease in antimicrobial peptides such as murine cathelin-related antimicrobial peptide and mouse β-defensin-2 (the murine homologues to human cathelicidin and β-defensin-2) [36]. Interestingly, concurrent treatment of mice with vehicle and hapten challenges was not able to reverse the expected decline in expression of antimicrobial peptides, while 20% urea normalized cathelin-related antimicrobial peptide and mouse β-defensin-2 expression. In addition, 10% and 20% urea significantly improved *stratum corneum* hydration and barrier function assessed as transepidermal water loss [36].

As already mentioned before, the urea content in the *stratum corneum* is significantly decreased in patients suffering from atopic dermatitis [2, 43]. An indirect approach to overcome this deficit was performed by Haustein and colleagues in a placebo-controlled, blinded study [43]. They treated 16 patients with chronic atopic eczema with either 2.5% arginine hydrochloride or the corresponding vehicle and compared urea content in *stratum corneum*, hydration, and transepidermal water loss before and after a 4 weeks twice daily treatment [43]. The rationale for this study is based on the fact that keratinocytes express an extrahepatic arginase, which allows keratinocytes to synthesize urea themselves from l-arginine [44]. Accordingly, a transient but significant increase of urea content within the *stratum corneum* in arginine hydrochloride but not in vehicle-treated patients with atopic eczema was observed. With regard to hydration and transepidermal water loss, verum treatment reached a significant increase already after 2 weeks, while vehicle treatment did not reach significance prior to 4 weeks.

In addition, it might be of value to combine low doses of urea such as 5% with other actives to improve skin physiology in patients suffering from dry skin. Accordingly, we could demonstrate that the improved skin hydration and the decreased transepidermal water loss obtained with a 5% urea oil-in-water cream could be significantly further increased when ceramides and vitamins have been added [45]. On a molecular level, both preparations caused in these 10 volunteers a significantly increased expression of the genes encoding involucrin, loricrin, and filaggrin [45].

The studies by Grether-Beck analyze the mechanism of action of urea from a new point of view and show that urea has more effects in the skin than previously thought. Its beneficial effects are not only due to a passive role as moisturizers but also due to its capacity to modulate keratinocyte gene expression and in that way to actively improve the properties of human skin. The effects and the mechanisms of action of urea on the skin are complex and need to be further investigated in future studies.

The mechanistic effects discussed above provide a rationale for the described action that urea reduces transepidermal water loss, an effect which cannot be explained by urea acting as a natural moisturizing factor.

Accordingly, 47 patients presenting with a dry skin were treated over 3 weeks with 3% and 10% urea cream. Both formulations were found efficient, resulting in improvement of hydration and reduction of scaling. Of interest, in skin treated with 10% urea cream, the transepidermal water loss decreased, indicating an improved water barrier function [31]. In double-blinded studies, moisturizers with urea have been shown to reduce transepidermal water loss in atopic and ichthyotic patients and to make skin less susceptible against irritation to sodium lauryl sulfate [1, 46–48]. Lodén evaluated the influence of different moisturizers on normal skin barrier properties by measuring transepidermal water loss, skin capacitance, and skin reactivity to the topically applied surfactant, sodium lauryl sulfate [47]. Treatment with two urea-containing moisturizers decreased transepidermal water loss and the irritant reactions after exposure to sodium lauryl sulfate. Skin capacitance increased after three applications of urea-containing moisturizers and was still increased after 10 days, but not after 20 days of this treatment [47]. Treatment for 20 days with two moisturizers without urea did not influence either transepidermal water loss or the susceptibility to irritation from sodium lauryl sulfate, but it increased the skin capacitance significantly [47]. In 1999, 15 patients with atopic dermatitis were treated twice daily for 20 days with a 5% urea cream. Skin capacitance and transepidermal water loss increased by the treatment, and the skin susceptibility to sodium lauryl sulfate was significantly reduced [49]. A non-detergent urea emulsion cleanser and a detergent cleanser with added moisturizers were compared for their effects on *stratum corneum* moisture, surface lipids, and transepidermal water loss of atopic skin [50]. Following a single wash with either cleanser, low corneometry and sebumetry values increased and elevated transepidermal water loss values decreased. The changes gradually return to their starting points after more than 6 h, but those induced by the urea emulsion lasted significantly longer than those caused by the detergent cleanser [50].

Topical urea can be used successfully in a variety of different preparations to improve the barrier function of the skin, alone or in combination. The application of the combination preparation containing urea, vitamins, and ceramides was significantly superior to the urea-only preparation in respect to reduction of transepidermal water loss and skin hydration levels [45]. In Fig. 34.2, most of the beneficial effects observed after urea treatment are depicted.

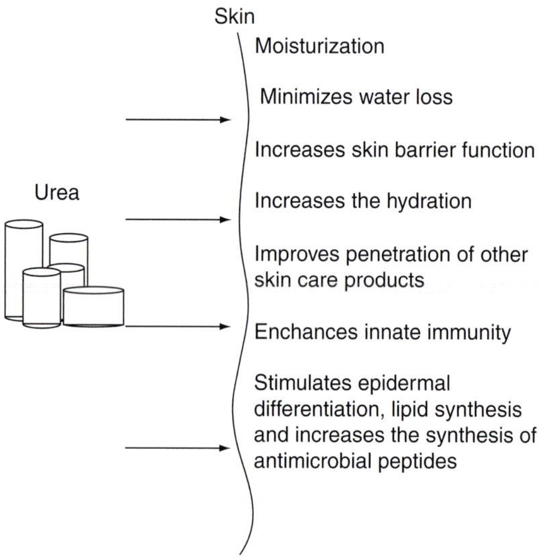

Fig. 34.2 Beneficial effects of urea. Urea is a natural moisturizing factor; creating a barrier that prevents transepidermal water loss urea helps to increase the hydration of the skin and the skin barrier function. Urea is a highly active substance; it possesses gene regulatory activities and affects mRNA expression of certain genes involved in keratinocyte differentiation which can be used to enhance barrier function and innate immunity of human skin. It stimulates epidermal differentiation and lipid synthesis and increases the synthesis of antimicrobial peptides in the epidermis which helps reinforce skin's immune system

Conclusion

Urea is a humectant which attracts water to the skin and plays an important role in maintaining the epidermal water level. It has the capacity to serve as natural moisturizing factor of the *stratum corneum* and to preserve its moisture. Creating a barrier that prevents transepidermal water loss urea helps to increase the hydration of the skin and the skin barrier function. The beneficial effects are numerous, and the mechanisms of action only partly known. However, recent findings provide a rational for the beneficial effects of urea and indicate that its effects are not exclusively due to a passive role as a moisturizer but to specific gene regulatory activities which affect mRNA expression of certain genes involved in keratinocyte differentiation. These later effects can be used to enhance barrier function and innate immunity of human skin especially in patients suffering from atopic dermatitis and other skin diseases. Accordingly, urea is much more than just a moisturizer; it is a highly active substance; it stimulates epidermal differentiation and lipid synthesis and increases the synthesis of antimicrobial peptides in the epidermis. These peptides help to reinforce skin's immune system and improve barrier function even in normal skin. Urea increased expression of the genes encoding transglutaminase 1, involucrin, loricrin, and filaggrin. This gene regulation is mediated by specific urea transporters. Additional but not yet identified transporters could also be involved. The effects and the mechanisms of action of urea on the skin are complex; the signal pathways involved in urea-induced changes in gene expression are currently still not completely known and need to be investigated in future studies; a further understanding of the mechanisms involved may help to fully exploit this extraordinary therapeutic agent for skin disorders.

Take Home Messages

- Urea is a humectant, a substance that attracts water to the skin and preserves its moisture.
- Urea is a natural moisturizing factor; however, its beneficial effects are not exclusively due to this passive role. Recent findings indicate that urea may have more pronounced effects in the skin than previously considered.
- Urea is a highly active substance; it possesses gene regulatory activities and affects mRNA expression of certain genes involved in keratinocyte differentiation which can be used to enhance barrier function and innate immunity of human skin especially in patients suffering from atopic dermatitis. It stimulates epidermal differentiation and lipid synthesis and increases the synthesis of antimicrobial peptides in the epidermis which helps reinforce skin's immune system.
- Urea-induced gene regulation is mediated by specific urea transporters.

Abbreviations

O/W emulsions	Oil-in-water emulsions
UT	Urea transporter

References

1. Loden M (2003) Role of topical emollients and moisturizers in the treatment of dry skin barrier disorders. Am J Clin Dermatol 4:771–788
2. Scheinfeld NS (2010) Urea: a review of scientific and clinical data. Skinmed 8:102–106
3. Cramers M, Thormann J (1981) Skin reactions to a urea-containing cream. Contact Dermatitis 7:189–191
4. Leite e Silva VR, Schulman MA, Ferelli C, Gimenis JM, Ruas GW, Baby AR, Velasco MV, Taqueda ME, Kaneko TM (2009) Hydrating effects of moisturizer active compounds incorporated into hydrogels: in vivo assessment and comparison between devices. J Cosmet Dermatol 8:32–39
5. Taube KM (1992) Moisture retaining effect and tolerance of urea-containing Externa in neurodermatitis patients. Hautarzt 43(Suppl 11):30–32
6. Savica S, Tamburic S, Savic M, Cekic N, Milic J, Vuleta G (2004) Vehicle-controlled effect of urea on normal and SLS-irritated skin. Int J Pharm 271:269–280

7. Puschmann M, Gogoll K (1989) Improvement of skin moisture and skin texture with urea therapy. Hautarzt 40(Suppl 9):67–70
8. Ademola J, Frazier C, Kim SJ, Theaux C, Saudez X (2002) Clinical evaluation of 40% urea and 12% ammonium lactate in the treatment of xerosis. Am J Clin Dermatol 3:217–222
9. Rizer R, Elias P, Mills OH (2006) Urea (40%) in an essential fatty acid vehicle improves barrier function in the stratum corneum. J Am Acad Dermatol 54:602
10. Kligman A, Stoudemayer S, Yaxian Zhen Y (2006) Improving chronically dry skin: clinical, patient, and laboratory evaluations. J Am Acad Dermatol 54:571
11. Bikowski J (2007) The treatment of xerosis with a new 40% urea foam. J Am Acad Dermatol 56:AB40
12. Gurge R (2007) Evaluation of the aesthetic attributes of topical products containing high concentrations of urea. J Am Acad Dermatol 56:AB45
13. Jacobi OK (1959) Moisture regulation in the skin. Drug Cosmet Ind 84:732–812
14. Jacobi OK (1970) The composition of normal human stratum corneum and callus. 3. Lactic acid, creatine, creatinine, urea and choline. Arch Dermatol Forsch 240:107–118
15. Loden M (1967) Natural moisturizing factors in skin. Am Perfum Cosmet 82:77–79
16. Loden M (2005) The clinical benefit of moisturizers. J Eur Acad Dermatol Venereol 19:672–688, quiz 686–677
17. Stüttgen G (1992) Results and consequences of long-term urea therapy for clinical practice. Hautarzt 43(Suppl 11):9–12
18. Gloor M, Gehring W (2003) Effects of emulsions on the stratum corneum barrier and hydration. Hautarzt 54:324–330
19. Fredriksson T, Gip L (1975) Urea creams in the treatment of dry skin and hand dermatitis. Int J Dermatol 14:442–444
20. Shemer A, Nathansohn N, Kaplan B, Weiss G, Newman N, Trau H (2000) Treatment of scalp seborrheic dermatitis and psoriasis with an ointment of 40% urea and 1% bifonazole. Int J Dermatol 39:532–534
21. Hagemann I, Proksch E (1996) Topical treatment by urea reduces epidermal hyperproliferation and induces differentiation in psoriasis. Acta Derm Venereol 76:353–356
22. Kuster W, Bohnsack K, Rippke F, Upmeyer HJ, Groll S, Traupe H (1998) Efficacy of urea therapy in children with ichthyosis. A multicenter randomized, placebo-controlled, double-blind, semilateral study. Dermatology 196:217–222
23. Pham HT, Exelbert L, Segal-Owens AC, Veves A (2002) A prospective, randomized, controlled double-blind study of a moisturizer for xerosis of the feet in patients with diabetes. Ostomy Wound Manage 48:30–36
24. Borelli C, Bielfeldt S, Borelli S, Schaller M, Korting HC (2011) Cream or foam in pedal skin care: towards the ideal vehicle for urea used against dry skin. Int J Cosmet Sci 33:37–43
25. Rattner H (1943) Use of urea in hand creams. Arch Dermatol Syph 48:47–49
26. Wiren K, Nohlgard C, Nyberg F, Holm L, Svensson M, Johannesson A, Wallberg P, Berne B, Edlund F, Loden M (2009) Treatment with a barrier-strengthening moisturizing cream delays relapse of atopic dermatitis: a prospective and randomized controlled clinical trial. J Eur Acad Dermatol Venereol 23:1267–1272
27. Loden M, Wiren K, Smerud K, Meland N, Honnas H, Mork G, Lützow-Holm C, Funk J, Meding B (2010) Treatment with a barrier-strengthening moisturizer prevents relapse of hand-eczema. An open, randomized, prospective, parallel group study. Acta Derm Venereol 90:602–606
28. Bonifaz A, Ibarra G (2000) Onychomycosis in children: treatment with bifonazole-urea. Pediatr Dermatol 17:310–314
29. Niewerth M, Korting HC (1999) Management of onychomycoses. Drugs 58:283–296
30. Grice K, Sattar H, Baker H (1973) Urea and retinoic acid in ichthyosis and their effect on transepidermal water loss and water holding capacity of stratum corneum. Acta Derm Venereol 53:114–118
31. Serup J (1992) A double-blind comparison of two creams containing urea as the active ingredient. Assessment of efficacy and side-effects by non-invasive techniques and a clinical scoring scheme. Acta Derm Venereol Suppl (Stockh) 177:34–43
32. Grether-Beck S, Felsner I, Brenden H, Reinhold K, Jaenicke T, Trullas C, Elias PM, Krutmann J (2009) Urea revisited: a well known molecule with previously unrecognized gene regulatory properties. J Invest Dermatol 129(S75):A449
33. Elias PM (2007) The skin barrier as an innate immune element. Semin Immunopathol 29:3–14
34. Candi E, Schmidt R, Melino G (2005) The cornified envelope: a model of cell death in the skin. Nat Rev Mol Cell Biol 6:328–340
35. Aberg KM, Man MQ, Gallo RL, Ganz T, Crumrine D, Brown BE, Choi EH, Kim DK, Schröder JM, Feingold KR, Elias PM (2008) Co-regulation and interdependence of the mammalian epidermal permeability and antimicrobial barriers. J Invest Dermatol 128: 917–925
36. Grether-Beck S, Felsner I, Brenden H, Kohne Z, Majora M, Marini A, Jaenicke J, Rodriguez-Martin M, Trullas C, Hupe M, Elias PM, Krutmann J Urea uptake enhances barrier function and antimicrobial defense in humans by regulating epidermal gene expression. J Invest Dermatol doi:10.1038/jid.2012.42
37. Rosette C, Karin M (1996) Ultraviolet light and osmotic stress: activation of the JNK cascade through multiple growth factor and cytokine receptors. Science 274:1194–1197
38. Schliess F, Reinehr R, Haussinger D (2007) Osmosensing and signaling in the regulation of mammalian cell function. FEBS J 274:5799–5803
39. Smith CP (2009) Mammalian urea transporters. Exp Physiol 94:180–185

40. Rojek A, Praetorius J, Frokiaer J, Nielsen S, Fenton RA (2008) A current view of the mammalian aquaglyceroporins. Annu Rev Physiol 70:301–327
41. Kim BE, Leung DY, Boguniewicz M, Howell MD (2008) Loricrin and involucrin expression is down-regulated by Th2 cytokines through STAT-6. Clin Immunol 126:332–337
42. Mildner M, Jin J, Eckhart L, Kezic S, Gruber F, Barresi C, Stremnitzer C, Buchberger M, Mlitz V, Ballaun C, Sterniczky B, Födinger D, Tschachler E (2010) Knockdown of filaggrin impairs diffusion barrier function and increases UV sensitivity in a human skin model. J Invest Dermatol 130:2286–2294
43. Nenoff P, Donaubauer K, Arndt T, Haustein UF (2004) Topically applied arginine hydrochloride. Effect on urea content of stratum corneum and skin hydration in atopic eczema and skin aging. Hautarzt 55:58–64
44. Wohlrab J, Siemes C, Marsch WC (2002) The influence of L-arginine on the regulation of epidermal arginase. Skin Pharmacol Appl Skin Physiol 15:44–54
45. Grether-Beck S, Muhlberg K, Brenden H, Krutmann J (2008) Urea plus ceramides and vitamins: improving the efficacy of a topical urea preparation by addition of ceramides and vitamins. Hautarzt 59:717–723
46. Loden M, Andersson AC, Andersson C, Frodin T, Oman H, Lindberg M (2001) Instrumental and dermatologist evaluation of the effect of glycerine and urea on dry skin in atopic dermatitis. Skin Res Technol 7:209–213
47. Loden M (1996) Urea-containing moisturizers influence barrier properties of normal skin. Arch Dermatol Res 288:103–107
48. Buraczewska I, Berne B, Lindberg M, Torma H, Loden M (2007) Changes in skin barrier function following long-term treatment with moisturizers, a randomized controlled trial. Br J Dermatol 156:492–498
49. Loden M, Andersson AC, Lindberg M (1999) Improvement in skin barrier function in patients with atopic dermatitis after treatment with a moisturizing cream (Canoderm). Br J Dermatol 140:264–267
50. Rudolph R, Kownatzki E (2004) Corneometric, sebumetric and TEWL measurements following the cleaning of atopic skin with a urea emulsion versus a detergent cleanser. Contact Dermatitis 50:354–358

The Influence of Climate on the Treatment of Dry Skin with Moisturizer

35

C. Stick and E. Proksch

35.1 Introduction

The climate influences the development of dry skin, and the treatment of dry skin must be adapted according to the climate. Therefore, it is important to know how the climate influences the development of xerosis. It is well known that dry skin most often occurs during winter at temperatures below freezing point. That means that dry skin occurs more often in the colder climate zones of the earth, well known from northern Europe, northern states of the USA, and Canada. Also, a high altitude predisposes to dry skin, not only high in the mountains, but also in the highland of Mexico. In the cold climate zones in Europe, often people have the impression that indoor radiator heating leads to dry skin, whereas heating by an old fashion oven as was often used in private homes until the 1970s was more pleasant to the skin. It is also known that strong winds lead to dryness of the skin. Also, artificial ventilation by air condition may lead to dry skin. Air condition may lead to a pronounced skin drying because it reduces the water content of the air. This is a desirable effect in hot and wet climate, for example, on the east cost of the USA in summer time, but it may lead to problems in desert zones like in the US southern mountain region (e.g., in Phoenix) where the relative humidity is low.

35.2 How Climate Can Cause Dry Skin

To answer the question why skin becomes dry and rough, why lips become chapped under certain climate conditions, one need to know some facts on air humidity on the one hand and on the properties of the skin's stratum corneum physiology on the other.

35.3 Water in the Air, Evaporation, and Condensation

Water is a constitutive component of the atmosphere that is not only involved in the physical processes, which make up weather and climate, but also influences the skin.

Contrary to the constant fractions of nitrogen and oxygen in dry air, the water vapor content of air is highly variable. There are several measures to quantify atmospheric moisture. With respect to

C. Stick • E. Proksch (✉)
Institute of Medical Climatology,
University of Kiel, Kiel, Germany
e-mail: eproksch@dermatology.uni-kiel.de

M. Lodén, H.I. Maibach (eds.), *Treatment of Dry Skin Syndrome*,
DOI 10.1007/978-3-642-27606-4_35,

the skin, however, the decisive ambient factor that acts on the hydration of the stratum corneum is relative humidity.

35.3.1 Changes in Relative Humidity Cause the Horny Layer to Expand or Contract

The outermost layer of the skin, the stratum corneum (horny layer), is in direct contact with the environment including the ambient air. The stratum corneum consists of protein-enriched cells, the corneocytes, and a lipid-enriched intercellular domain [1]. The hydrophobic intercellular lipid layer does not contain water. The corneocytes bind water by the so-called natural moisturizing factors which are, however, not well characterized [2]. Parts of the natural moisturizing factors are the filaggrin break down products pyrrolidone carbon acid and urocanic acid which may have hygroscopic properties [3]. The corneocytes and the entire stratum corneum layer shrink and expand depending on the environmental water content. It is well known that prolonged bathing or wearing occlusive gloves for hours leads to swelling of the skin, meaning the stratum corneum. Similar effects, less pronounced, occur in dry or humid ambient air. A water content of the stratum corneum of <10% leads to dry skin [4]. Shrinking of the corneocytes is visible in very dry skin. It is well known that in very dry skin on the lower legs, cracks occur called eczema craquele which resembles the cracking occurring in very dry soil [5, 6]. Shrinking of the corneocytes depends on the relative humidity of the air. A hair, for example, grows if the relative humidity is high, while it shrinks if the atmospheric relative humidity is low. This property of the horny substance is so pronounced that the change in the length of hair serves as a sensor to measure the relative humidity of the air. Instruments which use this principle are called hair hygrometers or hygrographs [7]. Stratum corneum behaves in a similar manner. It shrinks and becomes dry, rough and cracked when relative humidity is low. Shrinking of the corneocytes is an important feature of dry skin.

35.3.2 Relative Humidity and Dew Point Are Related to Each Other

Measurements of the relative humidity are frequently used to quantify the content of water vapor in the air. Why is it called relative humidity? Air cannot absorb an unlimited quantity of moisture, but rather is saturated at some point. The maximum water vapor content in the air is limited by the so-called saturation or dew point. Once the dew point is reached, any surplus of water vapor will begin to condense into liquid water. The atmospheric relative humidity is always related to the dew point.

To explain the situation of the skin under different climatic conditions and to define relative humidity, it is necessary to introduce another quantity, namely, water vapor pressure. Let us assume a closed vessel is partially filled with pure water (cf. Fig. 35.1). The space above the water may contain dry air at the beginning (Fig. 35.1a). With time, some water molecules will evaporate, that is, they will leave the liquid water and enter the gaseous phase. The evaporated water vapor exerts a certain pressure, which is called vapor pressure. The more water is evaporated and contained in a volume of gas, the higher is the vapor pressure (Fig. 35.1b). Net evaporation of water, however, will gradually be limited by the opposite process: condensation of water vapor to liquid water. The more molecules are in the gaseous phase, the more will change again into the liquid phase. Eventually, a steady state between evaporation and condensation is reached. In this state of equilibrium, the air is saturated with water (Fig. 35.1c). The pressure of the water vapor at this dew point is called saturation pressure, which cannot be exceeded at a given temperature.

The relative humidity is defined as a ratio of the actual vapor pressure in the air parcel to the saturated vapor pressure at the respective

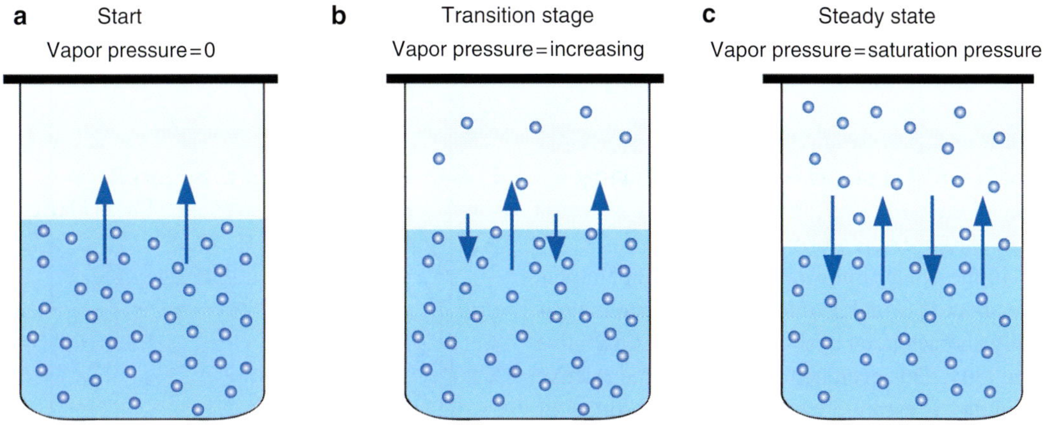

Fig. 35.1 (**a–c**) Evaporation, saturation

temperature. It is usually expressed as a percentage

35.3.3 Saturation Pressure Is Strongly Dependent upon Air Temperature

The saturation pressure is not constant, but rather strongly dependent upon temperature, meaning that temperature determines the maximum quantity of moisture the air can contain. The air can hold much more water at higher temperatures than at lower temperatures. The graph shown in Fig. 35.2 illustrates this relationship: The x-axis represents the temperature in the range from 0°C to 40°C. The vapor pressure expressed in mmHg is plotted on the left y-axis. The bold line (top curve) shows the saturation pressure corresponding to 100% relative humidity. This vapor pressure increases disproportionately with temperature. In the range between –10°C and 50°C, it roughly doubles with every 11°C temperature increase.

Beyond the borders of the range shown in the diagram of Fig. 35.2, the vapor pressure would reach 760 mmHg at 100°C, i.e., it would reach normal atmospheric pressure and water would begin to boil.

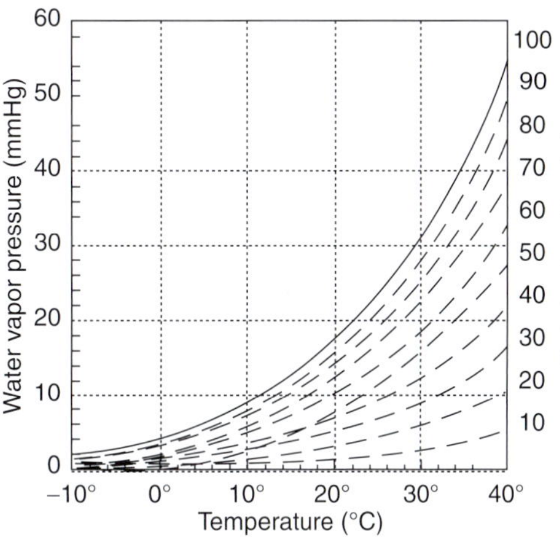

Fig. 35.2 The function of saturation pressure, i.e., 100% relative humidity, on temperature (*bold line*). The family of curves below shows the relative humidity in intervals of 10% [8]

The set of curves below the line showing the saturation pressure indicates relative humidity in increments of 10%. So, in accordance with the definition of relative humidity, these curves express the ratio between the vapor pressure and the saturation pressure in percent. For the sake of completeness, it should be noted that the curve shown here applies to the saturation pressure above a flat surface of pure water or ice, respectively.

35.4 High and Low Relative Humidity at the Same Vapor Pressure

Since in the moderate climates on mid-latitudes dryness of skin prevails or aggravates during the cold winter season, the situation may serve as examples.

In the wintertime when outdoor temperatures are about 0°C or 1°C, the indoor climate is typically characterized by a very low level of relative humidity. This even holds true when the relative humidity is extremely high outdoors with the air at 90% relative humidity or even higher, for example. What are the reasons for this low relative humidity in indoor environments? The attempt to improve the situation by replacing "dry" room air with "moist" air from outside through ventilation can serve as a suitable scenario to explain the mechanisms at work.

Figure 35.3 shows an enlarged detail of Fig. 35.2. Let us assume the outdoor air temperature is 1°C and the relative humidity 90%. At a temperature of 1°C, the saturation pressure is 4.9 mmHg. In such a scenario, a relative humidity of 90% would amount to an actual vapor pressure of 4.4 mmHg. If this outdoor air is heated up to 22°C in the indoor environment, for example, the vapor pressure as the absolute measure of water vapor contained in the air remains at a constant 4.4 mmHg, because the air flowing into the room through the open window will neither gain nor lose moisture. The saturation pressure, on the other hand, which is related to the relative humidity, is approximately five times higher at a temperature of 22°C than at 1°C (cf. Fig. 35.2). If the temperature is 22°C, the saturation pressure is 19.9 mmHg. Set in relation to this value, a pressure of 4.4 mmHg amounts to merely 22%. So, the relative humidity of the outdoor air, which still was 90% at 1°C, is only 22% once it is heated up to room temperature.

Given that the relative humidity of the air plays a decisive role in the expansion or contraction of the horny layer of the epidermis, as mentioned at the beginning, the conditions described above can easily make the skin become dry and rough.

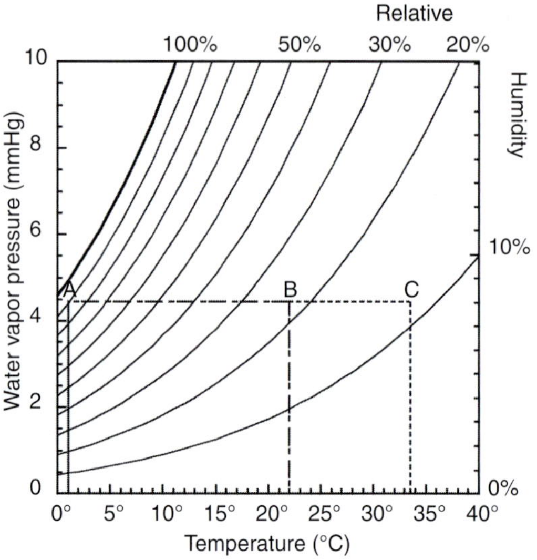

Fig. 35.3 Dependence of saturation pressure and relative humidity on temperature (enlarged detail from Fig. 35.2). The *vertical lines* mark the temperatures at the outset (point *A*) and the end of the scenarios assumed in the text (point *B*: ambient temperature in a room and *C*: mean skin temperature). Starting with an air temperature of 1°C and 90% relative humidity (*A*), the *broken, horizontal line* shows that the 4.4 mmHg vapor pressure remains constant when the cold air is heated. Due to the extreme increase in saturation pressure with rising temperatures, this *horizontal line* reaches the range of low relative humidity

Ventilating rooms in cold, wintry conditions actually does lead to a lowered humidity in heated rooms. On the one hand, air containing little moisture because of the low outdoor temperatures despite the high relative humidity is transported into the room. On the other hand, water vapor previously expelled indoors by plants and humans or other sources like kitchens and bathrooms is removed through the exchange of air.

The described situation becomes all the more pronounced, the greater the differences in indoor and outdoor temperatures. In principle, this effect also applies when the outside temperatures are below freezing (cf. Fig. 35.2). The saturation pressure above ice is even a little lower than above liquid water.

The scenario offers an explanation for the very low humidity that generally prevails in the indoor environment during wintertime. Not only does such low relative humidity affect the skin, which becomes dry and rough because its horny layer shrinks, it also has a detrimental effect on furniture, for example. (Dry cabin air that may cause discomfort to some people on long-haul flights can also be explained by this scenario.)

35.5 Clothing and Ventilation of the Boundary Layer Modify Skin Moisture

As far as the skin is concerned, at least two additional factors modify the situation, even though they act in opposite directions. On the one hand, skin temperature is normally higher than ambient room temperature. In thermal comfort conditions, the mean skin temperature would be in the range between 33°C and 34°C. At this temperature, the saturation pressure, which functions as the reference value for relative humidity, stands at 38–40 mmHg. In terms of the example given above, this would mean that relative humidity on the skin would be a mere 11–12% (cf. Fig. 35.3, point C).

But another factor actually counteracts this effect: There is an increased humidity very close to our skin due to the so-called perspiration insensibilis, i.e., imperceptible water evaporation from the skin, nowadays far better known as transepidermal water loss (TEWL). TEWL can easily determined by using a measurement device like the Tewameter®. It is well known that there are several inflammatory diseases with a high TEWL [1, 9]. TEWL is a marker of the inside-outside barrier. It is well accepted that in eczema and in psoriasis, the disrupted skin barrier is of importance for the pathophysiology of these diseases [1, 9]. The transport of this water vapor is inhibited by our clothing. So in fact, relative humidity in the boundary layer, which is the thin air layer right in contact with the surface of the skin, actually will not drop to the low levels calculated in our example and shown in Fig. 35.3. That means adequate clothing reduces the water loss and may prevent dry skin. This may explain why we often have dry skin in areas of the body which are not covered with clothes, the hands and the face. Excessive water loss is also prevented by greasy ointments, and it is well known that this prevents drying of the skin. Very occlusive wraps like latex gloves which nearly totally prevent water evaporation may, however, lead to hyperhydration which may irritate the skin together with the mechanical forces between glove and skin [1].

35.6 Outdoor Climate Is a Personal Matter as Well

We still need to clarify why our skin also becomes dry when we are staying outside under cold and wintry conditions even if relative humidity is quite high outdoors. Humans are only able to spend longer periods of time outdoors if they wear clothing to increase thermal insulation so that their mean skin temperature is in the neighborhood of 33°C once again. At the same time, local skin temperatures, particularly in the peripheral regions of the body, like hands, feet, ears, the nose, the face, etc., may be substantially lower. The skin temperature may also be slightly lower when an increased heat loss to the environment is compensated for by higher endogenous heat production. In a cold environment, people almost invariably generate such endogenous heat through physical activity. And yet, the decrease in average skin surface temperature is relatively low under these various conditions. The resulting situation, therefore, is more or less similar to the one described above: The cold air from the environment, which does in fact have a high relative humidity but low moisture content and hence low vapor pressure, is warmed up in the insulating layer of clothing by the heat produced by the body so that the temperatures reach app. 30°C across many areas of the skin. The saturation pressure is much higher at this temperature than at the low temperatures of the cold outdoor air. Consequently, the relative humidity of the skin decreases, and the horny layer shrinks and becomes cracked. As described above, the quantity of moisture evaporating from our skin is too low to increase the vapor pressure sufficiently to prevent this effect from happening. In principal, the scenario of ventilating a room and staying outside under cold and wintry conditions resembles each other.

Factors like wind or clothing ventilation through physical activity, for example, let water vapor escape from the boundary layer at the skin surface causing the skin to become even drier.

35.7 Direct Exposure to Cold Air Means Double the Stress for Your Skin

The skin temperatures of those parts of the body that are directly exposed to cold air, such as the hands or the face, may drop well below the average skin temperature, meaning that the difference between this temperature and the ambient air temperature is smaller than below the warming layer of clothing. On the other hand, clothing cannot fulfill its function of conserving moisture in the boundary layer of the skin in these circumstances. Thus, it is precisely this combination of wind and low air temperature which lets the skin exposed directly to the elements become dry.

The water vapor produced by the skin is transported through the boundary layer by a process called diffusion. Diffusion flow rate depends on the difference between the vapor pressure at the skin surface and the vapor pressure in the ambient air, and the thickness of the arrested air layer adjacent to the skin. So, in terms of water vapor transport, relative humidity is not the decisive factor but rather vapor pressure gradient between skin and ambient air. Since vapor pressure is always comparatively low at cold outside temperatures, the pressure gradients in the boundary layer are steeper in cold environments, and thus the discharge of water vapor from the skin is greater.

Wind intensifies water vapor diffusion through convection. The air currents reduce the thickness of the boundary layer of arrested air adjacent to the skin, resulting in a steeper vapor pressure gradient. Outside this boundary layer, water vapor is transported by way of turbulent air currents. As a result, two mechanisms contribute to skin dryness under direct exposure to cold air: reduced relative humidity due to the warming of the air and increased water vapor diffusion because of steep vapor pressure gradients between skin and ambient air.

Under summer conditions, i.e., at temperatures of about 20°C or 22°C, the vapor pressure is app. 10 mmHg even if relative humidity is only about 50–60%. In many places in moderate climates, the mean vapor pressure approximates or exceeds this value during the summer months. Compared to the conditions assumed for the wintry scenario discussed above (1°C, 90% relative humidity, 4.4 mmHg), this represents more than a twofold increase in vapor pressure, after all.

35.8 Physiological Reactions Intensify Itching

Let us discuss another observation. Many people feel that dry skin is particularly bothersome when they enter a warm room after having spent a longer period of time out in the cold. Vapor content and vapor pressure in the air do not change very much, as was described above. However, the higher indoor temperatures bring about a reduction in relative humidity, leading to the consequences we already discussed. Moreover, a physiological reaction occurs that intensifies these effects considerably: Cutaneous circulation which was reduced in the cold environment reacts to warm temperatures by increasing dramatically. The skin becomes flushed and skin temperature rises. Increased blood flow and higher transcapillary filtration make the skin plump up. The horny layer becomes dry and rough or cracked. In addition to the physical conditions, the physiological mechanism of reactive hyperemia thus helps create a situation which intensifies itching.

All in all, one can state that with respect to the skin, cold climate conditions always are dry conditions.

35.9 Dry and Hot Climates: The Wind Makes the Skin Go Dry

In hot and dry climates, skin is typically be moisturized by sweat that is secreted because of thermoregulation demands. Strong winds, however, may dry the skin as well, because the air currents carry the moisture away and by thinning the boundary layer steepen the gradient of water vapor pressure. This will increase water loss from the skin in particular on those areas that are unclothed and thus directly exposed to the dry and windy air. Wearing clothes in hot and dry climate conditions, which protect against solar radiation in the first instance, may also be helpful in protecting the skin from excessive loss of moisture.

35.10 Artificial Indoor Climate

A more modern climate influence on the skin is owed to the artificial cooling by air-conditioning devices. Keeping in mind the explanation made above that heating cold air decreases the relative humidity lets the statement that cooling air can make air dry as well seem to be paradoxical. Indeed, looking at the diagrams of Figs. 35.2 and 35.3, it becomes obvious that cooling humid air will increase the relative humidity. The fact that people staying in air-conditioned rooms nevertheless often suffer from dry skin is due to technical reasons regarding the construction of the air-conditioning devices. In order to cool a large volume of air, let us say the air of a common hotel room, by a small air conditioner, the temperature of the heat exchanger has to be very low. Indeed, the relative humidity increases as the air is cooled down by the heat exchanger, which takes up the heat of the air (cf. Fig. 35.4, points A and B). On most occasions, the air will eventually reach the dew point when cooled down. In this case, saturated vapor will condense at the surface of the heat exchanger. The condensed water drops from the cooler and is collected and drained from the air conditioner by a tube. This means that moisture is removed from the air, and thus the vapor pressure is reduced (Fig. 35.4, points B and C). The water deprived air returning from the cooler will be mixed with the air in the room and thus reheated to a certain amount. This again reduces the relative humidity. In total, this means that both absolute and relative humidity are lowered by the process of cooling the air.

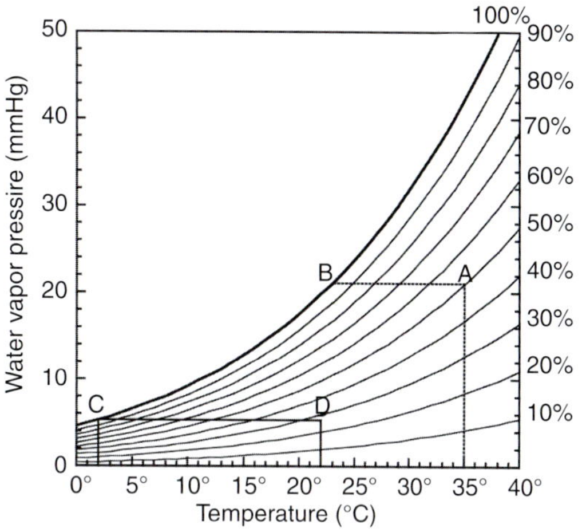

Fig. 35.4 Schematic diagram showing how air is dried at the heat exchanger of an air-conditioning plant. Let be the temperature of the uncooled air 35°C at 50% rel. humidity (point *A*), as the air is cooled down, the water vapor pressure remains constant while the relative humidity increases until the dew point is reached at point *B*. Continuing cooling the air water vapor will condensate following the saturation curve to point *C*. The condensation of water removes moisture from the air and thus reduces the vapor pressure. When the air is ventilated to the room and reheated to ambient temperature, the relative humidity decreases (point *D*). Actually, the relative humidity in the room depends on the temperature at the heat exchanger of the air-conditioning plant

Typically the air is recirculated between the room and the air conditioner in order to reach the desired room temperature and to compensate for the heat produced by persons and electrical devices being in the room and for the heat flowing from the walls, the windows, and so on into the air-conditioned room. This circulation will not only keep the room cool but will also remove some moisture from the air in the room again and again. Finally, the relative humidity in an air-conditioned room will mostly depend on the temperature at the heat exchanger and the ambient room temperature (Fig. 35.4, points C and D).

Moreover, the air condition needs fans for moving the air, which cause a draught of cool air. As mentioned above, air movement will increase the water loss of skin as well. All in all air-conditioning can have unpleasant and adverse effects by drying the skin.

35.11 Water Helps Dry Your Skin

So how can one protect the skin from this loss of moisture? Examples that point to the need and the possibility of skin protection actually seem to be somewhat paradoxical at first glance: Many people are quite familiar with the wintertime phenomenon that their skin starts to itch right after an intense exposure to water, during a swim in the pool, a stay in the sauna or a long shower, etc., even though one would think that the skin has become saturated with moisture on such occasions. But in fact, the water is diffused very rapidly from the horny layer and what is crucial in this connection is that this diffusion occurs especially fast because intense exposure to hot water and soap elutes lipids and possibly water binding compounds from the skin which would otherwise slow down and reduce the discharge of moisture. The demoisturizing, negative effect of too intense body care becomes particularly apparent when air humidity is low as is typically the case in the wintertime. Applying a lotion or cream or an occlusive ointment, on the other hand, is very useful to reduce water loss of the horny layers and to diminish shrinkage of the corneocytes.

The influence which the surface curvature of a human body has on the exchange of water might be a plausible explanation for the observation that convex formed skin areas suffer more from low humidity than concave ones. It is well known that dry skin occurs on the face, back of the hands, and the outside of extremities, whereas the body folds and the inside of the upper legs never get dry.

Taken all together, the symptoms of dry skin which one experiences in the wintertime can largely be explained by the basic properties of water vapor in the air. However, such general climate physiological considerations cannot clarify the issue of individual differences in sensitivity.

35.12 Treatment of Dry Skin Depending on the Climate Conditions

The treatment of the skin depends on the body region and on the climate conditions. In cold winter conditions and in people with very dry skin on legs and arms, greasy ointments can be applied. Under extreme weather conditions, greasy, water-free ointments like petrolatum or a mixture of different hydrocarbons can be used on the extremities. These ointments even can be used in the face to protect against harsh water conditions in windy and in very cold weather at temperature well below freezing temperature. A cream with high water content would possibly lead to freezing on the skin. On the other hand, at high temperature which leads to sweating, an occlusive ointment hinders water evaporation and leads to an unpleasant feeling. This may lead to irritation of the skin by hyperhydration. Chronic use of greasy ointment in the face, in particularly based on petrolatum, may also lead to a perioral or rosacea-like dermatitis. Therefore, even people with dry skin in the face must avoid chronic treatment with grease ointments in this region. Chronic use of greasy ointments may be suitable for the dry skin on the extremities. The use of creams with high water content may not be sufficient at those body areas.

35.13 Summary

The climate is of crucial importance for the development of dry skin conditions. Dry skin usually occurs in cold weather conditions in winter time and in the colder climate zones of the earth. Cold air can only bind a low amount of water because of a low dew point. Therefore, the outdoor climate leads to dry skin. The relative humidity is low indoors in winter time because of ventilation which leads to an influx of air with a low amount of water, and therefore the indoor climate in winter time may also lead to dry skin. Dry skin may even occur during summer time indoors if air condition reduces too much of the water. The draft by a fan from an air-conditioning device or outdoor wind aggravates dry skin. Treatment of dry skin must be performed according to the climate. A greasy ointment can be applied during winter time especially on the extremities. During summer time, in the face, an ointment may be too greasy and may lead to side effects. Therefore, a water-enriched cream is appropriate to treat dry skin during that season.

Take Home Messages

- The climate is of crucial importance for the development of dry skin.
- Dry skin occurs in cold weather conditions during winter time.
- Cold air can only bind a low amount of water.
- Outdoor and indoor climate in winter time lead to dry skin because of low absolute and relative low air water content, respectively.
- Strong wind and artificial ventilation aggravate dry skin.
- Air condition induced strong reduction of water content may also lead to dry skin.
- A greasy ointment should be applied during winter time especially on the extremities for the treatment of dry skin.
- A water-enriched cream is appropriate to treat dry skin during summer especially in the face.

References

1. Proksch E, Brandner JM, Jensen JM (2008) The skin: an indispensable barrier. Exp Dermatol 17:1063–1072
2. Johnsen GK, Norlen L, Martinsen OG, Grimnes S (2011) Sorption properties of the human stratum corneum. Skin Pharmacol Physiol 24:190–198
3. Kezic S, O'Regan GM, Yau N, Sandilands A, Chen H, Campbell LE, Kroboth K, Watson R, Rowland M, Irwin McLean WH, Irvine AD (2011) Levels of filaggrin degradation products are influenced by both filaggrin genotype and atopic dermatitis severity. Allergy 66:934–940
4. Papir YS, Hsu KH, Wildnauer RH (1975) The mechanical properties of stratum corneum. I. The effect of water and ambient temperature on the tensile properties of newborn rat stratum corneum. Biochim Biophys Acta 14(399):170–180
5. Proksch E, Lachapelle JM (2005) The management of dry skin with topical emollients–recent perspectives. J Dtsch Dermatol Ges 3:768–774
6. Proksch E (2008) The role of emollients in the management of diseases with chronic dry skin. Skin Pharmacol Physiol 21:75–80
7. World Meteorological Organisation (2008) Guide to meteorological instruments and methods of observation. Part I: measurement of meteorological variables. Chapter 4: measurement of humidity, WMO-No. 8, Geneva
8. Lide DR (1995) CRC handbook of chemistry and physics, 76th edn. CRC Press, Boca Raton
9. Proksch E, Fölster-Holst R, Bräutigam M, Sepehrmanesh M, Pfeiffer S, Jensen JM (2009) Role of the epidermal barrier in atopic dermatitis. J Dtsch Dermatol Ges 7:899–910

Emollient Therapy and Skin Barrier Function

36

Majella E. Lane

36.1 Introduction

The skin is the largest organ of the human body and serves the vital function of protection of human beings from excessive water loss in a terrestrial environment and from insult from xenobiotics. Disorders of the skin's finely tuned barrier function are associated with a variety of conditions including dermatitis and atopic eczema. Conventional treatment of such conditions involves the chronic application of emollients or moisturisers in order to replace the skin's water content and restore barrier integrity. However, a number of studies in the literature have also highlighted the ability of specific emollient products to compromise the skin's protective role. These studies are reviewed in this chapter, and the possible reasons underlying the effects of these products are considered.

36.2 Skin Structure and the Stratum Corneum

The skin represents, in adults, 10% of the total body mass with an average total surface area of 2 m^2 [1]. It is a complex living organ with a diverse cellular population and a range of physiological functions. In essence, the skin consists of three functional layers: the epidermis, the dermis and the subcutaneous tissue also known as the hypodermis. Appendages such as hair, follicles, sebaceous glands and sweat glands are also found in human skin. The outermost layer, the epidermis, is generally divided into two distinct layers: the stratum corneum (SC) and the viable epidermis (VE) (Fig. 36.1). The epidermis is a non-vascular tissue with a thickness that varies between 60 and 800 μm, depending on the body site. The VE is a multilayer tissue that is traditionally identified in terms of cell location and appearance: stratum basale, stratum spinosum, stratum granulosum and stratum lucidum. These layers represent the several stages of mitosis and keratinocyte differentiation, which ultimately contribute to the regeneration of the SC.

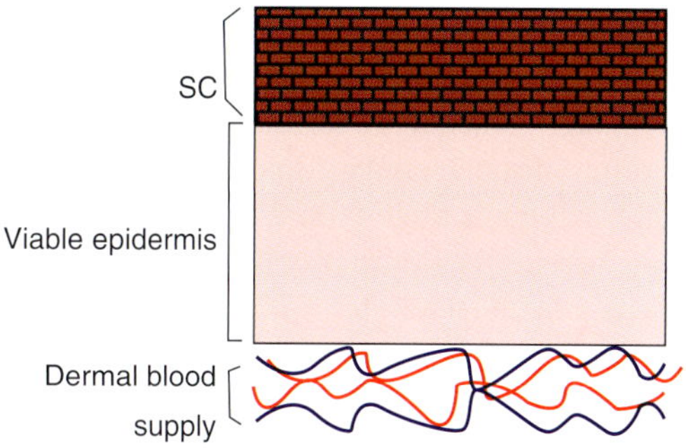

Fig. 36.1 Schematic representation of the stratum corneum and viable epidermis

The SC is the most superficial layer of the skin, and it is the principal barrier to percutaneous absorption of exogenous substances. Removal

M.E. Lane
Department of Pharmaceutics, School of Pharmacy, 29-39 Brunswick Square, WC1N 1AX London, UK
e-mail: majella.lane@btinternet.com

M. Lodén, H.I. Maibach (eds.), *Treatment of Dry Skin Syndrome*,
DOI 10.1007/978-3-642-27606-4_36, © Springer-Verlag Berlin Heidelberg 2012

of the SC by tape stripping increases the permeability of water and other compounds by approximately 1,000 times [2]. The water permeability of the SC is also much lower than most other biological membranes. Several factors contribute to the ability of the SC to control the loss of water and the permeation of exogenous compounds, such as high density, low hydration (15–20% w/w) and low surface area for diffusion (assuming that the main route is via the intercellular pathways) [3]. Constant renewal of the cells in this layer by desquamation/regeneration also maintains a very effective protection barrier [4].

Structurally, the SC is composed of 15–20 layers (with a thickness of 10–20 μm) of pentagonal or hexagonal, stacked and terminally differentiated corneocytes, surrounded by a complex mixture of intercellular lipids. A "brick and wall" analogy is usually used to describe the SC structure: the keratinised cells are the 'bricks' whereas the intercellular lipids are the 'mortar' [5]. Each cell is about 34–46 μm long, 25–36 μm wide and 0.5–1 μm thick [2]. These dimensions are subject to variation according to age, anatomical location and external factors (e.g. UV radiation) [2]. SC is mainly composed of intracorneocyte insoluble protein (~75% w/w), whereas the intercellular lipids account for 5–15% w/w and the cornified cell envelope represents ~5% w/w of the total dry weight [6, 7].

The cornified cell envelope is a 15–20-nm-thick protein shell that surrounds each cell. It is composed of ~15-nm layer of defined structural proteins and ~5-nm-thick layer of specialised lipids [8]. It results from the differentiation of the keratinocytes which originated in the stratum spinosum [9]. The cornified cell envelope has an important role in the organisation of the intercellular lipid domain, inter-corneocyte cohesion and resistance of the SC to proteolytic enzymes [2]. Michel et al. reported two types of CEs: polygonal mature rigid CEs and irregularly shaped immature fragile CEs [10]. Hirao et al. demonstrated that mature corneocytes are more hydrophobic than immature cells. While Nile Red is reported to stain the mature corneocytes, it can also stain immature cells [11]. A more specific measure of maturity involves immunostaining of the cornified envelope with antibodies specific for the precursor protein, e.g. 'involucrin' [11]. This allowed Hirao and colleagues to distinguish between the mature rigid CEs isolated from the outermost layer of SC and the fragile, less mature CEs which are present in deeper layers of the SC as well as in psoriatic and eczematous skin [11].

Between the cells (~75-nm gap), there is a complex matrix of lipids arranged in bilayers and in parallel orientation to the cells' surfaces [12]. The number of lipid bilayers varies between 4 and 20 [13]. These lipids are formed during the differentiation from the stratum granulosum and begin with the extrusion of the lamellar granules to the extracellular space. In this space, acid hydrolases break down the phospholipids into free fatty acids and convert glucosylceramides to ceramides [14, 15]. Additionally, following the extrusion of the lamellar granule contents, the stacks of lamellar membrane are rearranged edge to edge and then fuse to form continuous intercellular lamellae [16].

36.3 Skin Turnover and Desquamation

Skin turnover is a critical factor and plays a major role in skin barrier function. The cells of the SC (corneocytes) result from the differentiation of the keratinocytes from the stratum granulosum. The migration from this layer to the surface takes between 12 and 14 days, during which the cells differentiate and begin to die. The life span of the corneocytes in the SC is 2–3 weeks, as the superficial part of the SC is continuously desquamated at a balanced rate with the formation of new cell [17]. The terminally differentiated corneocytes are devoid of nuclei or other cellular organelles, but are filled with keratin intermediate filaments, cross linked by intermolecular disulfide bonds [18, 19].

In normal healthy skin, the process of stratum corneum (SC) maturation is finely regulated, and the loss of surface corneocytes is precisely balanced by the underlying rate of proliferation (Fig. 36.2). For desquamation to occur, the cohesive 'corneodesmosomes' which bind the corneocytes in the SC must be degraded by enzymes, i.e. proteases which catalyse peptide bond hydrolysis [20, 21]. Human tissue 'kallikreins (KLKs)' are a family of trypsin- or chymotrypsin-like-secreted serine proteases (KLK1-KLK15) found in a variety of tissues [22]. The KLKs have been suggested to function as an enzymatic cascade pathway [23–25]. Corneodesmosomes are broken down by several desquamatory-related serine proteases, such as KLK5, KLK6, KLK7, KLK8, KLK10, KLK11 and KLK13, present within the SC [26, 27]. As well as having a vital role in the proteolysis of the SC corneodesmosomes, KLKs are also reported to be involved in degradation of lipid-processing enzymes, such as β-glucocerebrosidase [28].

Reduced expression of tryptic (e.g. KLK5) and chymotryptic (e.g. KLK7) enzymes has been reported in the outer layers of the SC in dry skin [29]. In contrast, increased expression of KLK7 has been reported in two major chronic inflammatory diseases: psoriasis and atopic dermatitis [26, 30]. Alteration in the activity of serine proteases KLK5 and KLK7 appears to be associated with skin barrier disturbances [31–33]. This may partly be due to uncontrolled corneodesmolysis, which leads to weakening of the SC integrity and cohesion [28, 34].

Other enzymes such as plasmin, tryptase and urokinase are also reported to be present in the SC but are not necessarily involved in the desquamatory process. However, these enzymes may have an important role in skin inflammation [30, 35]. Several trypsin-like protease inhibitors, such as leupeptin, are reported to elevate barrier repair [36]. Leupeptin is reported to inhibit the activity of, e.g. plasmin [36, 37]. This suggests that increased activity of plasmin may impair barrier recovery. Tryptase concentration is reported to be high in those with allergic contact dermatitis [38].

Transepidermal water loss (TEWL) is a frequently used non-invasive technique for elucidation of skin barrier function [39]. When the skin barrier integrity is damaged, TEWL increases [39, 40]. The activity of certain proteases has been correlated with the TEWL. Kawai and colleagues showed that the activity of urokinase increased as TEWL increased in tape stripping from the cheeks of subjects with dry skin [41]. More recently, Voegeli et al. observed a positive correlation between the activity of trypsin-like KLKs, tryptase, plasmin and urokinase with SC barrier impairment [42]. However, chymotryptic-like enzymes showed no such correlation [42].

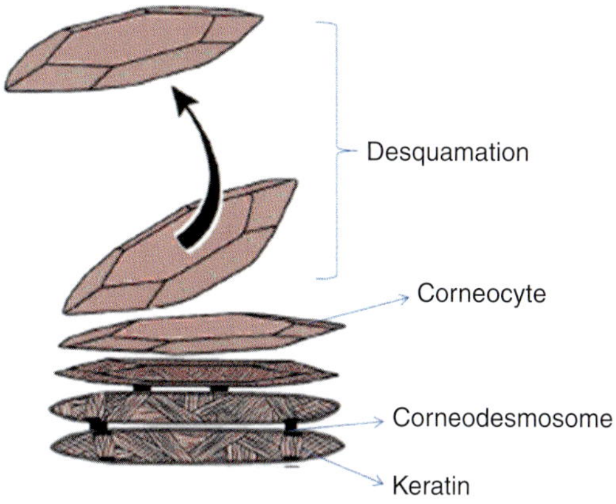

Fig. 36.2 The desquamation process (adapted from Milstone [21])

36.4 Biophysical and Pharmacodynamic Measurements of Skin Barrier Function

36.4.1 Transepidermal Water Loss (TEWL)

The SC receives water by diffusion mostly from the underlying tissues and also from the sweat glands with constant evaporation to the outside environment. The water that is constantly lost diffuses through the skin by a passive mode of transport, from the region of high water concentration inside the body to the low concentration at the surface. Transepidermal water loss (TEWL) corresponds to the steady-state water vapour flux density passing through the *SC* to the exterior (Fig. 36.3). Under these conditions, baseline TEWL can be described by Fick's first law of diffusion [43]:

$$J = -D\frac{\Delta c}{\Delta z} \quad (36.1)$$

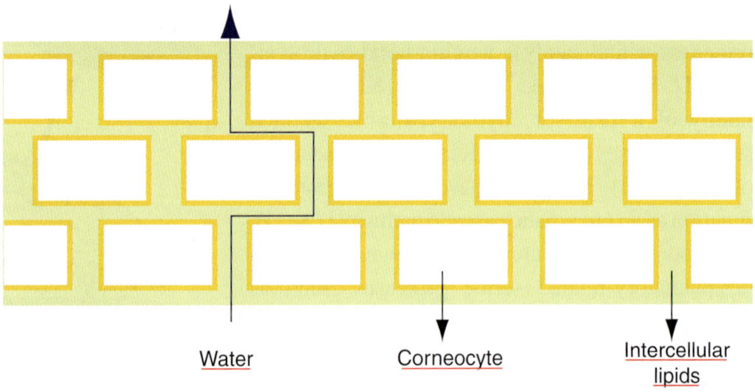

Fig. 36.3 Transepidermal water loss through intact *stratum corneum*

where:

J = water vapour flux density – TEWL (kg m^{-2} s^{-1})

D = diffusion coefficient of water in the *SC* (m^2 s^{-1})

Δc = positive concentration difference across the membrane (kg m^{-3})

Δz = membrane thickness (m)

TEWL measurements are regarded as an indicator of barrier function and allow an assessment of any macroscopic changes in the *SC* barrier function [43]. A range of instrumentation has been developed to measure TEWL, and both open and closed chamber devices are currently in use.

36.4.2 Skin Capacitance

As the dielectric constant of the skin will change with water content, the moisture content of the stratum corneum, i.e. hydration, may be measured using electrical capacitance. Instruments for hydration measurement generally use capacitance sensors to measure the dielectric constant of the skin [44]. Changes in the water content of the stratum corneum are converted to arbitrary units of hydration.

36.4.3 Skin Response to Vasoactive Compounds

After topical application, nicotinic acid derivatives are known to induce vasodilatation of the peripheral blood capillaries located in the dermal papillae, adjacent to the epidermis-dermis junction [45]. This pharmacological action has been used to characterise in vivo skin barrier function by a number of research groups [46, 47]. The most commonly used derivative to date is methyl nicotinate (Fig. 36.4a) which penetrates rapidly and causes the appearance of redness that fades away in a few hours (Fig. 36.4b) [48–50]. Hexyl nicotinate has also been used [51]. The proposed mechanism of action of the nicotinates involves receptor activation which leads to an increase of

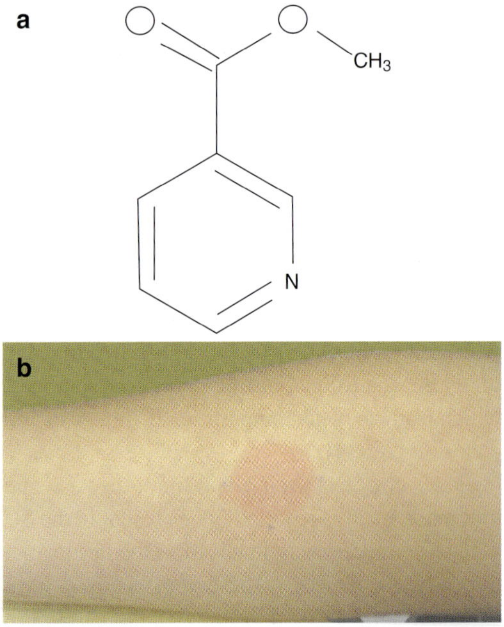

Fig. 36.4 (**a**) Methyl nicotinate. (**b**) Skin erythema caused by a 0.075% w/v methyl nicotinate solution applied for 20 s

the intercellular calcium. This induces the activation of a calcium-sensitive phospholipase A2 (PLA2) and the formation of arachidonic acid (AA) which is then metabolised to PGD2 and PGE2. Prostaglandins are able to induce vasodilation of the blood vessels in the upper layer of the dermis by activating their Gs-coupled receptors [45]. The induced erythema can be visually assessed by detecting its onset time or monitored using more objective methods such as Laser Doppler Velocimetry [LDV], chromametry and photoplethysmography.

36.5 Moisturisers and the Skin Barrier

Disorders or diseases of the skin must inevitably compromise aspects of its barrier properties. Extensive literature confirms that TEWL measurements in patients suffering from dry skin or atopic eczema have been reported to be higher compared with patients with healthy skin [52–55]. A rational approach to the problem of excessive water loss is therefore simply to restore water via application of a suitable formulation which either contains water or which artificially increases skin water content by occlusion. In some instances, however, the formulation components may themselves further aggravate or exacerbate the problem, and irritant skin reactions are commonly observed. In general, these reactions may be divided into three types: (1) stinging, a subjective and transient effect which appears and disappears within a short period (minutes) of moisturiser application; (2) inflammation with redness, oedema, elevated skin temperature and discomfort; and (3) damage to the skin barrier function resulting in dryness and scaling of the skin but not necessarily clinical symptoms [56]. This section considers specific case studies from the literature where the skin barrier is compromised following application of emollients. In some instances, the authors have also identified the mechanism by which the formulation is exerting these deleterious effects as well as the specific component(s) most likely to be responsible.

36.5.1 Locabase®

Locabase® is an emollient product containing white soft paraffin, liquid paraffin, cetostearyl alcohol, cetomacrogol 1,000 as well as preservatives and buffering agents. A study conducted by Halkier-Sørensen and Thestrup-Pedersen [57] indicated a general benefit associated with use of the product for workers exposed to water on a daily basis, as evaluated by electrical capacitance and clinical examination, but no changes were observed in TEWL. The product was also shown to be of benefit in the prevention and treatment of irritant contact dermatitis (ICD) [58].

In a later study on healthy skin, Held et al. [59] investigated the effects of application of Locabase® to the forearm of 20 healthy volunteers three times daily for 4 weeks, the other forearm acting as the untreated control. At the end of the study (day 28), both forearms were challenged with a patch test of sodium lauryl sulphate (SLS). TEWL and skin hydration measurements (electrical capacitance) were conducted to determine any changes in skin barrier function. Electrical capacitance increased significantly on the treated arm at days 14, 28 and 30 compared with the untreated site. No statistically significant differences in TEWL were observed for treated versus untreated sites. The authors also noted that the mean amount of moisturiser used in the study period did not affect the results. After challenge with SLS, TEWL was significantly higher on the arm treated with moisturizer than on the control arm ($p < 0.05$) suggesting that the moisturizer treatment might increase skin susceptibility to irritants. A study by the same group compared the short-term effects of Locabase® with another commercially available product (Decubal®) [60]. Decubal® contains water, isopropyl myristate, glycerol, sorbitan stearate, lanolin, dimethicone, cetyl alcohol, polysorbate 60 and sorbic acid and has a total lipid content of 38%. The products were applied to the upper arm/forearm of 19 healthy volunteers three times daily for 5 days while the other upper arm/forearm served as symmetrical control. After a 24-h washout period, the skin was challenged with a patch test of sodium lauryl sulphate. Skin reactions were evaluated using TEWL, electrical capacitance, laser Doppler flowmetry, chromametry and clinical scoring. The Locabase®-treated skin sites displayed more intense irritant reactions (TEWL and chromameter measurements) to SLS compared with untreated skin ($p < 0.05$) in line with the earlier findings, but these differences were not observed for the Decubal® product. The authors also speculated that the results might be a consequence of the relatively high lipid content in the Locabase® formulation compared with the other product (70% vs 30%).

The same workers evaluated the effect of Locabase® on skin susceptibility to nickel in volunteers with a known nickel allergy and in volunteers with no nickel allergy [61]. The product was applied to the forearm three times daily for 7 days prior to any allergy challenge. The other arm served as a symmetrical control. Electrical capacitance was measured prior to the study and at the end of the study for control and treated sites. At the end of the study, baseline values for TEWL, skin colour and skin thickness were measured at both sites, and filter discs with 1% $NiCl_2$ solution were subsequently applied for 24 h. Clinical scoring and measurements for TEWL, skin colour and dermal thickness were performed at the end of the 24-h period and at 72 h after application of the filter pads. In the nickel-allergic group, the strength of patch-test reactions was increased on the moisturizer-treated sites as evaluated by clinical scoring after 24 h and by TEWL and skin thickness after 72 h. In the control group, no significant differences were found. The authors suggested that the threshold values for elicitation of allergic reactions in nickel-sensitive individuals were influenced by moisturiser application.

Duval and co-workers compared Locabase® with a urea-containing cream [51]. A parallel, randomized and double blind study was conducted with 53 healthy volunteers. The participants were instructed to apply the cream twice daily for 3 weeks on the volar aspect of one of their forearms. The skin was then exposed to hexyl nicotinate to induce vasodilatation. The time course and magnitude of the microvascular skin changes in the two skin areas were monitored with laser Doppler flowmetry. A significantly shorter time to reach maximum blood flow was obtained for Locabase® compared with the untreated control sites. The findings were compatible with the earlier reports, i.e. the use of Locabase® appears to weaken the skin barrier to externally applied substances.

36.5.2 Aqueous Cream B.P.

Aqueous Cream B.P. is an oil-in-water emulsified cream which first appeared as a preparation of the British Pharmacopoeia in 1958, and its formulation, containing sodium lauryl sulphate (SLS), remains largely unchanged today [62]. The other components of the preparation are white soft paraffin, liquid paraffin, water, cetostearyl alcohol and a preservative. For the management of eczema and dry skin, the British National Formulary currently includes Aqueous Cream BP under the heading of 'emollients' which are further defined as 'preparations which soothe, smooth and hydrate the skin and are indicated for all dry or scaling disorders' [63]. Gloor et al. investigated the effects of Aqueous Cream B.P. and a range of other formulations on 29 healthy volunteers over a 7-day period [64]. Laser Doppler measurements were also conducted on 14 subjects. The products were applied on one arm twice daily, and the contralateral area was left untreated. TEWL and skin redness (chromameter) were measured before the start and at the end of each study. Significant increases in TEWL and laser Doppler readings were observed for treated versus untreated controls suggesting that the skin barrier had been compromised and an irritant response had been induced. At the end of the study, 15 subjects underwent a hydrocortisone blanching test where the hydrocortisone cream was applied under occlusion for 24 h. The blanching-induced decrease (chromameter) for treated sites was significantly greater than for non-treated sites suggesting that treatment with the cream increased penetration of hydrocortisone. After pretreatment with the cream, 14 subjects underwent the SLS irritation test. TEWL, chromameter and laser Doppler readings were obtained before and after this test. TEWL and chromameter values were significantly higher for the treated sites versus untreated sites compared with baseline measurements.

The problem of irritant reactions following the use of Aqueous Cream B.P. in the UK has been highlighted by Lapsley and by Cork et al. [65, 66]. An audit of adverse reactions to the use of Aqueous Cream B.P. in children was reported in the UK by the latter group. The notes of 100 children aged 1–16 with atopic eczema attending a paediatric dermatology clinic were assessed. Fifty-six percent of the episodes of exposure to Aqueous Cream B.P. were associated with an immediate cutaneous reaction. Several of the participants also reported that the cream caused irritancy when used for prolonged periods of time, i.e. as a 'leave on' emollient but not when used as a soap substitute. A later study by Tsang and Guy demonstrated a 20% increase ($p<0.0001$) in baseline TEWL for six healthy volunteers following topical treatment of the forearm with Aqueous Cream B.P. for 4 weeks [67]. Approximately 1.6 g of Aqueous Cream B.P. was applied to half of the forearm twice daily. SC thickness was also evaluated via measurement of TEWL and tape stripping [68] and was found to decrease by a mean value of 12% ($p=0.0015$).

In a more recent study by Mohammed et al. [69], the effects of Aqueous Cream B.P. at the molecular and cellular level were evaluated. The same study design used by Tsang and Guy was employed. At the end of the 28-day treatment period, the site was tape-stripped, and corneocyte maturity; corneocyte size and protease activity of the desquamatory kallikrein proteases, KLK5 and KLK7; and the inflammatory proteases tryptase and plasmin were measured. Protein content and TEWL were also measured. Corneocyte maturity (Fig. 36.5) and size (Table 36.1) decreased with increasing number of tape strips and were significantly lower in treated

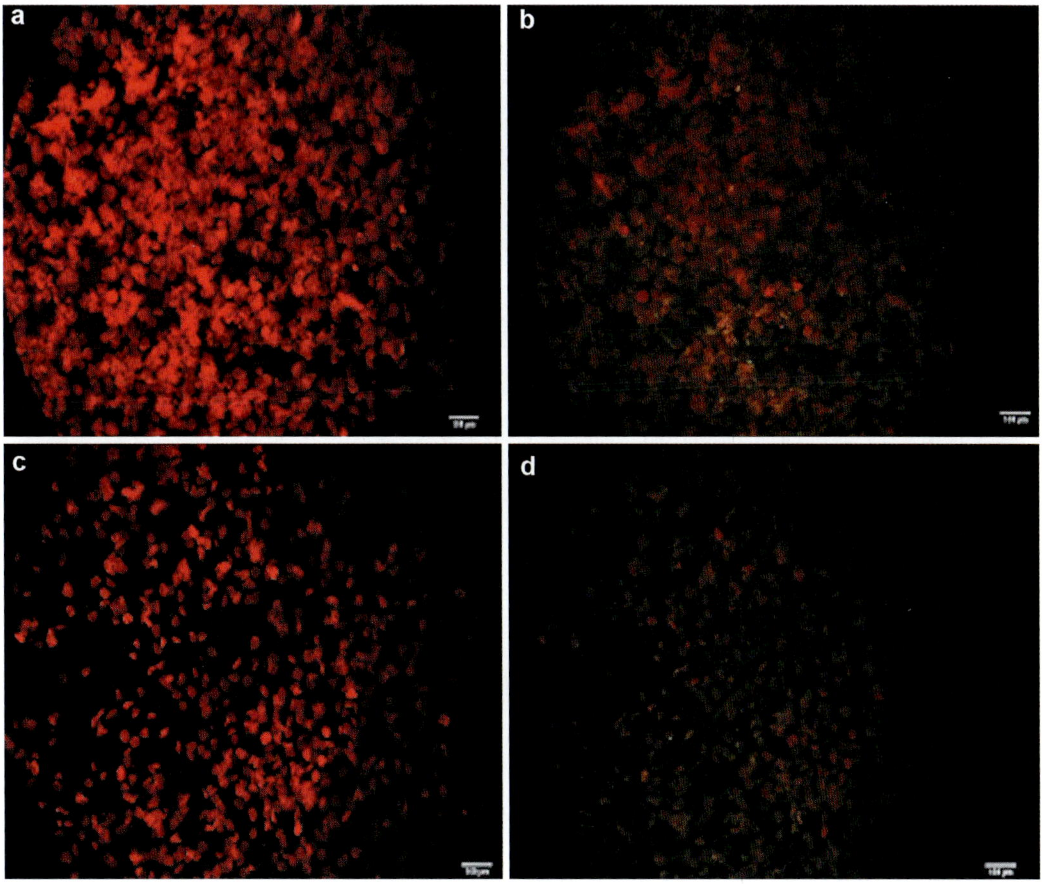

Fig. 36.5 Corneocyte maturity from tape 1 of the volar forearm. (**a**) and (**c**) Are control and treated, respectively, following nile red staining, (**b**) and (**d**) are immuno-stained control and treated sites

Table 36.1 Comparison of corneocyte surface area for control and treated sites with Aqueous Cream B.P. for sequential tape strippings ($n=6$; mean ± S.D.)

Tape strip number	Corneocyte surface area (μm²)	
	Non-treated	Treated
1	978.22 ± 155.15	864.99 ± 180.33
5	930.51 ± 161.76	842.32 ± 163.46
9	844.40 ± 133.02	774.32 ± 169.12
13	832.82 ± 129.77	768.44 ± 143.87
17	787.21 ± 138.13	712.75 ± 142.26

sites compared with untreated sites. Protease activity and TEWL values were higher ($p<0.05$) for the treated sites compared with untreated sites. The amount of protein removed from deeper layers of treated sites was significantly lower than from untreated sites. The application of Aqueous Cream appeared to disrupt the normal maturation process, i.e. the corneocytes did not mature fully because of exposure to the preparation, and this is also consistent with the observed increase in desquamatory protease activity (KLK5, KLK7). Elevated levels for the inflammatory enzymes also suggest inflammatory responses in sites treated with this preparation, and, indeed, the reduction in corneocyte surface area and maturity is entirely consistent with increased epidermal turnover. Increased TEWL values are consistent with this disturbance in corneocyte maturation during the treatment period. The results provide a mechanistic understanding for the observed thinning of the SC associated with use of Aqueous Cream B.P. and for the elevated TEWL and irritant effects reported following the use of this preparation in patients with atopic dermatitis and in healthy subjects [70]. Efforts by clinicians and patient groups in the UK are ongoing with a view to reclassification of this product as a soap replacement rather than an emollient.

36.6 Summary

The literature relating to two products which are commonly prescribed for the management of dry skin conditions has been reviewed. Locabase® is a lipid-rich formulation (70%) while Aqueous Cream is a water-in-oil cream containing a comparable amount of water. The effects of Aqueous Cream B.P. on skin function are thought to reflect the influence of one of the emulgents used in the formulation (SLS). However, further studies are needed to confirm this hypothesis. It is also important to note that sensitisation and irritation reactions have been reported to cetostearyl alcohol [71–73], a component of both Locabase® and Aqueous Cream B.P. With the increase in sensitivity and sophistication of measurement techniques, it should be possible to separate the different effects from the components that make up complex formulations. It may be possible to identify constituents which have an advantageous effect on the protease activity. This knowledge should allow the formulation of better emollients for the treatment of dry skin and atopic dermatitis, a problem that has increased significantly over the past decades [74].

Take Home Messages

- Conventional treatment of dry skin conditions involves the chronic application of emollients or moisturisers in order to replace the skin's water content and restore barrier integrity.
- The barrier function of the skin may be interrogated by a range of molecular and biophysical methods.
- A number of studies in the literature have highlighted the ability of specific emollient products to compromise the skin's protective role.
- Locabase® is a lipid-rich formulation and its use in patients with healthy skin and in patients with nickel allergy is associated with increased irritation in the former group and a lowering of allergy threshold in the latter group.
- Aqueous Cream B.P. is a water-rich formulation and its use in healthy volunteers is associated with elevated desquamatory and inflammatory protease

activity, increased transepidermal water loss and changes in corneocyte maturity and size indicative of accelerated skin turnover.

- In the management of dry skin and eczema, the prescription of emollients which are known to damage healthy skin must be firmly questioned.

References

1. Washington C, Washington N (1989) Drug delivery to the skin. In: Wilson CG, Washington N (eds) Physiological pharmaceutics: biological barriers to drug absorption. Ellis Horwood Limited, Chichester, pp 109–120
2. Walters KA, Roberts MS (2002) The structure and function of skin. In: Walters KA (ed) Dermatological and transdermal formulations. Marcel Dekker, Inc, New York, pp 1–39
3. Scheuplein RJ (1971) Permeability of the skin. Physiol Rev 51:702–747
4. Egelrud T (2000) Desquamation in the stratum corneum. Acta Derm Venereol Suppl (Stockh) 208:44–45
5. Michaels AS, Chandrasekaran SK, Shaw JE (1975) Drug permeation through human skin: theory and in vitro experimental measurement. AIChE J 21:985–996
6. Suhonen TM, Bouwstra JA, Urtti A (1999) Chemical enhancement of percutaneous absorption in relation to stratum corneum structural alterations. J Control Release 59:149–161
7. Kalinin AE, Kajava AV, Steinert PM (2002) Epithelial barrier function: assembly and structural features of the cornified cell envelope. Bioessays 24:789–800
8. Swartzendruber DC, Wertz PW, Madison KC, Downing DT (1987) Evidence that the corneocyte has a chemically bound lipid envelope. J Invest Dermatol 88:709–713
9. Kalinin A, Marekov LN, Steinert PM (2001) Assembly of the epidermal cornified cell envelope. J Cell Sci 114:3069–3070
10. Michel S, Schmidt R, Shroot B, Reichert U (1988) Morphological and biochemical characterization of the cornified envelopes from human epidermal keratinocytes of different origin. J Invest Dermatol 91:11–15
11. Hirao T, Denda M, Takahashi M (2001) Identification of immature cornified envelopes in the barrier-impaired epidermis by characterization of their hydrophobicity and antigenicities of the components. Exp Dermatol 10:35–44
12. Madison KC (2003) Barrier function of the skin: "La raison d'etre" of the epidermis. J Invest Dermatol 121:231–241
13. Bouwstra JA, Honeywell-Nguyen PL, Gooris GS, Ponec M (2003) Structure of the skin barrier and its modulation by vesicular formulations. Prog Lipid Res 42:1–36
14. Elias PM, Feingold KR, Tsai J, Thornfeldt C, Menon G (2003) Metabolic approach to transdermal drug delivery. In: Guy RH, Hadgraft J (eds) Transdermal drug delivery, 2nd edn, Revised and expanded. Marcel Dekker, New York, pp 285–305
15. Landmann L (1986) Epidermal permeability barrier: transformation of lamellar granule-disks into intercellular sheets by a membrane-fusion process, a freeze-fracture study. J Invest Dermatol 87: 202–209
16. Downing DT (1992) Lipid and protein structures in the permeability barrier of mammalian epidermis. J Lipid Res 33:301–313
17. Katz M, Poulsen BJ (1971) Absorption of drug through the skin. In: Brodie BB, Gilette JR (eds) Handbook of experimental pharmacology. Springer, Berlin, pp 103–174
18. Sun TT, Green H (1978) Keratin filaments of cultured human epidermal cells. Formation of intermolecular disulfide bonds during terminal differentiation. J Biol Chem 253:2053–2060
19. Kurihara-Bergstrom T, Good WR (1987) Skin development and permeability. J Control Release 6:51–58
20. Rawlings N, Barrett A (1999) MEROPS: the peptidase database. Nucleic Acids Res 27:325–331
21. Milstone LM (2004) Epidermal desquamation. J Dermatol Sci 36(3):131–140
22. Yousef GM, Diamandis EP (2001) The new human tissue kallikrein gene family: structure, function, and association to disease. Endocr Rev 22:184–204
23. Yousef GM, Diamandis EP (2002) Human tissue kallikreins: a new enzymatic cascade pathway? Biol Chem 383:1045–1057
24. Brattsand M, Stefansson K, Lundh C, Haasum Y, Egelrud T (2004) A proteolytic cascade of kallikreins in the stratum corneum. J Invest Dermatol 124: 198–203
25. Borgono CA, Michael IP, Diamandis EP (2004) Human tissue kallikreins: physiologic roles and applications in cancer. Mol Cancer Res 2:257–280
26. Komatsu N, Saijoh K, Toyama T, Ohka R, Otsuki N, Hussack G, Takehara K, Diamandis EP (2005) Multiple tissue kallikrein mRNA and protein expression in normal skin and skin diseases. Br J Dermatol 153:274–281
27. Suzuki Y, Nomura J, Hori J, Koyama J, Takahashi M, Horii I (1993) Detection and characterization of endogenous protease associated with desquamation of stratum corneum. Arch Dermatol Res 285:372–377
28. Hachem J-P, Man M-Q, Crumrine D, Uchida Y, Brown BE, Rogiers V, Roseeuw D, Feingold KR, Elias PM (2005) Sustained serine proteases activity

by prolonged increase in pH leads to degradation of lipid processing enzymes and profound alterations of barrier function and stratum corneum integrity. J Invest Dermatol 125:510–520
29. Overloop LV, Declercq L, Maes D (2001) Visual scaliness of human skin correlates to decreased ceramide levels and decreased stratum corneum protease activity. J Invest Dermatol 117:811
30. Voegeli R, Rawlings AV, Breternitz M, Doppler S, Schreier T, Fluhr JW (2009) Increased stratum corneum serine protease activity in acute eczematous atopic skin. Br J Dermatol 161:70–77
31. Egelrud T, Brattsand M, Kreutzmann P, Walden M, Vitzithum K, Marx UC, Forssmann WG, Mägert HJ (2005) hK5 and hK7, two serine proteinases abundant in human skin, are inhibited by LEKTI domain 6. Br J Dermatol 153:1200–1203
32. Hansson L, Stromqvist M, Backman A, Wallbrandt P, Carlstein A, Egelrud T (1994) Cloning, expression, and characterization of stratum corneum chymotryptic enzyme. A skin-specific human serine proteinase. J Biol Chem 269:19420–19426
33. Brattsand M, Egelrud T (1999) Purification, molecular cloning, and expression of a human stratum corneum trypsin-like serine protease with possible function in desquamation. J Biol Chem 274:30033–30040
34. Harding CR, Watkinson A, Rawlings AV, Scott IR (2000) Dry skin, moisturization and corneodesmolysis. Int J Cosmet Sci 22:21–52
35. Voegeli R, Rawlings AV, Doppler S, Heiland J, Schreier T (2007) Profiling of serine protease activities in human stratum corneum and detection of a stratum corneum tryptase-like enzyme. Int J Cosmet Sci 29:191–200
36. Denda M, Kitamura K, Elias PM, Feingold KK (1997) Trans-4-(aminomethyl)cyclohexane carboxylic acid (T-AMCHA), an anti-fibrinolytic agent, accelerates barrier recovery and prevents the epidermal hyperplasia induced by epidermal injury in hairless mice and humans. J Invest Dermatol 109:84–90
37. McConnell RM, York JL, Frizzell D, Ezell C (1993) Inhibition studies of some serine and thiol proteinases by new leupeptin analogs. J Med Chem 36:1084–1089
38. Brockow K, Abeck D, Hermann K, Ring J (1996) Tryptase concentration in skin blister fluid from patients with bullous skin conditions. Arch Dermatol Res 288:771–773
39. Endo K, Suzuki N, Yoshida O, Sato H, Fujikura Y (2007) The barrier component and the driving force component of transepidermal water loss and their application to skin irritant tests. Skin Res Technol 13:425–435
40. Farahmand S, Tien L, Hui X, Maibach HI (2009) Measuring transepidermal water loss: a comparative *in vivo* study of condenser-chamber, unventilated-chamber and open-chamber systems. Skin Res Technol 15:392–398
41. Kawai E, Kohno Y, Ogawa K, Sakuma K, Yoshikawa N, Aso D (2002) Can inorganic powders provide any biological benefit in stratum corneum, while residing on skin surface? IFSCC Mag 5(4):269–275
42. Voegeli R, Rawlings AV, Doppler S, Schreier T (2008) Increased basal transepidermal water loss leads to elevation of some but not all stratum corneum serine proteases. Int J Cosmet Sci 30:435–442
43. Imhof RE, De Jesus MEP, Xiao P, Ciortea LI, Berg EP (2009) New developments in skin barrier measurements. In: Rawlings AV, Leyden JJ (eds) Skin moisturization, 2nd edn, Cosmetic science and technology series. Informa Healthcare, New York, pp 463–479
44. Frödin T, Helander P, Molin L, Skogh M (1988) Hydration of human stratum corneum studied in vivo by optothermal infrared spectrometry, electrical capacitance measurement, and evaporimetry. Acta Derm Venereol 68(6):461–467
45. Bodor ET, Offermanns S (2008) Nicotinic acid: an old drug with a promising future. Br J Pharmacol 153(S1):S68–S75
46. Cronin E, Stoughton RB (1962) Percutaneous absorption. Regional variations and the effect of hydration and epidermal stripping. Br J Dermatol 74:265–272
47. Barrett CW, Hadgraft JW, Sarkany I (1964) The influence of vehicles on skin penetration. J Pharm Pharmacol 16(Suppl):104T–107T
48. Tur E, Guy RH, Tur M, Maibach HI (1983) Noninvasive assessment of local nicotinate pharmacodynamics by photoplethysmography. J Invest Dermatol 80:499–503
49. Leopold CS, Maibach HI (1996) Effect of lipophilic vehicles on in vivo skin penetration of methyl nicotinate in different races. Int J Pharm 139:161–167
50. Bonina FP, Montenegro L, Scrofani N, Esposito E, Cortesi R, Menegatti E, Nastruzzi C (1995) Effects of phospholipid based formulations on in vitro and in vivo percutaneous absorption of methyl nicotinate. J Control Release 34:53–63
51. Duval C, Lindberg M, Boman A, Johnsson S, Edlund F, Loden M (2003) Differences among moisturizers in affecting skin susceptibility to hexyl nicotinate measured as time to increase skin blood flow. Skin Res Technol 9:59–63
52. Thune P, Nilsen T, Hanstad IK, Gustavsen T, Lövig Dahl H, Thune P, Nilsen T, Hanstad IK, Gustavsen T, Lövig Dahl H (1988) The water barrier function of the skin in relation to the water content of stratum corneum, pH and skin lipids. The effect of alkaline soap and syndet on dry skin in elderly, non-atopic patients. Acta Derm Venereol 68(4):277–283
53. Lodén M (1995) Biophysical properties of dry atopic and normal skin with special reference to effects of skin care products. Acta Derm Venereol Suppl (Stockh) 192:1–48
54. Di Nardo A, Wertz P, Giannetti A, Seidenari S (1998) Ceramide and cholesterol composition of the skin of patients with atopic dermatitis. Acta Derm Venereol 78(1):27–30
55. Flohr C, England K, Radulovic S, McLean WH, Campbel LE, Barker J, Perkin M, Lack G (2010) Filaggrin loss-of-function mutations are associated with early-onset eczema, eczema severity and transepidermal water loss at 3 months of age. Br J Dermatol 163(6):1333–1336

56. Agner T, Held E, West W, Gray J (2000) Evaluation of an experimental patch test model for the detection of irritant skin reactions to moisturisers. Skin Res Technol 6:250–254
57. Halkier-Sørensen L, Thestrup-Pedersen K (1993) The efficacy of a moisturizer (Locobase) among cleaners and kitchen assistants during everyday exposure to water and detergents. Contact Dermatitis 29(5):266–271
58. Ramsing DW, Agner T (1997) Preventive and therapeutic effects of a moisturizer. An experimental study of human skin. Acta Derm Venereol 77(5):335–337
59. Held E, Sveinsdóttir S, Agner T (1999) Effect of long-term use of moisturizer on skin hydration, barrier function and susceptibility to irritants. Acta Derm Venereol 79(1):49–51
60. Held E, Agner T (2001) Effect of moisturizers on skin susceptibility to irritants. Acta Derm Venereol 81(2):104–107
61. Zachariae C, Held E, Johansen JD, Menné T, Agner T (2003) Effect of a moisturizer on skin susceptibility to $NiCl_2$. Acta Derm Venereol 83(2):93–97, ++
62. General Medical Council (Great Britain) (1958) British pharmacopoeia. The Pharmaceutical Press, London, pp 245–246, 1012 pp
63. British National Formulary 60. British Medical Association, Royal Pharmaceutical Society. Sept 2010:689–690
64. Gloor M, Hauth A, Gehring W (2003) O/W emulsions compromise the stratum corneum barrier and improve drug penetration. Pharmazie 58(10):709–715
65. Lapsley P (2000) Emollients – ADR concern (letter). Pharm J 265:555
66. Cork MJ, Timmins J, Holden C, Carr J, Berry V, Tazi-Ahnini R, Ward SJ (2003) An audit of adverse drug reactions to aqueous cream in children with atopic eczema. Pharm J 271:747–748
67. Tsang M, Guy RH (2010) Effect of Aqueous Cream BP on human stratum corneum in vivo. Br J Dermatol 163(5):954–958
68. Kalia YN, Pirot F, Guy RH (1996) Homogeneous transport in a heterogeneous membrane: water diffusion across human stratum corneum in vivo. Biophys J 71:2692–2700
69. Mohammed D, Matts PJ, Hadgraft J, Lane ME (2011) Influence of Aqueous Cream BP on corneocyte size, maturity, skin protease activity, protein content and transepidermal water loss. Br J Dermatol 164(6): 1304–1310
70. Danby SG, Al-Enezi T, Sultan A, Chittock J, Kennedy K, Cork MJ (2011) The effect of aqueous cream BP on the skin barrier in volunteers with a previous history of atopic dermatitis. Br J Dermatol 165(2):329–334
71. Pecegueiro M, Brandão M, Pinto J, Conçalo S (1987) Contact dermatitis to Hirudoid cream. Contact Dermatitis 17(5):290–293
72. Hannuksela M (1988) Skin contact allergy to emulsifiers. Int J Cosmet Sci 10:9–14
73. Wilson CL, Cameron J, Powell SM, Cherry G, Ryan TJ (1991) High incidence of contact dermatitis in leg-ulcer patients-implications for management. Clin Exp Dermatol 16(4):250–253
74. Plötz SG, Ring J (2010) What's new in atopic eczema? Expert Opin Emerg Drugs 15(2):249–267

Skin Barrier Responses to Moisturizers: Functional and Biochemical Changes

37

Izabela Buraczewska-Norin

37.1 Introduction

Moisturizers are often used as supplements to topical and/or systemic anti-inflammatory drugs in various types of skin conditions and disorders, such as contact dermatitis, atopic dermatitis, psoriasis, and ichthyosis, in order to bring relief and break a dry skin cycle (reviewed by Lodén [1, 2] and Proksch et al. [3]). Such skin conditions usually require long-lasting treatment with moisturizers, and in the case of atopic dermatitis, their use is recommended even when the eczema is cleared [4]. Use of moisturizers is also widespread among people who perceive their skin as dry or rough, for example, in the elderly, those living in a dry climate, or those in frequent contact with cleaning agents, and they use moisturizers to obtain relief and for smoothening of the skin. Moreover, skin protection creams (also called "barrier creams") are common at various workplaces to minimize the percutaneous penetration of chemicals. Moisturizers are also used in other situations, such as when they serve as carriers of substances that are supposed to be delivered on the skin in order to fulfill a special function, as in case of topical drugs, sunscreens, makeup products, or even hand sanitizers. Moisturizers are therefore common and used by a significant percentage of the population.

I. Buraczewska-Norin, Ph.D.
ACO HUD Nordic AB, Research & Development,
BOX 622, Upplands Väsby 19426, Sweden
e-mail: izabela.norin@aconordic.com

The primary function of a moisturizer is to smoothen the skin surface and to increase water content in the stratum corneum, i.e., to moisturize the skin. After application, water and other volatile ingredients gradually evaporate, which may even give a cooling or calming effect. Remaining ingredients form a semiocclusive deposit which stays on the skin surface for some time and smoothens it by filling the cracks. It may also influence skin surface pH, depending on applied ingredients. This deposit is usually removed from the skin surface within few hours due to washing, friction, and evaporation. During this time, some ingredients may also penetrate into the epidermis or even to the dermis and be uptaken by the body (Fig. 37.1).

The increase in water content is achieved by the water-binding properties of humectants, i.e., glycerin, urea, etc., and by formation of a semiocclusive layer on the skin surface which hampers water evaporation and increases water content in the upper epidermis. Moreover, an immediate increase in hydration of the stratum corneum may be caused by an uptake of water from the applied product. The increase in water content and the simultaneous filling of the fractures on the skin surface makes the skin more elastic and visibly and tactilely smoother as well as decreases itch and brings relief [1, 5, 6].

Studies on the impact of moisturizers on the skin barrier have mostly focused on short-term effects, showing that moisturizers are able to increase skin hydration by the mechanisms

M. Lodén, H.I. Maibach (eds.), *Treatment of Dry Skin Syndrome*,
DOI 10.1007/978-3-642-27606-4_37, © Springer-Verlag Berlin Heidelberg 2012

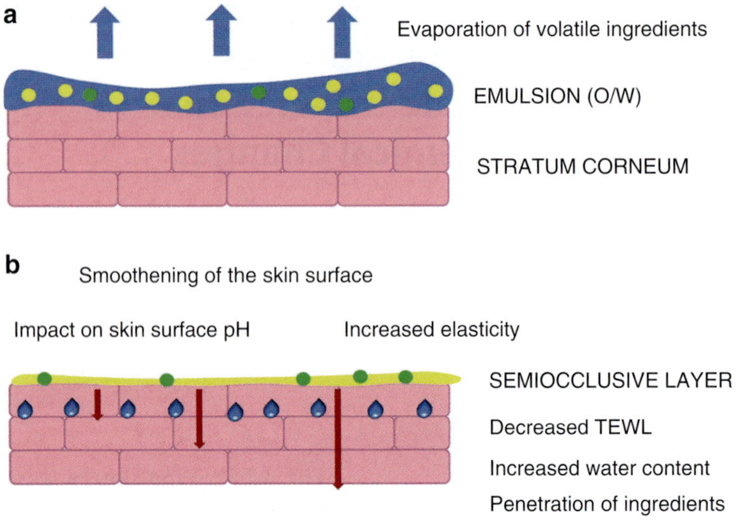

Fig. 37.1 Schematic representation of short-term effect of a moisturizer on the skin. (**a**) After application of a moisturizer, e.g., in the form of oil-in-water emulsion, water and other volatile ingredients evaporate. (**b**) Remaining ingredients form a semi-occlusive layer, which decreases TEWL. Skin surface became smoother. Skin surface pH may be altered temporarily, depending on ingredients applied. Water content in stratum corneum increases due to (i) hampered water evaporation, (ii) humectants, and (iii) uptake of water from moisturizer. Ingredients may penetrate into stratum corneum, lower layers of epidermis, and even to dermis and be uptaken by body. The semiocclusive layer is removed from the skin surface within few hours due to washing, friction, and evaporation

described above, decrease roughness and scaling, and improve the condition of dry skin (reviewed by Lodén et al. [1, 2, 6, 7]). However, little is known about the effects of their long-term use, lasting weeks, months, or even years, which better reflects the real-life situation. If moisturizers are used repeatedly over a long period, the consequences may be speculated upon: recurring application of various substances of exogenous origin on the skin, followed by such physicochemical changes as repeatable increase in water content in the stratum corneum or change in skin surface pH, may significantly influence the structure and function of the epidermis and, therefore, the skin barrier function.

The objective of the present chapter is to increase the understanding of the mechanisms by which long-term treatment with moisturizers influences the skin and its barrier function. The impact of formulation variables such as pH, lipid type, and humectants is presented. Skin barrier responses are discussed from the functional and biochemical perspectives.

37.2 Chemistry of Moisturizers

Moisturizers are formulated predominantly as oil-in-water (o/w) emulsions, where oil droplets are dispersed in water and stabilized by emulsifiers (Fig. 37.2). Reversed water-in-oil (w/o) emulsions are used less frequently due to their poor spreadability and the greasier feeling they leave on the skin; however, they can offer other attributes, for example, water resistance. Emulsions are categorized into creams or lotions, depending on their viscosity. Moisturizers may also be gels containing only hydrophilic material or ointments with only lipophilic ingredients. Other forms of moisturizers exist, but they are much less common, for example, multiple emulsions, silicone-in-water (si/w) emulsions, or suspensions. The choice moisturizer form depends on its desired effect and the ingredients that are supposed to be incorporated.

Moisturizers may either have a simple composition and contain only a few ingredients or be a complex mixture of many substances. In the case

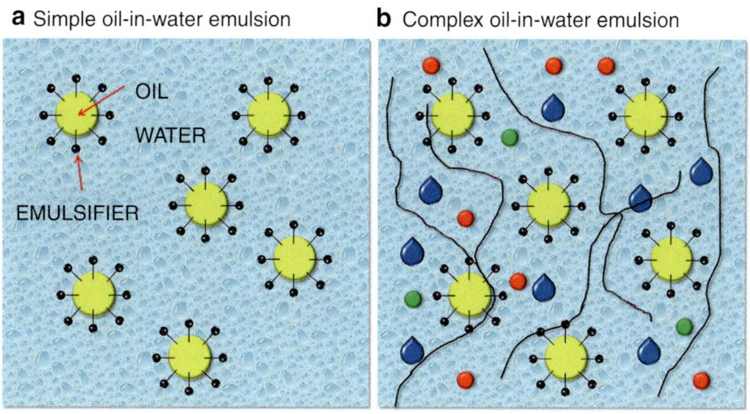

Fig. 37.2 Schematic representation of an oil-in-water emulsion. (**a**) Simple emulsion, containing only three ingredients: water as the continuous phase, dispersed oil droplets, and an emulsifier that stabilizes the droplets, so they do not coalesce. (**b**) Complex emulsion, containing more ingredients than simple emulsion, such as humectants, pH adjusters, preservatives, and thickeners (marked as *blue*, *green* and *red dots*, and *long lines*, respectively). This type of emulsion represents better real-life situation, as majority of moisturizers contain a big variety of ingredients in order to fulfill their function, have good cosmetic properties, and remain stable during declared shelf-life period

of o/w and w/o emulsions, the simplest possible moisturizer must contain three ingredients, namely, water, a lipid (oil), and an emulsifier.

Lipids can be of vegetable, animal, or mineral origin. Emulsifiers, which stabilize the lipid droplets in an emulsion, can be either low-molecular substances, for example, stearic acid, or long-chained polymers of large size, such as acrylates/C10–30 alkyl acrylate crosspolymer or carbomer. However, it is rare that emulsions contain only three ingredients, and usually, they are mixtures of at least 15–20 substances. Moisturizers with over 50–60 ingredients have also been encountered. Those additional ingredients allow achieving desired properties, efficacy, and stability of the product.

Moisturizers usually contain humectants, such as: (1) polyols, e.g., glycerin, propylene glycol, butylene glycol, and sorbitol; (2) alpha-hydroxy acids (AHAs) and their salts, e.g., glycolic acid, lactic acid, and sodium lactate; (3) low-molecular substances, e.g., urea, betaine, and amino acids; and/or (4) high-molecular polymers with water-binding capacity, e.g., sodium hyaluronate. Many ingredients used in moisturizers are the same as those found in the epidermis or on the skin surface: fatty acids, ceramides, vitamins, urea, lactic acid, pyrrolidone carboxylic acid (PCA), etc.

To increase stability of the emulsion and to adjust its rheology to either a cream or lotion form, viscosity-increasing agents must be added into the formulation, such as polymers (carbomer, acrylates copolymer, xanthan gum) and/or high-melting waxes (glyceryl stearate, cetearyl alcohol). Sensory properties may be modified with silicones, such as dimethicone and cyclohexasiloxane. Additionally, moisturizers may contain several other ingredients, such as preservatives, antioxidants, vitamins, herbal extracts, salts, and UV filters. Depending on the composition of a moisturizer, the pH is adjusted to between slightly acidic and slightly alkaline with typical ranges from 4 to 7, but in case of formulations containing stearic acid and zinc oxide, pH is slightly alkaline.

Since the majority of moisturizers contain several ingredients, identification of the parameters responsible for their effects on the skin barrier is difficult. Consequently, factors such as the concentration and type of lipids, humectants, and other ingredients, as well as pH adjustment, should be taken into account.

37.3 Methods Used for Evaluation of the Skin Barrier Function

Methods used for evaluation of the skin and its barrier function, including its responses to moisturizers, are numerous. Skin condition may be assessed visually, for example, for dryness, scaling, and redness. There are several instruments available for noninvasive assessments of the skin, where no skin sampling is necessary, as they measure the functional changes on the skin surface or within a defined skin depth, for example, TEWL, skin capacitance, blood flow, pH, surface topography, and elasticity. Such equipment is often portable and easy to use, and consequently, noninvasive measurements are a common tool in dermatological research. Today, assessment of TEWL is the most common method for evaluation of the skin barrier function. TEWL is increased when the skin barrier is impaired, for example, in dry skin disorders or after damage with an irritant, but also when the skin is excessively hydrated.

However, in order to investigate processes in the skin in greater detail, at the biochemical level, skin samples are required. They may be punch or shave biopsies or samples obtained by tape stripping. Studies utilizing such invasive methods are more complicated to perform and require more resources and assessment from ethical perspectives. Although they may be common in basic dermatological research, they have rarely been used in research about moisturizers and their effect on the skin barrier. It is also possible to perform studies in vivo on mice or in vitro on keratinocyte cultures or skin equivalents. However, results obtained from experiments performed using animal models or in vitro systems do not always correlate to the in vivo situation in humans. Analyses of human skin biopsies may give a lot of information about changes in epidermal structure, and gene and protein expression, as well as allowing for staining with antibodies against various proteins.

37.4 Functional and Biochemical Changes in the Skin Barrier After Long-Term Use of Moisturizers

The few studies which examined long-term treatment with moisturizers on normal and diseased human skin have shown functional changes in the skin barrier, as measured by noninvasive techniques. Both increases and decreases in skin barrier function, such as TEWL, skin capacitance, and susceptibility to an irritant, for example, SLS and nickel salts, were observed.

Improvement of the skin barrier function was reported after 2-, 3-, or 4-week treatments of normal or atopic skin with moisturizers containing urea, which decreased TEWL and susceptibility to sodium lauryl sulfate (SLS) or nickel [8–12]. Treatment with a moisturizer containing another widely used humectant, glycerine, seems to have a less pronounced impact on the skin barrier [12, 13], even if the clinical effects were similar to urea cream [14]. On the other hand, in studies by Held et al. [15, 16], a moisturizer containing a high lipid content (70%) impaired the barrier of normal skin after 5-day and 4-week treatments, measured as increased skin susceptibility to SLS, although no change in baseline TEWL of undamaged skin was found. The same cream also increased susceptibility to nickel in nickel-allergic volunteers after 7-day treatment [17]. In a study on patients with lamellar ichthyosis, an 8-week treatment with moisturizers containing high amounts of lactic acid significantly increased TEWL, while dryness and scaling decreased [18]. Moisturizers have also been shown to influence skin barrier recovery after exposure to a skin irritant [9, 19].

The described functional changes indicate that moisturizers may also have an impact on the epidermis at the molecular level, even if they do not contain any substance with known pharmacological activity, and that these functional and molecular changes may be linked to each other. Indeed, Short et al. [20] showed that a moisturizer containing high amounts of glycerin and silicones increased maximum epidermal thickness, decreased epidermal melanin content, and altered protein expressions of keratins 6, 10, and 16, as assessed with immunohistochemistry after a 4-week treatment. Moreover, all these changes were accompanied by decreased TEWL. Another study revealed that a 6-week treatment with a moisturizer containing glycerin and erythritol increased the number of keratinocytes with a well-matured cornified envelope; also, the interleukin-1 receptor agonist/interleukin-1α (IL-1ra/IL-1α) ratio in the epidermis was altered [21]. Of course, it may well be individual ingredients that affect the skin at a molecular level, i.e., not the moisturizer as a whole. Linoleic acid, found in certain vegetable oils commonly used in topical preparations, is a ligand of peroxisome proliferator-activated receptors (PPAR) which has been found to have effects comparable to a potent topical glucocorticoid in animal models [22]. Another substance, nicotinamide, was shown to increase levels of ceramides and free fatty acids and to decrease TEWL, as compared with placebo-treated skin [23].

These studies demonstrate that prolonged application of moisturizers may have a substantial impact on the skin and its barrier, from both a functional and biochemical perspective. However, factors responsible for the observed effects are unknown, especially since the studies were performed using moisturizers containing several ingredients. Therefore, in order to gain further understanding of the mechanism by which long-term treatment with moisturizers influences the skin in vivo, investigations should be performed in a way that allows identification of ingredients responsible, for example, using moisturizers containing as few ingredients as possible and carry out studies that are placebo controlled. Moreover, noninvasive techniques should be simultaneously coupled with other tools, allowing for investigation of the epidermis at the molecular and cellular level, to connect functional and biochemical changes to each other, if possible.

37.5 Effect of 7-Week Use of Moisturizers on the Skin Barrier

In order to find out more about the mechanisms by which moisturizers influence the skin, the investigations presented in this chapter were performed using very simple moisturizers, containing only few ingredients. Noninvasive techniques were performed as well as molecular analysis of skin biopsies, such as quantitative real-time polymerase chain reaction (QRT-PCR), immunofluorescence, immunohistochemistry, and histological evaluations.

To investigate the effect of long-term use of moisturizers, the duration of use was chosen to be 7 weeks, which is longer than the application time in the majority of similar studies performed to date. Moreover, this time is similar or slightly longer than the average turnover time of the epidermis, which is reported to be 40–45 days [24, 25].

37.5.1 Choice of Test Moisturizers

The three test moisturizers used in the investigation were formulated in such way as to minimize their complexity in order to diminish the number of possible confounding factors. They therefore contained only a few ingredients and are hereafter called "simple creams," in contrast to the majority of commercially available topical preparations that contain over a dozen substances. In addition, one moisturizer, called Complex cream, containing several ingredients and previously shown to influence the skin barrier in normal and atopic skin, was chosen as a reference for this investigation [10, 26].

The three simple creams were o/w emulsions containing 40% lipid phase consisting of either pure hydrophobic hydrocarbons derived from mineral oil (isohexadecane and paraffin = Hydrocarbon cream) or a more polar vegetable oil consisting of triglycerides and sterols (canola oil = Canola cream and Canola/urea cream). The Canola/urea cream contained additionally 5% urea. The simple creams were stabilized with a polymeric emulsifier, acrylates/C10–30 alkyl acrylate crosspolymer, which was not expected to penetrate or influence the skin barrier function due to its large molecular size. A gel, consisting of water and this polymer, was also investigated (Polymer gel). By contrast, Complex cream contained a mixture of lipids of various origins and was emulsified with a combination of polymers and low-molecular emulsifiers. Due to such choice of ingredients, the following factors were examined: (1) the impact of a humectant (urea); (2) difference between creams of minimum complexity (Hydrocarbon, Canola and Canola/urea creams) and a cream containing more ingredients (Complex cream); and (3) different types of lipids (hydrocarbons or vegetable oil). All test preparations had their pH adjusted to about 5 [27–29]. Table 37.1 presents detailed compositions along with the number of volunteers testing each preparation.

Table 37.1 Composition of the test moisturizers used for investigating the effect of their 7-week long use on the skin barrier in healthy human volunteers, their ingredients, and number of volunteers testing them

Test preparation	Lipids	Emulsifiers	Other ingredients	Urea	Number of volunteers and type of investigations
Complex cream[a]	20%	1.3%	Water, propylene glycol, glyceryl polymethacrylate, dimethicone, sodium lactate, methylparaben, propylparaben, lactic acid, citric acid	5%	15, functional changes [27]
	Capric/caprylic triglyceride, canola oil, cetearyl alcohol, paraffin, glyceryl stearate	PEG-100 stearate, carbomer, polysorbate 60			10, functional and biochemical changes [28, 29]
Hydrocarbon cream	40%	0.4%	Water	0%	16, functional changes [27]
	Isohexadecane[b] (20%), paraffin[c] (20%)	Acrylates/C10–30 alkyl acrylate crosspolymer[d]			10, functional and biochemical changes [28, 29]
Canola cream	40%	0.4%	Water	0%	15, functional changes [27]
	Canola oil[e]	Acrylates/C10–30 alkyl acrylate crosspolymer[d]			
Canola/urea cream	40%	0.4%	Water	5%	16, functional changes [27]
	Canola oil[e]	Acrylates/C10–30 alkyl acrylate crosspolymer[d]			
Polymer gel	0%	0.4%	Water, methylparaben[f]	0%	16, functional changes [27]
		Acrylates/C10–30 alkyl acrylate crosspolymer[d]			

Adapted from Buraczewska et al. [27], with permission
[a]Canoderm® kräm 5%, ACO HUD NORDIC AB, Stockholm, Sweden
[b]Arlamol HD, Uniqema, Gouda, The Netherlands
[c]Merkur White Oil Pharma, Merkur Vaseline, Hamburg, Germany
[d]Pemulen TR-2, Noveon Inc., Cleveland, OH, USA
[e]Akorex L, Karlshamns AB, Karlshamn, Sweden
[f]Nipagin M, Clariant International, Pontypridd, United Kingdom

37.5.2 Experimental Design

The studies were double blinded and randomized. Only volunteers with normal, healthy skin were used. They were allowed to wash normally, but not to use any skin care products on the test areas at least 3 days before, and during, the test period.

In the first study, only functional changes in the skin barrier were investigated. Volunteers treated one volar forearm twice daily for 7 weeks with one test preparation (Hydrocarbon cream, Canola cream, Canola/urea cream, Polymer gel, or Complex cream), leaving the other forearm to serve as the untreated control. After 7 weeks, both volar forearms, treated and control, were exposed to 1% aqueous solution SLS for 24 h. TEWL and blood flow were assessed on the SLS-exposed and undamaged skin on each forearm on day 1. Skin capacitance was also measured on undamaged skin [27].

In the following studies, both functional and biochemical changes in the skin after 7-week treatment were investigated. The volunteers applied one of the test preparations, Complex cream or Hydrocarbon cream, on one volar forearm and also on one buttock twice daily for 7 weeks, leaving the other forearm and buttock untreated to serve as control sites. Complex cream and Hydrocarbon cream were chosen for the additional investigations based on the results from the first study, which showed that these two moisturizers have an opposite effect on the skin barrier, as seen from functional changes [27]. After 7 weeks, one shave and one punch biopsy were taken from each buttock, preceded by TEWL measurements of the biopsy area. Biopsies were used for investigating the biochemical changes in the skin: the shave biopsies were used for gene expression analysis using quantitative real-time polymerase chain reaction (QRT-PCR) and the punch biopsies for histological and other molecular evaluations. Moreover, the skin of the forearms was investigated for functional changes, in a way similar to the first study, using noninvasive methods [28, 29].

37.5.3 Results

Twice-daily treatment of normal skin of volar forearms for 7 weeks with all test preparations examined in this research induced changes in the skin barrier function, as evaluated with noninvasive methods. Hydrocarbon cream, Canola cream, and Canola/urea cream appear to have a negative effect on the skin barrier, as their application resulted in elevated TEWL and increased skin susceptibility to SLS. Polymer gel, consisting of polymer and water, had similar effects. Moreover, Hydrocarbon cream decreased skin capacitance, indicating dryness. To the author's knowledge, it is the first reported case of skin dryness induced by a moisturizer. By contrast, treatment with Complex cream decreased TEWL and susceptibility to SLS (Figs. 37.3 and 37.4) [27]. Use of Hydrocarbon and Complex creams influenced TEWL of gluteal skin in a way similar to forearms [29].

Molecular analyses of skin biopsies after use of Hydrocarbon cream and Complex cream on normal skin for 7 weeks revealed that these two creams induced different effects on the mRNA expression of genes involved in the keratinocyte differentiation, corneocyte formation and desquamation, as well as lipid metabolism. Treatment with Hydrocarbon cream changed the expression of 11 out of 22 analyzed genes, while exposure to Complex cream affected expression of only two of them (Table 37.2). At the same time, the moisturizers had no effect on protein expression of three analyzed proteins: involucrin, transglutaminase 1, and filaggrin. Stratum corneum thickness, epidermal thickness, the size of corneocytes, and nonpolar lipid staining were also unaffected by the treatments [28, 29].

The studies therefore revealed that moisturizers have different effects on the barrier function of normal skin and that the changes were dependent on the composition of the moisturizer. The test preparations had an impact on the normal function and/or structure of the skin. The observed changes may be caused either by the ingredients of the test preparations (e.g., lipids, humectants, emulsifiers, or water), which have a direct or indi-

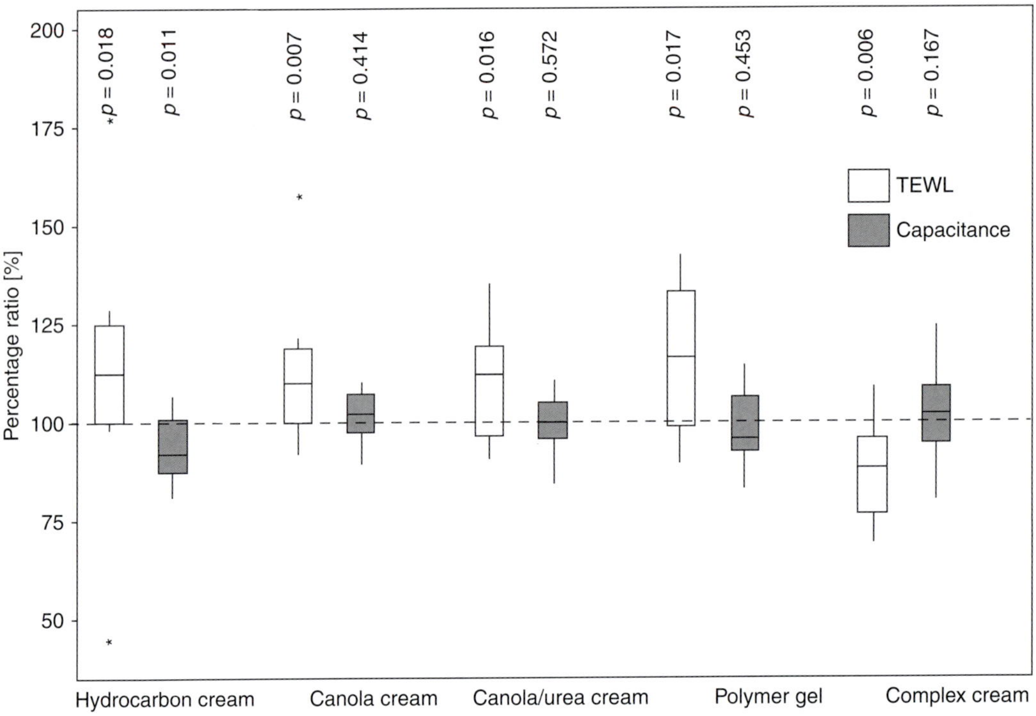

Fig. 37.3 TEWL and skin capacitance of undamaged skin treated with test preparations for 7 weeks. Values are presented as percentage ratio of the values obtained from the corresponding control areas, which serve as 100%. *P*-values relate to differences from control areas. The results are presented as *box* plots with the median value as a *line across* the box and the first quartile value at the *bottom* and the third at the *top*. The whiskers are lines that extend from the *top* and *bottom* of the box to the lowest and the highest observation within a defined region, with outliers plotted as *asterisks* outside this region. Reference line is given at 100%. $N=15$ for Canola cream and Complex cream and 16 for Canola/urea cream, Hydrocarbon cream, and Polymer gel (From Buraczewska et al. [27]. with permission)

rect effect on skin barrier components, or by the physical effects of moisturizers on the skin, such as occlusion or pH.

37.5.4 Possible Explanations of Observed Effects

Despite the apparent relationship between gene expression and the skin barrier function, it was not possible to ascertain whether the observed functional changes, such as increased/decreased TEWL, susceptibility to SLS or skin capacitance, were the effect of molecular changes in the epidermis or vice versa ("hen-and-egg" situation). The first possibility is that functional changes in the skin barrier, induced by moisturizers, could trigger epidermal keratinocytes to alter their gene expression. An example of such functional change may be the delivery of exogenous lipids from the moisturizers into the intercellular lipids of the stratum corneum, resulting in altered barrier function, or the impact of emulsifiers, humectants, or exposure to water.

37.5.4.1 Lipids

Lipids in moisturizers may remain on the skin surface or enter the skin [30], and more physiological lipids may penetrate into the epidermis and affect skin barrier structure and recovery [31–33]. Changes in lateral packing of stratum corneum lipids were observed in patients with atopic dermatitis and psoriasis after 3-week treatment with a moisturizer containing 10% petrola-

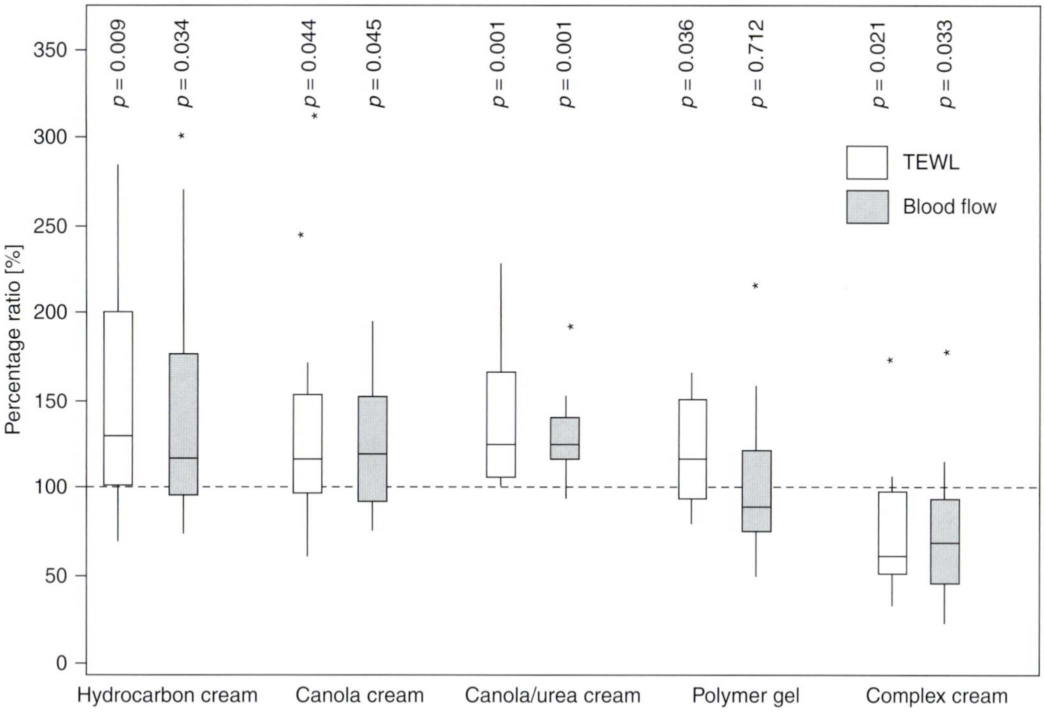

Fig. 37.4 TEWL and blood flow of SLS-exposed skin treated with test preparations, in relation to control areas (not treated with moisturizers but also exposed to SLS). For explanation of the graph, see Fig. 37.3 (From Buraczewska et al. [27], with permission)

tum [34]. Therefore, in our study, the possible penetration of lipids from test moisturizers could alter skin barrier properties.

The three simplified creams investigated, all of which had a negative effect on the skin barrier (Hydrocarbon cream, Canola cream, Canola/urea cream), contained high proportions of lipids, 40%, but the type of lipid (hydrocarbons or triglycerides) was of no importance to the effect. At the same time, Complex cream, containing 20% lipids, did not deteriorate the skin barrier. Effects similar to those for the simplified creams have been obtained with a moisturizer containing 70% lipids which made the skin more susceptible to SLS [15, 16]. These results suggest that differences in the lipid content or uptake rate may be important for the effect of moisturizers on the skin barrier function. As exogenous lipids may change the highly organized structure of intercellular lipid layers, TEWL or the ion flux may also be altered. Such changes may be recognized as barrier impairment by epidermal keratinocytes, initiating a repair process including altered gene expression.

37.5.4.2 Water

Penetration of lipids, however, cannot explain the impairment of the skin barrier obtained after treatment with Polymer gel, as it contains no lipids but much more water compared with other moisturizers, 99%. After application of a moisturizer, water, which is typically one of the main ingredients, evaporates within a short time [35, 36]. The effect on the skin barrier of twice-daily exposure to water for a few weeks is unknown. It has been shown that prolonged contact with water disrupts the intercellular lipid lamellar structure in the stratum corneum and may contribute to dryness and increased TEWL [37]. Moreover, changes in gene expression of epidermal enzymes and

Table 37.2 Summary of the gene expression analysis of skin biopsies after use of Hydrocarbon cream and Complex cream on normal skin for 7 weeks, presented in Buraczewska et al. [28, 29]

Function	Gene	Complex cream	Hydrocarbon cream
Proteins involved in keratinocyte differentiation	IVL	–	↑
	TGM1	–	↑
	FLG	–	–
	CDKN1A	↓	–
Enzymes involved in the process of desquamation	KLK5	–	↑
	KLK7	–	↑
Enzymes involved in ceramide synthesis	GBA	–	↑
	SPTLC2	–	↑
	SMPD1	–	↑
	UGCG	–	–
Enzymes involved in cholesterol synthesis	HMGCS1	–	↑
	HMGCR	–	–
Enzymes involved in fatty acid metabolism	ACACB	–	–
	FASN	–	–
	ACSL1	–	–
Nuclear hormone receptors	PPARA	–	–
	PPARB	–	–
	PPARG	↑	↓
	RXRA	–	–
Lipoxygenases	ALOX12B	–	↑
	ALOXE3	–	↑
Interleukin	IL1A	–	–

Molecular analyses revealed that these two creams induced different effects on the mRNA expression of genes involved in the keratinocyte differentiation, corneocyte formation and desquamation, as well as lipid metabolism. Treatment with Hydrocarbon cream changed the expression of 11 out of 22 analyzed genes, while exposure to Complex cream affected expression of only two of them

↑ increased messenger ribonucleic acid (mRNA) expression in comparison with untreated skin, ↓ decreased mRNA expression, – no difference, *ACACB* acetyl-CoA carboxylase beta, *ACSL1* acyl-CoA synthetase long-chain family member 1, *ALOX12B* arachidonate 12-lipoxygenase, 12R type, *ALOXE3* epidermal arachidonate lipoxygenase 3, *CDKN1A* cyclin-dependent kinase inhibitor 1A, *FASN* fatty acid synthase, *FLG* profilaggrin, *GBA* β-glucocerebrosidase, *HMGCR* HMG-CoA reductase, *HMGCS1* HMG-CoA synthase 1, *IL1A* interleukin-1α, *IVL* involucrin, *KLK5* kallikrein 5, *KLK7* kallikrein 7, *PPARA* PPAR-α, *PPARB* PPAR-β, *PPARG* PPAR-γ, *RXRA* RXR-α, *SMPD1* acid sphingomyelinase, *SPTLC2* serine palmitoyltransferase 2, *TGM1* transglutaminase 1, *UGCG* UDP-glucose ceramide glucosyltransferase

nonenzymatic proteins were found after exposure of skin to water (only) under occlusion [38]. It has also been suggested that the higher TEWL of the dorsal surface of hands, compared with the forearm and back, may be due to more frequent contact with water [39]. Increased TEWL and dryness of the skin could also be caused by contact with irritants, but the test preparations, including Polymer gel, were shown not to be irritant by an acute irritancy test and by blood flow measurements. Moreover, treatment with Hydrocarbon cream and Complex cream did not alter expression of IL1A, indicating lack of inflammation. Furthermore, though all simple creams and Complex cream contain similar amounts of water, around 60%, they induced different changes in the skin barrier.

37.5.4.3 Emulsifiers and Polymers

Emulsifiers are essential in moisturizers, as they stabilize the emulsion. Emulsifiers commonly used in o/w emulsions have been shown to influence the skin barrier function in normal and SLS-exposed skin [40]. Although the emulsifier used in the simple creams and Polymer gel, acrylates/C10–30 alkyl acrylate crosspolymer, was expected not to penetrate into the epidermis due to its large molecular size, in addition to the comments on water made above, its negative effect could have been caused by monomers which may be present at low concentrations. However, the Complex cream also contained a polymeric emulsifier, carbomer, which is similar in structure to acrylates/C10–30 alkyl acrylate crosspolymer, but lacked a negative impact on the skin barrier. Interestingly, it has been suggested that polymers themselves may have an effect on the skin barrier, as tested on mice, accelerating or delaying the barrier recovery [41]. Although this phenomenon is not fully understood, it is possible that polymers together with their counterions form an electric double layer on the skin surface, influencing the skin barrier [41].

37.5.4.4 Humectants

Humectants that are added to moisturizers, such as urea, glycerin, and propylene glycol, may penetrate into the skin [42, 43]. It has been suggested that the decreased TEWL and lower response to SLS after treatment with Complex cream was due to its urea content [10, 11, 26]. Moreover, it could be expected that the addition of urea to a moisturizer would be beneficial, as it has been reported that urea replaces water in the skin, leaving the physical properties of the stratum corneum intact [44]. However, the addition of urea to Canola/urea cream did not improve the skin barrier. It might be that in the Canola/urea cream, penetration of urea was different than in case of Complex cream due to the different emulsion system.

Urea has been reported to act as a keratolytic agent [45]; however, absence of a measurable thinning of the stratum corneum by the 5% urea in Complex cream in the present investigation [29] does not support keratolytic properties at a concentration commonly found in moisturizing creams.

Although treatment with Complex cream containing 5% urea significantly decreased TEWL and susceptibility to SLS, it had only minor effects on the mRNA expression of the analyzed genes. Therefore, the effect of urea on the barrier function may depend on the whole composition of the moisturizers, including the lipid content. Urea has also been found to diminish epidermal proliferation in psoriasis, measured as a decreased expression of involucrin and an increased expression of cytokeratins [46]. However, no difference in expression of proteins or the genes involved in keratinocyte differentiation and desquamation, apart from CDKN1A, was detected. Decreased expression of CDKN1A suggests influences in cell cycle progression after treatment with the urea-containing Complex cream, which could be interpreted as decrease in cell differentiation [47, 48], though not detectable by histological evaluations, since the thickness of the epidermis and the stratum corneum remained unchanged, as did corneocyte size.

37.5.4.5 Occlusion

As an alternative explanation, gene expression may be influenced by altered activity of various signaling pathways, resulting in a changed skin barrier function. However, it is still not clear what type of signal can trigger changes in gene expression: the changes could be due to ingredients included in the moisturizers or could have been indirectly induced by changes in ion or water flux. One possible signal may be a reduction in TEWL due to occlusion by the topically applied moisturizer, hypothetically resulting in water flux changes. It was previously shown that occlusion of the skin with a semipermeable membrane, mimicking the occlusion effect by a moisturizer, decreased TEWL and susceptibility to an irritant, in a group wearing the membrane 23 h a day for 3 weeks, suggesting changes in skin barrier function [49]. However, there is no evidence of a correlation between the occlusive properties of creams and their effects on the skin barrier, determined as the degree of irritation after SLS exposure, since Complex cream and a lipid-rich cream show similar occlusive capacity[49], but opposite effects on the skin barrier function [10, 11, 15, 16, 26]. Therefore, the detected difference in the effect on the skin barrier is more likely to have causes other than difference in occlusion between the creams. It is still not known whether a prolonged occlusion per se influences mRNA expression, since no investigation of this aspect has yet been performed. It is also worth noting that the semiocclusive layer formed by a moisturizer is usually removed from the skin within a few hours.

37.5.4.6 pH

The impact of the pH of topical preparations on the skin barrier is still not fully understood. A study investigating the effect of moisturizers of pH 4 and 7.5 showed that the pH of moisturizers seems not to be of major importance for their effects on the skin barrier: no difference in the impact on skin barrier recovery or susceptibility to an irritant was found [50]. The lack of difference in effect on skin barrier recovery of the moisturizers with acidic or alkaline pH values in our study disagrees with a previous study in mice, where barrier recovery was delayed after exposure to slightly alkaline pH [51]. However, the endogenous mechanisms involved in the formation of a pH gradient in the stratum corneum [52–56], as well as continuous exogenous excretion of sweat and sebum and NMF, could be expected to counteract the change in the skin surface pH induced by a topical application. It has been shown that after use of an alkaline soap, initially elevated skin surface pH decreases back toward acidic values [57], and therefore the same effect can be expected after a moisturizer. Moisturizers usually contain only small quantities of buffering ingredients, which make them unable to produce persistent changes in the skin surface pH, while the mentioned skin barrier recovery study on mice was performed using strong buffer systems [51]. Moreover, the majority of moisturizers have pH in a range of 4–6, which is in the range of the skin surface pH. However, it cannot be excluded that some ingredients of moisturizers may penetrate into the epidermis and influence the pH gradient there, which would have an effect on the skin barrier function.

37.5.5 Molecular Changes Induced by Hydrocarbon and Complex Creams

Regardless of the mechanisms involved, Hydrocarbon cream and Complex cream influenced the skin barrier in a way detectable by noninvasive measurements and molecular analyses of mRNA expression: the latter, however, were not confirmed at the protein level.

37.5.5.1 Effect of Hydrocarbon Cream on the Skin Barrier

Hydrocarbon cream appears to have a negative effect on the skin barrier since it elevates the TEWL and makes the skin more susceptible to SLS. Hydrocarbon cream increased the mRNA expression of genes responsible for the synthesis of ceramides and cholesterol, GBA, SPTLC2, SMPD1, and HMGCS1, but not the expression of free fatty acid-metabolizing enzymes. These results can be interpreted as an epidermal response to barrier damage. The results support such a hypothesis since Hydrocarbon cream increased also mRNA expression of IVL and TGM1, both being key proteins in formation of the cornified envelope. Other studies of skin barrier damage induced in mice by acetone, surfactant, tape stripping, or an essential fatty acid-deficient diet, also describe increased mRNA expressions or activities of lipid-processing enzymes [58–61]. However, in a recent study on healthy human volunteers, two creams containing 5% urea, the same amount as in Complex cream, increased mRNA expression of IVL, FLG, loricrin, and TGM1 after a 2-week treatment, which was also accompanied by a significant decrease in TEWL [62]. This gene expression profile is similar to the effect of Hydrocarbon cream, although the effect on TEWL is like that of Complex cream. This suggests that the relationship between mRNA expression and TEWL is not so straightforward and that the gene expression profile may change during treatment time.

37.5.5.2 Nuclear Receptors and Lipoxygenases

Hydrocarbon cream decreased the mRNA expression of PPARG as well as influenced mRNA expression of the two lipoxygenases, ALOX12B and ALOXE3. PPAR-γ and other PPARs are involved in the regulation of keratinocyte differentiation and expression of several of the lipid-processing enzymes. In skin equivalent models, activation of PPAR-α receptors by synthetic ligands resulted in an increase in the mRNA expression of lipid-metabolizing enzymes, three of which were the same as in our present study (GBA, SPTLC2, and HMGCS1) [63]. Although Hydrocarbon cream does not contain any known PPAR agonists, the elevated expressions of ALOX12B and ALOXE3, genes of lipoxygenases that produce derivatives acting as PPAR-α agonists [64], may suggest an endogenous formation of PPAR-α agonists by the Hydrocarbon cream treatment.

While Hydrocarbon cream decreased the mRNA expression of PPARG, Complex cream increased it. However, no difference in protein expression of PPAR-γ was found after use of any of the test preparations. Nevertheless, the opposite effect on the expression of PPARG and TEWL induced by Hydrocarbon and Complex cream, as well as a linear correlation between these two parameters in untreated skin, suggests an importance of PPAR-γ for the skin barrier function. Usually, PPAR-γ activation affects cell proliferation, cell differentiation, immune responses, and apoptosis in the skin. PPARγ signaling is triggered by various types of ligands, including linoleic acid (reviewed by Feingold [65], Schmuth et al. [66], and Sertznig et al. [67]). Although Complex cream contains a vegetable oil, which may contain a small fraction of free fatty acids, for example, linoleic acid, our present results do not suggest any activation of PPARs.

A linear correlation between TEWL and mRNA expression in untreated skin was found for ACACB. The enzyme encoded by this gene is involved in synthesis of fatty acids, and its importance for the skin barrier has been shown after barrier disruption in mice, which increased mRNA expression of this enzyme [59]. The regulation of ACACB in keratinocytes is unknown, but in mouse hepatocytes, it has been shown that the PPAR-α agonist WY-16,643 increases the expression of ACACB [68].

37.5.5.3 Enzymes and Proteins Involved in Keratinocyte Differentiation and Desquamation

Treatment with Hydrocarbon cream increased the mRNA level of INV and TGM1, but it was not accompanied by a corresponding increase in protein expression. This may indicate that the epidermis was preparing itself for possible repair of the impaired skin barrier or that the repair phase had already been completed, but there was still ongoing transcription. Another reason for the lack of correlation between mRNA and protein expression after treatment may be that the mRNA had not been translated into protein or that the protein turnover had increased for unknown reasons. The inhibition of mRNA translation has been shown to be caused by microRNA. For example, certain genes in the epidermis of psoriasis patients exhibit diminished translation due to the presence of certain microRNAs [69]. Furthermore, since protein and mRNA expressions were analyzed on a single occasion, after 7 weeks of treatment, it is possible that changes in protein levels occurred at another time, perhaps after a few days, but became "normalized" after a few weeks due to some adaptation mechanism. As already mentioned before, a recent study with two creams containing 5% urea showed mRNA expression profile of IVL, FLG, and TGM1 which differed from our study; however, the analysis was done after 2 weeks of treatment instead of 7 [62].

It is also possible that the analytical method used was not sufficiently sensitive to detect differences in protein expression. The mRNA expression increased by about 55% in the case of IVL and 120% in the case of TGM1, which may not be enough to show in detectable differences using an immunofluorescence technique. Other techniques, for example, western blot, may have been more powerful, but would have necessitated obtaining additional biopsies from the volunteers, which was not possible for ethical reasons. However, another study describes changes in mRNA expression of a magnitude similar to that seen in the present study, resulted in visible increased protein levels after 1–7 days after exposure to SLS [38]. This suggests that the effect of moisturizers at the protein level may also have occurred earlier.

Exposure to Hydrocarbon cream also increased the gene expression of KLK5 and KLK7, which may suggest an excessive desquamation, since these two proteases are involved in this process [70–73]. However, since the thickness of the stratum corneum remained unchanged, it could be possible that treatment with Hydrocarbon cream initially induced thickening of stratum corneum, but increased performance of kallikreins counteracted it. Another possibility is that both proliferation as well as desquamation increased simultaneously, which would end in unchanged thickness. However, the altered expression of kallikreins may also be due to other, not well-known, functions in the skin barrier since it has been shown that kallikrein 7 degrades some lipid-processing enzymes [74].

The altered expression of kallikreins may also be linked in some way to decreased skin capacitance after use of Hydrocarbon cream. This may indicate low skin hydration levels [75] since these enzymes have been found to have increased protein expression in psoriasis [76] and atopic dermatitis [77]. However, the protein expression of kallikreins was not assessed in the present study. Interestingly, decreased skin capacitance was not accompanied by any change in the mRNA expression of FLG or the protein expression of filaggrin, which degrades into free amino acids and PCA, the main components of NMF (reviewed by Rawlings et al. [78, 79]).

37.6 Conclusions and Future Perspectives

In the present investigation, after long-term treatment, moisturizers were examined for their effect on the skin barrier with regard to such factors as pH, lipid type, the presence of a humectant, as well as complexity of the product [27–29, 50]. Moisturizers are able to modify the skin barrier function, detected as changes in TEWL, skin capacitance, and susceptibility to an irritant, and also to change the mRNA expression of certain genes involved in the assembly, differentiation, and desquamation of the stratum corneum, as well as lipid metabolism. Therefore, moisturizers should not be perceived simply as inert topical preparations, even if they do not contain any substance with known pharmacological activity. However, the mechanisms behind the observed effects are still not fully understood. The observed outcome is most likely the combination of interplay and effects of several factors, rather than only one, which makes it more difficult to draw any firm conclusions. More research of this kind is needed to better understand the mechanism of action of moisturizers. Such research would aid in the treatment of various skin disorders through improved design of moisturizers, which can target specific skin problems and conditions both more efficiently and safely.

In the present investigations, traditional, noninvasive methods to investigate the skin barrier function were used, combined with invasive techniques allowing studying changes in the epidermis after use of moisturizers at the molecular and cellular level. Analysis of gene and protein expressions and histological evaluations lead to new hypotheses and answer more questions than noninvasive methods alone.

The investigation showed that treatment with moisturizers might change gene expression of a number of epidermal proteins, including structural proteins and enzymes. It was performed on selected genes known to be important for the skin barrier, and since their number was not very high, QRT-PCR was used for analyses. However, further investigations could also include cDNA microarrays, which allow for screening several thousands of genes at the same time. This would give a broader perspective over changes in gene expression in the epidermis and help to identify additional genes and proteins that should be investigated in more details.

Since the research investigated the effects of moisturizers after 7 weeks of treatment, one may consider exploring also their impact on the skin barrier at earlier time points. The course of gene and protein expression and histological changes may vary between shortly after application to after few-week use. It would also be interesting to continue the investigation for some time after use of a moisturizer is terminated, following the return of the skin barrier to the state from before the treatment.

Although molecular analyses provide plenty of information about the skin barrier, noninvasive evaluations should be utilized as well, as they do not require skin sampling and provide a different type of data, i.e., skin barrier function. The new types of noninvasive methods developed during recent years help us acquire detailed facts about the skin structure and function in vivo and may be used in studies investigating the effects of moisturizers. For example, Raman spectroscopy helps to evaluate the moisturizing effect by giving a detailed water profile in the epidermis and assess stratum corneum and epidermal thickness [80–82], as well as to follow drug penetration (reviewed by Wartewig et al. [83]). Multiphoton laser tomography [84] and confocal laser scanning microscopy (reviewed by Branzan et al. [85]) allow us to "look" inside the skin and may be exploited in various ways.

The results presented in this chapter as well as other studies demonstrate that the composition of moisturizers plays an essential role in their effects on the skin and its barrier function. Therefore, it would seem reasonable at first to systematically test various ingredients, combinations of ingredients, and complete moisturizers for their effects, in order to find those giving the desired efficacy, both in healthy and in diseased skin. However, taking into consideration that over 500 ingredients classified as humectants and about 1,500 emollients are available [86], the number of possible combinations is endless, even if the number of ingredients were limited to only those used more frequently. Therefore, it is more realistic to continue the research about these few ingredients, which are common in many moisturizers and for which some data is already available, regarding the effect of glycerin, urea, vegetable oils, and hydrocarbons.

As the knowledge about the effect of various ingredients and their combinations on the skin barrier is scarce, testing of complete moisturizers is currently the best way to assure benefits for the consumers. However, although clinical trials are mandatory for pharmaceuticals (over-the-counter or prescription drugs) to prove their efficacy, moisturizers available as cosmetic products are rarely evaluated for their effect on the skin barrier. Therefore, in theory, some commercially available moisturizers may have a negative impact on the skin, and their use could worsen the skin condition, facilitate penetration of irritants, and even lead to eczema. Consequently, the composition of a moisturizer should be an important issue when recommending it to a patient with skin problems since this choice may have an impact on the skin status and therefore on quality of life. Treatment with corticosteroids and other drugs improves the condition of the skin with eczema, but a relapse may only be a question of time. However, while the use of a moisturizer with the skin barrier-improving effect after corticosteroid therapy may increase an eczema-free period in comparison with no treatment [87], it is not known if use of a moisturizer with barrier-impairing properties causes an earlier relapse of eczema. This issue should be investigated further, as it may have a major impact on the approach to the treatment of dry skin disorders.

Improving or maintaining the skin status and quality of life may also involve more than choosing a proper moisturizer since compliance to treatment is also required. If a moisturizer is not attractive to a patient from a cosmetic perspective, for example, because it is too greasy and tacky, difficult to apply, has an unpleasant odor, or its package is impractical, there is a high probability that the patient will not use it according to guidelines and as a result will require more medical attention. The same problem may exist in the case of barrier creams, which are supposed to inhibit penetration of irritant substances. Therefore, the cosmetic properties of moisturizers must be taken into consideration during the early stages of the development, which is a challenge for researchers and formulating chemists, as various ingredients added to make a product more stable and attractive may weaken its performance or cause adverse reactions.

In conclusion, it is important to remember that moisturizers differ in their composition, which determines their impact on the skin barrier. A better understanding of the influence of moisturizers on the skin barrier, obtained by combination of noninvasive methods and molecular analyses, would facilitate in the design of skin care products adjusted to specific skin problems. It would also provide more efficient management of dry skin disorders and, hopefully, help to influence the development of moisturizers so that fewer products will have negative effects on the skin.

Take-Home Messages

- Use of moisturizers is widespread not only among people with dry skin but also with normal, healthy skin.
- Moisturizers are not inert topical preparations, and they are able to modify skin barrier function, even if they do not contain any substance with known pharmacological activity.
- Moisturizers may improve the skin barrier function, which can even lead to delay of eczema relapse, but also impair it, leading to increased susceptibility to irritants and dryness.
- Moisturizers differ in their composition, which determines their impact on the skin barrier.
- The mechanisms behind the impact of moisturizers on the skin barrier are still not fully understood.
- Development of moisturizers should encompass their effect on the skin barrier and be adjusted to specific skin problems.

Abbreviations

ACACB	Acetyl-CoA carboxylase beta
ACSL1	Acyl-CoA synthetase long-chain family member 1
ACTB	Actin beta (β-actin)
ALOX12B	Arachidonate 12-lipoxygenase 12R type
ALOXE3	Epidermal arachidonate lipoxygenase 3
ARCI	Autosomal recessive congenital ichthyosis
CDKN1A	Cyclin-dependent kinase inhibitor 1A
cDNA	Complementary deoxyribonucleic acid
CoA	Coenzyme A
DAPI	4′-6-Diamidino-2-phenylindole
FASN	Fatty acid synthase
FLG	Profilaggrin
GBA	Glucocerebrosidase beta; acid (β-glucocerebrosidase)
HMGCR	3-Hydroxy-3-methylglutaryl-CoA reductase (HMG-CoA reductase)
HMGCS1	3-Hydroxy-3-methylglutaryl-CoA synthase 1 (HMG-CoA synthase 1)
IL1A	Interleukin-1α
IVL	Involucrin
KLK5	Kallikrein 5
KLK7	Kallikrein 7
mRNA	Messenger ribonucleic acid
NMF	Natural moisturizing factor
o/w	Oil-in-water
PBS	Phosphate-buffered saline
PCA	Pyrrolidone carboxylic acid
PPARA	Peroxisome proliferator-activated receptor alpha (PPAR-α)
PPARB	Peroxisome proliferator-activated receptor beta (PPAR-β)
PPARG	Peroxisome proliferator-activated receptor gamma (PPAR-γ)
QRT-PCR	Quantitative real-time polymerase chain reaction
RT	Reverse transcription
RXRA	Retinoid X receptor alpha (RXR-α)
SLS	Sodium lauryl sulfate
SMPD1	Sphingomyelin phosphodiesterase 1 acid lysosomal (acid sphingomyelinase)
SPTLC2	Serine palmitoyltransferase long chain base subunit 2 (serine palmitoyltransferase 2)
TEWL	Transepidermal water loss
TGM1	Transglutaminase 1
UGCG	UDP-glucose ceramide glucosyltransferase

Acknowledgments I wish to express my sincere gratitude to my supervisors: Hans Törmä, Marie Lodén, Berit Berne, and Magnus Lindberg. The research presented in this chapter was financially supported by ACO HUD NORDIC AB, Uppsala University, and the Welander and Finsen Foundation.

References

1. Lodén M (2003) Role of topical emollients and moisturizers in the treatment of dry skin barrier disorders. Am J Clin Dermatol 4(11):771–788
2. Lodén M (2003) Do moisturizers work? J Cosmet Dermatol 2(3–4):141–149
3. Proksch E, Lachapelle JM (2005) The management of dry skin with topical emollients–recent perspectives. J Dtsch Dermatol Ges 3(10):768–774
4. Lewis-Jones S, Mugglestone MA (2007) Management of atopic eczema in children aged up to 12 years: summary of NICE guidance. BMJ 335(7632):1263–1264
5. Lodén M (1992) The increase in skin hydration after application of emollients with different amounts of lipids. Acta Derm Venereol 72(5):327–330
6. Lodén M (2005) The clinical benefit of moisturizers. J Eur Acad Dermatol Venereol 19(6):672–688; quiz 686–677
7. Lodén M, Lindberg M (1994) Product testing - testing of moisturizers. In: Elsner P, Berardesca E, Maibach H (eds) Bioengineering of the skin: water and the stratum corneum. CRC Press, Boca Raton, pp 275–289
8. Lodén M (1996) Urea-containing moisturizers influence barrier properties of normal skin. Arch Dermatol Res 288(2):103–107
9. Lodén M (1997) Barrier recovery and influence of irritant stimuli in skin treated with a moisturizing cream. Contact Dermatitis 36(5):256–260
10. Lodén M, Andersson AC, Lindberg M (1999) Improvement in skin barrier function in patients with atopic dermatitis after treatment with a moisturizing cream (Canoderm). Br J Dermatol 140(2):264–267
11. Lodén M, Kuzmina N, Nyren M, Edlund F, Emtestam L (2004) Nickel susceptibility and skin barrier function to water after treatment with a urea-containing moisturizer. Exogen Dermatol 3:99–105
12. Lodén M, Andersson AC, Andersson C, Frodin T, Oman H, Lindberg M (2001) Instrumental and dermatologist evaluation of the effect of glycerine and urea on dry skin in atopic dermatitis. Skin Res Technol 7(4):209–213
13. Lodén M, Wessman C (2001) The influence of a cream containing 20% glycerin and its vehicle on skin barrier properties. Int J Cosmet Sci 23:115–119
14. Lodén M, Andersson AC, Anderson C, Bergbrant IM, Frodin T, Ohman H, Sandstrom MH, Sarnhult T, Voog E, Stenberg B, Pawlik E, Preisler-Haggqvist A, Svensson A, Lindberg M (2002) A double-blind study comparing the effect of glycerin and urea on dry, eczematous skin in atopic patients. Acta Derm Venereol 82(1):45–47
15. Held E, Agner T (2001) Effect of moisturizers on skin susceptibility to irritants. Acta Derm Venereol 81(2):104–107
16. Held E, Sveinsdottir S, Agner T (1999) Effect of long-term use of moisturizer on skin hydration, barrier function and susceptibility to irritants. Acta Derm Venereol 79(1):49–51
17. Zachariae C, Held E, Johansen JD, Menne T, Agner T (2003) Effect of a moisturizer on skin susceptibility to NiCl2. Acta Derm Venereol 83(2):93–97
18. Ganemo A, Virtanen M, Vahlquist A (1999) Improved topical treatment of lamellar ichthyosis: a double-blind study of four different cream formulations. Br J Dermatol 141(6):1027–1032
19. Held E, Lund H, Agner T (2001) Effect of different moisturizers on SLS-irritated human skin. Contact Dermatitis 44(4):229–234
20. Short RW, Chan JL, Choi JM, Egbert BM, Rehmus WE, Kimball AB (2007) Effects of moisturization on epidermal homeostasis and differentiation. Clin Exp Dermatol 32(1):88–90, Epub 2006 Nov 27
21. Kikuchi K, Kobayashi H, Hirao T, Ito A, Takahashi H, Tagami H (2003) Improvement of mild inflammatory changes of the facial skin induced by winter environment with daily applications of a moisturizing cream. A half-side test of biophysical skin parameters, cytokine expression pattern and the formation of cornified envelope. Dermatology 207(3):269–275
22. Sheu MY, Fowler AJ, Kao J, Schmuth M, Schoonjans K, Auwerx J, Fluhr JW, Man MQ, Elias PM, Feingold KR (2002) Topical peroxisome proliferator activated receptor-alpha activators reduce inflammation in irritant and allergic contact dermatitis models. J Invest Dermatol 118(1):94–101
23. Tanno O, Ota Y, Kitamura N, Katsube T, Inoue S (2000) Nicotinamide increases biosynthesis of ceramides as well as other stratum corneum lipids to improve the epidermal permeability barrier. Br J Dermatol 143(3):524–531
24. Weinstein GD, McCullough JL, Ross P (1984) Cell proliferation in normal epidermis. J Invest Dermatol 82(6):623–628
25. Bergstresser PR, Taylor JR (1977) Epidermal 'turn-over time'–a new examination. Br J Dermatol 96(5):503–509
26. Lodén M, Barany E, Wessman C (2004) The influence of urea treatment on skin susceptibility to surfactant-induced irritation: a placebo-controlled and randomized study. Exogen Dermatol 3:1–6
27. Buraczewska I, Berne B, Lindberg M, Törmä H, Lodén M (2007) Changes in skin barrier function following long-term treatment with moisturizers, a randomized controlled trial. Br J Dermatol 156(3):492–498
28. Buraczewska I, Berne B, Lindberg M, Loden M, Torma H (2009) Moisturizers change the mRNA expression of enzymes synthesizing skin barrier lipids. Arch Dermatol Res 301(8):587–594. doi:10.1007/s00403-009-0958-2
29. Buraczewska I, Berne B, Lindberg M, Loden M, Torma H (2009) Long-term treatment with moisturizers affects the mRNA levels of genes involved in keratinocyte differentiation and desquamation. Arch Dermatol Res 301(2):175–181. doi:10.1007/s00403-008-0906-6

30. Ghadially R, Halkier-Sorensen L, Elias PM (1992) Effects of petrolatum on stratum corneum structure and function. J Am Acad Dermatol 26(3 Pt 2): 387–396
31. Man MQ, Feingold KR, Elias PM (1993) Exogenous lipids influence permeability barrier recovery in acetone-treated murine skin. Arch Dermatol 129(6): 728–738
32. Mao-Qiang M, Brown BE, Wu-Pong S, Feingold KR, Elias PM (1995) Exogenous nonphysiologic vs physiologic lipids. Divergent mechanisms for correction of permeability barrier dysfunction. Arch Dermatol 131(7):809–816
33. Wertz PW, Downing DT (1990) Metabolism of topically applied fatty acid methyl esters in BALB/C mouse epidermis. J Dermatol Sci 1(1):33–37
34. Pilgram GS, Vissers DC, van der Meulen H, Pavel S, Lavrijsen SP, Bouwstra JA, Koerten HK (2001) Aberrant lipid organization in stratum corneum of patients with atopic dermatitis and lamellar ichthyosis. J Invest Dermatol 117(3):710–717
35. Blichmann CW, Serup J, Winther A (1989) Effects of single application of a moisturizer: evaporation of emulsion water, skin surface temperature, electrical conductance, electrical capacitance, and skin surface (emulsion) lipids. Acta Derm Venereol 69(4): 327–330
36. Rietschel RL (1978) A method to evaluate skin moisturizers in vivo. J Invest Dermatol 70(3):152–155
37. Warner RR, Stone KJ, Boissy YL (2003) Hydration disrupts human stratum corneum ultrastructure. J Invest Dermatol 120(2):275–284
38. Törmä H, Lindberg M, Berne B (2008) Skin barrier disruption by sodium lauryl sulfate-exposure alters the expressions of involucrin, transglutaminase 1, profilaggrin, and kallikreins during the repair phase in human skin in vivo. J Invest Dermatol 128(5):1212–1219, Epub 2007 Nov 15
39. Lodén M, Olsson H, Axell T, Linde YW (1992) Friction, capacitance and transepidermal water loss (TEWL) in dry atopic and normal skin. Br J Dermatol 126(2):137–141
40. Barany E, Lindberg M, Lodén M (2000) Unexpected skin barrier influence from nonionic emulsifiers. Int J Pharm 195(1–2):189–195
41. Denda M, Nakanishi K, Kumazawa N (2005) Topical application of ionic polymers affects skin permeability barrier homeostasis. Skin Pharmacol Physiol 18(1):36–41
42. Wellner K, Wohlrab W (1993) Quantitative evaluation of urea in stratum corneum of human skin. Arch Dermatol Res 285(4):239–240
43. Brinkmann I, Muller-Goymann CC (2005) An attempt to clarify the influence of glycerol, propylene glycol, isopropyl myristate and a combination of propylene glycol and isopropyl myristate on human stratum corneum. Pharmazie 60(3):215–220
44. Costa-Balogh FO, Wennerstrom H, Wadso L, Sparr E (2006) How small polar molecules protect membrane systems against osmotic stress: the urea-water-phospholipid system. J Phys Chem B 110(47):23845–23852
45. Hellgren L, Larsson K (1974) On the effect of urea on human epidermis. Dermatologica 149(5):289–293
46. Hagemann I, Proksch E (1996) Topical treatment by urea reduces epidermal hyperproliferation and induces differentiation in psoriasis. Acta Derm Venereol 76(5):353–356
47. Weinberg WC, Denning MF (2002) P21Waf1 control of epithelial cell cycle and cell fate. Crit Rev Oral Biol Med 13(6):453–464
48. Chang BD, Watanabe K, Broude EV, Fang J, Poole JC, Kalinichenko TV, Roninson IB (2000) Effects of p21Waf1/Cip1/Sdi1 on cellular gene expression: implications for carcinogenesis, senescence, and age-related diseases. Proc Natl Acad Sci U S A 97(8): 4291–4296
49. Buraczewska I, Brostrom U, Lodén M (2007) Artificial reduction in transepidermal water loss improves skin barrier function. Br J Dermatol 157(1):82–86, Epub 2007 Jun 6
50. Buraczewska I, Lodén M (2005) Treatment of surfactant-damaged skin in humans with creams of different pH values. Pharmacology 73(1):1–7, Epub 2004 Sep 27
51. Mauro T, Holleran WM, Grayson S, Gao WN, Man MQ, Kriehuber E, Behne M, Feingold KR, Elias PM (1998) Barrier recovery is impeded at neutral pH, independent of ionic effects: implications for extracellular lipid processing. Arch Dermatol Res 290(4):215–222
52. Behne MJ, Barry NP, Hanson KM, Aronchik I, Clegg RW, Gratton E, Feingold K, Holleran WM, Elias PM, Mauro TM (2003) Neonatal development of the stratum corneum pH gradient: localization and mechanisms leading to emergence of optimal barrier function. J Invest Dermatol 120(6):998–1006
53. Behne MJ, Meyer JW, Hanson KM, Barry NP, Murata S, Crumrine D, Clegg RW, Gratton E, Holleran WM, Elias PM, Mauro TM (2002) NHE1 regulates the stratum corneum permeability barrier homeostasis. Microenvironment acidification assessed with fluorescence lifetime imaging. J Biol Chem 277(49): 47399–47406, Epub 2002 Sep 7
54. Fluhr JW, Behne MJ, Brown BE, Moskowitz DG, Selden C, Mao-Qiang M, Mauro TM, Elias PM, Feingold KR (2004) Stratum corneum acidification in neonatal skin: secretory phospholipase A2 and the sodium/hydrogen antiporter-1 acidify neonatal rat stratum corneum. J Invest Dermatol 122(2):320–329
55. Fluhr JW, Kao J, Jain M, Ahn SK, Feingold KR, Elias PM (2001) Generation of free fatty acids from phospholipids regulates stratum corneum acidification and integrity. J Invest Dermatol 117(1):44–51
56. Fluhr JW, Mao-Qiang M, Brown BE, Hachem JP, Moskowitz DG, Demerjian M, Haftek M, Serre G, Crumrine D, Mauro TM, Elias PM, Feingold KR (2004) Functional consequences of a neutral pH in neonatal rat stratum corneum. J Invest Dermatol 123(1):140–151

57. Korting HC, Kober M, Mueller M, Braun-Falco O (1987) Influence of repeated washings with soap and synthetic detergents on pH and resident flora of the skin of forehead and forearm. Results of a cross-over trial in health probationers. Acta Derm Venereol 67(1):41–47
58. Proksch E, Elias PM, Feingold KR (1990) Regulation of 3-hydroxy-3-methylglutaryl-coenzyme A reductase activity in murine epidermis. Modulation of enzyme content and activation state by barrier requirements. J Clin Invest 85(3):874–882
59. Harris IR, Farrell AM, Grunfeld C, Holleran WM, Elias PM, Feingold KR (1997) Permeability barrier disruption coordinately regulates mRNA levels for key enzymes of cholesterol, fatty acid, and ceramide synthesis in the epidermis. J Invest Dermatol 109(6):783–787
60. Holleran WM, Feingold KR, Man MQ, Gao WN, Lee JM, Elias PM (1991) Regulation of epidermal sphingolipid synthesis by permeability barrier function. J Lipid Res 32(7):1151–1158
61. Ottey KA, Wood LC, Grunfeld C, Elias PM, Feingold KR (1995) Cutaneous permeability barrier disruption increases fatty acid synthetic enzyme activity in the epidermis of hairless mice. J Invest Dermatol 104(3):401–404
62. Grether-Beck S, Muhlberg K, Brenden H, Krutmann J (2008) Urea plus ceramides and vitamins: Improving the efficacy of a topical urea preparation by addition of ceramides and vitamins. Hautarzt 6:6
63. Rivier M, Castiel I, Safonova I, Ailhaud G, Michel S (2000) Peroxisome proliferator-activated receptor-alpha enhances lipid metabolism in a skin equivalent model. J Invest Dermatol 114(4):681–687
64. Yu Z, Schneider C, Boeglin WE, Brash AR (2007) Epidermal lipoxygenase products of the hepoxilin pathway selectively activate the nuclear receptor PPARalpha. Lipids 42(6):491–497, Epub 2007 Apr 14
65. Feingold KR (2007) Thematic review series: skin lipids. The role of epidermal lipids in cutaneous permeability barrier homeostasis. J Lipid Res 48(12):2531–2546, Epub 2007 Sep 13
66. Schmuth M, Jiang YJ, Dubrac S, Elias PM, Feingold KR (2008) Thematic review series: skin lipids. Peroxisome proliferator-activated receptors and liver X receptors in epidermal biology. J Lipid Res 49(3):499–509, Epub 2008 Jan 8
67. Sertznig P, Seifert M, Tilgen W, Reichrath J (2008) Peroxisome proliferator-activated receptors (PPARs) and the human skin: importance of PPARs in skin physiology and dermatologic diseases. Am J Clin Dermatol 9(1):15–31
68. Guo L, Fang H, Collins J, Fan X, Dial S, Wong A, Mehta K, Blann E, Shi L, Tong W, Dragan YP (2006) Differential gene expression in mouse primary hepatocytes exposed to the peroxisome proliferator-activated receptor α agonists. BMC Bioinformatics 7(Suppl 2):S18
69. Sonkoly E, Wei T, Janson PC, Saaf A, Lundeberg L, Tengvall-Linder M, Norstedt G, Alenius H, Homey B, Scheynius A, Stahle M, Pivarcsi A (2007) MicroRNAs: novel regulators involved in the pathogenesis of Psoriasis? PLoS One 2(7):e610
70. Ekholm E, Egelrud T (2000) Expression of stratum corneum chymotryptic enzyme in relation to other markers of epidermal differentiation in a skin explant model. Exp Dermatol 9(1):65–70
71. Ekholm IE, Brattsand M, Egelrud T (2000) Stratum corneum tryptic enzyme in normal epidermis: a missing link in the desquamation process? J Invest Dermatol 114(1):56–63
72. Komatsu N, Saijoh K, Toyama T, Ohka R, Otsuki N, Hussack G, Takehara K, Diamandis EP (2005) Multiple tissue kallikrein mRNA and protein expression in normal skin and skin diseases. Br J Dermatol 153(2):274–281
73. Caubet C, Jonca N, Brattsand M, Guerrin M, Bernard D, Schmidt R, Egelrud T, Simon M, Serre G (2004) Degradation of corneodesmosome proteins by two serine proteases of the kallikrein family, SCTE/KLK5/hK5 and SCCE/KLK7/hK7. J Invest Dermatol 122(5):1235–1244
74. Hachem JP, Man MQ, Crumrine D, Uchida Y, Brown BE, Rogiers V, Roseeuw D, Feingold KR, Elias PM (2005) Sustained serine proteases activity by prolonged increase in pH leads to degradation of lipid processing enzymes and profound alterations of barrier function and stratum corneum integrity. J Invest Dermatol 125(3):510–520
75. Lodén M, Lindberg M (1991) The influence of a single application of different moisturizers on the skin capacitance. Acta Derm Venereol 71(1):79–82
76. Komatsu N, Saijoh K, Kuk C, Shirasaki F, Takehara K, Diamandis EP (2007) Aberrant human tissue kallikrein levels in the stratum corneum and serum of patients with psoriasis: dependence on phenotype, severity and therapy. Br J Dermatol 156(5):875–883
77. Komatsu N, Saijoh K, Kuk C, Liu AC, Khan S, Shirasaki F, Takehara K, Diamandis EP (2007) Human tissue kallikrein expression in the stratum corneum and serum of atopic dermatitis patients. Exp Dermatol 16(6):513–519
78. Rawlings AV, Matts PJ (2005) Stratum corneum moisturization at the molecular level: an update in relation to the dry skin cycle. J Invest Dermatol 124(6):1099–1110
79. Rawlings AV, Scott IR, Harding CR, Bowser PA (1994) Stratum corneum moisturization at the molecular level. J Invest Dermatol 103(5):731–741
80. Egawa M, Hirao T, Takahashi M (2007) In vivo estimation of stratum corneum thickness from water concentration profiles obtained with Raman spectroscopy. Acta Derm Venereol 87(1):4–8
81. Egawa M, Tagami H (2008) Comparison of the depth profiles of water and water-binding substances in the stratum corneum determined in vivo by Raman spectroscopy between the cheek and volar forearm skin:

effects of age, seasonal changes and artificial forced hydration. Br J Dermatol 158(2):251–260, Epub 2007 Nov 28
82. Crowther JM, Sieg A, Blenkiron P, Marcott C, Matts PJ, Kaczvinsky JR, Rawlings AV (2008) Measuring the effects of topical moisturizers on changes in stratum corneum thickness, water gradients and hydration in vivo. Br J Dermatol 159(3):567–577
83. Wartewig S, Neubert RH (2005) Pharmaceutical applications of Mid-IR and Raman spectroscopy. Adv Drug Deliv Rev 57(8):1144–1170
84. Koehler MJ, Hahn S, Preller A, Elsner P, Ziemer M, Bauer A, Konig K, Buckle R, Fluhr JW, Kaatz M (2008) Morphological skin ageing criteria by multiphoton laser scanning tomography: non-invasive in vivo scoring of the dermal fibre network. Exp Dermatol 17(6):519–523, Epub 2008 Jan 15
85. Branzan AL, Landthaler M, Szeimies RM (2007) In vivo confocal scanning laser microscopy in dermatology. Lasers Med Sci 22(2):73–82, Epub 2006 Nov 18
86. Gottschalck T, Bailey J (eds) (2008) International cosmetic ingredient dictionary and handbook, 12th edn. The Cosmetics, Toiletry, and Fragrance Association, Washington, DC
87. Wirén K, Nohlgård C, Nyberg F, Holm L, Svensson A, Johannesson A, Wallberg P, Berne B, Edlund F, Lodén M (2008) Treatment with a moisturizing cream delays recurrence of atopic eczema. Forum Nord Derm Ven 13(Suppl 15):35

Changes in Stratum Corneum Thickness, Water Gradients and Hydration by Moisturizers

38

Jonathan M. Crowther, Paul J. Matts, and Joseph R. Kaczvinsky

38.1 Introduction: Stratum Corneum Form and Function

As the outermost layer of skin, the stratum corneum (SC), plays the pivotal role in protecting our bodies. It is the first line of defense against the outside world, providing both mechanical and chemical protection and regulating the movement of water and other materials in and out, enabling the bodies' equilibrium to be maintained. Despite the relatively small dimensions of the SC over most of the body (its thickness is of the order of only 20 μm over a large portion of the body), it has a very complicated chemical and physical structure. Chemical concentrations and cellular structure change across its thickness, and these changes are responsible for the properties it possesses and for regulating the processes occurring within it. To better understand the role all of these components play within the SC, therefore, it is not only necessary to ask 'how much is there?', but also 'where is it located?' and 'how is it distributed?' While a number of techniques have been developed previously to analyze concentration gradients within the SC, until recently no single technique has been able to quantitatively assess different chemical components as a function of depth, rapidly and in vivo. Furthermore, as the use of topical cosmetic products has become more popular and widespread, especially in the anti-aging market, the ability to accurately monitor ingredients which are capable of penetrating into the skin is now a necessity. Also, it is becoming more and more important to demonstrate how topically applied products can improve the skin in clinical tests; therefore, new methods to assess the skin in greater and greater detail are constantly being explored.

The aim of this chapter is to review current research on assessment of chemical concentration gradients within the SC and provide an overview of the use of a relatively new technique, confocal Raman spectroscopy (CRS), for assessing these changes in vivo. We will also take this opportunity to share some of our recent findings of how the use of topical moisturizers can affect these chemical profiles and impact on changing SC thickness.

38.1.1 Concentration Gradients Within the SC

Despite its small size over most of the body (typically around 20 μm for most sites except the palms of the hands and soles of the feet), in cross section the SC itself is far from homogeneous. As

J.M. Crowther (✉) • P. J. Matts
Beauty and Grooming, Procter & Gamble Technical Centres Ltd., Rusham Park Technical Centre, Whitehall Lane, Egham, Surrey, TW20 9NW, UK
e-mail: crowther.j.1@pg.com; matts.pj@pg.com

J.R. Kaczvinsky
Clinical Research and Biometrics, The Procter and Gamble Company, Sharon Woods Technical Centre, 11510 Reed Hartman Highway, Cincinnati, OH 45241, USA
e-mail: kaczvinsky.jr@pg.com

M. Lodén, H.I. Maibach (eds.), *Treatment of Dry Skin Syndrome*,
DOI 10.1007/978-3-642-27606-4_38, © Springer-Verlag Berlin Heidelberg 2012

we move up from the basal layer where keratinocytes are birthed, we travel through regions where they mature and differentiate during their transition towards the surface, gradually flattening out to become the familiar, flat, 'squamous' corneocyte cells of the SC. These differentiating cells transition through a variety of chemical gradients as they move up through the SC, including water, natural moisturizing factors (NMF), lipids, urea, lactic acid and pH. This section outlines some of these gradient changes, why they are present and how they are currently assessed.

38.1.1.1 Water

At the surface of the skin, the SC is constantly losing water to the environment under normal conditions, while at the basal layer there is continual replenishment from the wet tissue of the viable epidermis. This ongoing process of loss at the surface and replenishment from beneath leads to the formation of a water gradient across the SC which decreases towards the outside of the body. Maintenance of a correct equilibrium state of SC hydration has enormous impact on its mechanical and optical properties, as well as helping to maintain skin barrier function and playing an important role in the regulation and activation of both intra- and extracellular enzymes which control the desquamation process [1, 2]. Deviations from the normal desquamation process fundamentally affect SC barrier function which in healthy individuals is most commonly expressed as 'dry skin' [3]. Even given the thinness of the SC, not all the water is present in the same state, typically being described as either free or bound [4]. Free, or 'unbound', water refers to the partially mobile molecules which can be easily lost if exposed to low humidity after exposure of the skin to an environment of high water activity. Bound water is held within corneocytes by both the polar groups within keratin proteins and a blend of NMF that increase the hygroscopicity of these cells.

The first attempt at determining true depth-resolved water profiling in skin was performed by Warner et al. in 1988 [5]. In this initial experiment, electron probe analysis was carried out on biopsied skin samples which had been cryo-sectioned and freeze-dried (the local dry mass of a freeze-dried cryo-section of skin being inversely related to its water content). This demonstrated how the surface of the SC was depleted in water with respect to the live tissue within the body and how a water gradient existed across its thickness. Further advancements were made to the technique making it simpler to perform [6] although this was still not a technique suitable for larger base size sample assessment.

Cryo-SEM has been used more recently to understand uptake and loss of water within the SC from salt solutions of different strengths by Richter et al. [7]. This demonstrated that there are three 'zones' which respond differently during the processes of hydration and dehydration, the behaviour of these zones being dependent on the osmotic potential of the hydrating solution. The concept of zones of hydration has also been examined before [8] showing that the central portion of the SC absorbed water strongly under conditions of high water activity, while the layers closest to the stratum granulosum showed no swelling under these conditions. The presence of a central zone capable of absorbing and holding water is in excellent agreement with the concentration of NMF, known to reach a maximum in the central portion of the SC [9]. Also, the layers closest to the stratum granulosum would not be expected to swell as much as the outer layers of the SC given the mechanical constraints placed on them by the surrounding cellular tissue. However, while cryo-SEM as a technique has been able to provide hydration profiles and detailed information on the hydration processes within the SC, the necessity for skin biopsies, along with the complexity of an analysis using cryo-sectioning and scanning electron microscopy (SEM), means that it is not a technique that it would be possible to deploy easily in a clinical environment for assessing the effects of topical moisturizer application on SC hydration.

Infrared spectroscopy has been used to examine water as a function of depth though combination with tape stripping [10] and Monte Carlo simulation [11]. However, like cryo-SEM, these methods require compromises to be taken in collection and analysis of the data. For example, in the work by Brancaleon et al. [10], the tape stripping approach used to sample incrementally into the skin was difficult to correlate with actual depth and, of course, was inherently destructive, thereby making it impossible to repeatedly reassess the same site over the course of a study. The Monte Carlo simulation by Arimoto et al. [11] relies on the assumption the water content varies linearly from 10% at the SC surface to 80% at the interface with the viable epidermis, despite the obviously more complex variation in structure across its thickness.

Confocal Raman spectroscopy has also been used to provide water profiles through the SC, and this will be discussed in more detail later on.

38.1.1.2 NMF and SC Lipids

Two key classes of materials are present within the SC in addition to the corneocyte cellular structure – the so-called natural moisturizing factors (NMF) and inter-cellular lipids present in the bilayer structure. Both of these classes of materials will have an impact on the amount and distribution of water within the skin. NMF comprises a collection of amino acids, salts and other small hygroscopic molecules which are present within the corneocytes. These are derived from proteolysis of epidermal filaggrin initiated a few cell layers above the stratum basale and as such are only present in the SC. These hygroscopic NMF components are efficient humectants, helping to bind water and assisting in maintaining skin hydration and flexibility [9]. However, because of their hydrophilic nature, they are readily removed from the surface of the SC during washing [12].

Confocal Raman spectroscopy has been used to measure concentration profiles of the different NMF components non-destructively and in vivo [13]. The concentration of most NMF components builds gradually from the stratum granulosum, peaking in the midportion of the SC and then showing a characteristic depletion near the surface. This seems to be associated with the water-labile nature of these components and their propensity to be washed out by, for example, daily cleansing. Lactate and urea, as sweat-derived NMF components, are more prevalent at the surface of the SC.

The ability of the SC to control the movement of molecules across it is mediated not only by the physical constraint of the corneocytes themselves but also chemically by the inter-cellular lipids. These are a mixture of ceramides, cholesterol and free fatty acids, as well as a small amount of non-polar liquids and cholesterol sulphates, and are organized along with a small amount of water, into a series of parallel lamellar membranes between the corneocytes. However, while some water is trapped in the lipid lamellar structure, most is actually held within the corneocytes themselves [14]. It is this series of lipid bilayer structures, together with the tightly stacked corneocytes, which provide a tight barrier against trans-epidermal water loss (TEWL), making it difficult for water to transfer across the SC structure.

Gradual removal of the SC results in an increase in TEWL; however, this does not occur at a constant rate as a function of depth. Most of the TEWL increase only occurs when about 75% of the barrier has been removed [15]. This suggests an anisotropic distribution of ingredients within the skin which are responsible for controlling the flow of water across it. It also suggests that people with thinner SC might have a greater lipid packing density in their tissue to provide the same amount of protection per percentage of depth.

Tape stripping has been used in combination with TEWL measurements to calculate SC thickness [16]. However, measurement methods which incorporate tape stripping are fundamentally destructive to the skin which makes them unsuitable for repeated assessment of the same area during a clinical trial.

38.1.1.3 pH

While the extracellular fluid within the body is maintained at a pH of approximately 7.4, the surface of the SC is more acidic with a pH typically between 4.5 and 6 [17, 18]. There is, therefore, a pH gradient across the SC. While this change in pH has been linked with a variety of skin functions, such as barrier function, desquamation and microbial defense, the mechanism responsible for its presence is not fully understood. However, it has been suggested that a build-up of trans-urocanic acid [19], carbon dioxide diffusion [20], the presence of free fatty acids [21], lactate and lactic acid produced as a by-product of sweating [22] or active regulation by a sodium-hydrogen anti-porter protein [23] are all linked with this observed acidic change towards the surface.

A number of techniques have been used to determine pH as a function of depth. Tape stripping measurements combined with pH assessment have shown the existence of this gradient [18, 24]. Once again, though, this is by its nature an inherently destructive technique and is not capable of discriminating between the intra- and intercellular components. Microscopy combined with a pH-sensitive fluorescent marker molecule has also been used to determine pH [25], and the advent of two photon and confocal imaging has pushed resolution down to submicron levels [26]. Confocal Raman spectroscopy has been used to measure concentration profiles of trans-urocanic acid and pyrrolidone carboxylic acid in vivo [13]. As with NMF, the concentration of these species is greatest in the middle portion of the SC, showing a gradual build up from the stratum granulosum layers and depletion near the surface.

38.1.1.4 Calcium

Calcium concentration varies across the entire epidermis, from high levels within the stratum granulosum down to low levels in the basal layer [27]. The calcium concentration is linked with regulation of epidermal keratinocyte proliferation and differentiation and skin structural integrity. It is also strongly linked with rate of SC barrier recovery after acute insult by detergents, tape stripping or organic solvents [28]. Analysis of calcium concentration as a function of depth has been carried out using scanning electron microscopy of biopsied samples [29].

38.1.1.5 Cosmetic Ingredients

Given the enormous expansion of the cosmetic product market in recent years, more attention is being focused on understanding how these products partition into and interact with the skin, both from an efficacy and a consumer safety point of view.

Infrared (IR) spectroscopy has been used to monitor the effects of cosmetic ingredients on SC chemical composition [30], and although this technique is capable of detecting changes in lipid packing and organization as a result of using different products, it is not a depth-profiling technique, and it is not certain from which depth data is collected. IR has been used in comparison with tape stripping to provide some measure of depth information on the penetration of ingredients from microemulsions into porcine skin; however, obviously, this is a destructive method and therefore not ideally suited to clinical testing [31]. Notingher et al. have used a modified version of IR spectroscopy to assess the delivery of topical components to the skin based on the principle of thermal emission delay from the surface after irradiation with an IR light source [32]; however, this technique requires complex modelling of the thermal properties of the extremely thin SC layers.

Confocal Raman spectroscopy has been used to monitor penetration of different lipid species into the SC and their corresponding effects on total skin lipid profiles and skin hydration [33]. Different lipid species were absorbed to different degrees, with petrolatum being most strongly absorbed, most likely due to a combination of its relatively short chain lengths and occlusive properties, resulting in destabilization of SC structure. Chrit et al. have used confocal Raman spectroscopy to assess the extent of skin hydration changes after using a glycerol-based moisturizing product in vivo [34] and were able to classify different hydrating products depending on their moisturizing effect on the skin. They showed that a polyphospholipid (poly [2-methacryoyloxy-lphosphorylcholine or pMPC]) was able to increase water levels in the skin, both in vivo and in vitro, although it should be noted that dosing of the products was not tightly controlled, with any excess product being removed after application and before analysis [35]. Recently, Förster et al. used confocal Raman microscopy to monitor the penetration of retinol into pig skin, and how formulation differences affect penetration [36]. In their work, they demonstrated that the nature of the surfactant used can have an impact on penetration.

With quantification of any component in the skin as a function of depth, the ideal clinical solution is determination of concentration in a non-destructive manner, without the need for complex modelling, especially when biopsies or other invasive procedures may not be viable (e.g. during testing of moisturizing products at different time points on large groups of panellists). As a technique for materials characterization, Raman spectroscopy has been used for many years; however, recently its use in the assessment of biological samples has become more widespread.

38.2 Raman Spectroscopy

It was in 1928 that the Indian physicist C. V. Raman first reported the new type of light-scattering phenomenon that would eventually bear his name. Raman reported that when a liquid was irradiated by light of a specific wavelength, while most of the re-emitted photons had not changed in energy (i.e. had been scattered elastically), an extremely small proportion of the reflected light had a wavelength which had shifted relative to the incident source. This shift in wavelength was directly related to the change in rotational and vibrational energy states of the molecules in the liquid, thereby providing information on the energy levels of the constituent molecules. Knowledge of these energy levels can be used to determine what chemical species are present. As the Raman phenomenon is very weak (occurring approximately once in a million photon interactions), a well-defined monochromatic light source is absolutely essential to achieving a good signal during measurement, and practical applications were not readily exploited until the development of the laser in the 1960s. Improvements in detection equipment such as photomultiplier tubes further enhanced the appeal and applicability of Raman, and it has since become a well-established material analysis technique. Raman spectroscopy is considered to be a complimentary technique to IR spectroscopy – molecular vibrations which are IR active are generally not Raman active and vice versa. In contrast with IR spectroscopy, Raman is relatively insensitive to the O-H vibrations in water, making it a more considered approach for analyzing skin (where with IR the high intensity of the water signal can mask other chemical species) – and indeed, a number of researchers in the last 15 years or so have reported varying degrees of success, principally using in vitro models [37–39].

The journey from measurement of in vitro systems to in vivo capture of Raman spectra on the surface of the SC presented many challenges [37, 40], specifically the low signal-to-noise ratio (based upon the safety needs requirements for relatively low laser power when used on live subjects, combined with the necessity of fast acquisition times to minimize the effects of subject movement). A huge leap forward in the use of in vivo Raman spectroscopy came with the instrumental design and research of Caspers et al. resulting in a system with very high optical efficiency, thus enabling rapid, non-invasive collection of Raman spectra [13].

38.2.1 In Vivo Confocal Raman Spectroscopy

The 'holy grail' of in vivo SC assessment is the measurement of different components within the skin as a function of depth in a non-destructive and rapid manner such that it can be routinely employed in a clinical environment. Recently, confocal Raman spectroscopy has been developed to the point where it can be used to obtain molecular concentration profiles real time and in vivo [13, 41–44]. Building on the success of their in vivo surface measurements, River Diagnostics designed and marketed the RD3100 in vivo confocal Raman spectrometer, capable of measuring skin chemical profiles by combining the principle of confocal microscopy with Raman spectroscopy. In operation, incident monochromatic laser light is focussed to a point on/within the skin tissue, which can be moved by changing the focal point of the microscope. When used to assess skin, this light enters the SC, and while most of it is scattered elastically without a change in energy and wavelength, a small proportion of this incident light becomes Raman-scattered photons. These leave the skin with minute shifts in their wavelength as a result of interacting with the molecules present and changing their vibrational state. On reaching the skin's surface, these scattered photons are re-emitted and some pass back through the microscope objective lens. Given the confocal nature of the microscope arrangement, only light re-entering the microscope from the focal plane will pass back through the pinhole – any photons re-emerging from other depths are excluded – hence, the chemical information is derived from specific depths within the skin. Collection and analysis of these Raman-scattered photons from different depths enable the construction of molecular concentration profiles for different components present as a function of depth within the SC. Using this technique, SC composition can be quantitatively measured by 'optically sectioning' skin tissue and expressing the relative chemical content as a function of depth, in a non-invasive, rapid and non-destructive manner. The combination of these properties makes it an ideal technique for implementation in a clinical environment for assessing chemical composition of the skin. For example, water concentration as it varies across the SC is calculated from ratioing the water signal against the combined signal from water and protein within the skin. This method has also been used to estimate differences in SC thickness in vivo at different body sites and during aging [45, 46] and to evaluate the effects of water and moisturizing ingredients on SC hydration, after both short-term treatment [34, 47] and long-term treatment [48].

The majority of current research which is using Raman to look at the skin focuses on the SC and upper layers of the viable epidermis, as light becomes increasingly scattered as it penetrates more deeply, reducing signal strength and making data collection more difficult. Nonetheless, Naito et al. have reported using a 1,064-nm light source to probe the dermal chemical structure [49]. The ability to measure deep within the skin opens up additional possibilities of, for example, probing the development of acne in teenagers, and the effects of aging on dermal chemical composition.

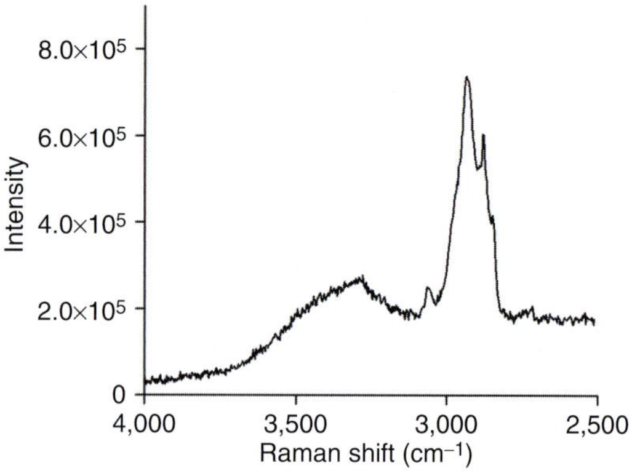

Fig. 38.1 Typical background-corrected Raman spectra from a single scan of human skin in vivo, collected at ~4 μm depth in the high wave number region (671-nm laser excitation, exposure 1 s)

The use of Raman spectroscopy for skin analysis relies on the fact that the chemical components of the skin possess different functional groups with unique vibrational frequencies. Water and protein contain different functional groups in their chemical structure which vibrate at distinctly different frequencies. It is these differences in vibrational frequency which enable the two species to be differentiated using Raman spectroscopy. To simplify the analysis of skin, the Raman spectra can be split into two distinct zones – the 'high wave number' and 'fingerprint' regions – which can be probed independently depending on the information required and the molecules being investigated. Information regarding total water content is contained within the 'high wave number' region, while levels of natural moisturizing factors (NMF), ceramides, cholesterol, cosmetic ingredients penetrating into the skin etc., can be derived from the information in the 'fingerprint' spectra. Scans in the high wave number region are used to calculate percentage hydration values by taking the ratio of the integrated signals of water (i.e. the O-H stretching vibration region between 3,350 and 3,550 cm^{-1}) to that of protein (i.e. the $-CH_3$ stretching vibration from 2,910 to 2,965 cm^{-1}) [41–44]. A typical skin spectra for the 'high wave number' spectral region showing the water and protein peaks collected at a single scan at an exposure time of 1 s is given in Fig. 38.1. During measurement of a depth profile, spectra like the one shown in Fig. 38.1 are captured at regular depth intervals from the surface of the SC down into the skin. On the River Diagnostics system, a correction factor, as determined by Caspers et al. [13], is used to normalize the spectral response of water and protein relative to their mass ratio. The normalized water-to-protein ratios obtained from each focal depth are plotted as % hydration as a function of depth. This, therefore, leads to a direct, semi-quantitative measure of amount of the water present within the SC as a function of depth. Although the signal intensity drops as the laser penetrates deeper into the skin, the fact that both the water and protein peaks are derived from the same scan enables hydration quantification throughout the range of analysis.

38.2.2 Calculation of SC Thickness

It has been understood for many years that SC thickness varies dynamically with its hydration state and in response to a variety of extrinsic factors. In order to analyze and interpret SC water concentration profiles properly, therefore, it is essential to take into account SC thickness, as well as any changes in thickness resulting from the treatment regime – after all, in a situation where SC thickness is varying dynamically, for example, during acute swelling due to exposure to wet environment, absolute static SC depths are of little meaning. It has been demonstrated in our own laboratories that SC thickness can be determined directly from water concentration profiles in a robust and clinically viable manner [48], and this procedure is described in more detail below. Other groups have also addressed the area of calculation of SC thickness, and while the work of Egawa et al. [45, 46] has clearly demonstrated the capability of CRS for deriving SC thickness estimates, these authors offered no formal validation data (establishing a direct relationship between their CRS-derived SC thickness data and values derived from other measurements). More recently, Bielfeldt et al. have reported SC thickness calculations based upon the concept of Fickian diffusion of water across the SC [50].

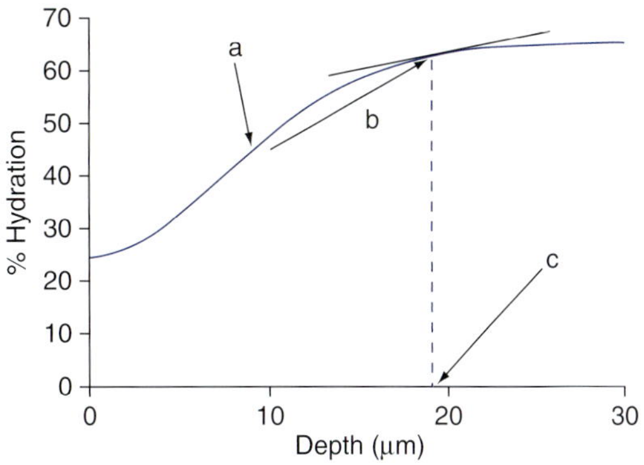

Fig. 38.2 Calculation of SC thickness from hydration curve. The algorithm calculates the point where the gradient equals 0.5, working from the middle of the curve (*a*) inwards (i.e. deeper in the tissue) (*b*). The depth at this point corresponds to the base of the SC (*c*)

We however used a different (and, we believe, a more rigorous) approach in calculating SC thickness from the water profile measurements and have validated it via correlation with values from a known objective measure of skin thickness (optical coherence tomography – OCT) which is discussed further later in the chapter.

The inherent biological variability of the skin, combined with the fact that Raman analysis is a point measure, means that a more accurate measure of thickness and hydration state can only be obtained through the use of an average water profile collected from a number of sites within the area of interest. After collecting a set of profiles, obvious outliers (arising, e.g. from scanning through heterogeneous structures, such as skin appendages including hair follicles, and sebaceous glands, or profiles recorded while the panellists were moving) are removed. Then, an average hydration profile is fitted through the remaining data, using a customized algorithm based on a 4-parameter Weibull curve. This curve is a well-accepted and widely used algorithm capable of accurately modelling a variety of profile shapes with the minimum number of parameters in the equation, producing model curves with very low RMS deviations from the mean data. The upper 'levelling off point' of each profile is determined via a gradient threshold method by calculating the location where the gradient reaches a value of 0.5 moving from the midpoint of the curve (Fig. 38.2). This point was originally hypothesized to be the theoretical boundary of the SC with the viable epidermis and serves as the deeper limit of the SC hydration profile. The area-under-the curve values (AUC) are determined by integrating each hydration profile from the skin surface ($x=0$ μm on the profile) to each individual SC boundary (point c in Fig. 38.2) and used to express the total SC hydration.

As work with CRS has progressed, the issue of refractive index changes within skin effecting absolute depth measures has been discussed [51]. It has been reported that the effects of the correction are small when the SC thickness is less than 20 μm [52]. In this circumstance, relative % changes from a baseline state would be a potential route to eliminate errors introduced from refractive index changes.

38.2.3 Validation of SC Thickness Measurements Using Confocal Raman Spectroscopy

While the control of the microscope movement can be done extremely accurately, interpreting where the base of the SC occurs from the water profile is not as simple a task. Without any form of validation of the thicknesses being measured, the value of the technique is drastically reduced. This section discusses how validation of the SC thickness measurement has been approached.

38.2.3.1 Correlation Between NMF and Hydration Profiles

Using the River Diagnostics RD3100 system and alternating the laser being used from 681 to 785 nm, thereby switching between the ‘high wave number’ and ‘fingerprint’ regions, it is possible to measure hydration and NMF profiles at exactly the same location on the skin while retaining the volar forearm on the window of the spectrometer. As can be seen in the example shown in Fig. 38.3, there is a strong correlation between the levelling off point location of the hydration profile and the position where the NMF profile starts to rise (profiles presented here are single scans from a specific location on the skin, which is why they are not presented as smooth average curves). This is to be expected, as NMF starts to be expressed a few microns above the base of the SC due to the breakdown of filaggrin, and this correlates well with the behaviour for NMF reported by Caspers [13]. While these observations provide increased confidence in the correlation between the levelling off point in the hydration profile and the location of the lower margin of the SC, it is not definitive proof. For example, external environmental variation can also be responsible for changes in the exact location of filaggrin hydrolysis. It was necessary, therefore, to validate empirically the levelling off point as the SC lower margin, using a separate objective measure of SC thickness.

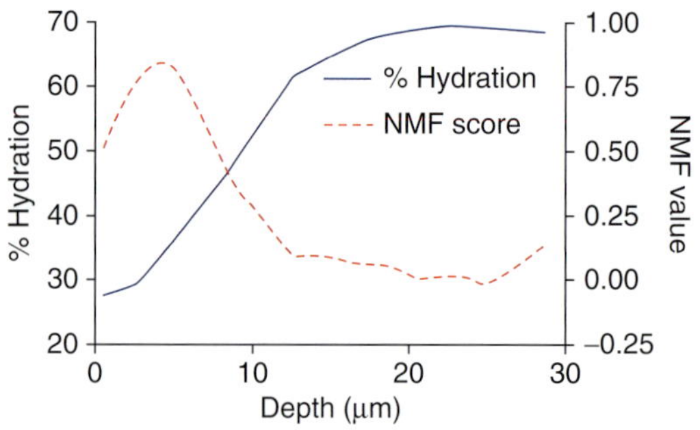

Fig. 38.3 Comparison of hydration and NMF profiles measured at the same point on the volar forearm

38.2.3.2 Correlation Between OCT and SC Hydration Profiles

OCT is a well-established technique for examining skin structure and thickness [53]. It is based on the principle that photons are backscattered from different structures within the skin. By using interferometry, the depth at which these backscattering events occur can be calculated, providing information on where different structures occur within the skin. During our validation, we measured sets of up to eight Raman profiles from each site and analyzed these together, rather than studying each water profile in isolation. Outlying scans were discarded, and the Weibull mathematical model applied to the remaining data point cloud representing each site, resulting in an ‘average’ hydration profile for that site. The location of the SC boundary as a function of the CRS water concentration

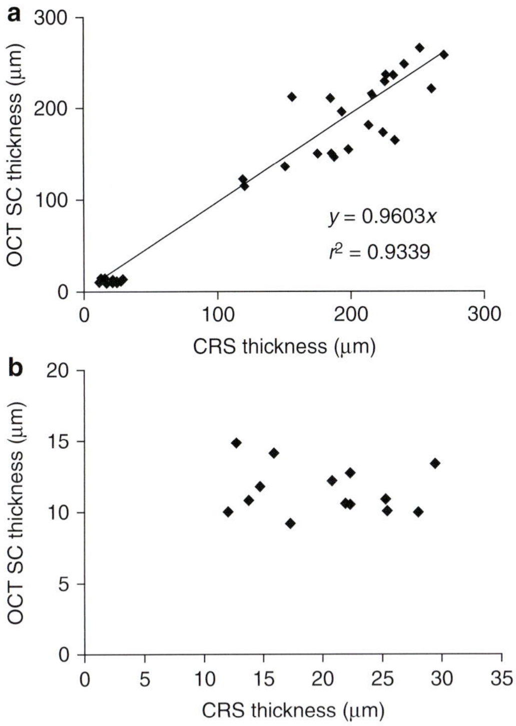

Fig. 38.4 (**a**) Comparison of OCT- and CRS-derived SC thicknesses at a variety of body sites. (**b**) Comparison of OCT- and CRS-derived SC thicknesses on volar forearm, cheek and outside of lower leg (complete dataset)

profiles was confirmed by comparing SC thicknesses from a number of different body sites obtained directly by OCT and CRS (Fig. 38.4a, b). Linear regression through the data shows a strong positive correlation between SC thickness derived from CRS and OCT (OCT thickness = 0.9603 × CRS thickness, $r^2 = 0.9339$; $p < 0.0001$). Expanding the area to the lower left of Fig. 38.4a, corresponding to the thinner skin sites of the body (volar forearm, cheek and outside of lower leg), shows how the dynamic range for OCT is compressed in this region (Fig. 38.4b). It can be seen that all of the OCT-derived SC thicknesses are between 9 and 15 μm, while the CRS-derived thicknesses vary between 12 and 30 μm. This is consistent with the expected behaviour of the OCT method in areas where the SC is relatively thin – the sensitivity of the OCT is limited by the pixel size of the detector (approximately 5 μm for the system used here). For sites with SC thickness in the region of 10–20 μm, therefore, this corresponds to only a few pixels. For panellists who had cheek, forearm and leg measures, CRS ranked the sites, in terms of SC thickness, as follows: cheek < forearm < leg (cheek 12.8 ± 0.9 μm, volar forearm 18.0 ± 3.9 μm, leg 22.0 ± 6.9 μm), whereas OCT gave very similar readings for these three different locations (cheek 11.1 ± 1.8 μm, volar forearm 10.4 ± 0.9 μm, leg 13.7 ± 1.4 μm). Of note, this ability to rank the sites in order of thickness gave further confidence that the new CRS method was giving accurate estimates of SC thickness, as it matched exactly the trends that which would be expected, based on known published values for these sites [54]. The limitations of OCT measurement of thinner skin sites have also been noted recently using in vivo laser scanning fluorescence microscopy [55, 56]. Overall, we believe that the results of this work demonstrate convincingly the capability of CRS in providing a new rapid, accurate and sensitive means of measuring SC thickness in vivo.

38.2.4 Effects of Acute Hydration on SC Water Content and Thickness

In order to demonstrate the ability of the CRS system to measure dynamic, rapid changes in SC water profiles, an initial simple study employing forced occlusion to drive maximal short-term acute hydration of the volar forearm was carried out. A set of hydration profiles were taken on a Caucasian volar forearm after equilibration in a standardized environment (Fig. 38.5a). The forearm was then covered in a wet towel soaked in de-ionized water. The towel was wrapped in Parafilm™ to help ensure complete saturation of the SC by occlusive hydration, and the arm site was left undisturbed for 90 min. After 90 min, the wrap and towel were removed, and any excess surface water removed by gentle patting with a dry towel. Sets of hydration profiles were then measured again using CRS over a time course (Fig. 38.5b). Given the complex nature of the shape of the hydration curve after this extreme treatment, the profiles here are represented as simple averages of the individual sets of scans rather

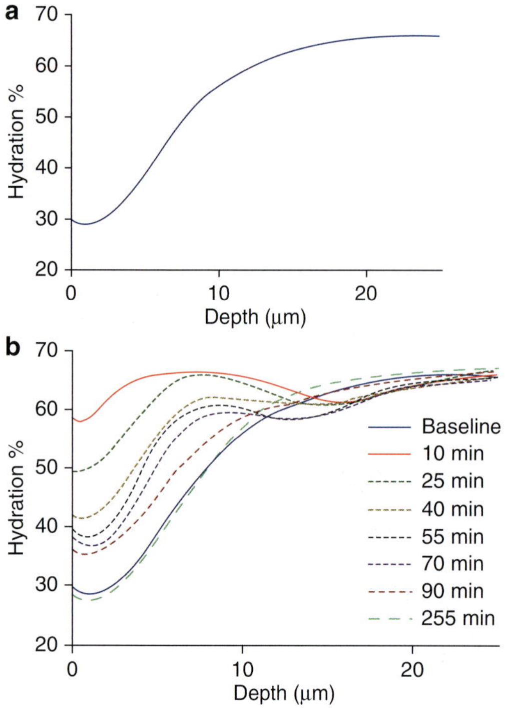

Fig. 38.5 (**a**) Baseline volar forearm SC hydration profile. (**b**) Hydration profiles of the volar forearm skin measured as a function of time after 90 min occlusion with a wet towel

than Weibull curve modelled fits. Between measurements, the arm was removed from the CRS optical window and allowed to acclimatize within the measurement room, and the window of the CRS cleaned with methanol to remove any residue left behind from the skin. The hydration profiles in Fig. 38.5b show the significant changes in SC hydration across its entire thickness, showing significant water uptake over the 90 min. Importantly, the point at which the hydration profile begins to level off after enforced hydration is further from the surface of the SC. From the OCT validation study described above, we now have confidence that this is because of SC swelling normal to its surface, driven by hydration. As observation only, it is interesting to note that the magnitude of this swelling is in the region of 25%, highly consistent with that noted by Norlen [57] in ex vivo models. It is also interesting that there appears to be a central portion of the SC which takes up more water than the upper or lower margins.

As the post-occlusion time course is followed and hydration profiles are measured over time, also it should be noted that surface hydration values fall fastest, while the 'hump' of hydration in the central portion of the SC falls the slowest. These observations are wholly consistent with presence of higher concentrations of hygroscopic NMF components in the central portion of the SC (the lower layers containing less because of the programmed hydrolysis of filaggrin and the upper layers containing less because of washout of these highly water-labile components by, e.g. daily cleansing). It is also probable that the corneocytes within the central portion of the SC are less physically constrained compared with those closer to the SC-stratum granulosum boundary (as discussed above) and, therefore, are potentially more readily capable of swelling when hydrated and increasing in thickness. This variance in swelling ability of the SC as a function of depth correlates with the work of Bouwstra et al. [8]. Remarkably, baseline conditions are only re-established after a period of some 4 h, demonstrating the efficient water-binding capacity of native, untreated SC.

Further in vitro validation of CRS has been reported by Wu and Polefka, where water content as measured using CRS was correlated with Karl Fischer assessment, along with water content increase for a moisturizing lotion, and decrease in water content after using bar soap [58]. While SC thickness changes as a result of the treatment, regimes were not taken into account, and the experiments were carried out on excised pig skin; this does demonstrate further the capability of the technique.

38.2.5 Effect of Long-Term Application of Moisturizers on SC Hydration Profiles

It might be expected that long-term application of moisturizers to the skin would increase SC water content and/or change the shape of the SC hydration profile. A comparison of the effect of long-term application of three moisturizers on SC hydration gradients has recently been reported by

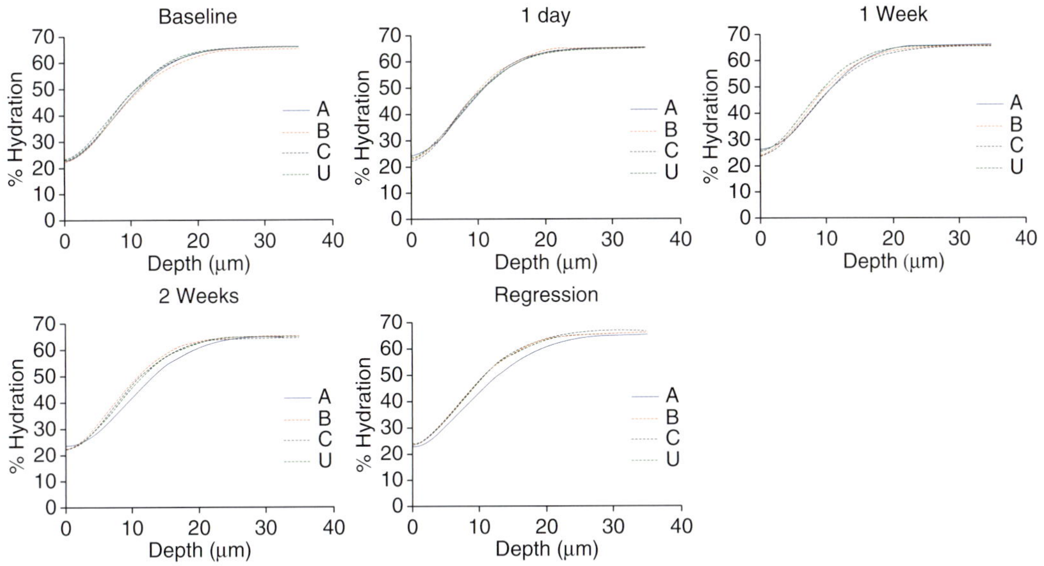

Fig. 38.6 Average hydration profiles for four different treatment regimes (*A*, *B*, *C* and *U*) over the course of a 3-week moisturizer usage study (2 weeks product usage and 1-week regression)

Crowther et al. [48]. To examine the effects of moisturizers on SC thickness, water gradients and total SC hydration CRS were used to compare the effects of a formulation containing niacinamide (A) which is known to improve SC barrier function and desquamation better than two other commercially available moisturizers (formulations B & C) [59].

For illustration, average hydration profiles from each treatment from this work are given in Fig. 38.6. All hydration profiles start at 20–30% hydration at 0 microns depth (i.e. the SC surface) and rise in a 'sigmoidal' type curve to 65–70% hydration, where they plateau. While all hydration profiles at baseline and 1-day treatment show the same shape, differences in shape start to appear after one week of treatment. By 2 weeks usage, notable differences are observed for formulation A, where a laterally 'stretched' water profile is evident, which is still present even after 1 week of regression. As a result of this stretching, the levelling off point of the water profile moved deeper in the skin indicating an increase in SC thickness. After 2 weeks treatment, the increase in SC thickness induced by formulation A was significantly different from the other two products being tested and the untreated control site ($p=0.0121$), and this difference remained at the 1 week regression time point ($p=0.0162$). The observed change corresponded to an approximate 10% increase in SC thickness. Total hydration in the SC can be calculated from the area under the profile (AUC; integration between $x=0$ μm and the calculated SC levelling off point). Concomitant with the increase in SC thickness, total skin hydration increased significantly following treatment with formulation A after 2 weeks product usage and the 1-week regression ($p=0.0275$ and $p=0.0435$, respectively).

While it is well accepted that all moisturizers have the effect of alleviating dry skin when formulated appropriately, it has become apparent in recent years that the nature of the formulation can impact its effects on the SC and the epidermis (for review see Loden [60]). Naturally, in the short-term, moisturizers will increase SC hydration given their relatively high water and humectant content [34, 43, 47, 59–61], and in the medium-term improve desquamation [62, 63]. However, in the longer term, it has become apparent that some can actually compromise SC barrier function [64–68], while others can strengthen it [59, 61, 69–71]. In vitro [7, 72–75] and in vivo [76, 77] studies have also demonstrated the ability of some moisturizing ingredients to influence SC thickness. Therefore, it is becoming increasingly apparent that not only is there a need for longer-term studies to evaluate the effect of moisturizers, but that the introduction of new measurements in addition to the more 'traditional' electrical parameter based devices is needed to understand their effects on skin more completely [67].

During the moisturizer study discussed in Crowther et al., on the first day after initial product application, little difference in CRS-derived hydration profiles is observed between any of the treatments or the untreated control site. After the first week of treatment though, there was a numerical diminution in SC thickness. While not statistically significant, it could have been be due to the osmotic effects of glycerol (which was present in all three formulations), or it could have been attributed to increased desquamation after a period without moisturizer usage. This type of behaviour has been reported before – Caussin et al. [75] reported that changes in SC swelling can occur when examining the effects of moisturizers on SC hydration and swelling. Lipophilic moisturizers increased SC thickness, whereas hydrophilic moisturizers tended to reduce SC thickness. This apparent SC thinning may, therefore, be due to osmotic effects of the moisturizing ingredients (used at high concentration), and the work of Fluhr et al. [78] describing the effect of glycerol on reducing corneocyte surface area would tend to support this hypothesis. However, inconsistencies remain where in vitro [75] and in vivo [76, 77] increased corneocyte swelling has been reported with glycerol solutions. Another possible explanation would be that during the first week of treatment, there was some activation of SC protease activity (simply by elevated water activity), resulting in more efficient desquamation and an ensuing reduction in SC thickness.

After 2 weeks of regular moisturizer usage, formulation A had induced a statistically significant increase in SC thickness (2 μm average increase, corresponding to an approximate 10% increase in thickness) unlike formulations B and C. As already discussed, water content measurements at absolute depths are simply not comparable between time points in a study where SC thickness may change or vary. It is, therefore, more meaningful to extract information from the profiles regarding total SC thickness and express water measurement derivatives as a function of this (e.g. our use of total SC water content). Considering SC thickness first of all, it can be seen that, after 2 weeks of treatment, formulation A produced a significantly greater increase in this parameter than the other two treatments and the untreated site ($p=0.0121$), and this difference remained at the 1-week regression time point ($p=0.0162$). Of note, increases in SC thickness have also been reported by Jacobson et al. [79] using a lipophilic niacin derivative.

Concomitant with this increase in SC thickness, total SC hydration as measured by CRS increased significantly with use of formulation A after 2 weeks treatment. Interestingly, this increase in total hydration level also remained at the 1-week regression time point. However, no such effect was observed for treatment with formulations B and C. These data did not, however, correspond with Corneometer® measurements taken at the same time points. Significantly, increased Corneometer® values were observed for all three products even after 1 day of application, and indeed, values remained elevated throughout the 2-week treatment phase. Corneometer® values also remained elevated for all treatments at the 1-week regression (although all values were significantly lower than those at the 2-week treatment time point – an effect observed in other regression studies [70, 80]). Considering the ingredients present in all three formulations, the capacitance effects noted may be attributable partially to the high dielectric constant of glycerol [81, 82]. It appears from the CRS hydration profiles presented herein and their relative difference to corresponding Corneometer® values, however, that measured changes in capacitance do not directly reflect total SC hydration. This raises the question as to where the capacitance signal is coming from within the skin and what moieties are driving changes in this parameter in the context of treatment with a moisturizer. These questions are the subject of ongoing research in our and other laboratories.

Our initial hypothesis was that it was niacinamide (nicotinamide, vitamin B3), present only in

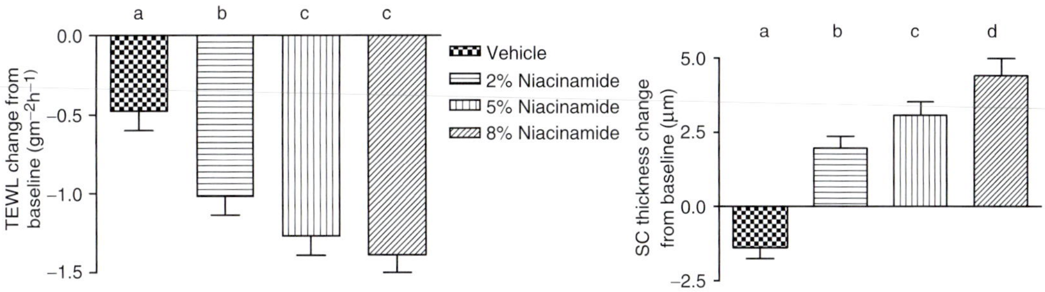

Fig. 38.7 Niacinamide dose response for stratum corneum thickness and TEWL change after 4 weeks regular product usage. *Letters* indicate statistical groupings at 95% confidence

formulation A, which was the agent responsible for these SC effects. Recent work has been undertaken to further examine the role of niacinamide in SC swelling using freshly prepared biopsy cross sections in a vehicle-controlled study [83]. Also, recently, a vehicle-controlled dose–response study was undertaken to demonstrate how the level of niacinamide formulated into a typical moisturizing product impacted both SC thickness changes and TEWL after 4 weeks of twice daily product usage, Fig. 38.7 [84]. A strong positive correlation was found between niacinamide level and both increases in SC thickness and barrier function improvement. We therefore believe this confirms our hypothesis regarding niacinamide as being the active ingredient in formulation A in our original work and demonstrates the validity or CRS for measuring and assessing the effects of topically applied cosmetic formulations on skin properties.

38.3 Conclusion and the Future

While there are a number of techniques currently available which are capable of providing information regarding distribution of different components within the skin, until recently, none have been capable of determining these non-destructively, rapidly and in vivo. As such, it has been difficult to incorporate these into routine clinical test protocols. The recent development of confocal Raman spectroscopy has enabled the assessment of changes in molecular concentration gradients in vivo for the first time for a variety of different chemical species. It is clear that CRS represents a powerful new class of measurement with significant advantage over traditional measurement techniques through its ability to assess these changes, both rapidly and in a non-destructive manner. The advent of this new technology seems timely as we consider the development of moisturizers that truly augment SC barrier function.

The capability of in vivo confocal Raman spectroscopy for probing chemical gradients within the skin has only been touched upon as the technique is still in its infancy. Even considering its relative youth, in vivo Raman spectroscopy of the skin has already provided a valuable new insight into SC behaviour and function and demonstrated its potential as a valuable tool for determining chemical concentration gradients in a clinical environment, both in relation to the use of cosmetic products and naturally occurring variation. As the technique becomes more established, its ability to measure these profiles within the skin will provide a deeper understanding of the interaction between chemical composition and location and skin health and function.

Acknowledgments The work was sponsored by Procter and Gamble Technical Centres Ltd.

References

1. Blank IH (1952) Factors which influence the water content of the stratum corneum. J Invest Dermatol 18:433–440
2. Grubauer G, Elias PM, Feingold KR (1989) Transepidermal water loss: the signal for recovery of barrier structure and function. J Lipid Res 30:323–333

3. Loden M (1995) Biophysical properties of dry atopic and normal skin with special reference to skin care products. Acta Derm Venereol Suppl (Stockholm) 192:1–48
4. Agache P (2004) Stratum corneum histopathology. In: Agache P, Humbert P (eds) Measuring the skin. Springer, Berlin
5. Warner RR, Myers MC, Taylor DA (1988) Electron probe analysis of human skin: determination of the water concentration profile. J Invest Dermatol 90: 218–244
6. Warner RR, Lilly NA (1994) Correlation of water content with ultrastructure in the stratum corneum. In: Elsner P, Berardesca E, Maibach HI (eds) Bioengineering of the skin: water and the stratum corneum. CRC Press Inc, Boca Raton
7. Richter T, Peuckert C, Sattler M et al (2004) Dead but highly dynamic – the stratum corneum is divided into three hydration zones. Skin Pharmacol Physiol 17:246–257
8. Bouwstra JA, de Graff A, Gooris GS et al (2003) Water distribution and related morphology in human stratum corneum at different hydration levels. J Invest Dermatol 120(5):750–758
9. Rawlings AV, Scott IR, Harding CR, Bowser P (1994) Stratum corneum moisturization at the molecular level. J Invest Dermatol 103:731–734
10. Brancaleon L, Bamberg MP, Sakamaki T, Kollias N (2001) Attenuated total reflection-Fourier transform infrared spectroscopy as a possible method to investigate biophysical parameters of stratum corneum in vivo. J Invest Dermatol 116:380–386
11. Arimoto H, Egawa M, Yamada Y (2005) Depth profile of diffuse reflectance near-infrared spectroscopy for measurement of water content in skin. Skin Res Technol 11:27–35
12. Robinson M, Visscher M, Laruffa A, Wickett R (2010) Natural moisturizing factors (NMF) in the stratum corneum (SC). II. Regeneration of NMF over time after soaking. J Cosmet Sci 61(1):23–29
13. Caspers PJ, Lucassen GW, Carter EA et al (2001) In vivo confocal Raman microspectrometer of the skin. Noninvasive determination of molecular concentration profiles. J Invest Dermatol 116:434–442
14. Wertz PW (2004) Stratum corneum lipids and water. Exogenous Dermatol 3:53–56
15. Kalia YN, Alberti I, Sekkat N et al (2000) Normalization of stratum corneum barrier function and transepidermal water loss in vivo. Pharma Res 17(9):1148–1150
16. Pirot F, Berardesca E, Kalia YN et al (1998) Stratum corneum thickness and apparent water diffusivity: facile and noninvasive quantification in vivo. Pharma Res 15(3):492–494
17. Dikstein S, Zlotogorski A (1994) Measurement of skin pH. Acta Dermatol Venereol (Stockholm) 185:18–20
18. Ohman H, Vahlquist A (1994) In vivo studies concerning a pH gradient in human stratum corneum and upper epidermis. Acta Dermatol Venereol (Stockholm) 74:375–379
19. Krien PM, Kermici M (2000) Evidence for the existence of self regulated enzymatic process within the human stratum corneum: an unexpected role for urocanic acid. J Invest Dermatol 115:414–420
20. Aberg C, Wennerstrom H, Sparr E (2008) Transport processes in responding lipid membranes: a possible mechanism for pH gradient in the stratum corneum. Langmuir 24:8061–8070
21. Lieckfeldt R, Villalain J, Gomez-Fernandez JC, Lee G (1995) Apparent pKa of the fatty acids within ordered mixtures of model human stratum corneum lipids. Pharmacol Res 12:1614–1617
22. Patterson MJ, Galloway SD, Nimmo NA (2000) Variations in regional sweat composition in normal human males. Exp Physiol 85:869–875
23. Behne M, Oda Y, Murata S et al (2000) Functional role of the sodium-hydrogen antiporter, NHE1, in the epidermis: pharmacologic and NHE1 null-allele mouse studies. J Invest Dermatol 114:797
24. Visscher MO, Chatterjee R, Munson KS et al (2000) Changes in diapered and nondiapered infant skin over the first month of life. Pediatr Dermatol 17:45–51
25. Hanson KM, Barry NP, Gratton E, Clegg RM (2000) Fluorescence lifetime imaging of pH in the stratum corneum. Biophys J Annu Meet Abstr:B588
26. Hanson KM, Behne MJ, Barry NP et al (2002) Two-photon fluorescence lifetime imaging of the skin stratum corneum pH gradient. Biophys J 83:1682–1690
27. Menon GK, Grayson S, Elias PM (1985) Ionic calcium reservoirs in mammalian epidermis: ultrastructural localization by ion-capture cytochemistry. J Invest Dermatol 84:508–512
28. Mauro T, Bench G, Sidderas-Haddad E et al (1998) Acute barrier perturbation abolishes the Ca^{2+} and K^{+} gradients in murine epidermis: quantitative measurement using PIXE. J Invest Dermatol 111:1198–1201
29. Elias PM, Ahn SK, Brown BE et al (2002) Origin of the epidermal calcium gradient: regulation by barrier status and role of active vs passive mechanisms. J Invest Dermatol 119:1269–1274
30. Prasch T, Knübel G, Schmidt-Fonk K et al (2000) Infrared spectroscopy of the skin: influencing the stratum corneum with cosmetic products. Int J Cosmet Sci 22:371–383
31. Hathout RM, Mansour S, Mortada ND et al (2010) Uptake of microemulsion components into the stratum corneum and their molecular effects on skin barrier function. Mol Pharm 7(4):1266–1273
32. Notingher I, Imhof RE (2004) Mid-infrared in vivo depth-profiling of topical chemicals on skin. Skin Res Technol 10:113–121
33. Stamatas GN, de Sterke J, Hauser M et al (2008) Lipid uptake and skin occlusion following topical application of oils on adult and infant skin. J Dermatol Sci 50:135–142
34. Chrit L, Bastien P, Sockalingum GD et al (2006) An in vivo randomized study of human skin moisturization by a new confocal Raman fiber-optic microprobe: assessment of a glycerol-based hydration cream. Skin Pharmacol Physiol 19(4):207–215

35. Chrit L, Bastien P, Biatry B et al (2006) In vitro and in vivo confocal Raman study of human skin hydration: assessment of anew moisturizing agent, pMPC. Biopolymers 85:359–369
36. Förster M, Bolzinger MA, Ach D et al (2011) Ingredients tracking of cosmetic formulations in the skin: a confocal Raman microscopy investigation. Pharm Res 28(4):858–872
37. Williams AC, Barry BW, Edwards HGM, Farwell DW (1993) A critical comparison of some Raman spectroscopic techniques for studies of human stratum corneum. Pharm Res 10:1642–1647
38. Williams AC, Edwards HGM, Barry BW (1992) Fourier transform Raman spectroscopy. A novel application for examining human stratum corneum. Int J Pharm 81:R11–R14
39. Lucassen GW, Caspers PJ, Puppels GJ (1998) In vivo infrared and Raman spectroscopy of human stratum corneum. Proc SPIE 3257:52–61
40. Shim MG, Wilson BC (1997) Development of an in vivo Raman spectroscopic system for diagnostic applications. J Raman Spectrosc 28:131–142
41. Caspers PJ, Lucassen GW, Wolthuis R et al (1998) In vitro and in vivo Raman spectroscopy of human skin. Biospectroscopy 4:S31–S39
42. Caspers PJ, Lucassen GW, Bruining HJ, Puppels GJ (2000) Automated depth-scanning confocal Raman microspectrometer for rapid in vivo determination of water concentration profiles in human skin. J Raman Spectrosc 31:813–818
43. Caspers PJ, Lucassen GW, Puppels GJ (2003) Combined in vivo confocal Raman spectroscopy and confocal microscopy of human skin. Biophys J 85:572–580
44. Chrit L, Hadjur C, Morel S et al (2005) In vivo chemical investigation of human skin using a confocal Raman fiber optic microprobe. J Biomed Opt 10(4):44007
45. Egawa M, Hirao T, Takahashi M (2007) In vivo estimation of stratum corneum thickness from water concentration profiles obtained with Raman spectroscopy. Acta Derm Venereol 87(1):4–8
46. Egawa M, Tagami H (2008) Comparison of the depth profiles of water and water binding substances in the stratum corneum determined by Raman spectroscopy between the cheek and volar forearm: effects of age, seasonal changes and artificial forced hydration. Br J Dermatol 158:251–260
47. Chrit L, Bastien P, Biatry B et al (2007) In vitro and in vivo confocal Raman study of human skin hydration: assessment of a new moisturizing agent, pMPC. Biopolymers 85(4):359–369
48. Crowther JM, Sieg A, Blenkiron P et al (2008) Measuring the effects of topical moisturizers on changes in stratum corneum thickness, water gradients and hydration in vivo. Br J Dermatol 159: 567–577
49. Naito S, Min YK, Osanai O et al (2008) In vivo measurement of human dermis by 1064 nm-excited fiber Raman spectroscopy. Skin Res Technol 14: 18–25
50. Bielfeldt S, Schoder V, Ely U et al (2009) Assessment of human stratum corneum thickness and its barrier properties by in-vivo confocal Raman spectroscopy. IFSCC Mag 12:9–15
51. Baldwin K, Batchelder D (2001) Confocal Raman microspectroscopy through a planar interface. Appl Spectrosc 55:517–524
52. Tfayli A, Piot O, Manfait M (2008) Confocal Raman microspectroscopy on excised human skin: uncertainties in depth profiling and mathematical correction applied to dermatological drug permeation. J Biophotonics 1:140–153
53. Welzel J (2001) Optical coherence tomography in dermatology: a review. Skin Res Technol 7:1–9
54. Ya-Xian Z, Suetake T, Tagami H (1999) Number of cell layers of the stratum corneum in normal skin – relationship to the anatomical locations on the body, age, sex and physical parameters. Arch Dermatol Res 291:555–559
55. Gambichler T, Boms S, Stacker M et al (2006) Epidermal thickness assessed by optical coherence tomography and routine histology: preliminary results of method comparison. J Eur Acad Dermatol Venereol 20(7):791–795
56. Lademann J, Otberg N, Richter H et al (2007) Application of optical non-invasive methods in skin physiology: a comparison of laser scanning microscopy and optical coherent tomography with histological analysis. Skin Res Technol 13(2): 119–132
57. Norlen L (2006) Stratum corneum keratin structure, function and formation – a comprehensive review. Int J Cosmet Sci 28(6):397–425
58. Wu J, Polefka TG (2008) Confocal Raman microspectroscopy of stratum corneum: a pre-clinical validation study. Int J Cosmet Sci 30:47–56
59. Matts PJ, Gray J, Rawlings AV (2005) The 'dry skin cycle' – a new model of dry skin and mechanisms for intervention (International congress and symposium series), vol 256. The Royal Society of Medicine Press Ltd, London, pp 1–38
60. Loden M (2005) The clinical benefit of moisturizers. JEADV 19:672–688
61. Breternitz M, Kowatski D, Langenauer M et al (2008) Placebo controlled, double blind, randomized prospective study of a glycerol-based emollient on eczematous skin in atopic dermatitis: biophysical and clinical evaluation. Skin Pharmacol Physiol 21: 39–45
62. Summers RS, Summers B, Chandar P et al (1996) The effect of lipids with and without humectants on skin xerosis. J Soc Cosmet Chem 47:27–39
63. Rawlings AV, Watkinson A, Hope J et al (1995) The effect of glycerol and humidity on desmosome degradation in stratum corneum. Arch Dermatol Res 287:457–464
64. Held E, Sveinsdottir S, Agner T (1999) Effect of long term use of moisturizer on skin hydration, barrier function and susceptibility to irritants. Acta Derm Venereol 79:49–51

65. Zachariae C, Held E, Johansen JD et al (2003) Effect of a moisturizer on skin susceptibility to NiCl2. Acta Derm Venereol 83:93–97
66. Berardesca E, Distante F, Vignoli GP et al (1997) Alpha hydroxyacids modulate stratum corneum barrier function. Br J Dermatol 137:934–938
67. Buraczewska I, Berne B, Lindberg M et al (2007) Changes in skin barrier function following long-term treatment with moisturizers, a randomized controlled trial. Br J Dermatol 156:492–498
68. Barany E, Lindberg M, Loden M (2000) Unexpected skin barrier influence from non-ionic emulsifiers. Int J Pharm 195:189–195
69. Fluhr JW, Gloor M, Lehmann L et al (1999) Glycerol accelerates recovery of barrier function in vivo. Acta Derm Venereol 79:418–421
70. Loden M, Andersson AC, Andersson C et al (2001) Instrumental and dermatologist evaluation of the effect of glycerine and urea on dry skin in atopic dermatitis. Skin Res Technol 7:209–213
71. Rawlings AV, Conti A, Verdejo P et al (1996) The effect of lactic acid isomers on epidermal lipid biosynthesis and stratum corneum barrier function. Arch Dermatol Res 288:383–390
72. Norlen L, Emilson A, Forslind B (1997) Stratum corneum swelling. Biophysical and computer assisted quantitative assessments. Arch Dermatol Res 289: 506–513
73. Richter T, Muller JH, Schwarz UD et al (2001) Investigation of the swelling of human skin cells in liquid media by tapping mode scanning force microscopy. Appl Phys A A72:S125–S128
74. Bouwstra JA, de Graaff A, Gooris GS et al (2003) Water distribution and related morphology in human stratum corneum at different hydration levels. J Invest Dermatol 120:750–758
75. Caussin J, Groenink HWW, de Graaff AM et al (2007) Lipophilic and hydrophilic moisturizers show different actions on human skin as revealed by cryo scanning electron microscopy. Exp Dermatol 16:891–898
76. Orth DS, Appa Y, Contard P et al (1995) Effect of high glycerin moisturizers on the ultrastructure of the stratum corneum. Poster at the 53rd annual meeting of the American Academy of Dermatology, New Orleans, Feb 1995
77. Orth DS, Appa Y (2000) Glycerine: a natural ingredient for moisturizing skin. In: Loden M, Maibach HI (eds) Dry skin and moisturizers: chemistry and function. CRC Press, Boca Raton
78. Fluhr JW, Bornkessel A, Berardesca E (2006) Glycerol-just a moisturizer? Biological & biophysical effects. In: Loden M, Maibach HI (eds) Dry skin and moisturizers, 2nd edn. CRC Press, Boca Raton
79. Jacobson EL, Kim H, Kim M et al (2007) A topical lipophilic niacin derivative increases NAD, epidermal differentiation and barrier function in photodamaged skin. Exp Dermatol 16(6):490–499
80. Loden M, Wessman C (2001) The influence of a cream containing 20% glycerin and its vehicle on skin barrier properties. Int J Cosmet Sci 23:115–119
81. Fluhr JW, Mao-Qiang M, Brown BE et al (2003) Glycerol regulates stratum corneum hydration in sebaceous gland deficient (Asebia) mice. J Invest Dermatol 120:728–737
82. Choi EH, Man MQ, Wang F et al (2005) Is endogenous glycerol a determinant of stratum corneum hydration in humans? J Invest Dermatol 125:288–293
83. Crowther JM, Matts PJ, publication in preparation
84. Kaczvinsky JR, publication in preparation

Skin Moisture and Heat Transfer

39

Jerrold Scott Petrofsky and Lee Berk

39.1 Introduction and Overview

A natural senescence of the skin occurs as a result of the aging process [65]. Over the life span of a human being, skin moisture and skin structure vary [65]. In the last few centuries, the human life span has nearly doubled, adding to the yearly chronology of stress on the skin and the deleterious effects of the aging process [79]. The skin serves as a protective immunological barrier between the outside world and the internal organs. As such, it is exposed to the environment including UV light and environmental toxins. In addition, stressors such as smoking and diet expose the skin to internal stresses from increasing concentrations of free radicals as we age [61].

While skin is a barrier, it is not a complete barrier and is permeable to oils, and to a lesser extent moisture. It can gain or lose moisture. The loss of moisture through the skin takes two forms, insensible water loss and sweat. Water loss is a means of removing heat from the body since the evaporation of 1 cc of water causes the loss of 540 cal from the body. While sweat is a major means of water loss, the insensible water loss, when added to moisture lost through respiration, is an important and significant means of removing heat from the body [27]. In addition to evaporation, there are three other ways that heat is lost through the body. These are radiation, convection, and conduction [27]. The skin is involved in all four to allow heat loss from the body.

Radiation involves the skin producing infrared light to lose heat from the body. The normal emissivity of human skin is 0.97 and is not influenced by race or skin color [115]. The intensity of the radiation emitted by the body can be viewed through a special camera called an infrared imager. In such a photograph, the temperature of the skin can be measured by infrared light intensity. In Fig. 39.1 below, for example, the intensity has been coded by color. The color white is used for "warmer" temperatures, and blue represents "cooler" temperatures. Temperatures in the middle are assigned to other colors such as red, yellow, and green [52].

The average person loses over 1,500,00 cal per day in heat from the body [57]. Much of this is lost through radiation (Fig. 39.2). But when body heat rises rapidly, as occurs during exercise, additional mechanisms are needed to cool the body. Thus, conduction and convection come into play and are also used in heat loss [130].

Conduction involves passive heat loss from the skin by direct contact to another media. For example, if a person sits on a chair with snow on it, heat moves from the skin into the snow eliciting a heat loss from the body. This mechanism works well for the skin when exposed to the environment. It is blunted with clothing since

J.S. Petrofsky, Ph.D., J.D. (✉) • L. Berk, DrPH
Department of Physical Therapy,
Loma Linda University,
Loma Linda, CA 92373, USA
e-mail: jpetrofsky@llu.edu

M. Lodén, H.I. Maibach (eds.), *Treatment of Dry Skin Syndrome*,
DOI 10.1007/978-3-642-27606-4_39, © Springer-Verlag Berlin Heidelberg 2012

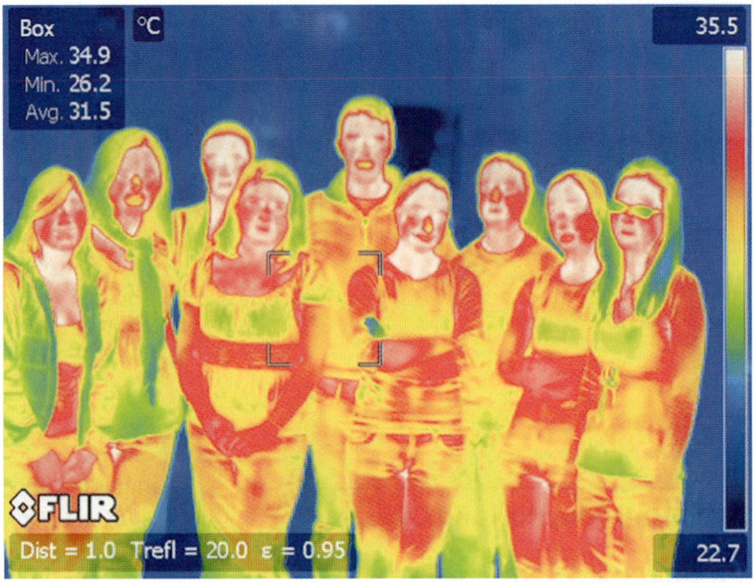

Fig. 39.1 An infrared picture of the skin in male and female subjects of various races

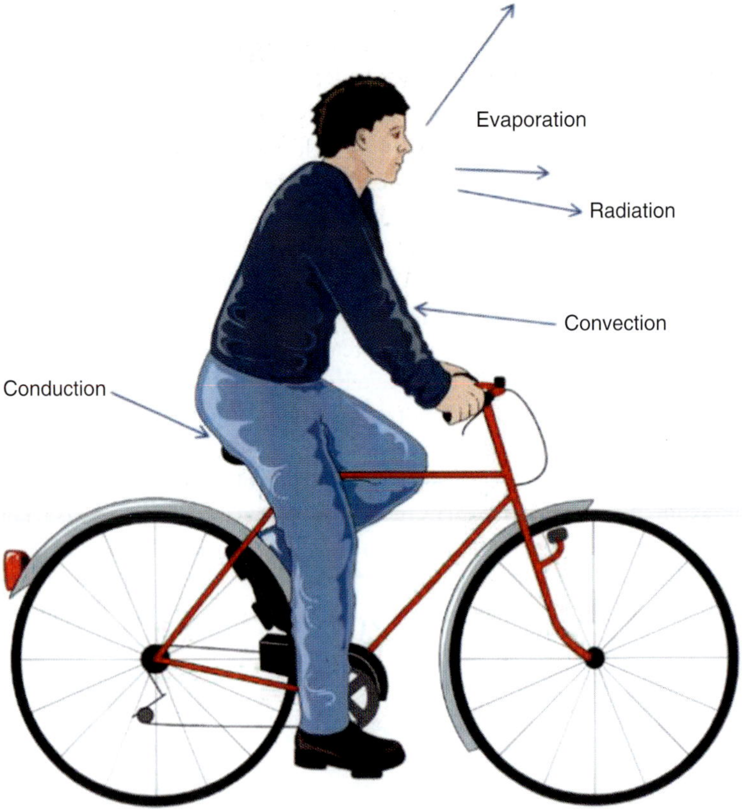

Fig. 39.2 The different mechanisms of heat loss from the body

heat cannot easily move through fabric due to its high air content [47]. Thus, the larger the surface area of the body that is in contact with a cooler object, the greater the heat loss.

Another mechanism is convection. Convective heat loss occurs when air moves over the exposed skin [44]. This causes a loss of calories directly from the skin. Finally, there is the mechanism of evaporation. Through sweating or insensible water loss, water changes from a liquid state to vapor and carries heat away from the body due to water changing from a state of liquid to gas. Each cc of water that evaporates causes the loss of 540 cal of heat [72]. But the reverse is also true. When water condenses on the skin, it gains 540 cal/cc of water that condenses. The average person sweats between 0.8 and 1.4 l/h. Thus, if all water was evaporated, it would lead to a heat loss of up to 750,000 cal/h. In fact, in athletes, even higher sweat losses have been reported [63].

All of these mechanisms rely on the skin being intact and circulation being normal. Aging is associated with an increase in tissue reactive oxygen species that damages multiple pathways [40]. Reactive oxygen species damage circulation, reducing radiation, convection, and conduction. Damage to nitric oxide release in sweat glands associated with aging also impairs sweating causing a reduction in evaporative loss [53].

These same reactive oxygen species can also damage cellular and nuclear membranes [40].

Skin structure can also alter heat transfer. With aging, cell proliferation in the skin decreases leading to a loss of skin integrity [112]. The skin dries and wrinkles with age [35]. Skin dryness has been reported with advancing age in over 95% of the people who were sampled in one study [59]. Skin thickness rises over the first 20 years of life [41] and then thins as age progresses [80, 110]. The epidermis may either become thin or cornified, and the dermis may thin as much as 50% or more with age [80, 131]. The loss of skin capillary density, called rarefaction [131], is paralleled with a loss of skin collagen and elastin [11]. The basement membrane also increases in thickness with age [129].

These generalized changes in moisture content and structure in the skin can be specifically addressed for each of the two major layers in the skin, the epidermis and dermis. The stratum corneum loses water content with age [43, 54, 67]. Part of this is due to a reduction in the amino acid composition of the epidermis, which reduces its capacity to bind water [54]. The integrity of the skin also depends on the lipid content of the epidermis. This decreases by as much as 65% with age [124]. These age-related changes reduce the ability of the skin to provide a barrier to protect the dermis below [30, 39].

The dermis also shows aging effects in terms of integrity and function much like the epidermis. Collagen, elastin, and hyaluronic acid in the dermis are all depleted with aging [32]. This weakens the integrity of the dermis [33]. Collagen turnover also changes. In young skin, the ratio of type I to type III collagen is 6:1. In older skin, this ratio drops by each decade of life [116]. Thus, the collagen becomes thicker with age. Increased collagen cross-links with age reduce skin elasticity [32]. Sensory transduction is also reduced with age. Additionally, a loss of Pacinian corpuscles and Meissner's corpuscles from the dermal layer in older skin reduces tactile sensation [26].

All of these changes lead to impaired convective and conductive heat transfer with age. Lower water content reduces the thermal coefficient of the skin making it easier to warm the skin when an external heat load is applied. Changes in the structural integrity also alter the skin thermal coefficient, so heat is not transferred as easily. Thus, heat going into or out of the skin is altered by aging. Since the blood flow is the most important consideration in heat loss, its control and the effects of aging and diabetes will be reviewed followed by the impact of skin moisture on skin circulation. Further, the effect of skin moisture on conductive heat transfer will also be reviewed more specifically.

39.2 Modeling of Heat Exchange Through the Skin

Heat exchange through the skin was first modeled by Pennes. The Pennes model predicted that there were two basic ways the skin can dissipate heat [81]. One of those was through conductive heat loss. Conductive heat loss, as described above, involves passive properties of the skin including skin fat content, moisture, and structure [64, 85]. The other way of moving heat is related to skin blood flow [81]. Pennes asserted that the primary site of temperature equilibration was the capillary bed and that all the blood perfusing of the skin starts at the core temperature of the body [81]. The Pennes' bioheat equation is:

$$h_b = V \rho_b C_b (1 - \kappa)(T_a - T)$$

where h_b is the rate of heat transfer per unit volume of tissue, V is the perfusion rate per unit volume of tissue, ρ_b is the density of blood, C_b is the specific heat of blood, κ is a factor that accounts for incomplete thermal equilibrium between blood and tissue, T_a is the temperature of arterial blood which is generally assumed to remain constant and equal to the core temperature of the body, and T is the local tissue temperature [135]. The basic premise is that heat in is equivalent to heat out; heat into the body is dissipated either into the blood or deeper tissues. Three major advantages of the model are that it is readily solvable for constant parameter values, gives two adjustable parameters (V and T_a), and requires no anatomical data [93]. On the downside, the model gives no prediction of actual details of vascular temperatures, the assumption of constant arterial temperature is not generally valid, and thermal equilibration occurs prior to the capillary bed. The Pennes model also did not take into consideration skin moisture and subcutaneous fat, both of which alter conductive heat exchange [82, 109]. In addition, aging and diabetes reduce skin blood flow [70, 71, 96] and may alter subcutaneous fat thickness and skin moisture, changing both conductive and blood-borne heat transfer.

39.2.1 Conductive Heat Loss Through the Skin

Conductive heat exchange through the skin is governed by the structure of the skin itself and the underlying tissues. When heat is rapidly applied to the skin, conductive heat exchange is the only means of heat removal. The circulation, as described below, is a much more efficient means of removing heat. However, there is a time delay after heat is applied to the skin before the circulation increases. Circulation takes seconds before it increases. Even after circulation increases, conductive heat loss is still important in the heat exchange process. Further, the conductive heat properties of the skin also govern heat loss and heat gain by radiation and convection as well.

The factors that determine the heat exchange properties of the skin are the coefficient of heat of the skin itself and the underlying tissue, namely fat. The coefficient of heat is the ease with which heat passes through a structure. For example, the coefficient of heat of water is 1.0. What this means is that 1 cal of heat will raise water 1°C. Iron on the other hand has a coefficient of heat of 0.09. One calorie will raise the temperature of iron about 10°C. Therefore, this is an important property of a material that determines how hot it gets when heat passes through it. A measure of the actual heat flow, which depends on the coefficient of heat, is the ability of heat to move laterally and deep below the skin. This is called thermal conductivity. This number shows the energy loss through a substance such as the skin.

For human skin, thermal conductivity has been determined [12]. While for water, it is 0.628 W/m^2. For fat, it is 0.33 and for blood plasma, it is 0.57 W/m^2. Thus, the greater the water content of the skin, the better the heat transfer. Some of heat applied to the skin moves laterally, while most heat moves into deep tissue. Thus, even if skin were very moist, the thickness of the subcutaneous fat layer would limit heat transfer out of the skin. If heat cannot leave the skin, the skin will get hot very quickly and can burn as predicted by Henriques [45, 75, 76]. The actual analysis of skin moisture and its role in heat transfer is complex since heat movement for conductive heat exchange varies in different layers of the skin. For example, in pig skin, a model of human skin, epidermal heat conductivity is 0.36, for the dermis it is 0.54, and for fat it is 0.21 [45, 75, 76]. Muscle is 0.064. Thus, the movement of heat involves a multicompartment model showing that any change in any layer will alter conductive heat movement across the skin. It can be predicted that changes in either oil or moisture content or thickness of any of these three layers would alter thermal conductivity, but it was not until recent years that these were examined as shown below.

Thus, in summary, the factors of importance for conductive heat transfer are:

1. The structure of the dermal and epidermal layer
2. The water content of the dermal and epidermal layer
3. The thickness of subcutaneous fat

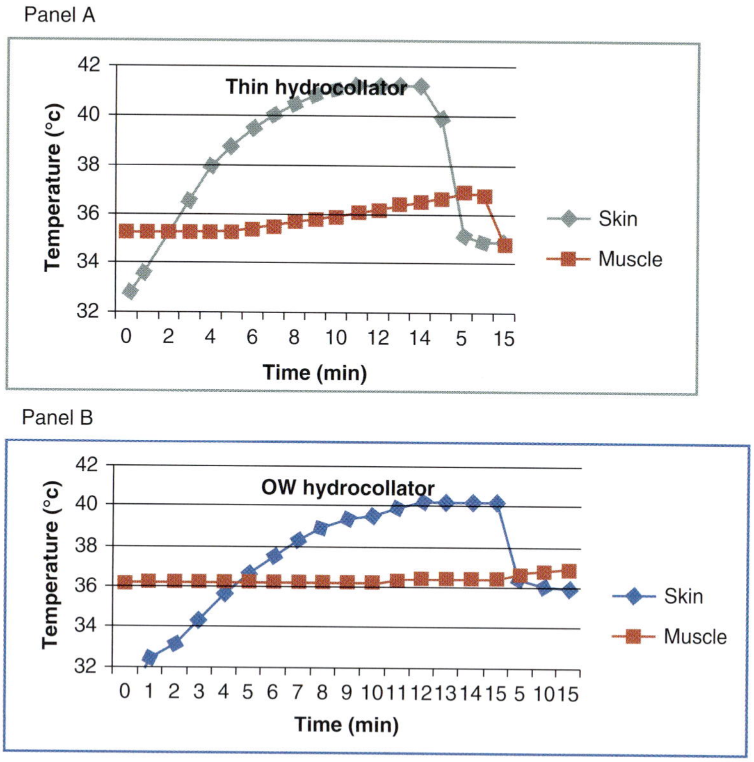

Fig. 39.3 The changes in skin and muscle temperature in the quadriceps muscle in a thin (*Panel A*) and overweight (*Panel B*) subject after immersion of the leg for 15 min in a water bath. *Each figure* shows the skin and muscle temperature. Skin temperature rises quickly, while muscle temperature is protected by the insulating capability of subcutaneous fat and the skin

39.2.1.1 Subcutaneous Fat

As stated previously, different thicknesses of subcutaneous fat and its effect on heat transfer were not taken into consideration by the Pennes model. Subcutaneous fat thickness has been shown to be greater in people who are older and who have diabetes compared to younger individuals [84, 101, 108]. Actual measurements of heat transfer in humans as a function of the thickness of the subcutaneous fat layer clearly show a slowing in heat transfer with increased fat so that the time constant which predicts heat dissipation into deeper layers is increased [108]. Thus, if subcutaneous fat is thickened, it is harder for muscle to lose heat outward to the skin, and if a heat load is applied to the skin, it impairs the ability of circulation to transfer heat into deeper tissues [103, 109]. This causes higher skin temperatures during both local and global heating [108, 134]. For example, Fig. 39.3 illustrates the data on two typical subjects who had their legs immersed in a water bath for 15 min. The skin and muscle temperatures were measured by thermocouples. The thermocouple was placed in the quadriceps muscle 2.5 cm below the surface of the skin, and a second thermocouple on the skin was just at the needle insertion site. After the leg was immersed in the bath water, skin temperature rapidly rose toward that of the water in both subjects. However, in the overweight subjects, there was a slower rise in muscle temperature compared to the thinner subject due to the subcutaneous fat. The same is true when energy is transferred from muscle to skin; subcutaneous fat acts as a barrier to energy movement. If a warm heat source is applied to the skin, the heat is kept in the skin in someone who is overweight causing skin temperature to rise faster and making the skin more susceptible to burns. But skin moisture also plays a critical role in conductive heat loss. Moisture content of subcutaneous fat is low. But as stated above, it is critical in heat transfer characteristics in the dermal layer.

39.2.1.2 Skin and Conductive Heat Transfer

Older people have thinner dermal layers than that found in younger people [69, 95, 106]. This impacts the ability of the skin to dissipate heat. Skin moisture is also less in older people. Previous studies indicate skin moisture content, as stated above, alters the ability of heat to passively transfer through skin [64]. Skin that is dry with low water content has a lower thermal index than moist skin causing small amounts of heat to greatly increase the temperature of the skin [14, 82, 119]. This can lead to skin damage and burns [117]. For example, in a recent study, when a constant heat source at 42°C was applied to the skin in the upper leg, older people required, in the first few seconds before skin blood flow could change, half the calories to heat the skin to the same temperature compared to younger people [7–9].

Further compounding the problems of dissipating heat in older people is diabetes. When compared to age-matched nondiabetic people, those with type II diabetes have thinner skin [10, 70, 96], thicker subcutaneous fat [10, 25], less skin moisture [69, 119], and reduced skin blood flow due to greater endothelial dysfunction compared to age matched controls [17, 18, 48–51, 58, 120]. When heat was applied to the skin of the leg in individuals with diabetes and the calories needed to increase skin temperature were measured, compared to age-matched controls, the skin required half the calories of the controls [7].

39.2.1.3 Skin Circulation and Heat Transfer

The skin circulation plays a major role in heat transfer. But the control of the circulation is complex and involves balancing many factors. When individuals are exposed to a thermally neutral environment, skin blood flow averages about 5% of their cardiac output [114]. However, during whole body heating, blood flow through the skin can increase to as much as 160% of cardiac output at rest, or about 8 l/min [114]. This provides a great potential for thermal cooling of the body. In glabrous (nonhairy) skin (e.g., palms, plantar aspects of the feet, and lips), cutaneous arterioles are innervated by only sympathetic adrenergic vasoconstrictor nerves [34, 64]. In addition to the sympathetic nerves, blood flow is also affected by local metabolites and effectors such as temperature and pressure on the skin [55, 56] In hairy (nonglabrous) skin, which is present over most of the body, three separate branches of the sympathetic nervous system control skin blood flow: adrenergic vasoconstrictor nerves that reduce (constrict) skin blood vessels [60] and cholinergic and nitrogenergic nerves that cause vasodilatation of blood vessels by releasing the neurotransmitters acetylcholine or nitric oxide, respectively [60, 87]. In addition, local effectors, such as metabolites and changes in local skin temperature or pressure, may mediate a change in skin blood flow [109]. Thus, the control of the circulation in the skin can be divided into generally two types of control: (1) the local response of vascular endothelial cells to metabolites and other effectors (such as local pressure or shear stress on the blood vessel wall) and (2) neurogenic control through the sympathetic nervous system. Both sympathetic synapses and local effectors mediate their effects through the thin layer of cells lining blood vessels, the vascular endothelial cells [94].

Using drugs that specifically block vasoconstriction (e.g., bretylium tosylate) and agents that inhibit vasodilatation by blocking acetylcholine (cholinergic antagonistic agents) has been used to confirm chemical mediators at neuronal synapses [109]. Sympathetic vasodilator and vasoconstrictor nerves innervate blood vessels by extensive terminal varicosities located on the surface of vascular endothelial cells [31]. The vascular endothelial cells, in turn, release fat soluble substances that cause the vascular smooth muscle surrounding it to relax or constrict, thereby mediating a change in skin blood flow. Stripping the inner layer of large conduit arteries (i.e., removing the endothelial layer) eliminates vasodilatation and vasoconstriction in vascular smooth muscle [31].

The most important vasodilator substance is nitric oxide. It is released from vascular endothelial cells due to a variety of stimuli including skin moisture content.

Nitric Oxide

A variety of different stressors can elicit an increase or decrease in skin blood flow in hairy skin. The blood flow response is controlled through a range of different mechanisms. In the

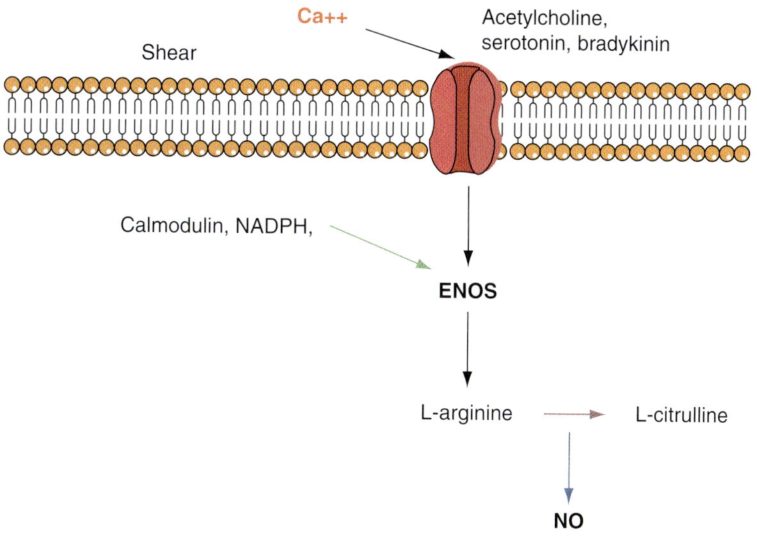

Fig. 39.4 Synthesis of nitric oxide

1990s, a number of research laboratories demonstrated an active role for nitric oxide as a mediator of vasodilatation in the skin [29, 58, 99]. Historically, it had been postulated that a substance released from vascular endothelial cells caused vascular smooth muscle to relax [98]. This substance, originally called endothelial cell-derived relaxation factor, is now known to be several different compounds, one of which is a fat-soluble chemical, nitric oxide [70].

Several lines of evidence indicate that nitric oxide is produced by endothelial cells in both humans and animal models and over a variety of species. Nitric oxide is produced from the amino acid L-arginine by the enzyme endothelial nitric oxide synthetase (Fig. 39.4). When LNAME (*N*-nitro-L-arginine methyl ester), an inhibitor of nitric oxide synthetase, is infused into the skin via microdialysis in both animals and humans, the increase in blood flow due to stressors such as heat is significantly attenuated, although not completely blocked [58]. During whole body heating, the bioavailability of nitric oxide increases in proportion to skin blood flow. However, nitric oxide may be generated from sources in addition to endothelial nitric oxide synthetase. For example, evidence exists that H1 histamine receptors on vascular endothelial cells generate nitric oxide during cutaneous active vasodilation [71]. It has also been suggested that the release of histamine from mast cells induced by VIP also could be involved because histamine increases the bioavailability of nitric oxide in the skin [71, 96].

Nitric oxide, once produced, diffuses both into the blood and into the surrounding vascular smooth muscle. In smooth muscle, nitric oxide activates the soluble enzyme in the cytoplasm, guanylate cyclase, which catalyzes the production of cyclic guanosine monophosphate (cyclic GMP) (Fig. 39.5).

Cyclic GMP has several biological actions which include decreasing calcium permeability, inhibiting actomyosin ATPase activity, and increasing potassium permeability in vascular smooth muscle. These three functions, taken together, have the combined effect of relaxing vascular smooth muscle.

Nitric oxide also has other effects on the endothelial cell and its environment. These autocrine and paracrine effects include nitric oxide being a potent anti-inflammatory agent on blood vessel walls, inhibiting leukocyte adhesion [89], platelet adhesion, and smooth muscle cell proliferation [104], promoting insulin release [97], and mediating the immune response to inflammation [88].

Nitric oxide also is involved in physiologic functions outside of the vascular endothelial cells. These include neuronal transmission

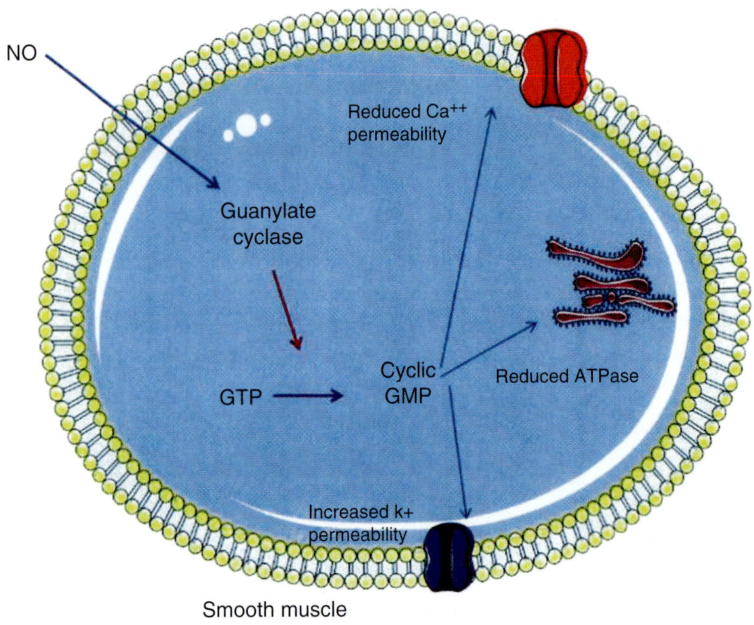

Fig. 39.5 The effect of nitric oxide on smooth muscle

[91, 123], pulmonary vascular remodeling [111], arterial sclerosis [86], and exercise-induced cardiac protection [105]. Impaired production or bioavailability of nitric oxide leads to endothelial dysfunction and is the root cause of much different cardiovascular pathology including diabetes, hypertension, heart failure, and coronary artery disease [92].

Nitric oxide is derived from the bioconversion of the amino acid, L-arginine, to the amino acid, L-citrulline. Like all amino acids, L-arginine and L-citrulline are nitrogen-bearing compounds. The L-arginine molecule has four nitrogens: when bioconverted to L-citrulline, it loses one atom of nitrogen and oxygen to form nitric oxide and yields another amino acid with three nitrogens, L-citrulline.

A family of enzymes called nitric oxide synthetases produce nitric oxide in various organ systems. The enzymes include neuronal nitric oxide synthetase (NOS), inducible nitric oxide synthetase (INOS), and endothelial nitric oxide synthetase (ENOS) [19]. ENOS is the predominant form of nitric oxide synthetase in the vasculature [128]. There are three subunits in ENOS, a central calmodulin-binding subunit and an oxidative and reductase end. In vascular endothelial cells, ENOS is normally inactive. It is activated through a complex sequence of chemical reactions that involve the binding of nicotinamide-adenine dinucleotide phosphate (NADPH), flavin mononucleotide, and flavin adenosine dinucleotide [128] to the enzyme. Mediated by flavin, electrons are transferred from the carboxylate (COOH) terminal bound to NADPH to the heme of the NH2 terminus. These electrons activate oxygen. L-Arginine is reduced to L-citrulline in two phases. In the first phase, L-arginine binds to ENOS. In the second phase, it is oxidized to L-citrulline and releases nitric oxide [19].

Intracellular calcium modulates the activity of ENOS through the calcium-binding subunit [37]. Intracellular calcium is mobilized through various signaling pathways, and ENOS is ultimately activated by phosphorylation at one of six phosphorylation sites [28]. Calcium-activated calmodulin increases the rate of transfer of electrons from NADPH to ENOS (Fig. 39.3). (The complex system of reactions used to increase calcium mobility from the extracellular to intracellular space is discussed in another section of this chapter.) Other substances, such as proteins and free fatty acids, can also modulate the activation of ENOS [13, 37].

Phosphorylation of ENOS via protein kinases is a critical step in its activation [127]. To date, six phosphorylation sites on ENOS have been identified, including serine 1,177, threonine 495, protein kinase b (pkb-akt) 939, adenosine monophosphate-activated kinase, protein kinase A, and protein kinase G [70, 107]. For example, the ENOS cascade can be activated by receptors for estrogen and glucocorticoids [95], insulin and vascular endothelial growth factor (VEGF) [4], and blood flow and laminar shear stress [3, 24].

The balance between nitric oxide production and degradation determines the bioavailability of nitric oxide. When nitric oxide bioavailability is reduced, heightened vasoconstriction occurs, as seen in hypertension, cardiovascular disease, and diabetes [38, 45].

Impairments of ENOS activity can affect nitric oxide production. For example, instability in ENOS may liberate oxygen instead of nitric oxide [4]. Decreased bioavailability of L-arginine may cause ENOS to reduce production of nitric oxide in vivo [21]. Oxidative stress causing reactive oxygen species also reduces nitric oxide bioavailability through degradation. These oxides and superoxides degrade nitric oxide, yielding molecules that bear three oxygen atoms, such as peroxynitrite [78]. These reactive oxygen species can in turn cause cellular damage. Oxidative stress potentially can be moderated via activating NADPH oxidases or xanthine oxidases in the vascular wall [28, 77].

Diabetes and cigarette smoking may not alter nitric oxide production via NOS enzymatic pathways yet still reduce nitric oxide bioavailability by increasing oxidative stress. The result is impaired vasodilatation [78]. This can raise cardiac work and blood pressure.

Other Vasodilators

Prostacyclin (PGI_2), a prostaglandin, is another vasodilator released by vascular endothelial cells [46]. In younger people, vasodilatation is mediated through the release of both nitric oxide and prostacyclin [46]. However, as individuals age, prostacyclin production is impaired, and nitric oxide becomes the predominant vasodilator [113]. One study of younger subjects revealed that at least 60% of acetylcholine-mediated vasodilatation was preserved after inhibition of both ENOS and cyclooxygenase (COX) [46]. Although this shows the importance of nitric oxide and prostacyclin in regulating cutaneous circulation, it points to other substances released by vascular endothelial cells, especially in younger individuals, that also mediate an increase in skin blood flow [46].

For example, in studies of chronic inflammation of the skin, neuropeptides such as substance P can be released from sympathetic nerve terminals [20]. Substance P binds to the endothelial cell on the NK-1 receptor [20]. In rats, administration of the NK-1 receptor antagonist CP-96–345 significantly reduced the blood flow increase which occurred during sympathetic nerve stimulation [20]. Thus, substance P may be responsible for the vasodilatation seen due to inflammation in the tissues in rats [6], and in response to direct electrical stimulation of sympathetic nerves [36], and other conditions such as electrical stimulation of the lumbar sympathetic trunk [20]. Substance P is normally expressed in small dorsal root ganglion neurons and in the skin and is upregulated in inflammatory conditions [137]. Nerve growth factors from inflamed tissue play a role in upregulating production of substance P [137]. Because sympathetic postganglionic neurons are affected by nerve growth factors from chronic inflammation, it has been hypothesized that upregulation of substance P alters the normal sympathetic combination of neurotransmitters released in sympathetic nerves [20].

39.2.2 The Effect of Heat on Circulation

It is well established that when heat is applied to the skin, there is an increase in skin blood flow [89, 101, 136]. Initially, warm thermoreceptors on skin tactile sensory nerves (TRPV1 receptors) sense the warmth and release substance P and calcitonin gene-related peptide which cause an increase in potassium permeability in vascular smooth muscle surrounding the endothelial cell [15, 16, 73]. This, in turn, causes an increase in blood flow by relaxing vascular smooth muscle. This is illustrated in Fig. 39.6.

Here, the data represents ten subjects with a 44°C heat source applied to their leg for 2 min.

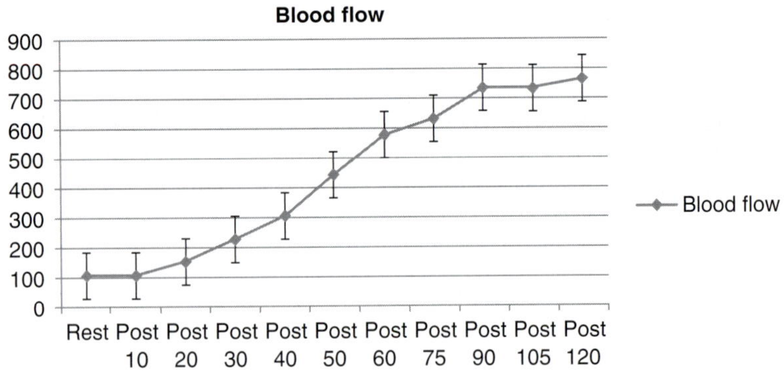

Fig. 39.6 The effect of locally applied heat at 44ºC on skin blood flow (flux) over a 120 seconds period

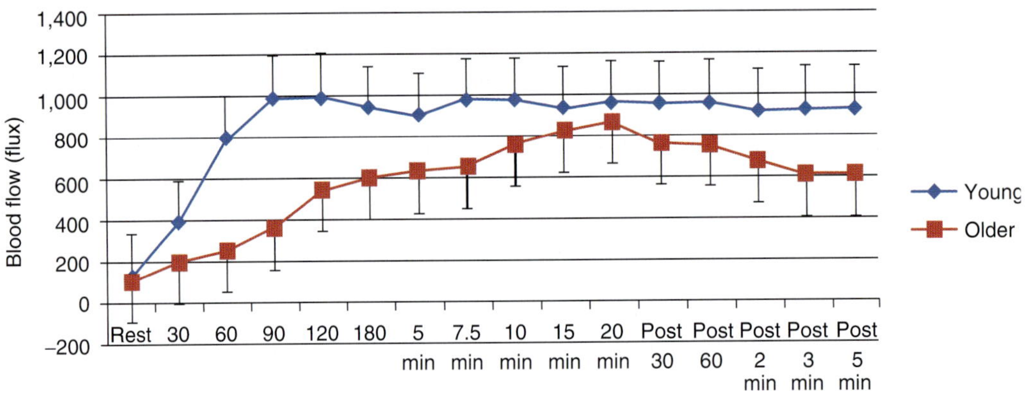

Fig. 39.7 Blood flow response to local heat and aging

The average data, shown in this figure in flux (units of blood flow from a laser Doppler imager) shows a time delay of a few seconds followed by a linear increase in skin blood flow that was starting to plateau after 2 min. This is a typical response in younger subjects (20–30 years old) and shows the delay in increase in circulation discussed by Pennes [81].

This increase in blood flow in the first 2 min is diminished with aging, showing an age effect on these same TRPV1 tactile sensors. In Fig. 39.7, the same experiment was conducted on individuals that were in the age range of 30–60 years. As shown in Fig. 39.7, the blood flow response was diminished and sluggish with the same heat stress on the skin.

The TRPV1 channels only elicit a vasodilatation that lasts a few minutes at best. A slower response that eventually becomes the predominant response to heat is mediated through warm receptors on endothelial cells themselves. These channels are TRPV4 voltage-gated calcium channels [132, 133]. Above a temperature of 35°C, these channels cause an exponential increase in calcium influx into the endothelial cell from the interstitial space thereby increasing activity of endothelial nitric oxide synthetase [136]. Nitric oxide then dilates vascular smooth muscle [16, 18, 73, 83, 84]. This is shown in Fig. 39.7. As seen here in younger and older subjects after 2 min of local heat exposure of 44°C on the skin above the quadriceps muscle, the sustained increase in circulation is maintained by TRPV4 calcium channels. However, the absolute blood flow is lesser in older people. This is believed to be due to increased free radicals in cells associated with aging. Free radicals in vascular endothelial cells impair production of both nitric oxide and also to the prostacyclin pathway, resulting in less blood flow in response to heat in older individuals [82]. The slower response to heat in older individuals as seen in this Fig. 39.7 may also be related to death of sensory nerves in the skin associated with aging, reducing the sensitivity to temperature in the skin [62].

Recent studies however have shown that the moisture content of skin may alter the response of vascular endothelial cells to changes in heat [90, 99, 102]. These studies show that if the skin is dry due to, for example, the application for the dry heat modality, the blood flow response is significantly less than if moist heat is used [90, 99, 102].

39.2.3 Skin Moisture, Heat, and Skin Blood Flow

The TRPV4 Ca^{++} channels in endothelial cells have receptor sites sensitive to multiple stimuli on the interior and exterior of the cell membrane. This receptor has multiple binding sites and senses such factors as temperature, pressure, and osmolarity [83, 95]. TRPV channels are expressed in smooth muscle cells, endothelial cells, as well as in perivascular nerves [5]. Thus, these cells, and the rest of the TRPV family of voltage-gated calcium channels, function as local cellular regulators that modify vascular function to respond to environmental and local stress on the cells [66]. They are used in many tissues in the body to maintain homeostasis. For example, in bone, they sense pressure and respond by activating [22]. Local pressure on bone causes osteoblasts to increase production of osteoprotegerin which, in turn, reduces activity of osteoclasts, allowing for less bone desorption and more bone generation [125]. In rat models, the pressure response of bone is altered by changing tissue osmolarity. Deletion of TRPV4 channels by removing the TRPV4 gene led to a lack of osmotically induced Ca^{++} release [22]. In the salivary gland, TRPV4 channels alter the response of aquaporin 5 channels. Thus, TRPV4 osmoreceptors aid in cell volume regulation in salivary glands and alter the response to multiple stimulate also effecting TRPV4 channels [2]. In skeletal muscle, TRPV4 channels also aid in the regulation and response of skeletal muscle [42]. Even the sympathetic response to low and high blood pressure is interrelated with TRPV4 osmoreceptors in the body [68]. The normal sympathetic response to a change in central arterial blood pressure is modulated by altering the osmotic pressure of blood. In TRPV4 knockout mice, hearing is impaired [126].

Therefore, because of the above, especially in the last few years, numerous papers have been published on the osmoreceptors and effect of dehydration and hyperhydration on the TRPV4 channels. The TRPV4 channels are multichannel sensing devices that have multiple input sites for everything from vertical and shear pressure to temperature, osmolarity, hydrogen ions, and other environmental factors, as well as the obvious response to substances, like acetylcholine, a neurotransmitter of the sympathetic nervous system, making these calcium gated channels a major part of most tissues in the body.

If the channels are activated, then calcium permeability in the extracellular membrane increases. In vascular endothelial cells, the influx of calcium causes calcium ions to bind to endothelial nitric oxide synthetase and increases production of nitric oxide and also elicits the production of prostaglandin I_2, another vasodilator. If the osmotic pressure is high in and around the cell, the calcium permeability is reduced, and endothelial nitric oxide synthetase is downregulated. Therefore, a positive stimulus that would increase blood flow in tissue can be blunted if a negative factor such as high osmolarity reduces calcium permeability.

An example is the effect of electrical stimulation of the skin on the blood flow. Normally, if the skin is cool, vasoconstriction predominates. If two electrodes are applied to the skin and stimulation is increased with square wave stimulation at a current of 20 milliamps and 40 pulses per second, the blood flow to the skin, as measured by laser Doppler imagers, does not change [1, 100, 121, 122]. However, if the skin or the room is warmed first to release the sympathetic vasoconstriction, then blood flow increases substantially during electrical stimulation of the skin and in the skin around wounds [1, 100, 121, 122].

This effect of dehydration causing diminished blood flow response was first seen almost 20 years ago (reference). Changing serum osmolarity, independent of changing blood volume, alters the skin blood flow response to global heat [23, 74].

Here, skin blood flow was reduced in response to whole body heating if the serum osmolarity was increased above normal. However, with TRPV4 receptors found all over the body, it was unknown what caused the effect. Was it blood vessels interaction of osmoreceptors on blood flow or a centrally mediated response in the hypothalamus since thirst receptors also use the same TRPV4 receptors [118]. More recent experiments have showed the effect of skin moisture on the local response to heat. This has been demonstrated by a simple experiment. If two layers of towels are placed around the arm and the arm is heated, blood flow under the towels can be measured with a laser Doppler flow meter. Plastic wrapped around the towels prevents moisture from entering or leaving. A thermocouple under the towels can be used to measure skin temperature, and then a feedback controller can turn an infrared lamp off and on to maintain constant skin temperatures.

Two such experiments were conducted. In one, dry rite (a drying agent) was placed between the towels, and in the second, the towels were moistened with water (Fig. 39.8). The skin was warmed with an infrared heat lamp to 38°C, 40°C, or 42°C for 30 min. Skin moisture was measured by a Corneometer (Courage+Khazaka electronic GmbH, Köln (Germany)). The Corneometer uses a 100-kHz sine wave signal to measure moisture content in the dermal layer; surface water has no effect on the readings. Before and after the exposure, there was constant skin moisture with dry heat but a doubling in skin moisture with moist heat. The skin moisture at each of the three temperatures is shown at the end of the 30-min heat exposure in Fig. 39.8 for moist and dry heat. As seen here, the skin moisture, in the same ten subjects, was substantially higher after the application of moist heat. In a similar manner, at each skin temperature, as shown in Fig. 39.9, the skin blood flow was significantly higher in the moist heat series than the dry heat series in the same subjects (age 20–32 years old).

This greater blood flow response to moist heat has several effects. First, skin warms faster with moist heat than dry heat. Part of this is due to the greater heat transfer properties of water than air, but part is due to self-heating of the skin by blood flow. Normally, skin temperature is almost 8°C below that of the core. This is due to the fact that the skin acts as a radiator to allow the transfer of heat from the core to the periphery to maintain a constant body temperature. The hands, for example, are normally between 29°C and 30°C.

This has the effect of warming the skin due to both the heat source and the faster perfusion of blood. To illustrate this concept, three series of experiments were conducted. One series assessed the change in skin temperature and blood flow during 6 min of heating of the skin. In the second series, the blood flow was occluded for the first minute and then released to observe the skin

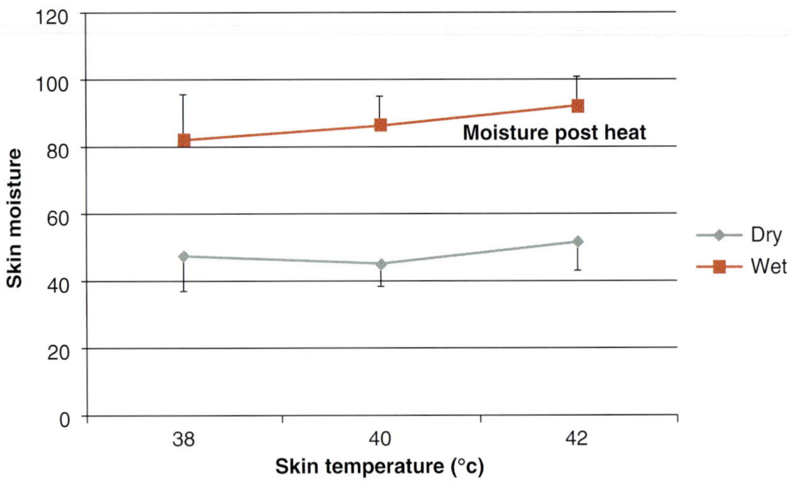

Fig. 39.8 Skin moisture of the arm after moist and dry heat applied for 30 min at skin temperatures of 38°C, 40°C, and 42°C. Skin Moisture is in arbitrary units

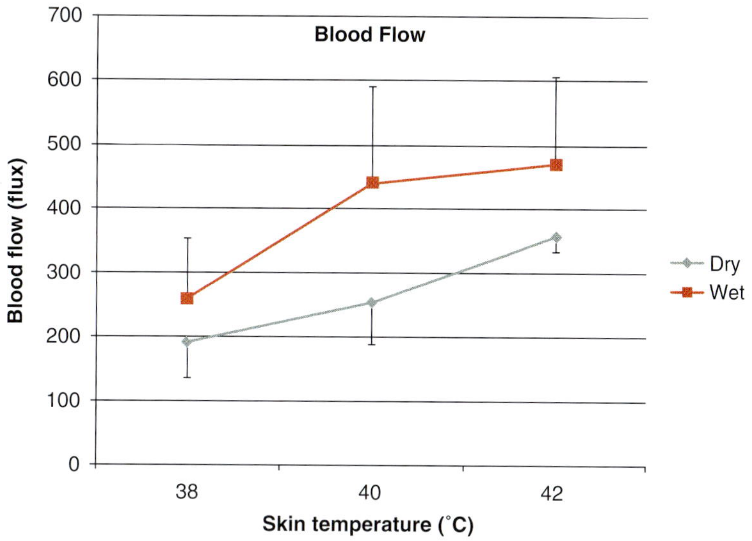

Fig. 39.9 The skin blood flow in ten subjects ± the standard deviation, measured by laser Doppler imager after 30 min of exposure to moist or dry heat. Skin temperature was clamped at 38°C, 40°C, or 42°C

temperature and caloric absorption of the skin with the skin cool and the heat source at 44°C. In the final series, the occlusion was maintained for 4 min so that the blood flow was interrupted until the skin temperature was at or above arterial blood temperature and then released. In this way, the effect of blood flow with the skin cool and warm could be differentially tested. Each of the experiments was conducted on a separate day with at least 24 h separating the experiments. The protocol was similar. A thermode, with water traversing it at 100 cc/min at a temperate of 44°C, was placed on the skin above the anterior surface of the forearm near the brachioradialis. The thermode was left on for a period of 6 min. During the time the thermode was left on, skin temperature was measured under the thermode, and blood flow was measured continuously through a hole in the center of thermode. In one series of experiments, the skin was simply heated the entire 6 min, and the parameters were measured. In a second series of experiments, occlusion was placed just above the center of the axilla with an arterial occlusion cuff inflated to 200 mmHg for the first minute that heat was applied; the cuff was then released and left off for the next 5 min. In the third series of experiments, occlusion remained on for the first 4 min and then was released for the last 2 min.

The results of the experiments are shown in Fig. 39.10.

As shown in Fig. 39.10, with or without occlusion, skin temperature changed at the same rate after application of the thermode. However, as shown in Fig. 39.11, when the calories needed to warm the skin were measured, the calories to warm the tissue were greater with occlusion for 1 or 4 min than were seen without occlusion, showing that part of the heat to warm the skin is from blood flow. With moist heat, the blood flow will even make the skin temperature rise quicker due to higher blood flows.

It can be predicted from this data that moist heat will increase skin temperature faster with deeper tissue penetration than was the case for dry heat. This was tested by applying thermocouples into the muscle in the quadriceps and then applying either dry or moist heat (Fig. 39.12).

When muscle temperature was measured over a 6-h application period of dry heat as shown in Fig. 39.13, skin temperature and muscle temperature rose slowly compared to that seen in moist heat in Fig. 39.14. With moist heat, the muscle temperature rose to similar or greater levels in 1 h than 6 h in dry heat in the same ten subjects. Thus, skin moisture has a strong influence ion not only blood flow in response to stress but also in transferring heat to deep tissue.

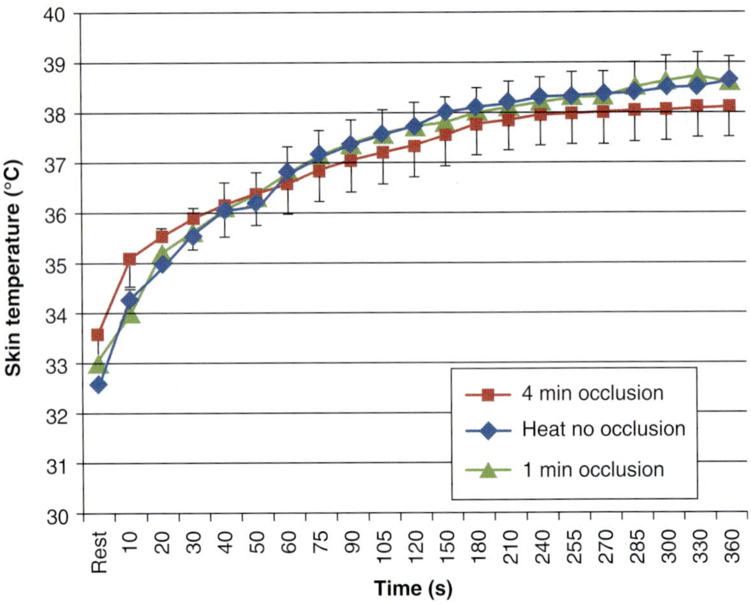

Fig. 39.10 Illustrated here is the average data on ten subjects ± the standard deviation showing the temperature of the skin over a 6-min period after a thermode was applied to the arm with no occlusion of the circulation, a 1-min occlusion of the circulation, and a 4-min occlusion of the circulation after the thermode was applied

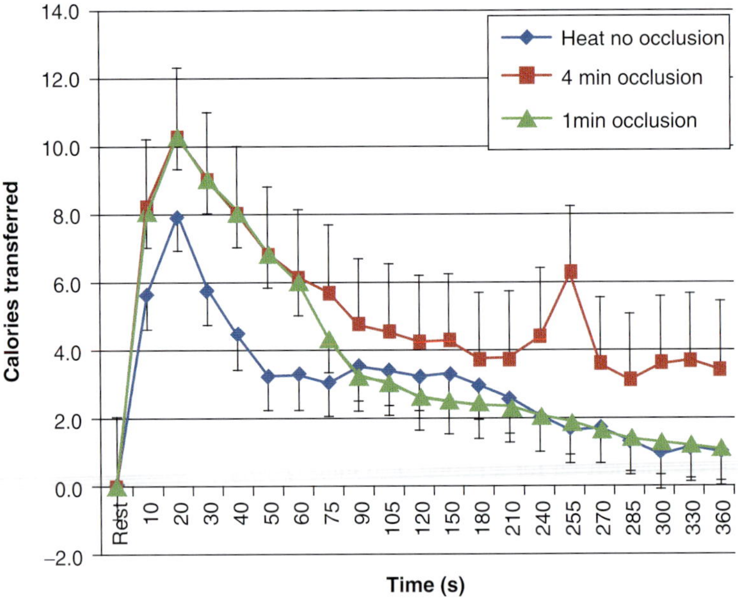

Fig. 39.11 Illustrated here is the average data on ten subjects ± the standard deviation showing the calories transferred to the skin over a 6-min period after a thermode was applied to the arm with no occlusion of the circulation, a 1-min occlusion of the circulation, and a 4-min occlusion of the circulation after the thermode was applied

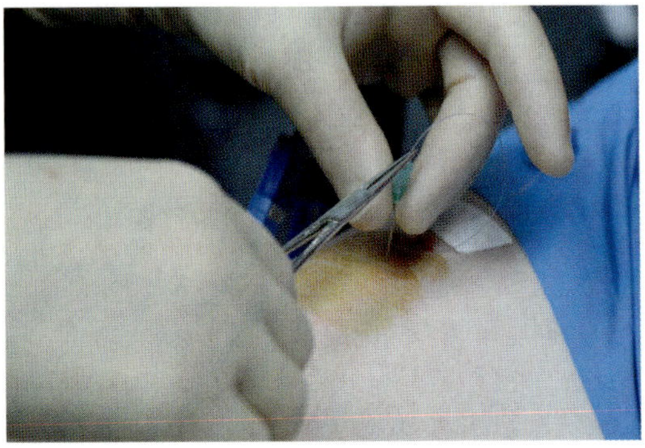

Fig. 39.12 The 21-gauge needle was used to insert 22-gauge thermocouples 2.5 cm into the quadriceps muscle

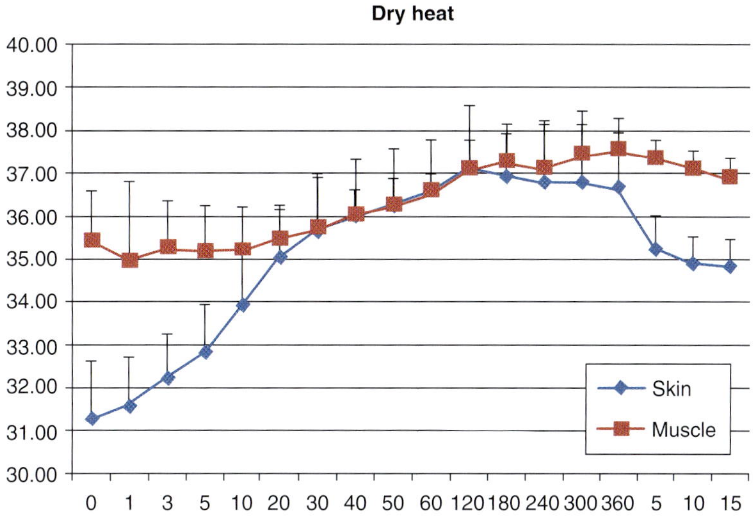

Fig. 39.13 The skin and muscle temperature in ten subjects after the application of dry heat to the quadriceps muscle ± the standard deviation. Skin temperatures are in degrees centigrade

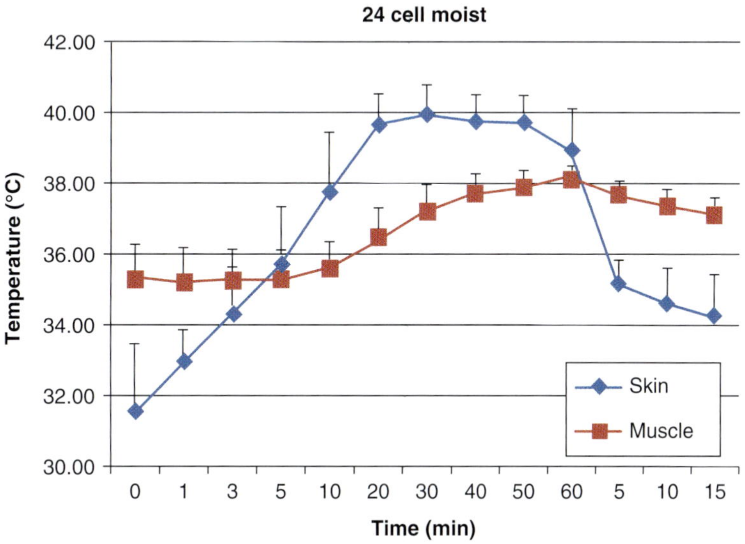

Fig. 39.14 The skin and muscle temperature in ten subjects after the application of moist heat to the quadriceps muscle ± the standard deviation

Conclusions

1. Skin moisture alters all modes of heat transfer in tissue including conduction, convection, radiation, and evaporation.
2. The majority of the influence of skin moisture on heat transfer is in the dermal layer of the skin.
3. This effect is exacerbated with aging and diabetes.

Take Home Messages

- The skin plays a major role in the exchange of heat.
- Heat can be transferred out of or into the skin by conduction, convection, radiation, and evaporation.

- Conduction, convection, evaporation, and radiation are all altered by the passive heat transfer properties of the skin and skin blood flow.
- The greater the moisture content of the skin, the greater the passive heat transfer, making it easier to lose heat from the body or dampen a heat source applied to the skin.
- High skin blood flow, the major mechanism used by the skin to move heat into the body or out of the body, is modulated by skin moisture; TRPV4 osmoreceptors reduce skin blood flow if the skin is dry.
- Thus, dry skin alters the ability of the skin to lose heat from the body and insulate the body from an external heat source.
- Older people and people with diabetes, as might be expected, have poor heat transfer in the skin due to dry skin and poor circulation.

References

1. Almalty AM, Petrofsky JS, Al-Naami B, Al-Nabulsi J (2009) An effective method for skin blood flow measurement using local heat combined with electrical stimulation. J Med Eng Technol 33:663–669
2. Aure MH, Roed A, Galtung HK (2010) Intracellular Ca2+ responses and cell volume regulation upon cholinergic and purinergic stimulation in an immortalized salivary cell line. Eur J Oral Sci 118:237–244
3. Aylin K, Arzu D, Sabri S, Handan TE, Ridvan A (2009) The effect of combined resistance and home-based walking exercise in type 2 diabetes patients. Int J Diabetes Dev Ctries 29:159–165
4. Bakolitsa C, Kumar A, Jin KK, McMullan D, Krishna SS, Miller MD, Abdubek P, Acosta C, Astakhova T, Axelrod HL, Burra P, Carlton D, Chen C, Chiu HJ, Clayton T, Das D, Deller MC, Duan L, Elias Y, Ellrott K, Ernst D, Farr CL, Feuerhelm J, Grant JC, Grzechnik A, Grzechnik SK, Han GW, Jaroszewski L, Johnson HA, Klock HE, Knuth MW, Kozbial P, Marciano D, Morse AT, Murphy KD, Nigoghossian E, Nopakun A, Okach L, Paulsen J, Puckett C, Reyes R, Rife CL, Sefcovic N, Tien HJ, Trame CB, Trout CV, van den Bedem H, Weekes D, White A, Xu Q, Hodgson KO, Wooley J, Elsliger MA, Deacon AM, Godzik A, Lesley SA, Wilson IA (2010) Structures of the first representatives of Pfam family PF06684 (DUF1185) reveal a novel variant of the Bacillus chorismate mutase fold and suggest a role in amino-acid metabolism. Acta Crystallogr Sect F Struct Biol Cryst Commun 66:1182–1189
5. Baylie RL, Brayden JE (2011) TRPV channels and vascular function. Acta Physiol (Oxf) 203(1):99–116. doi:10.1111/j.1748-1716.2010.02217.x, Epub 2010 Dec 9
6. Beysens D, Chatain D, Nikolayev VS, Ouazzani J, Garrabos Y (2010) Possibility of long-distance heat transport in weightlessness using supercritical fluids. Phys Rev E Stat Nonlin Soft Matter Phys 82: 061126
7. Blum K, Chen AL, Chen TJ, Prihoda TJ, Schoolfield J, Dinubile N, Waite RL, Arcuri V, Kerner M, Braverman ER, Rhoades P, Tung H (2008) The H-Wave device is an effective and safe non-pharmacological analgesic for chronic pain: a meta-analysis. Adv Ther 25: 644–657
8. Blum K, Ho CK, Chen AL, Fulton M, Fulton B, Westcott WL, Reinl G, Braverman ER, Dinubile N, Chen TJ (2008) The H-wave((R)) device induces NODependent augmented microcirculation and angiogenesis, providing both analgesia and tissue healing in sports injuries. Phys Sportsmed 36:103–114
9. Blumberg HP (2008) The next wave in neuroimaging research in pediatric bipolar disorder. J Am Acad Child Adolesc Psychiatry 47:483–485
10. Branchet MC, Boisnic S, Frances C, Robert AM (1990) Skin thickness changes in normal aging skin. Gerontology 36:28–35
11. Brincat M, Kabalan S, Studd JW et al (1987) A study of the decrease of skin collagen content, skin thickness, and bone mass in the post menopausal woman. Obstet Gynecol 70:840–845
12. Bronzino JD (2000) The biomedical engineering handbook. CRC Press, Boca Raton
13. Bui C, Petrofsky J, Berk L, Shavlik D, Remigio W, Montgomery S (2010) Acute effect of a single high-fat meal on forearm blood flow, blood pressure and heart rate in healthy male Asians and Caucasians: a pilot study. Southeast Asian J Trop Med Public Health 41:490–500
14. Carmeli E, Patish H, Coleman R (2003) The aging hand. J Gerontol A Biol Sci Med Sci 58:146–152
15. Charkoudian N, Eisenach JH, Atkinson JL, Fealey RD, Joyner MJ (2002) Effects of chronic sympathectomy on locally mediated cutaneous vasodilation in humans. J Appl Physiol 92:685–690
16. Charkoudian N, Fromy B, Saumet JL (2001) Reflex control of the cutaneous circulation after acute and chronic local capsaicin. J Appl Physiol 90:1860–1864
17. Charkoudian N, Johnson JM (1999) Reflex control of cutaneous vasoconstrictor system is reset by exogenous female reproductive hormones. J Appl Physiol 87:381–385
18. Charkoudian N, Rabbitts JA (2009) Sympathetic neural mechanisms in human cardiovascular health and disease. Mayo Clin Proc 84:822–830

19. Cheung K, Hume P, Maxwell L (2003) Delayed onset muscle soreness: treatment strategies and performance factors. Sports Med 33:145–164
20. Chu KL, Chandran P, Joshi SK, Jarvis MF, Kym PR, McGaraughty S (2011) TRPV1-related modulation of spinal neuronal activity and behavior in a rat model of osteoarthritic pain. Brain Res 1369:158–166
21. Claassen J, Hirsch LJ, Frontera JA, Fernandez A, Schmidt M, Kapinos G, Wittman J, Connolly ES, Emerson RG, Mayer SA (2006) Prognostic significance of continuous EEG monitoring in patients with poor-grade subarachnoid hemorrhage. Neurocrit Care 4:103–112
22. Clark AL, Votta BJ, Kumar S, Liedtke W, Guilak F (2010) Chondroprotective role of the osmotically sensitive ion channel transient receptor potential vanilloid 4: age- and sex-dependent progression of osteoarthritis in Trpv4-deficient mice. Arthritis Rheum 62:2973–2983
23. Coyle EF, Montain SJ (1992) Benefits of fluid replacement with carbohydrate during exercise. Med Sci Sports Exerc 24:S324–S330
24. Cristol DA, Brasso RL, Condon AM, Fovargue RE, Friedman SL, Hallinger KK, Monroe AP, White AE (2008) The movement of aquatic mercury through terrestrial food webs. Science 320:335
25. Dao H Jr, Kazin RA (2007) Gender differences in skin: a review of the literature. Gend Med 4:308–328
26. Duncan K, Leffell D (1997) Preoperative assessment of the elderly patient. Dermatol Clin 15:583–593
27. Edwards AM, Noakes TD (2009) Dehydration: cause of fatigue or sign of pacing in elite soccer? Sports Med 39:1–13
28. Evans CH, Karunaratne HB (1992) Exercise stress testing for the family physician: part I. Performing the test. Am Fam Physician 45:121–132
29. Evans WJ (1992) Exercise, nutrition and aging. J Nutr 122:796–801
30. Farage MA, Miller KW, Elsner P, Maibach HI (2008) Functional and physiological characteristics of the aging skin. Aging Clin Exp Res 20:195–200
31. Farage MA, Miller KW, Maibach HI (eds) (2010) Textbook of aging skin. Springer, Berlin/Heidelberg
32. Fenske NA, Lober CW (1986) Structural and functional changes of normal aging skin. J Am Acad Dermatol 15:571–585
33. Fisher G, Varani J, Voorhees J (2006) Looking older: fibroblast collapse and therapeutic implications. Arch Dermatol 144:666–672
34. Fox RH, Edholm OG (1963) Nervous control of the cutaneous circulation. Br Med Bull 19:110–114
35. Friedman O (2005) Changes associated with the aging face. Facial Plast Surg Clin North Am 13:371–380
36. Fu Y, Hou Y, Fu C, Gu M, Li C, Kong W, Wang X, Shyy JY, Zhu Y (2011) A novel mechanism of {gamma}/{delta} T-lymphocyte and endothelial activation by shear stress: the role of ecto-ATP synthase {beta} chain. Circ Res 108(4):410–417, Epub 2010 Dec 30
37. Gan SK, Kriketos AD, Ellis BA, Thompson CH, Kraegen EW, Chisholm DJ (2003) Changes in aerobic capacity and visceral fat but not myocyte lipid levels predict increased insulin action after exercise in overweight and obese men. Diabetes Care 26:1706–1713
38. Gapanhuk E, Henriques OB (1970) Kinins released from horse heat-acid-denaturated plasma by plasmin, plasma kallikrein, trypsin and Bothrops kininogenase. Biochem Pharmacol 19:2091–2096
39. Ghadially R, Brown BE, Sequeira-Martin SM, Feingold KR, Elias PM (1995) The aged epidermal permeability barrier structural, functional, and lipid biochemical abnormalities in humans and a senescent murine model. J Clin Invest 95:2281–2290
40. Ghersetich I, Troiano M, DeGiorgi V, Lotti T (2007) Receptors in skin ageing and antiageing agents. Dermatol Clin 25:655–662, xi
41. Grove G (1989) Physiologic changes in the older skin. Clin Geriatr Med 5:115–125
42. Guilak F, Leddy HA, Liedtke W (2010) Transient receptor potential vanilloid 4: the sixth sense of the musculoskeletal system? Ann N Y Acad Sci 1192:404–409
43. Harvell J, Maibach H (1994) Percutaneous absorption and inflammation in aged skin: a review. J Am Acad Dermatol 31(6):1015–1021
44. Haymes EM, Dickinson AL, Malville N, Ross RW (1982) Effects of wind on the thermal and metabolic responses to exercise in the cold. Med Sci Sports Exerc 14:41–45
45. Henriques FC, Moritz AR (1947) Studies of thermal injury: I. The conduction of heat to and through skin and the temperatures attained therein. A theoretical and an experimental investigation. Am J Pathol 23:530–549
46. Hirose L, Nosaka K, Newton M, Laveder A, Kano M, Peake J, Suzuki K (2004) Changes in inflammatory mediators following eccentric exercise of the elbow flexors. Exerc Immunol Rev 10:75–90
47. Holmer I (2000) Strategies for prevention of cold stress in the elderly. Int J Circumpolar Health 59: 267–272
48. Holowatz LA, Houghton BL, Wong BJ, Wilkins BW, Harding AW, Kenney WL, Minson CT (2003) Nitric oxide and attenuated reflex cutaneous vasodilation in aged skin. Am J Physiol Heart Circ Physiol 284:H1662–H1667
49. Holowatz LA, Kenney WL (2010) Peripheral mechanisms of thermoregulatory control of skin blood flow in aged humans. J Appl Physiol 109:1538–1544
50. Holowatz LA, Thompson-Torgerson C, Kenney WL (2010) Aging and the control of human skin blood flow. Front Biosci 15:718–739
51. Houghton BL, Meendering JR, Wong BJ, Minson CT (2006) Nitric oxide and noradrenaline contribute to the temperature threshold of the axon reflex response to gradual local heating in human skin. J Physiol 572:811–820
52. Huang J, Togawa T (1995) Improvement of imaging of skin thermal properties by successive thermographic measurements at a stepwise change in ambient radiation temperature. Physiol Meas 16:295–301

53. Hubing KA, Wingo JE, Brothers RM, del Coso J, Low DA, Crandall CG (2010) Nitric oxide synthase inhibition attenuates cutaneous vasodilation during postmenopausal hot flash episodes. Menopause 17:978–982
54. Jackson S, Williams M, Feingold K, Elias P (1993) Pathobiology of the stratum corneum. West J Med 158:279–289
55. Johnson JM (1986) Nonthermoregulatory control of human skin blood flow. J Appl Physiol 61:1613–1622
56. Johnson JM, Brengelmann GL, Hales JR, Vanhoutte PM, Wenger CB (1986) Regulation of the cutaneous circulation. Fed Proc 45:2841–2850
57. Johnson RK, Appel LJ, Brands M, Howard BV, Lefevre M, Lustig RH, Sacks F, Steffen LM, Wylie-Rosett J (2009) Dietary sugars intake and cardiovascular health: a scientific statement from the American Heart Association. Circulation 120: 1011–1020
58. Kellogg DL Jr, Crandall CG, Liu Y, Charkoudian N, Johnson JM (1998) Nitric oxide and cutaneous active vasodilation during heat stress in humans. J Appl Physiol 85:824–829
59. Kligman A, Koblenzer C (1997) Demographics and psychological implications for the aging population. Dermatol Clin 15:549–553
60. Koyama T, Hatanaka Y, Jin X, Yokomizo A, Fujiwara H, Goda M, Hobara N, Zamami Y, Kitamura Y, Kawasaki H (2010) Altered function of nitrergic nerves inhibiting sympathetic neurotransmission in mesenteric vascular beds of renovascular hypertensive rats. Hypertens Res 33:485–491
61. Langton AK, Sherratt MJ, Griffiths CE, Watson RE (2010) A new wrinkle on old skin: the role of elastic fibres in skin ageing. Int J Cosmet Sci 32(5):330–339. doi:10.1111/ics.2010.32.issue-5/issuetoc, Epub 2010 Oct
62. Libouton X, Barbier O, Plaghki L, Thonnard JL (2010) Tactile roughness discrimination threshold is unrelated to tactile spatial acuity. Behav Brain Res 208:473–478
63. Magalhaes FC, Passos RL, Fonseca MA, Oliveira KP, Ferreira-Junior JB, Martini AR, Lima MR, Guimaraes JB, Barauna VG, Silami-Garcia E, Rodrigues LO (2010) Thermoregulatory efficiency is increased after heat acclimation in tropical natives. J Physiol Anthropol 29:1–12
64. Maglinger PE, Sessler DI, Lenhardt R (2005) Cutaneous heat loss with three surgical drapes, one impervious to moisture. Anesth Analg 100:738–742, table of contents
65. Makrantonaki E, Zouboulis CC (2010) Dermato-endocrinology. Skin aging. Hautarzt 61:505–510
66. Malmberg AB, Bley KR (eds) (2005) Turning up the heat on pain: TRPV1 receptors in pain and inflammation. Birkhauser verlag, Basel/Boston/Berlin
67. McCallion R, Li Wan Po A (1993) Dry and photo-aged skin: manifestations and management. J Clin Pharm Ther 18:15–32
68. McHugh J, Keller NR, Appalsamy M, Thomas SA, Raj SR, Diedrich A, Biaggioni I, Jordan J, Robertson D (2010) Portal osmopressor mechanism linked to transient receptor potential vanilloid 4 and blood pressure control. Hypertension 55:1438–1443
69. McLellan K, Petrofsky JS, Bains G, Zimmerman G, Prowse M, Lee S (2009) The effects of skin moisture and subcutaneous fat thickness on the ability of the skin to dissipate heat in young and old subjects, with and without diabetes, at three environmental room temperatures. Med Eng Phys 31:165–172
70. McLellan K, Petrofsky JS, Zimmerman G, Lohman E, Prowse M, Schwab E, Lee S (2009) The influence of environmental temperature on the response of the skin to local pressure: the impact of aging and diabetes. Diabetes Technol Ther 11:791–798
71. McLellan K, Petrofsky JS, Zimmerman G, Prowse M, Bains G, Lee S (2009) Multiple stressors and the response of vascular endothelial cells: the effect of aging and diabetes. Diabetes Technol Ther 11:73–79
72. Mendes JC, Silva MC (2004) On the use of porous materials to simulate evaporation in the human sweating process. Eur J Appl Physiol 92:654–657
73. Minson CT, Berry LT, Joyner MJ (2001) Nitric oxide and neurally mediated regulation of skin blood flow during local heating. J Appl Physiol 91:1619–1626
74. Montain SJ, Coyle EF (1992) Influence of graded dehydration on hyperthermia and cardiovascular drift during exercise. J Appl Physiol 73:1340–1350
75. Moritz AR, Henriques FC Jr et al (1947) Studies of thermal injury; an exploration of the casualty-producing attributes of conflagrations; local and systemic effects of general cutaneous exposure to excessive circumambient (air) and circumradiant heat of varying duration and intensity. Arch Pathol (Chic) 43:466–488
76. Moritz AR, Henriques FC, McLean R (1945) The effects of inhaled heat on the Air passages and lungs: an experimental investigation. Am J Pathol 21:311–331
77. Muller AF, Batin P, Evans S, Hawkins M, Cowley AJ (1992) Regional blood flow in chronic heart failure: the reason for the lack of correlation between patients' exercise tolerance and cardiac output? Br Heart J 67:478–481
78. Muller AF, Hawkins M, Batin P, Evans S, Cowley AJ (1992) Food in chronic heart failure: improvement in central haemodynamics but deleterious effects on exercise tolerance. Eur Heart J 13:1460–1467
79. Oeppen J, Vaupel JW (2002) Demography. Broken limits to life expectancy. Science 296:1029–1031
80. Oriba H, Bucks D, Maibach H (1996) Percutaneous absorption of hydrocortisone and testosterone on the vulva and forearm: effect of the menopause and site. Br J Dermatol 134:229–233
81. Pennes HH (1948) Analysis of tissue and arterial blood temperatures in the resting human forearm. J Appl Physiol 1:93–122
82. Petrofsky J, Bains G, Prowse M, Gunda S, Berk L, Raju C, Ethiraju G, Vanarasa D, Madani P (2009) Does skin moisture influence the blood flow response

to local heat? A re-evaluation of the Pennes model. J Med Eng Technol 33:1–6
83. Petrofsky J, Bains G, Prowse M, Gunda S, Berk L, Raju C, Ethiraju G, Vanarasa D, Madani P (2009) Does skin moisture influence the blood flow response to local heat? A re-evaluation of the Pennes model. J Med Eng Technol 33:532–537
84. Petrofsky J, Bains G, Prowse M, Gunda S, Berk L, Raju C, Ethiraju G, Vanarasa D, Madani P (2009) Dry heat, moist heat and body fat: are heating modalities really effective in people who are overweight? J Med Eng Technol 33:361–369
85. Petrofsky J, Gunda S, Raju C, Bains GS, Bogseth MC, Focil N, Sirichotiratana M, Hashemi V, Vallabhaneni P, Kim Y, Madani P, Coords H, McClurg M, Lohman E (2010) Impact of hydrotherapy on skin blood flow: How much is due to moisture and how much is due to heat? Physiother Theory Pract 26:107–112
86. Petrofsky J, Hinds CM, Batt J, Prowse M, Suh HJ (2007) The interrelationships between electrical stimulation, the environment surrounding the vascular endothelial cells of the skin, and the role of nitric oxide in mediating the blood flow response to electrical stimulation. Med Sci Monit 13: CR391–CR397
87. Petrofsky J, Lee H, Trivedi M, Hudlikar AN, Yang CH, Goraksh N, Alshammari F, Mohanan M, Soni J, Agilan B, Pai N, Chindam T, Murugesan V, Yim JE, Katrak V (2010) The influence of ageing and diabetes on heat transfer characteristics of the skin to a rapidly applied heat source. Daibetes Technol Ther 12:1003–1010
88. Petrofsky J, Lee S, Cuneo ML (2005) Gait characteristics in patients with type 2 diabetes; improvement after administration of rosiglitazone. Med Sci Monit 11:PI43–PI51
89. Petrofsky J, Lohman E 3rd, Lee S, de la Cuesta Z, Labial L, Iouciulescu R, Moseley B, Korson R, Al Malty A (2007) Effects of contrast baths on skin blood flow on the dorsal and plantar foot in people with type 2 diabetes and age-matched controls. Physiother Theory Pract 23:189–197
90. Petrofsky J, Paluso D, Anderson D, Swan K, Alshammari F, Katrak V, Murugesan V, Hudlikar AN, Chindam T, Trivedi M, Lee H, Goraksh N, Yim J The ability of the skin to absorb heat from a locally applied heat source; the impact of diabetes. J med eng physics Diabetes Technol Ther. 2011 Mar;13(3):365-72. Epub 2011 Feb 3
91. Petrofsky J, Prowse M, Bain M, Ebilane E, Suh HJ, Batt J, Lawson D, Hernandez V, Abdo A, Yang TN, Mendoza E, Collins K, Laymon M (2008) Estimation of the distribution of intramuscular current during electrical stimulation of the quadriceps muscle. Eur J Appl Physiol 103:265–273
92. Petrofsky J, Schwab E, Lo T, Cuneo M, George J, Kim J, Al-Malty A (2005) Effects of electrical stimulation on skin blood flow in controls and in and around stage III and IV wounds in hairy and non hairy skin. Med Sci Monit 11:CR309–CR316
93. Petrofsky JS (2010) A device to measure heat flow through the skin in people with diabetes. Diabetes Technol Ther 12:737–743
94. Petrofsky JS, Al-Malty AM, Prowse M (2008) Relationship between multiple stimuli and skin blood flow. Med Sci Monit 14:CR399–CR405
95. Petrofsky JS, Bains G, Raju C, Lohman E, Berk L, Prowse M, Gunda S, Madani P, Batt J (2009) The effect of the moisture content of a local heat source on the blood flow response of the skin. Arch Dermatol Res 301:581–585
96. Petrofsky JS, Bains GS, Prowse M, Mc Lellan K, Ethiraju G, Lee S, Gunda S, Lohman E, Schwab E (2009) The influence of age and diabetes on the skin blood flow response to local pressure. Med Sci Monit 15:CR325–CR331
97. Petrofsky JS, Cuneo M, Lee S, Johnson E, Lohman E (2006) Correlation between gait and balance in people with and without Type 2 diabetes in normal and subdued light. Med Sci Monit 12:CR273–CR281
98. Petrofsky JS, Focil N, Prowse M, Kim Y, Berk L, Bains G, Lee S (2010) Autonomic stress and balance – the impact of age and diabetes. Diabetes Technol Ther 12:475–481
99. Petrofsky JS, Goraksh N, Alshammari F, Mohanan M, Soni J, Trivedi M, Lee H, Hudlikar AN, Yang C, Agilan B, Pai N, Katrak V, Chindam T, Murugesan V, Yim J (2011) The ability of the skin to absorb heat; the effect of repeated exposure and age. Med Sci Monit 17(1):CR1–CR8
100. Petrofsky JS, Lawson D, Berk L, Suh H (2010) Enhanced healing of diabetic foot ulcers using local heat and electrical stimulation for 30 min three times per week. J Diabetes 2:41–46
101. Petrofsky JS, Laymon M (2009) Heat transfer to deep tissue: the effect of body fat and heating modality. J Med Eng Technol 33:337–348
102. Petrofsky JS, Lee H, Trivedi M, Hudlikar AN, Yang C, Goraksh N, Alshammari F, Mohanan M, Soni J, Agilan B, Pai N, Chindam T, Murugesan V, Yim J, Katrak V (2010) The influence of ageing and diabetes on heat transfer characteristics of the skin to a rapidly applied heat source. Diabetes Technol Ther 12:1003–1010
103. Petrofsky JS, Lind AR (1975) Insulative power of body fat on deep muscle temperatures and isometric endurance. J Appl Physiol 39:639–642
104. Petrofsky JS, Lohman E 3rd, Lee S, de la Cuesta Z, Labial L, Iouciulescu R, Moseley B, Korson R, AlMalty A (2006) The influence of alterations in room temperature on skin blood flow during contrast baths in patients with diabetes. Med Sci Monit 12:CR290–CR295
105. Petrofsky JS, Lohman E 3rd, Suh HJ, Garcia J, Anders A, Sutterfield C, Khandge C (2006) The effect of aging on conductive heat exchange in the skin at two environmental temperatures. Med Sci Monit 12:CR400–CR408
106. Petrofsky JS, McLellan K (2009) Galvanic skin resistance – a marker for endothelial damage in diabetes. Diabetes Technol Ther 11:461–467

107. Petrofsky JS, Mclellan K, Bains GS, Prowse M, Ethiraju G, Lee S, Gunda S, Lohman E 3rd, Schwab E (2009) The influence of ageing on the ability of the skin to dissipate heat. Med Sci Monit 15:CR261–CR268
108. Petrofsky JS, McLellan K, Bains GS, Prowse M, Ethiraju G, Lee S, Gunda S, Lohman E, Schwab E (2008) Skin heat dissipation: the influence of diabetes, skin thickness, and subcutaneous fat thickness. Diabetes Technol Ther 10:487–493
109. Petrofsky JS, McLellan K, Prowse M, Bains G, Berk L, Lee S (2010) The effect of body fat, aging, and diabetes on vertical and shear pressure in and under a waist belt and its effect on skin blood flow. Diabetes Technol Ther 12:153–160
110. Petrofsky JS, Prowse M, Lohman E (2008) The influence of ageing and diabetes on skin and subcutaneous fat thickness in different regions of the body. J Appl Res Clin Exp Ther 8:55–61
111. Petrofsky JS, Suh HJ, Gunda S, Prowse M, Batt J (2008) Interrelationships between body fat and skin blood flow and the current required for electrical stimulation of human muscle. Med Eng Phys 30:931–936
112. Puizina-Ivic N (2008) Skin aging. Acta Dermatovenerol Alp Panonica Adriat 17:47–54
113. Reilly T, Ekblom B (2005) The use of recovery methods post-exercise. J Sports Sci 23:619–627
114. Rowell LB (1974) Human cardiovascular adjustments to exercise and thermal stress. Physiol Rev 54:75–159
115. Sanchez-Marin FJ, Calixto-Carrera S, Villasenor-Mora C (2009) Novel approach to assess the emissivity of the human skin. J Biomed Opt 14:024006
116. Savvas M, Bishop J, Laurent G, Watson N, Studd J (1993) Type III collagen content in the skin of postmenopausal women receiving oestradiol and testosterone implants. Br J Obstet Gynaecol 100:154–156
117. Shai A, Halevy S (2005) Direct triggers for ulceration in patients with venous insufficiency. Int J Dermatol 44:1006–1009
118. Sharif-Naeini R, Ciura S, Zhang Z, Bourque CW (2008) Contribution of TRPV channels to osmosensory transduction, thirst, and vasopressin release. Kidney Int 73:811–815
119. Siddappa K (2003) Dry skin conditions, eczema and emollients in their management. Indian J Dermatol Venereol Leprol 69:69–75
120. Stansberry KB, Peppard HR, Babyak LM, Popp G, McNitt PM, Vinik AI (1999) Primary nociceptive afferents mediate the blood flow dysfunction in nonglabrous (hairy) skin of type 2 diabetes: a new model for the pathogenesis of microvascular dysfunction. Diabetes Care 22:1549–1554
121. Suh H, Petrofsky J, Fish A, Hernandez V, Mendoza E, Collins K, Yang T, Abdul A, Batt J, Lawson D (2009) A new electrode design to improve outcomes in the treatment of chronic non-healing wounds in diabetes. Diabetes Technol Ther 11:315–322
122. Suh H, Petrofsky JS, Lo T, Lawson D, Yu T, Pfeifer TM, Morawski T (2009) The combined effect of a three-channel electrode delivery system with local heat on the healing of chronic wounds. Diabetes Technol Ther 11:681–688
123. Suhel P, Kralj B, Plevnik S (1978) Advances in non-implantable electrical stimulators for correction of urinary incontinence. J Life Sci 8:11–16
124. Suter-Widmer J, Elsner P (1996) The irritant contact dermatitis syndrome. CRC Press, Boca Raton
125. Ta HM, Nguyen GT, Jin HM, Choi J, Park H, Kim N, Hwang HY, Kim KK (2010) Structure-based development of a receptor activator of nuclear factor-{kappa}B ligand (RANKL) inhibitor peptide and molecular basis for osteopetrosis. Proc Natl Acad Sci U S A 107(47):20281–20286, Epub 2010 Nov 8
126. Tabuchi K, Suzuki M, Mizuno A, Hara A (2005) Hearing impairment in TRPV4 knockout mice. Neurosci Lett 382:304–308
127. Thompson D, Williams C, Garcia-Roves P, McGregor SJ, McArdle F, Jackson MJ (2003) Post-exercise vitamin C supplementation and recovery from demanding exercise. Eur J Appl Physiol 89: 393–400
128. Thompson PD (2003) Exercise and physical activity in the prevention and treatment of atherosclerotic cardiovascular disease. Arterioscler Thromb Vasc Biol 23:1319–1321
129. Vazquez F, Palacios S, Aleman N, Guerrero F (1996) Changes of the basement membrane and type iv collagen in human skin during aging. Maturitas 25: 209–215
130. Waligora JM, Michel EL (1968) Application of conductive cooling for working men in a thermally isolated environment. Aerosp Med 39:485–487
131. Waller J, Maibach H (2005) Age and skin structure and function, a quantitative approach (i): blood flow, ph, thickness and ultrasound echogenicity. Skin Res Technol 11:221–235
132. Watanabe H, Vriens J, Suh SH, Benham CD, Droogmans G, Nilius B (2002) Heat-evoked activation of TRPV4 channels in a HEK293 cell expression system and in native mouse aorta endothelial cells. J Biol Chem 277:47044–47051
133. Watanabe M, Toma S, Murakami M, Shimoyama I, Nakajima Y, Moriya H (2002) Assessment of mechanical and thermal thresholds of human C nociceptors during increases in skin sympathetic nerve activity. Clin Neurophysiol 113:1485–1490
134. Webb P (1992) Temperatures of skin, subcutaneous tissue, muscle and core in resting men in cold, comfortable and hot conditions. Eur J Appl Physiol Occup Physiol 64:471–476
135. Wissler EH (1998) Pennes' 1948 paper revisited. J Appl Physiol 85:35–41
136. Wong BJ, Fieger SM (2010) Transient receptor potential vanilloid type-1 (TRPV-1) channels contribute to cutaneous thermal hyperaemia in humans. J Physiol 588:4317–4326
137. Xiong J, Feng L, Yuan D, Fu C, Miao W (2010) Genome-wide identification and evolution of ATP-binding cassette transporters in the ciliate tetrahymena thermophila: a case of functional divergence in a multigene family. BMC Evol Biol 10:330

Appendix

Reference List of EEMCO Guidelines

Berardesca E (1997) EEMCO guidance for the assessment of stratum corneum hydration: electrical methods. Skin Res Technol 3:126–132

Berardesca E, Lévêque JL, Masson P (2002) EEMCO guidance for the measurement of skin microcirculation. Skin Pharmacol Appl Skin Physiol 15:442–456

Lévêque JL (1999) EEMCO guidance for the assessment of skin topography. The European Expert Group on efficacy measurement of cosmetics and other topical products. J Eur Acad Dermatol Venereol 12:103–114

Parra JL, Paye M (2003) EEMCO guidance for the in vivo assessment of skin surface pH. Skin Pharmacol Appl Skin Physiol 16:188–202

Piérard GE (1996) EEMCO guidance for the assessment of dry skin (xerosis) and ichthyosis: evaluation by stratum corneum shippings. Skin Res Technol 2:3–11

Piérard GE (1998) EMCO guidance for the assessment of skin colour. J Eur Acad Dermatol Venereol 10:1–11

Piérard GE (1999) EEMCO guidance to the in vivo assessment of tensile functional properties of the skin. Part 1: relevance to the structures and ageing of the skin and subcutaneous tissues. Skin Pharmacol Appl Skin Physiol 12:352–362

Piérard GE, Piérard-Franchimont C, Marks R, Paye M, Rogiers V (2000) EEMCO guidance for the in vivo assessment of skin greasiness. Skin Pharmacol Appl Skin Physiol 13:372–389

Rodrigues L (2001) EEMCO guidance to the in vivo assessment of tensile functional properties of the skin. Part 2: instrumentation and test modes. Skin Pharmacol Appl Skin Physiol 14:52–67

Rogiers V (2001) EEMCO guidance for the assessment of transepidermal water loss in cosmetic sciences. Skin Pharmacol Appl Skin Physiol 14:117–128

Serup J (1995) EEMCO guidance for the assessment of dry skin (xerosis) and ichthyosis: clinical scoring systems. Skin Res Technol 1:109–114

M. Lodén, H.I. Maibach (eds.), *Treatment of Dry Skin Syndrome*,
DOI 10.1007/978-3-642-27606-4,

Index

M. Lodén, H.I. Maibach (eds.), *Treatment of Dry Skin Syndrome*,
DOI 10.1007/978-3-642-27606-4, © Springer-Verlag Berlin Heidelberg 2012

D

O

P

Q

R

Printing and Binding: Stürtz GmbH, Würzburg